LEXI-COMP'S

D0150153

Drug Information Handbook FOR Oncology

Featuring
A Complete Guide to Combination Chemotherapy Regimens

5th Edition

Dominic A. Solimando, Jr., MA, BCOP
Senior Editor

LEXI-COMP'S

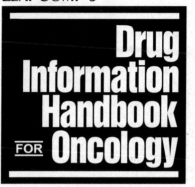

Drug Information Handbook

FOR **Oncology**

Featuring
**A Complete Guide to Combination
Chemotherapy Regimens**

5ᵗʰ Edition

Dominic A. Solimando, Jr, MA, BCOP
Senior Editor

Oncology Pharmacist
President, Oncology Pharmacy Services, Inc.
Arlington, VA

LEXI-COMP, INC

NOTICE

This handbook is intended to serve the user as a handy quick reference and not as a complete drug information resource. It does not include information on every therapeutic agent available. The publication covers commonly used drugs and is specifically designed to present certain important aspects of drug data in a more concise format than is generally found in medical literature or product material supplied by manufacturers.

Drug information is constantly evolving because of ongoing research and clinical experience and is often subject to interpretation. While great care has been taken to ensure the accuracy of the information presented, the reader is advised that the authors, editors, reviewers, contributors, and publishers cannot be responsible for the continued currency of the information or for any errors, omissions, or the application of this information, or for any consequences arising therefrom. Therefore, the author(s) and/or the publisher shall have no liability to any person or entity with regard to claims, loss, or damage caused, or alleged to be caused, directly or indirectly, by the use of information contained herein. Because of the dynamic nature of drug information, readers are advised that decisions regarding drug therapy must be based on the independent judgment of the clinician, changing information about a drug (eg, as reflected in the literature and manufacturer's most current product information), and changing medical practices. The editors are not responsible for any inaccuracy of quotation or for any false or misleading implication that may arise due to the text or formulas as used or due to the quotation of revisions no longer official.

The editors and contributors have written this book in their private capacities. No official support or endorsement by any federal agency or pharmaceutical company is intended or inferred.

If you have any suggestions or questions regarding any information presented in this handbook, please contact our drug information pharmacist at 1-800-837-LEXI (5394).

This manual was produced using the FormuLex™ Program —
a complete publishing service of Lexi-Comp, Inc.

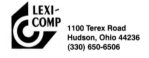

LEXI-COMP

1100 Terex Road
Hudson, Ohio 44236
(330) 650-6506

ISBN 1-59195-117-8

TABLE OF CONTENTS

TABLE OF CONTENTS *(Continued)*

ABOUT THE AUTHOR

Dominic A. Solimando, Jr, MA, FAPhA, FASHP, BCOP

Dominic Solimando is President of Oncology Pharmacy Services, Inc. He received a Bachelor of Science in Pharmacy from the Philadelphia College of Pharmacy and Science, and a Master of Arts in Management and Supervision, specializing in Health Care Administration, from Central Michigan University. Dominic is a Board Certified Oncology Pharmacist. He has practiced as an oncology pharmacist at Georgetown University Medical Center, Washington, DC, Thomas Jefferson University Hospital, Philadelphia; Walter Reed Army Medical Center, Washington, DC; Letterman Army Medical Center, San Francisco; and Tripler Army Medical Center, Honolulu.

Mr. Solimando is a contributing editor for *Hospital Pharmacy*, and was a member of the Editorial Board for *Drug Intelligence and Clinical Pharmacy* from 1984-1988, and the Journal of the American Pharmacists Association from 2000-2003. In addition to APhA and ASHP, Dominic is a member of the American College of Clinical Pharmacy, International Pharmaceutical Federation, International Society of Oncology Pharmacy Practitioners, Hematology/Oncology Pharmacists Association, American Institute of the History of Pharmacy, the Virginia Pharmacists Association, and the Washington Metropolitan Area Society of Health-System Pharmacists. His interests include safety precautions in handling parenteral medications, drug preparation and administration procedures, pain control, antiemetic therapy, and drug-induced toxicities.

EDITORIAL ADVISORY PANEL

Harold L. Crossley, DDS, PhD
Associate Professor of Pharmacology
Baltimore College of Dental Surgery
Dental School
University of Maryland Baltimore
Baltimore, Maryland

Wayne R. DeMott, MD
Consultant in Pathology and Laboratory Medicine
Shawnee Mission, Kansas

Samir Desai, MD
Assistant Professor of Medicine
Department of Medicine
Baylor College of Medicine
Houston, Texas
Staff Physician
Veterans Affairs Medical Center
Houston, Texas

Andrew J. Donnelly, PharmD, MBA
Director of Pharmacy
and
Clinical Professor of Pharmacy Practice
University of Illinois Medical Center at Chicago
Chicago, Illinois

Thom C. Dumsha, DDS
Associate Professor and Chair
Dental School
University of Maryland Baltimore
Baltimore, Maryland

Michael S. Edwards, PharmD, MBA
Assistant Director, Weinberg Pharmacy
Johns Hopkins Hospital
Baltimore, Maryland

Vicki L. Ellingrod-Ringold, PharmD, BCPP
Assistant Professor
University of Iowa
Iowa City, Iowa

Margaret A. Fitzgerald, MS, APRN, BC, NP-C, FAANP
President
Fitzgerald Health Education Associates, Inc.
North Andover, Massachusetts
Family Nurse Practitioner
Greater Lawrence Family Health Center
Lawrence, Massachusetts

Matthew A. Fuller, PharmD, BCPS, BCPP, FASHP
Clinical Pharmacy Specialist, Psychiatry
Cleveland Department of Veterans Affairs Medical Center
Brecksville, Ohio
Associate Clinical Professor of Psychiatry
Clinical Instructor of Psychology
Case Western Reserve University
Cleveland, Ohio
Adjunct Associate Professor of Clinical Pharmacy
University of Toledo
Toledo, Ohio

EDITORIAL ADVISORY PANEL *(Continued)*

Rebecca T. Horvat, PhD
Assistant Professor of Pathology and Laboratory Medicine
University of Kansas Medical Center
Kansas City, Kansas

Collin A. Hovinga, PharmD
Neuropharmacologist
Miami Children's Hospital
Miami, Florida

Darrell T. Hulisz, PharmD
Department of Family Medicine
Case Western Reserve University
Cleveland, Ohio

Sana Isa-Pratt, MD
Attending Physician
Department of Medicine
Overlake Hospital
Bellevue, Washington

David S. Jacobs, MD
President, Pathologists Chartered
Consultant in Pathology and Laboratory Medicine
Overland Park, Kansas

Bernard L. Kasten, Jr, MD, FCAP
Vice-President/Chief Medical Officer
Quest Diagnostics Inc
Teteroboro, New Jersey

Polly E. Kintzel, PharmD, BCPS, BCOP
Clinical Pharmacy Specialist-Oncology
Spectrum Health
Grand Rapids, Michigan

Jill Kolesar, PharmD, FCCP, BCPS
Associate Professor of Pharmacy
University of Wisconsin
Madison, Wisconsin

Donna M. Kraus, PharmD, FAPhA
Associate Professor of Pharmacy Practice
Departments of Pharmacy Practice and Pediatrics
Pediatric Clinical Pharmacist
University of Illinois
Chicago, Illinois

Daniel L. Krinsky, RPh, MS
Director, Pharmacotherapy Sales and Marketing
Lexi-Comp, Inc
Hudson, Ohio

Kay Kyllonen, PharmD
Clinical Specialist
The Cleveland Clinic Children's Hospital
Cleveland, Ohio

EDITORIAL ADVISORY PANEL *(Continued)*

Vincent F. Mauro, BS, PharmD, FCCP
Associate Professor of Clinical Pharmacy
Department of Pharmacy Practice
College of Pharmacy
The University of Toledo
Adjunct Associate Professor of Medicine
Department of Medicine
Medical College of Ohio
Toledo, Ohio

Timothy F. Meiller, DDS, PhD
Professor
Diagnostic Sciences and Pathology
Baltimore College of Dental Surgery
Professor of Oncology
Greenebaum Cancer Center
University of Maryland Baltimore
Baltimore, Maryland

Franklin A. Michota, Jr, MD
Head, Section of Hospital and Preoperative Medicine
Department of General Internal Medicine
The Cleveland Clinic Foundation
Cleveland, Ohio

Michael A. Militello, PharmD, BCPS
Clinical Cardiology Specialist
Department of Pharmacy
The Cleveland Clinic Foundation
Cleveland, Ohio

J. Robert Newland, DDS, MS
Professor
Department of Diagnostic Sciences
University of Texas Health Science Center
Houston, Texas

Cecelia O'Keefe, PharmD
Pharmacotherapy Specialist
Lexi-Comp, Inc.
Hudson, Ohio

Eugene S. Olsowka, MD, PhD
Pathologist
Institute of Pathology PC
Saginaw, Michigan

Dwight K. Oxley, MD
Consultant in Pathology and Laboratory Medicine
Wichita, Kansas

Frank P. Paloucek, PharmD, DABAT
Clinical Associate Professor in Pharmacy Practice
Director, Residency Programs
University of Illinois
Chicago, Illinois

Christopher J. Papasian, PhD
Director of Diagnostic Microbiology and Immunology Laboratories
Truman Medical Center
Kansas City, Missouri

EDITORIAL ADVISORY PANEL *(Continued)*

Liz Tomsik, PharmD, BCPS
Pharmacotherapy Specialist
Lexi-Comp, Inc
Hudson, Ohio

Beatrice B. Turkoski, RN, PhD
Associate Professor, Graduate Faculty,
Advanced Pharmacology
College of Nursing
Kent State University
Kent, Ohio

Dave Weinstein, PhD
Pharmacotherapy Specialist
Lexi-Comp, Inc.
Hudson, Ohio

Anne Marie Whelan, PharmD
College of Pharmacy
Dalhouise University
Halifax, Nova Scotia

Richard L. Wynn, PhD
Professor of Pharmacology
Baltimore College of Dental Surgery
Dental School
University of Maryland Baltimore
Baltimore, Maryland

PREFACE

The *Drug Information Handbook for Oncology* was designed to meet the needs of all oncology professionals involved in prescribing, preparing, and administering therapy. Presented in a concise and uniform format, this book contains 239 monographs with information pertaining to both antineoplastic agents and ancillary medications. This handbook serves as a portable quick reference while providing comprehensive oncology-related drug information. Organized like a dictionary for ease-of-use, a drug can be quickly located by generic name.

The Chemotherapy Regimen section provides a comprehensive presentation of cancer chemotherapy regimens. The regimens are listed alphabetically by regimen name (acronym). An index lists regimens by indication. In addition, a special Combination Chemotherapy Regimen field in each drug monograph will link you to the applicable regimens.

A special topics section addresses issues regarding Cancer Treatment-Related Complications (eg, fertility and cancer therapy, management of nausea and vomiting, management of infections, etc); Cancer-Related Complications (eg, hypercalcemia, pain); Bone Marrow Transplantation; Drug Development, Approval, and Distribution; Investigational Drug Service; and Safe Handling of Hazardous Drugs

The appendix section includes information related to conversions, renal function, and adult reference values. A pharmacologic category index provides a practical approach to categorizing drugs by their respective therapeutic classification.

We know you will find this handbook to be a valuable source of information and we welcome comments or suggestions to further improve future editions.

ACKNOWLEDGMENTS

The *Drug Information Handbook for Oncology* exists in its present form as the result of the concerted efforts of the following individuals: Robert D. Kerscher, publisher and president of Lexi-Comp, Inc; Mark Bonfiglio, PharmD, director of pharmacotherapy resources; Stacy S. Robinson, editorial manager; Barbara F. Kerscher, production manager; David C. Marcus, director of information systems; Cecelia O'Keefe, PharmD and Jeff Lewis, PharmD, pharmacotherapy specialists; Leslie Jo Hoppes, pharmacology database manager; Dawn Conover, project manager; Katie Seabeck, product manager; Tracey J. Henterly, graphic designer; and Julian I. Graubart, American Pharmacists Association (APhA), Director of Books and Electronic Products.

Special acknowledgement to all Lexi-Comp staff for their contributions ot this handbook.

Much of the material contained in this book was a result of pharmacy contributors throughout the United States and Canada. Lexi-Comp has assisted many medical institutions to develop hospital-specific formulary manuals that contain clinical drug information as well as dosing. Working with these clinical pharmacists, hospital pharmacy and therapeutics committees, and hospital drug information centers, Lexi-Comp has developed an evolutionary drug database that reflects the practice of pharmacy in these major institutions.

USE OF THE DRUG INFORMATION HANDBOOK FOR ONCOLOGY

The *Drug Information Handbook for Oncology* is divided into five sections.

The first section is a compilation of introductory text pertinent to the use of this book.

The drug information section of the handbook, in which all drugs are listed alphabetically, details information pertinent to each drug. Extensive cross-referencing is provided by brand names and synonyms.

The Chemotherapy Regimen section provides a comprehensive presentation of cancer chemotherapy regimens. The regimens are listed alphabetically by regimen name (acronym). An index lists regimens by indications. In addition, a special Combination Chemotherapy Regimen field in each drug monograph will link you to the applicable regimens.

The Special Topics section contains important cancer-related issues (ie, pain management, bone marrow transplantation, managing infections, and safe handling of hazardous drugs). These issues are discussed in detail.

The fifth section is an invaluable appendix section with charts, tables, nomograms, algorithms, and guidelines.

The last section of this handbook is an index listing drugs in their unique pharmacologic category.

Alphabetical Listing of Drugs

Drug information is presented in a consistent format and provides the following:

Generic Name	U.S. adopted name
Pronunciation Guide	Phonetic pronunciation
Medication Safety Issues	In an effort to promote the safe use of medications, this field is intended to highlight possible sources of medication errors such as look-alike/sound-alike drugs or highly concentrated formulations which require vigilance on the part of healthcare professionals. In addition, medications which have been associated with severe consequences in the event of a medication error are also identified in this field.
Related Information	Cross-reference to other pertinent drug information found elsewhere in this handbook
U.S. Brand Names	Trade names (manufacturer-specific) found in the United States. The symbol [DSC] appears after trade names that have been recently discontinued.
Canadian Brand Names	Trade names found in Canada
Generic Available	Specifies whether a generic equivalent is available
Synonyms	Other names or accepted abbreviations of the generic drug
Pharmacologic Category	Unique systematic classification of medications
Pregnancy Risk Factor	Five categories established by the FDA to indicate the potential of a systemically absorbed drug for causing birth defects
Lactation	Information describing characteristics of using the drug while breast-feeding

Use	Information pertaining to appropriate FDA-approved indications of the drug.
Unlabeled/Investigational Use	Information pertaining to non-FDA approved and investigational indications of the drug.
Mechanism of Action	How the drug works in the body to elicit a response
Restrictions	The controlled substance classification from the Drug Enforcement Agency (DEA). U.S. schedules are I-V. Schedules vary by country and sometimes state (ie, Massachusetts uses I-VI). May also include restricted availability information.
Labeled Contraindications	Information pertaining to inappropriate use of the drug
Warnings/Precautions	Precautionary considerations, hazardous conditions related to use of the drug, and disease states or patient populations in which the drug should be cautiously used
Adverse Reactions	Side effects are grouped by percentage of incidence (if known) and/or body system
Vesicant	Indicates whether the drug is considered to be a vesicant and likely to cause significant morbidity if the infusion infiltrates soft tissues
Emetic Potential	Likelihood that the drug will cause nausea or vomiting
Overdosage/Toxicology	Comments and/or considerations are offered when appropriate and include signs or symptoms of excess drug and suggested management of the patient
Drug Interactions	
Cytochrome P450 Effect	Describes which cytochrome P450 enzymes are responsible for metabolizing the drug and/or which enzymes might be induced or inhibited by the drug.
Increased Effect/Toxicity	Drug combinations that result in an increased or toxic therapeutic effect between the drug listed in the monograph and other drugs or drug classes
Decreased Effect	Drug combinations that result in a decreased therapeutic effect between the drug listed in the monograph and other drugs or drug classes.
Ethanol/Nutrition/Herb Interactions	Information regarding potential interactions with food, nutritionals, herbal products, vitamins, or ethanol
Storage/Stability	Information regarding storage of product. Provides the time and conditions for which a solution or mixture will maintain full potency. For example, some solutions may require refrigeration after reconstitution while stored at room temperature prior to preparation.
Reconstitution	Includes comments on solution choice with time or conditions for the mixture to maintain full potency before administration
Compatibility	Whether drug is compatible, Y-site compatible, or incompatible with other drugs
Pharmacodynamics/ Kinetics	The magnitude of a drug's effect depends on the drug concentration at the site of action. The pharmacodynamics are expressed in terms of onset of action and duration of action. Pharmacokinetics are expressed in terms of absorption, distribution (including appearance in breast milk and crossing of the placenta), protein binding, metabolism, bioavailability, half-life, time to peak serum concentration, and elimination.

USE OF THE DRUG INFORMATION HANDBOOK FOR ONCOLOGY *(Continued)*

Dosage	The amount of the drug to be typically given or taken during therapy for children and adults; also includes any dosing adjustment for renal impairment or hepatic failure
Combination Regimens	List of combination chemotherapy regimens in which the drug is a component
Administration	Information regarding the recommended final concentrations, rates of administration for parenteral drugs, or other guidelines when giving the medication
Dosage Forms	Information with regard to form, strength, and availability of the drug
High Dose Considerations	Special information regarding high dose chemotherapy use, such as transplantation of autologous or allogeneic bone marrow or peripheral blood cells to facilitate hematopoietic recovery after myeloablative chemotherapy (autologous, allogeneic), and replace a diseased hematopoietic system (allogeneic)
High Dose	Chemotherapy doses 1.5- to 30-fold greater than standard dosages. Nonhematologic adverse reactions are dose-limiting.
Unique Toxicities	Nonhematologic adverse reactions that occur commonly with, or are unique to, high-dose chemotherapy administration.
Comments	Additional information
Monitoring Parameters	Suggested monitoring parameters are listed
Dietary Considerations	Specific dietary modifications and/or restrictions
Patient Information	Specific information pertinent for the patient
Additional Information	Pertinent information about specific brands
Special Geriatric Considerations	Pertinent information specific to the elderly population
Extemporaneous Preparations	Directions for preparing oral or rectal suppositories or liquid formulations from solid drug products. May include stability information and references.
Selected Readings	Recommended for additional information

Chemotherapy Regimens

The Chemotherapy Regimen section provides a comprehensive presentation of cancer chemotherapy regimens. The regimens are listed alphabetically by regimen name (acronym). An index lists regimens by indications. In addition, a special Combination Chemotherapy Regimen field in each drug monograph will link you to the applicable regimens.

Special Topics

Important cancer-related issues (ie, pain management, bone marrow transplantation, managing infections, safe handling of hazardous drugs) are discussed in detail.

Appendix

The appendix offers a compilation of tables, guidelines, nomograms, algorithms, and conversion information which can often be helpful when considering patient care.

Pharmacologic Category Index

This index provides a useful listing of drugs by their pharmacologic classification.

FDA PREGNANCY CATEGORIES

Throughout this book there is a field labeled Pregnancy Risk Factor and the letter A, B, C, D, or X immediately following the field name which signifies a category. The FDA has established these five categories to indicate the potential of a systemically absorbed drug for causing birth defects. The key differentiation among the categories rests upon the reliability of documentation and the risk:benefit ratio. Pregnancy Category X is particularly notable in that if any data exists that may implicate a drug as a teratogen and the risk:benefit ratio is clearly negative, the drug is contraindicated during pregnancy.

These categories are summarized as follows:

A   Controlled studies in pregnant women fail to demonstrate a risk to the fetus in the first trimester with no evidence of risk in later trimesters. The possibility of fetal harm appears remote.

B   Either animal-reproduction studies have not demonstrated a fetal risk but there are no controlled studies in pregnant women, or animal-reproduction studies have shown an adverse effect (other than a decrease in fertility) that was not confirmed in controlled studies in women in the first trimester and there is no evidence of a risk in later trimesters.

C   Either studies in animals have revealed adverse effects on the fetus (teratogenic or embryocidal effects or other) and there are no controlled studies in women, or studies in women and animals are not available. Drugs should be given only if the potential benefits justify the potential risk to the fetus.

D   There is positive evidence of human fetal risk, but the benefits from use in pregnant women may be acceptable despite the risk (eg, if the drug is needed in a life-threatening situation or for a serious disease for which safer drugs cannot be used or are ineffective).

X   Studies in animals or human beings have demonstrated fetal abnormalities or there is evidence of fetal risk based on human experience, or both, and the risk of the use of the drug in pregnant women clearly outweighs any possible benefit. The drug is contraindicated in women who are or may become pregnant.

REDUCING PRESCRIBING ERRORS

Antineoplastic drugs have a low therapeutic index and therefore carry a high risk for toxicity. Even modest deviations in dosage can produce under- or overdosage. Medication errors often occur during prescribing or order writing. The field of oncology is filled with acronyms that may serve as a source of medication error. While acronyms are useful and convenient, they may prove to be an obstacle to those less familiar with antineoplastic therapy, leading to possible misinterpretation. The newspapers have been quick to report fatal antineoplastic orders that resulted from poor prescribing habits and misinterpretation. Standardizing prescribing vocabulary in your institution is one way of reducing the risk for error. The following guidelines outline strategies for error reduction in medication prescribing. These guidelines can be applied to either written treatment protocols or treatment plans as well as written medication orders.

DRUG NAME

Use only approved generic names (United States Adopted Names [USAN]). The use of abbreviations is a source of potential error. This is especially true because abbreviations may stand for more than one drug. Common abbreviations such as "MTX", "CTX", "HN$_2$", "VCR", and "CDDP" can easily be misinterpreted and should be avoided. Even using terms such as "platinum" may cause confusion between cisplatin, carboplatin, or oxaliplatin. Drugs with similar names and actions, but different toxicities and dosage requirements, have been involved in medication errors. Continuing the use of drug name abbreviations that were once utilized when the drug product was investigational is also a problem. Abbreviations such as "VP-16", "VM-26", "CBDCA", "2-Cda", and "FK506" should no longer be used. Abbreviations for current investigational drugs should also be avoided. If your institution utilizes some abbreviations, they should be listed so that everyone has access to them and they are applied consistently.

NUMBERS AND DOSAGE UNITS

The use of zeros in drug doses is a source of error, especially with regard to the use of decimal points. Leading zeros should **always** be used before a decimal point (eg, 0.4 mg) but trailing zeros should **never** be used (eg, 7 mg **NOT** 7.0 mg). The word "units" should always be spelled out rather than abbreviated as "U". A "U" can be mistaken for a zero. The Greek letter mu (μ) should not be used; use "mcg" instead. The use of numbers within drug names should also be avoided. For example, fluorouracil instead of 5-fluorouracil, thioguanine instead of 6-thioguanine, mercaptopurine instead of 6-mercaptopurine.

DOSE, TOTAL DOSE, AND DURATION

The description of dose and duration is complicated and often left to interpretation because of nonstandard language in treatment plans and protocols. For example, "cisplatin 100 mg/m^2 continuously infused days 1-4" has been misinterpreted as cisplatin 100 mg/m^2/day for 4 days, dispensed and administered, resulting in the death of the patient. Providing clear dose and duration instructions will prevent errors that occur due to interpretation of the author's meaning. Treatment plans and medication orders should include the dose based on patient parameters (body surface area, body weight, pharmacokinetic parameters), the calculated dose with any dosage reduction, how many hours or days the dose is to be administered, which specific days the dose should be administered, and the total dose per treatment course or cycle.

REDUCING PRESCRIBING ERRORS *(Continued)*

Example: Patient is 1.8 m^2. ABC 50 mg/m^2/day I.V. push for 3 days = 90 mg I.V.
push on days 3, 4, and 5
(total dose per cycle = 270 mg).

Some would argue that each institution should standardize the calculations for body surface area and creatinine clearance.

VERIFYING DOSES/PROTOCOLS

Each institution should develop policies for as many independent dose checks as possible. The pharmacist should review the treatment protocol. If there is no treatment protocol, or the treatment plan is from a published article, the pharmacist should verify the doses from additional sources due to the possibility of errors in the literature.

STANDARDIZED ORDER FORMS

Many prescribing errors can be eliminated by the use of preprinted order forms. Pharmacists should be involved in the development of a form in their institution. The format of the form can vary. Three common formats have been suggested. First, a blank form that includes preprinted areas for premedications, antineoplastic drugs with doses in mg/m^2 or mg/kg, an area for the duration and dates of therapy, and an area for posttreatment drugs. Second, a preprinted form that is specific to a treatment protocol and contains preprinted drug doses. Third, a form that includes preprinted names of all antineoplastic drugs with check-off boxes and fill-ins for doses and routes. Whichever form is adapted for use, it is important that the form is easily distinguished from other order forms and is readily available at the point when and where antineoplastic orders are written.

COMMUNICATION

Communication is an important part of preventing medication errors from occurring. Pharmacists should be involved in writing or editing treatment protocols within institutions along with other healthcare providers. Pharmacists may participate in national study group committees that review dosing guidelines in protocols. Educating patients and families on their antineoplastic therapy will encourage them to question healthcare providers and become part of the error prevention process.

CONCLUSION

It is possible for anyone to make a mistake. A systematic method for preventing medication prescribing errors includes policies on drug names, use of abbreviations, stating duration and days of therapy, and total dose per cycle. The addition of preprinted order forms and communication among all disciplines during the protocol development process provides additional tools for preventing errors. It is important to remember that this is only one part of an entire process that contributes to potential medication errors.

Selected Readings

"ASHP Guidelines on Preventing Medication Errors in Hospitals," *Am J Hosp Pharm*, 1993, 50(2):305-14.

Attilio RM, "Strategies for Reducing Chemotherapy-Related Medication Errors: Improving the Chemotherapy Prescribing, Dispensing, and Administration Process, and the Patient's Role in Ensuring Safety," *Hosp Pharm*, 1997, 32(Suppl 1):S14-20.

Cohen MR, Anderson RW, Attilio RM, et al, "Preventing Medication Errors in Cancer Chemotherapy," *Am J Health Syst Pharm*, 1996, 53(7):737-46.

Kohler DR, Montello MJ, Green L, et al, "Standardizing the Expression and Nomenclature of Cancer Treatment Regimens," *Am J Health Syst Pharm*, 1998; 55(2):137-44.

ALPHABETICAL LISTING OF DRUGS

♦ **1370-999-397** *see* Anagrelide *on page 82*

Abarelix (a ba REL iks)

U.S. Brand Names Plenaxis™

Generic Available No

Synonyms PPI-149; R-3827

Pharmacologic Category Gonadotropin Releasing Hormone Antagonist

Pregnancy Risk Factor X

Lactation Excretion in breast milk unknown/not indicated in women

Use Palliative treatment of advanced symptomatic or metastatic prostate cancer; treatment is limited to men who are not candidates for LHRH therapy, refuse surgical castration, and have one or more of the following complications due to metastases or local encroachment: 1) risk of neurological compromise, 2) ureteral or bladder outlet obstruction, or 3) severe bone pain (persisting despite narcotic analgesia)

Mechanism of Action Competes with naturally occurring GnRH for binding on receptors of the pituitary. Suppresses LH and FSH, resulting in decreased testosterone.

Restrictions Abarelix is not distributed through retail pharmacies. Prescribing and distribution of abarelix is limited to physicians and hospital pharmacies participating in the Plenaxis™ PLUS program. See Additional Information, or contact Praecis Pharmaceuticals at www.plenaxisplus.com or by calling 1-877-772-3247.

Labeled Contraindications Hypersensitivity to abarelix or any component of the formulation

Warnings/Precautions Hazardous agent - use appropriate precautions for handling and disposal. See Safe Handling of Hazardous Drugs *on page 1034* in the Appendix. Has been associated with immediate-onset allergic reactions; may occur with initial dose and risk increases with duration of treatment. Observe for signs/symptoms of allergic reactions (which may include hypotension and/or syncope) for at least 30 minutes following each injection. Abarelix may cause prolongation of the QT interval; consider risk:benefit in patients with baseline QT_c values >450 msec or patients receiving concurrent medications which prolong the QT_c interval (class Ia and class III antiarrhythmics). Efficacy may diminish during prolonged treatment, particularly in patients weighing >225 pounds; monitor serum testosterone levels to identify treatment failures. Monitor transaminase levels and hepatic function during therapy. Extended treatment may result in a decrease in bone mineral density. Not indicated for use in women or children.

Adverse Reactions

>10%:

Cardiovascular: Hot flushes (79%), peripheral edema (15%)

Central nervous system: Sleep disturbance (44%), pain (31%), dizziness (12%), headache (12%)

Endocrine & metabolic: Breast enlargement (30%), nipple discharge/tenderness (20%)

Gastrointestinal: Constipation (15%), diarrhea (11%)

Neuromuscular & skeletal: Back pain (17%)

Respiratory: Upper respiratory infection (12%)

1% to 10%:

Central nervous system: Fatigue (10%)

Endocrine & metabolic: Serum triglycerides increased (10%)

Gastrointestinal: Nausea (10%)

Genitourinary: Dysuria (10%), micturition frequency (10%), urinary retention (10%), urinary tract infection (10%)

Hepatic: Transaminases increased (2% to 8%)

Miscellaneous: Allergic reactions (urticaria, pruritus, syncope, hypotension): risk increases with prolonged treatment

Vesicant No

Emetic Potential Low (10%)

Overdosage/Toxicology No experience in overdose. Treatment is symptomatic and supportive.

Drug Interactions

Increased Effect/Toxicity: When used with other QT_c-prolonging agents, additive QT_c prolongation may occur. Life-threatening ventricular arrhythmias may result; example drugs include class Ia and class III antiarrhythmics, cisapride, selected quinolones, erythromycin, pimozide, mesoridazine, and thioridazine.

Storage/Stability Store at room temperature: 25°C (77°F), excursions permitted to 15°C to 30°C (58°F to 86°F). Reconstituted solution is stable for at least 8 hours at 30°C.

Reconstitution Reconstitute vial with 2.2 mL of NS; reconstituted solutions contain abarelix 50 mg/mL.

Pharmacodynamics/Kinetics

Distribution: V_d: 4040 L (± 1607)

Metabolism: Hepatic, via peptide hydrolysis

Half-life elimination: 13 days

Time to peak, serum: 3 days (following I.M. administration)

Excretion: Urine (13% unchanged drug)

Dosage I.M.: Male prostate cancer: 100 mg administered on days 1, 15, 29 (week 4), then every 4 weeks

Administration Administer intramuscularly (to the buttock).

Dosage Forms Injection, powder for reconstitution [preservative free]: 113 mg [provides 100 mg/2 mL depot suspension when reconstituted; packaged with diluent and syringe]

Monitoring Parameters Signs/symptoms of allergic reaction (for at least 30 minutes after each injection). Obtain transaminase levels at baseline and periodically during treatment. Serum testosterone (to identify treatment failure) just prior to abarelix administration, beginning on day 29 and every 8 weeks thereafter. PSA and bone mineral density may be monitored as needed.

Additional Information Prior to distribution, Praecis Pharmaceuticals must enroll prescribing physicians and/or hospital pharmacies in the Plenaxis™ user safety program (Plenaxis™ PLUS). A Physician Attestation form must be used to document the physician's qualifications and acceptance of responsibilities concerning patient education and adverse effect reporting. Physicians must obtain the patient's signature and personally cosign the two-part Plenaxis™ Patient Information leaflet. The original signed copy should be retained in the patient's medical record while the other copy should be given to the patient. Hospital pharmacies must submit a hospital pharmacy agreement form to allow dispensing, which will be limited to physicians enrolled in the prescriber's registry. Confirmation of physician enrollment may be obtained by calling 1-866-753-6294. All doses must be dispensed with a Patient Information (Continued)

Abarelix *(Continued)*

leaflet. Distributors must restrict shipment to physicians or hospital pharmacies enrolled in the Plenaxis™ prescribing program. Additional details and/or forms may be obtained through Praecis Pharmaceuticals at www.plenaxisplus.com or by calling 1-877-772-3247.

Selected Readings

"Abarelix: Abarelix-depot-F, Abarelix-depot-M, Abarelix-L, PPI 149, R 3827," *Drugs R D*, 2003, 4(3):161-6.

McLeod D, Zinner N, Tomera K, et al, "A Phase 3, Multicenter, Open-Label, Randomized Study of Abarelix Versus Leuprolide Acetate in Men With Prostate Cancer," *Urology*, 2001, 58(5):756-61.

Trachtenberg J, Gittleman M, Steidle C, et al, "A Phase 3, Multicenter, Open Label, Randomized Study of Abarelix Versus Leuprolide Plus Daily Antiandrogen in Men With Prostate Cancer," *J Urol*, 2002, 167(4):1670-4.

Wong SL, Lau DR, Baughman SA, et al, "Pharmacokinetics and Pharmacodynamics of Abarelix, a Gonadotropin-Releasing Hormone Antagonist, After Subcutaneous Continuous Infusion in Patients With Prostate Cancer," *Clin Pharmacol Ther*, 2003, 73(4):304-11.

- ♦ **Abbott-43818** *see* Leuprolide *on page 500*
- ♦ **ABCD** *see* Amphotericin B Cholesteryl Sulfate Complex *on page 66*
- ♦ **Abelcet®** *see* Amphotericin B (Lipid Complex) *on page 73*
- ♦ **ABLC** *see* Amphotericin B (Lipid Complex) *on page 73*
- ♦ **Abraxane™** *see* Paclitaxel (Protein Bound) *on page 644*
- ♦ **9-AC** *see* Aminocamptothecin *on page 59*
- ♦ **Acetoxymethylprogesterone** *see* MedroxyPROGESTERone *on page 524*
- ♦ **Aciclovir** *see* Acyclovir *on page 26*
- ♦ **4-(9-Acridinylamino) Methanesulfon-m-Anisidide** *see* Amsacrine *on page 80*
- ♦ **Acridinyl Anisidide** *see* Amsacrine *on page 80*
- ♦ **ACT** *see* Dactinomycin *on page 245*
- ♦ **Act-D** *see* Dactinomycin *on page 245*
- ♦ **Actimmune®** *see* Interferon Gamma-1b *on page 477*
- ♦ **Actinomycin** *see* Dactinomycin *on page 245*
- ♦ **Actinomycin Cl** *see* Dactinomycin *on page 245*
- ♦ **Actinomycin D** *see* Dactinomycin *on page 245*
- ♦ **Actiq®** *see* Fentanyl *on page 335*
- ♦ **Activase®** *see* Alteplase *on page 46*
- ♦ **Activase® rt-PA (Can)** *see* Alteplase *on page 46*
- ♦ **ACV** *see* Acyclovir *on page 26*
- ♦ **Acycloguanosine** *see* Acyclovir *on page 26*

Acyclovir *(ay SYE kloe veer)*

Medication Safety Issues

Sound-alike/look-alike issues:

Zovirax® may be confused with Zostrix®, Zyvox™

Related Information

Management of Infections *on page 978*

U.S. Brand Names Zovirax®

Canadian Brand Names Alti-Acyclovir; Apo-Acyclovir®; Gen-Acyclovir; Nu-Acyclovir; ratio-Acyclovir; Zovirax®

Generic Available Yes: Excludes cream, ointment

Synonyms Aciclovir; ACV; Acycloguanosine

Pharmacologic Category Antiviral Agent

Pregnancy Risk Factor B

Lactation Enters breast milk/use with caution (AAP rates "compatible")

Use Treatment of genital herpes simplex virus (HSV), herpes labialis (cold sores), herpes zoster (shingles), HSV encephalitis, neonatal HSV, mucocutaneous HSV, varicella-zoster (chickenpox)

Unlabeled/Investigational Use Prevention of HSV reactivation in HIV positive patients; prevention of HSV reactivation in hematopoietic stem cell transplant (HSCT); prevention of CMV infection after bone marrow transplants in HSV and CMV seropositive individuals

Mechanism of Action Acyclovir is converted to acyclovir monophosphate by virus-specific thymidine kinase then further converted to acyclovir triphosphate by other cellular enzymes. Acyclovir triphosphate inhibits DNA synthesis and viral replication by competing with deoxyguanosine triphosphate for viral DNA polymerase and being incorporated into viral DNA.

Labeled Contraindications Hypersensitivity to acyclovir, valacyclovir, or any component of the formulation

Warnings/Precautions Use with caution in immunocompromised patients; thrombocytopenic purpura/hemolytic uremic syndrome (TTP/HUS) has been reported. Use caution in the elderly, pre-existing renal disease or in those receiving other nephrotoxic drugs. Maintain adequate hydration during I.V. therapy. Use I.V. preparation with caution in patients with underlying neurologic abnormalities, serious hepatic or electrolyte abnormalities, or substantial hypoxia.

Chickenpox: Treatment should begin within 24 hours of appearance of rash; oral route not recommended for routine use in otherwise healthy children with varicella, but may be effective in patients at increased risk of moderate to severe infection (>12 years of age, chronic cutaneous or pulmonary disorders, long-term salicylate therapy, corticosteroid therapy).

Genital herpes: Physical contact should be avoided when lesions are present; transmission may also occur in the absence of symptoms. Treatment should begin with the first signs or symptoms.

Herpes labialis: For external use only to the lips and face; do not apply to eye or inside the mouth or nose. Treatment should begin with the first signs or symptoms.

Herpes zoster: Acyclovir should be started within 72 hours of appearance of rash to be effective.

Adverse Reactions

Systemic: Oral:

1% to 10%:

Central nervous system: Lightheadedness, headache

Gastrointestinal: Diarrhea, nausea, vomiting, abdominal pain

Systemic: Parenteral:

>10%:

Central nervous system: Lightheadedness

Gastrointestinal: Anorexia

1% to 10%:

Dermatologic: Hives, itching, rash

Gastrointestinal: Nausea, vomiting

(Continued)

Acyclovir *(Continued)*

   Hepatic: Liver function tests increased
   Local: Inflammation at injection site or phlebitis
   Renal: Acute renal failure, BUN increased, creatinine increased

Topical:
   >10%: Mild pain, burning, or stinging
   1% to 10%: Itching

All forms: <1%, postmarketing, and/or case reports: Abdominal pain, aggression, agitation, alopecia, anaphylaxis, anemia, angioedema, anorexia, ataxia, coma, confusion, consciousness decreased, delirium, diarrhea, dizziness, dysarthria, encephalopathy, erythema multiforme, fatigue, fever, gastrointestinal distress, hallucinations, hematuria, hepatitis, hyperbilirubinemia, insomnia, jaundice, leukocytoclastic vasculitis, leukopenia, local tissue necrosis (following extravasation), mental depression, myalgia, paresthesia, peripheral edema, photosensitization, pruritus, psychosis, renal failure, seizure, somnolence, sore throat, Stevens-Johnson syndrome, thrombocytopenia, thrombocytopenic purpura/hemolytic uremic syndrome (TTP/HUS), toxic epidermal necrolysis, tremor, urticaria, visual disturbances

Vesicant No

Emetic Potential Very low (<10%)

Overdosage/Toxicology Symptoms of overdose include seizures, somnolence, confusion, elevated serum creatinine, and renal failure. In the event of overdose, sufficient urine flow must be maintained to avoid drug precipitation within renal tubules. Hemodialysis has resulted in up to 60% reduction in serum acyclovir levels.

Drug Interactions
   Increased Effect/Toxicity: Increased CNS side effects when taken with zidovudine or probenecid.

Ethanol/Nutrition/Herb Interactions Food: Does not appear to affect absorption of acyclovir.

Storage/Stability
   Capsule, tablet: Store at controlled room temperature of 15°C to 25°C (59°F to 77°F); protect from moisture.
   Cream, suspension: Store at controlled room temperature of 15°C to 25°C (59°F to 77°F).
   Ointment: Store at controlled room temperature of 15°C to 25°C (59°F to 77°F) in a dry place.
   Injection: Store powder at controlled room temperature of 15°C to 25°C (59°F to 77°F). Reconstituted solutions remain stable for 12 hours at room temperature. Do not refrigerate reconstituted solutions as they may precipitate. Once diluted for infusion, use within 24 hours.

Reconstitution Powder for injection: Reconstitute acyclovir 500 mg with SWFI 10 mL; do not use bacteriostatic water containing benzyl alcohol or parabens. For intravenous infusion, dilute to a final concentration of ≤7 mg/mL. Concentrations >10 mg/mL increase the risk of phlebitis.

Compatibility Incompatible with blood products and protein-containing solutions
   Stable in D_5W, D_5NS, $D_51/4NS$, $D_51/2NS$, LR, NS.
   Y-site administration: Compatible: Allopurinol, amikacin, amphotericin B cholesteryl sulfate complex, ampicillin, cefamandole, cefazolin, cefoperazone, cefotaxime, cefoxitin, ceftazidime, ceftizoxime, ceftriaxone,

cefuroxime, chloramphenicol, cimetidine, clindamycin, co-trimoxazole, dexamethasone, dimenhydrinate, diphenhydramine, docetaxel, doxorubicin liposome, doxycycline, erythromycin lactobionate, etoposide, famotidine, filgrastim, fluconazole, gatifloxacin, gentamicin, granisetron, heparin, hydrocortisone sodium succinate, hydromorphone, imipenem/cilastatin, linezolid, lorazepam, magnesium sulfate, melphalan, methylprednisolone sodium succinate, metoclopramide, metronidazole, multivitamins, nafcillin, oxacillin, paclitaxel, penicillin G potassium, pentobarbital, perphenazine, piperacillin, potassium chloride, propofol, ranitidine, remifentanil, sodium bicarbonate, tacrolimus, teniposide, theophylline, thiotepa, ticarcillin, tobramycin, vancomycin, zidovudine. **Incompatible:** Amifostine, amsacrine, aztreonam, cefepime, dobutamine, dopamine, fludarabine, foscarnet, gemcitabine, idarubicin, levofloxacin, ondansetron, piperacillin/tazobactam, sargramostim, vinorelbine. **Variable (consult detailed reference):** Cisatracurium, diltiazem, meperidine, meropenem, morphine, TPN.

Compatibility when admixed: Compatible: Fluconazole. **Incompatible:** Dobutamine, dopamine. **Variable (consult detailed reference):** Meropenem.

Pharmacodynamics/Kinetics

Absorption: Oral: 15% to 30%

Distribution: V_d: 0.8 L/kg (63.6 L): Widely (ie, brain, kidney, lungs, liver, spleen, muscle, uterus, vagina, CSF)

Protein binding: <30%

Metabolism: Hepatic (small amounts)

Half-life elimination: Terminal: Neonates: 4 hours; Children 1-12 years: 2-3 hours; Adults: 3 hours

Time to peak, serum: Oral: Within 1.5-2 hours; I.V.: Within 1 hour

Excretion: Urine (30% to 90% as unchanged drug)

Dosage Note: Obese patients should be dosed using ideal body weight

Genital HSV:

I.V.: Children ≥12 years and Adults (immunocompetent): Initial episode, severe: 5 mg/kg every 8 hours for 5-7 days

Oral:

Children:

Initial episode (unlabeled use): 40-80 mg/kg/day divided into 3-4 doses for 5-10 days (maximum: 1 g/day)

Chronic suppression (unlabeled use; limited data): 80 mg/kg/day in 3 divided doses (maximum: 1 g/day), re-evaluate after 12 months of treatment

Adults:

Initial episode: 200 mg every 4 hours while awake (5 times/day) for 10 days (per manufacturer's labeling); 400 mg 3 times/day for 5-10 days has also been reported

Recurrence: 200 mg every 4 hours while awake (5 times/day) for 5 days (per manufacturer's labeling; begin at earliest signs of disease); 400 mg 3 times/day for 5 days has also been reported

Chronic suppression: 400 mg twice daily or 200 mg 3-5 times/day, for up to 12 months followed by re-evaluation (per manufacturer's labeling); 400-1200 mg/day in 2-3 divided doses has also been reported

(Continued)

Acyclovir *(Continued)*

Topical: Adults (immunocompromised): Ointment: Initial episode: $1/2$" ribbon of ointment for a 4" square surface area every 3 hours (6 times/day) for 7 days

Herpes labialis (cold sores): Topical: Children ≥12 years and Adults: Cream: Apply 5 times/day for 4 days

Herpes zoster (shingles):

Oral: Adults (immunocompetent): 800 mg every 4 hours (5 times/day) for 7-10 days

I.V.:

Children <12 years (immunocompromised): 20 mg/kg/dose every 8 hours for 7 days

Children ≥12 years and Adults (immunocompromised): 10 mg/kg/dose or 500 mg/m^2/dose every 8 hours for 7 days

HSV encephalitis: I.V.:

Children 3 months to 12 years: 20 mg/kg/dose every 8 hours for 10 days (per manufacturer's labeling); dosing for 14-21 days also reported

Children ≥12 years and Adults: 10 mg/kg/dose every 8 hours for 10 days (per manufacturer's labeling); 10-15 mg/kg/dose every 8 hours for 14-21 days also reported

Mucocutaneous HSV:

I.V.:

Children <12 years (immunocompromised): 10 mg/kg/dose every 8 hours for 7 days

Children ≥12 years and Adults (immunocompromised): 5 mg/kg/dose every 8 hours for 7 days (per manufacturer's labeling); dosing for up to 14 days also reported

Oral: Adults (immunocompromised, unlabeled use): 400 mg 5 times a day for 7-14 days

Topical: Ointment: Adults (nonlife-threatening, immunocompromised): $1/2$" ribbon of ointment for a 4" square surface area every 3 hours (6 times/day) for 7 days

Neonatal HSV: I.V.: Neonate: Birth to 3 months: 10 mg/kg/dose every 8 hours for 10 days (manufacturer's labeling); 15 mg/kg/dose or 20 mg/kg/dose every 8 hours for 14-21 days has also been reported

Varicella-zoster (chickenpox): Begin treatment within the first 24 hours of rash onset:

Oral:

Children ≥2 years and ≤40 kg (immunocompetent): 20 mg/kg/dose (up to 800 mg/dose) 4 times/day for 5 days

Children >40 kg and Adults (immunocompetent): 800 mg/dose 4 times a day for 5 days

I.V.:

Children <1 year (immunocompromised, unlabeled use): 10 mg/kg/dose every 8 hours for 7-10 days

Children ≥1 year and Adults (immunocompromised, unlabeled use): 1500 mg/m^2/day divided every 8 hours or 10 mg/kg/dose every 8 hours for 7-10 days

Prevention of HSV reactivation in HIV-positive patients, for use only when recurrences are frequent or severe (unlabeled use): Oral:
Children: 80 mg/kg/day in 3-4 divided doses
Adults: 200 mg 3 times/day or 400 mg 2 times/day

Prevention of HSV reactivation in HSCT (unlabeled use): Note: Start at the beginning of conditioning therapy and continue until engraftment or until mucositis resolves (~30 days)
Oral: Adults: 200 mg 3 times/day
I.V.:
Children: 250 mg/m^2/dose every 8 hours or 125 mg/m^2/dose every 6 hours
Adults: 250 mg/m^2/dose every 12 hours

Bone marrow transplant recipients (unlabeled use): I.V.: Children and Adults: Allogeneic patients who are HSV and CMV seropositive: 500 mg/m^2/dose (10 mg/kg) every 8 hours; for clinically-symptomatic CMV infection, consider replacing acyclovir with ganciclovir

Dosing adjustment in renal impairment:
Oral:
Cl_{cr} 10-25 mL/minute: Normal dosing regimen 800 mg every 4 hours: Administer 800 mg every 8 hours
Cl_{cr} <10 mL/minute:
Normal dosing regimen 200 mg every 4 hours, 200 mg every 8 hours, or 400 mg every 12 hours: Administer 200 mg every 12 hours
Normal dosing regimen 800 mg every 4 hours: Administer 800 mg every 12 hours
I.V.:
Cl_{cr} 25-50 mL/minute: Administer recommended dose every 12 hours
Cl_{cr} 10-25 mL/minute: Administer recommended dose every 24 hours
Cl_{cr} <10 mL/minute: Administer 50% of recommended dose every 24 hours
Hemodialysis: Administer dose after dialysis
Peritoneal dialysis: No supplemental dose needed
CAVH: 3.5 mg/kg/day
CVVHD/CVVH: Adjust dose based upon Cl_{cr} 30 mL/minute

Administration
Oral: May be administered with or without food.
I.V.: Avoid rapid infusion; infuse over 1 hour to prevent renal damage; maintain adequate hydration of patient; check for phlebitis and rotate infusion sites
Topical: Not for use in the eye. Apply using a finger cot or rubber glove to avoid transmission to other parts of the body or to other persons.

Dosage Forms
Capsule: 200 mg
Cream, topical: 5% (2 g)
Injection, powder for reconstitution, as sodium: 500 mg, 1000 mg
Zovirax®: 500 mg
Injection, solution, as sodium [preservative free]: 25 mg/mL (20 mL, 40 mL); 50 mg/mL (10 mL, 20 mL)
Ointment, topical: 5% (15 g)
Suspension, oral: 200 mg/5 mL (480 mL) [banana flavor]
Tablet: 400 mg, 800 mg
(Continued)

Acyclovir *(Continued)*

Monitoring Parameters Urinalysis, BUN, serum creatinine, liver enzymes, CBC

Dietary Considerations May be taken with or without food. Acyclovir 500 mg injection contains sodium ~50 mg (~2 mEq).

Patient Information This is not a cure for herpes (recurrences tend to continually reappear every 3-6 months after original infection), nor will this medication reduce the risk of transmission to others when lesions are present; avoid sexual intercourse when visible lesions are present. Take as directed for full course of therapy; do not discontinue even if feeling better. Oral doses may be taken with food.

Special Geriatric Considerations Calculate creatinine clearance. Dose adjustment may be necessary depending on renal function.

Selected Readings

Almond MK, Fan S, Dhillon S, et al, "Avoiding Acyclovir Neurotoxicity in Patients With Chronic Renal Failure Undergoing Haemodialysis," *Nephron*, 1995, 69(4):428-32.

American Academy of Pediatrics Committee on Infectious Diseases, "The Use of Oral Acyclovir in Otherwise Healthy Children With Varicella," *Pediatrics*, 1993, 91(3):674-6.

Arndt KA, "Adverse Reactions to Acyclovir: Topical, Oral, and Intravenous," *J Am Acad Dermatol*, 1988, 18(1 Pt 2):188-90.

Englund JA, Fletcher CV, and Balfour HH Jr, "Acyclovir Therapy in Neonates," *J Pediatr*, 1991, 119(1 Pt 1):129-35.

McKendrick MW, McGill JI, White JE, et al, "Oral Acyclovir in Acute Herpes Zoster," *Br Med J [Clin Res Ed]*, 1986, 293:1529-32.

Whitley RJ and Gnann JW Jr, "Acyclovir: A Decade Later," *N Engl J Med*, 1992, 327(11):782-3.

- ◆ **AD3L** *see* Valrubicin *on page 808*
- ◆ **ADR** *see* DOXOrubicin *on page 280*
- ◆ **Adria** *see* DOXOrubicin *on page 280*
- ◆ **Adriamycin® (Can)** *see* DOXOrubicin *on page 280*
- ◆ **Adriamycin PFS®** *see* DOXOrubicin *on page 280*
- ◆ **Adriamycin RDF®** *see* DOXOrubicin *on page 280*
- ◆ **Adrucil®** *see* Fluorouracil *on page 359*
- ◆ **Advate** *see* Antihemophilic Factor (Recombinant) *on page 92*
- ◆ **AG** *see* Aminoglutethimide *on page 63*
- ◆ **Agrylin®** *see* Anagrelide *on page 82*
- ◆ **AGT** *see* Aminoglutethimide *on page 63*
- ◆ **AHF (Human)** *see* Antihemophilic Factor (Human) *on page 87*
- ◆ **AHF (Porcine)** *see* Antihemophilic Factor (Porcine) *on page 90*
- ◆ **AHF (Recombinant)** *see* Antihemophilic Factor (Recombinant) *on page 92*
- ◆ **A-hydroCort** *see* Hydrocortisone *on page 419*
- ◆ **AK-Pred®** *see* PrednisoLONE *on page 679*
- ◆ **AKTob®** *see* Tobramycin *on page 771*
- ◆ **Alcomicin® (Can)** *see* Gentamicin *on page 398*

Aldesleukin *(al des LOO kin)*

Medication Safety Issues

Sound-alike/look-alike issues:

Aldesleukin may be confused with oprelvekin

Proleukin® may be confused with oprelvekin

Related Information

Safe Handling of Hazardous Drugs *on page 1034*

U.S. Brand Names Proleukin®

Canadian Brand Names Proleukin®

Generic Available No

Synonyms Epidermal Thymocyte Activating Factor; ETAF; IL-2; Inter-leukin-2; Lymphocyte Mitogenic Factor; NSC-373364; T-Cell Growth Factor; TCGF; Thymocyte-Stimulating Factor

Pharmacologic Category Biological Response Modulator

Pregnancy Risk Factor C

Lactation Enters breast milk/contraindicated

Use Treatment of metastatic renal cell cancer, melanoma

Unlabeled/Investigational Use Investigational: Multiple myeloma, HIV infection, and AIDS; may be used in conjunction with lympho-kine-activated killer (LAK) cells, tumor-infiltrating lymphocyte (TIL) cells, interleukin-1, and interferons; colorectal cancer; non-Hodgkin's lymphoma

Mechanism of Action Aldesleukin promotes proliferation, differentiation, and recruitment of T and B cells, natural killer (NK) cells, and thymocytes; causes cytolytic activity in a subset of lymphocytes and subsequent inter-actions between the immune system and malignant cells; can stimulate lymphokine-activated killer (LAK) cells and tumor-infiltrating lymphocytes (TIL) cells.

Labeled Contraindications Hypersensitivity to aldesleukin or any component of the formulation; patients with abnormal thallium stress or pulmonary function tests; patients who have had an organ allograft; retreatment in patients who have experienced sustained ventricular tach-ycardia (≥5 beats), refractory cardiac rhythm disturbances, recurrent chest pain with ECG changes consistent with angina or myocardial infarc-tion, intubation ≥72 hours, pericardial tamponade, renal dialysis for ≥72 hours, coma or toxic psychosis lasting ≥48 hours, repetitive or refractory seizures, bowel ischemia/perforation, GI bleeding requiring surgery

Warnings/Precautions Hazardous agent - use appropriate precautions for handling and disposal. See Safe Handling of Hazardous Drugs *on page 1034* in the Appendix. Has been associated with capillary leak syndrome (CLS) resulting in hypotension and reduced organ perfusion which may be severe and can result in death. Therapy should be restricted to patients with normal cardiac and pulmonary functions as defined by thallium stress and formal pulmonary function testing. Extreme caution should be used in patients with a history of prior cardiac or pulmonary disease.

May exacerbate pre-existing or initial presentation of autoimmune diseases and inflammatory disorders. Patients should be evaluated and treated for CNS metastases and have a negative scan prior to treatment. Mental status changes (irritability, confusion, depression) can occur and may indicate bacteremia, hypoperfusion, CNS malignancy, or CNS toxicity.

Adverse Reactions

>10%:

Cardiovascular: Hypotension (85%), dose-limiting, possibly fatal; sinus tachycardia (70%); arrhythmia (22%); edema (47%); angina

Central nervous system: Mental status changes (transient memory loss, confusion, drowsiness) (73%); dizziness (17%); cognitive changes, (Continued)

Aldesleukin *(Continued)*

fatigue, malaise, somnolence and disorientation (25%); headaches, insomnia, paranoid delusion

Dermatologic: Macular erythematous rash (100% of patients on high-dose therapy); pruritus (48%); erythema (41%); rash (26%); exfoliative dermatitis (14%); dry skin (15%)

Endocrine & metabolic: Fever and chills (89%); low electrolyte levels (magnesium, calcium, phosphate, sodium) (1% to 15%)

Gastrointestinal: Nausea and vomiting (87%); diarrhea (76%); stomatitis (32%); GI bleeding (13%); weight gain (23%), anorexia (27%)

Hematologic: Anemia (77%); thrombocytopenia (64%); leukopenia (34%) - may be dose-limiting; coagulation disorders (10%)

Hepatic: Transient elevations of bilirubin (64%) and enzymes (56%); jaundice (11%)

Neuromuscular & skeletal: Weakness; rigors - respond to acetaminophen, diphenhydramine, an NSAID, or meperidine

Renal: Oliguria/anuria (63%, severe in 5% to 6%), proteinuria (12%); renal failure (dose-limiting toxicity) manifested as oliguria noted within 24-48 hours of initiation of therapy; marked fluid retention, azotemia, and increased serum creatinine seen, which may return to baseline within 7 days of discontinuation of therapy; hypophosphatemia

Respiratory: Congestion (54%); dyspnea (27% to 52%)

Miscellaneous: Pain (54%), infection (including sepsis and endocarditis) due to neutrophil impairment (23%)

1% to 10%:

Cardiovascular: Capillary leak syndrome, including peripheral edema, ascites, pulmonary infiltration, and pleural effusion (2% to 4%), may be dose-limiting and potentially fatal; MI (2%)

Central nervous system: Seizures (1%)

Endocrine & metabolic: Hypo- and hyperglycemia (2%); increased electrolyte levels (magnesium, calcium, phosphate, potassium, sodium) (1%), hypothyroidism

Hepatic: Ascites (4%)

Neuromuscular & skeletal: Arthralgia (6%), myalgia (6%)

Renal: Hematuria (9%), increased creatinine (5%)

Respiratory: Pleural effusions, edema (10%)

<1%: CHF, coma, alopecia, pancreatitis, allergic reactions, injection site reactions (SubQ doses)

Vesicant No

Emetic Potential Highly emetogenic (60% to 90%, dose-related)

Overdosage/Toxicology Side effects following the use of aldesleukin are dose related. Administration of more than the recommended dose has been associated with a more rapid onset of expected dose-limiting toxicities. Adverse reactions generally will reverse when the drug is stopped particularly because of its short serum half-life. Provide supportive treatment of any continuing symptoms. Life-threatening toxicities have been ameliorated by the I.V. administration of dexamethasone, but may decrease the therapeutic effect of aldesleukin.

Drug Interactions

Increased Effect/Toxicity: Aldesleukin may affect central nervous function; therefore, interactions could occur following concomitant administration of psychotropic drugs (eg, narcotics, analgesics, antiemetics, sedatives, tranquilizers).

Concomitant administration of drugs possessing nephrotoxic (eg, aminoglycosides, indomethacin), myelotoxic (eg, cytotoxic chemotherapy), cardiotoxic (eg, doxorubicin), or hepatotoxic effects with aldesleukin may increase toxicity in these organ systems.

Beta-blockers and other antihypertensives may potentiate the hypotension seen with aldesleukin.

Decreased Effect: Corticosteroids have been shown to decrease toxicity of aldesleukin, but may reduce the efficacy of the lymphokine.

Ethanol/Nutrition/Herb Interactions Ethanol: May increase CNS adverse effects

Storage/Stability Store vials of lyophilized injection in a refrigerator at 2°C to 8°C (36°F to 46°F). Reconstituted vials and solutions diluted for infusion are stable for 48 hours at room temperature or refrigerated, per the manufacturer. Solution diluted with D_5W to a concentration of 220 mg/mL and repackaged into tuberculin syringes was reported to be stable for 14 days refrigerated.

Reconstitution Reconstitute vials with 1.2 mL SWFI. Gently swirl; do not shake. Further dilute with 50 mL of D_5W. Smaller volumes of D_5W should be used for doses <1.5 mg; avoid concentrations <30 mcg/mL and >70 mcg/mL (an increased variability in drug delivery has been seen). Concentrations <30 mcg/mL **OR** concentrations between ≥30-70 mcg/mL for infusion via ambulatory infusion pump require addition of albumin (final albumin concentration: 0.1%), see table.

Final Dilution Concentration (mcg/mL)	Final Dilution Concentration (10^6 int. units/mL)	Stability
<30	<0.49	Albumin must be added to bag **prior to addition** of aldesleukin at a final concentration of 0.1% (1 mg/mL) albumin; stable at room temperature or at ≥32°C (89°F) for 6 days[1,2]
≥30 to ≤70	≥0.49 to ≤1.1	Stable at room temperature at 6 days without albumin added or at ≥32°C (89°F) for 6 days only if albumin is added (0.1%)[1,2]
70-100	1.2-1.6	Unstable; avoid use
>100-500	1.7-8.2	Stable at room temperature and at ≥32°C (89°F) for 6 days[1,2]

[1]These solutions do not contain a preservative; use for more than 24 hours may not be advisable.

[2]Continuous infusion via ambulatory infusion device raises aldesleukin to this temperature.

Note: Filtration will result in significant loss of bioactivity.

Compatibility Stable in D_5W

Y-site administration: Compatible: Amikacin, amphotericin B, calcium gluconate, co-trimoxazole, diphenhydramine, dopamine, fat emulsion 20%, fluconazole, foscarnet, gentamicin, heparin, magnesium sulfate, metoclopramide, morphine, ondansetron, piperacillin, potassium chloride, ranitidine, thiethylperazine, ticarcillin, tobramycin, vancomycin. **Incompatible:** Ganciclovir, lorazepam, pentamidine, prochlorperazine edisylate, promethazine

Pharmacodynamics/Kinetics

Distribution: V_d: 4-7 L; primarily in plasma and then in the lymphocytes

Bioavailability: I.M.: 37%

(Continued)

Aldesleukin *(Continued)*

Half-life elimination: Initial: 6-13 minutes; Terminal: 80-120 minutes

Dosage Refer to individual protocols.

I.V.:

Renal cell carcinoma: 600,000 int. units/kg every 8 hours for a maximum of 14 doses; repeat after 9 days for a total of 28 doses per course. Retreat if needed 7 weeks after previous course.

Melanoma:

Single-agent use: 600,000 int. units/kg every 8 hours for a maximum of 14 doses; repeat after 9 days for a total of 28 doses per course. Retreat if needed 7 weeks after previous course.

In combination with cytotoxic agents: 24 million int. units/m^2 days 12-16 and 19-23

SubQ:

Single-agent doses: 3-18 million int. units/day for 5 days each week, up to 6 weeks

In combination with interferon:

5 million int. units/m^2 3 times/week

1.8 million int. units/m^2 twice daily 5 days/week for 6 weeks

Investigational regimen: SubQ: 11 million int. units (flat dose) daily for 4 days per week for 4 consecutive weeks; repeat every 6 weeks

Combination Regimens

Melanoma:

Dacarbazine-Carboplatin-Aldesleukin- Interferon *on page 871*

IL-2 + IFN *on page 902*

Renal cell cancer:

Interleukin 2-Interferon Alfa 2 *on page 902*

Interleukin 2-Interferon Alfa 2-Fluorouracil *on page 903*

Administration Administer as I.V. infusion over 15 minutes; may be administered by SubQ injection

Management of symptoms related to vascular leak syndrome:

If actual body weight increases >10% above baseline, or rales or rhonchi are audible:

Administer furosemide at dosage determined by patient response

Administer dopamine hydrochloride 2-4 mcg/kg/minute to maintain renal blood flow and urine output

If patient has dyspnea at rest: Administer supplemental oxygen by face mask

If patient has severe respiratory distress: Intubate patient and provide mechanical ventilation; administer ranitidine (as the hydrochloride salt), 50 mg I.V. every 8-12 hours as prophylaxis against stress ulcers

Dosage Forms Injection, powder for reconstitution: 22 x 10^6 int. units [18 million int. units/mL = 1.1 mg/mL when reconstituted]

Monitoring Parameters

The following clinical evaluations are recommended for all patients prior to beginning treatment and then frequently during drug administration:

Standard hematologic tests including CBC, differential, and platelet counts; blood chemistries including electrolytes, renal and hepatic function tests

Chest x-rays

Monitoring during therapy should include vital signs (temperature, pulse, blood pressure, and respiration rate) and weight; in a patient with a decreased blood pressure, especially <90 mm Hg, cardiac monitoring for rhythm should be conducted. If an abnormal complex or rhythm is seen, an ECG should be performed; vital signs in these hypotension patients should be taken hourly and central venous pressure (CVP) checked.

During treatment, pulmonary function should be monitored on a regular basis.

Additional Information

1 Cetus unit = 6 int. units

1.1 mg = 18×10^6 int. units (or 3×10^6 Cetus units)

1 Roche unit (Teceleukin) = 3 int. units

Selected Readings

Atkins MB, Lotze MT, Dutcher JP, et al, "High-Dose Recombinant Interleukin 2 Therapy for Patients With Metastatic Melanoma: Analysis of 270 Patients Treated Between 1985 and 1993," *J Clin Oncol*, 1999, 17(7):2105-16.

Foa R, "Interleukin 2 in the Management of Acute Leukaemia," *Br J Haematol*, 1996, 92(1):1-8.

Kintzel PE and Calis KA, "Recombinant Interleukin-2: Biological Response Modifier," *Clin Pharm*, 1991, 10(2):110-28.

Sundin DJ and Wolin MJ, "Toxicity Management in Patients Receiving Low-Dose Aldesleukin Therapy," *Ann Pharmacother*,1998, 32(12):1344-52.

Whittington R and Faulds D, "Interleukin-2: A Review of Its Pharmacological Properties and Therapeutic Use in Patients With Cancer," *Drugs*, 1993, 46(3):446-514.

Yang JC, Topalian SL, Parkinson D, et al, "Randomized Comparison of High-Dose and Low-Dose Intravenous Interleukin-2 for the Therapy of Metastatic Renal Cell Carcinoma: An Interim Report," *J Clin Oncol*, 1994, 12(8):1572-6.

Alemtuzumab (ay lem TU zoo mab)

U.S. Brand Names Campath®

Generic Available No

Synonyms Campath-1H; DNA-Derived Humanized Monoclonal Antibody; Humanized IgG1 Anti-CD52 Monoclonal Antibody

Pharmacologic Category Antineoplastic Agent, Monoclonal Antibody

Pregnancy Risk Factor C

Lactation Excretion in breast milk unknown/contraindicated

Use Treatment of B-cell chronic lymphocytic leukemia (B-CLL)

Unlabeled/Investigational Use Treatment of refractory T-cell prolymphocytic leukemia (T-PLL); rheumatoid arthritis; graft versus host disease; multiple myeloma

Mechanism of Action Binds to CD52, a nonmodulating antigen present on the surface of B and T lymphocytes, a majority of monocytes, macrophages, NK cells and a subpopulation of granulocytes. After binding to $CD52^+$ cells, an antibody-dependent lysis occurs.

Labeled Contraindications Known type 1 hypersensitivity or anaphylactic reaction to alemtuzumab or any component of the formulation; hypersensitivity to another monoclonal antibody; active systemic infections; underlying immunodeficiency (eg, seropositive for HIV)

Warnings/Precautions Prophylactic therapy against *Pneumocystis carinii* pneumonia and herpes viral infections is recommended upon initiation of therapy and for at least 2 months following last dose or until $CD4^+$ counts ≥200 cells/µL. Gradual escalation to the recommended maintenance dose is required at initiation and after interruption of therapy for ≥7 days to minimize infusion-related reactions. Patients should not be immunized with live, viral vaccines during or recently after treatment. Safety and efficacy have not been established in pediatric patients. (Continued)

Alemtuzumab *(Continued)*

Adverse Reactions

>10%:

Cardiovascular: Hypotension (15% to 32%, infusion-related), peripheral edema (13%), hypertension (11%), tachycardia/SVT (11%)

Central nervous system: Drug-related fever (83%, infusion-related), fatigue (22% to 34%, infusion-related), headache (13% to 24%), dysthesias (15%), dizziness (12%), neutropenic fever (10%)

Dermatologic: Rash (30% to 40%, infusion-related), urticaria (22% to 30%, infusion-related), pruritus (14% to 24%, infusion-related)

Gastrointestinal: Nausea (47% to 54%), vomiting (33% to 41%), anorexia (20%), diarrhea (13% to 22%), stomatitis/mucositis (14%), abdominal pain (11%)

Hematologic: Lymphopenia, severe neutropenia (64% to 70%); severe anemia (38% to 47%) and severe thrombocytopenia (50% to 52%) may be prolonged and dose-limiting

Neuromuscular & skeletal: Rigors (89%, infusion-related), skeletal muscle pain (24%), weakness (13%), myalgia (11%)

Respiratory: Dyspnea (17% to 26%, infusion-related), cough (25%), bronchitis/pneumonitis (21%), pharyngitis (12%)

Miscellaneous: Infection (43% including sepsis, pneumonia, opportunistic infection; received PCP pneumonia and herpes prophylaxis); diaphoresis (19%)

1% to 10%:

Cardiovascular: Chest pain (10%)

Central nervous system: Insomnia (10%), malaise (9%), depression (7%), temperature change sensation (5%), somnolence (5%)

Dermatologic: Purpura (8%)

Gastrointestinal: Dyspepsia (10%), constipation (9%)

Hematologic: Pancytopenia/marrow hypoplasia (6%), positive Coombs' test without hemolysis (2%), autoimmune thrombocytopenia (2%), autoimmune hemolytic anemia (1%)

Neuromuscular & skeletal: Back pain (10%), tremor (7%)

Respiratory: Bronchospasm (9%), epistaxis (7%), rhinitis (7%)

<1%: Abnormal gait, abnormal thinking, acidosis, acute renal failure, agranulocytosis, alkaline phosphatase elevation, allergic reactions, anaphylactoid reactions, angina pectoris, angioedema, anuria, apathy, aphasia, arthritis, arthritis exacerbation, arthropathy, ascites, asthma, biliary pain, bone fracture, bone marrow aplasia, bronchitis, bullous eruption, capillary fragility, cardiac arrest, cardiac failure, cellulitis, cerebral hemorrhage, cerebrovascular disorder, cervical dysplasia, coagulation abnormality, colitis, coma, confusion, COPD, decreased haptoglobin, deep vein thrombosis, dehydration, diabetes mellitus exacerbation, disseminated intravascular coagulation, duodenal ulcer, endophthalmitis, esophagitis, facial edema, fluid overload, gingivitis, gastroenteritis, gastrointestinal hemorrhage, hallucinations, hearing loss, hematemesis, hematoma, hematuria, hemolysis, hemolytic anemia, hemoptysis, hemorrhoids, hepatic failure, hepatocellular damage, hyperbilirubinemia, hyperglycemia, hyperkalemia, hyperthyroidism, hypoalbuminemia, hypoglycemia, hyponatremia, hypovolemia, hypoxia, influenza-like syndrome, interstitial pneumonitis, intestinal obstruction, intestinal perforation, intracranial hemorrhage, lymphadenopathy, malignant lymphoma, malignant testicular neoplasm, marrow

depression, melena, meningitis, mouth edema, MI, myositis, muscle atrophy, muscle weakness, nervousness, osteomyelitis, pancreatitis, paralysis, paralytic ileus, paroxysmal nocturnal hemoglobinuria-like monocytes, peptic ulcer, pericarditis, peritonitis, plasma cell dyscrasia, phlebitis, pleural effusion, pleurisy, pneumothorax, polymyositis, progressive multifocal leukoencephalopathy, prostate cancer, pseudo-membranous colitis, pulmonary edema, pulmonary embolism, pulmonary fibrosis, pulmonary infiltration, purpuric rash, renal dysfunction, respiratory alkalosis, respiratory depression, respiratory insufficiency, secondary leukemia, seizure (grand mal), sinusitis, splenic infarction, splenomegaly, squamous cell carcinoma, stridor, subarachnoid hemorrhage, syncope, taste loss, toxic nephropathy, transformation to aggressive lymphoma, transformation to prolymphocytic leukemia, thrombocythemia, thrombophlebitis, throat tightness, ureteric obstruction, urinary retention, ventricular arrhythmia, ventricular tachycardia

Vesicant No

Emetic Potential Moderate (30% to 60%)

Overdosage/Toxicology Symptoms are likely to be extensions of adverse events (may include respiratory distress, bronchospasm, anuria, tumor lysis syndrome). Treatment is symptom-directed and supportive.

Storage/Stability Prior to dilution, store at 2°C to 8°C (36°F to 46°F). Do not freeze. Following dilution, use within 8 hours. Store at room temperature or refrigerate; protect from light.

Reconstitution Do not shake prior to use. Dilute with 100 mL NS or D$_5$W.

Compatibility Medications should not be added to the solution or simultaneously infused through the same I.V. line.

Pharmacodynamics/Kinetics

Distribution: V$_d$: 0.18 L/kg

Metabolism: Clearance decreases with repeated dosing (due to loss of CD52 receptors in periphery), resulting in a sevenfold increase in AUC.

Half-life elimination: Initial: 11 hours; 6 days following repeated dosing

Dosage Note: Dose escalation is required; usually accomplished in 3-7 days. Do not exceed single doses >30 mg or cumulative doses >90 mg/week.

I.V. infusion: Adults: B-CLL:

Initial: 3 mg/day (I.V. or SubQ); increase to 10 mg/day, then to 30 mg/day as tolerated

Maintenance: 30 mg/day (I.V. or SubQ) 3 times/week on alternate days for up to 12 weeks

Dosage adjustment for hematologic toxicity (severe neutropenia or thrombocytopenia, not autoimmune):

First occurrence: ANC <250/µL and/or platelet count ≤25,000/µL: Hold therapy; resume at same dose when ANC ≥500/µL and platelet count ≥50,000/µL. If delay between dosing is ≥7 days, restart at 3 mg/day and escalate as tolerated.

Second occurrence: ANC <250/µL and/or platelet count ≤25,000/µL: Hold therapy; resume at 10 mg/day when ANC ≥500/µL and platelet count ≥50,000/µL. If delay between dosing is ≥7 days, restart at 3 mg/day and escalate as tolerated.

Third occurrence: ANC <250/µL and/or platelet count ≤25,000/µL: Permanently discontinue therapy

(Continued)

Alemtuzumab (Continued)

Patients with a baseline ANC ≤500/µL and/or a baseline platelet count ≤25,000/µL at initiation of therapy: If ANC and/or platelet counts decreased to ≤50% of the baseline value, hold therapy. When ANC and/or platelet count return to baseline, resume therapy. If delay between dosing is ≥7 days, restart at 3 mg/day and escalate as tolerated.

Administration Administer by I.V. infusion only over 2 hours. Premedicate with diphenhydramine and acetaminophen 30 minutes before initiation of infusion. Start anti-infective prophylaxis. Other drugs should not be added to or simultaneously infused through the same I.V. line. Do not give I.V. bolus or push.

Dosage Forms [DSC] = Discontinued product
Injection, solution [ampul]: 10 mg/mL (3 mL)
Injection, solution [vial]: 30 mg/mL (1 mL) [DSC]

Monitoring Parameters Vital signs; carefully monitor BP especially in patient with ischemic heart disease or on antihypertensive medications; CBC and platelets; signs and symptoms of infection; CD4⁺ lymphocyte counts. Monitor closely for infusion reactions (including hypotension, rigors, fever, shortness of breath, bronchospasm, chills, and/or rash).

Patient Information You will need frequent laboratory tests during course of therapy. Do not use any prescription or OTC medications unless approved by your prescriber. Maintain adequate hydration (2-3 L/day unless otherwise instructed) and nutrition (frequent small meals will help). You may experience abdominal pain, mouth sores, nausea, or vomiting (small frequent meals, good mouth care with soft toothbrush or swabs, sucking lozenges or chewing gum, and avoidance of spicy or salty foods may help). Report unresolved gastrointestinal problems, persistent fever, chills, muscle pain, skin rash, unusual bleeding or bruising, signs of infection (mouth sores, sore throat, white plaques in mouth or perianal area, burning on urination); swelling of extremities; difficulty breathing; chest pain or palpitations; or other persistent adverse reactions.

Selected Readings

Dearden CE, Matutes E, and Catovsky D, "Alemtuzumab in T-Cell Malignancies," *Med Oncol*, 2002, 19(Suppl):27-32.

Dumont FJ, "CAMPATH (Alemtuzumab) for the Treatment of Chronic Lymphocytic Leukemia and Beyond," *Expert Rev Anticancer Ther*, 2002, 2(1):23-35.

Ferrajoli A, O'Brien S, and Keating MJ, "Alemtuzumab: A Novel Monoclonal Antibody," *Expert Opin Biol Ther*, 2001, 1(6):1059-65.

Hale G, "Alemtuzumab in Stem Cell Transplantation," *Med Oncol*, 2002, 19(Suppl):33-47.

Kennedy B and Hillmen P, "Immunological Effects and Safe Administration of Alemtuzumab (MabCampath) in Advanced B-cLL," *Med Oncol*, 2002, 19(Suppl):49-55.

Lundin J, Kimby E, Bjorkholm M, et al, "Phase II Trial of Subcutaneous Anti-CD52 Monoclonal Antibody Alemtuzumab (Campath-1H) as First-line Treatment for Patients With B-cell Chronic Lymphocytic Leukemia (B-CLL)," *Blood*, 2002, 100(3):768-73.

Lundin J, Osterborg A, Brittinger G, et al, "CAMPATH-1H Monoclonal Antibody in Therapy for Previously Treated Low-Grade Non-Hodgkin's Lymphomas: A Phase II Multicenter Study. European Study Group of CAMPATH-1H Treatment in Low-Grade Non-Hodgkin's Lymphoma," *J Clin Oncol*, 1998, 16(10):3257-63.

Osterborg A, Dyer MJ, Bunjes D, et al, "Phase II Multicenter Study of Human CD52 Antibody in Previously Treated Chronic Lymphocytic Leukemia. European Study Group of CAMPATH-1H Treatment in Chronic Lymphocytic Leukemia," *J Clin Oncol*, 1997, 15(4):1567-74.

Osterborg A, Fassas AS, Anagnostopoulos A, et al, "Humanifed CD52 Monoclonal Antibody Campath-1H as First-Line Treatment in Chronic Lymphocytic Leukaemia," *Br J Haematol*, 1996, 93(1):151-3.

Osterborg A, Mellstedt H, and Keating M, "Clinical Effects of Alemtuzumab (Campath-1H) in B-cell Chronic Lymphocytic Leukemia," *Med Oncol*, 2002, 19(Suppl):21-6.

Rai K and Hallek M, "Future Prospects for Alemtuzumab (MabCampath)," *Med Oncol*, 2002, 19(Suppl):57-63.

♦ **Alimta**® *see* Pemetrexed *on page 655*

Alitretinoin (a li TRET i noyn)

Medication Safety Issues
Sound-alike/look-alike issues:
Panretin® may be confused with pancreatin

Related Information
Safe Handling of Hazardous Drugs *on page 1034*

U.S. Brand Names Panretin®

Canadian Brand Names Panretin®

Generic Available No

Pharmacologic Category Antineoplastic Agent, Miscellaneous

Pregnancy Risk Factor D

Lactation Excretion in breast milk unknown/not recommended

Use Orphan drug: Topical treatment of cutaneous lesions in AIDS-related Kaposi's sarcoma

Unlabeled/Investigational Use Cutaneous T-cell lymphomas

Mechanism of Action Binds to retinoid receptors to inhibit growth of Kaposi's sarcoma

Labeled Contraindications Hypersensitivity to alitretinoin, other retinoids, or any component of the formulation; pregnancy

Warnings/Precautions Do not use concurrently with topical products containing DEET (a common component of insect repellent products). Safety in pediatric patients or geriatric patients has not been established.

Adverse Reactions
>10%:
Central nervous system: Pain (0% to 34%)
Dermatologic: Rash (25% to 77%), pruritus (8% to 11%)
Neuromuscular & skeletal: Paresthesia (3% to 22%)
5% to 10%:
Cardiovascular: Edema (3% to 8%)
Dermatologic: Exfoliative dermatitis (3% to 9%), skin disorder (0% to 8%)

Emetic Potential Very low (<10%)

Overdosage/Toxicology There has been no experience with human overdosage of alitretinoin, and overdose is unlikely following topical application. Treatment is symptomatic and supportive.

Drug Interactions
Increased Effect/Toxicity: Increased toxicity of DEET may occur if products containing this compound are used concurrently with alitretinoin. Due to limited absorption after topical application, interaction with systemic medications is unlikely.

Storage/Stability Store at room temperature.

Pharmacodynamics/Kinetics Absorption: Not extensive

Dosage Topical: Apply gel twice daily to cutaneous lesions

Administration Do not use occlusive dressings.

Dosage Forms Gel: 0.1% (60 g tube)

Patient Information For external use only; avoid UV light exposure (sun or sunlamps) of treated areas; avoid DEET-containing products

♦ **Alkeran**®   *see* Melphalan *on page 530*

Allopurinol (al oh PURE i nole)
Medication Safety Issues
Sound-alike/look-alike issues:
Allopurinol may be confused with Apresoline
Zyloprim® may be confused with Xylo-Pfan®, ZORprin®
Related Information
Investigational Drug Service *on page 1031*
Tumor Lysis Syndrome *on page 1002*
U.S. Brand Names Aloprim™; Zyloprim®
Canadian Brand Names Apo-Allopurinol®; Zyloprim®
Generic Available Yes
Synonyms Allopurinol Sodium
Pharmacologic Category Xanthine Oxidase Inhibitor
Pregnancy Risk Factor C
Lactation Enters breast milk/use caution (AAP rates "compatible")
Use
Oral: Prevention of attack of gouty arthritis and nephropathy; treatment of secondary hyperuricemia which may occur during treatment of tumors or leukemia; prevention of recurrent calcium oxalate calculi
I.V.: Treatment of elevated serum and urinary uric acid levels when oral therapy is not tolerated in patients with leukemia, lymphoma, and solid tumor malignancies who are receiving cancer chemotherapy

Mechanism of Action Allopurinol inhibits xanthine oxidase, the enzyme responsible for the conversion of hypoxanthine to xanthine to uric acid. Allopurinol is metabolized to oxypurinol which is also an inhibitor of xanthine oxidase; allopurinol acts on purine catabolism, reducing the production of uric acid without disrupting the biosynthesis of vital purines.

Labeled Contraindications Hypersensitivity to allopurinol or any component of the formulation

Warnings/Precautions Do not use to treat asymptomatic hyperuricemia. Discontinue at first signs of rash. Reduce dosage in renal insufficiency. Reinstate with caution in patients who have had a previous mild allergic reaction. Monitor liver function and complete blood counts before initiating therapy and periodically during therapy. Use with caution in patients taking diuretics concurrently. Risk of skin rash may be increased in patients receiving amoxicillin or ampicillin. The risk of hypersensitivity may be increased in patients receiving thiazides, and possibly ACE inhibitors. Use caution with mercaptopurine or azathioprine; dosage adjustment required.

Adverse Reactions The most common adverse reaction to allopurinol is a skin rash (usually maculopapular; however, more severe reactions, including Stevens-Johnson syndrome, have also been reported). While some studies cite an incidence of these reactions as high as >10% of cases (often in association with ampicillin or amoxicillin), the product labeling cites a much lower incidence, reflected below. Allopurinol should be discontinued at the first appearance of a rash or other sign of hypersensitivity.
>1%:
Dermatologic: Rash (1.5%)
Gastrointestinal: Nausea (1.3%), vomiting (1.2%)
Renal: Renal failure/impairment (1.2%)

<1%: Hypersensitivity syndrome, increased alkaline phosphatase or hepatic transaminases, granulomatous hepatitis, dyspepsia, pancreatitis, gynecomastia, agranulocytosis, aplastic anemia, acute tubular necrosis, interstitial nephritis, nephrolithiasis, vasculitis, toxic epidermal necrolysis, exfoliative dermatitis, Stevens-Johnson syndrome, granuloma annulare, toxic pustuloderma, peripheral neuropathy, neuritis, paresthesia, bronchospasm, cataracts, macular retinitis, angioedema, epistaxis

Vesicant No

Emetic Potential Very low (<10%)

Overdosage/Toxicology If significant amounts of allopurinol have been absorbed, it is theoretically possible that oxypurinol stones could form, but no record of such occurrence exists. Alkalinization of urine and forced diuresis can help prevent potential xanthine stone formation.

Drug Interactions

Increased Effect/Toxicity: Allopurinol may increase the effects of azathioprine, chlorpropamide, mercaptopurine, theophylline, and oral anticoagulants. An increased risk of bone marrow suppression may occur when given with myelosuppressive agents (cyclophosphamide, possibly other alkylating agents). Amoxicillin/ampicillin, ACE inhibitors, and thiazide diuretics have been associated with hypersensitivity reactions when combined with allopurinol (rare), and the incidence of rash may be increased with penicillins (ampicillin, amoxicillin). Urinary acidification with large amounts of vitamin C may increase kidney stone formation.

Decreased Effect: Ethanol decreases effectiveness.

Ethanol/Nutrition/Herb Interactions

Ethanol: Avoid ethanol (may decrease effectiveness).

Iron supplements: Hepatic iron uptake may be increased.

Vitamin C: Large amounts of vitamin C may acidify urine and increase kidney stone formation.

Storage/Stability

Powder for injection: Store at controlled room temperature of 15°C to 30°C (59°F to 86°F). Following reconstitution, intravenous solutions should be stored at 20°C to 25°C. Do not refrigerate reconstituted and/or diluted product. Must be administered within 10 hours of solution preparation.

Tablet: Store at controlled room temperature of 15°C to 25°C (59°F to 77°F).

Reconstitution Allopurinol injection must be reconstituted and diluted. Each 30 mL vial should be reconstituted with 25 mL sterile water for injection, USP. It may then be added to NS or D_5W. A final concentration of no greater than 6 mg/mL is recommended.

Compatibility Stable in D_5W, NS, sterile water for injection

Y-site administration: Compatible: Acyclovir, aminophylline, aztreonam, bleomycin, bumetanide, buprenorphine, butorphanol, calcium gluconate, carboplatin, cefazolin, cefoperazone, cefotetan, ceftazidime, ceftizoxime, ceftriaxone, cefuroxime, cisplatin, co-trimoxazole, cyclophosphamide, dactinomycin, dexamethasone sodium phosphate, doxorubicin liposome, enalaprilat, etoposide, famotidine, fluconazole, fludarabine, fluorouracil, furosemide, ganciclovir, granisetron, heparin, hydrocortisone sodium phosphate, hydrocortisone sodium succinate, (Continued)

Allopurinol *(Continued)*

hydromorphone, ifosfamide, lorazepam, mannitol, mesna, methotrexate, metronidazole, mitoxantrone, morphine, piperacillin,
plicamycin, potassium chloride, ranitidine, teniposide, thiotepa, ticarcillin, ticarcillin/clavulanate, vancomycin, vinblastine, vincristine, zidovudine. **Incompatible:** Amikacin, amphotericin B, carmustine, cefotaxime,
chlorpromazine, cimetidine, clindamycin, cytarabine, dacarbazine,
daunorubicin, diphenhydramine, doxorubicin, doxycycline, droperidol,
floxuridine, gentamicin, haloperidol, hydroxyzine, idarubicin, imipenem/
cilastatin, mechlorethamine, meperidine, methylprednisolone sodium
succinate, metoclopramide, minocycline, nalbuphine, netilmicin, ondansetron, prochlorperazine edisylate, promethazine, sodium bicarbonate,
streptozocin, tobramycin, vinorelbine

Pharmacodynamics/Kinetics

Onset of action: Peak effect: 1-2 weeks

Absorption: Oral: ~80%; Rectal: Poor and erratic

Distribution: V_d: ~1.6 L/kg; V_{ss}: 0.84-0.87 L/kg; enters breast milk

Protein binding: <1%

Metabolism: ~75% to active metabolites, chiefly oxypurinol

Bioavailability: 49% to 53%

Half-life elimination:

Normal renal function: Parent drug: 1-3 hours; Oxypurinol: 18-30 hours

End-stage renal disease: Prolonged

Time to peak, plasma: Oral: 30-120 minutes

Excretion: Urine (76% as oxypurinol, 12% as unchanged drug)

Allopurinol and oxypurinol are dialyzable

Dosage

Oral: Doses >300 mg should be given in divided doses.

Children ≤10 years: Secondary hyperuricemia associated with chemotherapy: 10 mg/kg/day in 2-3 divided doses **or** 200-300 mg/m²/day in
2-4 divided doses, maximum: 800 mg/24 hours

Alternative (manufacturer labeling): <6 years: 150 mg/day in 3 divided
doses; 6-10 years: 300 mg/day in 2-3 divided doses

Children >10 years and Adults:

Secondary hyperuricemia associated with chemotherapy: 600-800
mg/day in 2-3 divided doses for prevention of acute uric acid
nephropathy for 2-3 days starting 1-2 days before chemotherapy

Gout: Mild: 200-300 mg/day; Severe: 400-600 mg/day; to reduce the
possibility of acute gouty attacks, initiate dose at 100 mg/day and
increase weekly to recommended dosage.

Recurrent calcium oxalate stones: 200-300 mg/day in single or
divided doses

Elderly: Initial: 100 mg/day, increase until desired uric acid level is
obtained

I.V.: Hyperuricemia secondary to chemotherapy: Intravenous daily dose
can be given as a single infusion or in equally divided doses at 6-, 8-, or
12-hour intervals. A fluid intake sufficient to yield a daily urinary output
of at least 2 L in adults and the maintenance of a neutral or, preferably,
slightly alkaline urine are desirable.

Children ≤10 years: Starting dose: 200 mg/m²/day

Children >10 years and Adults: 200-400 mg/m²/day (max: 600 mg/day)

Dosing adjustment in renal impairment: Must be adjusted due to accumulation of allopurinol and metabolites:

Oral: Removed by hemodialysis; adult maintenance doses of allopurinol (mg) based on creatinine clearance (mL/minute): See table.

Adult Maintenance Doses of Allopurinol[1]

Creatinine Clearance (mL/min)	Maintenance Dose of Allopurinol (mg)
140	400 daily
120	350 daily
100	300 daily
80	250 daily
60	200 daily
40	150 daily
20	100 daily
10	100 every 2 days
0	100 every 3 days

[1]This table is based on a standard maintenance dose of 300 mg of allopurinol per day for a patient with a creatinine clearance of 100 mL/min.

Hemodialysis: Administer dose posthemodialysis or administer 50% supplemental dose

I.V.:
Cl_{cr} 10-20 mL/minute: 200 mg/day
Cl_{cr} 3-10 mL/minute: 100 mg/day
Cl_{cr} <3 mL/minute: 100 mg/day at extended intervals

Administration

Oral: Should administer oral forms after meals with plenty of fluid.

I.V.: The rate of infusion depends on the volume of the infusion. Whenever possible, therapy should be initiated at 24-48 hours before the start of chemotherapy known to cause tumor lysis (including adrenocorticosteroids). I.V. daily dose can be administered as a single infusion or in equally divided doses at 6-, 8-, or 12-hour interval.

Dosage Forms

Injection, powder for reconstitution, as sodium (Aloprim™): 500 mg
Tablet (Zyloprim®): 100 mg, 300 mg

Monitoring Parameters CBC, serum uric acid levels, I & O, hepatic and renal function, especially at start of therapy

Dietary Considerations Should administer oral forms after meals with plenty of fluid. Fluid intake should be administered to yield neutral or slightly alkaline urine and an output of ~2 L (in adults).

Patient Information Take after meals with plenty of fluid (at least 10-12 glasses of fluids per day); discontinue the drug and contact prescriber at first sign of rash, painful urination, blood in urine, irritation of the eyes, or swelling of the lips or mouth; may cause drowsiness; alcohol decreases effectiveness

Special Geriatric Considerations Adjust dose based on renal function.

Extemporaneous Preparations Crush tablets to make a 5 mg/mL suspension in simple syrup; stable 14 days under refrigeration

Nahata MC and Hipple TF, *Pediatric Drug Formulations*, 1st ed, Harvey Whitney Books Co, 1990.

(Continued)

Allopurinol *(Continued)*

Selected Readings

Allen LV and Erickson MA 3d, "Stability of Acetazolamide, Allopurinol, Azathioprine, Clonazepam, and Flucytosine in Extemporaneously Compounded Oral Liquids," *Am J Health Syst Pharm*, 1996, 53(16):1944-9.

"American Academy of Pediatrics Committee on Drugs. The Transfer of Drugs and Other Chemicals Into Human Milk," *Pediatrics*, 2001, 108(3):776-89.

Appelbaum SJ, Mayersohn M, Dorr RT, et al, "Allopurinol Kinetics and Bioavailability. Intravenous, Oral and Rectal Administration," *Cancer Chemother Pharmacol*, 1982, 8(1):93-8.

Bennett WM, Aronoff GR, Golper TA, et al, *Drug Prescribing in Renal Failure*, Philadelphia, PA: American College of Physicians, 1987.

Day RO, Birkett DJ, Hicks, M, et al, "New Uses for Allopurinol," *Drugs*, 1994, 48(3):399-44.

Elasy T, Kaminsky D, Tracy M, et al, "Allopurinol Hypersensitivity Syndrome Revisited," *West J Med*, 1995, 162(4):360-1.

Emmerson BT, "The Management of Gout," *N Engl J Med*, 1996, 334(7):445-51.

Ferner RE, Simmonds HA, and Bateman DN, "Allopurinol Kinetics After Massive Overdose," *Hum Toxicol*, 1988, 7(3):293-4.

Hande KR and Garrow GC, "Acute Tumor Lysis Syndrome in Patients With High-Grade Non-Hodgkin's Lymphoma," *Am J Med*, 1993, 94(2):133-9.

Krakoff IH and Murphy ML, "Hyperuricemia in Neoplastic Disease in Children: Prevention With Allopurinol, A Xanthine Oxidase Inhibitor," *Pediatrics*, 1968, 41(1):52-6.

McInnes GT, Lawson DH, and Jick H, "Acute Adverse Reactions Attributed to Allopurinol in Hospitalized Patients," *Ann Rheum Dis*, 1981, 40(3):245-9.

Murrell GA and Rapeport WG, "Clinical Pharmacokinetics of Allopurinol," *Clin Pharmacokinet*, 1986, 11(5):343-53.

Parra E, Gota R, Gamen A, et al, "Granulomatous Interstitial Nephritis Secondary to Allopurinol Treatment," *Clin Nephrol*, 1995, 43(5):350.

Vinciullo C, "Allopurinol Hypersensitivity," *Med J Aust*, 1984, 141(7):449-50.

♦ **Allopurinol Sodium** *see* Allopurinol *on page 42*

♦ **All-*trans*-Retinoic Acid** *see* Tretinoin (Oral) *on page 792*

♦ **Alophen® [OTC]** *see* Bisacodyl *on page 133*

♦ **Aloprim™** *see* Allopurinol *on page 42*

♦ **Aloxi™** *see* Palonosetron *on page 648*

♦ **Alphanate®** *see* Antihemophilic Factor (Human) *on page 87*

♦ **AlphaNine® SD** *see* Factor IX *on page 327*

Alteplase *(AL te plase)*

Medication Safety Issues

Sound-alike/look-alike issues:

Alteplase may be confused with Altace®

"tPA" abbreviation should not be used when writing orders for this medication; has been misread as TNKase (tenecteplase)

U.S. Brand Names Activase®; Cathflo™ Activase®

Canadian Brand Names Activase® rt-PA; Cathflo™ Activase®

Generic Available No

Synonyms Alteplase, Recombinant; Alteplase, Tissue Plasminogen Activator, Recombinant; tPA

Pharmacologic Category Thrombolytic Agent

Pregnancy Risk Factor C

Lactation Excretion in breast milk unknown

Use Management of acute myocardial infarction for the lysis of thrombi in coronary arteries; management of acute massive pulmonary embolism (PE) in adults

Acute myocardial infarction (AMI): Chest pain ≥20 minutes, ≤12-24 hours; S-T elevation ≥0.1 mV in at least two ECG leads

Acute pulmonary embolism (APE): Age ≤75 years: Documented massive pulmonary embolism by pulmonary angiography or echocardiography or high probability lung scan with clinical shock

Cathflo™ Activase®: Restoration of central venous catheter function

Unlabeled/Investigational Use Acute peripheral arterial occlusive disease

Mechanism of Action Initiates local fibrinolysis by binding to fibrin in a thrombus (clot) and converts entrapped plasminogen to plasmin

Labeled Contraindications Hypersensitivity to alteplase or any component of the formulation

Treatment of acute MI or PE: Active internal bleeding; history of CVA; recent intracranial or intraspinal surgery or trauma; intracranial neoplasm; arteriovenous malformation or aneurysm; known bleeding diathesis; severe uncontrolled hypertension

Treatment of acute ischemic stroke: Evidence of intracranial hemorrhage or suspicion of subarachnoid hemorrhage on pretreatment evaluation; recent (within 3 months) intracranial or intraspinal surgery; prolonged external cardiac massage; suspected aortic dissection; serious head trauma or previous stroke; history of intracranial hemorrhage; uncontrolled hypertension at time of treatment (eg, >185 mm Hg systolic or >110 mm Hg diastolic); seizure at the onset of stroke; active internal bleeding; intracranial neoplasm; arteriovenous malformation or aneurysm; known bleeding diathesis including but not limited to: current use of anticoagulants or an INR >1.7, administration of heparin within 48 hours preceding the onset of stroke and an elevated aPTT at presentation, platelet count <100,000/mm³.

Other exclusion criteria (NINDS recombinant tPA study): Stroke or serious head injury within 3 months, major surgery or serious trauma within 2 weeks, GI or urinary tract hemorrhage within 3 weeks, aggressive treatment required to lower blood pressure, glucose level <50 mg/dL or >400 mg/dL, arterial puncture at a noncompressible site or lumbar puncture within 1 week, clinical presentation suggesting post-MI pericarditis, pregnancy; breast-feeding.

Warnings/Precautions Concurrent heparin anticoagulation may contribute to bleeding. Monitor all potential bleeding sites. Doses >150 mg are associated with increased risk of intracranial hemorrhage. Intramuscular injections and nonessential handling of the patient should be avoided. Venipunctures should be performed carefully and only when necessary. If arterial puncture is necessary, use an upper extremity vessel that can be manually compressed. If serious bleeding occurs then the infusion of alteplase and heparin should be stopped.

For the following conditions the risk of bleeding is higher with use of alteplase and should be weighed against the benefits of therapy: recent major surgery (eg, CABG, obstetrical delivery, organ biopsy, previous puncture of noncompressible vessels), cerebrovascular disease, recent gastrointestinal or genitourinary bleeding, recent trauma, hypertension (systolic BP >175 mm Hg and/or diastolic BP >110 mm Hg), high likelihood of left heart thrombus (eg, mitral stenosis with atrial fibrillation), acute pericarditis, subacute bacterial endocarditis, hemostatic defects including ones caused by severe renal or hepatic dysfunction, significant hepatic dysfunction, pregnancy, diabetic hemorrhagic retinopathy or other hemorrhagic ophthalmic conditions, septic thrombophlebitis or
(Continued)

Alteplase *(Continued)*

occluded AV cannula at seriously infected site, advanced age (eg, >75 years), patients receiving oral anticoagulants, any other condition in which bleeding constitutes a significant hazard or would be particularly difficult to manage because of location.

Coronary thrombolysis may result in reperfusion arrhythmias. In treatment of patients with acute ischemic stroke more than 3 hours after symptom onset is not recommended; treatment of patients with minor neurological deficit or with rapidly improving symptoms is not recommended.

Cathflo™ Activase®: When used to restore catheter function, use Cathflo™ cautiously in those patients with known or suspected catheter infections. Evaluate catheter for other causes of dysfunction before use. Avoid excessive pressure when instilling into catheter. Use of Cathflo™ in children <2 years of age (or weighing <10 kg) has not been studied.

Adverse Reactions As with all drugs which may affect hemostasis, bleeding is the major adverse effect associated with alteplase. Hemorrhage may occur at virtually any site. Risk is dependent on multiple variables, including the dosage administered, concurrent use of multiple agents which alter hemostasis, and patient predisposition. Rapid lysis of coronary artery thrombi by thrombolytic agents may be associated with reperfusion-related atrial and/or ventricular arrhythmia. **Note:** Lowest rate of bleeding complications expected with dose used to restore catheter function.

1% to 10%:

Cardiovascular: Hypotension

Central nervous system: Fever

Dermatologic: Bruising (1%)

Gastrointestinal: GI hemorrhage (5%), nausea, vomiting

Genitourinary: GU hemorrhage (4%)

Local: Bleeding at catheter puncture site (15.3%, accelerated administration)

Hematologic: Bleeding (0.5% major, 7% minor: GUSTO trial)

<1% (Limited to important or life-threatening): Intracranial hemorrhage (0.4% to 0.87% when dose is ≤100 mg), retroperitoneal hemorrhage, pericardial hemorrhage, gingival hemorrhage, epistaxis, allergic reactions: anaphylaxis, anaphylactoid reactions, laryngeal edema, rash, and urticaria (<0.02%).

Additional cardiovascular events associated **with use in MI:** AV block, cardiogenic shock, heart failure, cardiac arrest, recurrent ischemia/infarction, myocardial rupture, electromechanical dissociation, pericardial effusion, pericarditis, mitral regurgitation, cardiac tamponade, thromboembolism, pulmonary edema, asystole, ventricular tachycardia, bradycardia, ruptured intracranial AV malformation, seizure, hemorrhagic bursitis, cholesterol crystal embolization

Additional events associated **with use in pulmonary embolism:** Pulmonary re-embolization, pulmonary edema, pleural effusion, thromboembolism

Additional events associated **with use in stroke:** Cerebral edema, cerebral herniation, seizure, new ischemic stroke

Overdosage/Toxicology Increased incidence of intracranial bleeding.

Drug Interactions

Increased Effect/Toxicity: The potential for hemorrhage with alteplase is increased by oral anticoagulants (warfarin), heparin, low molecular weight heparins, and drugs which affect platelet function (eg, NSAIDs, dipyridamole, ticlopidine, clopidogrel, IIb/IIIa antagonists). Concurrent use with aspirin and heparin may increase the risk of bleeding. However, aspirin and heparin were used concomitantly with alteplase in the majority of patients in clinical studies.

Decreased Effect: Aminocaproic acid (an antifibrinolytic agent) may decrease the effectiveness of thrombolytic therapy. Nitroglycerin may increase the hepatic clearance of alteplase, potentially reducing lytic activity (limited clinical information).

Ethanol/Nutrition/Herb Interactions Herb/Nutraceutical: Avoid cat's claw, dong quai, evening primrose, feverfew, red clover, horse chestnut, garlic, green tea, ginseng, ginkgo (all have additional antiplatelet activity).

Storage/Stability

Activase®: The lyophilized product may be stored at room temperature (not to exceed 30°C/86°F), or under refrigeration; once reconstituted it should be used within 8 hours

Cathflo™ Activase®: Store lyophilized product in refrigerator. Once reconstituted, store at 2°C to 30°C (36°F to 86°F).

Reconstitution

Activase®:

50 mg vial: Use accompanying diluent (50 mL sterile water for injection); do not shake; final concentration: 1 mg/mL

100 mg vial: Use transfer set with accompanying diluent (100 mL vial of sterile water for injection); no vacuum is present in 100 mg vial; final concentration: 1 mg/mL

Cathflo™ Activase®: Add 2.2 mL SWFI to vial; do not shake. Final concentration: 1 mg/mL

Compatibility Stable in NS, sterile water for injection; not stable with bacteriostatic water; **variable stability (consult detailed reference)** in D_5W

Y-site administration: Compatible: Lidocaine, metoprolol, propranolol. **Incompatible:** Dobutamine, dopamine, heparin, nitroglycerin

Compatibility when admixed: Compatible: Lidocaine, morphine, nitroglycerin. **Incompatible:** Dobutamine, dopamine, heparin

Pharmacodynamics/Kinetics

Duration: >50% present in plasma cleared ~5 minutes after infusion terminated, ~80% cleared within 10 minutes

Excretion: Clearance: Rapidly from circulating plasma (550-650 mL/minute), primarily hepatic; >50% present in plasma is cleared within 5 minutes after the infusion is terminated, ~80% cleared within 10 minutes

Dosage

I.V.:

Coronary artery thrombi: Front loading dose (weight-based):

Patients >67 kg: Total dose: 100 mg over 1.5 hours; infuse 15 mg over 1-2 minutes. Infuse 50 mg over 30 minutes. See "Note."

Patients ≤67 kg: Total dose: 1.25 mg/kg; infuse 15 mg I.V. bolus over 1-2 minutes, then infuse 0.75 mg/kg (not to exceed 50 mg) over next 30 minutes, followed by 0.5 mg/kg over next 60 minutes (not to exceed 35 mg). See "Note."

(Continued)

Alteplase *(Continued)*

Note: Concurrently, begin heparin 60 units/kg bolus (maximum: 4000 units) followed by continuous infusion of 12 units/kg/hour (maximum: 1000 units/hour) and adjust to aPTT target of 1.5-2 times the upper limit of control. Infuse remaining 35 mg of alteplase over the next hour.

Acute pulmonary embolism: 100 mg over 2 hours.

Acute ischemic stroke: Doses should be given within the first 3 hours of the onset of symptoms; recommended total dose: 0.9 mg/kg (maximum dose should not exceed 90 mg) infused over 60 minutes.

Load with 0.09 mg/kg (10% of the 0.9 mg/kg dose) as an I.V. bolus over 1 minute, followed by 0.81 mg/kg (90% of the 0.9 mg/kg dose) as a continuous infusion over 60 minutes. Heparin should not be started for 24 hours or more after starting alteplase for stroke.

Intracatheter: Central venous catheter clearance: Cathflo™ Activase®:

Patients ≥10 to <30 kg: 110% of the internal lumen volume of the catheter (≤2 mg [1 mg/mL]); retain in catheter for 30 minutes to 2 hours; may instill a second dose if catheter remains occluded

Patients ≥30 kg: 2 mg (1 mg/mL); retain in catheter for 30 minutes to 2 hours; may instill a second dose if catheter remains occluded

Intra-arterial: Acute peripheral arterial occlusive disease (unlabeled use): 0.02-0.1 mg/kg/hour for up to 36 hours

Advisory Panel to the Society for Cardiovascular and Interventional Radiology on Thrombolytic Therapy recommendation: ≤2 mg/hour and subtherapeutic heparin (aPTT <1.5 times baseline)

Administration

Activase®: Acute MI: Accelerated infusion:

Bolus dose may be prepared by one of three methods:

1) removal of 15 mL reconstituted (1 mg/mL) solution from vial
2) removal of 15 mL from a port on the infusion line after priming
3) programming an infusion pump to deliver a 15 mL bolus at the initiation of infusion

Remaining dose may be administered as follows:

50 mg vial: Either PVC bag or glass vial and infusion set

100 mg vial: Insert spike end of the infusion set through the same puncture site created by transfer device and infuse from vial

If further dilution is desired, may be diluted in equal volume of 0.9% sodium chloride or D_5W to yield a final concentration of 0.5 mg/mL AD

Cathflo™ Activase®: Intracatheter: Instill dose into occluded catheter. Do not force solution into catheter. After a 30-minute dwell time, assess catheter function by attempting to aspirate blood. If catheter is functional, aspirate 4-5 mL of blood to remove Cathflo™ Activase® and residual clots. Gently irrigate the catheter with NS. If catheter remains nonfunctional, let Cathflo™ Activase® dwell for another 90 minutes (total dwell time: 120 minutes) and reassess function. If catheter function is not restored, a second dose may be instilled.

Dosage Forms Injection, powder for reconstitution, recombinant:

Activase®: 50 mg [29 million int. units]; 100 mg [58 million int. units]

Cathflo™ Activase®: 2 mg

Monitoring Parameters

When using for central venous catheter clearance: Assess catheter function by attempting to aspirate blood.

When using for management of acute myocardial infarction: Assess for evidence of cardiac reperfusion through resolution of chest pain, resolution of baseline ECG changes, preserved left ventricular function, cardiac enzyme washout phenomenon, and/or the appearance of reperfusion arrhythmias; assess for bleeding potential through clinical evidence of GI bleeding, hematuria, gingival bleeding, fibrinogen levels, fibrinogen degradation products, prothrombin times, and partial thromboplastin times.

Selected Readings

Gerlach AT and Pickworth KK, "Use of Alteplase in Peripheral Arterial Occlusions: Outcomes and Complications," Abstracts of the American College of Clinical Pharmacy Annual Meeting, Los Angeles, 2000, November 5-8; Abs No 47.

Ponec D, Irwin D, Haire WD, et al, "Recombinant Tissue Plasminogen Activator (Alteplase) for Restoration of Flow in Occluded Central Venous Access Devices: A Double-Blind Placebo-Controlled Trial - The Cardiovascular Thrombolytic to Open Occluded Lines (COOL) Efficacy Trial," *J Vasc Interv Radiol*, 2001, 12(8):951-5.

Sugimoto K, Hofmann LV, Razavi MK, et al, "The Safety, Efficacy, and Pharmacoeconomics of Low-Dose Alteplase Compared With Catheter-Directed Thrombolysis of Arterial and Venous Occlusions," *J Vasc Surg*, 2003, 37(3):512-7.

Zacharias JM, Weatherston CP, Spewak CR, et al, "Alteplase Versus Urokinase for Occluded Hemodialysis Catheters," *Ann Pharmacother*, 2003, 37(1):27-33.

- **Alteplase, Recombinant** see Alteplase on page 46
- **Alteplase, Tissue Plasminogen Activator, Recombinant** see Alteplase on page 46
- **Alti-Acyclovir (Can)** see Acyclovir on page 26
- **Alti-CPA (Can)** see Cyproterone on page 227
- **Alti-MPA (Can)** see MedroxyPROGESTERone on page 524

Altretamine (al TRET a meen)

Related Information

Safe Handling of Hazardous Drugs on page 1034

U.S. Brand Names Hexalen®

Canadian Brand Names Hexalen®

Generic Available No

Synonyms Hexamethylmelamine; HEXM; HMM; HXM; NSC-13875

Pharmacologic Category Antineoplastic Agent, Miscellaneous

Pregnancy Risk Factor D

Lactation Excretion in breast milk unknown

Use Palliative treatment of persistent or recurrent ovarian cancer

Mechanism of Action Although altretamine's clinical antitumor spectrum resembles that of alkylating agents, the drug has demonstrated activity in alkylator-resistant patients. The drug selectively inhibits the incorporation of radioactive thymidine and uridine into DNA and RNA, inhibiting DNA and RNA synthesis; reactive intermediates covalently bind to microsomal proteins and DNA; can spontaneously degrade to demethylated melamines and formaldehyde which are also cytotoxic.

Labeled Contraindications Hypersensitivity to altretamine or any component of the formulation; pre-existing severe bone marrow suppression or severe neurologic toxicity; pregnancy

Warnings/Precautions The U.S. Food and Drug Administration (FDA) currently recommends that procedures for proper handling and disposal of antineoplastic agents be considered. Use with caution in patients previously treated with other myelosuppressive drugs or with pre-existing (Continued)

Altretamine *(Continued)*

neurotoxicity. Use with caution in patients with renal or hepatic dysfunction.

Adverse Reactions

>10%:

Central nervous system: Peripheral sensory neuropathy, neurotoxicity (21%; may be progressive and dose-limiting)

Gastrointestinal: Nausea/vomiting (50% to 70%), anorexia (48%), diarrhea (48%)

Hematologic: Anemia, thrombocytopenia (31%), leukopenia (62%), neutropenia

1% to 10%:

Central nervous system: Seizures

Gastrointestinal: Stomach cramps

Hepatic: Alkaline phosphatase increased

<1%: Alopecia, depression, dizziness, hepatotoxicity, rash, tremor

Vesicant No

Emetic Potential Moderate (30% to 60%)

Overdosage/Toxicology Symptoms of overdose include nausea, vomiting, peripheral neuropathy, severe bone marrow suppression. Treatment is supportive.

Drug Interactions

Increased Effect/Toxicity: Altretamine may cause severe orthostatic hypotension when administered with MAO inhibitors. Cimetidine may decrease metabolism of altretamine.

Decreased Effect: Phenobarbital may increase metabolism of altretamine which may decrease the effect.

Pharmacodynamics/Kinetics

Absorption: Well absorbed (75% to 89%)

Distribution: Highly concentrated hepatically and renally; low in other organs

Metabolism: Hepatic; rapid and extensive demethylation; active metabolites

Half-life elimination: 13 hours

Time to peak, plasma: 0.5-3 hours

Excretion: Urine (<1% as unchanged drug)

Dosage Refer to individual protocols. Oral:

Adults: 4-12 mg/kg/day in 3-4 divided doses for 21-90 days

Alternatively: 240-320 mg/m^2/day in 3-4 divided doses for 21 days, repeated every 6 weeks

Alternatively: 260 mg/m^2/day for 14-21 days of a 28-day cycle in 4 divided doses

Alternatively: 150 mg/m^2/day in 3-4 divided doses for 14 days of a 28-day cycle

Administration Administer total daily dose as 3-4 divided doses after meals and at bedtime.

Dosage Forms Gelcap: 50 mg [contains lactose]

Dietary Considerations Should be taken after meals at bedtime.

Patient Information Report any numbness or tingling in extremities; nausea and vomiting may occur

Selected Readings

Ames MM, "Hexamethylmelamine: Pharmacology and Mechanism of Action," *Cancer Treat Rev*, 1991, 18(Suppl A):3-14.

Bruckner HW and Schleifer SJ, "Orthostatic Hypotension as a Complication of Hexamethylmelamine Antidepressant Interaction," *Cancer Treat Rep*, 1983, 67:516.

Damia G and D'Incalci M, "Clinical Pharmacokinetics of Altretamine," *Clin Pharmacokinet*, 1995, 28(6):439-48.

Hahn DA and Black C, "Hexamethylamine: A Review," *Drug Intell Clin Pharm*, 1980, 14:541-7.

Hansen LA and Hughes TE, "Altretamine," *DICP*, 1991, 25(2):146-52.

Lee CR and Faulds D, "Altretamine. A Review of Its Pharmacodynamic and Pharmacokinetic Properties, and Therapeutic Potential in Cancer Chemotherapy," *Drugs*, 1995, 49(6):932-53.

Manetta A, Mac Neill C, Lyter JA, et al, "Hexamethylmelamine as a Single Second-Line Agent in Ovarian Cancer," *Gynecol Oncol*, 1990, 36(1):93-6.

Sutton GP, "Secondary Therapy for Epithelial Ovarian Cancer - 1994," *Semin Oncol*, 1994, 21(4 Suppl 7):32-6.

Thigpen JT, Vance RB, and Khansur T, "Second-Line Chemotherapy for Recurrent Carcinoma of the Ovary," *Cancer*, 1993, 71(4 Suppl):1559-64.

♦ **AmBisome**® *see* Amphotericin B (Liposomal) *on page 76*

♦ **A-Methapred** *see* MethylPREDNISolone *on page 558*

♦ **Amethopterin** *see* Methotrexate *on page 549*

♦ **Amicar**® *see* Aminocaproic Acid *on page 61*

Amifostine (am i FOS teen)

Medication Safety Issues

Sound-alike/look-alike issues:

Ethyol® may be confused with ethanol

Related Information

Safe Handling of Hazardous Drugs *on page 1034*

U.S. Brand Names Ethyol®

Canadian Brand Names Ethyol®

Generic Available No

Synonyms Ethiofos; Gammaphos; NSC-296961; WR-2721; YM-08310

Pharmacologic Category Adjuvant, Chemoprotective Agent (Cytoprotective); Antidote

Pregnancy Risk Factor C

Lactation Excretion in breast milk unknown/contraindicated

Use Reduce the incidence of moderate to severe xerostomia in patients undergoing postoperative radiation treatment for head and neck cancer, where the radiation port includes a substantial portion of the parotid glands. Reduce the cumulative renal toxicity associated with repeated administration of cisplatin in patients with advanced ovarian cancer or nonsmall cell lung cancer.

Mechanism of Action Prodrug that is dephosphorylated by alkaline phosphatase in tissues to a pharmacologically active free thiol metabolite. The free thiol is available to bind to, and detoxify, reactive metabolites of cisplatin; and can also act as a scavenger of free radicals that may be generated in tissues.

Labeled Contraindications Hypersensitivity to aminothiol compounds, mannitol, or any component of the formulation

Warnings/Precautions Patients who are hypotensive or in a state of dehydration should not receive amifostine. Interrupt antihypertensive (Continued)

53

Amifostine *(Continued)*

therapy for 24 hours before amifostine. Patients receiving antihypertensive therapy that cannot be stopped for 24 hours preceding amifostine treatment also should not receive amifostine.

It is recommended that antiemetic medication, including dexamethasone 20 mg I.V. and a serotonin 5-HT$_3$ receptor antagonist be administered prior to and in conjunction with amifostine. Rare hypersensitivity reactions, including anaphylaxis and severe cutaneous reaction, have been reported with a higher frequency in patients receiving amifostine as a radioprotectant. Discontinue if allergic reaction occurs; do not rechallenge.

Reports of clinically relevant hypocalcemia are rare, but serum calcium levels should be monitored in patients at risk of hypocalcemia, such as those with nephrotic syndrome.

Adverse Reactions

>10%:

    Cardiovascular: Flushing; hypotension (62%)

    Central nervous system: Chills, dizziness, somnolence

    Gastrointestinal: Nausea/vomiting (may be severe)

    Respiratory: Sneezing

    Miscellaneous: Feeling of warmth/coldness, hiccups

<1%, postmarketing, and/or case reports: Apnea, anaphylactoid reactions, anaphylaxis, arrhythmia, atrial fibrillation, cardiac arrest, erythema multiforme, exfoliative dermatitis; hypersensitivity reactions (fever, rash, hypoxia, dyspnea, laryngeal edema); hypocalcemia, mild rash, myocardial ischemia, rigors, seizure, Stevens-Johnson syndrome, toxic epidermal necrolysis, toxoderma

Vesicant No

Emetic Potential High (60% to 90%)

Overdosage/Toxicology Symptoms of overdose include hypotension, nausea, and vomiting. Treatment includes supportive measures as clinically indicated.

Drug Interactions

Increased Effect/Toxicity: Special consideration should be given to patients receiving antihypertensive medications or other drugs that could potentiate hypotension.

Storage/Stability Reconstitute with 9.7 mL of sterile 0.9% sodium chloride. Reconstituted solutions (500 mg/10 mL) are chemically stable for up to 5 hours at room temperature (25°C) or up to 24 hours under refrigeration 2°C to 8°C. Amifostine should be further diluted in 0.9% sodium chloride to a concentration of 5-40 mg/mL

Reconstitution Reconstitute with 9.7 mL of 0.9% sodium chloride injection. For I.V. infusion, dilute in 50-250 mL of 0.9% sodium chloride. For SubQ administration, reconstitute with 2.4 mL NS or SWFI.

Compatibility Stable in NS

Y-site administration: Compatible: Amikacin, aminophylline, ampicillin, ampicillin/sulbactam, aztreonam, bleomycin, bumetanide, buprenorphine, butorphanol, calcium gluconate, carboplatin, carmustine, cefazolin, cefotaxime, cefotetan, cefoxitin, ceftazidime, ceftizoxime, ceftriaxone, cefuroxime, cimetidine, ciprofloxacin, clindamycin, co-trimoxazole, cyclophosphamide, cytarabine, dacarbazine, dactino-mycin, daunorubicin, dexamethasone sodium phosphate, diphenhydra-mine, dobutamine, docetaxel, dopamine, doxorubicin, doxycycline, droperidol, enalaprilat, etoposide, famotidine, floxuridine, fluconazole, fludarabine, fluorouracil, furosemide, gemcitabine, gentamicin, granise-tron, haloperidol, heparin, hydrocortisone sodium phosphate, hydrocor-tisone sodium succinate, hydromorphone, idarubicin, ifosfamide, imipenem/cilastatin, leucovorin, lorazepam, magnesium sulfate, mannitol, mechlorethamine, meperidine, mesna, methotrexate, methyl-prednisolone sodium succinate, metoclopramide, metronidazole, mito-mycin, mitoxantrone, morphine, nalbuphine, netilmicin, ondansetron, piperacillin, plicamycin, potassium chloride, promethazine, ranitidine, sodium bicarbonate, streptozocin, teniposide, thiotepa, ticarcillin, ticar-cillin/clavulanate, tobramycin, trimetrexate, vancomycin, vinblastine, vincristine, zidovudine. **Incompatible:** Acyclovir, amphotericin B, cefo-perazone, chlorpromazine, cisplatin, ganciclovir, hydroxyzine, minocy-cline, prochlorperazine edisylate

Pharmacodynamics/Kinetics

Distribution: V_d: 3.5 L

Metabolism: Hepatic dephosphorylation to two metabolites (active-free thiol and disulfide)

Half-life elimination: 9 minutes

Excretion: Urine

Clearance, plasma: 2.17 L/minute

Dosage Note: It is recommended that antiemetic medication including dexamethasone 20 mg I.V. and a serotonin 5-HT_3 receptor antagonist be administered prior to and in conjunction with amifostine.

Adults:

Cisplatin-induced renal toxicity, reduction: I.V.: 740-910 mg/m² once daily 30 minutes prior to cytotoxic therapy

Note: Doses >740 mg/m² are associated with a higher incidence of hypotension and may require interruption of therapy or dose modifi-cation for subsequent cycles. For 910 mg/m² doses, the manufac-turer suggests the following blood pressure-based adjustment schedule:

The infusion of amifostine should be interrupted if the systolic blood pressure decreases significantly from baseline, as defined below:

Decrease of 20 mm Hg if baseline systolic blood pressure <100

Decrease of 25 mm Hg if baseline systolic blood pressure 100-119

Decrease of 30 mm Hg if baseline systolic blood pressure 120-139

Decrease of 40 mm Hg if baseline systolic blood pressure 140-179

Decrease of 50 mm Hg if baseline systolic blood pressure ≥180

If the blood pressure returns to normal within 5 minutes (assisted by fluid administration and postural management) and the patient is asymptomatic, the infusion may be restarted so that the full dose of amifostine may be administered. If the full dose of amifostine cannot be administered, the dose of amifostine for subsequent cycles should be 740 mg/m².

Xerostomia from head and neck cancer, reduction:

I.V.: 200mg/m²/day during radiation therapy **or**

SubQ: 500 mg/day during radiation therapy

(Continued)

Amifostine *(Continued)*

Administration

I.V.: Administer over 3-15 minutes; administration as a longer infusion is associated with a higher incidence of side effects. **Note:** SubQ administration has been used.

Dosage Forms Injection, powder for reconstitution: 500 mg

Monitoring Parameters Blood pressure should be monitored every 5 minutes during the infusion

Patient Information This medication is given to help reduce side effects of your cancer therapy. Report immediately lightheadedness, dizziness, fainting, or any nausea; you will be given medication. Report chills, severe dizziness, tremors or shaking, or sudden onset of hiccups.

Additional Information Mean onset of hypotension is 14 minutes into the 15-minute infusion and the mean duration was 6 minutes.

Selected Readings

Anne PR and Curran WJ Jr, "A Phase II Trial of Subcutaneous Amifostine and Radiation Therapy in Patients With Head and Neck Cancer," *Semin Radiat Oncol*, 2002, 12(1 Suppl 1):18-9.

Capizzi RL and Oster W, "Chemoprotective and Radioprotective Effects of Amifostine: An Update of Clinical Trials," *Int J Hematol*, 2000, 72(4):425-35.

Culy CR and Spencer CM, "Amifostine: An Update on Its Clinical Status as a Cytoprotectant in Patients With Cancer Receiving Chemotherapy or Radiotherapy and Its Potential Therapeutic Application in Myelodysplastic Syndrome," *Drugs*, 2001, 61(5):641-84.

Koukourakis MI, "Amifostine in Clinical Oncology: Current Use and Future Applications," *Anticancer Drugs*, 2002, 13(3):181-209.

Koukourakis MI, Kyrias G, and Kakolyris S, "Subcutaneous Administration of Amifostine During Fractionated Radiotherapy: A Randomized Phase II Study," *J Clin Oncol*, 2000, 18(11):2226-33.

Spencer CM and Goa KL, "Amifostine. A Review of Its Pharmacodynamic and Pharmacokinetic Properties, and Therapeutic Potential as a Radioprotector and Cytotoxic Chemoprotector," *Drugs*, 1995, 50(6):1001-31.

Wasserman TH and Brizel DM, "The Role of Amifostine as a Radioprotector," *Oncology (Huntingt)*, 2001, 15(10):1349-54.

Amikacin *(am i KAY sin)*

Medication Safety Issues

Sound-alike/look-alike issues:

Amikacin may be confused with Amicar®, anakinra

Amikin® may be confused with Amicar®

U.S. Brand Names Amikin®

Canadian Brand Names Amikin®

Generic Available Yes

Synonyms Amikacin Sulfate

Pharmacologic Category Antibiotic, Aminoglycoside

Pregnancy Risk Factor D

Lactation Enters breast milk/compatible

Use Treatment of serious infections due to organisms resistant to gentamicin and tobramycin including *Pseudomonas*, *Proteus*, *Serratia*, and other gram-positive bacilli (bone infections, respiratory tract infections, endocarditis, and septicemia); documented infection of mycobacterial organisms susceptible to amikacin

Mechanism of Action Inhibits protein synthesis in susceptible bacteria by binding to 30S ribosomal subunits

Labeled Contraindications Hypersensitivity to amikacin sulfate or any component of the formulation; cross-sensitivity may exist with other aminoglycosides

Warnings/Precautions Dose and/or frequency of administration must be monitored and modified in patients with renal impairment. Drug should be discontinued if signs of ototoxicity, nephrotoxicity, or hypersensitivity occur. Ototoxicity is proportional to the amount of drug given and the duration of treatment. Tinnitus or vertigo may be indications of vestibular injury and impending bilateral **irreversible** damage. Renal damage is usually reversible. May contain sulfites, use with caution in patients with asthma.

Adverse Reactions
1% to 10%:
  Central nervous system: Neurotoxicity
  Otic: Ototoxicity (auditory), ototoxicity (vestibular)
  Renal: Nephrotoxicity
<1%: Hypotension, headache, drowsiness, drug fever, rash, nausea, vomiting, eosinophilia, paresthesia, tremor, arthralgia, weakness, dyspnea, allergic reaction

Vesicant No

Emetic Potential Very low (<10%)

Overdosage/Toxicology Symptoms of overdose include ototoxicity, nephrotoxicity, and neuromuscular toxicity. Treatment of choice following a single acute overdose appears to be maintenance of urine output of at least 3 mL/kg/hour during the acute treatment phase. Dialysis is of questionable value in enhancing aminoglycoside elimination. If required, hemodialysis is preferred over peritoneal dialysis in patients with normal renal function.

Drug Interactions
  Increased Effect/Toxicity: Amikacin may increase or prolong the effect of neuromuscular blocking agents. Concurrent use of amphotericin (or other nephrotoxic drugs) may increase the risk of amikacin-induced nephrotoxicity. The risk of ototoxicity from amikacin may be increased with other ototoxic drugs.

Storage/Stability Stable for 24 hours at room temperature and 2 days at refrigeration when mixed in D_5W, $D_5{}^1/_4NS$, $D_5{}^1/_2NS$, NS, LR.

Compatibility Stable in dextran 75 6% in NS, D_5LR, $D_5{}^1/_4NS$, $D_5{}^1/_3NS$, $D_5{}^1/_2NS$, D_5NS, $D_{10}NS$, D_5W, $D_{10}W$, $D_{20}W$, mannitol 20%, $^1/_4NS$, $^1/_2NS$, NS; **variable stability (consult detailed reference)** in peritoneal dialysis solutions

  Y-site administration: Compatible: Acyclovir, alatrofloxacin, amifostine, amiodarone, amsacrine, aztreonam, cefpirome, cisatracurium, cyclophosphamide, dexamethasone sodium phosphate, diltiazem, docetaxel, enalaprilat, esmolol, etoposide, filgrastim, fluconazole, fludarabine, foscarnet, furosemide, gatifloxacin, gemcitabine, granisetron, idarubicin, IL-2, labetalol, levofloxacin, linezolid, lorazepam, magnesium sulfate, melphalan, midazolam, morphine, ondansetron, paclitaxel, perphenazine, remifentanil, sargramostim, teniposide, thiotepa, vinorelbine, warfarin, zidovudine. **Incompatible:** Allopurinol, amphotericin B cholesteryl sulfate complex, hetastarch, propofol

  Compatibility in syringe: Compatible: Clindamycin, doxapram. **Incompatible:** Heparin

(Continued)

Amikacin *(Continued)*

Compatibility when admixed: Compatible: Amobarbital, ascorbic acid injection, bleomycin, calcium chloride, calcium gluconate, cefepime, cefoxitin, chloramphenicol, chlorpheniramine, cimetidine, ciprofloxacin, clindamycin, colistimethate, dimenhydrinate, diphenhydramine, epinephrine, ergonovine, fluconazole, furosemide, hyaluronidase, hydrocortisone sodium phosphate, hydrocortisone sodium succinate, lincomycin, metaraminol, metronidazole, metronidazole with sodium bicarbonate, norepinephrine, pentobarbital, phenobarbital, phytonadione, polymyxin B sulfate, prochlorperazine edisylate, promethazine, ranitidine, sodium bicarbonate, succinylcholine, vancomycin, verapamil. **Incompatible:** Amphotericin B, ampicillin, cefazolin, chlorothiazide, heparin, phenytoin, thiopental, vitamin B complex with C. **Variable (consult detailed reference):** Aminophylline, dexamethasone sodium phosphate, oxacillin, penicillin G potassium, potassium chloride

Pharmacodynamics/Kinetics

Absorption: I.M.: May be delayed in the bedridden patient

Distribution: Primarily into extracellular fluid (highly hydrophilic); penetrates blood-brain barrier when meninges inflamed; crosses placenta

Relative diffusion of antimicrobial agents from blood into CSF: Good only with inflammation (exceeds usual MICs)

CSF:blood level ratio: Normal meninges: 10% to 20%; Inflamed meninges: 15% to 24%

Half-life elimination (renal function and age dependent):

Infants: Low birth weight (1-3 days): 7-9 hours; Full-term >7 days: 4-5 hours

Children: 1.6-2.5 hours

Adults: Normal renal function: 1.4-2.3 hours; Anuria/end-stage renal disease: 28-86 hours

Time to peak, serum: I.M.: 45-120 minutes

Excretion: Urine (94% to 98%)

Dosage Individualization is critical because of the low therapeutic index

Use of ideal body weight (IBW) for determining the mg/kg/dose appears to be more accurate than dosing on the basis of total body weight (TBW)

In morbid obesity, dosage requirement may best be estimated using a dosing weight of IBW + 0.4 (TBW - IBW)

Initial and periodic peak and trough plasma drug levels should be determined, particularly in critically-ill patients with serious infections or in disease states known to significantly alter aminoglycoside pharmacokinetics (eg, cystic fibrosis, burns, or major surgery)

Infants, Children, and Adults: I.M., I.V.: 5-7.5 mg/kg/dose every 8 hours

Some clinicians suggest a daily dose of 15-20 mg/kg for all patients with normal renal function. This dose is at least as efficacious with similar, if not less, toxicity than conventional dosing.

Dosing interval in renal impairment: Some patients may require larger or more frequent doses if serum levels document the need (ie, cystic fibrosis or febrile granulocytopenic patients)

Cl_{cr} ≥60 mL/minute: Administer every 8 hours

Cl_{cr} 40-60 mL/minute: Administer every 12 hours

Cl_{cr} 20-40 mL/minute: Administer every 24 hours

Cl_{cr} <20 mL/minute: Loading dose, then monitor levels

Hemodialysis: Dialyzable (50% to 100%); administer dose postdialysis or administer $2/3$ normal dose as a supplemental dose postdialysis and follow levels

Peritoneal dialysis: Dose as Cl_{cr} <20 mL/minute: Follow levels

Continuous arteriovenous or venovenous hemodiafiltration effects: Dose as for Cl_{cr} 10-40 mL/minute and follow levels

Administration Administer I.M. injection in large muscle mass

Dosage Forms Injection, solution, as sulfate: 50 mg/mL (2 mL, 4 mL); 62.5 mg/mL (8 mL); 250 mg/mL (2 mL, 4 mL) [contains metabisulfite]

Monitoring Parameters Urinalysis, BUN, serum creatinine, appropriately timed peak and trough concentrations, vital signs, temperature, weight, I & O, hearing parameters

Dietary Considerations Sodium content of 1 g: 29.9 mg (1.3 mEq)

Patient Information Report loss of hearing, ringing or roaring in the ears, or feeling of fullness in head

Additional Information Aminoglycoside levels measured from blood taken from Silastic® central catheters can sometimes give falsely high readings (draw levels from alternate lumen or peripheral stick, if possible)

Special Geriatric Considerations Adjust dose based on renal function.

Selected Readings

Begg EJ and Barclay ML, "Aminoglycosides - 50 Years On," *Br J Clin Pharmacol*, 1995, 39(6):597-603.

Cunha BA, "Aminoglycosides: Current Role in Antimicrobial Therapy," *Pharmacotherapy*, 1988, 8(6):334-50.

Edson RS and Terrell CL, "The Aminoglycosides," *Mayo Clin Proc*, 1999, 74(5):519-28.

Gilbert DN, "Once-Daily Aminoglycoside Therapy," *Antimicrob Agents Chemother*, 1991, 35(3):399-405.

Lortholary O, Tod M, Cohen Y, et al, "Aminoglycosides," *Med Clin North Am*, 1995, 79(4):761-87.

Preston SL and Briceland LL, "Single Daily Dosing of Aminoglycosides," *Pharmacotherapy*, 1995, 15(3):297-316.

Vogelstein B, Kowarski A, and Lietman PS, "The Pharmacokinetics of Amikacin in Children," *J Pediatr*, 1977, 91(2):333-9.

Yasuhara H, Kobayashi S, Sakamoto K, et al, "Pharmacokinetics of Amikacin and Cephalothin in Bedridden Elderly Patients," *J Clin Pharmacol*, 1982, 22(8-9):403-9.

♦ **Amikacin Sulfate** *see* Amikacin *on page 56*

♦ **Amikin**® *see* Amikacin *on page 56*

♦ **2-Amino-6-Mercaptopurine** *see* Thioguanine *on page 762*

Aminocamptothecin (a min o camp to THE sin)

Related Information

Investigational Drug Service *on page 1031*

Safe Handling of Hazardous Drugs *on page 1034*

Generic Available No

Synonyms 9-AC; 9-Aminocamptothecin; NSC-603071

Pharmacologic Category Antineoplastic Agent, DNA Binding Agent; Enzyme Inhibitor, Topoisomerase I Inhibitor

Unlabeled/Investigational Use Phase II trials: Relapsed lymphoma, refractory breast cancer, nonsmall cell lung cancer, untreated colorectal carcinoma

Mechanism of Action Aminocamptothecin binds to topoisomerase I, stabilizing the cleavable DNA-topoisomerase I complex, resulting in arrest of the replication fork and inhibition of DNA synthesis.

Restrictions Not available in U.S./Investigational

(Continued)

Aminocamptothecin *(Continued)*

Labeled Contraindications Hypersensitivity to aminocamptothecin or any component of the formulation

Warnings/Precautions Hazardous agent - use appropriate precautions for handling and disposal. See Safe Handling of Hazardous Drugs *on page 1034* in the Appendix.

Adverse Reactions Frequency not defined.

Central nervous system: Fatigue

Dermatologic: Alopecia

Gastrointestinal: Nausea, vomiting, diarrhea, mucositis, anorexia

Hematologic: Neutropenia (may be dose-limiting), thrombocytopenia (reversible, but may be dose-limiting), anemia

Vesicant No

Emetic Potential Moderate (30% to 60%)

Drug Interactions

Decreased Effect: Anticonvulsants may decrease aminocamptothecin levels.

Storage/Stability Store ampuls at room temperature. Diluted solutions are stable for 28 hours at room temperature. Undiluted aminocamptothecin should not contact plastic items.

Reconstitution Contents of ampul are added to vial (supplied) containing 24.5 mL of special diluent. Resulting aminocamptothecin concentration is 100 mcg/mL. Further dilutions with special diluent for administration via syringe pump is acceptable. May further dilute with NS if resulting concentration is <1 mcg/mL. Undiluted aminocamptothecin should not come in contact with plastics.

Pharmacodynamics/Kinetics Ratio of lactone to total drug is 8.7 ± 4.7% because of instability of aminocamptothecin lactone in plasma.

Distribution: V_d: 46-92 L

Metabolism: None identified

Half-life elimination: Terminal: 8-17 hours for total aminocamptothecin

Excretion: Urine (32% of total drug delivered)

Dosage I.V.: Adults: 45-59 mcg/m^2/hour for 72 hours as a continuous infusion; repeat every 2 weeks **or** 35 mcg/m^2/hour as a 72-hour continuous infusion

Administration Administer by continuous I.V. infusion.

Dosage Forms Injection: 5 mg ampul

Monitoring Parameters WBC with differential, platelet count

Selected Readings

Grossman SA, Hochberg F, Fisher J, et al, "Increased 9-Aminocamptothecin Dose Requirements in Patients on Oral Anticonvulsants. NAPTT CNS Consortium. The New Approaches to Brain Tumor Therapy," *Cancer Chemother Pharmacol*, 1998, 42(2):118-26.

Iyer L and Ratain MJ, "Clinical Pharmacology of Camptothecins," *Cancer Chemother Pharmacol*, 1998, 42(Suppl):31-43.

Potmesil M, Arbuck SG, Takimoto CH, et al, "9-Aminocamptothecin and Beyond. Preclinical and Clinical Studies," *Ann N Y Acad Sci*, 1996, 803:231-46.

Takimota CH, Wright J, and Arbuck SG, "Clinical Applications of the Camptothecins," *Biochim Biophys Acta*, 1998, 1400(1-3):107-19.

♦ **9-Aminocamptothecin** *see* Aminocamptothecin *on page 59*

Aminocaproic Acid (a mee noe ka PROE ik AS id)

Medication Safety Issues
Sound-alike/look-alike issues:
Amicar® may be confused with amikacin, Amikin®

U.S. Brand Names Amicar®

Canadian Brand Names Amicar®

Generic Available Yes: Syrup, tablet

Synonyms Epsilon Aminocaproic Acid

Pharmacologic Category Hemostatic Agent

Pregnancy Risk Factor C

Lactation Excretion in breast milk unknown/use caution

Use Treatment of excessive bleeding from fibrinolysis

Unlabeled/Investigational Use Treatment of traumatic hyphema; control bleeding in thrombocytopenia; control oral bleeding in congenital and acquired coagulation disorders

Mechanism of Action Competitively inhibits activation of plasminogen to plasmin, also, a lesser antiplasmin effect

Labeled Contraindications Hypersensitivity to aminocaproic acid or any component of the formulation; disseminated intravascular coagulation (without heparin); evidence of an intravascular clotting process

Warnings/Precautions Avoid rapid I.V. administration; may induce hypotension, bradycardia, or arrhythmia. Aminocaproic acid may accumulate in patients with decreased renal function. Intrarenal obstruction may occur secondary to glomerular capillary thrombosis or clots in the renal pelvis and ureters. Do not use in hematuria of upper urinary tract origin unless possible benefits outweigh risks. Use with caution in patients with cardiac, renal, or hepatic disease. Do not administer without a definite diagnosis of laboratory findings indicative of hyperfibrinolysis. Inhibition of fibrinolysis may promote clotting or thrombosis; more likely due in the presence of DIC. Subsequently, use with great caution in patients with or at risk for veno-occlusive disease of the liver. Benzyl alcohol is used as a preservative in the injection, therefore, these products should not be used in the neonate. Do not administer with factor IX complex concentrates or anti-inhibitor coagulant complexes.

Adverse Reactions Frequency not defined.
Cardiovascular: Arrhythmia, bradycardia, hypotension, peripheral ischemia, syncope, thrombosis

Central nervous system: Confusion, delirium, dizziness, fatigue, hallucinations, headache, intracranial hypertension, malaise, seizure, stroke

Dermatologic: Rash, pruritus

Gastrointestinal: Abdominal pain, anorexia, cramps, diarrhea, GI irritation, nausea

Genitourinary: Dry ejaculation

Hematologic: Agranulocytosis, bleeding time increased, leukopenia, thrombocytopenia

Neuromuscular & skeletal: CPK increased, myalgia, myositis, myopathy, rhabdomyolysis (rare), weakness

Ophthalmic: Watery eyes, vision decreased

Otic: Tinnitus

Renal: Failure (rare), myoglobinuria (rare)

Respiratory: Dyspnea, nasal congestion, pulmonary embolism

Vesicant No

(Continued)

Aminocaproic Acid *(Continued)*

Emetic Potential Very low (<10%)

Overdosage/Toxicology Symptoms of overdose include acute renal failure, delirium, diarrhea, hepatic necrosis, nausea, seizures, transient hypotension, and thromboembolism. Aminocaproic acid may be removed by hemodialysis.

Drug Interactions

Increased Effect/Toxicity: Increased risk of hypercoagulability with oral contraceptives, estrogens. Should not be administered with factor IX complex concentrated or anti-inhibitor complex concentrates due to an increased risk of thrombosis.

Storage/Stability Store at 15°C to 30°C (59°F to 86°F).

Reconstitution Dilute I.V. solution (1 g/50 mL of diluent) with D_5W, 0.9% sodium chloride, or lactated Ringer's.

Compatibility Stable in D_5W, NS

Compatibility when admixed: Compatible: Netilmicin

Pharmacodynamics/Kinetics

Onset of action: ~1-72 hours

Distribution: Widely through intravascular and extravascular compartments;

V_d: Oral: 23 L, I.V.: 30 L

Metabolism: Minimally hepatic

Half-life elimination: 2 hours

Time to peak: Oral: Within 2 hours

Excretion: Urine (65% as unchanged drug, 11% as metabolite)

Dosage

Acute bleeding syndrome:

Children (unlabeled use): Oral, I.V.: 100-200 mg/kg during the first hour, followed by continuous infusion at 33.3 mg/kg/hour or 100 mg/kg (I.V. or Oral) every 6 hours

Adults: Oral, I.V.: 4-5 g during the first hour, followed by 1 g/hour for 8 hours or until bleeding controlled (maximum daily dose: 30 g)

Control bleeding in thrombocytopenia (unlabeled use): Adults:

Initial: I.V.: 0.1 g/kg over 30-60 minutes

Maintenance: Oral: 1-3 g every 6 hours

Control oral bleeding in congenital and acquired coagulation disorder (unlabeled use): Adults: Oral: 50-60 mg/kg every 4 hours

Traumatic hyphema (unlabeled use): Children and Adults: Oral: 100 mg/kg/dose every 4 hours (maximum daily dose: 30 g)

Dosing adjustment in renal impairment: May accumulate in patients with decreased renal function.

Administration I.V.: May be given over 30-60 minutes or by continuous infusion; rapid I.V. injection (IVP) should be avoided due to possible hypotension, bradycardia, and arrhythmia.

Dosage Forms

Injection, solution: 250 mg/mL (20 mL) [contains benzyl alcohol]

Syrup: 1.25 g/5 mL (240 mL, 480 mL)

Amicar®: 1.25 g/5 mL (480 mL) [raspberry flavor]

Tablet [scored]: 500 mg, 1000 mg

Monitoring Parameters Fibrinogen, fibrin split products, creatine phosphokinase (with long-term therapy)

Patient Information Report any signs of bleeding; change positions slowly to minimize dizziness

Selected Readings

Bartholomew JR, Salgia R, and Bell WR, "Control of Bleeding in Patients With Immune and Nonimmune Thrombocytopenia With Aminocaproic Acid," *Arch Intern Med*, 1989, 149(9):1959-61.

Gardner FH and Helmer RE 3rd, "Aminocaproic Acid. Use in Control of Hemorrhage in Patients With Amegakaryocytic Thrombocytopenia," *JAMA*, 1980, 243(1):35-7.

Mannucci P, "Hemostatic Drugs," *N Engl J Med*, 1998, 339(4):245-53.

Pieramici DJ, Goldberg MF, Melia M, et al, "A Phase III, Multicenter, Randomized, Placebo-Controlled Clinical Trial of Topical Aminocaproic Acid (Caprogel) in the Management of Traumatic Hyphema," *Ophthalmology*, 2003, 110(11):2106-12.

Aminoglutethimide (a mee noe gloo TETH i mide)

Medication Safety Issues

Sound-alike/look-alike issues:

Cytadren® may be confused with cytarabine

U.S. Brand Names Cytadren®

Generic Available No

Synonyms AG; AGT; BA-16038; Elipten

Pharmacologic Category Antineoplastic Agent, Aromatase Inhibitor; Aromatase Inhibitor; Enzyme Inhibitor; Hormone Antagonist, Anti-Adrenal; Nonsteroidal Aromatase Inhibitor

Pregnancy Risk Factor D

Lactation Excretion in breast milk unknown/contraindicated

Use Suppression of adrenal function in selected patients with Cushing's syndrome

Unlabeled/Investigational Use Treatment of breast and prostate cancer (androgen synthesis inhibitor)

Mechanism of Action Blocks the enzymatic conversion of cholesterol to delta-5-pregnenolone, thereby reducing the synthesis of adrenal glucocorticoids, mineralocorticoids, estrogens, aldosterone, and androgens

Labeled Contraindications Hypersensitivity to aminoglutethimide, glutethimide, or any component of the formulation; pregnancy; breast-feeding

Warnings/Precautions Monitor blood pressure in all patients at appropriate intervals. Hypothyroidism may occur. **Mineralocorticoid replacement is necessary in up to 50% of patients.** Glucocorticoid replacement is necessary in most patients.

Adverse Reactions Most adverse effects will diminish in incidence and severity after the first 2-6 weeks

>10%:

Central nervous system: Headache, dizziness, drowsiness, lethargy, clumsiness

Dermatologic: Skin rash

Gastrointestinal: Nausea, anorexia

Hepatic: Cholestatic jaundice

Neuromuscular & skeletal: Myalgia

Renal: Nephrotoxicity

Respiratory: Pulmonary alveolar damage

1% to 10%:

Cardiovascular: Hypotension, tachycardia, orthostasis

Dermatologic: Hirsutism, pruritus

Endocrine & metabolic: Adrenocortical insufficiency

(Continued)

Aminoglutethimide *(Continued)*

Gastrointestinal: Vomiting

<1%: Adrenal suppression, hepatotoxicity, hypercholesterolemia, hyperkalemia, hypothyroidism, goiter, masculinization of females, pulmonary hypersensitivity, urticaria; rare cases of neutropenia, leukopenia, thrombocytopenia, pancytopenia, agranulocytosis have been reported

Emetic Potential Very low (<10%)

Overdosage/Toxicology Symptoms of overdose include ataxia, somnolence, lethargy, dizziness, distress, fatigue, coma, hyperventilation, respiratory depression, hypovolemia, and shock. Treatment is supportive.

Drug Interactions

Cytochrome P450 Effect: Induces CYP1A2 (strong), 2C19 (strong), 3A4 (strong)

Decreased Effect: Aminoglutethimide may decrease therapeutic effect of dexamethasone, digitoxin (after 3-8 weeks), warfarin, medroxyprogesterone, megestrol, and tamoxifen. Aminoglutethimide may decrease the levels/effects of aminophylline, benzodiazepines, calcium channel blockers, citalopram, clarithromycin, cyclosporine, diazepam, erythromycin, estrogens, fluvoxamine, methsuximide, mirtazapine, nateglinide, nefazodone, nevirapine, phenytoin, proton pump inhibitors, protease inhibitors, ropinirole, sertraline, tacrolimus, theophylline, venlafaxine, voriconazole and other drugs metabolized by CYP1A2, 2C19, or 3A4.

Storage/Stability Store at controlled room temperature not >30°C (86°F).

Pharmacodynamics/Kinetics

Onset of action: Adrenal suppression: 3-5 days; following withdrawal of therapy, adrenal function returns within 72 hours

Absorption: 90%

Protein binding, plasma: 20% to 25%

Metabolism: Major metabolite is N-acetylaminoglutethimide; induces its own metabolism

Half-life elimination: 7-15 hours; shorter following multiple doses

Excretion: Urine (34% to 50% as unchanged drug, 25% as metabolites)

Dosage Oral: Adults:

Adrenal suppression: 250 mg every 6 hours may be increased at 1- to 2-week intervals to a total of 2 g/day

Breast and prostate cancer (unlabeled use): 250 mg 4 times/day

Dosing adjustment in renal impairment: Dose reduction may be necessary

Administration Oral: Every 6 hours to reduce incidence of nausea and vomiting.

Dosage Forms Tablet [scored]: 250 mg

Monitoring Parameters Follow adrenal cortical response by careful monitoring of plasma cortisol until the desired level of suppression is achieved. Mineralocorticoid (fludrocortisone) replacement therapy may be necessary in up to 50% of patients. If glucocorticoid replacement therapy is necessary, 20-30 mg hydrocortisone orally in the morning will replace endogenous secretion.

Selected Readings

Lonning PE and Kvinnsland S, "Mechanisms of Action of Aminoglutethimide as Endocrine Therapy of Breast Cancer," *Drugs*, 1988, 35(6):685-710.

Robinson MR, "Aminoglutethimide: Medical Adrenalectomy in the Management of Carcinoma of the Prostate. A review After 6 Years," *Br J Urol*, 1980, 52(4):328-9.

Roseman BJ, Budzar AU, and Singletary SE, "Use of Aromatase Inhibitors in Postmenopausal Women With Advanced Breast Cancer," *J Surg Oncol*, 1997, 66(3):215-20.

Russell CA, Green SJ, O'Sullivan J, et al, "Megestrol Acetate and Aminoglutethimide/ Hydrocortisone in Sequence or in Combination as Second-Line Endocrine Therapy of Estrogen Receptor-Positive Metastatic Breast Cancer: A Southwest Oncology Group Phase III Trial," *J Clin Oncol*, 1997, 15(7):2494-501.

Sanford EJ, Drago JR, Rohner TJ Jr, et al, "Aminoglutethimide medical adrenalectomy for advanced prostatic carcinoma," *J Urol*, 1976, 115(2):170-4.

Santen RJ and Misbin RI, "Aminoglutethimide: Review of Pharmacology and Clinical Use," *Pharmacotherapy*, 1981, 1(2):95-120.

◆ **AMJ 9701** *see* Palifermin *on page 646*

Amonafide (a MON a fide)

Related Information

Investigational Drug Service *on page 1031*
Safe Handling of Hazardous Drugs *on page 1034*

Generic Available No

Synonyms Amonafide Hydrochloride; Benzisoquinolinedione; BIDA; M-FA-142; Nafidimide; NSC-308847

Pharmacologic Category Antineoplastic Agent, DNA Binding Agent; Enzyme Inhibitor, Topoisomerase II Inhibitor

Unlabeled/Investigational Use Breast, prostate, renal cell, ovarian, pancreatic, and nonsmall cell lung cancers

Mechanism of Action Amonafide acts as a DNA intercalator, stabilizing DNA to thermal denaturation and producing single-strand DNA breaks.

Labeled Contraindications Hypersensitivity to amonafide or any component of the formulation; pregnancy

Warnings/Precautions Hazardous agent - use appropriate precautions for handling and disposal. See Safe Handling of Hazardous Drugs *on page 1034* in the Appendix. Amonafide should be used cautiously in bone marrow transplant patients and patients with existing bone marrow suppression, hepatic dysfunction, arrhythmias, conduction problems, congestive heart failure, or seizures or other neurological disorders. Amonafide toxicity, particularly hematologic, correlates with the patient's acetylator status. If possible, determination of acetylator type (fast vs slow) should be considered prior to beginning therapy.

Adverse Reactions

>10%:

Gastrointestinal: Nausea and vomiting (mild)

Hematologic: Granulocytopenia, possibly dose-limiting; nadir occurs at days 12-15, recovery by day 21

1% to 10%:

Cardiovascular: Chest pain

Central nervous system: Dizziness, fatigue, headache

Dermatologic: Skin rash, exfoliative dermatitis, alopecia

Local: Inflammatory reactions

Otic: Tinnitus

Neuromuscular & skeletal: Myoclonic jerking, weakness

<1%: CHF, hypotension, taste alteration, thrombocytopenia

Vesicant No

Emetic Potential Moderate (30% to 60%)

Storage/Stability Store intact vials under refrigeration at 2°C to 8°C (36°F to 46°F). Reconstituted vials and solutions for infusion are stable for up to 14 days at room temperature or under refrigeration.

(Continued)

Amonafide *(Continued)*

Reconstitution Vials may be reconstituted with SWFI or 0.9% sodium chloride.

Compatibility Incompatible: Dextrose solutions

Pharmacodynamics/Kinetics

Distribution: V_d: 370-530 L/m^2

Protein binding: High

Half-life:

Elimination: 3.5-11 hours

Terminal: 3-6 hours

Metabolism: Hepatic, primarily by oxidation and N-acetylation. N-acetylamonafide (active) and amonafide-N'-oxide are the major metabolites. Clearance depends on whether the patient is a fast or slow acetylator. Fast acetylators may experience greater toxicity from the drug.

Excretion: Urine (3% to 22% as unchanged drug)

Dosage Adults (refer to individual protocols):

Breast cancer: 800 mg/m^2 over 3 hours every 28 days

Renal cell, ovarian, pancreatic cancer: Up to 450 mg/m^2 over 1 hour on days 1-5 every 21 days

Nonsmall cell lung cancer: 1600 mg/m^2 by continuous infusion over 24 hours every 21 days

Dosage adjustment in hepatic impairment: May be required but specific guidelines have not been established.

Administration May be administered by short (1-3 hours) infusion or continuous (24-hour) infusion.

Dosage Forms Powder for injection, lyophilized: 500 mg

Selected Readings

Kornek G, Raderer M, Depisch D, et al, "Amonafide as First-Line Chemotherapy for Metastatic Breast Cancer," *Eur J Cancer*, 1994, 30A(3):398-400.

Kreis W, Chan K, Budman DR, et al, "Clinical Pharmacokinetics of Amonafide (NSC-308847) in 62 Patients," *Cancer Invest*, 1996, 14(4):320-7.

Leaf AN, Neuberg D, Schwartz EL, et al, "An ECOG Phase II Study of Amonafide in Unresectable or Recurrent Carcinoma of the Head and Neck (PB390). Eastern Cooperative Oncology Group," *Invest New Drugs*, 1997, 15(2):165-72.

Marshall ME, Blumenstein B, Crawford ED, et al, "Phase II Trial of Amonafide for the Treatment of Advanced, Hormonally Refractory Carcinoma of the Prostate," *Am J Clin Oncol*, 1994, 17(6):514-5.

Ratain MJ, Rosner G, Allen SL, et al, "Population Pharmacodynamic Study of Amonafide: A Cancer and Leukemia Group B Study," *J Clin Oncol*, 1995, 13(3):741-7.

♦ **Amonafide Hydrochloride** *see* Amonafide *on page 65*

♦ **Amphadase™** *see* Hyaluronidase *on page 417*

♦ **Amphocin®** *see* Amphotericin B (Conventional) *on page 69*

♦ **Amphotec®** *see* Amphotericin B Cholesteryl Sulfate Complex *on page 66*

Amphotericin B Cholesteryl Sulfate Complex

(am foe TER i sin bee kole LES te ril SUL fate KOM plecks)

Medication Safety Issues

Safety issues:

Lipid-based amphotericin formulations (Amphotec®) may be confused with conventional formulations (Amphocin®, Fungizone®)

Large overdoses have occurred when conventional formulations were dispensed inadvertently for lipid-based products. Single daily doses of conventional amphotericin formulation never exceed 1.5 mg/kg.

Related Information
Management of Infections *on page 978*

U.S. Brand Names Amphotec®

Canadian Brand Names Amphotec®

Generic Available No

Synonyms ABCD; Amphotericin B Colloidal Dispersion

Pharmacologic Category Antifungal Agent, Parenteral

Pregnancy Risk Factor B

Lactation Excretion in breast milk unknown/contraindicated

Use Treatment of invasive aspergillosis in patients who have failed amphotericin B deoxycholate treatment, or who have renal impairment or experience unacceptable toxicity which precludes treatment with amphotericin B deoxycholate in effective doses.

Unlabeled/Investigational Use Effective in patients with serious *Candida* species infections

Mechanism of Action Binds to ergosterol altering cell membrane permeability in susceptible fungi and causing leakage of cell components with subsequent cell death. Proposed mechanism suggests that amphotericin causes an oxidation-dependent stimulation of macrophages (Lyman, 1992).

Labeled Contraindications Hypersensitivity to amphotericin B or any component of the formulation

Warnings/Precautions Anaphylaxis has been reported. Facilities for cardiopulmonary resuscitation should be available. Infusion reactions, sometimes severe, usually subside with continued therapy.

Adverse Reactions
>10%: Central nervous system: Chills, fever
1% to 10%:
  Cardiovascular: Hypotension, tachycardia
  Central nervous system: Headache
  Dermatologic: Rash
  Endocrine & metabolic: Hypokalemia, hypomagnesemia
  Gastrointestinal: Nausea, diarrhea, abdominal pain
  Hematologic: Thrombocytopenia
  Hepatic: LFT change
  Neuromuscular & skeletal: Rigors
  Renal: Elevated creatinine
  Respiratory: Dyspnea

Note: Amphotericin B colloidal dispersion has an improved therapeutic index compared to conventional amphotericin B, and has been used safely in patients with amphotericin B-related nephrotoxicity; however, continued decline of renal function has occurred in some patients.

Overdosage/Toxicology Symptoms of overdose include renal dysfunction, anemia, thrombocytopenia, granulocytopenia, fever, nausea, and vomiting. Treatment is supportive.

Drug Interactions
Increased Effect/Toxicity: Toxic effect with other nephrotoxic drugs (eg, cyclosporine and aminoglycosides) may be additive. Corticosteroids may increase potassium depletion caused by amphotericin. (Continued)

Amphotericin B Cholesteryl Sulfate Complex
(Continued)

Amphotericin B may predispose patients receiving digitalis glycosides or neuromuscular blocking agents to toxicity secondary to hypokalemia.

Decreased Effect: Pharmacologic antagonism may occur with azole antifungals (eg, ketoconazole, miconazole).

Compatibility Stable in D_5W; **incompatible** with NS

Y-site administration: Compatible: Acyclovir, aminophylline, cefoxitin, ceftizoxime, clindamycin, dexamethasone sodium phosphate, fentanyl, furosemide, ganciclovir, granisetron, hydrocortisone sodium succinate, ifosfamide, lorazepam, mannitol, methotrexate, methylprednisolone sodium succinate, nitroglycerin, sufentanil, trimethoprim/sulfamethoxazole, vinblastine, vincristine, zidovudine. **Incompatible:** Alfentanil, amikacin, ampicillin, ampicillin/sulbactam, atenolol, aztreonam, bretylium, buprenorphine, butorphanol, calcium chloride, calcium gluconate, carboplatin, cefazolin, cefepime, cefoperazone, ceftazidime, ceftriaxone, chlorpromazine, cimetidine, cisatracurium, cisplatin, cyclophosphamide, cyclosporine, cytarabine, diazepam, digoxin, diphenhydramine, dobutamine, dopamine, doxorubicin, doxorubicin liposome, droperidol, enalaprilat, esmolol, famotidine, fluconazole, fluorouracil, gatifloxacin, gentamicin, haloperidol, heparin, hydromorphone, hydroxyzine, imipenem/cilastatin, labetalol, leucovorin, lidocaine, magnesium sulfate, meperidine, mesna, metoclopramide, metoprolol, metronidazole, midazolam, mitoxantrone, morphine, nalbuphine, naloxone, ofloxacin, ondansetron, paclitaxel, pentobarbital, phenobarbital, phenytoin, piperacillin, piperacillin/tazobactam, potassium chloride, prochlorperazine, promethazine, propranolol, ranitidine, remifentanil, sodium bicarbonate, ticarcillin, ticarcillin/clavulanate, tobramycin, vancomycin, vecuronium, verapamil, vinorelbine

Pharmacodynamics/Kinetics

Distribution: V_d: Total volume increases with higher doses, reflects increasing uptake by tissues (with 4 mg/kg/day = 4 L/kg); predominantly distributed in the liver; concentrations in kidneys and other tissues are lower than observed with conventional amphotericin B

Half-life elimination: 28-29 hours; prolonged with higher doses

Dosage Children and Adults: I.V.:

Premedication: For patients who experience chills, fever, hypotension, nausea, or other nonanaphylactic infusion-related immediate reactions, premedicate with the following drugs, 30-60 minutes prior to drug administration: a nonsteroidal (eg, ibuprofen, choline magnesium trisalicylate) with or without diphenhydramine; or acetaminophen with diphenhydramine; or hydrocortisone 50-100 mg. If the patient experiences rigors during the infusion, meperidine may be administered.

Range: 3-4 mg/kg/day (infusion of 1 mg/kg/hour); maximum: 7.5 mg/kg/day

Dosage Forms Injection, powder for reconstitution: 50 mg, 100 mg

Monitoring Parameters Liver function tests, electrolytes, BUN, Cr, temperature, CBC, I/O, signs of hypokalemia (muscle weakness, cramping, drowsiness, ECG changes)

Additional Information Controlled trials which compare the original formulation of amphotericin B to the newer liposomal formulations (ie, Amphotec®) are lacking. Thus, comparative data discussing differences among the formulations should be interpreted cautiously. Although the risk of nephrotoxicity and infusion-related adverse effects may be less with Amphotec®, the efficacy profiles of Amphotec® and the original amphotericin formulation are comparable. Consequently, Amphotec® should be restricted to those patients who cannot tolerate or fail a standard amphotericin B formulation.

Special Geriatric Considerations The pharmacokinetics and dosing of amphotericin have not been studied in the elderly. It appears that use is similar to young adults. Caution should be exercised and renal function and desired effect monitored closely.

Selected Readings

Edwards JE Jr, Bodey GP, Bowden RA, et al, "International Conference for the Development of a Consensus on the Management and Prevention of Severe Candidal Infections," *Clin Infect Dis*, 1997, 25(1):43-59.

Eggimann P, Francioli P, Bille J, et al, "Fluconazole Prophylaxis Prevents Intra-Abdominal Candidiasis in High-Risk Surgical Patients," *Crit Care Med*, 1999, 27(6):1066-72.0n

Fichtenbaum CJ, Zackin R, Rajicic N, et al, "Amphotericin B Oral Suspension for Fluconazole-Refractory Oral Candidiasis in Persons With HIV Infection. Adult AIDS Clinical Trials Group Study Team 295," *AIDS*, 2000, 14(7):845-52.

Hiemenz JW and Walsh TJ, "Lipid Formulations of Amphotericin B: Recent Progress and Future Directions," *Clin Infect Dis*, 1996, 22(Suppl 2):133-44.

Lister J, "Amphotericin B Lipid Complex (Abelcet®) in the Treatment of Invasive Mycoses: The North American Experience," *Eur J Haematol Suppl*, 1996, 57:18-23.

Lyman CA and Walsh TJ, "Systemically Administered Antifungal Agents. A Review of Their Clinical Pharmacology and Therapeutic Applications," *Drugs*, 1992, 44(1):9-35.

Mora-Duarte J, Betts R, Rotstein C, et al, "Comparison of Caspofungin and Amphotericin B for Invasive Candidiasis," *N Engl J Med*, 2002, 347(25):2020-9.

Patel R, "Antifungal Agents. Part I. Amphotericin B Preparations and Flucytosine," *Mayo Clin Proc*, 1998, 73(12):1205-25.

Prentice HG, Hann IM, Herbrecht R, et al, "A Randomized Comparison of Liposomal Versus Conventional Amphotericin B for the Treatment of Pyrexia of Unknown Origin in Neutropenic Patients," *Br J Haematol*, 1997, 98(3):711-8.

Rex JH, Bennett JE, Sugar AM, "A Randomized Trial Comparing Fluconazole With Amphotericin B for the Treatment of Candidemia in Patients Without Neutropenia. Candidemia Study Group and the National Institute," *N Engl J Med*, 1994, 331(20):1325-30.

Rex JH, Pappas PG, Karchmer AW, et al, "A Randomized and Blinded Multicenter Trial of High-Dose Fluconazole Plus Placebo Versus Fluconazole Plus Amphotericin B as Therapy for Candidemia and Its Consequences in Nonneutropenic Subjects," *Clin Infect Dis*, 2003, 36(10):1221-8.

Rex JH, Walsh TJ, Sobel JD, et al, "Practice Guidelines for the Treatment of Candidiasis. Infectious Diseases Society of America," *Clin Infect Dis*, 2000, 30(4):662-78.

Slain D, "Lipid-Based Amphotericin B for the Treatment of Fungal Infections," *Pharmacotherapy*, 1999, 19(3):306-23.

♦ **Amphotericin B Colloidal Dispersion** *see* Amphotericin B Cholesteryl Sulfate Complex *on page 66*

Amphotericin B (Conventional)
(am foe TER i sin bee con VEN sha nal)

Medication Safety Issues

Safety issues:

Conventional amphotericin formulations (Amphocin®, Fungizone®) may be confused with lipid-based formulations (AmBisome®, Abelcet®, Amphotec®).

Large overdoses have occurred when conventional formulations were dispensed inadvertently for lipid-based products. Single daily doses of conventional amphotericin formulation never exceed 1.5 mg/kg.

Related Information

Management of Infections *on page 978*

U.S. Brand Names Amphocin®; Fungizone®

(Continued)

Amphotericin B (Conventional) *(Continued)*

Canadian Brand Names Fungizone®

Generic Available Yes: Powder for reconstitution

Synonyms Amphotericin B Desoxycholate

Pharmacologic Category Antifungal Agent, Parenteral; Antifungal Agent, Topical

Pregnancy Risk Factor B

Lactation Excretion in breast milk unknown/contraindicated

Use Treatment of severe systemic and central nervous system infections caused by susceptible fungi such as *Candida* species, *Histoplasma capsulatum*, *Cryptococcus neoformans*, *Aspergillus* species, *Blastomyces dermatitidis*, *Torulopsis glabrata*, and *Coccidioides immitis*; fungal peritonitis; irrigant for bladder fungal infections; and topically for cutaneous and mucocutaneous candidal infections; used in fungal infection in patients with bone marrow transplantation, amebic meningoencephalitis, ocular aspergillosis (intraocular injection), candidal cystitis (bladder irrigation), chemoprophylaxis (low-dose I.V.), immunocompromised patients at risk of aspergillosis (intranasal/nebulized), refractory meningitis (intrathecal), coccidioidal arthritis (intra-articular/I.M.).

Low-dose amphotericin B has been administered after bone marrow transplantation to reduce the risk of invasive fungal disease.

Mechanism of Action Binds to ergosterol altering cell membrane permeability in susceptible fungi and causing leakage of cell components with subsequent cell death. Proposed mechanism suggests that amphotericin causes an oxidation-dependent stimulation of macrophages (Lyman, 1992).

Labeled Contraindications Hypersensitivity to amphotericin or any component of the formulation

Warnings/Precautions Avoid use with other nephrotoxic drugs. Monitor BUN and serum creatinine, potassium, and magnesium levels every 2-4 days, and daily in patients at risk for acute renal dysfunction. Topical preparations may stain clothing. The standard dosage of lipid-based amphotericin B formulations, including amphotericin B cholesteryl sulfate (Amphotec®), amphotericin B lipid complex (Abelcet®), and liposomal amphotericin B (AmBisome®) is many fold greater than the dosage of conventional amphotericin B. To prevent inadvertent overdose, the product name and dosage must be verified for any amphotericin B dosage exceeding 1.5 mg/kg. Amphotericin B has been administered to pregnant women without obvious deleterious effects to the fetus, but the number of cases reported is small. Use during pregnancy only if absolutely necessary.

Adverse Reactions

>10%:

Central nervous system: Fever, chills, headache, malaise, generalized pain

Endocrine & metabolic: Hypokalemia, hypomagnesemia

Gastrointestinal: Anorexia

Hematologic: Anemia

Renal: Nephrotoxicity

1% to 10%:

Cardiovascular: Hypotension, hypertension, flushing

Central nervous system: Delirium, arachnoiditis, pain along lumbar nerves

Gastrointestinal: Nausea, vomiting

Genitourinary: Urinary retention

Hematologic: Leukocytosis

Local: Thrombophlebitis

Neuromuscular & skeletal: Paresthesia (especially with I.T. therapy)

Renal: Renal tubular acidosis, renal failure

<1%: Cardiac arrest, bone marrow suppression, convulsions, maculopapular rash, coagulation defects, thrombocytopenia, agranulocytosis, leukopenia, acute liver failure, vision changes, hearing loss, anuria, dyspnea

Vesicant No

Emetic Potential Very low (<10%)

Overdosage/Toxicology Symptoms of overdose include renal dysfunction, cardiac arrest, anemia, thrombocytopenia, granulocytopenia, fever, nausea, and vomiting. Treatment is supportive.

Drug Interactions

Increased Effect/Toxicity: Use of amphotericin with other nephrotoxic drugs (eg, cyclosporine and aminoglycosides) may result in additive toxicity. Amphotericin may increase the toxicity of flucytosine. Antineoplastic agents may increase the risk of amphotericin-induced nephrotoxicity, bronchospasms, and hypotension. Corticosteroids may increase potassium depletion caused by amphotericin. Amphotericin B may predispose patients receiving digitalis glycosides or neuromuscular-blocking agents to toxicity secondary to hypokalemia.

Decreased Effect: Pharmacologic antagonism may occur with azole antifungal agents (ketoconazole, miconazole).

Storage/Stability Store intact vials under refrigeration; protect from light. Reconstituted vials are stable, protected from light, for 24 hours at room temperature and 1 week when refrigerated. Parenteral admixtures are stable, protected from light, for 24 hours at room temperature and 2 days under refrigeration.

Reconstitution Add 10 mL of SWFI (without a bacteriostatic agent) to each vial of amphotericin B. Further dilute with 250-500 mL of D_5W; final concentration should not exceed 0.1 mg/mL (peripheral infusion) or 0.25 mg/mL (central infusion).

Compatibility Solution compatibility:

Compatible: Heparin sodium, hydrocortisone, sodium bicarbonate

Incompatible: Ampicillin, calcium gluconate, carbenicillin, cimetidine, dopamine, gentamicin, lidocaine, potassium chloride, sodium chloride, tetracycline, verapamil

Pharmacodynamics/Kinetics

Distribution: Minimal amounts enter the aqueous humor, bile, CSF (inflamed or noninflamed meninges), amniotic fluid, pericardial fluid, pleural fluid, and synovial fluid

Protein binding, plasma: 90%

Half-life elimination: Biphasic: Initial: 15-48 hours; Terminal: 15 days

Time to peak: Within 1 hour following a 4- to 6-hour dose

Excretion: Urine (2% to 5% as biologically active form); ~40% eliminated over a 7-day period and may be detected in urine for at least 7 weeks after discontinued use

(Continued)

Amphotericin B (Conventional) *(Continued)*

Dosage

I.V.: Premedication: For patients who experience infusion-related immediate reactions, premedicate with the following drugs, 30-60 minutes prior to drug administration: a nonsteroidal with or without diphenhydramine; or acetaminophen with diphenhydramine; or hydrocortisone 50-100 mg. If the patient experiences rigors during the infusion, meperidine may be administered.

Infants and Children:

Test dose: I.V.: 0.1 mg/kg/dose to a maximum of 1 mg; infuse over 30-60 minutes. Many clinicians believe a test dose is unnecessary.

Maintenance dose: 0.25-1 mg/kg/day given once daily; infuse over 2-6 hours. Once therapy has been established, amphotericin B can be administered on an every-other-day basis at 1-1.5 mg/kg/dose; cumulative dose: 1.5-2 g over 6-10 week.

Adults:

Test dose: 1 mg infused over 20-30 minutes. Many clinicians believe a test dose is unnecessary.

Maintenance dose: Usual: 0.25-1.5 mg/kg/day; 1-1.5 mg/kg over 4-6 hours every other day may be given once therapy is established; aspergillosis, mucormycosis, rhinocerebral phycomycosis often require 1-1.5 mg/kg/day; do not exceed 1.5 mg/kg/day

Duration of therapy varies with nature of infection: Usual duration is 4-12 weeks or cumulative dose of 1-4 g

I.T.: Meningitis, coccidioidal or cryptococcal:

Children.: 25-100 mcg every 48-72 hours; increase to 500 mcg as tolerated

Adults: Initial: 25-300 mcg every 48-72 hours; increase to 500 mcg to 1 mg as tolerated; maximum total dose: 15 mg has been suggested

Oral: 1 mL (100 mg) 4 times/day

Topical: Apply to affected areas 2-4 times/day for 1-4 weeks of therapy depending on nature and severity of infection

Bladder irrigation: Candidal cystitis: Irrigate with 50 mcg/mL solution instilled periodically or continuously for 5-10 days or until cultures are clear

Dosing adjustment in renal impairment: If renal dysfunction is due to the drug, the daily total can be decreased by 50% or the dose can be given every other day; I.V. therapy may take several months

Dialysis: Poorly dialyzed; no supplemental dosage necessary when using hemo- or peritoneal dialysis or continuous arteriovenous or venovenous hemodiafiltration effects

Administration in dialysate: Children and Adults: 1-2 mg/L of peritoneal dialysis fluid either with or without low-dose I.V. amphotericin B (a total dose of 2-10 mg/kg given over 7-14 days). Precipitate may form in ionic dialysate solutions.

Dosage Forms

Cream (Fungizone®): 3% (20 g)

Injection, powder for reconstitution, as desoxycholate (Amphocin®; Fungizone®): 50 mg

Lotion (Fungizone®): 3% (30 mL)

Monitoring Parameters Renal function (monitor frequently during therapy), electrolytes (especially potassium and magnesium), liver function tests, temperature, PT/PTT, CBC; monitor input and output; monitor for signs of hypokalemia (muscle weakness, cramping, drowsiness, ECG changes, etc)

Patient Information Amphotericin cream may slightly discolor skin and stain clothing; good personal hygiene may reduce the spread and recurrence of lesions; avoid covering topical applications with occlusive bandages; most skin lesions require 1-3 weeks of therapy; report any cramping, muscle weakness, or pain at or near injection site

Additional Information Premedication with diphenhydramine and acetaminophen may reduce the severity of acute infusion-related reactions. Meperidine reduces the duration of amphotericin B-induced rigors and chilling. Hydrocortisone may be used in patients with severe or refractory infusion-related reactions. Bolus infusion of normal saline immediately preceding, or immediately preceding and following amphotericin B may reduce drug-induced nephrotoxicity. Risk of nephrotoxicity increases with amphotericin B doses >1 mg/kg/day. Infusion of admixtures more concentrated than 0.25 mg/mL should be limited to patients absolutely requiring volume restriction. Amphotericin B does not have a bacteriostatic constituent, subsequently admixture expiration is determined by sterility more than chemical stability.

Special Geriatric Considerations Caution should be exercised and renal function and desired effect monitored closely in older adults.

Selected Readings

Benson JM and Nahata MC, "Pharmacokinetics of Amphotericin B in Children," *Antimicrob Agents Chemother*, 1989, 33(11):1989-93.

Gallis HA, Drew RH, and Pickard WW, "Amphotericin B: 30 Years of Clinical Experience," *Rev Infect Dis*, 1990, 12(2):308-29.

Kauffman CA and Carver PL, "Antifungal Agents in the 1990s. Current Status and Future Developments," *Drugs*, 1997, 53(4):539-49.

Kintzel PE and Smith GH, "Practical Guidelines for Preparing and Administering Amphotericin B," *Am J Hosp Pharm*, 1992, 49(5):1156-64.

Koren G, Lau A, Klein J, et al, "Pharmacokinetics and Adverse Effects of Amphotericin B in Infants and Children," *J Pediatr*, 1988, 113(3):559-63.

Lyman CA and Walsh TJ, "Systemically Administered Antifungal Agents. A Review of Their Clinical Pharmacology and Therapeutic Applications," *Drugs*, 1992, 44(1):9-35.

Patel R, "Antifungal Agents. Part I. Amphotericin B Preparations and Flucytosine," *Mayo Clin Proc*, 1998, 73(12):1205-25.

♦ **Amphotericin B Desoxycholate** *see* Amphotericin B (Conventional) *on page 69*

Amphotericin B (Lipid Complex)
(am foe TER i sin bee LIP id KOM pleks)

Medication Safety Issues

Safety issues:

Lipid-based amphotericin formulations (Abelcet®) may be confused with conventional formulations (Amphocin®, Fungizone®)

Large overdoses have occurred when conventional formulations were dispensed inadvertently for lipid-based products. Single daily doses of conventional amphotericin formulation never exceed 1.5 mg/kg.

Related Information

Management of Infections *on page 978*

U.S. Brand Names Abelcet®

Canadian Brand Names Abelcet®

Generic Available No

Synonyms ABLC

Pharmacologic Category Antifungal Agent, Parenteral

(Continued)

Amphotericin B (Lipid Complex) *(Continued)*

Pregnancy Risk Factor B

Lactation Enters breast milk/contraindicated

Use Treatment of aspergillosis or any type of progressive fungal infection in patients who are refractory to or intolerant of conventional amphotericin B therapy

Unlabeled/Investigational Use Effective in patients with serious *Candida* species infections

Mechanism of Action Binds to ergosterol altering cell membrane permeability in susceptible fungi and causing leakage of cell components with subsequent cell death. Proposed mechanism suggests that amphotericin causes an oxidation-dependent stimulation of macrophages.

Labeled Contraindications Hypersensitivity to amphotericin or any component of the formulation

Warnings/Precautions Anaphylaxis has been reported with amphotericin B-containing drugs. If severe respiratory distress occurs, the infusion should be immediately discontinued. During the initial dosing, the drug should be administered under close clinical observation. Acute reactions (including fever and chills) may occur 1-2 hours after starting an intravenous infusion. These reactions are usually more common with the first few doses and generally diminish with subsequent doses.

Adverse Reactions Nephrotoxicity and infusion-related hyperpyrexia, rigor, and chilling are reduced relative to amphotericin deoxycholate.

>10%:

Central nervous system: Chills, fever

Renal: Increased serum creatinine

1% to 10%:

Cardiovascular: Hypotension, cardiac arrest

Central nervous system: Headache, pain

Dermatologic: Rash

Endocrine & metabolic: Bilirubinemia, hypokalemia, acidosis

Gastrointestinal: Nausea, vomiting, diarrhea, gastrointestinal hemorrhage, abdominal pain

Renal: Renal failure

Respiratory: Respiratory failure, dyspnea, pneumonia

Vesicant No

Emetic Potential Very low (<10%)

Drug Interactions

Increased Effect/Toxicity: See Drug Interactions - Increased Effect/Toxicity in Amphotericin B (Conventional) *on page 69.*

Decreased Effect: See Drug Interactions - Decreased Effect in Amphotericin B (Conventional) *on page 69.*

Storage/Stability 100 mg vials in 20 mL of suspension in single-use vials (no preservative is present). Intact vials should be stored at 2°C to 8°C (35°F to 46°F) and protected from exposure to light; do not freeze intact vials. Solutions for infusion are stable for 48 hours under refrigeration and 6 hours at room temperature.

Reconstitution Shake vial gently to disperse yellow sediment at bottom of container. Dilute with D_5W to 1-2 mg/mL. Protect from light.

Compatibility Do not admix or Y-site with any blood products, intravenous drugs, or intravenous fluids other than D_5W.

Pharmacodynamics/Kinetics

Distribution: V_d: Increases with higher doses; reflects increased uptake by tissues (131 L/kg with 5 mg/kg/day)

Half-life elimination: ~24 hours

Excretion: Clearance: Increases with higher doses (5 mg/kg/day): 400 mL/hour/kg

Dosage Children and Adults: I.V.:

Premedication: For patients who experience infusion-related immediate reactions, premedicate with the following drugs, 30-60 minutes prior to drug administration: A nonsteroidal anti-inflammatory agent ± diphenhydramine; or acetaminophen with diphenhydramine; or hydrocortisone 50-100 mg. If the patient experiences rigors during the infusion, meperidine may be administered.

Range: 2.5-5 mg/kg/day as a single infusion

Dosing adjustment in renal impairment: None necessary; effects of renal impairment are not currently known

Hemodialysis: No supplemental dosage necessary

Peritoneal dialysis: No supplemental dosage necessary

Continuous arteriovenous or venovenous hemofiltration: No supplemental dosage necessary

Administration

Patients who experience nonanaphylactic infusion-related reactions, premedication 30-60 minutes prior to drug administration with a nonsteroidal anti-inflammatory agent ± diphenhydramine; acetaminophen with diphenhydramine or hydrocortisone 50-100 mg. If the patient experiences rigors during the infusion, meperidine may be administered.

Invert infusion container several times prior to administration and every 2 hours during infusion.

Dosage Forms Injection, suspension: 5 mg/mL (20 mL)

Monitoring Parameters Renal function (monitor frequently during therapy), electrolytes (especially potassium and magnesium), liver function tests, temperature, PT/PTT, CBC; monitor input and output; monitor for signs of hypokalemia (muscle weakness, cramping, drowsiness, ECG changes, etc)

Additional Information As a modification of dimyristoyl phosphatidylcholine:dimyristoyl phosphatidylglycerol 7:3 (DMPC:DMPG) liposome, amphotericin B lipid-complex has a higher drug to lipid ratio and the concentration of amphotericin B is 33 M. ABLC is a ribbon-like structure, not a liposome.

Controlled trials which compare the original formulation of amphotericin B to the newer liposomal formulations (ie, Abelcet®) are lacking. Thus, comparative data discussing differences among the formulations should be interpreted cautiously. Although the risk of nephrotoxicity and infusion-related adverse effects may be less with Abelcet®, the efficacy profiles of Abelcet® and the original amphotericin formulation are comparable. Consequently, Abelcet® should be restricted to those patients who cannot tolerate or fail a standard amphotericin B formulation.

Special Geriatric Considerations Caution should be exercised and renal function and desired effect monitored closely in older adults.

Selected Readings

De Marie S, "Clinical Use of Liposomal and Lipid-Complexed Amphotericin B," *J Antimicrob Chemother*, 1994, 33(5):907-16.

(Continued)

Amphotericin B (Lipid Complex) *(Continued)*

Hiemenz JW and Walsh TJ, "Lipid Formulations of Amphotericin B: Recent Progress and Future Directions," *Clin Infect Dis*, 1996, 22(Suppl 2):133-44.

Lyman CA and Walsh TJ, "Systemically Administered Antifungal Agents. A Review of Their Clinical Pharmacology and Therapeutic Applications," *Drugs*, 1992, 44(1):9-35.

Patel R, "Antifungal Agents. Part I. Amphotericin B Preparations and Flucytosine," *Mayo Clin Proc*, 1998, 73(12):1205-25.

Rapp RP, Gubbins PO, and Evans ME, "Amphotericin B Lipid Complex," *Ann Pharmacother*, 1997, 31(10):1174-86.

Slain D, "Lipid-Based Amphotericin B for the Treatment of Fungal Infections," *Pharmacotherapy*, 1999, 19(3):306-23.

Amphotericin B (Liposomal)

(am foe TER i sin bee lye po SO mal)

Medication Safety Issues

Safety issues:

Lipid-based amphotericin formulations (AmBisome®) may be confused with conventional formulations (Amphocin®, Fungizone®)

Large overdoses have occurred when conventional formulations were dispensed inadvertently for lipid-based products. Single daily doses of conventional amphotericin formulation never exceed 1.5 mg/kg.

Related Information

Management of Infections *on page 978*

U.S. Brand Names AmBisome®

Canadian Brand Names AmBisome®

Generic Available No

Synonyms L-AmB

Pharmacologic Category Antifungal Agent, Parenteral

Pregnancy Risk Factor B

Lactation Excretion in breast milk unknown/contraindicated

Use Empirical therapy for presumed fungal infection in febrile, neutropenic patients. Treatment of patients with *Aspergillus* species, *Candida* species and/or *Cryptococcus* species infections refractory to amphotericin B desoxycholate, or in patients where renal impairment or unacceptable toxicity precludes the use of amphotericin B desoxycholate. Treatment of cryptococcal meningitis in HIV-infected patients. Treatment of visceral leishmaniasis.

Unlabeled/Investigational Use Effective in patients with serious *Candida* species infections

Mechanism of Action Binds to ergosterol altering cell membrane permeability in susceptible fungi and causing leakage of cell components with subsequent cell death. Proposed mechanism suggests that amphotericin causes an oxidation-dependent stimulation of macrophages (Lyman, 1992).

Labeled Contraindications Hypersensitivity to amphotericin B or any component of the formulation

Warnings/Precautions Although amphotericin B (liposomal) has been shown to be significantly less toxic than amphotericin B desoxycholate, adverse events may still occur. Patients should be under close clinical observation during initial dosing. As with other amphotericin B-containing products, anaphylaxis has been reported. Facilities for cardiopulmonary resuscitation should be available during administration. Acute reactions (including fever and chills) may occur 1-2 hours after starting infusions; reactions are more common with the first few doses and generally diminish with subsequent doses. Immediately discontinue infusion if severe respiratory distress occurs; the patient should not receive further infusions. Safety and efficacy have not been established in patients <1 year of age.

Adverse Reactions Percentage of adverse reactions is dependent upon population studied and may vary with respect to premedications and underlying illness. Incidence of decreased renal function and infusion-related events are lower than rates observed with amphotericin B deoxycholate.

>10%:

Cardiovascular: Peripheral edema (15%), edema (12% to 14%), tachycardia (9% to 18%), hypotension (7% to 14%), hypertension (8% to 20%), chest pain (8% to 12%), hypervolemia (8% to 12%)

Central nervous system: Chills (29% to 48%), insomnia (17% to 22%), headache (9% to 20%), anxiety (7% to 14%), pain (14%), confusion (9% to 13%)

Dermatologic: Rash (5% to 25%), pruritus (11%)

Endocrine & metabolic: Hypokalemia (31% to 51%), hypomagnesemia (15% to 50%), hyperglycemia (8% to 23%), hypocalcemia (5% to 18%), hyponatremia (8% to 12%)

Gastrointestinal: Nausea (16% to 40%), vomiting (10% to 32%), diarrhea (11% to 30%), abdominal pain (7% to 20%), constipation (15%), anorexia (10% to 14%)

Hematologic: Anemia (27% to 48%), blood transfusion reaction (9% to 18%), leukopenia (15% to 17%), thrombocytopenia (6% to 13%)

Hepatic: Increased alkaline phosphatase (7% to 22%), increased BUN (7% to 21%), bilirubinemia (9% to 18%), increased ALT (15%), increased AST (13%), abnormal liver function tests (not specified) (4% to 13%)

Local: Phlebitis (9% to 11%)

Neuromuscular & skeletal: Weakness (6% to 13%), back pain (12%)

Renal: Increased creatinine (18% to 40%), hematuria (14%)

Respiratory: Dyspnea (18% to 23%), lung disorder (14% to 18%), increased cough (2% to 18%), epistaxis (8% to 15%), pleural effusion (12%), rhinitis (11%)

Miscellaneous: Sepsis (7% to 14%), infection (11% to 12%)

2% to 10%:

Cardiovascular: Arrhythmia, atrial fibrillation, bradycardia, cardiac arrest, cardiomegaly, facial swelling, flushing, postural hypotension, valvular heart disease, vascular disorder

Central nervous system: Agitation, abnormal thinking, coma, convulsion, depression, dysesthesia, dizziness (7% to 8%), hallucinations, malaise, nervousness, somnolence

Dermatologic: Alopecia, bruising, cellulitis, dry skin, maculopapular rash, petechia, purpura, skin discoloration, skin disorder, skin ulcer, urticaria, vesiculobullous rash

Endocrine & metabolic: Acidosis, increased amylase, fluid overload, hypernatremia (4%), hyperchloremia, hyperkalemia, hypermagnesemia, hyperphosphatemia, hypophosphatemia, hypoproteinemia, increased lactate dehydrogenase, increased nonprotein nitrogen

Gastrointestinal: Constipation, dry mouth, dyspepsia, enlarged abdomen, eructation, fecal incontinence, flatulence, gastrointestinal

(Continued)

Amphotericin B (Liposomal) *(Continued)*

hemorrhage (10%), hematemesis, hemorrhoids, gum/oral hemorrhage, ileus, mucositis, rectal disorder, stomatitis, ulcerative stomatitis

Genitourinary: Vaginal hemorrhage

Hematologic: Coagulation disorder, hemorrhage, decreased prothrombin, thrombocytopenia

Hepatic: Hepatocellular damage, hepatomegaly, veno-occlusive liver disease

Local: Injection site inflammation

Neuromuscular & skeletal: Arthralgia, bone pain, dystonia, myalgia, neck pain, paresthesia, rigors, tremor

Ocular: Conjunctivitis, dry eyes, eye hemorrhage

Renal: Abnormal renal function, acute kidney failure, dysuria, kidney failure, toxic nephropathy, urinary incontinence

Respiratory: Asthma, atelectasis, cough, dry nose, hemoptysis, hyperventilation, lung edema, pharyngitis, pneumonia, respiratory alkalosis, respiratory insufficiency, respiratory failure, sinusitis, hypoxia (6% to 8%)

Miscellaneous: Allergic reaction, cell-mediated immunological reaction, flu-like syndrome, graft versus host disease, herpes simplex, hiccup, procedural complication (8% to 10%), diaphoresis (7%)

Postmarketing and/or case reports: Angioedema, erythema, urticaria, cyanosis/hypoventilation, pulmonary edema, agranulocytosis, hemorrhagic cystitis

Overdosage/Toxicology The toxicity due to overdose has not been defined. Repeated daily doses up to 7.5 mg/kg have been administered in clinical trials with no reported dose-related toxicity. If overdosage should occur, cease administration immediately. Symptomatic supportive measures should be instituted. Particular attention should be given to monitoring renal function.

Drug Interactions

Increased Effect/Toxicity: Drug interactions have not been studied in a controlled manner; however, drugs that interact with conventional amphotericin B may also interact with amphotericin B liposome for injection. See Drug Interactions - Increased Effect/Toxicity in Amphotericin B (Conventional) monograph.

Storage/Stability Unopened vials should be refrigerated at 2°C to 8°C (36°F to 46°F). Vials reconstituted with SWFI are stable for 24 hours under refrigeration. Infusion solutions in D_5W should be used within 6 hours of preparation.

Reconstitution

1. Add 12 mL SWFI to vial. The use of any solution other than those recommended, or the presence of a bacteriostatic agent in the solution, may cause precipitation.

2. **Shake the vial vigorously** for 30 seconds.

Filtration and Dilution:

3. The 5 micron filter should be on the syringe used to remove the reconstituted AmBisome®.

4. Dilute to a final concentration of 1-2 mg/mL (0.2-0.5 mg/mL for infants and small children).

Compatibility Compatible: Stable in D_5W. **Incompatible:** NS, ½NS, other saline-containing solutions, or preservatives

Pharmacodynamics/Kinetics

Distribution: V_d: 131 L/kg

Half-life elimination: Terminal: 174 hours

Dosage Children and Adults: I.V.:

Note: Premedication: For patients who experience nonanaphylactic infusion-related immediate reactions, premedicate with the following drugs, 30-60 minutes prior to drug administration: A nonsteroidal anti-inflammatory agent ± diphenhydramine; or acetaminophen with diphenhydramine; or hydrocortisone 50-100 mg. If the patient experiences rigors during the infusion, meperidine may be administered.

Empiric therapy: Recommended initial dose: 3 mg/kg/day

Systemic fungal infections (*Aspergillus, Candida, Cryptococcus*): Recommended initial dose of 3-5 mg/kg/day

Cryptococcal meningitis in HIV-infected patients: 6 mg/kg/day

Treatment of visceral leishmaniasis:

Immunocompetent patients: 3 mg/kg/day on days 1-5, and 3 mg/kg/day on days 14 and 21; a repeat course may be given in patients who do not achieve parasitic clearance

Immunocompromised patients: 4 mg/kg/day on days 1-5, and 4 mg/kg/day on days 10, 17, 24, 31, and 38

Dosing adjustment in renal impairment: None necessary; effects of renal impairment are not currently known

Hemodialysis: No supplemental dosage necessary

Peritoneal dialysis effects: No supplemental dosage necessary

Continuous arteriovenous or venovenous hemofiltration: No supplemental dosage necessary

Administration Intravenous infusion, over a period of approximately 2 hours. Infusion time may be reduced to approximately 1 hour in patients in whom the treatment is well-tolerated. If the patient experiences discomfort during infusion, the duration of infusion may be increased. Administer at a rate of 2.5 mg/kg/hour. Existing intravenous line should be flushed with D_5W prior to infusion (if not feasible, administer through a separate line). An in-line membrane filter (not less than 1 micron) may be used.

Dosage Forms Injection, powder for reconstitution: 50 mg

Monitoring Parameters Renal function (monitor frequently during therapy), electrolytes (especially potassium and magnesium), liver function tests, temperature, PT/PTT, CBC; monitor input and output; monitor for signs of hypokalemia (muscle weakness, cramping, drowsiness, ECG changes, etc)

Additional Information Amphotericin B (liposomal) is a true single bilayer liposomal drug delivery system. Liposomes are closed, spherical vesicles created by mixing specific proportions of amphophilic substances such as phospholipids and cholesterol so that they arrange themselves into multiple concentric bilayer membranes when hydrated in aqueous solutions. Single bilayer liposomes are then formed by microemulsification of multilamellar vesicles using a homogenizer. Amphotericin B (liposomal) consists of these unilamellar bilayer liposomes with amphotericin B intercalated within the membrane. Due to the nature and quantity of amphophilic substances used, and the lipophilic moiety in the amphotericin B molecule, the drug is an integral part of the overall structure of the amphotericin B liposomal liposomes. (Continued)

Amphotericin B (Liposomal) *(Continued)*

Amphotericin B (liposomal) contains true liposomes that are <100 nm in diameter.

Selected Readings

Emminger W, Graninger W, Emminger-Schmidmeir W, et al, "Tolerance of High Doses of Amphotericin B by Infusion of a Liposomal Formulation in Children With Cancer," *Ann Hematol*, 1994, 68:27-31.

Hiemenz JW and Walsh TJ, "Lipid Formulations of Amphotericin B: Recent Progress and Future Directions," *Clin Infect Dis*, 1996, 22(Suppl 2):133-44.

Lyman CA and Walsh TJ, "Systemically Administered Antifungal Agents. A Review of Their Clinical Pharmacology and Therapeutic Applications," *Drugs*, 1992, 44(1):9-35.

Patel R, "Antifungal Agents. Part I. Amphotericin B Preparations and Flucytosine," *Mayo Clin Proc*, 1998, 73(12):1205-25.

Ringden O, Andstrom E, Remberger M, et al, "Safety of Liposomal Amphotericin B (AmBisome®) In 187 Transplant Recipients Treated With Cyclosporin," *Bone Marrow Transplant*, 1994, 14(Suppl 5):10-4.

Slain D, "Lipid-Based Amphotericin B for the Treatment of Fungal Infections," *Pharmacotherapy*, 1999, 19(3):306-23.

♦ **AMSA** *see Amsacrine on page 80*

Amsacrine *(AM sah kreen)*

Related Information

Investigational Drug Service *on page 1031*
Safe Handling of Hazardous Drugs *on page 1034*

Generic Available No

Synonyms 4-(9-Acridinylamino) Methanesulfon-m-Anisidide; Acridinyl Anisidide; AMSA; m-AMSA; NSC-249992

Pharmacologic Category Antineoplastic Agent

Unlabeled/Investigational Use Investigational: Refractory acute lymphocytic and nonlymphocytic leukemias, Hodgkin's disease, and non-Hodgkin's lymphomas; head and neck tumors

Mechanism of Action Amsacrine has been shown to inhibit DNA synthesis by binding to, and intercalating with, DNA; inhibits topoisomerase II activity.

Restrictions Not available in the U.S./Investigational

Labeled Contraindications Hypersensitivity to amsacrine or any component of the formulation; hypokalemia

Warnings/Precautions Procedures for proper handling and disposal of antineoplastic agents should be considered. The drug should be used cautiously in patients who have underlying cardiac disease, severe renal or hepatic dysfunction, or who have received high cumulative doses of anthracyclines. **Do not administer amsacrine if serum potassium <4 mEq/L.**

Adverse Reactions

>10%:

Cardiovascular: ECG changes (T-wave flattening, S-T wave alterations) consistent with anterolateral ischemia, ventricular fibrillation, ventricular extrasystoles, atrial tachycardia and fibrillation, CHF, cardiac arrest. Patients with hypokalemia, who have received >400 mg/m² of doxorubicin or daunorubicin (or the equivalent), >200 mg/m² of amsacrine within 48 hours, or a total dose of anthracycline + amsacrine >900 mg/m² have an increased risk of cardiac toxicity.

Dermatologic: Alopecia

Gastrointestinal: Nausea and vomiting (30%), diarrhea (30%), dose-limiting stomatitis (32%), oral ulceration (10%)

Genitourinary: Orange-red discoloration of the urine

Hematologic: Leukopenia (nadir at 10 days); thrombocytopenia (nadir at 12-14 days), with recovery at 21-25 days

Hepatic: Hyperbilirubinemia (30%), increased liver enzymes (10%)

Local: Phlebitis

1% to 10%:

Central nervous system: Headache, dizziness, confusion, convulsions

Hematologic: Anemia

Neuromuscular & skeletal: Paresthesias

Ocular: Blurred vision

<1%: Allergic reactions (0.4%), sperm production decreased

Vesicant Yes; see Management of Drug Extravasations *on page 965.*

Emetic Potential Moderate (30% to 60%)

Storage/Stability Intact vials are stored at controlled room temperature 15°C to 30°C (59°F to 86°F). Reconstituted vials may be stored at room temperature for up to 48 hours. Solutions diluted for administration are stable for up to 48 hours at room temperature. The addition of 1 mEq/L of sodium bicarbonate increases the stability to 96 hours.

Note: Use of glass syringes and avoidance of plastic filters to draw up undiluted amsacrine solutions is recommended since the N,N-dimethylacetamide solvent has been reported to dissolve plastic syringes and filters. The solution may be mixed in plastic bags when diluted for infusion.

Reconstitution 1.5 mL of the drug solution is added to 13.5 mL of lactic acid diluent (provided with the drug) to form a 5 mg/mL solution.

Compatibility Stable in D_5W; **Incompatible:** BNS, D_5NS, $D_5^{1}/_4NS$, $D_5^{1}/_2NS$, D_5LR, $D_{10}NS$, NSS, LR, chloride ion. Amsacrine forms an immediate precipitate in the presence of chloride ion; do not mix with drugs that are chloride or hydrochloride salts.

Y-site administration: Compatible: Amikacin, chlorpromazine, clindamycin, cytarabine, dexamethasone, diphenhydramine, famotidine, fludarabine, gentamicin, granisetron, haloperidol, hydrocortisone sodium succinate, hydromorphone, lorazepam, morphine, prochlorperazine, promethazine, ranitidine, sodium bicarbonate, tobramycin, vancomycin. **Incompatible:** Acyclovir, amphotericin, aztreonam, calcium chloride, ceftazidime, ceftriaxone, cephalothin, cimetidine, cisplatin, filgrastim, furosemide, ganciclovir, heparin, methylprednisolone, metoclopramide, ondansetron, potassium chloride, sargramostim

Compatibility when admixed: Compatible: Sodium bicarbonate, bleomycin

Pharmacodynamics/Kinetics

Distribution: V_d: 1.67 L/kg; minimal CNS penetration

Protein binding: 96% to 98%

Metabolism: Hepatic, to inactive metabolites (major metabolite is 5′ glutathione conjugate)

Half-life elimination: 1.4-5 hours; Terminal: 5.6-7.8 hours

Excretion: Bile; urine (2% to 10% as unchanged drug)

Dosage Refer to individual protocols. I.V.:

Children: 125-150 mg/m²/day for 5 days

Adults: 60-160 mg/m²/day every 3-4 weeks; 5- to 7-day I.V. infusions of 40-120 mg/m²/day every 3-4 weeks have also been reported.

(Continued)

Amsacrine *(Continued)*

Dosage adjustment in renal impairment: BUN >20 or S_{cr} >1.5: Administer 25% of normal dose.

Dosage adjustment in hepatic impairment: Bilirubin >2 mg/dL: Administer 75% of normal dose.

Administration I.V.: Administer as a 30- to 90-minute infusion or a 24-hour continuous infusion. Use of glass syringes and avoidance of plastic filters to draw up undiluted amsacrine solutions is recommended since the N,N-dimethylacetamide solvent has been reported to dissolve plastic syringes and filters. The solution can be placed in plastic bags when diluted for I.V. infusion.

Dosage Forms Injection, solution [preservative free]: 50 mg/1.5 mL (supplied with L-lactic acid 0.0353 M 13.5 mL)

Patient Information This drug may cause darkening or discoloration of the urine for 24-48 hours. Watch for fever, malaise, bleeding, bruising, sore throat or mouth, difficulty swallowing, or for pain, redness, or swelling at the injection site.

Selected Readings

Arlin ZA, "A Special Role for Amsacrine in the Treatment of Acute Leukemia," *Cancer Invest*, 1989, 7(6):607-9.

Hornedo J and Van Echo DA, "Amsacrine (m-AMSA): A New Antineoplastic Agent. Pharmacology, Clinical Activity and Toxicity," *Pharmacotherapy*, 1985, 5(2):78-90.

Louie AC and Issell BF, "Amsacrine (AMSA) - A Clinical Review," *J Clin Oncol*, 1985, 3(4):562-92.

Van Mouwerik TJ, Caines PM, and Ballentine R, "Amsacrine Evaluation," *Drug Intell Clin Pharm*, 1987, 21(4):330-4.

Anagrelide *(an AG gre lide)*

Related Information

Safe Handling of Hazardous Drugs *on page 1034*

U.S. Brand Names Agrylin®

Canadian Brand Names Agrylin®

Generic Available No

Synonyms 1370-999-397; Anagrelide Hydrochloride; BL4162A; 6,7-Dichloro-1,5-Dihydroimidazo [2,1b] Quinazolin-2(3H)-one Monohydrochloride

Pharmacologic Category Phospholipase A_2 Inhibitor

Pregnancy Risk Factor C

Lactation Excretion in breast milk unknown/not recommended

Use Treatment of essential thrombocythemia (ET) and thrombocythemia associated with chronic myelogenous leukemia (CML), polycythemia vera, and other myeloproliferative disorders

Mechanism of Action Anagrelide appears to inhibit cyclic nucleotide phosphodiesterase and the release of arachidonic acid from phospholipase, possibly by inhibiting phospholipase A_2. It also causes a dose-related reduction in platelet production, which results from decreased megakaryocyte hypermaturation. The drug disrupts the postmitotic phase of maturation.

Labeled Contraindications Hypersensitivity to anagrelide or any component of the formulation; severe hepatic impairment

Warnings/Precautions Use caution in patients with known or suspected heart disease; palpitations, orthostatic hypotension, and congestive heart failure have been reported. Use caution in patients with renal dysfunction (serum creatinine ≥2 mg/dL) or hepatic dysfunction (measures of liver function >1.5 times ULN).

Adverse Reactions

>10%:

Cardiovascular: Palpitations (27%), edema (other than peripheral: 21%),

Central nervous system: Headache (44%), dizziness (15%), pain (15%),

Gastrointestinal: Diarrhea (26%), nausea (17%), abdominal pain (16%)

Neuromuscular & skeletal: Weakness (23%)

Respiratory: Dyspnea (12%)

1% to 10%:

Cardiovascular: Angina, arrhythmias, cardiovascular disease, chest pain (8%), CHF, hypertension, orthostatic hypotension, peripheral edema (9%), syncope, tachycardia (7%), thrombosis, vasodilatation

Central nervous system: Amnesia, chills, confusion, depression, fever (9%), insomnia, malaise (6%), migraine, nervousness, somnolence

Dermatologic: Alopecia, photosensitivity, pruritus (6%), rash (8%), urticaria

Endocrine & skeletal: Dehydration

Gastrointestinal: Anorexia (8%), aphthous stomatitis, constipation, dyspepsia (5%), eructation, flatulence (10%), gastritis, GI distress, GI hemorrhage, melena, vomiting (10%)

Hematologic: Anemia, ecchymosis, hemorrhage, lymphadenoma, thrombocytopenia

Hepatic: Liver enzymes increased

Neuromuscular & skeletal: Arthralgia, back pain (6%), leg cramps, myalgia, paresthesia (6%)

Ocular: Amblyopia, diplopia , tinnitus, visual field abnormality

Renal: Dysuria, hematuria, renal failure

Respiratory: Asthma, bronchitis, cough (6%), epistaxis, pharyngitis (7%), pneumonia, rhinitis, sinusitis

Miscellaneous: Flu-like syndrome

Frequency not defined: Atrial fibrillation, cardiomegaly, cardiomyopathy, cerebrovascular accident, complete heart block, gastric/duodenal ulceration, leukocyte count increased, MI, pancreatitis, pericarditis, pericardial effusion, pleural effusion, pulmonary fibrosis, pulmonary infiltrates, pulmonary hypertension, seizure

Emetic Potential Low (10% to 30%)

Overdosage/Toxicology

There are no reports of human overdosage with anagrelide. Platelet reduction from anagrelide therapy is dose-related; therefore, thrombocytopenia, which can potentially cause bleeding, is expected from overdosage.

Should overdosage occur, cardiac and central nervous system toxicity can also be expected. In the case of overdosage, close clinical supervision of the patient is required; this especially includes monitoring of the platelet count for thrombocytopenia. Dosage should be decreased or stopped, as appropriate, until the platelet count returns to within the normal range.

(Continued)

Anagrelide *(Continued)*

Drug Interactions

Cytochrome P450 Effect: Substrate of CYP1A2 (minor)

Increased Effect/Toxicity: Antiplatelet agents may enhance the adverse/toxic effects of drotrecogin alfa. Concurrent use of NSAIDs, salicylates, or treprostinil may enhance the adverse/toxic effects of antiplatelet agents.

Ethanol/Nutrition/Herb Interactions

Ethanol: May increase CNS adverse effects.

Food: No clinically significant effect on absorption.

Pharmacodynamics/Kinetics

Duration: 6-24 hours

Metabolism: Hepatic

Half-life elimination, plasma: 1.3 hours

Time to peak, serum: 1 hour

Excretion: Urine (<1% as unchanged drug)

Dosage Note: Maintain for ≥1 week, then adjust to the lowest effective dose to reduce and maintain platelet count <600,000/µL ideally to the normal range; the dose must not be increased by >0.5 mg/day in any 1 week; maximum dose: 10 mg/day or 2.5 mg/dose

Oral:

Children: Initial: 0.5 mg/day (range: 0.5 mg 1-4 times/day)

Adults: 0.5 mg 4 times/day or 1 mg twice daily

Elderly: There are no special requirements for dosing in the elderly

Dosage adjustment in hepatic impairment:

Moderate impairment: Initial: 0.5 mg once daily; maintain for 1 week with careful monitoring of cardiovascular status

Severe impairment: Contraindicated

Administration Orally, in 2-4 divided doses daily initially, then once or twice daily

Dosage Forms Capsule: 0.5 mg, 1 mg

Monitoring Parameters Anagrelide therapy requires close supervision of the patient. Because of the positive inotropic effects and side effects of anagrelide, a pretreatment cardiovascular examination is recommended along with careful monitoring during treatment; while the platelet count is being lowered (usually during the first 2 weeks of treatment), blood counts (hemoglobin, white blood cells), liver function test (AST, ALT) and renal function (serum creatinine, BUN) should be monitored. Platelet counts should be performed every 2 days during the first week of treatment and at least weekly until the maintenance dose is reached.

Selected Readings

Anagrelide Study Group, "Anagrelide, a Therapy for Thrombocythemic States: Experience in 577 Patients," *Am J Med*, 1992, 92:69-76.

Brooks WG, Stanley DD, and Goode JV, "Role of Anagrelide in the Treatment of Thrombocytosis," *Ann Pharmacother*, 1999, 33(10):1116-8, 1121.

Dingli D and Tefferi A, "Anagrelide: An Update on its Mechanisms of Action and Therapeutic Potential," *Expert Rev Anticancer Ther*, 2004, 4(4):533-41.

Pescatore SL and Lindley C, "Anagrelide: A Novel Agent for the Treatment of Myeloproliferative Disorders," *Expert Opin Pharmacother*, 2000, 1(3):537-46.

Petitt RM, Silverstein MN, and Petrone ME, "Anagrelide for Control of Thrombocythemia in Polycythemia and Other Myeloproliferative Disorders," *Semin Hematol*, 1997, 34(1):51-4.

Spencer CM and Brogden RN, "Anagrelide. A Review of Its Pharmacodynamic and Pharmacokinetic Properties, and Therapeutic Potential in the Treatment of Thrombocythaemia," *Drugs*, 1994, 47(5):809-22.

♦ **Anagrelide Hydrochloride** *see* Anagrelide *on page 82*

♦ **Anandron® (Can)** *see* Nilutamide *on page 608*

Anastrozole (an AS troe zole)

Related Information

Safe Handling of Hazardous Drugs *on page 1034*

U.S. Brand Names Arimidex®

Canadian Brand Names Arimidex®

Generic Available No

Synonyms ICI-D1033; ZD1033

Pharmacologic Category Antineoplastic Agent, Miscellaneous

Pregnancy Risk Factor D

Lactation Excretion in breast milk unknown/use caution

Use Treatment of locally-advanced or metastatic breast cancer (ER-positive or hormone receptor unknown) in postmenopausal women; treatment of advanced breast cancer in postmenopausal women with disease progression following tamoxifen therapy; adjuvant treatment of early ER-positive breast cancer in postmenopausal women

Mechanism of Action Potent and selective nonsteroidal aromatase inhibitor. By inhibiting aromatase, the conversion of androstenedione to estrone, and testosterone to estradiol, is prevented. Anastrozole causes an 85% decrease in estrone sulfate levels.

Labeled Contraindications Hypersensitivity to anastrozole or any component of the formulation; pregnancy

Warnings/Precautions Use with caution in patients with hyperlipidemias; total cholesterol and LDL-cholesterol increase in patients receiving anastrozole. Exclude pregnancy before initiating therapy. Anastrozole may be associated with a reduction in bone mineral density. Safety and efficacy in premenopausal women or pediatric patients have not been established.

Adverse Reactions

>10%:

Cardiovascular: Vasodilatation (25% to 35%)

Central nervous system: Pain (11% to 15%), headache (9% to 13%), depression (5% to 11%)

Endocrine & metabolic: Hot flashes (12% to 35%)

Neuromuscular & skeletal: Weakness (16% to 17%), arthritis (14%), arthralgia (13%), back pain (8% to 12%), bone pain (5% to 11%)

Respiratory: Cough increased (7% to 11%), pharyngitis (6% to 12%)

1% to 10%:

Cardiovascular: Peripheral edema (5% to 10%), hypertension (5% to 9%), chest pain (5% to 7%)

Central nervous system: Insomnia (6% to 9%), dizziness (6%), anxiety (5%), lethargy (1%), fever, malaise, confusion, nervousness, somnolence

Dermatologic: Rash (6% to 10%), alopecia, pruritus

Endocrine & metabolic: Hypercholesteremia (7%)

Gastrointestinal: Vomiting (8% to 9%), constipation (7% to 9%), abdominal pain (7% to 8%), diarrhea (7% to 8%), anorexia (5% to 7%), xerostomia (6%), dyspepsia (5%), weight gain (2% to 8%), weight loss

(Continued)

Anastrozole *(Continued)*

Genitourinary: Urinary tract infection (6%), vulvovaginitis (6%), vaginal bleeding (5%) leukorrhea (2%), vaginal hemorrhage (2%), vaginal dryness (2%)

Hematologic: Anemia, leukopenia

Hepatic: Liver function tests increased, alkaline phosphatase increased

Local: Deep vein thrombosis, thrombophlebitis

Neuromuscular & skeletal: Osteoporosis (7%), fracture (7%), arthrosis (6%), paresthesia (5% to 6%), hypertonia (3%), myalgia, arthralgia

Ocular: Cataracts (4%)

Respiratory: Dyspnea (6% to 10%), sinusitis, bronchitis, rhinitis

Miscellaneous: Lymph edema (9%), infection (7%), flu-like syndrome (5% to 7%), diaphoresis (2% to 4%)

<1%: Angina pectoris, CVA, cerebral ischemia, cerebral infarct, endometrial cancer, erythema multiforme, MI, myocardial ischemia, pulmonary embolus, retinal vein thrombosis, Stevens-Johnson syndrome, thrombophlebitis

Postmarketing and/or case reports: Anaphylaxis, angioedema, joint pain, joint stiffness, urticaria

Emetic Potential Very low (<10%)

Overdosage/Toxicology Symptoms of overdose include severe irritation to the stomach (necrosis, gastritis, ulceration, and hemorrhage). There is no specific antidote; treatment must be symptomatic. Dialysis may be helpful because anastrozole is not highly protein bound.

Drug Interactions

Cytochrome P450 Effect: Inhibits CYP1A2 (weak), 2C8/9 (weak), 3A4 (weak)

Decreased Effect:

Estrogens: May decrease efficacy of anastrozole

Tamoxifen: May decrease plasma concentrations of anastrozole

Ethanol/Nutrition/Herb Interactions Herb/Nutraceutical: Avoid black cohosh, hops, licorice, red clover, thyme, and dong quai.

Storage/Stability Store at 20°C to 25°C (68°F to 77°F).

Pharmacodynamics/Kinetics

Onset of estradiol reduction: 24 hours

Duration of estradiol reduction: 6 days

Absorption: Well absorbed (80%); not affected by food

Protein binding, plasma: 40%

Metabolism: Extensively hepatic (85%) via N-dealkylation, hydroxylation, and glucuronidation; primary metabolite inactive

Half-life elimination: 50 hours

Excretion: Urine (10% as unchanged drug; 60% as metabolites)

Dosage Breast cancer: Adults: Oral (refer to individual protocols): 1 mg once daily

Dosage adjustment in renal impairment: Dosage adjustment not necessary

Dosage adjustment in hepatic impairment: Plasma concentrations in subjects with stable hepatic cirrhosis were within the range concentrations in normal subjects across all clinical trials; therefore, no dosage adjustment is needed

Dosage Forms Tablet: 1 mg

Selected Readings

Boeddinghaus IM and Dowsett M, "Comparative Clinical Pharmacology and Pharmacokinetic Interactions of Aromatase Inhibitors," *J Steroid Biochem Mol Biol*, 2001, 79(1-5):85-91.

Buzdar AU, Robertson JF, Eiermann W, et al, "An Overview of the Pharmacology and Pharmacokinetics of the Newer Generation Aromatase Inhibitors Anastrozole, Letrozole, and Exemestane," *Cancer*, 2002, 95(9):2006-16.

Higa GM and AlKhouri N, "Anastrozole: A Selective Aromatase Inhibitor for the Treatment of Breast Cancer," *Am J Health Syst Pharm*, 1998, 1;55(5):445-52.

Koberle D and Thurlimann B, "Anastrozole: Pharmacological and Clinical Profile in Postmenopausal Women With Breast Cancer," *Expert Rev Anticancer Ther*, 2001, 1(2):169-76.

Lonning PE, Geisler J, and Dowsett M, "Pharmacological and Clinical Profile of Anastrozole," *Breast Cancer Res Treat*, 1998, 49(Suppl 1):53-7.

Njar VC and Brodie AM, "Comprehensive Pharmacology and Clinical Efficacy of Aromatase Inhibitors," *Drugs*, 1999, 58(2):233-55.

- ◆ **Ancobon®** *see* Flucytosine *on page 354*
- ◆ **Androcur® (Can)** *see* Cyproterone *on page 227*
- ◆ **Androcur® Depot (Can)** *see* Cyproterone *on page 227*
- ◆ **Anti-CD20 Monoclonal Antibody** *see* Rituximab *on page 709*
- ◆ **Anti-CD20-Murine Monoclonal Antibody I-131** *see* Tositumomab and Iodine I 131 Tositumomab *on page 781*

Antihemophilic Factor (Human)

(an tee hee moe FIL ik FAK tor HYU man)

U.S. Brand Names Alphanate®; Hemofil® M; Humate-P®; Koāte®-DVI; Monarc® M; Monoclate-P®

Canadian Brand Names Hemofil® M; Humate-P®

Generic Available Yes

Synonyms AHF (Human); Factor VIII (Human)

Pharmacologic Category Antihemophilic Agent; Blood Product Derivative

Pregnancy Risk Factor C

Lactation Excretion in breast milk unknown/use caution

Use Management of hemophilia A for patients in whom a deficiency in factor VIII has been demonstrated; can be of significant therapeutic value in patients with acquired factor VIII inhibitors not exceeding 10 Bethesda units/mL

Humate-P®: In addition, indicated as treatment of spontaneous bleeding in patients with severe von Willebrand disease and in mild and moderate von Willebrand disease where desmopressin is known or suspected to be inadequate

Orphan status: Alphanate®: Management of von Willebrand disease

Mechanism of Action Protein (factor VIII) in normal plasma which is necessary for clot formation and maintenance of hemostasis; activates factor X in conjunction with activated factor IX; activated factor X converts prothrombin to thrombin, which converts fibrinogen to fibrin, and with factor XIII forms a stable clot

Labeled Contraindications Hypersensitivity to any component of the formulation or to mouse protein (Monoclate-P®, Hemofil® M)

Warnings/Precautions Risk of viral transmission is not totally eradicated. Because antihemophilic factor is prepared from pooled plasma, it may contain the causative agent of viral hepatitis and other viral (Continued)

Antihemophilic Factor (Human) *(Continued)*

diseases. Hepatitis B vaccination is recommended for all patients. Hepatitis A vaccination is also recommended for seronegative patients. Antihemophilic factor contains trace amounts of blood groups A and B isohemagglutinins and when large or frequently repeated doses are given to individuals with blood groups A, B, and AB, the patient should be monitored for signs of progressive anemia and the possibility of intravascular hemolysis should be considered. Natural rubber latex is a component of Hemofil® M packaging. Products vary by preparation method; final formulations contain human albumin.

Adverse Reactions <1%: Acute hemolytic anemia, allergic reactions (rare), anaphylaxis (rare), anemia, blurred vision, chest tightness, chills, edema, fever, headache, hyperfibrinogenemia, increased bleeding tendency, itching, jittery feeling, lethargy, nausea, paresthesia, pruritus, somnolence, stinging at the infusion site, stomach discomfort, tachycardia, tingling, vasomotor reactions with rapid infusion, vomiting

Overdosage/Toxicology Massive doses have been reported to cause acute hemolytic anemia, increased bleeding tendency, or hyperfibrinogenemia. Occurrence is rare.

Storage/Stability Store under refrigeration, 2°C to 8°C (36°F to 46°F); avoid freezing. Use within 3 hours of reconstitution. Do not refrigerate after reconstitution, precipitation may occur.

   Alphanate®: May be stored at room temperature for ≤2 months.

   Hemofil® M: May be stored at room temperature for ≤12 months.

   Humate-P®, Koāte®-DVI; Monoclate-P®: May also be stored at room temperature for ≤6 months.

If refrigerated, the dried concentrate and diluent should be warmed to room temperature before reconstitution.

Reconstitution Gently agitate or rotate vial after adding diluent; do not shake vigorously

Pharmacodynamics/Kinetics Half-life elimination: Mean: 12-17 hours with hemophilia A; consult specific product labeling

Dosage Children and Adults: I.V.: Individualize dosage based on coagulation studies performed prior to treatment and at regular intervals during treatment; 1 AHF unit is the activity present in 1 mL of normal pooled human plasma; dosage should be adjusted to actual vial size currently stocked in the pharmacy. (General guidelines presented; consult individual product labeling for specific dosing recommendations.)

Dosage based on desired factor VIII increase (%):

   To calculate dosage needed based on desired factor VIII increase (%):

   Body weight (kg) x 0.5 int. units/kg x desired factor VIII increase (%) = int. units factor VIII required

   For example:

      50 kg x 0.5 int. units/kg x 30 (% increase) = 750 int. units factor VIII

Dosage based on expected factor VIII increase (%):

   It is also possible to calculate the **expected** % factor VIII increase:

   (# int. units administered x 2%/int. units/kg) divided by body weight (kg) = expected % factor VIII increase

   For example:

      (1400 int. units x 2%/int. units/kg) divided by 70 kg = 40%

General guidelines:
 Minor Hemorrhage: Required peak postinfusion AHF level: 20% to 40%
  (10-20 int. units/kg), repeat dose every 12-24 hours for 1-3 days until
  bleeding is resolved or healing achieved; mild superficial or early
  hemorrhages may respond to a single dose
 Moderate hemorrhage: Required peak postinfusion AHF level: 30% to
  60% (15-30 int. units/kg): Infuse every 12-24 hours for ≥3 days until
  pain and disability are resolved
  Alternatively, a loading dose to achieve 50% (25 int. units/kg) may be
   given, followed by 10-15 int. units/kg dose given every 8-12 hours;
   may be needed for >7 days
 Severe/life-threatening hemorrhage: Required peak postinfusion AHF
  level: 60% to 100% (30-50 int. units/kg): Infuse every 8-24 hours until
  threat is resolved
  Alternatively, a loading dose to achieve 80% to 100% (40-50 int.
   units/kg) may be given, followed by 20-25 int. units/kg dose given
   every 8-12 hours for ≥14 days
 Minor surgery: Required peak postinfusion AHF level: 30% to 80%
  (15-40 int. units/kg): Highly dependent upon procedure and specific
  product recommendations; for some procedures, may be administered as a single infusion plus oral antifibrinolytic therapy within 1
  hour; in other procedures, may repeat dose every 12-24 hours as
  needed
 Major surgery: Required peak pre- and postsurgery AHF level: 80% to
  100% (40-50 int. units/kg): Administer every 6-24 hours until healing
  is complete (10-14 days)
 Prophylaxis: May also be given on a regular schedule to prevent
  bleeding
 If bleeding is not controlled with adequate dose, test for presence of
 inhibitor. It may not be possible or practical to control bleeding if inhibitor titers >10 Bethesda units/mL; antihemophilic factor (porcine) may
 be considered as an alternative

von Willebrand disease:
 Treatment of hemorrhage in von Willebrand disease (Humate-P®): 1 int.
  units of factor VIII per kg of body weight would be expected to raise
  circulating vWF:RC of approximately 3.5-4 int. units/dL
 Type 1, mild (if desmopressin is not appropriate): Major hemorrhage:
  Loading dose: 40-60 int. units/kg
  Maintenance dose: 40-50 int. units/kg every 8-12 hours for 3 days,
   keeping vWF:RC of nadir >50%; follow with 40-50 int. units/kg daily
   for up to 7 days
 Type 1, moderate or severe:
  Minor hemorrhage: 40-50 int. units/kg for 1-2 doses
  Major hemorrhage:
   Loading dose: 50-75 int. units/kg
   Maintenance dose: 40-60 int. units/kg daily for up to 7 days
 Types 2 and 3:
  Minor hemorrhage: 40-50 int. units/kg for 1-2 doses
  Major hemorrhage:
   Loading dose: 60-80 int. units/kg
   Maintenance dose: 40-60 int. units/kg every 8-12 hours for 3 days,
    keeping vWF:RC of nadir >50%; follow with 40-60 int. units/kg
    daily for up to 7 days
(Continued)

Antihemophilic Factor (Human) *(Continued)*

Elderly: Response in the elderly is not expected to differ from that of younger patients; dosage should be individualized

Administration I.V.: Over 5-10 minutes (maximum: 10 mL/minute); infuse Monoclate-P® at 2 mL/minute

Dosage Forms Injection, human [single-dose vial]: Labeling on cartons and vials indicates number of int. units

Monitoring Parameters Heart rate and blood pressure (before and during I.V. administration); AHF levels prior to and during treatment; in patients with circulating inhibitors, the inhibitor level should be monitored; hematocrit; monitor for signs and symptoms of intravascular hemolysis; bleeding

Patient Information This medication can only be given intravenously. Report sudden-onset headache, rash, chest or back pain, wheezing, or respiratory difficulties, hives, itching, low grade fever, nausea, vomiting, tiredness, decreased appetite to prescriber. Wear identification indicating that you have a hemophilic condition.

Selected Readings

Ablidgaard CF, Simone JV, Corrigan JJ, et al, "Treatment of Hemophilia With Glycine-precipitated Factor VIII," *N Engl J Med*, 1966, 275(9):471-5.

Berntorp E, "Impact of Replacement Therapy on the Evolution of HIV Infection in Hemophiliacs," *Thromb Haemost*, 1994, 71(6):678-83.

Berntorp E, "Plasma Product Treatment in Various Types of von Willebrand Disease," *Haemostasis*, 1994, 24(5):287-97.

Lusher JM, "Transfusion Therapy in Congenital Coagulopathies," *Hematol Oncol Clin North Am*, 1994, 8(6):1167-80.

Manucci PM, "Impact of Recombinant Factor VIII on Hemophilia Care," *Vox Sang*, 1994, 67(Suppl 3):49-52.

Nisson IM, Berntorp E, Lofqvist T, et al, "Twenty-five Years' Experience of Prophylactic Treatment in Severe Haemophilia A and B," *J Intern Med*, 1992, 232(1):25-32.

Peterson CW, "Treating Hemophilia," *Am Pharm*, 1994, NS34(8):57-67.

Scharrer I, Vigh T, and Aygoren-Purun E, "Experience With Haemate P in von Willebrand Disease," *Haemostasis*, 1994, 24(5):298-303.

Antihemophilic Factor (Porcine)

(an tee hee moe FIL ik FAK ter POR seen)

U.S. Brand Names Hyate:C®

Generic Available No

Synonyms AHF (Porcine); Factor VIII (Porcine)

Pharmacologic Category Antihemophilic Agent

Pregnancy Risk Factor C

Lactation Excretion in breast milk unknown/use caution

Use Management of hemophilia A in patients with antibodies to human factor VIII (consider use of human factor VIII in patients with antibody titer of <5 Bethesda units/mL); management of previously nonhemophilic patients with spontaneously-acquired inhibitors to human factor VIII, regardless of initial antihuman inhibitor titer

Mechanism of Action Factor VIII is the coagulation portion of the factor VIII complex in plasma. Factor VIII acts as a cofactor for factor IX to activate factor X in the intrinsic pathway of blood coagulation.

Labeled Contraindications Hypersensitivity to porcine or any component of the formulation

Warnings/Precautions Rarely administration has been associated with anaphylaxis; use caution when administering. Infusion may be followed by a rise in plasma levels of antibody to both human and porcine factor VIII. Inhibitor levels should be monitored both pre- and post-treatment.

Adverse Reactions Reactions tend to lessen in frequency and severity as further infusions are given; hydrocortisone and/or antihistamines may help to prevent or alleviate side effects and may be prescribed as precautionary measures.

1% to 10%:
    Central nervous system: Fever, headache, chills
    Dermatologic: Rashes
    Gastrointestinal: Nausea, vomiting
<1% and case reports: Anaphylaxis, thrombocytopenia

Overdosage/Toxicology Massive doses of antihemophilic factor (human) have been reported to cause acute hemolytic anemia, increased bleeding tendency, or hyperfibrinogenemia. Occurrence is rare.

Storage/Stability Store at -15°C to -20°C (5°F to -4°F); warm to 20°C to 37°C (68°F to 98.6°F) prior to reconstitution; use within 3 hours of mixing.

Pharmacodynamics/Kinetics Half-life elimination: 10-11 hours (patients without detectable inhibitors)

Dosage
Initial dose:
    Antibody level to human factor VIII <50 Bethesda units/mL: 100-150 porcine units/kg (body weight) is recommended
    Antibody level to human factor VIII >50 Bethesda units/mL: Activity of the antibody to antihemophilic (porcine) should be determined; **an antiporcine antibody level** >20 Bethesda units/mL indicates that the patient is unlikely to benefit from treatment; for lower titers, a dose of 100-150 porcine units/kg is recommended
    The initial dose may also be calculated using the following method:
    1. Determine patient's antibody titer against porcine factor VIII
    2. Calculate average plasma volume:
        (body weight kg) (average blood volume) (1 - hematocrit) = plasma volume
        (body weight kg) (80 mL/kg) (1 - hematocrit) = plasma volume
        Note: A hematocrit of 50% = 0.5 for the equation
    3. Neutralizing dose:
        (plasma volume mL) (antibody titer Bethesda units/mL) = neutralizing dose units
        This is the predicted dose required to neutralize the circulating antibodies. An incremental dose must be added to the neutralizing dose in order to increase the plasma factor VIII to the desired level.
    4. Incremental dose:
        (desired plasma factor VIII level) (body weight) divided by 1.5 = incremental dose units
    5. Total dose = neutralizing dose + incremental dose = total dose units
    If a patient has previously been treated with Hyate:C®, this may provide a guide to his likely response and, therefore, assist in estimation of the preliminary dose

Subsequent doses: Following administration of the initial dose, if the recovery of factor VIII in the patient's plasma is not sufficient, another larger dose should be administered; if recovery after the second dose is still insufficient, a third and larger dose may prove effective. Once
(Continued)

Antihemophilic Factor (Porcine) *(Continued)*

appropriate factor VIII levels are achieved, dosing can be repeated every 6-8 hours.

Administration I.V. infusion 2-5 mL/minute

Dosage Forms Injection, powder for reconstitution: 400-700 porcine units [to be reconstituted with 20 mL SWFI]

Monitoring Parameters Factor VIII levels pre- and postinfusion; inhibitor levels to human and/or porcine factor VIII pre- and postinfusion; heart rate and blood pressure (before and during I.V. administration); bleeding

Antibody levels to human factor VIII >50 Bethesda units/mL: Activity of the antibody to antihemophilic factor (porcine) should be determined

Antiporcine antibody level >20 Bethesda units/mL: Patient may not benefit from treatment

Patient Information This medication can only be given intravenously. Report sudden-onset headache, rash, chest or back pain, or respiratory difficulties to prescriber. Wear identification indicating that you have a hemophilic condition.

Additional Information Sodium ion concentration is not more than 200 mmol/L. The assayed amount of activity is stated on the label, but may vary depending on the type of assay and hemophilic substrate plasma used.

Antihemophilic Factor (Recombinant)

(an tee hee moe FIL ik FAK tor ree KOM be nant)

U.S. Brand Names Advate; Helixate® FS; Kogenate® FS; Recombinate™; ReFacto®

Canadian Brand Names Helixate® FS; Kogenate®; Kogenate® FS; Recombinate™; ReFacto®

Generic Available No

Synonyms AHF (Recombinant); Factor VIII (Recombinant); rAHF

Pharmacologic Category Antihemophilic Agent

Pregnancy Risk Factor C

Lactation Excretion in breast milk unknown/use caution

Use Management of hemophilia A (classic hemophilia) for patients in whom a deficiency in factor VIII has been demonstrated; prevention and control of bleeding episodes; perioperative management of hemophilia A; can be of significant therapeutic value in patients with acquired factor VIII inhibitors not exceeding 10 Bethesda units/mL

Mechanism of Action Protein (factor VIII) in normal plasma which is necessary for clot formation and maintenance of hemostasis; activates factor X in conjunction with activated factor IX; activated factor X converts prothrombin to thrombin, which converts fibrinogen to fibrin, and with factor XIII forms a stable clot

Labeled Contraindications Hypersensitivity to mouse or hamster protein (Advate, Helixate® FS, Kogenate® FS); hypersensitivity to mouse, hamster, or bovine protein (Recombinate™, ReFacto®); hypersensitivity to any component of the formulation

Warnings/Precautions Monitor for signs of formation of antibodies to factor VIII; may occur at anytime but more common in young children with severe hemophilia. Monitor for allergic hypersensitivity reactions. Products vary by preparation method. Recombinate™ is stabilized using human albumin. Helixate® FS and Kogenate® FS are stabilized with sucrose.

Adverse Reactions <1%, postmarketing, and/or case reports: Acne, allergic reactions, increased aminotransferase, anaphylaxis, angina pectoris, asthenia, bilirubin increased, chest discomfort, chills, cold feet, constipation, cough, increased CPK, depersonalization, diaphoresis, diarrhea, dizziness, dysgeusia, dyspnea, epistaxis, facial flushing, fatigue, fever, headache, hot flashes, hypotension (slight), injection site reactions (burning, pruritus, erythema), lethargy, nausea, perspiration increased, pruritus, rash, rhinitis, somnolence, sore throat, tachycardia, unusual taste, urticaria, vasodilation, abnormal vision, venous catheter access complications, vomiting

Overdosage/Toxicology Massive doses of antihemophilic factor (human) have been reported to cause acute hemolytic anemia, increased bleeding tendency, or hyperfibrinogenemia. Occurrence is rare.

Storage/Stability Store under refrigeration, 2°C to 8°C (36°F to 46°F); avoid freezing. Use within 3 hours of reconstitution. Do not refrigerate after reconstitution, a precipitation may occur.

Advate: May also be stored at room temperature for up to 6 months.

Kogenate® FS: Avoid prolonged exposure to light during storage.

Recombinate™, ReFacto®: May also be stored at room temperature for up to 3 months; avoid prolonged exposure to light during storage

If refrigerated, the dried concentrate and diluent should be warmed to room temperature before reconstitution.

Reconstitution Gently agitate or rotate vial after adding diluent, do not shake vigorously.

Pharmacodynamics/Kinetics Half-life elimination: Mean: 14-16 hours

Dosage Children and Adults: I.V.: Individualize dosage based on coagulation studies performed prior to treatment and at regular intervals during treatment; 1 AHF unit is the activity present in 1 mL of normal pooled human plasma; dosage should be adjusted to actual vial size currently stocked in the pharmacy. (General guidelines presented; consult individual product labeling for specific dosing recommendations.)

Dosage based on desired factor VIII increase (%):

To calculate dosage needed based on desired factor VIII increase (%):
Body weight (kg) x 0.5 int. units/kg x desired factor VIII increase (%) = int. units factor VIII required

For example:
50 kg x 0.5 int. units/kg x 30 (% increase) = 750 int. units factor VIII

Dosage based on expected factor VIII increase (%):

It is also possible to calculate the **expected** % factor VIII increase:
(# int. units administered x 2%/int. units/kg) divided by body weight (kg) = expected % factor VIII increase

For example:
(1400 int. units x 2%/int. units/kg) divided by 70 kg = 40%

General guidelines:

Minor hemorrhage: Required peak postinfusion AHF level: 20% to 40% (10-20 int. units/kg); mild superficial or early hemorrhages may respond to a single dose; may repeat dose every 12-24 hours for 1-3 days until bleeding is resolved or healing achieved

Moderate hemorrhage/minor surgery: Required peak postinfusion AHF level: 30% to 60% (15-30 int. units/kg); repeat dose at 12-24 hours if

(Continued)

Antihemophilic Factor (Recombinant) *(Continued)*

needed; some products suggest continuing for ≥3 days until pain and disability are resolved

Severe/life-threatening hemorrhage: Required peak postinfusion AHF level: Initial dose: 80% to 100% (40-50 int. units/kg); maintenance dose: 40% to 50% (20-25 int. units/kg) every 8-12 hours until threat is resolved

Major surgery: Required peak pre- and postsurgery AHF level: ~100% (50 int. units/kg) give first dose prior to surgery and repeat every 6-12 hours until healing complete (10-14 days)

Prophylaxis: May also be given on a regular schedule to prevent bleeding

If bleeding is not controlled with adequate dose, test for presence of inhibitor. It may not be possible or practical to control bleeding if inhibitor titers >10 Bethesda units/mL; antihemophilic factor (porcine) may be considered as an alternative

Elderly: Response in the elderly is not expected to differ from that of younger patients; dosage should be individualized

Administration I.V. infusion over 5-10 minutes (maximum: 10 mL/minute)

Advate: Infuse over ≤5 minutes (maximum: 10 mL/minute)

Dosage Forms

Injection, powder for reconstitution, recombinant [preservative free]:

Advate: 250 int. units, 500 int. units, 1000 int. units, 1500 int. units [plasma/albumin free]

Helixate® FS, Kogenate® FS: 250 int. units, 500 int. units, 1000 int. units [contains sucrose 28 mg/vial]

Recombinate™: 250 int. units, 500 units, 1000 int. units [contains human albumin 12.5 mg/mL; packaging contains natural rubber latex]

ReFacto®: 250 int. units, 500 int. units, 1000 int. units, 2000 int. units [contains sucrose]

Monitoring Parameters Heart rate and blood pressure (before and during I.V. administration); AHF levels prior to and during treatment; development of factor VIII inhibitors; bleeding

Patient Information This medication can only be given intravenously. Report hives, itching, wheezing, sudden-onset headache, rash, chest or back pain, or other respiratory difficulties to prescriber. Wear identification indicating that you have a hemophilic condition.

Selected Readings

Abildgaard CF, Simone JV, Corrigan JJ, et al, "Treatment of Hemophilia With Glycine-precipitated Factor VIII," *N Engl J Med*, 1966, 275(9):471-5.

Manucci PM, "Impact of Recombinant Factor VIII on Hemophilia Care," *Vox Sang*, 1994, 67(Suppl 3):49-52.

Nisson IM, Berntorp E, Lofqvist T, et al, "Twenty-five Years' Experience of Prophylactic Treatment in Severe Haemophilia A and B," *J Intern Med*, 1992, 232(1):25-32.

Peterson CW, "Treating Hemophilia," *Am Pharm*, 1994, NS34(8):57-67.

Antithrombin III *(an tee THROM bin three)*

U.S. Brand Names Thrombate III®

Canadian Brand Names Thrombate III®

Generic Available No

Synonyms AT III; Heparin Cofactor I

Pharmacologic Category Anticoagulant; Blood Product Derivative

Pregnancy Risk Factor B

Lactation Excretion in breast milk unknown/use caution

Use Treatment of hereditary antithrombin III deficiency in connection with surgical or obstetrical procedures; thromboembolism

Unlabeled/Investigational Use Acquired antithrombin III deficiencies related to disseminated intravascular coagulation (DIC)

Mechanism of Action Antithrombin III is the primary physiologic inhibitor of *in vivo* coagulation. It is an alpha$_2$-globulin. Its principal actions are the inactivation of thrombin, plasmin, and other active serine proteases of coagulation, including factors IXa, Xa, XIa, XIIa, and VIIa. The inactivation of proteases is a major step in the normal clotting process. The strong activation of clotting enzymes at the site of every bleeding injury facilitates fibrin formation and maintains normal hemostasis. Thrombosis in the circulation would be caused by active serine proteases if they were not inhibited by antithrombin III after the localized clotting process.

Labeled Contraindications Hypersensitivity to any component of the formulation

Warnings/Precautions Product is prepared from pooled human plasma; may contain the causative agents of viral diseases.

Adverse Reactions
1% to 10%: Central nervous system: Dizziness (2%)
<1%: Abdominal cramps, bowel fullness, chest pain, chest tightness, chills, cramps, fever, film over eye, foul taste, hematoma formation, hives, lightheadedness, nausea

Vesicant No

Emetic Potential Very low (<1%)

Drug Interactions
Increased Effect/Toxicity: Heparin's anticoagulant effects are potentiated by antithrombin III (half-life of antithrombin III is decreased by heparin). Risk of hemorrhage with antithrombin III may be increased by drotrecogin, thrombolytic agents, oral anticoagulants (warfarin), and drugs which affect platelet function (eg, aspirin, NSAIDs, dipyridamole, ticlopidine, clopidogrel, and IIb/IIIa antagonists).

Storage/Stability Store vials under refrigeration at 2°C to 8°C (36°F to 46°F); avoid freezing. Bring to room temperature prior to reconstitution. Administer within 3 hours of mixing.

Reconstitution Reconstitute with sterile water for injection. Do not shake; swirl to mix to avoid foaming. Filter through sterile filter needle provided prior to administration.

Pharmacodynamics/Kinetics Half-life elimination: Biologic: 2.5 days (immunologic assay); 3.8 days (functional AT-III assay)

Dosage Adults:
Initial dose: Dosing is individualized based on pretherapy AT-III levels. The initial dose should raise antithrombin III levels (AT-III) to 120% and may be calculated based on the following formula:
Initial dosage (int. units) = [desired AT-III level % - baseline AT-III level %] x body weight (kg) divided by 1.4%/int. units/kg (eg, if a 70 kg adult patient had a baseline AT-III level of 57%, the initial dose would be (120% - 57%) x 70/1.4%/int. units/kg = 3150 int. units).
Maintenance dose: Subsequent dosing should be targeted to keep levels between 80% to 120% which may be achieved by administering 60% of the initial dose every 24 hours. Adjustments may be made by adjusting dose or interval. Maintain level within normal range for 2-8 days depending on type of surgery or procedure.
(Continued)

Antithrombin III (Continued)

Administration I.V.: Infuse over 10-20 minutes

Dosage Forms Injection, powder for reconstitution [preservative free]: 500 int. units, 1000 int. units [contains heparin; packaged with diluent]

Monitoring Parameters Monitor antithrombin III levels (preinfusion and 20 minutes postinfusion for each dose); liver function tests

Dietary Considerations Contains sodium 110-210 mEq/L

Selected Readings
Schwartz RS, Bauer KA, Rosenberg RD, et al, "Clinical Experience With Antithrombin III Concentrate in Treatment of Congenital and Acquired Deficiency of Antithrombin. The Antithrombin III Study Group," *Am J Med*, 1989, 87(3B):53S-60S.

Antithymocyte Globulin (Equine)

(an te THY moe site GLOB yu lin, E kwine)

Medication Safety Issues
Sound-alike/look-alike issues:
Atgam® may be confused with Ativan®

U.S. Brand Names Atgam®

Canadian Brand Names Atgam®

Generic Available No

Synonyms Antithymocyte Immunoglobulin; ATG; Horse Antihuman Thymocyte Gamma Globulin; Lymphocyte Immune Globulin

Pharmacologic Category Immunosuppressant Agent

Pregnancy Risk Factor C

Lactation Excretion in breast milk unknown/use caution

Use Prevention and treatment of acute renal allograft rejection; treatment of moderate to severe aplastic anemia in patients not considered suitable candidates for bone marrow transplantation

Unlabeled/Investigational Use Prevention and treatment of other solid organ allograft rejection; prevention of graft-versus-host disease following bone marrow transplantation

Mechanism of Action May involve elimination of antigen-reactive T-lymphocytes (killer cells) in peripheral blood or alteration of T-cell function

Labeled Contraindications Hypersensitivity to lymphocytic immune globulin, any component of the formulation, or other equine gamma globulins

Warnings/Precautions For I.V. use only. Must be administered via central line due to chemical phlebitis. Should only be used by physicians experienced in immunosuppressive therapy or management of solid organ or bone marrow transplant patients. Adequate laboratory and supportive medical resources must be readily available in the facility for patient management. Rash, dyspnea, hypotension, or anaphylaxis precludes further administration of the drug. Discontinue if severe and unremitting thrombocytopenia and/or leukopenia occur. Dose must be administered over at least 4 hours. Patient may need to be pretreated with an antipyretic, antihistamine, and/or corticosteroid.

Adverse Reactions
>10%:
Central nervous system: Fever, chills
Dermatologic: Pruritus, rash, urticaria
Hematologic: Leukopenia, thrombocytopenia

1% to 10%:

Cardiovascular: Bradycardia, chest pain, CHF, edema, encephalitis, hyper-/hypotension, myocarditis, tachycardia

Central nervous system: Agitation, headache, lethargy, lightheadedness, listlessness, seizure

Gastrointestinal: Diarrhea, nausea, stomatitis, vomiting

Hepatic: Hepatosplenomegaly, liver function tests abnormal

Local: Pain at injection site, phlebitis, thrombophlebitis, burning soles/palms

Neuromuscular & skeletal: Myalgia, back pain, arthralgia

Ocular: Periorbital edema

Renal: Abnormal renal function tests

Respiratory: Dyspnea, respiratory distress

Miscellaneous: Anaphylaxis, serum sickness, viral infection, night sweats, diaphoresis, lymphadenopathy

<1%: Dizziness, epigastric pain, faintness, herpes simplex reactivation, hiccups, hyperglycemia, iliac vein obstruction, infection, laryngospasm, malaise, paresthesia, pulmonary edema, renal artery thrombosis, serum sickness, toxic epidermal necrosis, weakness, wound dehiscence

Postmarketing and/or case reports: Acute renal failure, anemia, aplasia, confusion, cough, deep vein thrombosis, disorientation, GI bleeding, granulocytopenia, hemolysis, kidney enlarged, neutropenia, nosebleed, pancytopenia, vasculitis

Vesicant No

Emetic Potential Very low (<10%)

Storage/Stability Ampuls must be refrigerated; do not freeze. Diluted solution is stable for 24 hours (including infusion time) at refrigeration.

Reconstitution Dilute into inverted bottle of sterile vehicle to ensure that undiluted lymphocyte immune globulin does not contact air. Gently rotate or swirl to mix. Final concentration should be 4 mg/mL. May be diluted in NS, $D_5$1/4NS, $D_5$1/2NS.

Pharmacodynamics/Kinetics

Distribution: Poorly into lymphoid tissues; binds to circulating lymphocytes, granulocytes, platelets, bone marrow cells

Half-life elimination, plasma: 1.5-12 days

Excretion: Urine (~1%)

Dosage An intradermal skin test is recommended prior to administration of the initial dose of ATG; use 0.1 mL of a 1:1000 dilution of ATG in normal saline. A positive skin reaction consists of a wheal ≥10 mm in diameter. If a positive skin test occurs, the first infusion should be administered in a controlled environment with intensive life support immediately available. The absence of a reaction does **not** preclude the possibility of an immediate sensitivity reaction.

Premedication with diphenhydramine, hydrocortisone, and acetaminophen is recommended prior to first dose.

Children: I.V.:

Aplastic anemia protocol: 10-20 mg/kg/day for 8-14 days; then administer every other day for 7 more doses; addition doses may be given every other day for 21 total doses in 28 days

Renal allograft: 5-25 mg/kg/day

(Continued)

Antithymocyte Globulin (Equine) *(Continued)*

Adults: I.V.:

Aplastic anemia protocol: 10-20 mg/kg/day for 8-14 days, then administer every other day for 7 more doses, for a total of 21 doses in 28 days

Renal allograft:

Rejection prophylaxis: 15 mg/kg/day for 14 days followed by 14 days of alternative day therapy at the same dose; the first dose should be administered within 24 hours before or after transplantation

Rejection treatment: 10-15 mg/kg/day for 14 days, then administer every other day for 10-14 days up to 21 doses in 28 days

Administration Infuse dose over at least 4 hours. Epinephrine and resuscitative equipment should be nearby. Patient may need to be pretreated with an antipyretic, antihistamine, and/or corticosteroid. Infuse into a vascular shunt, arterial venous fistula, or high-flow central vein through a 0.2-1 micron in-line filter

First dose: Premedicate with diphenhydramine orally 30 minutes prior to and hydrocortisone I.V. 15 minutes prior to infusion and acetaminophen 2 hours after start of infusion.

Dosage Forms Injection, solution: 50 mg/mL (5 mL)

Monitoring Parameters Lymphocyte profile, CBC with differential and platelet count, vital signs during administration

Antithymocyte Globulin (Rabbit)

(an te THY moe site GLOB yu lin (RAB bit)

Related Information

Transplantation *on page 1019*

U.S. Brand Names Thymoglobulin®

Generic Available No

Synonyms Antithymocyte Immunoglobulin; ATG

Pharmacologic Category Immune Globulin

Use Treatment of renal transplant acute rejection in conjunction with concomitant immunosuppression

Mechanism of Action May involve elimination of antigen-reactive T-lymphocytes (killer cells) in peripheral blood or alteration of T-cell function

Labeled Contraindications Patients with history of allergy or anaphylaxis to rabbit proteins, or who have an acute viral illness

Warnings/Precautions Should only be used by physicians experienced in immunosuppressive therapy for the treatment of transplant patients. Chronic immunosuppression increases the risk of opportunistic infections and secondary malignancies.

Adverse Reactions

>10%:

Central nervous system: Fever, chills, headache

Dermatologic: Rash

Endocrine & metabolic: Hyperkalemia

Gastrointestinal: Abdominal pain, diarrhea

Hematologic: Leukopenia, thrombocytopenia

Neuromuscular & skeletal: Weakness

Respiratory: Dyspnea

Miscellaneous: Systemic infection, pain

1% to 10%:
Gastrointestinal: Gastritis
Respiratory: Pneumonia
Miscellaneous: Sensitivity reactions: Anaphylaxis (hypotension, respiratory distress, serum sickness, viral infection)

Vesicant No

Emetic Potential Very low (<10%)

Pharmacodynamics/Kinetics Half-life elimination, plasma: 2-3 days

Dosage I.V.: 1.5 mg/kg/day for 7-14 days

Administration For I.V. use only; administer via central line; use of high flow veins will minimize the occurrence of phlebitis and thrombosis; administer by slow I.V. infusion through an in-line filter with pore size of 0.2 micrometer over a minimum of 6 hours for the first infusion and over at least 4 hours on subsequent days of therapy.

Dosage Forms Injection, powder for reconstitution: 25 mg vial [packaged with diluent]

Monitoring Parameters Lymphocyte profile, CBC with differential and platelet count, vital signs during administration; any severe systemic reaction to the skin test (eg, generalized rash, tachycardia, dyspnea, hypotension, or anaphylaxis) should preclude further therapy; T-lymphocyte count prior to retreatment (verify T-cell depletion).

♦ **Apo-Metronidazole® (Can)** *see* Metronidazole *on page 568*

♦ **Apo-Oflox® (Can)** *see* Ofloxacin *on page 618*

♦ **Apo-Prednisone® (Can)** *see* PredniSONE *on page 683*

♦ **Apo-Prochlorperazine® (Can)** *see* Prochlorperazine *on page 691*

♦ **Apo-Sulfatrim® (Can)** *see* Sulfamethoxazole and Trimethoprim *on page 727*

♦ **Apo-Tamox® (Can)** *see* Tamoxifen *on page 743*

♦ **Apo-Tobramycin® (Can)** *see* Tobramycin *on page 771*

♦ **Apo-Trimethoprim® (Can)** *see* Trimethoprim *on page 797*

Aprepitant (ap RE pi tant)

U.S. Brand Names Emend®

Generic Available No

Synonyms L 754030; MK 869

Pharmacologic Category Antiemetic; Substance P/Neurokinin 1 Receptor Antagonist

Pregnancy Risk Factor B

Lactation Excretion in breast milk unknown/not recommended

Use Prevention of acute and delayed nausea and vomiting associated with highly-emetogenic chemotherapy in combination with a corticosteroid and 5-HT$_3$ receptor antagonist

Mechanism of Action Prevents acute and delayed vomiting by selectively inhibiting the substance P/neurokinin 1 (NK$_1$) receptor.

Labeled Contraindications Hypersensitivity to aprepitant or any component of the formulation; use with cisapride or pimozide

Warnings/Precautions Use caution with agents primarily metabolized via CYP3A4. Use caution with hepatic impairment. Not intended for treatment of nausea and vomiting or for chronic continuous therapy. Safety and efficacy in pediatric patients have not been established.

Adverse Reactions

>10%:
  Central nervous system: Fatigue (18%)
  Gastrointestinal: Nausea (13%)
  Neuromuscular & skeletal: Weakness (18%)
  Miscellaneous: Hiccups (11%)

1% to 10%:
  Central nervous system: Dizziness (7%)
  Endocrine & metabolic: Dehydration (6%)
  Gastrointestinal: Diarrhea (10%), abdominal pain (5%), epigastric discomfort (4%), gastritis (4%)
  Hepatic: ALT increased (6%), AST increased (3%)
  Renal: BUN increased (5%), proteinuria (7%), serum creatinine increased (4%)

>0.5%: Acid reflux, alkaline phosphatase increased, alopecia, anemia, anxiety, appetite decreased, confusion, cough, deglutition disorder, depression, diabetes mellitus, diaphoresis, DVT, dysgeusia, dyspepsia, dysphagia, dyspnea, dysuria, edema, erythrocyturia, febrile neutropenia, flatulence, flushing, hyperglycemia, hyper-/hypotension, hypokalemia, hyponatremia, leukocytes increased, leukocyturia, malaise, MI, muscular weakness, musculoskeletal pain, myalgia, nasal secretion,

obstipation, pelvic pain, peripheral neuropathy, pharyngitis, pneumonitis, pulmonary embolism, rash, renal insufficiency, respiratory infection, salivation, sensory neuropathy, septic shock, tachycardia, taste disturbance, thrombocytopenia, vocal disturbance, weight loss

Postmarketing and/or case reports: Angioedema, bradycardia, disorientation, duodenal ulcer (perforating), Stevens-Johnson syndrome, urticaria

Overdosage/Toxicology Single doses up to 600 mg were well-tolerated, drowsiness was noted at a dose of 1440 mg. In case of overdose, treatment should be symptom-directed and supportive. Not removed by hemodialysis.

Drug Interactions

Cytochrome P450 Effect: Substrate of CYP1A2 (minor), 2C19 (minor), 3A4 (major); **Inhibits** CYP2C8/9 (weak), 2C19 (weak), 3A4 (moderate); **Induces** CYP2C9 (weak), 3A4 (weak)

Increased Effect/Toxicity: Use with cisapride or pimozide is contraindicated. CYP3A4 inhibitors may increase the levels/effects of aprepitant; example inhibitors include azole antifungals, ciprofloxacin, clarithromycin, diclofenac, diltiazem, doxycycline, erythromycin, imatinib, isoniazid, nefazodone, nicardipine, propofol, protease inhibitors, quinidine, and verapamil. Aprepitant may increase the bioavailability of corticosteroids; dose adjustment of dexamethasone and methylprednisolone is needed. Aprepitant may increase the levels/effects of CYP3A4 substrates; example substrates include benzodiazepines, calcium channel blockers, ergot derivatives, mirtazapine, nateglinide, nefazodone, tacrolimus, and venlafaxine.

Decreased Effect: CYP3A4 inducers may decrease the levels/effects of aprepitant; example inducers include aminoglutethimide, carbamazepine, nafcillin, nevirapine, phenobarbital, phenytoin, and rifamycins. Metabolism of warfarin may be induced; monitor INR following the start of each cycle. Efficacy of oral contraceptives may be decreased (plasma levels of ethinyl estradiol and norethindrone decreased with concomitant use). Plasma levels of both paroxetine and aprepitant are decreased with concomitant use.

Ethanol/Nutrition/Herb Interactions

Food: Aprepitant serum concentration may be increased when taken with grapefruit juice; avoid concurrent use.

Herb/Nutraceutical: St John's wort may decrease aprepitant levels.

Storage/Stability Store at controlled room temperature of 20°C to 25°C (68°F to 77°F).

Pharmacodynamics/Kinetics

Distribution: V_d: 70 L; crosses the blood brain barrier

Protein binding: >95%

Metabolism: Extensively hepatic via CYP3A4 (major); CYP1A2 and CYP2C19 (minor); forms seven metabolites (weakly active)

Bioavailability: 60% to 65%

Half-life elimination: Terminal: 9-13 hours

Time to peak, plasma: 4 hours

Dosage Oral: Adults: 125 mg on day 1, followed by 80 mg on days 2 and 3

Dosage adjustment in renal impairment: No dose adjustment necessary in patients with renal disease or end-stage renal disease maintained on hemodialysis.

(Continued)

Aprepitant *(Continued)*

Dosage adjustment in hepatic impairment:
Mild to moderate impairment (Child-Pugh score 5-9): No adjustment necessary

Severe impairment (Child-Pugh score >9): No data available

Administration Oral: With or without food. First dose should be given 1 hour prior to antineoplastic therapy; subsequent doses should be given in the morning.

Dosage Forms
Capsule: 80 mg, 125 mg

Combination package: Capsule 80 mg (2s), capsule 125 mg (1s)

Dietary Considerations May be taken with or without food.

Patient Information May be taken with or without food. Common side effects include diarrhea, hiccups, loss of appetite, tiredness or weakness. This medicine may not mix well with other medicines; check medicines with prescriber.

Special Geriatric Considerations In two studies by the manufacturer, with a total of 544 patients, 31% were >65 years of age, while 5% were >75 years. No differences in safety and efficacy were noted between elderly subjects and younger adults. No dosing adjustment is necessary.

- ◆ **Aquacort**® **(Can)** *see* Hydrocortisone *on page 419*
- ◆ **AquaMEPHYTON**® **(Can)** *see* Phytonadione *on page 664*
- ◆ **Aquanil**™ **HC [OTC]** *see* Hydrocortisone *on page 419*
- ◆ **Arabinosylcytosine** *see* Cytarabine *on page 229*
- ◆ **Ara-C** *see* Cytarabine *on page 229*
- ◆ **Aredia**® *see* Pamidronate *on page 650*
- ◆ **Arimidex**® *see* Anastrozole *on page 85*
- ◆ **Aromasin**® *see* Exemestane *on page 324*

Arsenic Trioxide (AR se nik tri OKS id)

Related Information
Safe Handling of Hazardous Drugs *on page 1034*

U.S. Brand Names Trisenox™

Generic Available No

Synonyms NSC-706363

Pharmacologic Category Antineoplastic Agent, Miscellaneous

Pregnancy Risk Factor D

Lactation Excretion in breast milk unknown/contraindicated

Use Induction of remission and consolidation in patients with acute promyelocytic leukemia (APL) which is specifically characterized by t(15;17) translocation or PML/RAR-alpha gene expression.

Orphan drug: Treatment of myelodysplastic syndrome; multiple myeloma; chronic myeloid leukemia (CML); acute myelocytic leukemia (AML)

Mechanism of Action Not fully understood; causes *in vitro* morphological changes and DNA fragmentation to NB4 human promyelocytic leukemia cells; also damages or degrades the fusion protein PML-RAR alpha

Labeled Contraindications Hypersensitivity to arsenic or any component of the formulation; pregnancy

Warnings/Precautions The U.S. Food and Drug Administration (FDA) currently recommends that procedures for proper handling and disposal of antineoplastic agents be considered. For use only by physicians experienced with the treatment of acute leukemia. A baseline 12-lead ECG, serum electrolytes (potassium, calcium, magnesium), and creatinine should be obtained. Correct electrolyte abnormalities prior to treatment and monitor potassium and magnesium levels during therapy (potassium should stay >4 mEq/dL and magnesium >1.8 mg/dL). Correct QT_c >500 msec prior to treatment. Discontinue therapy and hospitalize patient if QT_c >500 msec, syncope or irregular heartbeats develop during therapy. May prolong the QT interval. May lead to torsade de pointes or complete AV block. Risk factors for torsade de pointes include CHF, a history of torsade de pointes, pre-existing QT interval prolongation, patients taking potassium-wasting diuretics, and conditions which cause hypokalemia or hypomagnesemia. If possible, discontinue all medications known to prolong the QT interval. May cause retinoic-acid-acute promyelocytic leukemia (RA-APL) syndrome or APL differentiation syndrome (high-dose steroids have been used for treatment). May lead to the development of hyperleukocytosis. Use with caution in renal impairment. Safety and efficacy in children <5 years of age have not been established (limited experience with children 5-16 years of age).

Adverse Reactions

>10%:

Cardiovascular: Tachycardia (55%), edema (40%), QT interval >500 msec (38%), chest pain (25%), hypotension (25%)

Central nervous system: Fatigue (63%), fever (63%), headache (60%), insomnia (43%), anxiety (30%), dizziness (23%), depression (20%), pain (15%)

Dermatologic: Dermatitis (43%), pruritus (33%), bruising (20%), dry skin (13%)

Endocrine & metabolic: Hypokalemia (50%), hyperglycemia (45%), hypomagnesemia (45%), hyperkalemia (18%)

Gastrointestinal: Nausea (75%), abdominal pain (58%), vomiting (58%), diarrhea (53%), sore throat (40%), constipation (28%), anorexia (23%), decreased appetite (15%), weight gain (13%)

Genitourinary: Vaginal hemorrhage (13%)

Hematologic: Leukocytosis (50%), APL differentiation syndrome (23%), thrombocytopenia (19%), anemia (14%), febrile neutropenia (13%)

Hepatic: Elevated ALT (20%), elevated AST (13%)

Local: Injection site: Pain (20%), erythema (13%)

Neuromuscular & skeletal: Rigors (38%), arthralgia (33%), paresthesia (33%), myalgia (25%), bone pain (23%), back pain (18%), limb pain (13%), neck pain (13%), tremor (13%)

Respiratory: Cough (65%), dyspnea (53%), epistaxis (25%), hypoxia (23%), pleural effusion (20%), sinusitis (20%), postnasal drip (13%), upper respiratory tract infection (13%), wheezing (13%)

Miscellaneous: Herpes simplex (13%)

1% to 10%:

Cardiovascular: Hypotension (10%), flushing (10%), pallor (10%), palpitation (10%), facial edema (8%), abnormal ECG (not QT prolongation) (7%)

Central nervous system: Convulsion (8%), somnolence (8%), agitation (5%), coma (5%), confusion (5%)

(Continued)

Arsenic Trioxide *(Continued)*

Dermatologic: Erythema (10%), hyperpigmentation (8%), petechia (8%), skin lesions (8%), urticaria (8%), local exfoliation (5%)

Endocrine & metabolic: Hypocalcemia (10%), hypoglycemia (8%), acidosis (5%)

Gastrointestinal: Dyspepsia (10%), loose stools (10%), abdominal distension (8%), abdominal tenderness (8%), dry mouth (8%), fecal incontinence (8%), gastrointestinal hemorrhage (8%), hemorrhagic diarrhea (8%), oral blistering (8%), weight loss (8%), oral candidiasis (5%)

Genitourinary: Intermenstrual bleeding (8%), incontinence (5%)

Hematologic: Neutropenia (10%), DIC (8%), hemorrhage (8%), lymphadenopathy (8%)

Neuromuscular & skeletal: Weakness (10%)

Ocular: Blurred vision (10%), eye irritation (10%), dry eye (8%), eyelid edema (5%), painful eye (5%)

Otic: Earache (8%), tinnitus (5%)

Renal: Renal failure (8%), renal impairment (8%), oliguria (5%)

Respiratory: Crepitations (10%), decreased breath sounds (10%), rales (10%), hemoptysis (8%), rhonchi (8%), tachypnea (8%), nasopharyngitis (5%)

Miscellaneous: Diaphoresis increased (10%), injection site edema (10%), bacterial infection (8%), herpes zoster (8%), night sweats (8%), hypersensitivity (5%), sepsis (5%)

Vesicant No

Emetic Potential High (60% to 90%)

Overdosage/Toxicology Symptoms of arsenic toxicity include convulsions, muscle weakness, and confusion. Discontinue treatment and begin chelation therapy. One suggested adult protocol: Dimercaprol 3 mg/kg I.M. every 4 hours, continue until life-threatening toxicity has subsided; follow with penicillamine 250 mg orally up to 4 times/day (total daily dose ≤1 g).

Drug Interactions

Increased Effect/Toxicity: Use caution with medications causing hypokalemia or hypomagnesemia (ampho B, aminoglycosides, diuretics, cyclosporin). Use caution with medications that prolong the QT interval, avoid concurrent use if possible; includes type Ia and type III antiarrhythmic agents, selected quinolones (sparfloxacin, gatifloxacin, moxifloxacin, grepafloxacin), cisapride, thioridazine, and other agents.

Ethanol/Nutrition/Herb Interactions

Food: Avoid seafood (due to presence of arsenic as arsenobetaine and arsenocholine).

Herb/Nutraceutical: Avoid homeopathic products (arsenic is present in some homeopathic medications).

Storage/Stability Store at room temperature, 25°C (77°F); do not freeze. Following dilution, stable for 24 hours at room temperature or 48 hours when refrigerated.

Reconstitution Dilute in 100-250 mL D_5W or 0.9% NaCl. Discard unused portion.

Pharmacodynamics/Kinetics

Metabolism: Hepatic; pentavalent arsenic is reduced to trivalent arsenic (active) by arsenate reductase; trivalent arsenic is methylated to monomethylarsinic acid, which is then converted to dimethylarsinic acid via methyltransferases

Excretion: Urine (as methylated metabolite); disposition not yet studied

Dosage I.V.: Children >5 years and Adults:

Induction: 0.15 mg/kg/day; administer daily until bone marrow remission; maximum induction: 60 doses

Consolidation: 0.15 mg/kg/day starting 3-6 weeks after completion of induction therapy; maximum consolidation: 25 doses over 5 weeks

Dosage adjustment in renal impairment: Safety and efficacy have not been established; use with caution due to renal elimination

Dosage adjustment in hepatic impairment: Safety and efficacy have not been established

Elderly: Safety and efficacy have not been established; clinical trials included patients ≤72 years of age; use with caution due to the increased risk of renal impairment in the elderly

Administration I.V. infusion over 1-2 hours. If acute vasomotor reactions occur, infuse over a maximum of 4 hours. Does not require administration via a central venous catheter.

Dosage Forms Injection, solution [preservative free]: 1 mg/mL (10 mL)

Monitoring Parameters Baseline then weekly 12-lead ECG, baseline then twice weekly serum electrolytes, hematologic and coagulation profiles at least twice weekly; more frequent monitoring may be necessary in unstable patients

Patient Information Check other medications with prescriber. Some medications may not mix well. Avoid homeopathic, herbal, or over-the-counter medications during treatment without approval of prescriber. You may not be alert. Avoid driving, doing other tasks or hobbies until response to drug is known. May cause fatigue, fever, nausea, vomiting, diarrhea, cough, or headache. Contact prescriber immediately for unexplained fever, shortness of breath, lightheadedness, passing out, rapid heartbeats, or weight gain. ECG and blood tests will be performed regularly during treatment.

Additional Information Arsenic is stored in liver, kidney, heart, lung, hair, and nails. Arsenic trioxide is a human carcinogen.

Selected Readings

Chen Z, Chen GQ, Shen ZX, et al, "Expanding the Use of Arsenic Trioxide: Leukemias and Beyond," *Semin Hematol*, 2002, 39(2 Suppl 1):22-6.

Davison K, Mann KK, and Miller WH Jr, "Arsenic Trioxide: Mechanisms of Action," *Semin Hematol*, 2002, 39(2 Suppl 1):3-7.

Evens AM, Tallman MS, and Gartenhaus RB, "The Potential of Arsenic Trioxide in the Treatment of Malignant Disease: Past, Present, and Future," *Leuk Res*, 2004, 28(9):891-900.

Hussein MA, "Arsenic Trioxide: A New Immunomodulatory Agent in the Management of Multiple Myeloma," *Med Oncol*, 2001, 18(4):239-42.

Liu P and Han ZC, "Treatment of Acute Promyelocytic Leukemia and Other Hematologic Malignancies With Arsenic Trioxide: Review of Clinical and Basic Studies," *Int J Hematol*, 2003, 78(1):32-9.

Mathews V, Chandy M, and Srivastava A, "Arsenic Trioxide in the Management of Acute Promyelocytic Leukaemia," *Natl Med J India*, 2001, 14(4):215-22.

Miller WH Jr, Schipper HM, Lee JS, et al, "Mechanisms of Action of Arsenic Trioxide," *Cancer Res*, 2002, 62(14):3893-903.

Vey N, "Arsenic Trioxide for the Treatment of Myelodysplastic Syndromes," *Expert Opin Pharmacother*, 2004, 5(3):613-21.

(Continued)

Arsenic Trioxide *(Continued)*

Zhang TD, Chen GQ, Wang ZG, et al, "Arsenic Trioxide, a Therapeutic Agent for APL," *Oncogene*, 2001, 20(49):7146-53.

Asparaginase *(a SPEAR a ji nase)*

Medication Safety Issues
Sound-alike/look-alike issues:
Asparaginase may be confused with pegaspargase

Related Information
Safe Handling of Hazardous Drugs *on page 1034*

U.S. Brand Names Elspar®

Canadian Brand Names Elspar®; Kidrolase®

Generic Available No

Synonyms *E. coli* Asparaginase; *Erwinia* Asparaginase; L-asparaginase; NSC-106977 (*Erwinia*); NSC-109229 (*E. coli*)

Pharmacologic Category Antineoplastic Agent, Miscellaneous

Pregnancy Risk Factor C

Lactation Excretion in breast milk unknown

Use Treatment of acute lymphocytic leukemia, lymphoma

Mechanism of Action Asparaginase inhibits protein synthesis by hydrolyzing asparagine to aspartic acid and ammonia. Leukemia cells, specially lymphoblasts, require exogenous asparagine; normal cells can synthesize asparagine. Asparaginase is cycle-specific for the G_1 phase.

Labeled Contraindications Hypersensitivity to asparaginase or any component of the formulation; history of anaphylaxis to asparaginase; pancreatitis (active or any history of); if a reaction occurs to Elspar®, pegaspargase may be used cautiously

Warnings/Precautions Hazardous agent - use appropriate precautions for handling and disposal. See Safe Handling of Hazardous Drugs *on page 1034* in the Appendix. Monitor for severe allergic reactions. May alter hepatic function. Use cautiously in patients with an underlying coagulopathy. Up to 33% of patients who have an allergic reaction to *E. coli* asparaginase will also react to the *Erwinia* form or pegaspargase.

A test dose is often recommended prior to the first dose of asparaginase, or prior to restarting therapy after a hiatus of several days. **False-negative rates of up to 80% to test doses of 2-50 units are reported.** Desensitization may be performed in patients found to be hypersensitive by the intradermal test dose or who have received previous courses of therapy with the drug.

Adverse Reactions Note: Immediate effects: Fever, chills, nausea, and vomiting occur in 50% to 60% of patients.

>10%:
Central nervous system: Fatigue, somnolence, depression, hallucinations, agitation, disorientation or convulsions (10% to 60%), stupor, confusion, coma (25%)

Endocrine & metabolic: Fever, chills (50% to 60%), hyperglycemia (10%)

Gastrointestinal: Nausea, vomiting (50% to 60%), anorexia, abdominal cramps (70%), acute pancreatitis (15%, may be severe in some patients)

Hematologic: Hypofibrinogenemia and depression of clotting factors V and VIII, variable decreased in factors VII and IX, severe protein C deficiency and decrease in antithrombin III (may be dose-limiting or fatal)

Hepatic: Transaminases, bilirubin, and alkaline phosphatase increased (transient)

Hypersensitivity: Acute allergic reactions (fever, rash, urticaria, arthralgia, hypotension, angioedema, bronchospasm, anaphylaxis (15% to 35%); may be dose-limiting in some patients, may be fatal)

Renal: Azotemia (66%)

1% to 10%:

Endocrine & metabolic: Hyperuricemia

Gastrointestinal: Stomatitis

<1%: Acute renal failure, albumin decreased, coma, cough, disorientation, drowsiness, fibrinogen decreased, hallucinations, hyperthermia, hypotension, insulin-dependent diabetes, ketoacidosis, laryngospasm, venous thrombosis, Parkinsonian symptoms (including tremor and increased muscle tone), pruritus, rash, seizure, serum cholesterol decreased, urticaria, weight loss; mild to moderate myelosuppression, leukopenia, anemia, thrombocytopenia (Onset: 7 days, Nadir: 14 days, Recovery: 21 days)

Vesicant No

Emetic Potential Moderate (30% to 60%)

Overdosage/Toxicology Symptoms of overdose include nausea and diarrhea.

Drug Interactions

Increased Effect/Toxicity: Increased toxicity has been noticed when asparaginase is administered with vincristine (neuropathy) and prednisone (hyperglycemia). Decreased metabolism when used with cyclophosphamide. Increased hepatotoxicity when used with mercaptopurine.

Decreased Effect: Asparaginase terminates methotrexate action.

Storage/Stability Intact vials of powder should be refrigerated (<8°C); reconstituted solutions are stable 1 week at room temperature. Solutions for I.V. infusion are stable for 8 hours at room temperature or under refrigeration.

Reconstitution Lyophilized powder should be reconstituted with 1-5 mL sterile water or NS for I.V. administration; NS for I.M. use. Use of a 5 micron filter has been suggested to remove fiber-like particles. Shake well but not too vigorously; use of a 5 micron in-line filter is recommended to remove fiber-like particles in the solution (not 0.2 micron filter - has been associated with some loss of potency).

Standard I.M./SubQ dilution: 2000, 5000, or 10,000 units/mL: 2 mL/ syringe

Standard I.V. dilution: 50-250 mL NS or D_5W

Compatibility Stable in D_5W, NS

Y-site administration: Compatible: Methotrexate, sodium bicarbonate

Pharmacodynamics/Kinetics

Absorption: I.M.: Produces peak blood levels 50% lower than those from I.V. administration

Distribution: V_d: 4-5 L/kg; 70% to 80% of plasma volume; does not penetrate CSF

Metabolism: Systemically degraded

Half-life elimination: 8-30 hours

Excretion: Urine (trace amounts)

(Continued)

Asparaginase *(Continued)*

Clearance: Unaffected by age, renal or hepatic function

Dosage Refer to individual protocols.

Children:

I.V.:

Infusion for induction: 1000 units/kg/day for 10 days

Consolidation: 6000-10,000 units/m^2/day for 14 days

I.M.: 6000 units/m^2 on days 4, 7, 10, 13, 16, 19, 22, 25, 28

Adults:

I.V. infusion single agent for induction:

200 units/kg/day for 28 days **or**

5000-10,000 units/m^2/day for 7 days every 3 weeks **or**

10,000-40,000 units every 2-3 weeks

I.M. as single agent: 6000-12,000 units/m^2; reconstitution to 10,000 units/mL may be necessary

Some institutions recommended the following precautions for asparaginase administration: Have parenteral epinephrine, diphenhydramine, and hydrocortisone available at the bedside. Have a freely running I.V. in place. Have a physician readily accessible. Monitor the patient closely for 30-60 minutes. Avoid administering the drug at night.

Some practitioners recommend a desensitization regimen for patients who react to a test dose, or are being retreated following a break in therapy. Doses are doubled and given every 10 minutes until the total daily dose for that day has been administered. See table.

Asparaginase Desensitization

Injection No.	Elspar Dose (int. units)	Accumulated Total Dose
1	1	1
2	2	3
3	4	7
4	8	15
5	16	31
6	32	63
7	64	127
8	128	255
9	256	511
10	512	1023
11	1024	2047
12	2048	4095
13	4096	8191
14	8192	16,383
15	16,384	32,767
16	32,768	65,535
17	65,536	131,071
18	131,072	262,143

For example, if a patient was to receive a total dose of 4000 units, he/she would receive injections 1 through 12 during the desensitization

Combination Regimens
Leukemia, acute lymphocytic:
Larson Regimen *on page 904*
Linker Protocol *on page 904*
PVA (POG 8602) *on page 932*
PVA (POG 9005) *on page 934*
PVDA *on page 936*
Leukemia, acute myeloid: CA *on page 849*

Administration May be administered I.M., I.V., or SubQ

I.M.: Doses should be given as a deep intramuscular injection into a large muscle

Note: I.V. administration greatly increases the risk of allergic reactions and should be avoided if possible.

I.V.: I.V. infusion in 50-250 mL of D_5W or NS over at least 60 minutes. The manufacturer recommends a test dose (0.1 mL of a dilute 20 units/ mL solution) prior to initial administration and when given after an interval of 7 days or more. Institutional policies vary.

Gelatinous fiber-like particles may develop on standing; filtration through a 5-micron filter during administration will remove the particles with no loss of potency

Dosage Forms Injection, powder for reconstitution: 10,000 units

Monitoring Parameters Vital signs during administration, CBC, urinalysis, amylase, liver enzymes, prothrombin time, renal function tests, urine dipstick for glucose, blood glucose, uric acid. Be prepared to treat anaphylaxis at each administration; monitor for onset of abdominal pain and mental status changes.

Patient Information This medication can be given I.M., I.V., or subcutaneously. It is vital to maintain good hydration (2-3 L/day of fluids unless instructed to restrict fluid intake) and good nutritional status (small frequent meals may help). You may experience acute gastric disturbances (eg, nausea or vomiting); frequent mouth care or lozenges may help or antiemetic may be prescribed. Report any respiratory difficulty, skin rash, or acute anxiety immediately. Report unusual fever or chills, confusion, agitation, depression, yellowing of skin or eyes, unusual bleeding or bruising, unhealed sores, or vaginal discharge. Contraceptive measures are recommended during therapy.

Additional Information The *E. coli* and the *Erwinia* strains of asparaginase differ slightly in their gene sequencing, and have slight differences in their enzyme characteristics. Both are highly specific for asparagine and have <10% activity for the D-isomer. The *E. coli* form is most commonly used.

Selected Readings
Capizzi RL, "Asparaginase Revisited," *Leukemia & Lymphoma*, 1993, 10(Suppl):147-50.
Ettinger LJ, Ettinger AG, Avramis VI, et al, "Acute Lymphoblastic Leukemia: A Guide to Asparaginase and Pegaspargase Therapy," *BioDrugs*, 1997, 7:30-9.
Gallagher MP, Marshall RD, and Wilson R, "Asparaginase as a Drug for Treatment of Acute Lymphoblastic Leukemia," *Essays Biochem*, 1989, 24:1-40.
Keating MJ, Holmes R, Lerner S, et al, "L-Asparaginase and PEG Asparaginase - Past, Present, and Future," *Leukemia & Lymphoma*, 1993, 10(Suppl):153-7.
Muller HJ and Boos J,"Use of L-Asparaginase in Childhood ALL," *Crit Rev Oncol Hematol*, 1998, 28(2):97-113.

♦ **Astramorph/PF**™ *see* Morphine Sulfate *on page 588*

♦ **Atarax**® *see* HydrOXYzine *on page 436*

♦ **ATG** *see* Antithymocyte Globulin (Equine) *on page 96*

- ◆ **ATG** *see* Antithymocyte Globulin (Rabbit) *on page 98*
- ◆ **Atgam**® *see* Antithymocyte Globulin (Equine) *on page 96*
- ◆ **AT III** *see* Antithrombin III *on page 94*
- ◆ **Ativan**® *see* Lorazepam *on page 517*
- ◆ **ATRA** *see* Tretinoin (Oral) *on page 792*
- ◆ **Avastin**™ *see* Bevacizumab *on page 124*
- ◆ **Avinza**™ *see* Morphine Sulfate *on page 588*
- ◆ **AY-25650** *see* Triptorelin *on page 801*

Azacitidine (ay za SYE ti deen)

Related Information
Investigational Drug Service *on page 1031*
Safe Handling of Hazardous Drugs *on page 1034*

U.S. Brand Names Vidaza™

Generic Available No

Synonyms AZA-CR; 5-Azacytidine; 5-AZC; Ladakamycin; NSC-102816

Pharmacologic Category Antineoplastic Agent, Antimetabolite (Pyrimidine)

Pregnancy Risk Factor D

Lactation Excretion in breast milk unknown/not recommended

Use Treatment of myelodysplastic syndrome (MDS)

Unlabeled/Investigational Use Investigational: Refractory acute lymphocytic and myelogenous leukemia

Mechanism of Action Antineoplastic effects may be a result of azacitidine's ability to promote hypomethylation of DNA leading to direct toxicity of abnormal hematopoietic cells in the bone marrow.

Labeled Contraindications Hypersensitivity to azacitidine, mannitol, or any component of the formulation; advanced malignant hepatic tumors; pregnancy

Warnings/Precautions Hazardous agent - use appropriate precautions for handling and disposal. See Safe Handling of Hazardous Drugs *on page 1034* in the Appendix. Azacitidine may be hepatotoxic, use caution with hepatic impairment. Progressive hepatic coma leading to death has been reported (rare) in patients with extensive tumor burden, especially those with a baseline albumin <30 g/L. Use caution with renal impairment; dose adjustment may be required. **Solutions for injection have very limited stability and must be prepared immediately prior to each dose.**

Adverse Reactions Note: Percentages reported following SubQ administration unless otherwise noted:

>10%:
Cardiovascular: Hypotension (7%; I.V. 6% to 66% - incidence may be related to dose and rate of infusion), chest pain (16%), pallor (15%), peripheral edema (19%), pitting edema (14%)

Central nervous system: Pyrexia (52%), fatigue (13% to 36%), headache (22%), dizziness (19%), anxiety (13%), depression (12%), insomnia (11%), malaise (11%), pain (11%)

Dermatologic: Alopecia (I.V. 20%), bruising (30%), petechiae (24%), erythema (17%), skin lesion (14%); rash (14%), redness, irritation, and induration at injection site (80%)

Gastrointestinal: Nausea (58% to 85%; more common/more severe with I.V. administration), vomiting (54%; more common/more severe with I.V. administration), mucositis (I.V. 23% to 45%), diarrhea (36%), constipation (34%), anorexia (21%), weight loss (16%), abdominal pain (15%), appetite decreased (13%), abdominal tenderness (12%)

Hematologic: Anemia (70%), thrombocytopenia (66%), leukopenia (48%), neutropenia (32%), febrile neutropenia (16%)

Nadir: Day 10-17

Recovery: Day 28-31

Hepatic: Hepatic enzymes increased (I.V. 37%)

Local: Injection site:

I.V.: Redness, irritation, and induration (80%)

SubQ: Erythema (35%), pain (23%), bruising (14%)

Neuromuscular & skeletal: Weakness (30%), rigors (26%), arthralgia (22%), limb pain (20%), back pain (19%), myalgia (16%)

Respiratory: Cough (30%), dyspnea (5% to 30%), pharyngitis (20%), epistaxis (16%), nasopharyngitis (14%), upper respiratory tract infection (13%), productive cough (11%), pneumonia (11%)

Miscellaneous: Contusion (19%)

5% to 10%:

Cardiovascular: Cardiac murmur (10%), tachycardia (9%) peripheral swelling (7%), syncope (6%), chest wall pain (5%), hypoesthesia (5%), postprocedural pain (5%)

Central nervous system: Lethargy (8%)

Dermatologic: Cellulitis (8%), urticaria (6%), dry skin (5%), skin nodule (5%)

Gastrointestinal: Upper abdominal pain (10%), gingival bleeding (9%), oral mucosal petechiae (8%), stomatitis (8%), dyspepsia (7%), hemorrhoids (7%), abdominal distension (6%), loose stools (5%), dysphagia (5%), tongue ulceration (5%)

Genitourinary: Dysuria (8%), urinary tract infection (8%)

Hematologic: Hematoma (9%), postprocedural hemorrhage (6%)

Local: Injection site: Pruritus (7%), granuloma (5%), pigmentation change (5%), swelling (5%)

Neuromuscular & skeletal: Muscle cramps (6%)

Respiratory: Crackles (10%), rhinorrhea (10%), wheezing (9%), breath sounds decreased (8%), pleural effusion (6%), postnasal drip (6%), rhonchi (6%), nasal congestion (5%), atelectasis (5%), sinusitis (5%)

Miscellaneous: Diaphoresis (10%), lymphadenopathy (9%), herpes simplex (9%), night sweats (9%), transfusion reaction (7%), mouth hemorrhage (5%)

<5% (Limited to important or life-threatening): Agranulocytosis, anaphylactic shock, bone marrow depression, CHF, convulsions, dehydration, diverticulitis, hypersensitivity reaction, pyoderma gangrenosum, splenomegaly; myalgia, weakness, and lethargy progressing to somnolence, stupor, or coma (<1%)

Vesicant No. Subcutaneous injection of undissolved crystals may cause localized reactions.

Emetic Potential Moderate (30% to 60%)

Overdosage/Toxicology Diarrhea, nausea, and vomiting were reported following a single I.V. dose of 290 mg/m². Treatment should be supportive.

Storage/Stability

SubQ: Prior to reconstitution, store powder at room temperature of 15°C to 30°C (59°F to 86°F). Following reconstitution, suspension may be (Continued)

Azacitidine *(Continued)*

stored at room temperature for up to 1 hour, or immediately refrigerated at 2°C to 8°C (36°F to 46°F) and stored for up to 8 hours.

I.V.: **Solutions for injection have very limited stability and must be prepared fresh immediately prior to each dose.** Solutions (≥2 mg/mL) in lactated Ringer's injection are stable for 3 hours; solutions in 5% dextrose in water or 0.9% sodium chloride injection are only stable for ~1 hour.

Reconstitution

SubQ: Slowly add 4 mL SWFI to each vial. Invert vial 2-3 times and gently rotate until a suspension is formed.

I.V.: Reconstitute vial with 19.9 mL of lactated Ringer's injection, 0.9% sodium chloride, or 5% dextrose to form a 5 mg/mL solution. Mix in 50-250 mL (final concentration ≥2 mg/mL) lactated Ringer's injection for infusion.

Pharmacodynamics/Kinetics

Absorption: SubQ: Rapid and complete

Bioavailability: SubQ: 89%

Distribution: V_d: 76 ± 26 L; does not cross blood-brain barrier

Metabolism: Hepatic; hydrolysis to several metabolites

Half-life elimination: ~4 hours

Time to peak concentration: 30 minutes

Excretion: Urine (50% to 85%); feces (minor)

Dosage

I.V. (unlabeled use, doses reported in combination regimens):

Children:

Pediatric AML and ANLL: 250 mg/m^2 days 4 and 5 every 4 weeks

Pediatric AML induction: 300 mg/m^2 days 5 and 6

Adults:

Acute leukemia:

50-150 mg/m^2 days 1 through 5 of induction

200 mg/m^2 CIVI days 7 through 9 of induction

CML (accelerated phase and blast crisis): 50-150 mg/m^2 days 1 through 5 of induction

AML induction: 150 mg/m^2 days 3 through 5 and 8 through 10, **then** 150 mg/m^2 days 1 through 5 and 8 through 10 (cycle 2 consolidation)

AML consolidation: 150 mg/m^2 CIVI days 1 through 7 for 3 cycles

AML maintenance: 150 mg/m^2 days 1 through 3 every 6 weeks

MDS: 75-150 mg/m^2 CIVI days 1 through 7 every 4 weeks

SubQ: MDS: 75 mg/m^2/day for 7 days repeated every 4 weeks. Dose may be increased to 100 mg/m^2/day if no benefit is observed after 2 cycles and no toxicity other than nausea and vomiting have occurred. Treatment is recommended for at least 4 cycles.

Dosage adjustment based on hematology: Adults: SubQ:

For baseline WBC ≥3.0 x 10^9/L, ANC ≥1.5 x 10^9/L, and platelets ≥75 x 10^9/L:

Nadir count: ANC <0.5 x 10^9/L and platelets <25 x 10^9/L: Administer 50% of dose during next treatment course

Nadir count: ANC 0.5-1.5 x 10^9/L and platelets 25-50 x 10^9/L: Administer 67% of dose during next treatment course

Nadir count: ANC >1.5 x 10^9/L and platelets >50 x 10^9/L: Administer 100% of dose during next treatment course

For baseline WBC <3 x 10^9/L, ANC 1.5 x 10^9/L, or platelets <75 x 10^9/L: Adjust dose as follows based on nadir counts and bone marrow biopsy cellularity at the time of nadir, unless clear improvement in differentiation at the time of the next cycle:

WBC or platelet nadir decreased 50% to 75% from baseline and bone marrow biopsy cellularity at time of nadir 30% to 60%: Administer 100% of dose during next treatment course

WBC or platelet nadir decreased 50% to 75% from baseline and bone marrow biopsy cellularity at time of nadir 15% to 30%: Administer 50% of dose during next treatment course

WBC or platelet nadir decreased 50% to 75% from baseline and bone marrow biopsy cellularity at time of nadir <15%: Administer 33% of dose during next treatment course

WBC or platelet nadir decreased >75% from baseline and bone marrow biopsy cellularity at time of nadir 30% to 60%: Administer 75% of dose during next treatment course

WBC or platelet nadir decreased >75% from baseline and bone marrow biopsy cellularity at time of nadir 15% to 30%: Administer 50% of dose during next treatment course

WBC or platelet nadir decreased >75% from baseline and bone marrow biopsy cellularity at time of nadir <15%: Administer 33% of dose during next treatment course

Note: If a nadir defined above occurs, administer the next treatment course 28 days after the start of the preceding course as long as WBC and platelet counts are >25% above the nadir and rising. If a >25% increase above the nadir is not seen by day 28, reassess counts every 7 days. If a 25% increase is not seen by day 42, administer 50% of the scheduled dose.

Dosage adjustment based on serum electrolytes: The manufacturer recommends that if serum bicarbonate falls to <20 mEq/L (unexplained decrease), reduce dose by 50% for next treatment course

Dosage adjustment in renal impairment: If increases in BUN or serum creatinine occur, delay next cycle until values reach baseline or normal, then reduce dose by 50% for next treatment course.

Administration

I.V.: Administer I.V. via bolus (15 minutes to 2 hours) or continuous infusion (24 hours). Due to limited stability, the dose for continuous infusion should be divided by $1/2$, and a freshly prepared dose, using a freshly reconstituted vial, should be started every 12 hours.

SubQ: Doses >50 mg (2 mL) may be divided into 2 syringes. Rotate site for each injection (thigh, abdomen, or upper arm). Allow refrigerated suspensions to come to room temperature prior to injection. Resuspend by gently rolling the syringe between the palms for 30 seconds.

Dosage Forms Injection, powder for suspension: 100 mg [contains mannitol 100 mg]

Monitoring Parameters Liver function tests, electrolytes, CBC, renal function tests (BUN and serum creatinine) should be obtained prior to initiation of therapy. Electrolytes, renal function (BUN and creatinine), CBC should be monitored periodically to monitor response and toxicity. At a minimum, CBC should be repeated prior to each cycle.

Special Geriatric Considerations Monitor renal function

(Continued)

Azacitidine *(Continued)*

Selected Readings

Aparicio A and Weber JS, "Review of the Clinical Experience With 5-Azacytidine and 5-Aza-2′-deoxycytidine in Solid Tumors," *Curr Opin Investig Drugs*, 2002, 3(4):627-33.

Beran M, "Intensive Chemotherapy for Patients With High-Risk Myelodysplastic Syndrome," *Int J Hematol*, 2000, 72(2):139-50.

Cheson BD, Zwiebel JA, Dancey J, et al, "Novel Therapeutic Agents for the Treatment of Myelodysplastic Syndromes," *Semin Oncol*, 2000, 27(5):560-77.

Christman JK, "5-Azacytidine and 5-aza-2′-deoxycytidine as Inhibitors of DNA Methylation: Mechanistic Studies and Their Implications for Cancer Therapy," *Oncogene*, 2002, 21(35):5483-95.

Dutcher JP, Eudey L, Wiernik PH, et al, "Phase II Study of Mitoxantrone and 5-Azacytidine for Accelerated and Blast Crisis of Chronic Myelogenous Leukemia: A Study of the Eastern Cooperative Oncology Group," *Leukemia*, 1992, 6(8):770-5.

Goldberg J, Gryn J, Raza A, et al, "Mitoxantrone and 5-Azacytidine for Refractory/Relapsed ANLL or CML in Blast Crisis: A Leukemia Intergroup Study," *Am J Hematol*, 1993, 43(4):286-90.

Holcombe E, Grier HE, Gelber RD, et al, "Intensive Sequential Chemotherapy for Children With Acute Myelogenous Leukemia: VAPA, 80-035, and HI-C-Daze," *Leukemia*, 1992, (6 Suppl 2):48-51.

Hurwitz CA, Krance R, Schell MJ, et al, "Current Strategies for Treatment of Acute Myeloid Leukemia at St Jude Children's Research Hospital," *Leukemia*, 1992, (6 Suppl 2):39-43.

Jehn U, "Long-term Outcome of Postremission Chemotherapy for Adults With Acute Myeloid Leukemia Using Different Dose-Intensities," *Leuk Lymphoma*, 1994, 15(1-2):99-112.

Jehn U, Zittoun R, Suciu S, et al, "A Randomized Comparison of Intensive Maintenance Treatment for Adult Acute Myelogenous Leukemia Using Either Cyclic Alternating Drugs or Repeated Courses of the Induction-Type Chemotherapy: AML-6 Trial of the EORTC Leukemia Cooperative Group," *Haematol Blood Transfus*, 1990, 33:277-84.

Kornblith AB, Herndon JE 2nd, Silverman LR, et al, "Impact of Azacytidine on the Quality of Life of Patients With Myelodysplastic Syndrome Treated in a Randomized Phase III Trial: A Cancer and Leukemia Group B Study," *J Clin Oncol*, 2002, 20(10):2441-52.

Kritz AD, Raptis G, Menendez-Botet C, et al, "Pilot Study of 5-Azacytidine (5-AZA) and Carboplatin (CBDCA) in Patients With Relapsed/Refractory Leukemia," *Am J Hematol*, 1996, 51(2):117-21.

Rees JK, Gray RG, and Wheatley K, "Dose Intensification in Acute Myeloid Leukaemia: Greater Effectiveness at lower cost. Principal Report of the Medical Research Council's AML9 Study. MRC Leukaemia in Adults Working Party," *Br J Haematol*, 1996, 94(1):89-98.

Silverman LR, Demakos EP, Peterson BL, et al, "Randomized Controlled Trial of Azacitidine in Patients With the Myelodysplastic Syndrome: A Study of the Cancer and Leukemia Group B," *J Clin Oncol*, 2002, 20(10):2429-40.

Silverman LR, Holland JF, Weinberg RS, et al, "Effects of Treatment With 5-Azacytidine on the *in vivo* and *in vitro* Hematopoiesis in Patients With Myelodysplastic Syndromes," *Leukemia*, 1993, (7 Suppl 1):21-9.

Steuber CP, Krischer J, Holbrook T, et al, "Therapy of Refractory or Recurrent Childhood Acute Myeloid Leukemia Using Amsacrine and Etoposide With or Without Azacitidine: A Pediatric Oncology Group Randomized Phase II Study," *J Clin Oncol*, 1996, 14(5):1521-5.

Steuber CP, Holbrook T, Camitta B, et al, "Toxicity Trials of Amsacrine (AMSA) and Etoposide ± Azacitidine (AZ) in Childhood Acute Non-Lymphocytic Leukemia (ANLL): A Pilot Study," *Invest New Drugs*, 1991, 9(2):181-4.

Volger WR, Weiner RS, Moore JO, et al, "Long-term Follow-up of a Randomized Post-Induction Therapy Trial in Acute Myelogenous Leukemia (A Southeastern Cancer Study Group Trial)," *Leukemia*, 1995, 9(9):1456-60.

♦ **AZA-CR** *see* Azacitidine *on page 110*

♦ **Azactam**® *see* Aztreonam *on page 115*

♦ **5-Azacytidine** *see* Azacitidine *on page 110*

♦ **5-AZC** *see* Azacitidine *on page 110*

♦ **Azthreonam** *see* Aztreonam *on page 115*

Aztreonam (AZ tree oh nam)
Medication Safety Issues
Sound-alike/look-alike issues:
Aztreonam may be confused with azidothymidine
Related Information
Management of Infections *on page 978*
U.S. Brand Names Azactam®
Canadian Brand Names Azactam®
Generic Available No
Synonyms Azthreonam
Pharmacologic Category Antibiotic, Miscellaneous
Pregnancy Risk Factor B
Lactation Enters breast milk/not recommended (AAP rates "compatible")
Use Treatment of patients with urinary tract infections, lower respiratory tract infections, septicemia, skin/skin structure infections, intra-abdominal infections, and gynecological infections caused by susceptible gram-negative bacilli
Mechanism of Action Inhibits bacterial cell wall synthesis by binding to one or more of the penicillin binding proteins (PBPs); which in turn inhibits the final transpeptidation step of peptidoglycan synthesis in bacterial cell walls, thus inhibiting cell wall biosynthesis. Bacteria eventually lyse due to ongoing activity of cell wall autolytic enzymes (autolysins and murein hydrolases) while cell wall assembly is arrested. Monobactam structure makes cross-allergenicity with beta-lactams unlikely.
Labeled Contraindications Hypersensitivity to aztreonam or any component of the formulation
Warnings/Precautions Rare cross-allergenicity to penicillins and cephalosporins has been reported. Use caution in renal impairment; dosing adjustment required.
Adverse Reactions As reported in adults:
1% to 10%:
Dermatologic: Rash
Gastrointestinal: Diarrhea, nausea, vomiting
Local: Thrombophlebitis, pain at injection site
<1%: Abdominal cramps, abnormal taste, anaphylaxis, anemia, angioedema, aphthous ulcer, breast tenderness, bronchospasm, *C. difficile*-associated diarrhea, chest pain, confusion, diaphoresis, diplopia, dizziness, dyspnea, eosinophilia, erythema multiforme, exfoliative dermatitis, fever, flushing, halitosis, headache, hepatitis, hypotension, insomnia, jaundice, leukopenia, liver enzymes increased, muscular aches myalgia, neutropenia, numb tongue, pancytopenia, paresthesia, petechiae, pruritus, pseudomembranous colitis, purpura, seizure, sneezing, thrombocytopenia, tinnitus, toxic epidermal necrolysis, urticaria, vaginitis, vertigo, weakness, wheezing
Vesicant No
Emetic Potential Very low (<10%)
Overdosage/Toxicology Symptoms of overdose include seizures. Treatment is supportive. If necessary, dialysis can reduce the drug concentration in the blood.
Drug Interactions
Decreased Effect: Avoid antibiotics that induce beta-lactamase production (cefoxitin, imipenem).
(Continued)

Aztreonam *(Continued)*

Storage/Stability Prior to reconstitution, store at room temperature. Avoid excessive heat. Use reconstituted solutions and I.V. solutions (in NS and D_5W) within 48 hours if kept at room temperature (25°C) or 7 days if kept in refrigerator (4°C). Solution for infusion may be frozen at <-2°C (<-4°F) for up to 3 months. Thawed solution should be used within 24 hours if thawed at room temperature or within 72 hours if thawed under refrigeration. **Do not refreeze.**

Reconstitution Reconstituted solutions are colorless to light yellow straw and may turn pink upon standing without affecting potency.

I.M.: Reconstitute with at least 3 mL SWFI, sterile bacteriostatic water for injection, NS, or bacteriostatic sodium chloride.

I.V.:

Bolus injection: Reconstitute with 6-10 mL SWFI. The final concentration should not exceed 20 mg/mL.

Infusion: Reconstitute to a final concentration ≤2%.

Compatibility Solution for infusion: D_5LR, $D_5^1/_4NS$, $D_5^1/_2NS$, D_5NS, D_5W, $D_{10}W$, mannitol 5%, mannitol 10%, LR, NS; **variable stability (consult detailed reference)** in peritoneal dialysis solution

Y-site administration: Compatible: Allopurinol, amifostine, amikacin, aminophylline, ampicillin, ampicillin/sulbactam, bleomycin, bumetanide, buprenorphine, butorphanol, calcium gluconate, carboplatin, carmustine, cefazolin, cefepime, cefoperazone, cefotaxime, cefotetan, cefoxitin, ceftazidime, ceftizoxime, ceftriaxone, cefuroxime, cimetidine, ciprofloxacin, cisatracurium, cisplatin, clindamycin, co-trimoxazole, cyclophosphamide, cytarabine, dacarbazine, dactinomycin, dexamethasone sodium phosphate, diltiazem, diphenhydramine, dobutamine, docetaxel, dopamine, doxorubicin, doxorubicin liposome, doxycycline, droperidol, enalaprilat, etoposide, etoposide phosphate, famotidine, filgrastim, floxuridine, fluconazole, fludarabine, fluorouracil, foscarnet, furosemide, gatifloxacin, gemcitabine, gentamicin, granisetron, haloperidol, heparin, hydrocortisone sodium phosphate, hydrocortisone sodium succinate, hydromorphone, hydroxyzine, idarubicin, ifosfamide, imipenem/cilastatin, insulin (regular), leucovorin, linezolid, magnesium sulfate, mannitol, mechlorethamine, melphalan, meperidine, mesna, methotrexate, methylprednisolone sodium succinate, metoclopramide, minocycline, morphine, nalbuphine, netilmicin, ondansetron, piperacillin, piperacillin/tazobactam, plicamycin, potassium chloride, promethazine, propofol, ranitidine, remifentanil, sargramostim, sodium bicarbonate, teniposide, theophylline, thiotepa, ticarcillin, ticarcillin/clavulanate, tobramycin, vinblastine, vincristine, vinorelbine, zidovudine. **Incompatible:** Acyclovir, alatrofloxacin, amphotericin B, amphotericin B cholesteryl sulfate complex, amsacrine, chlorpromazine, daunorubicin, ganciclovir, lorazepam, metronidazole, mitomycin, mitoxantrone, prochlorperazine edisylate, streptozocin. **Variable (consult detailed reference):** Vancomycin

Compatibility in syringe: Compatible: Clindamycin

Compatibility when admixed: Compatible: Ampicillin/sulbactam, cefazolin, ciprofloxacin, clindamycin, gentamicin, linezolid, tobramycin. **Incompatible:** Metronidazole, nafcillin. **Variable (consult detailed reference):** Ampicillin, cefoxitin, vancomycin

Pharmacodynamics/Kinetics

Absorption: I.M.: Well absorbed; I.M. and I.V. doses produce comparable serum concentrations

Distribution: Widely to most body fluids and tissues; crosses placenta; enters breast milk

V_d: Children: 0.2-0.29 L/kg; Adults: 0.2 L/kg

Relative diffusion of antimicrobial agents from blood into CSF: Good only with inflammation (exceeds usual MICs)

CSF:blood level ratio: Meninges: Inflamed: 8% to 40%; Normal: ~1%

Protein binding: 56%

Metabolism: Hepatic (minor %)

Half-life elimination:

Children 2 months to 12 years: 1.7 hours

Adults: Normal renal function: 1.7-2.9 hours

End-stage renal disease: 6-8 hours

Time to peak: I.M., I.V. push: Within 60 minutes; I.V. infusion: 1.5 hours

Excretion: Urine (60% to 70% as unchanged drug); feces (~13% to 15%)

Dosage

Children >1 month: I.M., I.V.:

Mild-to-moderate infections: 30 mg/kg every 8 hours

Moderate-to-severe infections: 30 mg/kg every 6-8 hours; maximum: 120 mg/kg/day (8 g/day)

Cystic fibrosis: 50 mg/kg/dose every 6-8 hours (ie, up to 200 mg/kg/day); maximum: 8 g/day

Adults:

Urinary tract infection: I.M., I.V.: 500 mg to 1 g every 8-12 hours

Moderately-severe systemic infections: 1 g I.V. or I.M. or 2 g I.V. every 8-12 hours

Severe systemic or life-threatening infections (especially caused by *Pseudomonas aeruginosa*): I.V.: 2 g every 6-8 hours; maximum: 8 g/day

Dosing adjustment in renal impairment: Adults: Following initial dose, maintenance doses should be given as follows:

Cl_{cr} 10-30 mL/minute: 50% of usual dose at the usual interval

Cl_{cr} <10 mL/minute: 25% of usual dosage at the usual interval

Hemodialysis: Moderately dialyzable (20% to 50%); $^1/_8$ of initial dose after each hemodialysis session (given in addition to the maintenance doses)

Peritoneal dialysis: Administer as for Cl_{cr} <10 mL/minute

Continuous arteriovenous or venovenous hemofiltration: Dose as for Cl_{cr} 10-30 mL/minute

Administration Doses >1 g should be administered I.V.

I.M.: Administer by deep injection into large muscle mass, such as upper outer quadrant of gluteus maximus or the lateral part of the thigh

I.V.: Administer by slow I.V. push over 3-5 minutes or by intermittent infusion over 20-60 minutes.

Dosage Forms

Infusion [premixed]: 1 g (50 mL); 2 g (50 mL)

Injection, powder for reconstitution: 500 mg, 1 g, 2 g

Monitoring Parameters Periodic liver function test; monitor for signs of anaphylaxis during first dose

Additional Information Although marketed as an agent similar to aminoglycosides, aztreonam is a monobactam antimicrobial with almost
(Continued)

Aztreonam *(Continued)*

pure gram-negative aerobic activity. It cannot be used for gram-positive infections. Aminoglycosides are often used for synergy in gram-positive infections.

Special Geriatric Considerations Adjust dose relative to renal function.

Selected Readings

Bosso JA and Black PG, "The Use of Aztreonam in Pediatric Patients: A Review," *Pharmacotherapy*, 1991, 11(1):20-5.

Brogden RN and Heel RC, "Aztreonam. A Review of Its Antibacterial Activity, Pharmacokinetic Properties and Therapeutic Use," *Drugs*, 1986, 31(2):96-130.

Creasey WA, Platt TB, Frantz M, et al, "Pharmacokinetics of Aztreonam in Elderly Male Volunteers," *Br J Clin Pharmacol*, 1985, 19:233-7.

Hellinger WC and Brewer NS, "Carbapenems and Monobactams: Imipenem, Meropenem, and Aztreonam," *Mayo Clin Proc*, 1999, 74(4):420-34.

Johnson DH and Cunha BA, "Aztreonam," *Med Clin North Am*, 1995, 79(4):733-43.

+ **B1** *see* Tositumomab and Iodine I 131 Tositumomab *on page 781*
+ **B1 Antibody** *see* Tositumomab and Iodine I 131 Tositumomab *on page 781*
+ **BA-16038** *see* Aminoglutethimide *on page 63*
+ **Bacillus Calmette-Guérin (BCG) Live** *see* BCG Vaccine *on page 120*
+ **Bactrim**™ *see* Sulfamethoxazole and Trimethoprim *on page 727*
+ **Bactrim**™ **DS** *see* Sulfamethoxazole and Trimethoprim *on page 727*

Basiliximab *(ba si LIK si mab)*

U.S. Brand Names Simulect®

Canadian Brand Names Simulect®

Generic Available No

Pharmacologic Category Monoclonal Antibody

Pregnancy Risk Factor B (manufacturer)

Lactation Excretion in breast milk unknown/not recommended

Use Prophylaxis of acute organ rejection in renal transplantation

Mechanism of Action Chimeric (murine/human) monoclonal antibody which blocks the alpha-chain of the interleukin-2 (IL-2) receptor complex; this receptor is expressed on activated T lymphocytes and is a critical pathway for activating cell-mediated allograft rejection

Labeled Contraindications Hypersensitivity basiliximab, murine proteins, or any component of the formulation

Warnings/Precautions To be used as a component of immunosuppressive regimen which includes cyclosporine and corticosteroids.

The incidence of lymphoproliferative disorders and/or opportunistic infections may be increased by immunosuppressive therapy. Severe hypersensitivity reactions, occurring within 24 hours, have been reported. Reactions, including anaphylaxis, have occurred both with the initial exposure and/or following re-exposure after several months. Use caution during re-exposure to a subsequent course of therapy in a patient who has previously received basiliximab. Discontinue the drug permanently if a reaction occurs. Medications for the treatment of hypersensitivity reactions should be available for immediate use. Treatment may result in the development of human antimurine antibodies (HAMA); however, limited evidence suggesting the use of muromonab-CD3 or other murine products is not precluded.

Adverse Reactions Administration of basiliximab did not appear to increase the incidence or severity of adverse effects in clinical trials. Adverse events were reported in 96% of both the placebo and basiliximab groups.

>10%:

Cardiovascular: Peripheral edema, hypertension, atrial fibrillation

Central nervous system: Fever, headache, insomnia, pain

Dermatologic: Wound complications, acne

Endocrine & metabolic: Hypokalemia, hyperkalemia, hyperglycemia, hyperuricemia, hypophosphatemia, hypercholesterolemia

Gastrointestinal: Constipation, nausea, diarrhea, abdominal pain, vomiting, dyspepsia

Genitourinary: Urinary tract infection

Hematologic: Anemia

Neuromuscular & skeletal: Tremor

Respiratory: Dyspnea, infection (upper respiratory)

Miscellaneous: Viral infection

3% to 10%:

Cardiovascular: Chest pain, cardiac failure, hypotension, arrhythmia, tachycardia, generalized edema, abnormal heart sounds, angina pectoris

Central nervous system: Hypoesthesia, neuropathy, agitation, anxiety, depression, malaise, fatigue, rigors, dizziness

Dermatologic: Cyst, hypertrichosis, pruritus, rash, skin disorder, skin ulceration

Endocrine & metabolic: Dehydration, diabetes mellitus, fluid overload, hypercalcemia, hyperlipidemia, hypoglycemia, hypomagnesemia, acidosis, hypertriglyceridemia, hypocalcemia, hyponatremia

Gastrointestinal: Flatulence, gastroenteritis, GI hemorrhage, gingival hyperplasia, melena, esophagitis, stomatitis, enlarged abdomen, moniliasis, ulcerative stomatitis, weight gain

Genitourinary: Impotence, genital edema, albuminuria, bladder disorder, hematuria, urinary frequency, oliguria, abnormal renal function, renal tubular necrosis, ureteral disorder, urinary retention, dysuria

Hematologic: Hematoma, hemorrhage, purpura, thrombocytopenia, thrombosis, polycythemia, leukopenia

Neuromuscular & skeletal: Arthralgia, arthropathy, cramps, fracture, hernia, myalgia, paresthesia, weakness, back pain, leg pain

Ocular: Cataract, conjunctivitis, abnormal vision

Respiratory: Bronchitis, bronchospasm, pneumonia, pulmonary edema, sinusitis, rhinitis, cough, pharyngitis

Miscellaneous: Accidental trauma, facial edema, sepsis, infection, increased glucocorticoids, herpes infection

Postmarketing and/or case reports: Severe hypersensitivity reactions, including anaphylaxis, have been reported. Symptoms may include hypotension, tachycardia, cardiac failure, dyspnea, bronchospasm, pulmonary edema, urticaria, rash, pruritus, sneezing, capillary leak syndrome, and respiratory failure.

Vesicant No

Emetic Potential Very low (<10%)

Overdosage/Toxicology There have been no reports of overdose.

(Continued)

Basiliximab *(Continued)*

Drug Interactions

Increased Effect/Toxicity: Basiliximab is an immunoglobulin; specific drug interactions have not been evaluated, but are not anticipated.

Decreased Effect: Basiliximab is an immunoglobulin; specific drug interactions have not been evaluated, but are not anticipated. It is not known if the immune response to vaccines will be impaired during or following basiliximab therapy.

Storage/Stability
Store vials under refrigeration 2°C to 8°C (36°F to 46°F). Reconstituted vials are stable under refrigeration for 24 hours, but only 4 hours at room temperature.

Reconstitution
Reconstitute vials with sterile water for injection. Dilute reconstituted contents in normal saline or 5% dextrose.

Pharmacodynamics/Kinetics

Duration: Mean: 36 days (determined by IL-2R alpha saturation)

Distribution: Mean: V_d: Children: 5.2 ± 2.8 L; Adults: 8.6 ± 4.1 L

Half-life elimination: Children: 9.4 days; Adults: Mean: 7.2 days

Excretion: Clearance: Children: 20 mL/hour; Adults: Mean: 41 mL/hour

Dosage Note: Patients previously administered basiliximab should only be re-exposed to a subsequent course of therapy with extreme caution.

I.V.:

Children <35 kg: Renal transplantation: 10 mg within 2 hours prior to transplant surgery, followed by a second 10 mg dose 4 days after transplantation; the second dose should be withheld if complications occur (including severe hypersensitivity reactions or graft loss)

Children ≥35 kg and Adults: Renal transplantation: 20 mg within 2 hours prior to transplant surgery, followed by a second 20 mg dose 4 days after transplantation; the second dose should be withheld if complications occur (including severe hypersensitivity reactions or graft loss)

Dosing adjustment/comments in renal or hepatic impairment: No specific dosing adjustment recommended

Administration
Intravenous infusion over 20-30 minutes

Dosage Forms
Injection, powder for reconstitution: 10 mg, 20 mg

Monitoring Parameters
Signs and symptoms of acute rejection

♦ **Bayer 205** *see* Suramin *on page 733*

♦ **BayRho-D® Full-Dose** *see* Rh$_o$(D) Immune Globulin *on page 705*

♦ **BayRho-D® Mini-Dose** *see* Rh$_o$(D) Immune Globulin *on page 705*

♦ **BCG, Live** *see* BCG Vaccine *on page 120*

BCG Vaccine *(bee see jee vak SEEN)*

Related Information
Safe Handling of Hazardous Drugs *on page 1034*

U.S. Brand Names TheraCys®; TICE® BCG

Canadian Brand Names ImmuCyst®; Oncotice™; Pacis™

Generic Available No

Synonyms Bacillus Calmette-Guérin (BCG) Live; BCG, Live

Pharmacologic Category Biological Response Modulator; Vaccine

Pregnancy Risk Factor C

Use Immunization against tuberculosis and immunotherapy for cancer; treatment and prophylaxis of carcinoma *in situ* of the urinary bladder;

prophylaxis of primary or recurrent superficial papillary tumors following transurethral resection

BCG vaccine is not routinely recommended for use in the U.S. for prevention of tuberculosis

BCG vaccine is strongly recommended for infants and children with negative tuberculin skin tests who:

are at high risk of intimate and prolonged exposure to persistently untreated or ineffectively treated patients with infectious pulmonary tuberculosis, and

cannot be removed from the source of exposure, and

cannot be placed on long-term preventive therapy

are continuously exposed with tuberculosis who have bacilli resistant to isoniazid and rifampin

BCG is also recommended for tuberculin-negative infants and children in groups in which the rate of new infections exceeds 1% per year and for whom the usual surveillance and treatment programs have been attempted but are not operationally feasible

Mechanism of Action BCG live is an attenuated strain of bacillus Calmette-Guérin used as a biological response modifier; BCG live, when used intravesicular for treatment of bladder carcinoma *in situ*, is thought to cause a local, chronic inflammatory response involving macrophage and leukocyte infiltration of the bladder. By a mechanism not fully understood, this local inflammatory response leads to destruction of superficial tumor cells of the urothelium. Evidence of systemic immune response is also commonly seen, manifested by a positive PPD tuberculin skin test reaction, however, its relationship to clinical efficacy is not well-established. BCG is active immunotherapy which stimulates the host's immune mechanism to reject the tumor.

Labeled Contraindications Hypersensitivity to BCG vaccine or any component of the formulation; immunocompromised, AIDS, and burn patients; tuberculin-positive individual

Warnings/Precautions Hazardous agent - use appropriate precautions for handling and disposal. See Safe Handling of Hazardous Drugs *on page 1034* in the Appendix. Protection against tuberculosis is only relative, not permanent, nor entirely predictable; systemic reactions have been reported in patients treated as immunotherapy for bladder cancer

BCG should be administered with caution to persons in groups at high risk for HIV infection or persons known to be severely immunocompromised. Although limited data suggest that the vaccine may be safe for use in asymptomatic children infected with HIV, BCG vaccination is not recommended for HIV infected adults or for persons with symptomatic disease. Until further research can clearly define the risks and benefits of BCG vaccination for this population, vaccination should be restricted to persons at exceptionally high risk for tuberculosis infection. HIV-infected persons thought to be infected with *Mycobacterium tuberculosis* should be strongly recommended for tuberculosis preventive therapy.

Adverse Reactions All serious adverse reactions must be reported to the U.S. Department of Health and Human Services (DHHS) Vaccine Adverse Event Reporting System (VAERS) 1-800-822-7967.
>10%:

Gastrointestinal: Nausea and vomiting (3% to 16%)

Genitourinary: Dysuria (62%), polyuria (42%), hematuria (26% to 40%), cystitis (6% to 30%), urinary urgency (6% to 18%)

(Continued)

BCG Vaccine *(Continued)*

    Miscellaneous: Flu-like syndrome including fever, chills (42%)

   1% to 10%:

    Central nervous system: Fatigue, headache, dizziness

    Gastrointestinal: Anorexia, diarrhea

    Genitourinary: Urinary incontinence (2% to 6%)

   <1%: Abscesses, anemia, bladder irritation, coagulation abnormalities, hepatitis, hepatic granuloma, leukopenia, prostatitis, rash, skin ulceration, thrombocytopenia

Vesicant No

Emetic Potential Low (10% to 30%)

Storage/Stability Refrigerate; protect from light.

   TICE® BCG: Use within 2 hours of mixing

Reconstitution

   TheraCys®: Reconstitute with 3 mL of diluent provided and shake gently. Add contents to 50 mL of 0.9% NaCl (preservative free) provided.

   TICE® BCG: Reconstitute with 1 mL 0.9% NaCl (preservative free). Mix by drawing and expelling solution into ampul 3 times. Dilute with 50 mL of 0.9% NaCl.

Dosage Children >1 month and Adults:

   Immunization against tuberculosis (TICE® BCG): 0.2-0.3 mL percutaneous; initial lesion usually appears after 10-14 days consisting of small red papule at injection site and reaches maximum diameter of 3 mm in 4-6 weeks; conduct postvaccinal tuberculin test (ie, 5 TU of PPD) in 2-3 months; if test is negative, repeat vaccination

   Immunotherapy for bladder cancer:

    TheraCys®: One dose instilled into bladder weekly for 6 weeks followed by one treatment at 3, 6, 12, 18, and 24 months after initial treatment

    TICE® BCG: One dose instilled into the bladder once weekly for 6 weeks followed by once monthly for 6-12 months

Administration Should only be given intravesicularly or percutaneously; **do not administer I.V., SubQ, or intradermally;** can be used for bladder irrigation

Dosage Forms Injection, powder for reconstitution, intravesical:

   TheraCys®: 81 mg [with diluent]

   TICE® BCG: 50 mg

Additional Information When used for immunization against tuberculosis, Federal law requires that the date of administration, the vaccine manufacturer, lot number of vaccine, and the administering person's name, title and address be entered into the patient's permanent medical record.

Selected Readings

Alexandroff AB, Jackson AM, O'Donnell MA, et al, "BCG Immunotherapy of Bladder Cancer: 20 Years On," *Lancet*, 1999, 353(9165):1689-94.

Badalament RA and Farah RN, "Treatment of Superficial Bladder Cancer With Intravesicle Chemotherapy," *Semin Surg Oncol*, 1997, 13(5):335-41.

Bassi P, "BCG (Bacillus of Calmette Guerin) Therapy of High-Risk Superficial Bladder Cancer," *Surg Oncol*, 2002, 11(1-2):77-83.

Centers for Disease Control, "Recommendations of the Advisory Committee on Immunization Practices (ACIP): General Recommendations on Immunization," *MMWR Recomm Rep*, 2002, 51(RR-2):1-36.

Lamm DL, Steg A, Boccon-Gibod L, et al, "Complications of Bacillus Calmette-Guérin Immunotherapy: Review of 2602 Patients and Comparison of Chemotherapy Complications," *Prog Clin Biol Res*, 1989, 310:335-55.

Martinez-Pineiro JA and Martinez-Pineiro L, "BCG Update: Intravesical Therapy," *Eur Urol*, 1997, 31(Suppl 1):31-41.

Meyer JP, Persad R, and Gillatt DA, "Use of Bacille Calmette-Guerin in Superficial Bladder Cancer," *Postgrad Med J*, 2002, 78(922):449-54.

Nathanson L, "Use of BCG in the Treatment of Human Neoplasms: A Review," *Semin Oncol*, 1974, 1(4):337-50.

Nseyo UO and Lamm DL, "Immunotherapy of Bladder Cancer," *Semin Surg Oncol*, 1997, 13(5):342-9.

Rischmann P, Desgrandchamps F, Malavaud B, et al, "BCG Intravesical Instillations: Recommendations for Side-Effects Management," *Eur Urol*, 2000, 37(Suppl 1):33-6.

♦ **BCNU** *see* Carmustine *on page 154*

♦ **Bebulin® VH** *see* Factor IX Complex (Human) *on page 330*

♦ **BeneFix®** *see* Factor IX *on page 327*

♦ **Benzisoquinolinedione** *see* Amonafide *on page 65*

♦ **Benzmethyzin** *see* Procarbazine *on page 688*

Benzydamine (ben ZID a meen)

Canadian Brand Names Apo-Benzydamine®; Dom-Benzydamine; Novo-Benzydamine; PMS-Benzydamine; ratio-Benzydamine; Sun-Benz®; Tantum®

Generic Available Yes

Synonyms Benzydamine Hydrochloride

Pharmacologic Category Local Anesthetic, Oral

Lactation Excretion in breast milk unknown/use caution

Use Symptomatic treatment of pain associated with acute pharyngitis; treatment of pain associated with radiation-induced oropharyngeal mucositis

Mechanism of Action Local anesthetic and anti-inflammatory, reduces local pain and inflammation. Does not interfere with arachidonic acid metabolism.

Restrictions Not available in U.S.

Labeled Contraindications Hypersensitivity to benzydamine or any component of the formulation

Warnings/Precautions May cause local irritation and/or burning sensation in patients with altered mucosal integrity. Dilution (1:1 in warm water) may attenuate this effect. Use caution in renal impairment. Safety and efficacy have not been established in children ≤5 years of age.

Adverse Reactions
Central nervous system: Drowsiness, headache
Gastrointestinal: Nausea and/or vomiting (2%), dry mouth
Local: Numbness (10%), burning/stinging sensation (8%)
Respiratory: Pharyngeal irritation, cough

Drug Interactions
Cytochrome P450 Effect: Substrate (minor) of CYP1A2, 2C19, 2D6, 3A4
Increased Effect/Toxicity: No interactions established.
Decreased Effect: No interactions established.

Storage/Stability Store at 15°C to 30°C. Protect from freezing.

Pharmacodynamics/Kinetics
Absorption: Oral rinse may be absorbed, at least in part, through the oral mucosa
Excretion: Urine (primarily as unchanged drug)
(Continued)

Benzydamine *(Continued)*

Dosage Oral rinse: Adults:

Mucositis: 15 mL of undiluted solution as a gargle or rinse 3-4 times/day; contact between the liquid and the oral mucosa should be maintained for at least 30 seconds, followed by expulsion from the mouth. Patient should not swallow the liquid. Begin treatment 1 day prior to initiation of radiation therapy and continue daily during treatment.

Acute pharyngitis: Gargle with 15 mL of undiluted solution every 1.5-3 hours until symptoms resolve. Patient should expel solution from mouth following use; solution should not be swallowed.

Dosage adjustment in renal impairment: No adjustment required.

Dosage Forms Oral rinse, as hydrochloride: 0.15% (100 mL, 250 mL)

Selected Readings

Epstein JB, Silverman S Jr, Paggiarino DA, et al, "Benzydamine HCl for Prophylaxis of Radiation-Induced Oral Mucositis: Results From a Multicenter, Randomized, Double-Blind, Placebo-Controlled Clinical Trial," *Cancer*, 2001, 92(4):875-85.

♦ **Benzydamine Hydrochloride** *see* Benzydamine *on page 123*
♦ **Beta-HC®** *see* Hydrocortisone *on page 419*

Bevacizumab *(be vuh SIZ uh mab)*

U.S. Brand Names Avastin™

Generic Available No

Synonyms Anti-VEGF Monoclonal Antibody; rhuMAb-VEGF

Pharmacologic Category Antineoplastic Agent, Monoclonal Antibody; Vascular Endothelial Growth Factor (VEGF) Inhibitor

Pregnancy Risk Factor C

Lactation Excretion in breast milk unknown/not recommended

Use Treatment of metastatic colorectal cancer

Unlabeled/Investigational Use Breast cancer, malignant mesothelioma, prostate cancer

Mechanism of Action Bevacizumab is a recombinant, humanized monoclonal antibody which binds to, and neutralizes, vascular endothelial growth factor (VEGF), preventing its association with endothelial receptors. VEGF binding initiates angiogenesis (endothelial proliferation and the formation of new blood vessels). The inhibition of microvascular growth is believed to retard the growth of all tissues (including metastatic tissue).

Labeled Contraindications Hypersensitivity to bevacizumab, murine products, or any component of the formulation

Warnings/Precautions Gastrointestinal perforation, intra-abdominal abscess, and wound dehiscence have been reported in patients receiving bevacizumab; monitor patients for signs/symptoms of abdominal pain, constipation or vomiting. Permanent discontinuation is recommended in patients who develop these complications. The appropriate intervals between administration of bevacizumab and surgical procedures to avoid impairment in wound healing has not been established. Do not initiate therapy within 28 days of major surgery and only following complete healing of the incision. Bevacizumab should be discontinued prior to elective surgery and the estimated half-life (20 days) should be considered.

Avoid use in patients with recent hemoptysis; significant pulmonary bleeding has been reported in patients receiving bevacizumab (primarily in patients with nonsmall cell lung cancer). Avoid use in patients with CNS metastases; patients with CNS metastases were excluded from clinical trials due to concerns for bleeding. Other serious bleeding events may occur, but with a lower frequency; discontinuation of treatment is recommended in all patients with serious hemorrhage.

An increased risk for arterial thromboembolic events (eg, stroke, MI, TIA, angina) is associated with bevacizumab use with combination chemotherapy. History of arterial thromboembolism or ≥65 years of age may present an even greater risk; permanently discontinue if serious arterial thromboembolic events occur.

May cause CHF and/or potentiate cardiotoxic effects of anthracyclines. Use with caution in patients with cardiovascular disease; patients with significant cardiovascular disease were excluded from clinical trials. Bevacizumab may cause and/or worsen hypertension; use caution in patients with pre-existing hypertension and monitor BP closely in all patients. Permanent discontinuation is recommended in patients who experience a hypertensive crisis. Temporarily discontinue in patients who develop uncontrolled hypertension. Interrupt therapy in patients experiencing severe infusion reactions; there are no data to address reinstitution of therapy in patients who experience CHF and/or severe infusion reactions. Proteinuria and/or nephrotic syndrome has been associated with bevacizumab; discontinuation of therapy is recommended in patients with nephrotic syndrome. Safety and efficacy in pediatric patients have not been established.

Adverse Reactions No data are available concerning the frequency of adverse reactions to bevacizumab alone. The frequencies noted below are from two controlled clinical trials of bevacizumab in combination with irinotecan, fluorouracil, and leucovorin (IFL). These frequencies, where noted, are compared to the incidence in the placebo-controlled arms of the trials.

>10%:

Cardiovascular: Hypertension (23% to 34% vs 14%, severe/life-threatening 12% vs 2%); hypotension (7% to 15% vs 7%); thromboembolism (18% vs 15%)

Central nervous system: Pain (61% to 62% vs 55%, severe 8% vs 5%); abdominal pain (50% to 61% vs 55%, severe/life-threatening 8% vs 5%); headache (26% vs 19%); dizziness (19% to 26% vs 20%)

Dermatologic: Alopecia (6% to 32% vs 26%), dry skin (7% to 20% vs 7%), exfoliative dermatitis (3% to 19% vs 3%), skin discoloration (2% to 16% vs 3%)

Endocrine & metabolic: Weight loss (15% to 16% vs 10%), hypokalemia (12% to 16% vs 11%)

Gastrointestinal: Diarrhea (severe/life-threatening 34% vs 25%); vomiting (47% to 52% vs 47%); anorexia (35% to 43% vs 30%); constipation (29% to 40% vs 29%, severe/life-threatening 4% vs 2%); stomatitis (30% to 32% vs 18%); dyspepsia (17% to 24% vs 15%); flatulence (11% to 19% vs 10%); taste disorder (14% to 21% vs 9%)

Hematologic: Leukopenia (severe/life-threatening 37% vs 31%), epistaxis (32% to 35% vs 10%), gastrointestinal hemorrhage (19% to 24% vs 6%), neutropenia (severe/life-threatening 21% vs 14%)

Neuromuscular & skeletal: Weakness (73% to 74% vs 70%, severe/life-threatening 10% vs 7%); myalgia (8% to 15% vs 7%)

Ocular: Tearing increased (6% to 18% vs 2%)

(Continued)

Bevacizumab *(Continued)*

Renal: Proteinuria includes nephrotic syndrome in some patients (36% vs 24%)

Respiratory: Upper respiratory infection (40% to 47% vs 39%), dyspnea (25% to 26% vs 15%)

1% to 10%:

Cardiovascular: DVT (6% to 9% vs 3%, severe/life-threatening 9% vs 5%); intra-arterial thrombosis (severe/life-threatening 3% vs 1%), syncope (severe/life-threatening 3% vs 1%)

Central nervous system: Confusion (1% to 6% vs 1%), abnormal gait (1% to 5% vs 0%)

Dermatologic: Skin ulcer (6% vs 1%), nail disorders (2% to 8% vs 3%)

Endocrine & metabolic: Infusion reactions (<3%)

Gastrointestinal: Dry mouth (4% to 7% vs 2%), colitis (1% to 6% vs 1%)

Hematologic: Thrombocytopenia (5% vs 0%)

Hepatic: Bilirubinemia (1% to 6% vs 0%)

Renal: Urinary frequency/urgency (3% to 6% vs 1%)

Respiratory: Voice alteration (6% to 9% vs 2%)

<1% (Limited to important or life-threatening): Anastomotic ulceration, hypertensive encephalopathy, hyponatremia, intestinal necrosis, intestinal obstruction, mesenteric venous occlusion, pancytopenia, polyserositis, subarachnoid hemorrhage, ureteral stricture

Vesicant No

Emetic Potential Very low <10%

Drug Interactions

Increased Effect/Toxicity: Bevacizumab may potentiate the cardiotoxic effects of anthracyclines. Serum concentrations of irinotecan's active metabolite may be increased by bevacizumab; an approximate 33% increase has been observed.

Storage/Stability Store vials at 2°C to 8°C (36°F to 46°F). Protect from light; do not freeze or shake. Diluted solutions are stable for up to 8 hours under refrigeration.

Reconstitution Prior to infusion, dilute prescribed dose of bevacizumab in 100 mL NS. Do not mix with dextrose-containing solutions.

Pharmacodynamics/Kinetics

Distribution: V_d: 46 mL/kg

Half-life elimination: 20 days (range: 11-50 days)

Excretion: Clearance: 2.75-5 mL/kg/day

Dosage I.V.: Adults:

Colorectal cancer: 5-10 mg/kg every 2 weeks

Breast cancer (unlabeled use): 3 mg/kg or 10 mg/kg or 20 mg/kg every 2 weeks

Head and neck cancer (unlabeled use): 5 mg/kg or 10 mg/kg, or 15 mg/kg every 3 weeks

Prostate cancer (unlabeled use): 10 mg/kg every 2 weeks

Renal cell cancer (unlabeled use): 3 mg/kg or 10 mg/kg every 2 weeks

Dosage adjustment for toxicity: Temporary suspension is recommended in moderate-to-severe proteinuria or in patients with severe hypertension which is not controlled with medical management. Permanent discontinuation is recommended (by the manufacturer) in patients who develop wound dehiscence requiring intervention, gastrointestinal perforation, hypertensive crisis, serious bleeding, or nephrotic syndrome.

Administration I.V. infusion, usually after the other antineoplastic agents. Infuse the initial dose over 90 minutes. Infusion may be shortened to 60 minutes if the initial infusion is well tolerated. The third and subsequent infusions may be shortened to 30 minutes if the 60 minute infusion is well tolerated. Monitor closely during the infusion for signs/symptoms of an infusion reaction.

Dosage Forms Injection, solution [preservative free]: 25 mg/mL (4 mL, 16 mL)

Monitoring Parameters Monitor closely during the infusion for signs/symptoms of an infusion reaction. Monitor CBC with differential; signs/symptoms of gastrointestinal perforation or abscess (including abdominal pain, constipation and vomiting); signs/symptoms of bleeding, including hemoptysis, gastrointestinal, and/or CNS bleeding, and/or epistaxis. Monitor blood pressure every 2-3 weeks. Monitor for proteinuria/nephrotic syndrome.

Patient Information Report any signs and symptoms of abdominal pain, unusual bleeding, or delayed wound healing.

Special Geriatric Considerations Elderly patients ≥65 years of age had an increased incidence of arterial thromboembolic events; other serious adverse events occurring often include weakness, sepsis, hyper-/hypotension, CHF, constipation, anorexia, anemia, hyper-/hypokalemia, and diarrhea.

Selected Readings

Bevacizumab, "Anti-VEGF Monoclonal Antibody, Avastin, Rhumab-VEGF," *Drugs R D*, 2002, 3(1):28-30.

Ignoffo RJ, "Overview of Bevacizumab: A New Cancer Therapeutic Strategy Targeting Vascular Endothelial Growth Factor," *Am J Health Syst Pharm*, 2004, 61(21 Suppl 5):S21-6.

Zondor SD and Medina PJ, "Bevacizumab: An Angiogenesis Inhibitor With Efficacy in Colorectal and Other Malignancies," *Ann Pharmacother*, 2004, 38(7-8):1258-64.

Bexarotene (beks AIR oh teen)

Related Information

Safe Handling of Hazardous Drugs *on page 1034*

U.S. Brand Names Targretin®

Canadian Brand Names Targretin®

Generic Available No

Pharmacologic Category Antineoplastic Agent, Miscellaneous

Pregnancy Risk Factor X

Lactation Excretion in breast milk unknown/contraindicated

Use

Oral: Treatment of cutaneous manifestations of cutaneous T-cell lymphoma in patients who are refractory to at least one prior systemic therapy

Topical: Treatment of cutaneous lesions in patients with refractory cutaneous T-cell lymphoma (stage 1A and 1B) or who have not tolerated other therapies

Mechanism of Action The exact mechanism is unknown. Binds and activates retinoid X receptor subtypes. Once activated, these receptors function as transcription factors that regulate the expression of genes which control cellular differentiation and proliferation. Bexarotene inhibits (Continued)

Bexarotene *(Continued)*

the growth *in vitro* of some tumor cell lines of hematopoietic and squamous cell origin.

Labeled Contraindications Hypersensitivity to bexarotene or any component of the formulation; pregnancy

Warnings/Precautions Pregnancy test needed 1 week before initiation and every month thereafter. Effective contraception must be in place one month before initiation, during therapy, and for at least 1 month after discontinuation. Male patients with sexual partners who are pregnant, possibly pregnant, or who could become pregnant, must use condoms during sexual intercourse during treatment and for 1 month after last dose. Induces significant lipid abnormalities in a majority of patients (triglyceride, total cholesterol, and HDL); reversible on discontinuation. Use extreme caution in patients with underlying hypertriglyceridemia. Pancreatitis secondary to hypertriglyceridemia has been reported. Monitor for liver function test abnormalities and discontinue drug if tests are three times the upper limit of normal values for AST (SGOT), ALT (SGPT) or bilirubin. Hypothyroidism occurs in about a third of patients. Monitor for signs and symptoms of infection about 4-8 weeks after initiation (leukopenia may occur). Any new visual abnormalities experienced by the patient should be evaluated by an ophthalmologist (cataracts can form, or worsen, especially in the geriatric population). May cause photosensitivity. Safety and efficacy are not established in the pediatric population. Avoid use in hepatically impaired patients. Limit additional vitamin A intake to <15,000 int. units/day. Use caution with diabetic patients.

Adverse Reactions First percentage is at a dose of 300 mg/m²/day; the second percentage is at a dose >300 mg/m²/day.

>10%:

  Cardiovascular: Peripheral edema (13% to 11%)

  Central nervous system: Headache (30% to 42%), chills (10% to 13%)

  Dermatologic: Rash (17% to 23%), exfoliative dermatitis (10% to 28%)

  Endocrine & metabolic: Hyperlipidemia (about 79% in both dosing ranges), hypercholesteremia (32% to 62%), hypothyroidism (29% to 53%)

  Hematologic: Leukopenia (17% to 47%)

  Neuromuscular & skeletal: Weakness (20% to 45%)

  Miscellaneous: Infection (13% to 23%)

<10%:

  Cardiovascular: Hemorrhage, hypertension, angina pectoris, right heart failure, tachycardia, cerebrovascular accident, syncope

  Central nervous system: Fever (5% to 17%), insomnia (5% to 11%), subdural hematoma, depression, agitation, ataxia, confusion, dizziness, hyperesthesia

  Dermatologic: Dry skin (about 10% for both dosing ranges), alopecia (4% to 11%), skin ulceration, acne, skin nodule, maculopapular rash, serous drainage, vesicular bullous rash, cheilitis

  Endocrine & metabolic: Hypoproteinemia, hyperglycemia, weight loss/gain, serum amylase (elevated), breast pain

  Gastrointestinal: Abdominal pain (11% to 4%), nausea (16% to 8%), diarrhea (7% to 42%), vomiting (4% to 13%), anorexia (2% to 23%), constipation, xerostomia, flatulence, colitis, dyspepsia, gastroenteritis, gingivitis, melena, pancreatitis,

Genitourinary: Albuminuria, hematuria, urinary incontinence, urinary tract infection, urinary urgency, dysuria, kidney function abnormality

Hematologic: Hypochromic anemia (4% to 13%), anemia (6% to 25%), eosinophilia, thrombocythemia, coagulation time increased, lymphocytosis, thrombocytopenia

Hepatic: LDH increase (7% to 13%), hepatic failure

Neuromuscular & skeletal: Back pain (2% to 11%), arthralgia, myalgia, bone pain, myasthenia, arthrosis, neuropathy

Ocular: Dry eyes, conjunctivitis, blepharitis, corneal lesion, visual field defects, keratitis

Otic: Ear pain, otitis externa

Renal: Creatinine (elevated)

Respiratory: Pharyngitis, rhinitis, dyspnea, pleural effusion, bronchitis, increased cough, lung edema, hemoptysis, hypoxia

Miscellaneous: Flu-like syndrome (4% to 13%), bacterial infection (1% to 13%)

Topical:

Cardiovascular: Edema (10%)

Central nervous system: Headache (14%), weakness (6%), pain (30%)

Dermatologic: Rash (14% to 72%), pruritus (6% to 40%), contact dermatitis (14%), exfoliative dermatitis (6%)

Hematologic: Leukopenia (6%), lymphadenopathy (6%)

Neuromuscular & skeletal: Paresthesia (6%)

Respiratory: Cough (6%), pharyngitis (6%)

Miscellaneous: Diaphoresis (6%), infection (18%)

Emetic Potential Low (10% to 30%)

Overdosage/Toxicology Doses up to 1000 mg/m^2/day have been used in humans without acute toxic effects. Any overdose should be treated with supportive care focused on the symptoms exhibited.

Drug Interactions

Cytochrome P450 Effect: Substrate of CYP3A4 (minor); **Induces** CYP3A4 (weak)

Increased Effect/Toxicity: Bexarotene plasma concentrations may be increased by gemfibrozil. Bexarotene may increase the toxicity of DEET.

Decreased Effect: Bexarotene may decrease the plasma levels of hormonal contraceptives and tamoxifen.

Ethanol/Nutrition/Herb Interactions

Food: Take with a fat-containing meal. Bexarotene serum levels may be increased by grapefruit juice; avoid concurrent use.

Herb/Nutraceutical: Avoid dong quai, St John's wort (may also cause photosensitization). St John's wort may decrease bexarotene levels. Additional vitamin A supplements may lead to vitamin A toxicity (dry skin, irritation, arthralgias, myalgias, abdominal pain, hepatic changes).

Storage/Stability Store at 2°C to 25°C (36°F to 77°F). Protect from light.

Pharmacodynamics/Kinetics

Absorption: Significantly improved by a fat-containing meal

Protein binding: >99%

Metabolism: Hepatic via CYP3A4 isoenzyme; four metabolites identified; further metabolized by glucuronidation

Half-life elimination: 7 hours

(Continued)

Bexarotene *(Continued)*

Time to peak: 2 hours

Excretion: Primarily feces; urine (<1% as unchanged drug and metabolites)

Dosage

Oral: 300-400 mg/m^2/day taken as a single daily dose

Topical: Apply once every other day for first week, then increase on a weekly basis to once daily, 2 times/day, 3 times/day, and finally 4 times/day, according to tolerance

Dosing adjustment in renal impairment: No studies have been conducted; however, renal insufficiency may result in significant protein binding changes and alter pharmacokinetics of bexarotene

Dosing adjustment in hepatic impairment: No studies have been conducted; however, hepatic impairment would be expected to result in decreased clearance of bexarotene due to the extensive hepatic contribution to elimination

Administration

Oral: Administer capsule following a fat-containing meal.

Topical: Allow gel to dry before covering with clothing. Avoid application to normal skin. Use of occlusive dressings is not recommended.

Dosage Forms

Capsule: 75 mg

Gel: 1% (60 g)

Monitoring Parameters If female, pregnancy test 1 week before initiation then monthly while on bexarotene; lipid panel before initiation, then weekly until lipid response established and then at 8-week intervals thereafter; baseline LFTs, repeat at 1, 2, and 4 weeks after initiation then at 8-week intervals thereafter if stable; baseline and periodic thyroid function tests; baseline CBC with periodic monitoring

Dietary Considerations It is preferable to take the oral capsule following a fat-containing meal.

Patient Information

Oral: Take with a fat-containing meal. Get pregnancy test before starting therapy and then every month thereafter while on the medicine. Do not get pregnant while taking this medicine. Use 2 forms of birth control 1 month before, during, and for at least a month after completion of therapy. For male patients, protect your partner against pregnancy by wearing a condom. Continue using protection for 1 month after last dose. Take at a similar time daily. Call your prescriber if you have a fever, chills, or any signs of infection. You are at risk of infections: stay away from crowds and people with viruses. Wash your hands frequently. Check vitamin A intake with your prescriber. You should avoid large amounts of vitamin A.

Topical gel: Allow gel to dry before covering. Avoid applying to normal skin or mucous membranes. Do not use occlusive dressings.

Selected Readings

Farol LT and Hymes KB, "Bexarotene: A Clinical Review," *Expert Rev Anticancer Ther*, 2004, 4(2):180-8.

Hurst RE, "Bexarotene Ligand Pharmaceuticals," *Curr Opin Investig Drugs*, 2000, 1(4):514-23.

Lowe MN and Plosker GL, "Bexarotene," *Am J Clin Dermatol*, 2000, 1(4):245-50.

Martin AG, "Bexarotene Gel: A New Skin-Directed Treatment Option for Cutaneous T-Cell Lymphomas," *J Drugs Dermatol*, 2003, 2(2):155-67.

♦ **Bexxar**® *see* Tositumomab and Iodine I 131 Tositumomab *on page 781*

♦ **BI-007** *see* Paclitaxel (Protein Bound) *on page 644*

Bicalutamide (bye ka LOO ta mide)

Related Information

Safe Handling of Hazardous Drugs *on page 1034*

U.S. Brand Names Casodex®

Canadian Brand Names Casodex®

Generic Available No

Synonyms CDX; ICI-176334

Pharmacologic Category Antineoplastic Agent, Antiandrogen

Pregnancy Risk Factor X

Lactation Excretion in breast milk unknown

Use In combination therapy with LHRH agonist analogues in treatment of advanced prostatic carcinoma

Mechanism of Action Pure nonsteroidal antiandrogen that binds to androgen receptors; specifically a competitive inhibitor for the binding of dihydrotestosterone and testosterone; prevents testosterone stimulation of cell growth in prostate cancer

Labeled Contraindications Hypersensitivity to bicalutamide or any component of the formulation; pregnancy

Warnings/Precautions Rare cases of death or hospitalization due to hepatitis have been reported postmarketing. Use with caution in moderate to severe hepatic dysfunction. Hepatotoxicity generally occurs within the first 3-4 months of use. Baseline liver function tests should be obtained and repeated regularly during the first 4 months of treatment, and periodically thereafter. Additionally, patients should be monitored for signs and symptoms of liver dysfunction. Bicalutamide should be discontinued if patients have jaundice or ALT is two times the upper limit of normal. May cause gynecomastia in a high percentage of patients.

Adverse Reactions

>10%: Endocrine & metabolic: Hot flashes (8% to 24% in combination with LHRH agonists), gynecomastia (23% to 62%), breast tenderness (25% to 60%)

≥2% to <5%:

Cardiovascular: Angina pectoris, CHF, edema

Central nervous system: Anxiety, depression, confusion, somnolence, nervousness, fever, chills

Dermatologic: Dry skin, pruritus, alopecia

Endocrine & metabolic: Breast pain, diabetes mellitus, decreased libido, dehydration, gout

Gastrointestinal: Anorexia, dyspepsia, rectal hemorrhage, xerostomia, melena, weight gain

Genitourinary: Polyuria, urinary impairment, dysuria, urinary retention, urinary urgency

Hepatic: Alkaline phosphatase increased

Neuromuscular & skeletal: Myasthenia, arthritis, myalgia, leg cramps, pathological fracture, neck pain, hypertonia, neuropathy

Renal: Creatinine increased

Respiratory: Cough increased, pharyngitis, bronchitis, pneumonia, rhinitis, lung disorder

Miscellaneous: Sepsis, neoplasma

<1%: Diarrhea

Emetic Potential Very low (<10%)

(Continued)

Bicalutamide *(Continued)*

Overdosage/Toxicology Symptoms of overdose include hypoactivity, ataxia, anorexia, vomiting, slow respiration, and lacrimation. Management is supportive. Dialysis is of no benefit.

Drug Interactions

Increased Effect/Toxicity: Bicalutamide may displace warfarin from protein binding sites which may result in an increased anticoagulant effect, especially when bicalutamide therapy is started after the patient is already on warfarin.

Storage/Stability Store at room temperature.

Pharmacodynamics/Kinetics

Absorption: Rapid and complete

Protein binding: 96%

Metabolism: Extensively hepatic; stereospecific metabolism

Half-life elimination: Up to 10 days; active enantiomer 5.8 days

Excretion: Urine and feces (as unchanged drug and metabolites)

Dosage Adults: Oral: 50-150 mg/day

Dosage adjustment in renal impairment: None necessary as renal impairment has no significant effect on elimination

Dosage adjustment in liver impairment: Discontinue if ALT >2 times ULN or patient develops jaundice

Combination Regimens

Prostate cancer: Bicalutamide + LHRH-A *on page 848*

Administration Dose should be taken at the same time each day with or without food.

Dosage Forms Tablet: 50 mg

Monitoring Parameters CBC, ECG, echocardiograms, and serum testosterone and luteinizing hormone (periodically). Liver function tests should be obtained at baseline and repeated regularly during the first 4 months of treatment, and periodically thereafter; monitor for signs and symptoms of liver dysfunction. (discontinue if jaundice is noted or ALT is two or more times the upper limit of normal).

Dietary Considerations May be taken with or without food.

Patient Information Take as directed and do not alter dose or discontinue without consulting prescriber. Take with or without food. Diabetics should monitor serum glucose closely and notify prescriber of changes; this medication can alter hypoglycemic requirements. You may lose your hair and experience impotency. May cause dizziness, confusion, or drowsiness (use caution when driving or engaging in tasks that require alertness until response to drug is known); nausea or vomiting (small frequent meals, frequent mouth care, sucking lozenges, or chewing gum may help); or constipation (increased dietary fiber, fruit, or fluid and increased exercise may help). Report easy bruising or bleeding; yellowing of skin or eyes; change in color of urine or stool; unresolved CNS changes (nervousness, chills, insomnia, somnolence); skin rash, redness, or irritation; chest pain or palpitations; difficulty breathing; urinary retention or inability to void; muscle weakness, tremors, or pain; persistent nausea, vomiting, diarrhea, or constipation; or other unusual signs or adverse reactions.

Special Geriatric Considerations Renal impairment has no clinically significant changes in elimination of the parent compound or active metabolite; therefore, no dosage adjustment is needed in the elderly. In dosage studies, no difference was found between young adults and elderly with regard to steady-state serum concentrations for bicalutamide and its active R-enantiomer metabolite.

Selected Readings
Cockshott ID, "Bicalutamide: Clinical Pharmacokinetics and Metabolism," *Clin Pharmacokinet*, 2004, 43(13):855-78.

Iversen P, "Bicalutamide Monotherapy for Early Stage Prostate Cancer: An Update," *J Urol*, 2003, 170(6 Pt 2):S48-52.

Schellhammer PF, "An Evaluation of Bicalutamide in the Treatment of Prostate Cancer," *Expert Opin Pharmacother*, 2002, 3(9):1313-28.

Schellhammer PF and Davis JW, "An Evaluation of Bicalutamide in the Treatment of Prostate Cancer," *Clin Prostate Cancer*, 2004, 2(4):213-9.

♦ **BiCNu**® *see Carmustine on page 154*

♦ **BIDA** *see Amonafide on page 65*

♦ **Bio-Statin**® *see Nystatin on page 613*

♦ **Bisac-Evac**™ **[OTC]** *see Bisacodyl on page 133*

Bisacodyl (bis a KOE dil)

Medication Safety Issues
Sound-alike/look-alike issues:
Doxidan® may be confused with doxepin
Modane® may be confused with Matulane®, Moban®

U.S. Brand Names Alophen® [OTC]; Bisac-Evac™ [OTC]; Bisacodyl Uniserts® [OTC]; Correctol® Tablets [OTC]; Doxidan® *(reformulation)* [OTC]; Dulcolax® [OTC]; Femilax™ [OTC]; Fleet® Bisacodyl Enema [OTC]; Fleet® Stimulant Laxative [OTC]; Gentlax® [OTC]; Modane Tablets® [OTC]; Veracolate [OTC]

Canadian Brand Names Apo-Bisacodyl®; Carter's Little Pills®; Dulcolax®

Generic Available Yes: Excludes enema

Pharmacologic Category Laxative, Stimulant

Pregnancy Risk Factor C

Use Treatment of constipation; colonic evacuation prior to procedures or examination

Mechanism of Action Stimulates peristalsis by directly irritating the smooth muscle of the intestine, possibly the colonic intramural plexus; alters water and electrolyte secretion producing net intestinal fluid accumulation and laxation

Labeled Contraindications Hypersensitivity to bisacodyl or any component of the formulation; abdominal pain, obstruction, nausea or vomiting

Adverse Reactions <1%:
Central nervous system: Vertigo
Endocrine & metabolic: Electrolyte and fluid imbalance (metabolic acidosis or alkalosis, hypocalcemia)
Gastrointestinal: Mild abdominal cramps, nausea, vomiting, rectal burning

Emetic Potential Very low (<10%)

Drug Interactions
Decreased Effect: Milk or antacids may decrease the effect of bisacodyl. Bisacodyl may decrease the effect of warfarin.

Ethanol/Nutrition/Herb Interactions Food: Milk or dairy products may disrupt enteric coating, increasing stomach irritation.

Pharmacodynamics/Kinetics
Onset of action: Oral: 6-10 hours; Rectal: 0.25-1 hour
Absorption: Oral, rectal: Systemic, <5%
(Continued)

Bisacodyl *(Continued)*

Dosage
Children:
Oral: >6 years: 5-10 mg (0.3 mg/kg) at bedtime or before breakfast
Rectal suppository:
<2 years: 5 mg as a single dose
>2 years: 10 mg

Adults:
Oral: 5-15 mg as single dose (up to 30 mg when complete evacuation of bowel is required)
Rectal suppository: 10 mg as single dose

Administration Administered with glass of water on empty stomach for rapid effect. Do not administer within 1 hour of milk, any dairy products, or taking an antacid, to protect the coating.

Dosage Forms
Enema (Fleet® Bisacodyl Enema): 10 mg/30 mL (37 mL)
Suppository, rectal (Bisac-Evac™, Bisacodyl Uniserts®; Dulcolax®): 10 mg
Tablet, enteric coated (Alophen®; Bisac-Evac™, Correctol®, Dulcolax®, Femilax™, Fleet® Stimulant Laxative, Gentlax®, Modane®, Veracolate): 5 mg
Tablet, delayed release (Doxidan®): 5 mg

Dietary Considerations Should not be administered within 1 hour of milk, any dairy products, or taking an antacid, to protect the coating; should be administered with glass of water on empty stomach for rapid effect.

♦ **Bisacodyl Uniserts® [OTC]** *see Bisacodyl on page 133*
♦ **bis-chloronitrosourea** *see Carmustine on page 154*
♦ **BL4162A** *see Anagrelide on page 82*
♦ **Blenoxane®** *see Bleomycin on page 134*
♦ **Bleo** *see Bleomycin on page 134*

Bleomycin *(blee oh MYE sin)*

Medication Safety Issues
Sound-alike/look-alike issues:
Bleomycin may be confused with Cleocin®

Related Information
Fertility and Cancer Therapy *on page 962*
Safe Handling of Hazardous Drugs *on page 1034*

U.S. Brand Names Blenoxane®
Canadian Brand Names Blenoxane®
Generic Available Yes
Synonyms Bleo; Bleomycin Sulfate; BLM; NSC-125066
Pharmacologic Category Antineoplastic Agent, Antibiotic
Pregnancy Risk Factor D
Lactation Excretion in breast milk unknown/not recommended
Use Treatment of squamous cell carcinomas, melanomas, sarcomas, testicular carcinoma, Hodgkin's lymphoma, and non-Hodgkin's lymphoma
Orphan drug: Sclerosing agent for malignant pleural effusion
Mechanism of Action Inhibits synthesis of DNA; binds to DNA leading to single- and double-strand breaks

Labeled Contraindications Hypersensitivity to bleomycin sulfate or any component of the formulation; severe pulmonary disease; pregnancy

Warnings/Precautions Hazardous agent - use appropriate precautions for handling and disposal. See Safe Handling of Hazardous Drugs *on page 1034* in the Appendix. Occurrence of pulmonary fibrosis is higher in elderly patients and in those receiving >400 units total and in smokers and patients with prior radiation therapy. A severe idiosyncratic reaction consisting of hypotension, mental confusion, fever, chills, and wheezing is possible.

Adverse Reactions

>10%:

Cardiovascular: Raynaud's phenomenon

Dermatologic: Pain at the tumor site, phlebitis. About 50% of patients develop erythema, induration, hyperkeratosis, and peeling of the skin, particularly on the palmar and plantar surfaces of the hands and feet. Hyperpigmentation (50%), alopecia, nailbed changes may also occur. These effects appear dose related and reversible with discontinuation of the drug.

Gastrointestinal: Stomatitis and mucositis (30%), anorexia, weight loss

Respiratory: Tachypnea, rales, acute or chronic interstitial pneumonitis and pulmonary fibrosis (5% to 10%), hypoxia and death (1%). Symptoms include cough, dyspnea, and bilateral pulmonary infiltrates. The pathogenesis is not certain, but may be due to damage of pulmonary, vascular, or connective tissue. Response to steroid therapy is variable and somewhat controversial.

Miscellaneous: Acute febrile reactions (25% to 50%); anaphylactoid reactions characterized by hypotension, confusion, fever, chills, and wheezing. Onset may be immediate or delayed for several hours.

1% to 10%:

Dermatologic: Rash (8%), skin thickening, diffuse scleroderma, onycholysis

Miscellaneous: Acute anaphylactoid reactions

<1%: Angioedema, cerebrovascular accident, hepatotoxicity, MI, nausea, vomiting; Myelosuppressive (rare); Onset: 7 days, Nadir: 14 days, Recovery: 21 days

Vesicant No

Emetic Potential Very low (<10%)

Overdosage/Toxicology Symptoms of overdose include chills, fever, pulmonary fibrosis, and hyperpigmentation. Treatment is supportive.

Drug Interactions

Increased Effect/Toxicity: Cisplatin may decrease bleomycin elimination.

Decreased Effect: Bleomycin may decrease plasma levels of digoxin. Concomitant therapy with phenytoin results in decreased phenytoin levels.

Storage/Stability Refrigerate intact vials of powder; intact vials are stable for up to one month at 45°C. Solutions for infusion are stable for 96 hours at room temperature and 14 days under refrigeration.

Reconstitution Reconstitute powder with 1-5 mL BWFI or BNS which is stable at room temperature or under refrigeration for 28 days.

Standard I.V. dilution: Dose/50-1000 mL NS or D_5W

Compatibility Stable in NS; **variable stability (consult detailed reference)** in D_5W

(Continued)

Bleomycin *(Continued)*

Y-site administration: Compatible: Allopurinol, amifostine, aztreonam, cefepime, cisplatin, cyclophosphamide, doxorubicin, doxorubicin liposome, droperidol, etoposide phosphate, filgrastim, fludarabine, fluorouracil, gemcitabine, granisetron, heparin, leucovorin, melphalan, methotrexate, metoclopramide, mitomycin, ondansetron, paclitaxel, piperacillin/tazobactam, sargramostim, teniposide, thiotepa, vinblastine, vincristine, vinorelbine

Compatibility in syringe: Compatible: Cisplatin, cyclophosphamide, doxorubicin, droperidol, fluorouracil, furosemide, heparin, leucovorin, methotrexate, metoclopramide, mitomycin, vinblastine, vincristine

Compatibility when admixed: Compatible: Amikacin, dexamethasone sodium phosphate, diphenhydramine, fluorouracil, gentamicin, heparin, hydrocortisone sodium phosphate, phenytoin, streptomycin, tobramycin, vinblastine, vincristine. **Incompatible:** Aminophylline, ascorbic acid injection, cefazolin, diazepam, hydrocortisone sodium succinate, methotrexate, mitomycin, nafcillin, penicillin G sodium, terbutaline

Pharmacodynamics/Kinetics

Absorption: I.M. and intrapleural administration: 30% to 50% of I.V. serum concentrations; intraperitoneal and SubQ routes produce serum concentrations equal to those of I.V.

Distribution: V_d: 22 L/m^2; highest concentrations in skin, kidney, lung, heart tissues; lowest in testes and GI tract; does not cross blood-brain barrier

Protein binding: 1%

Metabolism: Via several tissues including hepatic, GI tract, skin, pulmonary, renal, and serum

Half-life elimination: Biphasic (renal function dependent):
  Normal renal function: Initial: 1.3 hours; Terminal: 9 hours
  End-stage renal disease: Initial: 2 hours; Terminal: 30 hours

Time to peak, serum: I.M.: Within 30 minutes

Excretion: Urine (50% to 70% as active drug)

Dosage Refer to individual protocols; 1 unit = 1 mg

May be administered I.M., I.V., SubQ, or intracavitary

Children and Adults:

Test dose for lymphoma patients: I.M., I.V., SubQ: Because of the possibility of an anaphylactoid reaction, ≤2 units of bleomycin for the first 2 doses; monitor vital signs every 15 minutes; wait a minimum of 1 hour before administering remainder of dose; if no acute reaction occurs, then the regular dosage schedule may be followed. **Note:** Test doses may produce false-negative results.

Single-agent therapy:

I.M./I.V./SubQ: Squamous cell carcinoma, lymphoma, testicular carcinoma: 0.25-0.5 units/kg (10-20 units/m^2) 1-2 times/week

CIV: 15 units/m^2 over 24 hours daily for 4 days

Combination-agent therapy:

I.M./I.V.: 3-4 units/m^2

I.V.: ABVD: 10 units/m^2 on days 1 and 15

Maximum cumulative lifetime dose: 400 units

Pleural sclerosing: 60-240 units as a single infusion. Dose may be repeated at intervals of several days if fluid continues to accumulate (mix in 50-100 mL of D$_5$W, NS, or SWFI); may add lidocaine 100-200 mg to reduce local discomfort.

Dosing adjustment in renal impairment:
Cl_{cr} 10-50 mL/minute: Administer 75% of normal dose
Cl_{cr} <10 mL/minute: Administer 50% of normal dose

Combination Regimens

Head and neck cancer: CABO *on page 849*

Lymphoma, Hodgkin's:
ABVD *on page 843*
BEACOPP *on page 846*
CAD/MOPP/ABV *on page 850*
MOPP/ABV Hybrid *on page 913*
MOPP/ABVD *on page 913*
Stanford V *on page 937*

Lymphoma, non-Hodgkin's:
CEPP(B) *on page 857*
COP-BLAM *on page 866*
MACOP-B *on page 908*
m-BACOD *on page 908*
Pro-MACE-CytaBOM *on page 931*

Melanoma: BOLD *on page 849*

Ovarian cancer:
BEP (Ovarian) *on page 847*
BEP (Ovarian, Testicular) *on page 847*

Testicular cancer:
BEP (Ovarian, Testicular) *on page 847*
BEP (Testicular) *on page 847*
PVB *on page 935*
VBP *on page 945*

Administration I.V. doses should be administered slowly (manufacturer recommends giving over a period of 10 minutes); I.M. or SubQ may cause pain at injection site

Dosage Forms Injection, powder for reconstitution, as sulfate: 15 units, 30 units

Monitoring Parameters Pulmonary function tests (total lung volume, forced vital capacity, carbon monoxide diffusion), renal function, chest x-ray, temperature initially; check body weight at regular intervals

Patient Information You may experience loss of appetite, nausea, vomiting, mouth sores; small frequent meals, frequent mouth care with soft swab, frequent mouth rinses, sucking lozenges, or chewing gum may help; if unresolved, notify prescriber. You may experience fever or chills (will usually resolve); redness, peeling, or increased color of skin, or loss of hair (reversible after cessation of therapy). Report any change in respiratory status; difficulty breathing; wheezing; air hunger; increased secretions; difficulty expectorating secretions; confusion; unresolved fever or chills; sores in mouth; vaginal itching, burning, or discharge; sudden onset of dizziness; or acute headache. Contraceptive measures are recommended during therapy.

Special Geriatric Considerations Pulmonary toxicity has been reported more frequently in geriatric patients (>70 years of age).

♦ **Bleomycin Sulfate** *see* Bleomycin *on page 134*

♦ **BLM** *see* Bleomycin *on page 134*

♦ **Body Surface Area** *see page 1047*

♦ **Bonefos® (Can)** *see* Clodronate *on page 199*

Bortezomib (bore TEZ oh mib)

U.S. Brand Names Velcade™

Generic Available No

Synonyms LDP-341; MLN341; PS-341

Pharmacologic Category Antineoplastic Agent; Proteasome Inhibitor

Pregnancy Risk Factor D

Lactation Excretion in breast milk unknown/not recommended

Use Treatment of multiple myeloma in patients who have had at least one prior therapy

Mechanism of Action Bortezomib inhibits proteasomes, enzyme complexes which regulate protein homeostasis within the cell. Specifically, it reversibly inhibits chymotrypsin-like activity at the 26S proteasome, leading to activation of signaling cascades, cell-cycle arrest and apoptosis.

Labeled Contraindications Hypersensitivity to bortezomib, boron, mannitol, or any component of the formulation; pregnancy

Warnings/Precautions Hazardous agent - use appropriate precautions for handling and disposal. See Safe Handling of Hazardous Drugs *on page 1034* in the Appendix. May cause peripheral neuropathy (usually sensory but may be mixed sensorimotor); risk may be increased with previous use of neurotoxic agents or pre-existing peripheral neuropathy; adjustment of dose and schedule may be required. May cause orthostatic/postural hypotension; use caution with dehydration, history of syncope or medications associated with hypotension. Has been associated with the development or exacerbation of congestive heart failure; use caution in patients with risk factors or existing heart disease. May cause tumor lysis syndrome; risk is increased in patients with large tumor burden prior to treatment. Hematologic toxicity with severe thrombocytopenia may occur; risk is increased in patients with pretreatment platelet counts <75,000 µL; frequent monitoring is required throughout treatment. Use caution with hepatic or renal impairment. Safety and efficacy have not been established in pediatric patients.

Adverse Reactions

>10%:

Cardiovascular: Edema (25%), hypotension (12%)

Central nervous system: Pyrexia (36%), psychiatric disturbance (35%), headache (28%), insomnia (27%), dizziness (21%, excludes vertigo), anxiety (14%)

Dermatologic: Rash (21%), pruritus (11%)

Endocrine & metabolic: Dehydration (18%)

Gastrointestinal: Nausea (64%), diarrhea (51%), appetite decreased (43%), constipation (43%), vomiting (36%), abdominal pain (13%), abnormal taste (13%), dyspepsia (13%)

Hematologic: Thrombocytopenia (43%, Grade 3: 27%, Grade 4: 3%; Nadir: Day 11); anemia (32%, Grade 3: 9%); neutropenia (24%, Grade 3: 13%, Grade 4: 3%)

Neuromuscular & skeletal: Asthenic conditions (65%, Grade 3: 18% - includes fatigue, malaise, weakness); peripheral neuropathy (37%, Grade 3: 14%); arthralgia (26%); limb pain (26%); paresthesia and dysesthesia (23%); bone pain (16%); back pain (14%); muscle cramps (14%); myalgia (14%); rigors (12%)

Ocular: Blurred vision (11%)

Respiratory: Dyspnea (22%), upper respiratory tract infection (18%), cough (17%), lower respiratory infection (15%), nasopharyngitis (14%)

Miscellaneous: Herpes zoster (11%)

1% to 10%: Respiratory: Pneumonia (10%)

Frequency not defined (serious adverse events reported in trials relationship to drug not established): Acute respiratory distress syndrome, agitation, allergic reaction, anaphylaxis, angina, ascites, aspergillosis, ataxia, atelectasis, atrial fibrillation, atrial flutter, AV block, bacteremia, bladder spasm, bradycardia, cardiac amyloidosis, cardiogenic shock, cerebral hemorrhage, CHF, cholestasis, coma, confusion, cranial palsy, deep venous thrombosis, diplopia, duodenitis (hemorrhagic), dysarthria, dysautonomia, dysphagia, dyspnea, edema (facial), encephalopathy, embolism, epistaxis, fecal impaction, fracture, gastritis (hemorrhagic), gastroenteritis, hearing impaired, hematemesis, hematuria, hemoptysis, hemorrhagic cystitis, hepatitis, hydronephrosis, hyperbilirubinemia, hyper-/hypoglycemia, hyper-/hypokalemia, hyper-/hyponatremia, hyperuricemia, hypocalcemia, hypoxia, immune complex hypersensitivity, injection site erythema, intestinal obstruction, intestinal perforation, listeriosis, melena, MI, myocardial ischemia, neuralgia, oral candidiasis, oral mucosal petechiae, pancreatitis, paralytic ileus, paraplegia, pericardial effusion, pericarditis, peritonitis, pleural effusion, pneumonia, pneumonitis, portal vein thrombosis, proliferative glomerular nephritis, pulmonary edema, pulmonary embolism, pulmonary hypertension, psychosis, renal calculus, renal failure, seizure, septic shock, spinal cord compression, stomatitis, stroke (hemorrhagic), stroke, subdural hematoma, suicidal ideation, torsade de pointes, toxoplasmosis, transient ischemic attack, urinary incontinence, urinary retention, urinary tract infection, urticaria, ventricular tachycardia, vertigo

Postmarketing and/or case reports: Cardiac tamponade, ischemic colitis, deafness, disseminated intravascular coagulation, tumor lysis syndrome

Overdosage/Toxicology In case of overdose, treatment should be symptom directed and supportive.

Drug Interactions

Cytochrome P450 Effect: Substrate of CYP1A2 (minor), 2C8/9 (minor), 2C19 (minor), 2D6 (minor), 3A4 (major); **Inhibits** CYP1A2 (weak), 2C8/9 (weak), 2C19 (moderate), 2D6 (weak), 3A4 (weak)

Increased Effect/Toxicity: Bortezomib may increase the levels/effects citalopram, diazepam, methsuximide, phenytoin, propranolol, sertraline, and other CYP2C19 substrates. Levels/effects of bortezomib may be increased by azole antifungals, ciprofloxacin, clarithromycin, diclofenac, doxycycline, erythromycin, imatinib, isoniazid, nefazodone, nicardipine, propofol, protease inhibitors, quinidine, telithromycin, verapamil, and other CYP3A4 inhibitors.

Decreased Effect: Levels/effects of bortezomib may be decreased by aminoglutethimide, carbamazepine, nafcillin, nevirapine, phenobarbital, phenytoin, rifamycins, and other CYP3A4 inducers.

Storage/Stability Prior to reconstitution, store at controlled room temperature, 15°C to 30°C (59°F to 86°F). Protect from light. Once reconstituted, may be stored at room temperature for up to 8 hours in vial or 3 hours in syringe; solution should be administered within 8 hours

(Continued)

Bortezomib *(Continued)*

Reconstitution Dilute each 3.5 mg vial with 3.5 mL NS.

Pharmacodynamics/Kinetics

Protein binding: ~83%

Metabolism: Hepatic via CYP 1A2, 2C9, 2C19, 2D6, 3A4; forms metabolites (inactive)

Half-life elimination: 9-15 hours

Dosage I.V.: Adults: Multiple myeloma: 1.3 mg/m² twice weekly for 2 weeks on days 1, 4, 8, 11, every 21 days. Consecutive doses should be separated by at least 72 hours.

Dosage adjustment in renal impairment: Specific guidelines are not available; studies did not include patients with Cl_{cr} <13 mL/minute and patients on hemodialysis. Monitor closely for toxicity.

Dosage adjustment in hepatic impairment: Specific guidelines are not available; clearance may be decreased; monitor closely for toxicity

Dosage adjustment for toxicity:

Grade 3 nonhematological (excluding neuropathy) or Grade 4 hematological toxicity: Withhold until toxicity resolved; may reinitiate at a 25% reduced dose

Neuropathic pain and/or peripheral sensory neuropathy:

Grade 1 without pain or loss of function: No action needed

Grade 1 with pain or Grade 2 interfering with function but not activities of daily living: Reduce dose to 1 mg/m²

Grade 2 with pain or Grade 3 interfering with activities of daily living: Withhold until toxicity resolved, may reinitiate at 0.7 mg/m² once weekly

Grade 4: Discontinue therapy

Administration Administer via rapid I.V. push (<1 minute)

Dosage Forms Injection, powder for reconstitution [preservative free]: 3.5 mg [contains mannitol 35 mg]

Monitoring Parameters Signs/symptoms of peripheral neuropathy, dehydration, or hypotension; CBC; platelets should be monitored frequently throughout therapy

Additional Information Bortezomib was FDA approved under an accelerated approval program. Clinical trials have shown safety and efficacy as well as a decrease in tumor size. Studies addressing clinical benefit (including impact on survival) are ongoing.

Selected Readings

Adams J, "Proteasome Inhibition in Cancer: Development of PS-341," *Semin Oncol*, 2001, 28(6):613-9.

Aghajanian C, Soignet S, Dizon DS, et al, "A Phase I Trial of the Novel Proteasome Inhibitor PS341 in Advanced Solid Tumor Malignancies," *Clin Cancer Res*, 2002, 8(8):2505-11.

Orlowski RZ, Stinchcombe TE, Mitchell BS, et al, "Phase I Trial of the Proteasome Inhibitor PS-341 in Patients With Refractory Hematologic Malignancies," *J Clin Oncol*, 2002, 20(22):4420-7.

Teicher BA, Ara G, Herbst R, et al, "The Proteasome Inhibitor PS-341 in Cancer Therapy," *Clin Cancer Res*, 1999, 5(9):2638-45.

Terpos E, Politou M, and Rahemtulla A, "Tumour Lysis Syndrome in Multiple Myeloma After Bortezomib (VELCADE) Administration," *J Cancer Res Clin Oncol*, 2004, 130(10):623-5.

♦ **BRL 43694** *see* Granisetron *on page 405*

♦ **Bubbli-Pred™** *see* PrednisoLONE *on page 679*

Busulfan (byoo SUL fan)

Medication Safety Issues

Sound-alike/look-alike issues:

Busulfan may be confused with Butalan®

Myleran® may be confused with melphalan, Mylicon®

Related Information

Fertility and Cancer Therapy *on page 962*

Safe Handling of Hazardous Drugs *on page 1034*

Transplantation *on page 1019*

U.S. Brand Names Busulfex®; Myleran®

Canadian Brand Names Busulfex®; Myleran®

Generic Available No

Pharmacologic Category Antineoplastic Agent, Alkylating Agent

Pregnancy Risk Factor D

Lactation Contraindicated

Use

Oral: Chronic myelogenous leukemia; conditioning regimens for bone marrow transplantation

I.V.: Combination therapy with cyclophosphamide as a conditioning regimen prior to allogeneic hematopoietic progenitor cell transplantation for chronic myelogenous leukemia

Unlabeled/Investigational Use Oral: Bone marrow disorders, such as polycythemia vera and myeloid metaplasia; thrombocytosis

Mechanism of Action Reacts with N-7 position of guanosine and interferes with DNA replication and transcription of RNA. Busulfan has a more marked effect on myeloid cells than on lymphoid cells. The drug is also very toxic to hematopoietic stem cells. Busulfan exhibits little immunosuppressive activity. Interferes with the normal function of DNA by alkylation and cross-linking the strands of DNA.

Labeled Contraindications Hypersensitivity to busulfan or any component of the formulation; failure to respond to previous courses; pregnancy

Warnings/Precautions Hazardous agent - use appropriate precautions for handling and disposal. See Safe Handling of Hazardous Drugs *on page 1034* in the Appendix. May induce severe bone marrow hypoplasia. Use caution in patients predisposed to seizures. Discontinue if lung toxicity develops. Busulfan has been causally related to the development of secondary malignancies (tumors and acute leukemias). Busulfan has been associated with ovarian failure (including failure to achieve puberty) in females. High busulfan area under the concentration versus time curve (AUC) values (>1500 μM/minute) are associated with increased risk of hepatic veno-occlusive disease during conditioning for allogenic BMT.

Adverse Reactions

>10%: Hematologic: Severe pancytopenia, leukopenia, thrombocytopenia, anemia, and bone marrow suppression

Myelosuppressive:

WBC: Moderate

Platelets: Moderate

Onset: 7-10 days

Nadir: 14-21 days

Recovery: 28 days

(Continued)

Busulfan *(Continued)*

1% to 10%:

Dermatologic: Hyperpigmentation skin (busulfan tan), urticaria, erythema, alopecia

Endocrine & metabolic: Amenorrhea

Gastrointestinal: Nausea, vomiting, diarrhea; drug has little effect on the GI mucosal lining

Neuromuscular & skeletal: Weakness

<1%:

Cardiovascular: Endocardial fibrosis

Endocrine & metabolic: Adrenal suppression, gynecomastia, hyperuricemia

Genitourinary: Isolated cases of hemorrhagic cystitis have been reported; sterility; ovarian supression, testicular atrophy, malignant tumors

Hepatic: Hepatic dysfunction

Ocular: Blurred vision, cataracts

Respiratory: After long-term or high-dose therapy, a syndrome known as "busulfan lung" may occur. This syndrome is manifested by a diffuse interstitial pulmonary fibrosis and persistent cough, fever, rales, and dyspnea associated with cumulative lifetime doses. May be relieved by corticosteroids.

Vesicant No

Emetic Potential Low (<10%)

Overdosage/Toxicology Symptoms of overdose include leukopenia and thrombocytopenia. Induction of vomiting or gastric lavage with charcoal is indicated for recent ingestion; the effects of dialysis are unknown.

Drug Interactions

Cytochrome P450 Effect: Substrate of CYP3A4 (major)

Increased Effect/Toxicity: CYP3A4 inhibitors may increase the levels/ effects of busulfan; example inhibitors include azole antifungals, ciprofloxacin, clarithromycin, diclofenac, doxycycline, erythromycin, imatinib, isoniazid, nefazodone, nicardipine, propofol, protease inhibitors, quinidine, and verapamil. Metronidazole may increase busulfan plasma levels.

Decreased Effect: CYP3A4 inducers may decrease the levels/effects of busulfan; example inducers include aminoglutethimide, carbamazepine, nafcillin, nevirapine, phenobarbital, phenytoin, and rifamycins.

Ethanol/Nutrition/Herb Interactions

Ethanol: Avoid ethanol due to GI irritation.

Food: No clear or firm data on the effect of food on busulfan bioavailability.

Herb/Nutraceutical: St John's wort may decrease busulfan levels.

Storage/Stability Store unopened ampuls (injection) under refrigeration (2°C to 8°C). Final solution is stable for up to 8 hours at room temperature (25°C); the infusion must also be completed within that 8-hour time frame. Dilution of busulfan injection in 0.9% sodium chloride is stable for up to 12 hours at refrigeration (2°C to 8°C) but the infusion must also be completed within that 12-hour time frame.

Reconstitution Dilute in 0.9% NaCl injection or dextrose 5% in water. The dilution volume should be 10 times the volume of busulfan injection, ensuring that the final concentration of busulfan is 0.5 mg/mL.

Compatibility Variable stability (consult detailed reference) in D_5W, NS

Pharmacodynamics/Kinetics

Duration: 28 days

Absorption: Rapid and complete

Distribution: V_d: ~1 L/kg; into CSF and saliva with levels similar to plasma

Protein binding: ~14%

Metabolism: Extensively hepatic (may increase with multiple doses)

Half-life elimination: After first dose: 3.4 hours; After last dose: 2.3 hours

Time to peak, serum: Oral: Within 4 hours; I.V.: Within 5 minutes

Excretion: Urine (10% to 50% as metabolites) within 24 hours (<2% as unchanged drug)

Dosage

Children:

For remission induction of CML: Oral: 0.06-0.12 mg/kg/day **OR** 1.8-4.6 mg/m^2/day; titrate dosage to maintain leukocyte count above 40,000/ mm^3; reduce dosage by 50% if the leukocyte count reaches 30,000-40,000/mm^3; discontinue drug if counts fall to ≤20,000/mm^3

BMT marrow-ablative conditioning regimen:

Oral: 1 mg/kg/dose (ideal body weight) every 6 hours for 16 doses

I.V.:

≤12 kg: 1.1 mg/kg/dose (ideal body weight) every 6 hours for 16 doses

>12 kg: 0.8 mg/kg/dose (ideal body weight) every 6 hours for 16 doses

Adjust dose to desired AUC [1125 μmol(min)] using the following formula:

Adjusted dose (mg) = Actual dose (mg) x [target AUC μmol(min) / actual AUC μmol(min)]

Adults:

For remission induction of CML: Oral: 4-8 mg/day (may be as high as 12 mg/day); Maintenance doses: 1-4 mg/day to 2 mg/week to maintain WBC 10,000-20,000 cells/mm^3

BMT marrow-ablative conditioning regimen:

Oral: 1 mg/kg/dose (ideal body weight) every 6 hours for 16 doses

I.V.: 0.8 mg/kg (ideal body weight or actual body weight, whichever is lower) every 6 hours for 4 days (a total of 16 doses)

Polycythemia vera (unlabeled use): Oral: 2-6 mg/day

Thrombocytosis (unlabeled use): Oral: 4-6 mg/day

Administration Intravenous busulfan should be administered as a 2-hour infusion, every 6 hours for 4 consecutive days for a total of 16 doses.

BMT only: To facilitate ingestion of high oral doses, insert multiple tablets into gelatin capsules.

Dosage Forms

Injection, solution (Busulfex®): 6 mg/mL (10 mL)

Tablet (Myleran®): 2 mg

High Dose Considerations

High Dose: Note: Generally combined with other high-dose chemotherapeutic drugs or total body irradiation.

Oral:

0.875-1 mg/kg/dose every 6 hours for 16 doses; total dose: 12-16 mg/ kg

(Continued)

Busulfan *(Continued)*

37.5 mg/m^2 every 6 hours for 16 doses; total dose: 600 mg/m^2 (studied primarily in pediatric patients)

150 mg/m^2 daily for 4 days; total dose: 600 mg/m^2 (studied primarily in pediatric patients)

I.V.: 0.8 mg/kg every 6 hours for 16 doses (4 days)

Unique Toxicities:

Central nervous system: Generalized or myoclonic seizures and loss of consciousness, abnormal electroencephalographic findings

Gastrointestinal: Mucositis, anorexia, moderately emetogenic

Hepatic: Veno-occlusive disease (VOD), hyperbilirubinemia

Respiratory: Idiopathic pneumonia syndrome

Miscellaneous: Transient pain at tumor sites, transient autoimmune disorders

Comments: Phenytoin or clonazepam should be administered prophylactically during and for at least 48 hours following completion of busulfan. Risk of seizures is increased in patients with sickle cell disease. Increased risk of VOD when busulfan AUC >3000 µmol(min)/L (mean AUC, 2012 µmol(min)/L). Increased risk of failure to engraft for allogeneic BMT patients when AUC is <900 µmol (min)/L. To facilitate ingestion of high doses, multiple tablets may be inserted into gelatin capsules. Ursodiol 9-12 mg/kg/day may reduce the risk of hepatotoxicity.

Monitoring Parameters CBC with differential and platelet count, hemoglobin, liver function tests

Patient Information Take oral medication as directed with chilled liquids. Maintain adequate hydration (2-3 L/day of fluids unless instructed to restrict fluid intake) to help prevent kidney complications. Avoid alcohol, acidic or spicy foods, aspirin, or OTC medications unless approved by prescriber. Brush teeth with soft toothbrush or cotton swab. You may lose head hair or experience darkening of skin color (reversible when medication is discontinued), amenorrhea, sterility, or skin rash. You may experience nausea, vomiting, anorexia, or constipation (small frequent meals, increased exercise, and increased dietary fruit or fiber may help). You will be more susceptible to infection (avoid crowds or contagious persons, and do not receive any vaccinations unless approved by prescriber). Report palpitations or chest pain, excessive dizziness, confusion, respiratory difficulty, numbness or tingling of extremities, unusual bruising or bleeding, pain or changes in urination, or other adverse effects. Contraceptive measures are recommended during therapy.

Special Geriatric Considerations Toxicity to immunosuppressives is increased in the elderly. Start with lowest recommended adult doses. Signs of infection, such as fever and rise in WBCs, may not occur. Lethargy and confusion may be more prominent signs of infection.

Selected Readings

Buggia I, Locatelli F, Regazzi MB, et al, "Busulfan," *Ann Pharmacother*, 1994, 28(9):1055-62.

Heard BE and Cooke RA, "Busulphan Lung," *Thorax*, 1968, 23(2):187-93.

Regazzi MB, Locatelli F, Buggia I, et al, "Disposition of High-Dose Busulfan in Pediatric Patients Undergoing Bone Marrow Transplantation," *Clin Pharmacol Ther*, 1993, 54(1):45-52.

Shaw PJ, Nath C, Berry A, et al, "Busulphan Given as Four Single Daily Doses of 150 mg/m^2 is Safe and Effective in Children of All Ages," *Bone Marrow Transplant*, 2004, 34(3):197-205.

Vassal G, Gouyette A, Hartmann O, et al, "Pharmacokinetics of High-Dose Busulfan in Children," *Cancer Chemother Pharmacol*, 1989, 24(6):386-90.

♦ **Busulfex®** *see* Busulfan *on page 141*

♦ **C2B8** *see* Rituximab *on page 709*

♦ **C2B8 Monoclonal Antibody** *see* Rituximab *on page 709*

♦ **C225** *see* Cetuximab *on page 172*

♦ **Caelyx® (Can)** *see* DOXOrubicin (Liposomal) *on page 286*

♦ **Calcimar® (Can)** *see* Calcitonin *on page 145*

Calcitonin (kal si TOE nin)

Medication Safety Issues
Sound-alike/look-alike issues:
Calcitonin may be confused with calcitriol
Miacalcin® may be confused with Micatin®

U.S. Brand Names Miacalcin®

Canadian Brand Names Calcimar®; Caltine®; Miacalcin® NS

Generic Available No

Synonyms Calcitonin (Salmon)

Pharmacologic Category Antidote

Pregnancy Risk Factor C

Lactation Excretion in breast milk unknown

Use Calcitonin (salmon): Treatment of Paget's disease of bone (osteitis deformans); adjunctive therapy for hypercalcemia; used in postmenopausal osteoporosis and osteogenesis imperfecta

Mechanism of Action Structurally similar to human calcitonin; it directly inhibits osteoclastic bone resorption; promotes the renal excretion of calcium, phosphate, sodium, magnesium and potassium by decreasing tubular reabsorption; increases the jejunal secretion of water, sodium, potassium, and chloride

Labeled Contraindications Hypersensitivity to salmon protein or gelatin diluent

Warnings/Precautions A skin test should be performed prior to initiating therapy of calcitonin salmon in patients with suspected sensitivity. Have epinephrine immediately available for a possible hypersensitivity reaction. Use caution with renal insufficiency, pernicious anemia.

Adverse Reactions
>10%:
Cardiovascular: Facial flushing
Gastrointestinal: Nausea, diarrhea, anorexia
Local: Edema at injection site
1% to 10%:
Genitourinary: Polyuria
Neuromuscular & skeletal: Back/joint pain
Respiratory: Nasal bleeding/crusting (following intranasal administration)
<1% (Limited to important or life-threatening): Allergic-type reactions (including anaphylactic shock); dyspnea

Vesicant No

Emetic Potential Moderate (30% to 60%); nausea and vomiting are generally mild

Overdosage/Toxicology Symptoms of overdose include nausea, vomiting, hypocalcemia, and hypocalcemic tetany. Treat symptomatically. (Continued)

Calcitonin *(Continued)*

Drug Interactions
Decreased Effect: Calcitonin may be antagonized by calcium and vitamin D in treating hypercalcemia.
Ethanol/Nutrition/Herb Interactions Ethanol: Avoid ethanol (may increase risk of osteoporosis).

Storage/Stability Salmon calcitonin:
Injection: Store under refrigeration at 2°C to 6°C (36°F to 43°F); stable for up to 2 weeks at room temperature.
Nasal: Store unopened bottle under refrigeration at 2°C to 8°C. Once the pump has been activated, store at room temperature.

Reconstitution Salmon calcitonin: Injection: NS has been recommended for the dilution to prepare a skin test in patients with suspected sensitivity.

Pharmacodynamics/Kinetics
Hypercalcemia:
Onset of action: ~2 hours
Duration: 6-8 hours
Distribution: Does not cross placenta
Half-life elimination: SubQ: 1.2 hours
Excretion: Urine (as inactive metabolites)

Dosage Salmon calcitonin:
Children: Dosage not established
Adults:
Paget's disease: I.M., SubQ: Initial: 100 units/day; maintenance: 50 units/day or 50-100 units every 1-3 days
Hypercalcemia: Initial: I.M., SubQ: 4 units/kg every 12 hours; may increase up to 8 units/kg every 12 hours to a maximum of every 6 hours
Osteogenesis imperfecta: I.M., SubQ: 2 units/kg 3 times/week
Postmenopausal osteoporosis:
I.M., SubQ: 100 units/day
Intranasal: 200 units (1 spray)/day

Administration I.V., SubQ, Nasal inhalation: The intramuscular route is recommended over the subcutaneous route when the volume of calcitonin to be injected exceeds 2 mL. Such volumes should be given in divided injections.

Dosage Forms
Injection, solution, calcitonin-salmon: 200 int. units/mL (2 mL)
Solution, nasal spray, calcitonin-salmon: 200 int. units/0.09 mL (3.7 mL) [contains benzalkonium chloride]

Monitoring Parameters Serum electrolytes and calcium; alkaline phosphatase and 24-hour urine collection for hydroxyproline excretion (Paget's disease); serum calcium

Dietary Considerations Adequate vitamin D and calcium intake is essential for osteoporosis. Patients with Paget's disease and hypercalcemia should follow a low calcium diet as prescribed.

Patient Information Nasal spray: Notify prescriber if you develop significant nasal irritation. To activate the pump, hold the bottle upright and depress the two white side arms toward the bottle six times until a faint spray is emitted. The pump is activated once this first faint spray has been emitted; at this point, firmly place the nozzle into the bottle. It is not

necessary to reactivate the pump before each daily use. Alternate nostrils with the spray formulation.

Special Geriatric Considerations Calcitonin may be the drug of choice for postmenopausal women unable to take estrogens to increase bone density and reduce fractures. Calcium and vitamin D supplements should also be given. Calcitonin may also be effective in steroid-induced osteoporosis and other states associated with high bone turnover.

Selected Readings

Bergqvist E, Sjoberg HE, Hjern B, et al, "Calcitonin in the Treatment of Hypercalcaemic Crisis," *Acta Med Scand*, 1972, 192(5):385-9.

Reginster JY, "Calcitonin for Prevention and Treatment of Osteoporosis," *Am J Med*, 1993, 95(5A):44S-47S.

Silverman SL, "Calcitonin," *Endocrinol Metab Clin North Am*, 2003, 32(1):273-84.

Silverman SL, "Calcitonin," *Rheum Dis Clin North Am*, 2001, 27(1):187-96.

Zaidi M, Inzerillo AM, Moonga BS, et al, "Forty Years of Calcitonin - Where Are We Now? A Tribute to the Work of Iain Macintyre, FRS," *Bone*, 2002, 30(5):655-63.

♦ **Calcitonin (Salmon)** *see* Calcitonin *on page 145*
♦ **Calcium Leucovorin** *see* Leucovorin *on page 497*
♦ **Caldecort® [OTC]** *see* Hydrocortisone *on page 419*
♦ **Caltine® (Can)** *see* Calcitonin *on page 145*
♦ **Campath®** *see* Alemtuzumab *on page 37*
♦ **Campath-1H** *see* Alemtuzumab *on page 37*
♦ **Camptosar®** *see* Irinotecan *on page 478*
♦ **Camptothecin-11** *see* Irinotecan *on page 478*
♦ **Cancidas®** *see* Caspofungin *on page 159*
♦ **Candistatin® (Can)** *see* Nystatin *on page 613*
♦ **Canesten® Topical (Can)** *see* Clotrimazole *on page 203*
♦ **Canesten® Vaginal (Can)** *see* Clotrimazole *on page 203*

Capecitabine (ka pe SITE a been)

Related Information
Safe Handling of Hazardous Drugs *on page 1034*
U.S. Brand Names Xeloda®
Canadian Brand Names Xeloda®
Generic Available No
Pharmacologic Category Antineoplastic Agent, Antimetabolite
Pregnancy Risk Factor D
Lactation Excretion in breast milk unknown/not recommended
Use Treatment of metastatic colorectal cancer, metastatic breast cancer
Mechanism of Action Capecitabine is a prodrug of fluorouracil. It undergoes hydrolysis in the liver and tissues to form fluorouracil which is the active moiety. Fluorouracil is a fluorinated pyrimidine antimetabolite that inhibits thymidylate synthetase, blocking the methylation of deoxyuridylic acid to thymidylic acid, interfering with DNA, and to a lesser degree, RNA synthesis. Fluorouracil appears to be phase specific for the G_1 and S phases of the cell cycle.
Labeled Contraindications Hypersensitivity to capecitabine, fluorouracil, or any component of the formulation; known deficiency of dihydropyrimidine dehydrogenase (DPD); severe renal impairment (Cl_{cr} <30 mL/minute); pregnancy
Warnings/Precautions Hazardous agent - use appropriate precautions for handling and disposal. See Safe Handling of Hazardous Drugs *on page 1034* in the Appendix. Use with caution in patients with bone
(Continued)

Capecitabine *(Continued)*

marrow suppression, poor nutritional status, on warfarin therapy, ≥80 years of age, or renal or hepatic dysfunction. Use with caution in patients who have received extensive pelvic radiation or alkylating therapy. Use cautiously with warfarin; altered coagulation parameters and bleeding have been reported.

Capecitabine can cause severe diarrhea; median time to first occurrence is 31 days; subsequent doses should be reduced after grade 3 or 4 diarrhea

If grade 2 or 3 hand-and-foot syndrome occurs, interrupt administration of capecitabine until the event resolves or decreases in intensity to grade 1. Following grade 3 hand-and-foot syndrome, decrease subsequent doses of capecitabine.

Use caution in patients with coronary artery disease. Cardiotoxicity has been associated with fluorinated pyrimidine therapy, including myocardial infarction, angina, dysrhythmias, cardiogenic shock, sudden death, and ECG changes (increased risk in CAD).

Adverse Reactions Frequency listed derived from monotherapy trials.

>10%:

Cardiovascular: Edema (9% to 15%)

Central nervous system: Fatigue (~40%), fever (12% to 18%), pain (colorectal cancer: 12%)

Dermatologic: Palmar-plantar erythrodysesthesia (hand-and-foot syndrome) (~55%, may be dose limiting), dermatitis (27% to 37%)

Gastrointestinal: Diarrhea (~55%, may be dose limiting), mild to moderate nausea (43% to 53%), vomiting (27% to 37%), stomatitis (~25%), decreased appetite (colorectal cancer: 26%), anorexia (23%), abdominal pain (20% to 35%), constipation (~15%)

Hematologic: Lymphopenia (94%), anemia (72% to 80%; Grade 3/4: <1% to 3%), neutropenia (13% to 26%; Grade 3/4: 1% to 2%), thrombocytopenia (24%; Grade 3/4: 1% to 3%)

Hepatic: Increased bilirubin (22% to 48%)

Neuromuscular & skeletal: Paresthesia (21%)

Ocular: Eye irritation (~15%)

Respiratory: Dyspnea (colorectal cancer: 14%)

5% to 10%:

Cardiovascular: Venous thrombosis (colorectal cancer: 8%), chest pain (colorectal cancer: 6%)

Central nervous system: Headache (~10%), dizziness (~8%), insomnia (8%), mood alteration (colorectal cancer: 5%), depression (colorectal cancer: 5%)

Dermatologic: Nail disorders (7%), skin discoloration (colorectal cancer: 7%), alopecia (colorectal cancer: 6%)

Endocrine & metabolic: Dehydration (7%)

Gastrointestinal: Motility disorder (colorectal cancer: 10%), oral discomfort (colorectal cancer: 10%), dyspepsia (8%), upper GI inflammatory disorders (colorectal cancer: 8%), hemorrhage (colorectal cancer: 6%), ileus (colorectal cancer: 6%), taste disturbance (colorectal cancer: 6%)

Neuromuscular & skeletal: Back pain (colorectal cancer: 10%), myalgia (9%), neuropathy (colorectal cancer: 10%), arthralgia (colorectal cancer: 8%), limb pain (colorectal cancer: 6%)

Respiratory: Cough (7%), sore throat (2%), epistaxis (3%)

Ocular: Abnormal vision (colorectal cancer: 5%)

Miscellaneous: Viral infection (colorectal cancer: 5%)

<5%: Abdominal distension, angina, appetite increased, arthritis, ascites, asthma, ataxia, atrial fibrillation, bronchitis, bone pain, bradycardia, bronchopneumonia, bronchospasm, cachexia, cardiac arrest, cardiac failure, cardiomyopathy, cerebral vascular accident, cholestasis, colitis, confusion, conjunctivitis, deep vein thrombosis, diaphoresis increased, duodenitis, dysarthria, dysphagia, dysrhythmia, ecchymoses, ECG changes, encephalopathy, esophagitis, fibrosis, fungal infection, gastric ulcer, gastritis, gastroenteritis, GI hemorrhage, hematemesis, hemoptysis, hepatitis, hepatic failure, hepatic fibrosis, hoarseness, hot flushes, hypokalemia, hypomagnesemia, hypotension, hypersensitivity, hypertension, hypertriglyceridemia, idiopathic thrombocytopenia purpura, ileus, impaired balance, infection, influenza-like illness, intestinal obstruction ($\sim$1%), irritability, joint stiffness, keratoconjunctivitis, laryngitis, leukopenia, loss of consciousness, lymphedema, MI, myocardial ischemia, myocarditis, necrotizing enterocolitis, nocturia, oral candidiasis, pericardial effusion, thrombocytopenic purpura, pancytopenia, photosensitivity reaction, pneumonia, proctalgia, pruritus, pulmonary embolism, radiation recall syndrome, renal impairment, respiratory distress, sedation, sepsis, skin ulceration, toxic dilation of intestine, tachycardia, thirst, thrombophlebitis, tremor, weight gain, ventricular extrasystoles, vertigo

Emetic Potential Moderate (30% to 60%)

Overdosage/Toxicology Symptoms of overdose include myelosuppression, nausea, vomiting, diarrhea, and alopecia. No specific antidote exists. Monitor hematologically for at least 4 weeks. Treatment is supportive.

Drug Interactions

Increased Effect/Toxicity: Response to warfarin may be increased by capecitabine.

Ethanol/Nutrition/Herb Interactions Food: Food reduced the rate and extent of absorption of capecitabine.

Storage/Stability Store tablets at room temperature of 25°C (77°F).

Pharmacodynamics/Kinetics

Absorption: Rapid and extensive

Protein binding: <60%; 35% to albumin

Metabolism: Hepatic: Inactive metabolites: 5'-deoxy-5-fluorocytidine, 5'-deoxy-5-fluorouridine; Tissue: Active metabolite: Fluorouracil

Half-life elimination: 0.5-1 hour

Time to peak: 1.5 hours; Fluorouracil: 2 hours

Excretion: Urine (96%, 50% as α-fluoro-β-alanine)

Dosage Oral:

Adults: 2500 mg/m^2/day in 2 divided doses ($\sim$12 hours apart) for 2 weeks every 21-28 days

Elderly: The elderly may be pharmacodynamically more sensitive to the toxic effects of fluorouracil. Insufficient data are available to provide dosage modifications.

Dosing adjustment in renal impairment:

Cl_{cr} 50-80 mL/minute: No adjustment of initial dose

Cl_{cr} 30-50 mL/minute: Reduce dose by 25%

Cl_{cr} <30 mL/minute: Do not use

(Continued)

Capecitabine *(Continued)*

Dosing adjustment in hepatic impairment:

Mild to moderate impairment: No starting dose adjustment is necessary; however, carefully monitor patients

Severe hepatic impairment: Patients have not been studied

Combination Regimens

Colorectal cancer: XelOx *on page 949*

Pancreatic cancer: Gemcitabine/Capecitabine *on page 895*

Administration Capecitabine is administered orally, usually in two divided doses taken 12 hours apart. Doses should be taken after meals with water.

Dosage Forms Tablet: 150 mg, 500 mg

Monitoring Parameters Renal function should be estimated at baseline to determine initial dose; during therapy, CBC with differential, hepatic function, and renal function should be monitored

Dietary Considerations Because current safety and efficacy data are based upon administration with food, it is recommended that capecitabine be administered with food. In all clinical trials, patients were instructed to administer capecitabine within 30 minutes after a meal.

Patient Information Take with food or within 30 minutes after meal. Avoid use of antacids within 2 hours of taking capecitabine. Do not crush, chew, or dissolve tablets. You will need frequent blood tests while taking this medication. Maintain adequate hydration (2-3 L/day of fluids unless instructed to restrict fluid intake). You may experience lethargy, dizziness, visual changes, confusion, anxiety (avoid driving or engaging in tasks requiring alertness until response to drug is known). For nausea, vomiting, loss of appetite, or dry mouth, small, frequent meals, chewing gum, or sucking lozenges may help. You may experience loss of hair (will grow back when treatment is discontinued). You may experience photosensitivity (use sunscreen, wear protective clothing and eyewear, and avoid direct sunlight). You may experience dry, itchy, skin, and dry or irritated eyes (avoid contact lenses). You will be more susceptible to infection; avoid crowds or infected persons. Report chills or fever, confusion, persistent or violent vomiting or stomach pain, persistent diarrhea, respiratory difficulty, chest pain or palpitations, unusual bleeding or bruising, bone pain, muscle spasms/tremors, or vision changes immediately.

Special Geriatric Considerations Patients ≥80 years of age may experience a greater incidence of grade 3 or 4 adverse events (diarrhea, hand-and-foot syndrome, nausea/vomiting).

Selected Readings

Budman DR, "Capecitabine," *Invest New Drugs*, 2000, 18(4):355-63.

Dooley M and Goa KL, "Capecitabine," *Drugs*, 1999, 58(1):69-76.

Ishitsuka H, "Capecitabine: Preclinical Pharmacology Studies," *Invest New Drugs*, 2000, 18(4):343-54.

Johnston PG and Kaye S, "Capecitabine: A Novel Agent for the Treatment of Solid Tumors," *Anticancer Drugs*, 2001, 12(8):639-46.

McGavin JK and Goa KL, "Capecitabine: A Review of Its Use in the Treatment of Advanced or Metastatic Colorectal Cancer," *Drugs*, 2001, 61(15):2309-26.

Schilsky RL, "Pharmacology and Clinical Status of Capecitabine," *Oncology*, 2000, 14(9):1297-306.

♦ **Carac**™ *see Fluorouracil on page 359*

Carboplatin (KAR boe pla tin)

Medication Safety Issues

Sound-alike/look-alike issues:

Carboplatin may be confused with cisplatin

Paraplatin® may be confused with Platinol®

Related Information

Management of Nausea and Vomiting *on page 982*

Safe Handling of Hazardous Drugs *on page 1034*

Transplantation *on page 1019*

U.S. Brand Names Paraplatin®

Canadian Brand Names Paraplatin-AQ

Generic Available Yes

Synonyms CBDCA

Pharmacologic Category Antineoplastic Agent, Alkylating Agent

Pregnancy Risk Factor D

Lactation Excretion in breast milk unknown/contraindicated

Use Treatment of ovarian cancer

Unlabeled/Investigational Use Lung cancer, head and neck cancer, endometrial cancer, esophageal cancer, bladder cancer, breast cancer, cervical cancer, CNS tumors, germ cell tumors, osteogenic sarcoma, and high-dose therapy with stem cell/bone marrow support

Mechanism of Action Carboplatin is an alkylating agent which covalently binds to DNA; possible cross-linking and interference with the function of DNA

Labeled Contraindications History of severe allergic reaction to cisplatin, carboplatin, other platinum-containing formulations, mannitol, or any component of the formulation; pregnancy

Warnings/Precautions Hazardous agent - use appropriate precautions for handling and disposal. See Safe Handling of Hazardous Drugs *on page 1034* in the Appendix. High doses have resulted in severe abnormalities of liver function tests. Bone marrow suppression, which may be severe, and vomiting are dose related; reduce dosage in patients with bone marrow suppression and impaired renal function. Increased risk of allergic reactions in patients previously exposed to platinum therapy. When administered as sequential infusions, taxane derivatives (docetaxel, paclitaxel) should be administered before the platinum derivatives (carboplatin, cisplatin) to limit myelosuppression and to enhance efficacy.

Adverse Reactions

>10%:

Dermatologic: Alopecia

Endocrine & metabolic: Hypomagnesemia, hypokalemia, hyponatremia, hypocalcemia; less severe than those seen after cisplatin (usually asymptomatic)

Gastrointestinal: Nausea, vomiting, stomatitis

Hematologic: Myelosuppression (dose related and dose-limiting); thrombocytopenia (37% to 80%); leukopenia (27% to 38%)

Nadir: ~21 days following a single dose

Hepatic: Alkaline phosphatase increased, AST increased (usually mild and reversible)

Otic: Hearing loss at high tones (above speech ranges, up to 19%); clinically-important ototoxicity is not usually seen

(Continued)

Carboplatin *(Continued)*

Renal: Increases in creatinine and BUN have been reported

1% to 10%:

Gastrointestinal: Diarrhea, anorexia

Hematologic: Hemorrhagic complications

Local: Pain at injection site

Neuromuscular & skeletal: Peripheral neuropathy (4% to 6%; up to 10% in older and/or previously-treated patients)

Otic: Ototoxicity

<1% (Limited to important or life-threatening): Neurotoxicity, urticaria, rash, nephrotoxicity, secondary malignancies, anaphylaxis, malaise, hypertension

Vesicant No

Emetic Potential Moderate (30% to 60%)

Overdosage/Toxicology Symptoms of overdose include bone marrow suppression and hepatic toxicity. Treatment is symptomatic and supportive.

Drug Interactions

Increased Effect/Toxicity: Nephrotoxic drugs; aminoglycosides increase risk of ototoxicity. When administered as sequential infusions, observational studies indicate a potential for increased toxicity when platinum derivatives (carboplatin, cisplatin) are administered before taxane derivatives (docetaxel, paclitaxel).

Ethanol/Nutrition/Herb Interactions Herb/Nutraceutical: Avoid black cohosh, dong quai in estrogen-dependent tumors.

Storage/Stability Store intact vials at room temperature of 15°C to 30°C (59°F to 86°F); protect from light. Further dilution to a concentration as low as 0.5 mg/mL is stable at room temperature (25°C) or under refrigeration for 8 days in D_5W.

Powder for reconstitution: Reconstituted to a final concentration of 10 mg/mL is stable for 5 days at room temperature (25°C).

Solution for injection: Multidose vials are stable for up to 14 days after opening when stored at room temperature.

Reconstitution Reconstitute powder to yield a final concentration of 10 mg/mL; reconstituted carboplatin 10 mg/mL should be further diluted to a final concentration of 0.5-2 mg/mL with D_5W or NS for administration

Compatibility Stable in $D_5{}^1/_4NS$, $D_5{}^1/_2NS$, D_5NS, D_5W, NS

Y-site administration: Compatible: Allopurinol, amifostine, aztreonam, cefepime, cladribine, doxorubicin liposome, etoposide phosphate, filgrastim, fludarabine, gatifloxacin, gemcitabine, granisetron, linezolid, melphalan, ondansetron, paclitaxel, piperacillin/tazobactam, propofol, sargramostim, teniposide, thiotepa, topotecan, vinorelbine. **Incompatible:** Amphotericin B cholesteryl sulfate complex

Compatibility when admixed: Compatible: Cisplatin, etoposide, floxuridine, ifosfamide, ifosfamide with etoposide, paclitaxel. **Incompatible:** Fluorouracil, mesna

Pharmacodynamics/Kinetics

Distribution: V_d: 16 L/kg; Into liver, kidney, skin, and tumor tissue

Protein binding: 0%; platinum is 30% irreversibly bound

Metabolism: Minimally hepatic to aquated and hydroxylated compounds

Half-life elimination: Terminal: 22-40 hours; Cl_{cr} >60 mL/minute: 2.5-5.9 hours

Excretion: Urine (~60% to 90%) within 24 hours

Dosage Refer to individual protocols: **Note: Doses are usually determined by the AUC using the Calvert formula. IVPB, I.V. infusion, intraperitoneal:**

Children:

Solid tumor: 300-600 mg/m² once every 4 weeks

Brain tumor: 175 mg/m² weekly for 4 weeks every 6 weeks, with a 2-week recovery period between courses

Adults:

Ovarian cancer: 300-360 mg/m² I.V. every 3-4 weeks

Autologous BMT: I.V.: 1600 mg/m² (total dose) divided over 4 days

Dosing adjustment in renal impairment: No guidelines are available.

Dosing adjustment in hepatic impairment: No guidelines are available.

Intraperitoneal: 200-650 mg/m² in 2 L of dialysis fluid have been administered into the peritoneum of ovarian cancer patients

Combination Regimens

Adenocarcinoma, unknown primary:

Carbo-Tax (Adenocarcinoma) *on page 851*

Paclitaxel, Carboplatin, Etoposide *on page 926*

Bladder cancer: PC (Bladder Cancer) *on page 927*

Head and neck cancer: CF *on page 858*

Lung cancer (nonsmall cell):

Carbo-Tax (Nonsmall Cell Lung Cancer) *on page 851*

CaT (Nonsmall Cell Lung Cancer) *on page 852*

EC (Nonsmall Cell Lung Cancer) *on page 876*

Gemcitabine-Carboplatin *on page 896*

PC (Nonsmall Cell Lung Cancer) *on page 927*

Lung cancer (small cell): EC (Small Cell Lung Cancer) *on page 876*

Lymphoma, non-Hodgkin's:

ICE (Lymphoma, non-Hodgkin's) *on page 899*

Melanoma: Dacarbazine-Carboplatin-Aldesleukin-Interferon *on page 871*

Neuroblastoma:

CE (Neuroblastomas) *on page 856*

CE-CAdO *on page 856*

CI (Neuroblastomas) *on page 860*

Osteosarcoma: ICE (Sarcoma) *on page 899*

Ovarian cancer:

Carbo-Tax (Ovarian Cancer) *on page 852*

CaT (Ovarian Cancer) *on page 853*

CC *on page 854*

Prostate cancer:

Estramustine + Docetaxel + Carboplatin *on page 882*

Paclitaxel + Estramustine + Carboplatin *on page 926*

Retinoblastoma: CE (Retinoblastoma) *on page 856*

Rhabdomyosarcoma: CEV *on page 857*

Sarcoma, soft tissue:

ICE (Sarcoma) *on page 899*

ICE-T *on page 900*

Administration I.V.: Over 15 minutes up to 24 hours; may also be administered intraperitoneally

Dosage Forms

Injection, powder for reconstitution: 50 mg, 150 mg, 450 mg

Injection, solution: 10 mg/mL (5 mL, 15 mL, 45 mL, 60 mL)

(Continued)

Carboplatin (Continued)

High Dose Considerations

High Dose: I.V.: $1.2\text{-}2.4$ g/m^2 administered as 3-4 divided doses every 24-48 hours; generally infused over at least 60 minutes; 400 mg/m^2 has been infused over 15-30 minutes; generally combined with other high-dose chemotherapeutic drugs.

Unique Toxicities:

Dermatologic: Alopecia

Endocrine & metabolic: Hypokalemia, hypomagnesemia

Gastrointestinal: Nausea, vomiting, mucositis

Hepatic: Elevated liver function tests

Renal: Nephrotoxicity

Comments: Observe serum creatinine. Carboplatin is nephrotoxic and drug accumulation occurs with decreased creatinine clearance.

Monitoring Parameters CBC (with differential and platelet count), serum electrolytes, creatinine clearance, liver function tests

Patient Information Maintain adequate nutrition (frequent small meals may help) and adequate hydration (2-3 L/day of fluids unless instructed to restrict fluid intake). Nausea and vomiting may be severe; request antiemetic. You will be susceptible to infection; avoid crowds or exposure to infection. Report sore throat, fever, chills, unusual fatigue or unusual bruising/bleeding, difficulty breathing, muscle cramps or twitching, or change in hearing acuity. Contraceptive measures are recommended during therapy.

Special Geriatric Considerations Peripheral neuropathy is more frequent in patients >65 years of age.

Selected Readings

Duffull SB and Robinson BA, "Clinical Pharmacokinetics and Dose Optimisation of Carboplatin," *Clin Pharmacokinet*, 1997, 33(3):161-83.

Lokich J, "What is the "Best" Platinum: Cisplatin, Carboplatin, or Oxaliplatin," *Cancer Invest*, 2001, 19(7):756-60.

Lokich J and Anderson N, "Carboplatin Versus Cisplatin in Solid Tumors: An Analysis of the Literature," *Ann Oncol*, 1998, 9(1):13-21.

Lovett D, Kelsen D, Eisenberger M, et al, "A Phase II Trial of Carboplatin and Vinblastine in the Treatment of Advanced Squamous Cell Carcinoma of the Esophagus," *Cancer*, 1991, 67(2):354-6.

Murry DJ, "Comparative Clinical Pharmacology of Cisplatin and Carboplatin," *Pharmacotherapy*, 1997, 17(5 Pt 2):140S-145S.

Oguri S, Sakakibara T, Mase H, et al, "Clinical Pharmacokinetics of Carboplatin," *J Clin Pharmacol*, 1988, 28(3):208-15.

Reece PA, Stafford I, Abbott RI, et al, "Two- Versus 24-Hour Infusion of Cisplatin: Pharmacokinetic Considerations," *J Clin Oncol*, 1989, 7(2):270-5.

Zeltzer PM, Epport K, Nelson MD Jr, et al, "Prolonged Response to Carboplatin in an Infant With Brain Stem Glioma," *Cancer*, 1991, 67(1):43-7.

♦ **Carimune™ [DSC]** *see* Immune Globulin (Intravenous) *on page 458*

♦ **Carimune™ NF** *see* Immune Globulin (Intravenous) *on page 458*

Carmustine (kar MUS teen)

Related Information

Safe Handling of Hazardous Drugs *on page 1034*

Transplantation *on page 1019*

U.S. Brand Names BiCNu®; Gliadel®

Canadian Brand Names BiCNu®

Generic Available No

Synonyms BCNU; bis-chloronitrosourea; Carmustinum; NSC-409962; WR-139021

Pharmacologic Category Antineoplastic Agent; Antineoplastic Agent, Alkylating Agent (Nitrosourea); Antineoplastic Agent, DNA Adduct-Forming Agent; Antineoplastic Agent, DNA Binding Agent

Pregnancy Risk Factor D

Lactation Excretion in breast milk unknown/contraindicated

Use

Injection: Treatment of brain tumors (glioblastoma, brainstem glioma, medulloblastoma, astrocytoma, ependymoma, and metastatic brain tumors), multiple myeloma, Hodgkin's disease, non-Hodgkin's lymphomas, melanoma, lung cancer, colon cancer

Wafer (implant): Adjunct to surgery in patients with recurrent glioblastoma multiforme; adjunct to surgery and radiation in patients with high-grade malignant glioma

Mechanism of Action Interferes with the normal function of DNA by alkylation and cross-linking the strands of DNA, and by possible protein modification

Labeled Contraindications Hypersensitivity to carmustine or any component of the formulation; myelosuppression; pregnancy

Warnings/Precautions Hazardous agent - use appropriate precautions for handling and disposal. See Safe Handling of Hazardous Drugs *on page 1034* in the Appendix. Administer with caution to patients with renal or hepatic impairment. Diluent contains significant amounts of ethanol; use caution with aldehyde dehydrogenase-2 deficiency or history of "alcohol flushing syndrome."

Adverse Reactions

>10%:

Cardiovascular: Hypotension with high dose therapy, due to the alcohol content of the diluent

Central nervous system: Dizziness, ataxia; Wafers: Seizures (54%) postoperatively

Dermatologic: Pain and burning at the injection site; phlebitis

Gastrointestinal: Severe nausea and vomiting, usually begins within 2-4 hours of drug administration and lasts for 4-6 hours. Patients should receive a prophylactic antiemetic regimen.

Hematologic: Myelosuppression - cumulative, dose related, delayed, thrombocytopenia is usually more common and more severe than leukopenia

Onset (days): 7-14

Nadir (days): 21-35

Recovery (days): 42-56

Hepatic: Reversible increases in bilirubin, alkaline phosphatase, and SGOT occur in 20% to 25% of patients

Ocular: Ocular toxicities (transient conjunctival flushing and blurred vision), retinal hemorrhages

Respiratory: Interstitial fibrosis occurs in up to 50% of patients receiving a cumulative dose >1400 mg/m^2, or bone marrow transplantation doses; may be delayed up to 3 years; rare in patients receiving lower doses. A history of lung disease or concomitant bleomycin therapy may increase the risk of this reaction. Patients with forced vital capacity (FVC) or carbon monoxide diffusing capacity of the lungs (DLCO) <70% of predicted are at higher risk.

(Continued)

Carmustine *(Continued)*

1% to 10%:

Central nervous system: Wafers: Amnesia, aphasia, ataxia, cerebral edema, confusion, convulsion, depression, diplopia, dizziness, headache, hemiplegia, hydrocephalus, insomnia, meningitis, somnolence, stupor

Dermatologic: Facial flushing, probably due to the alcohol diluent; alopecia

Gastrointestinal: Anorexia, constipation, diarrhea, stomatitis

Hematologic: Anemia

<1%: Azotemia, cerebral hemorrhage infarction (wafer formulation), dermatitis, hepatic coma, hyperpigmentation, painless jaundice, subacute hepatitis

Vesicant No; the alcohol-based diluent may be an irritant, especially with high doses.

Emetic Potential Very high (>90%)

Overdosage/Toxicology Symptoms of overdose include nausea, vomiting, thrombocytopenia, and leukopenia. Treatment is symptomatic and supportive.

Drug Interactions

Increased Effect/Toxicity: Carmustine given in combination with cimetidine is reported to cause bone marrow depression. Carmustine given in combination with etoposide is reported to cause severe hepatic dysfunction with hyperbilirubinemia, ascites, and thrombocytopenia. Diluent for infusion contains alcohol; avoid concurrent use of medications that inhibit aldehyde dehydrogenase-2 or cause disulfiram-like reactions.

Ethanol/Nutrition/Herb Interactions Ethanol: Avoid ethanol.

Storage/Stability

Injection: Store intact vials under refrigeration; vials are stable for 36 days at room temperature. Reconstituted solutions are stable for 8 hours at room temperature (25°C) and 24 hours under refrigeration (2°C to 8°C) and protected from light. Further dilution in D_5W or NS is stable for 8 hours at room temperature (25°C) and 48 hours under refrigeration (4°C) in glass or Excel® protected from light.

Wafer: Store at or below -20°C (-4°F). May be kept at room temperature for up to 6 hours.

Reconstitution Injection: Initially, dilute with 3 mL of absolute alcohol. Further dilute with SWFI (27 mL) to a concentration of 3.3 mg/mL; protect from light; may further dilute with D_5W or NS.

Compatibility Compatible with D_5W, NS, SWFI, dacarbazine

Y-site administration: Compatible: Amifostine, aztreonam, cefepime, filgrastim, fludarabine, gemcitabine, granisetron, ondansetron, piperacillin/tazobactam, sargramostim, teniposide, thiotepa, vinorelbine.

Incompatible: Allopurinol, sodium bicarbonate

Pharmacodynamics/Kinetics

Distribution: Readily crosses blood-brain barrier producing CSF levels equal to 15% to 70% of blood plasma levels; enters breast milk; highly lipid soluble

Metabolism: Rapidly hepatic

Half-life elimination: Biphasic: Initial: 1.4 minutes; Secondary: 20 minutes (active metabolites: plasma half-life of 67 hours)

Excretion: Urine (~60% to 70%) within 96 hours; lungs (6% to 10% as CO_2)

Dosage

I.V. (refer to individual protocols):

Children: 200-250 mg/m^2 every 4-6 weeks as a single dose

Adults: Usual dosage (per manufacturer labeling): 150-200 mg/m^2 every 6 weeks as a single dose or divided into daily injections on 2 successive days

Alternative regimens:

75-120 mg/m^2 days 1 and 2 every 6-8 weeks **or**

50-80 mg/m^2 days 1,2,3 every 6-8 weeks

Primary brain cancer:

150-200 mg/m^2 every 6-8 weeks as a single dose **or**

75-120 mg/m^2 days 1 and 2 every 6-8 weeks **or**

20-65 mg/m^2 every 4-6 weeks **or**

0.5-1 mg/kg every 4-6 weeks **or**

40-80 mg/m^2/day for 3 days every 6-8 weeks

Autologous BMT: ALL OF THE FOLLOWING DOSES ARE FATAL WITHOUT BMT

Combination therapy: Up to 300-900 mg/m^2

Single-agent therapy: Up to 1200 mg/m^2 (fatal necrosis is associated with doses >2 g/m^2)

Implantation (wafer): Adults: Recurrent glioblastoma multiforme, malignant glioma: Up to 8 wafers may be placed in the resection cavity (total dose 62.6 mg); should the size and shape not accommodate 8 wafers, the maximum number of wafers allowed should be placed

Hemodialysis: Supplemental dosing is not required

Dosing adjustment in hepatic impairment: Dosage adjustment may be necessary; however, no specific guidelines are available

Combination Regimens

Lymphoma, Hodgkin's: mini-BEAM *on page 910*

Melanoma:

CCDT (Melanoma) *on page 855*

Dartmouth Regimen *on page 872*

Multiple myeloma:

M-2 *on page 906*

VBAP *on page 944*

VBMCP *on page 945*

Administration Injection: Significant absorption to PVC containers - should be administered in either glass or Excel® container. I.V. infusion over 1-2 hours is recommended; infusion through a free-flowing saline or dextrose infusion, or administration through a central catheter can alleviate venous pain/irritation

High-dose carmustine: Maximum rate of infusion of ≤3 mg/m^2/minute to avoid excessive flushing, agitation, and hypotension; infusions should run over at least 2 hours; some investigational protocols dictate shorter infusions.

Dosage Forms

Injection, powder for reconstitution (BiCNu®): 100 mg [packaged with 3 mL of absolute alcohol as diluent]

Wafer (Gliadel®): 7.7 mg (8s)

(Continued)

Carmustine *(Continued)*

High Dose Considerations

High Dose: I.V.: 300-800 mg/m^2 infused over at least 2 hours; may be divided into two doses administered every 12 hours; generally combined with other high-dose chemotherapeutic drugs.

Unique Toxicities:

Cardiovascular: Hypotension (infusion-related), arrhythmias (infusion-related)

Central nervous system: Encephalopathy, ethanol intoxication, seizures, fever

Endocrine & metabolic: Hyperprolactinemia and hypothyroidism in patients with brain tumors treated with radiation

Gastrointestinal: Severe nausea and vomiting

Hepatic Hepatitis, hepatic veno-occlusive disease

Pulmonary: Dyspnea

Comments: Due to risk of hypotension, patients receiving high-dose carmustine must be supine and may require the Trendelenburg position, fluid support, and vasopressor support. Vital signs must be monitored frequently during the infusion of high-dose carmustine.

Infusion-related cardiovascular effects are primarily due to concomitant ethanol and acetaldehyde. Use with great caution in patients with aldehyde dehydrogenase-2 deficiency or history of "alcohol flushing syndrome". Avoid concurrent use of medications that inhibit aldehyde dehydrogenase-2 or cause disulfiram-like reactions. Acute lung injury tends to occur 1-3 months following carmustine infusion. Patients must be counseled to contact their BMT physician for dyspnea, cough, or fever following carmustine. Acute lung injury is managed with a course of corticosteroids.

Fatal doses if not followed by bone marrow or peripheral stem cell infusions.

Monitoring Parameters CBC with differential and platelet count, pulmonary function, liver function, and renal function tests; monitor blood pressure during administration

Wafer: Complications of craniotomy (seizures, intracranial infection, brain edema)

Patient Information Limit oral intake for 4-6 hours before therapy. Do not use alcohol, aspirin-containing products, and OTC medications without consulting prescriber. You may experience nausea or vomiting (frequent small meals, frequent mouth care, sucking lozenges, or chewing gum may help). If this is ineffective, consult prescriber for antiemetic medication. You may experience loss of hair (reversible). You will be more susceptible to infection (avoid crowds and exposure to infection as much as possible). You will be more sensitive to sunlight; use sunblock, wear protective clothing and dark glasses, or avoid direct exposure to sunlight. Frequent mouth care with soft toothbrush or cotton swabs and frequent mouth rinses may help relieve mouth sores. Report fever, chills, unusual bruising or bleeding, signs of infection, excessive fatigue, yellowing of eyes or skin, or change in color of urine or stool. Contraceptive measures are recommended during therapy.

Additional Information Accidental skin contact may cause transient burning and brown discoloration of the skin. Delayed onset pulmonary fibrosis occurring up to 17 years after treatment has been reported in patients who received cumulative >1400 mg/m^2.

Selected Readings

Buzaid AC and Murren J, "Chemotherapy for Advanced Malignant Melanoma," *Int J Clin Lab Res*, 1992, 21(3):205-9.

Durando X, Lemaire JJ, Tortochaux J, et al, "High-Dose BCNU Followed by Autologous Hematopoietic Stem Cell Transplantation in Supratentorial High-Grade Malignant Gliomas: A Retrospective Analysis of 114 Patients," *Bone Marrow Transplant*, 2003, 31(7):559-64.

Fleming AB and Saltzman WM, "Pharmacokinetics of the Carmustine Implant," *Clin Pharmacokinet*, 2002, 41(6):403-19.

Lesser GJ and Grossman SA, "The Chemotherapy of Adult Primary Brain Tumors," *Cancer Treat Rev*, 1993, 19(3):261-81.

Mahendra P, Johnson D, Scott MA, et al, "Peripheral Blood Progenitor Cell Transplantation: A Single Centre Experience Comparing Two Mobilisation Regimens in 67 Patients," *Bone Marrow Transplant*, 1996, 17(4):503-7.

Weingart JD and Brem H, "Carmustine Implants: Potential in the Treatment of Brain Tumors," *CNS Drugs*, 1996, 4:263-9.

Weiss RB and Issell BF, "The Nitrosoureas: Carmustine (BCNU) and Lomustine (CCNU)," *Cancer Treat Rev*, 1982, 9(3):313-30.

♦ **Carmustinum** *see* Carmustine *on page 154*

♦ **Carter's Little Pills® (Can)** *see* Bisacodyl *on page 133*

♦ **Casodex®** *see* Bicalutamide *on page 131*

Caspofungin (kas poe FUN jin)

U.S. Brand Names Cancidas®

Canadian Brand Names Cancidas®

Generic Available No

Synonyms Caspofungin Acetate

Pharmacologic Category Antifungal Agent, Parenteral

Pregnancy Risk Factor C

Lactation Excretion in breast milk unknown/use caution

Use Treatment of invasive *Aspergillus* infections in patients who are refractory or intolerant of other therapy; treatment of candidemia and other *Candida* infections (intra-abdominal abscesses, esophageal, peritonitis, pleural space); empirical treatment for presumed fungal infections in febrile neutropenic patient

Mechanism of Action Inhibits synthesis of β(1,3)-D-glucan, an essential component of the cell wall of susceptible fungi. Highest activity in regions of active cell growth. Mammalian cells do not require β(1,3)-D-glucan, limiting potential toxicity.

Labeled Contraindications Hypersensitivity to caspofungin or any component of the formulation

Warnings/Precautions Concurrent use of cyclosporine should be limited to patients for whom benefit outweighs risk, due to a high frequency of hepatic transaminase elevations observed during concurrent use. Limited data are available concerning treatment durations longer than 4 weeks; however, treatment appears to be well tolerated. Use caution in hepatic impairment; dosage reduction required in moderate impairment. Safety and efficacy in pediatric patients have not been established.

Adverse Reactions

>10%:

Central nervous system: Headache (up to 11%), fever (3% to 26%), chills (up to 14%)

Endocrine & metabolic: Hypokalemia (4% to 11%)

(Continued)

Caspofungin *(Continued)*

Hematologic: Hemoglobin decreased (1% to 12%)

Hepatic: Serum alkaline phosphatase (3% to 11%) increased, transaminases increased (up to 13%)

Local: Infusion site reactions (2% to 12%), phlebitis/thrombophlebitis (up to 16%)

1% to 10%:

Cardiovascular: Flushing (2% to 3%), facial edema (up to 3%), hypertension (1% to 2%), tachycardia (1% to 2%), hypotension (1%)

Central nervous system: Dizziness (2%), pain (1% to 5%), insomnia (1%)

Dermatologic: Rash (<1% to 6%), pruritus (1% to 3%), erythema (1% to 2%)

Gastrointestinal: Nausea (2% to 6%), vomiting (1% to 4%), abdominal pain (1% to 4%), diarrhea (1% to 4%), anorexia (1%)

Hematologic: Eosinophils increased (3%), neutrophils decreased (2% to 3%), WBC decreased (5% to 6%), anemia (up to 4%), platelet count decreased (2% to 3%)

Hepatic: Bilirubin increased (3%)

Local: Induration (up to 3%)

Neuromuscular & skeletal: Myalgia (up to 3%), paresthesia (1% to 3%), tremor (≤2%)

Renal: Nephrotoxicity (8%)*, proteinuria (5%), hematuria (2%), serum creatinine increased (<1% to 4%), urinary WBCs increased (up to 8%), urinary RBCs increased (1% to 4%), blood urea nitrogen increased (1%)

*Nephrotoxicity defined as serum creatinine ≥2X baseline value or ≥1 mg/dL in patients with serum creatinine above ULN range (patients with Cl_{cr} <30 mL/minute were excluded)

Miscellaneous: Flu-like syndrome (3%), diaphoresis (up to 3%)

<1%: Adult respiratory distress syndrome (ARDS), jaundice, pulmonary edema, renal insufficiency, serum bicarbonate decreased, tachypnea; histamine-mediated reactions (including facial swelling, bronchospasm, sensation of warmth) have been reported

Postmarketing and/or case reports: Anaphylaxis, dyspnea, dystonia, hepatic dysfunction, hypercalcemia, peripheral edema, swelling, stridor

Overdosage/Toxicology No experience with overdosage has been reported. Caspofungin is not dialyzable. Treatment is symptomatic and supportive.

Drug Interactions

Increased Effect/Toxicity: Concurrent administration of cyclosporine may increase caspofungin concentrations; hepatic serum transaminases may be observed.

Decreased Effect: Caspofungin may decrease blood concentrations of tacrolimus. Dosage adjustment of caspofungin to 70 mg is required for patients on rifampin.

Storage/Stability Store vials at 2°C to 8°C (36°F to 46°F). Reconstituted solution may be stored at less than 25°C (77°F) for 1 hour prior to preparation of infusion solution. Infusion solutions may be stored at less than 25°C (77°F) and should be used within 24 hours; up to 48 hours if stored at 2°C to 8°C (36°F to 46°F).

Reconstitution Bring refrigerated vial to room temperature. Reconstitute vials using 0.9% sodium chloride for injection, SWFI, or bacteriostatic water for injection. Mix gently until clear solution is formed; do not use if cloudy or contains particles. Solution should be further diluted with 0.9%, 0.45%, or 0.225% sodium chloride or LR. Do not mix with dextrose-containing solutions. Do not coadminister with other medications.

Compatibility Compatible in NS, ½NS, ¼NS, LR. Do not mix with dextrose-containing solutions.

Pharmacodynamics/Kinetics

Protein binding: 97% to albumin

Metabolism: Slowly, via hydrolysis and *N*-acetylation as well as by spontaneous degradation, with subsequent metabolism to component amino acids. Overall metabolism is extensive.

Half-life elimination: Beta (distribution): 9-11 hours; Terminal: 40-50 hours

Excretion: Urine (41% as metabolites, 1% to 9% unchanged) and feces (35% as metabolites)

Dosage I.V.:

Children: Safety and efficacy in pediatric patients have not been established

Adults: **Note:** Duration of caspofungin treatment should be determined by patient status and clinical response. Empiric therapy should be given until neutropenia resolves. In patients with positive cultures, treatment should continue until 14 days after last positive culture. In neutropenic patients, treatment should be given at least 7 days after both signs and symptoms of infection **and** neutropenia resolve.

Empiric therapy: Initial dose: 70 mg on day 1; subsequent dosing: 50 mg/day; may increase up to 70 mg/day if tolerated, but clinical response is inadequate

Invasive *Aspergillus*, candidiasis: Initial dose: 70 mg on day 1; subsequent dosing: 50 mg/day

Esophageal candidiasis: 50 mg/day; **Note:** The majority of patients studied for this indication also had oropharyngeal involvement.

Concomitant use of an enzyme inducer:

Patients receiving rifampin: 70 mg caspofungin daily

Patients receiving carbamazepine, dexamethasone, efavirenz, nevirapine, **or** phenytoin (and possibly other enzyme inducers) may require an increased daily dose of caspofungin (70 mg/day).

Elderly: The number of patients >65 years of age in clinical studies was not sufficient to establish whether a difference in response may be anticipated.

Dosage adjustment in renal impairment: No specific dosage adjustment is required; supplemental dose is not required following dialysis

Dosage adjustment in hepatic impairment:

Mild hepatic insufficiency (Child-Pugh score 5-6): No adjustment necessary

Moderate hepatic insufficiency (Child-Pugh score 7-9): 35 mg/day; initial 70 mg loading dose should still be administered in treatment of invasive infections

Severe hepatic insufficiency (Child-Pugh score >9): No clinical experience

Administration Infuse slowly, over 1 hour; monitor during infusion; isolated cases of possible histamine-related reactions have occurred during clinical trials (rash, flushing, pruritus, facial edema)

(Continued)

Caspofungin *(Continued)*

Dosage Forms Injection, powder for reconstitution, as acetate: 50 mg [contains sucrose 39 mg], 70 mg [contains sucrose 54 mg]

Patient Information This medication can only be administered by infusion. Report immediately any pain, burning, or swelling at infusion site, or any signs of allergic reaction (eg, difficulty breathing or swallowing, back pain, chest tightness, rash, hives, or swelling of lips or mouth). Report nausea, vomiting, abdominal pain, or diarrhea.

Selected Readings

Mora-Duarte J, Betts R, Rotstein C, et al, "Comparison of Caspofungin and Amphotericin B for Invasive Candidiasis," *N Engl J Med*, 2002, 347(25):2020-9.

Pappas PG, Rex JH, Sobel JD, et al, "Guidelines for Treatment of Candidiasis," *Clin Infect Dis*, 2004, 38:161-89.

Stone EA, Fung HB, and Kirschenbaum HL, "Caspofungin: An Echinocandin Antifungal Agent," *Clin Ther*, 2002, 24(3):351-77.

- ◆ **Caspofungin Acetate** *see* Caspofungin *on page 159*
- ◆ **Cathflo™ Activase®** *see* Alteplase *on page 46*
- ◆ **CB-1348** *see* Chlorambucil *on page 175*
- ◆ **CBDCA** *see* Carboplatin *on page 151*
- ◆ **CCNU** *see* Lomustine *on page 514*
- ◆ **2-CdA** *see* Cladribine *on page 196*
- ◆ **CDDP** *see* Cisplatin *on page 190*
- ◆ **CDX** *see* Bicalutamide *on page 131*
- ◆ **CeeNU®** *see* Lomustine *on page 514*

Cefepime *(SEF e pim)*

U.S. Brand Names Maxipime®

Canadian Brand Names Maxipime®

Generic Available No

Synonyms Cefepime Hydrochloride

Pharmacologic Category Antibiotic, Cephalosporin (Fourth Generation)

Pregnancy Risk Factor B

Lactation Enters breast milk/use caution

Use Treatment of uncomplicated and complicated urinary tract infections, including pyelonephritis caused by typical urinary tract pathogens; monotherapy for febrile neutropenia; uncomplicated skin and skin structure infections caused by *Streptococcus pyogenes*; moderate to severe pneumonia caused by pneumococcus, *Pseudomonas aeruginosa*, and other gram-negative organisms; complicated intra-abdominal infections (in combination with metronidazole). Also active against methicillin-susceptible staphylococci, *Enterobacter* sp, and many other gram-negative bacilli.

Children 2 months to 16 years: Empiric therapy of febrile neutropenia patients, uncomplicated skin/soft tissue infections, pneumonia, and uncomplicated/complicated urinary tract infections.

Mechanism of Action Inhibits bacterial cell wall synthesis by binding to one or more of the penicillin-binding proteins (PBPs) which in turn inhibits the final transpeptidation step of peptidoglycan synthesis in bacterial cell walls, thus inhibiting cell wall biosynthesis. Bacteria eventually lyse due to ongoing activity of cell wall autolytic enzymes (autolysis and murein hydrolases) while cell wall assembly is arrested.

Labeled Contraindications Hypersensitivity to cefepime, any component of the formulation, or other cephalosporins

Warnings/Precautions Modify dosage in patients with severe renal impairment; prolonged use may result in superinfection; use with caution in patients with a history of penicillin or cephalosporin allergy, especially IgE-mediated reactions (eg, anaphylaxis, urticaria). May cause antibiotic-associated colitis or colitis secondary to *C. difficile*. Use in patients <2 months of age has not been established.

Adverse Reactions

>10%: Hematologic: Positive Coombs' test without hemolysis

1% to 10%:

Central nervous system: Fever (1%), headache (1%)

Dermatologic: Rash, pruritus

Gastrointestinal: Diarrhea, nausea, vomiting

Local: Pain, erythema at injection site

<1%: Anaphylactic shock, anaphylaxis, agranulocytosis, coma, encephalopathy, hallucinations, leukopenia, myoclonus, neuromuscular excitability, neutropenia, seizure, thrombocytopenia

Reactions reported with other cephalosporins include aplastic anemia, erythema multiforme, hemolytic anemia, hemorrhage, pancytopenia, prolonged PT, renal dysfunction, Stevens-Johnson syndrome, superinfection, toxic epidermal necrolysis, toxic nephropathy, vaginitis

Overdosage/Toxicology Symptoms of overdose include neuromuscular hypersensitivity and CNS toxicity (including hallucinations, confusion, seizures, and coma). Many beta-lactam containing antibiotics have the potential to cause neuromuscular hyperirritability or convulsive seizures. Hemodialysis may be helpful to aid in removal of the drug from blood; otherwise, treatment is supportive and symptom-directed.

Drug Interactions

Increased Effect/Toxicity: High-dose probenecid decreases clearance and increases effect of cefepime. Aminoglycosides increase nephrotoxic potential when taken with cefepime.

Compatibility Stable in D_5LR, D_5NS, D_5W, $D_{10}W$, NS, bacteriostatic water, sterile water for injection; **variable stability (consult detailed reference)** in peritoneal dialysis solutions

Y-site administration: Compatible: Ampicillin/sulbactam, aztreonam, bleomycin, bumetanide, buprenorphine, butorphanol, calcium gluconate, carboplatin, carmustine, co-trimoxazole, cyclophosphamide, cytarabine, dactinomycin, dexamethasone sodium phosphate, docetaxel, doxorubicin liposome, fluconazole, fludarabine, fluorouracil, furosemide, granisetron, hydrocortisone sodium phosphate, hydrocortisone sodium succinate, hydromorphone, imipenem/cilastatin, leucovorin, lorazepam, melphalan, mesna, methotrexate, methylprednisolone sodium succinate, metronidazole, paclitaxel, piperacillin/tazobactam, ranitidine, sargramostim, sodium bicarbonate, thiotepa, ticarcillin/clavulanate, zidovudine. **Incompatible:** Acyclovir, amphotericin B, amphotericin B cholesteryl sulfate complex, chlordiazepoxide, chlorpromazine, cimetidine, ciprofloxacin, cisplatin, dacarbazine, daunorubicin, diazepam, diphenhydramine, dobutamine, dopamine, doxorubicin, droperidol, enalaprilat, etoposide, etoposide phosphate, famotidine, filgrastim, floxuridine, ganciclovir, haloperidol, hydroxyzine, idarubicin, ifosfamide, magnesium sulfate, mannitol,

(Continued)

Cefepime *(Continued)*

mechlorethamine, meperidine, metoclopramide, mitomycin, mitoxantrone, morphine, nalbuphine, ofloxacin, ondansetron, plicamycin, prochlorperazine edisylate, promethazine, streptozocin, vancomycin, vinblastine, vincristine

Compatibility when admixed: Compatible: Amikacin, clindamycin, heparin, potassium chloride, theophylline, vancomycin. **Incompatible:** Aminophylline, gentamicin, netilmicin, tobramycin. **Variable (consult detailed reference):** Ampicillin, metronidazole

Pharmacodynamics/Kinetics

Absorption: I.M.: Rapid and complete

Distribution: V_d: Adults: 14-20 L; penetrates into inflammatory fluid at concentrations ~80% of serum levels and into bronchial mucosa at levels ~60% of those reached in the plasma; crosses blood-brain barrier

Protein binding, plasma: 16% to 19%

Metabolism: Minimally hepatic

Half-life elimination: 2 hours

Time to peak: 0.5-1.5 hours

Excretion: Urine (85% as unchanged drug)

Dosage

Children:

Febrile neutropenia: I.V.: 50 mg/kg every 8 hours for 7-10 days

Uncomplicated skin/soft tissue infections, pneumonia, and complicated/uncomplicated UTI: I.V.: 50 mg/kg twice daily

Adults:

Most infections: I.V.: 1-2 g every 12 hours for 7-10 days; higher doses or more frequent administration may be required in pseudomonal infections

Urinary tract infections, mild to moderate: I.M., I.V.: 500-1000 mg every 12 hours

Monotherapy for febrile neutropenic patients: I.V.: 2 g every 8 hours for 7 days or until the neutropenia resolves

Dosing adjustment in renal impairment: Adults: Recommended maintenance schedule based on creatinine clearance (mL/minute), compared to normal dosing schedule: See table.

Cefepime Hydrochloride

Creatinine Clearance (mL/minute)	Recommended Maintenance Schedule			
>60 Normal recommended dosing schedule	500 mg every 12 hours	1 g every 12 hours	2 g every 12 hours	2 g every 8 hours
30-60	500 mg every 24 hours	1 g every 24 hours	2 g every 24 hours	2 g every 12 hours
11-29	500 mg every 24 hours	500 mg every 24 hours	1 g every 24 hours	2 g every 24 hours
<11	250 mg every 24 hours	250 mg every 24 hours	500 mg every 24 hours	1 g every 24 hours

Hemodialysis: Initial: 1 g (single dose) on day 1. Maintenance: 500 mg once daily (1 g once daily in febrile neutropenic patients). Dosage should be administered after dialysis on dialysis days.

Peritoneal dialysis: Removed to a lesser extent than hemodialysis; administer 250 mg every 48 hours

Continuous arteriovenous or venovenous hemofiltration: Dose as normal Cl_{cr} (eg, >30 mL/minute)

Administration May be administered either I.M. or I.V.

Dosage Forms Injection, powder for reconstitution, as hydrochloride: 500 mg, 1 g, 2 g

Monitoring Parameters Obtain specimen for culture and sensitivity prior to the first dose; monitor for signs of anaphylaxis during first dose

Patient Information Report side effects such as diarrhea, dyspepsia, headache, blurred vision, and lightheadedness.

Special Geriatric Considerations Adjust dose for changes in renal function.

Selected Readings

Barradell LB and Bryson HM, "Cefepime. A Review of Its Antibacterial Activity, Pharmacokinetic Properties, and Therapeutic Use," *Drugs*, 1994, 47(3):471-505.

Cunha BA and Gill MV, "Cefepime," *Med Clin North Am*, 1995, 79(4):721-32.

Okamoto MP, Nakahiro RK, Chin A, et al, "Cefepime: A New Fourth-Generation Cephalosporin," *Am J Hosp Pharm*, 1994, 51(4):463-77.

Sanders CC, "Cefepime: The Next Generation?" *Clin Infect Dis*, 1993, 17(3):369-79.

Wynd MA and Paladino JA, "Cefepime: A Fourth-Generation Parenteral Cephalosporin," *Ann Pharmacother*, 1996, 30(12):1414-24.

♦ **Cefepime Hydrochloride** *see* Cefepime *on page 162*

Ceftazidime (SEF tay zi deem)

Medication Safety Issues

Sound-alike/look-alike issues:

Ceftazidime may be confused with ceftizoxime

Ceptaz® may be confused with Septra®

Tazicef® may be confused with Tazidime®

Tazidime® may be confused with Tazicef®

Related Information

Management of Infections *on page 978*

U.S. Brand Names Ceptaz® [DSC]; Fortaz®; Tazicef®

Canadian Brand Names Fortaz®

Generic Available No

Pharmacologic Category Antibiotic, Cephalosporin (Third Generation)

Pregnancy Risk Factor B

Lactation Enters breast milk (small amounts)/use caution (AAP rates "compatible")

Use Treatment of documented susceptible *Pseudomonas aeruginosa* infection and infections due to other susceptible aerobic gram-negative organisms; empiric therapy of a febrile, granulocytopenic patient

Mechanism of Action Inhibits bacterial cell wall synthesis by binding to one or more of the penicillin-binding proteins (PBPs) which in turn inhibits the final transpeptidation step of peptidoglycan synthesis in bacterial cell walls, thus inhibiting cell wall biosynthesis. Bacteria eventually lyse due to ongoing activity of cell wall autolytic enzymes (autolysins and murein hydrolases) while cell wall assembly is arrested.

Labeled Contraindications Hypersensitivity to ceftazidime, any component of the formulation, or other cephalosporins

(Continued)

Ceftazidime *(Continued)*

Warnings/Precautions Modify dosage in patients with severe renal impairment; prolonged use may result in superinfection; use with caution in patients with a history of penicillin allergy especially IgE-mediated reactions (eg, anaphylaxis, urticaria). May cause antibiotic-associated colitis or colitis secondary to *C. difficile*.

Adverse Reactions

1% to 10%:

Gastrointestinal: Diarrhea (1%)

Local: Pain at injection site (1%)

Miscellaneous: Hypersensitivity reactions (2%)

<1%: Anaphylaxis, angioedema, asterixis, BUN increased, candidiasis, creatinine increased, dizziness, encephalopathy, eosinophilia, erythema multiforme, fever, headache, hemolytic anemia, hyperbilirubinemia, jaundice, leukopenia, myoclonus, nausea, neuromuscular excitability, paresthesia, phlebitis, pruritus, pseudomembranous colitis, rash, Stevens-Johnson syndrome, thrombocytosis, toxic epidermal necrolysis, transaminases increased, vaginitis, vomiting

Reactions reported with other cephalosporins include seizure, urticaria, serum-sickness reactions, renal dysfunction, interstitial nephritis, toxic nephropathy, elevated BUN, elevated creatinine, cholestasis, aplastic anemia, hemolytic anemia, pancytopenia, agranulocytosis, colitis, prolonged PT, hemorrhage, superinfection

Vesicant No

Emetic Potential Very low (<10%)

Overdosage/Toxicology Symptoms of overdose include neuromuscular hypersensitivity and convulsions. Many beta-lactam containing antibiotics have the potential to cause neuromuscular hyperirritability or convulsive seizures. Hemodialysis may be helpful to aid in removal of the drug from blood; otherwise, treatment is supportive or symptom-directed.

Drug Interactions

Increased Effect/Toxicity: Probenecid may decrease cephalosporin elimination. Aminoglycosides: *in vitro* studies indicate additive or synergistic effect against some strains of Enterobacteriaceae and *Pseudomonas aeruginosa*. Furosemide, aminoglycosides in combination with ceftazidime may result in additive nephrotoxicity.

Reconstitution Reconstituted solution and I.V. infusion in NS or D$_5$W solution are stable for 24 hours at room temperature, 10 days when refrigerated, or 12 weeks when frozen. After freezing, thawed solution is stable for 24 hours at room temperature or 4 days when refrigerated. After mixing for 96 hours refrigerated.

Compatibility

Stable in D$_5$NS, D$_5$W, NS, sterile water for injection; **variable stability (consult detailed reference)** in peritoneal dialysis solutions

Y-site administration: Compatible: Acyclovir, allopurinol, amifostine, aminophylline, aztreonam, ciprofloxacin, diltiazem, docetaxel, enalaprilat, esmolol, etoposide phosphate, famotidine, filgrastim, fludarabine, foscarnet, gatifloxacin, gemcitabine, granisetron, heparin, hydromorphone, labetalol, linezolid, melphalan, meperidine, morphine, ondansetron, paclitaxel, propofol, ranitidine, remifentanil, tacrolimus, teniposide, theophylline, thiotepa, vinorelbine, zidovudine. **Incompatible:** Alatrofloxacin, amphotericin B cholesteryl sulfate complex, amsacrine, doxorubicin liposome, fluconazole, idarubicin, midazolam, pentamidine, warfarin. **Variable (consult detailed reference):** Cisatracurium, sargramostim, vancomycin.

Compatibility in syringe: Compatible: Hydromorphone.

Compatibility when admixed: Compatible: Ciprofloxacin, clindamycin, fluconazole, linezolid, metronidazole, ofloxacin. **Incompatible:** Aminophylline, ranitidine. **Variable (consult detailed reference):** Vancomycin.

Pharmacodynamics/Kinetics

Distribution: Widely throughout the body including bone, bile, skin, CSF (higher concentrations achieved when meninges are inflamed), endometrium, heart, pleural and lymphatic fluids

Protein binding: 17%

Half-life elimination: 1-2 hours, prolonged with renal impairment; Neonates <23 days: 2.2-4.7 hours

Time to peak, serum: I.M.: ~1 hour

Excretion: Urine (80% to 90% as unchanged drug)

Dosage

Infants and Children 1 month to 12 years: I.V.: 30-50 mg/kg/dose every 8 hours; maximum dose: 6 g/day

Adults: I.M., I.V.: 500 mg to 2 g every 8-12 hours

Urinary tract infections: 250-500 mg every 12 hours

Dosing interval in renal impairment:

Cl_{cr} 30-50 mL/minute: Administer every 12 hours

Cl_{cr} 10-30 mL/minute: Administer every 24 hours

Cl_{cr} <10 mL/minute: Administer every 48-72 hours

Hemodialysis: Dialyzable (50% to 100%)

Continuous arteriovenous or venovenous hemodiafiltration effects: Dose as for Cl_{cr} 30-50 mL/minute

Administration Any carbon dioxide bubbles that may be present in the withdrawn solution should be expelled prior to injection; administer around-the-clock to promote less variation in peak and trough serum levels; ceftazidime can be administered deep I.M. into large mass muscle, IVP over 3-5 minutes, or I.V. intermittent infusion over 15-30 minutes; do not admix with aminoglycosides in same bottle/bag; final concentration for I.V. administration should not exceed 100 mg/mL

Dosage Forms [DSC] = Discontinued product

Infusion, as sodium [premixed iso-osmotic solution] (Fortaz®): 1 g (50 mL); 2 g (50 mL)

Injection, powder for reconstitution:

Ceptaz® [DSC]: 10 g [L-arginine formulation]

Fortaz®: 500 mg, 1 g, 2 g, 6 g [contains sodium carbonate]

Tazicef®: 1 g, 2 g, 6 g [contains sodium carbonate]

Monitoring Parameters Observe for signs and symptoms of anaphylaxis during first dose

Dietary Considerations Sodium content of 1 g: 2.3 mEq

Additional Information With some organisms, resistance may develop during treatment (including *Enterobacter* spp and *Serratia* spp); consider combination therapy or periodic susceptibility testing for organisms with inducible resistance

Special Geriatric Considerations Changes in renal function associated with aging and corresponding alterations in pharmacokinetics result in every 12-hour dosing being an adequate dosing interval. Adjust dose based on renal function.

(Continued)

Ceftazidime *(Continued)*

Selected Readings

McCracken GH Jr, Threlkeld N, and Thomas ML, "Pharmacokinetics of Ceftazidime in Newborn Infants," *Antimicrob Agents Chemother*, 1984, 26(4):583-4.

Rains CP, Bryson HM, and Peters DH, "Ceftazidime. An Update of Its Antibacterial Activity, Pharmacokinetic Properties and Therapeutic Efficacy," *Drugs*, 1995, 49(4):577-617.

Ceftriaxone *(sef trye AKS one)*

Medication Safety Issues

Sound-alike/look-alike issues:

Rocephin® may be confused with Roferon®

U.S. Brand Names Rocephin®

Canadian Brand Names Rocephin®

Generic Available No

Synonyms Ceftriaxone Sodium

Pharmacologic Category Antibiotic, Cephalosporin (Third Generation)

Pregnancy Risk Factor B

Lactation Enters breast milk/use caution (AAP rates "compatible")

Use Treatment of lower respiratory tract infections, acute bacterial otitis media, skin and skin structure infections, bone and joint infections, intra-abdominal and urinary tract infections, pelvic inflammatory disease (PID), uncomplicated gonorrhea, bacterial septicemia, and meningitis; used in surgical prophylaxis

Unlabeled/Investigational Use Treatment of chancroid, epididymitis, complicated gonococcal infections; sexually-transmitted diseases (STD); periorbital or buccal cellulitis; salmonellosis or shigellosis; atypical community-acquired pneumonia; Lyme disease; used in chemoprophylaxis for high-risk contacts and persons with invasive meningococcal disease; sexual assault

Mechanism of Action Inhibits bacterial cell wall synthesis by binding to one or more of the penicillin-binding proteins (PBPs) which in turn inhibits the final transpeptidation step of peptidoglycan synthesis in bacterial cell walls, thus inhibiting cell wall biosynthesis. Bacteria eventually lyse due to ongoing activity of cell wall autolytic enzymes (autolysins and murein hydrolases) while cell wall assembly is arrested.

Labeled Contraindications Hypersensitivity to ceftriaxone sodium, any component of the formulation, or other cephalosporins; **do not use in hyperbilirubinemic neonates**, particularly those who are premature since ceftriaxone is reported to displace bilirubin from albumin binding sites

Warnings/Precautions Modify dosage in patients with severe renal impairment, prolonged use may result in superinfection. Use with caution in patients with a history of penicillin allergy, especially IgE-mediated reactions (eg, anaphylaxis, urticaria). May cause antibiotic-associated colitis or colitis secondary to *C. difficile*. Discontinue in patients with signs and symptoms of gallbladder disease.

Adverse Reactions

1% to 10%:

Dermatologic: Rash (2%)

Gastrointestinal: Diarrhea (3%)

Hematologic: Eosinophilia (6%), thrombocytosis (5%), leukopenia (2%)

Hepatic: Transaminases increased (3.1% to 3.3%)

Local: Pain, induration at injection site (I.V. 1%); warmth, tightness, induration (5% to 17%) following I.M. injection

Renal: BUN increased (1%)

<1%: Agranulocytosis, allergic pneumonitis, anaphylaxis, anemia, basophilia, bronchospasm, candidiasis, chills, colitis, diaphoresis, dizziness, dysgeusia, flushing, gallstones, glycosuria, headache, hematuria, hemolytic anemia, jaundice, leukocytosis, lymphocytosis, lymphopenia, monocytosis, nausea, neutropenia, phlebitis, prolonged or decreased PT, pruritus, pseudomembranous colitis, renal stones, seizure, serum sickness, thrombocytopenia, urinary casts, vaginitis, vomiting; increased alkaline phosphatase, bilirubin, and creatinine

Postmarketing and/or case reports: Nephrolithiasis, renal precipitations

Reactions reported with other cephalosporins include angioedema, aplastic anemia, asterixis, cholestasis, encephalopathy, erythema multiforme, hemorrhage, interstitial nephritis, neuromuscular excitability, pancytopenia, paresthesia, renal dysfunction, Stevens-Johnson syndrome, superinfection, toxic epidermal necrolysis, toxic nephropathy

Vesicant No

Emetic Potential Very low (<10%)

Overdosage/Toxicology Symptoms of overdose include neuromuscular hypersensitivity and convulsions. Many beta-lactam containing antibiotics have the potential to cause neuromuscular hyperirritability or convulsive seizures. Hemodialysis may be helpful to aid in removal of the drug from blood; otherwise, treatment is supportive or symptom-directed.

Drug Interactions

Increased Effect/Toxicity: Cephalosporins may increase the anticoagulant effect of coumarin derivatives (eg, dicumarol, warfarin).

Decreased Effect: Uricosuric agents (eg, probenecid, sulfinpyrazone) may decrease the excretion of cephalosporin; monitor for toxic effects.

Storage/Stability

Powder for injection: Prior to reconstitution, store at room temperature of 25°C (77°F); protect from light.

Premixed solution (manufacturer premixed): Store at -20°C; once thawed, solutions are stable for 3 days at room temperature of 25°C (77°F) or for 21 days refrigerated at 5°C (41°F). Do not refreeze.

Stability of reconstituted solutions:

10-40 mg/mL: Reconstituted in D_5W or NS: Stable for 2 days at room temperature of 25°C (77°F) or for 10 days when refrigerated at 5°C (41°F).

100 mg/mL:

Reconstituted in D_5W or NS: Stable for 2 days at room temperature of 25°C (77°F) or for 10 days when refrigerated at 5°C (41°F). Stable for 26 weeks when frozen at -20°C. Once thawed, solutions are stable for 2 days at room temperature of 25°C (77°F) or for 10 days when refrigerated at 5°C (41°F); does not apply to manufacturer's premixed bags. Do not refreeze.

Reconstituted in lidocaine 1% solution: Stable for 24 hours at room temperature of 25°C (77°F) or for 10 days when refrigerated at 5°C (41°F).

250-350 mg/mL: Reconstituted in D_5W, NS, lidocaine 1% solution, or SWFI: Stable for 24 hours at room temperature of 25°C (77°F) or for 3 days when refrigerated at 5°C (41°F).

(Continued)

Ceftriaxone *(Continued)*

Reconstitution

I.M. injection: Vials should be reconstituted with appropriate volume of diluent (including D_5W, NS, or 1% lidocaine) to make a final concentration of 250 mg/mL or 350 mg/mL.

Volume to add to create a **250 mg/mL** solution:
250 mg vial: 0.9 mL
500 mg vial: 1.8 mL
1 g vial: 3.6 mL
2 g vial: 7.2 mL

Volume to add to create a **350 mg/mL** solution:
500 mg vial: 1.0 mL
1 g vial: 2.1 mL
2 g vial: 4.2 mL

I.V. infusion: Infusion is prepared in two stages: Initial reconstitution of powder, followed by dilution to final infusion solution.

Vials: Reconstitute powder with appropriate I.V. diluent (including SWFI, D_5W, NS) to create an initial solution of ~100 mg/mL. Recommended volume to add:
250 mg vial: 2.4 mL
500 mg vial: 4.8 mL
1 g vial: 9.6 mL
2 g vial: 19.2 mL

Note: After reconstitution of powder, further dilution into a volume of compatible solution (eg, 50-100 mL of D_5W or NS) is recommended.

Piggyback bottle: Reconstitute powder with appropriate I.V. diluent (D_5W or NS) to create a resulting solution of ~100 mg/mL. Recommended initial volume to add:
1 g bottle:10 mL
2 g bottle: 20 mL

Note: After reconstitution, to prepare the final infusion solution, further dilution to 50 mL or 100 mL volumes with the appropriate I.V. diluent (including D_5W or NS) is recommended.

Compatibility Stable in D_5W with KCl 10 mEq, $D_5^{1}/_{4}$NS with KCl 20 mEq, $D_5^{1}/_{2}$ NS, D_5W, $D_{10}W$, NS, mannitol 5%, mannitol 10%, sodium bicarbonate 5%, bacteriostatic water, sterile water for injection; **variable stability (consult detailed reference)** in LR, peritoneal dialysis solutions

Y-site administration: Compatible: Acyclovir, allopurinol, amifostine, aztreonam, cisatracurium, diltiazem, docetaxel, doxorubicin liposome, etoposide phosphate, famotidine, fludarabine, foscarnet, gatifloxacin, gemcitabine, granisetron, heparin, linezolid, melphalan, meperidine, methotrexate, morphine, paclitaxel, propofol, remifentanil, sargramostim, sodium bicarbonate, tacrolimus, teniposide, theophylline, thiotepa, warfarin, zidovudine. **Incompatible:** Alatrofloxacin, amphotericin B cholesteryl sulfate complex, amsacrine, filgrastim, fluconazole, labetalol, pentamidine, vinorelbine. **Variable (consult detailed reference):** Vancomycin

Compatibility in syringe: Variable (consult detailed reference): Lidocaine

Compatibility when admixed: Compatible: Metronidazole. **Incompatible:** Aminophylline, clindamycin, linezolid, theophylline. **Variable (consult detailed reference):** Metronidazole, vancomycin

Pharmacodynamics/Kinetics

Absorption: I.M.: Well absorbed

Distribution: Widely throughout the body including gallbladder, lungs, bone, bile, CSF (higher concentrations achieved when meninges are inflamed); crosses placenta; enters amniotic fluid and breast milk

Protein binding: 85% to 95%

Half-life elimination: Normal renal and hepatic function: 5-9 hours

Time to peak, serum: I.M.: 1-2 hours

Excretion: Urine (33% to 65% as unchanged drug); feces

Dosage

Infants and Children:

Usual dose: I.M., I.V.:

Mild-to-moderate infections: 50-75 mg/kg/day in 1-2 divided doses every 12-24 hours (maximum: 2 g/day); continue until at least 2 days after signs and symptoms of infection have resolved

Serious infections: 80-100 mg/kg/day in 1-2 divided doses (maximum: 4 g/day)

Gonococcal infection, uncomplicated: I.M.: 125 mg in a single dose

Gonococcal conjunctivitis, complicated (unlabeled use): I.M.:

<45 kg: 50 mg/kg in a single dose (maximum: 1 g)

>45 kg: 1 g in a single dose

Gonococcal endocarditis (unlabeled use):

<45 kg: I.M., I.V.: 50 mg/kg/day every 12 hours (maximum: 2 g/day) for at least 28 days

>45 kg: I.V.: 1-2 g every 12 hours, for at least 28 days

Gonococcal infection, disseminated (unlabeled use): I.M., I.V.:

<45 kg: 25-50 mg/kg once daily (maximum: 1 g)

>45 kg: 1 g once daily for 7 days

Meningitis: I.M., I.V.:

Uncomplicated: Loading dose of 100 mg/kg (maximum: 4 g), followed by 100 mg/kg/day divided every 12-24 hours (maximum: 4 g/day); usual duration of treatment is 7-14 days

Gonococcal, complicated:

<45 kg: 50 mg/kg/day given every 12 hours (maximum: 2 g/day); usual duration of treatment is 10-14 days

>45 kg: I.V.: 1-2 g every 12 hours; usual duration of treatment is 10-14 days

Otitis media: I.M., I.V.:

Acute: 50 mg/kg in a single dose (maximum: 1 g)

Persistent or relapsing (unlabeled use): 50 mg/kg once daily for 3 days

STD, sexual assault (unlabeled uses): 125 mg in a single dose

Children >8 years (≥45 kg) and Adolescents (unlabeled use): Epididymitis, acute: I.M.: 125 mg in a single dose

Children ≤15 years: Chemoprophylaxis for high-risk contacts and persons with invasive meningococcal disease (unlabeled use): I.M.: 125 mg in a single dose. Children >15 years: Refer to Adults dosing.

Adults: Usual dose: I.M., I.V.: 1-2 g every 12-24 hours, depending on the type and severity of infection

Gonococcal conjunctivitis, complicated (unlabeled use): I.M.: 1 g in a single dose

Gonococcal endocarditis (unlabeled use): I.M., I.V.: 1-2 g every 12 hours for at least 28 days

(Continued)

Ceftriaxone *(Continued)*

Gonococcal infection, disseminated (unlabeled use): I.M., I.V.: 1 g once daily for 7 days

Gonococcal infection, uncomplicated: I.M.: 125-250 mg in a single dose

PID: I.M.: 250 mg in a single dose

Surgical prophylaxis: I.V.: 1 g 30 minutes to 2 hours before surgery

Epididymitis, acute (unlabeled use): I.M.: 250 mg in a single dose

Chemoprophylaxis for high-risk contacts and persons with invasive meningococcal disease (unlabeled use): I.M.: 250 mg in a single dose

Dosage adjustment in renal/hepatic impairment: No adjustment necessary

Hemodialysis: Not dialyzable (0% to 5%); administer dose postdialysis

Peritoneal dialysis effects: Administer 750 mg every 12 hours

Continuous arteriovenous or venovenous hemofiltration: Removes 10 mg of ceftriaxone of liter of filtrate per day

Dosage Forms Note: Contains sodium 83 mg (3.6 mEq) per ceftriaxone 1 g

Infusion [premixed in dextrose]: 1 g (50 mL); 2 g (50 mL)

Injection, powder for reconstitution: 250 mg, 500 mg, 1 g, 2 g, 10 g

Monitoring Parameters Observe for signs and symptoms of anaphylaxis

Dietary Considerations Sodium contents: 83 mg (3.6 mEq) per ceftriaxone 1 g

Special Geriatric Considerations No adjustment for changes in renal function necessary.

Selected Readings

Bradley JS, Compogiannis LS, Murray WE, et al, "Pharmacokinetics and Safety of Intramuscular Injection of Concentrated Ceftriaxone in Children," *Clin Pharm,* 1992, 11(11):961-4.

Richards DM, Heel RC, Brogden RN, et al, "Ceftriaxone: A Review of Its Antibacterial Activity, Pharmacological Properties and Therapeutic Use," *Drugs,* 1984, 27(6):469-527.

Schaad UB, Suter S, Gianella-Borradori A, et al, "A Comparison of Ceftriaxone and Cefuroxime for the Treatment of Bacterial Meningitis in Children," *N Engl J Med,* 1990, 322(3):141-7.

♦ **Ceftriaxone Sodium** *see* Ceftriaxone *on page 168*

♦ **CellCept®** *see* Mycophenolate *on page 598*

♦ **Ceptaz® [DSC]** *see* Ceftazidime *on page 165*

♦ **Cerubidine®** *see* DAUNOrubicin Hydrochloride *on page 250*

♦ **Cetacort®** *see* Hydrocortisone *on page 419*

Cetuximab *(se TUK see mab)*

U.S. Brand Names Erbitux™

Generic Available No

Synonyms C225; IMC-C225

Pharmacologic Category Antineoplastic Agent, Monoclonal Antibody; Epidermal Growth Factor Receptor (EGFR) Inhibitor

Pregnancy Risk Factor C

Lactation Excretion in breast milk is unknown/not recommended

Use Treatment of metastatic colorectal carcinoma

Unlabeled/Investigational Use Breast cancer, head and neck cancer, tumors overexpressing EGFR

Mechanism of Action Recombinant human/mouse chimeric monoclonal antibody which binds specifically to the epidermal growth factor receptor

(EGFR, HER1, c-ErbB-1) and competitively inhibits the binding of epidermal growth factor (EGF) and other ligands. Binding to the EGFR blocks phosphorylation and activation of receptor-associated kinases, resulting in inhibition of cell growth, induction of apoptosis, and decreased matrix metalloproteinase and vascular endothelial growth factor production.

Labeled Contraindications Hypersensitivity to cetuximab, murine proteins, or any component of the formulation

Warnings/Precautions Severe infusion reactions have been reported in ~3% of patients; ~90% with the first infusion despite the use of prophylactic antihistamines. **Note:** Although a 20 mg test dose was used in some studies, it did not reliably predict the risk of an infusion reaction, and is not recommended. In case of severe reaction, treatment should be stopped and permanently discontinued. Immediate treatment for anaphylactic/anaphylactoid reactions should be available during administration. Interstitial lung disease (ILD) has been reported; use caution with pre-existing lung disease. Dermatologic toxicities have been reported, including a 90% incidence of acneform rash; sunlight may exacerbate skin reactions. Non-neutralizing anticetuximab antibodies were detected in 5% of evaluable patients. Relationship between the appearance of antibodies and the safety or antitumor activity of the molecule is unknown. Safety and efficacy have not been established in pediatric patients.

Adverse Reactions

>10%:

Central nervous system: Malaise (49%), fever (33%), headache (25%), pain (19%)

Dermatologic: Acneform rash (90%; ~10% severe), nail disorder (16%)

Gastrointestinal: Nausea (mild-to-moderate 29%), constipation (28%), diarrhea (28%), abdominal pain (25%), vomiting (25%), anorexia (25%), stomatitis (11%)

Neuromuscular & skeletal: Back pain (11%), weakness (49%)

Respiratory: Dyspnea (20%)

Miscellaneous: Infusion reaction (25%; ~3% severe; ~90% with first infusion), infection (11%)

1% to 10%:

Cardiovascular: Peripheral edema (10%)

Central nervous system: Insomnia (10%), depression (9%)

Dermatologic: Pruritus (10%), alopecia (5%), skin disorder (5%)

Endocrine & metabolic: Dehydration (9%)

Gastrointestinal: Weight loss (9%), dyspepsia (7%)

Hematologic: Anemia (10%), leukopenia (1%)

Hepatic: Alkaline phosphatase increased (5% to 10%), transaminases increased (5% to 10%)

Ocular: Conjunctivitis (7%)

Renal: Kidney failure (2%)

Respiratory: Cough increased (10%), pulmonary embolus (1%)

Miscellaneous: Sepsis (3%)

<1%: Interstitial lung disease (occurred between the fourth and eleventh doses)

Vesicant No

Emetic Potential Low (10% to 30%)

(Continued)

Cetuximab *(Continued)*

Overdosage/Toxicology There is no experience with overdosage in human clinical trials. Treatment is symptom-directed and supportive.

Drug Interactions

Increased Effect/Toxicity: Interactions have not been evaluated in clinical trials.

Storage/Stability Store unopened vials under refrigeration at 2°C to 8°C (36°F to 46°F). Do not freeze. Preparations in infusion containers are stable for up to 12 hours under refrigeration at 2°C to 8°C (36°F to 46°F) and up to 8 hours at controlled room temperature of 20°C to 25°C (68°F to 77°F).

Reconstitution Reconstitution is not required. Appropriate dose should be added to sterile evacuated container.

Pharmacodynamics/Kinetics

Distribution: V_d: ~2-3 L/m^2

Half-life elimination: 114 hours (range: 75-188 hours)

Dosage I.V.: Adults:

Colorectal cancer:

Initial loading dose: 400 mg/m^2 infused over 120 minutes

Maintenance dose: 250 mg/m^2 infused over 60 minutes

Breast cancer (unlabeled use): 50-200 mg/m^2 weekly for 6 weeks

Head and neck cancer (unlabeled use):

Loading dose: 100-500 mg/m^2

Maintenance dose: 100-250 mg/m^2 weekly for 7 weeks

or

200-400 mg/m^2 weekly (no loading dose)

Tumors overexpressing EGFR (unlabeled use):

5-100 mg/m^2 weekly

or

Loading dose: 100-500 mg/m^2

Maintenance dose: 5-400 mg/m^2 weekly

Elderly: Refer to Adults dosing.

Dosage adjustment for toxicity:

Mild-to-moderate (grade 1 or 2) infusion reactions: Permanently reduce the infusion rate by 50% and continue to use prophylactic antihistamines

Severe (grade 3 or 4) infusion reactions: Immediately and permanently discontinue treatment

Mild-to-moderate skin toxicity: No dosage modification required

Severe acneform rash:

First occurrence: Delay cetuximab infusion 1-2 weeks

If improvement, continue at 250 mg/m^2

If no improvement, discontinue therapy

Second occurrence: Delay cetuximab infusion 1-2 weeks

If improvement, continue at 200 mg/m^2

If no improvement, discontinue therapy

Third occurrence: Delay cetuximab infusion 1-2 weeks

If improvement, continue at 150 mg/m^2

If no improvement, discontinue therapy

Fourth occurrence: Delay cetuximab infusion 1-2 weeks

Discontinue therapy

Dosage adjustment for renal/hepatic impairment: No adjustment required.

Administration Administer via I.V. infusion over 1-2 hours. Do not administer as I.V. push or bolus. Do not shake or dilute. May be administered via infusion pump or syringe pump. "Piggyback" into the patient's infusion line. Following the infusion, a 1-hour observation period is recommended. Premedication with antihistamines is recommended. The maximum infusion rate is 5 mL/minute. Administer through a low protein-binding 0.22 micrometer in-line filter and low-sorbing (nonPVC) tubing. Use 0.9% NaCl to flush line at the end of infusion.

Dosage Forms Injection, solution [preservative free]: 2 mg/mL (50 mL)

Monitoring Parameters Vital signs during infusion and observe for 1 hour postinfusion. Patients developing dermatologic toxicities should be monitored for the development of complications.

Patient Information Patients should wear sunscreen and limit sun exposure as sunlight can exacerbate skin reactions.

Additional Information Premedication with an H_1 antagonist (eg, diphenhydramine 50 mg I.V.) is recommended.

Selected Readings

Baselga J, "The EGFR as a Target for Anticancer Therapy - Focus on Cetuximab," *Eur J Cancer*, 2001, 37(Suppl 4):16-22.

Kies MS and Harari PM, "Cetuximab (Imclone/Merck/Bristol-Myers Squibb)," *Curr Opin Investig Drugs*, 2002, 3(7):1092-1100.

Reynolds NA and Wagstaff AJ, "Cetuximab: In the Treatment of Metastatic Colorectal Cancer," *Drugs*, 2004, 64(1):109-18.

♦ **CGP-42446** *see* Zoledronic Acid *on page 834*

♦ **CGP 57148B** *see* Imatinib *on page 449*

♦ **Chemotherapy and Pregnancy** *see page 960*

Chlorambucil (klor AM byoo sil)

Medication Safety Issues

Sound-alike/look-alike issues:

Chlorambucil may be confused with Chloromycetin®

Leukeran® may be confused with Alkeran®, leucovorin, Leukine®

Related Information

Fertility and Cancer Therapy *on page 962*

Safe Handling of Hazardous Drugs *on page 1034*

U.S. Brand Names Leukeran®

Canadian Brand Names Leukeran®

Generic Available No

Synonyms CB-1348; Chlorambucilum; Chloraminophene; Chlorbutinum; NSC-3088; WR-139013

Pharmacologic Category Antineoplastic Agent, Alkylating Agent

Pregnancy Risk Factor D

Lactation Excretion in breast milk unknown

Use Management of chronic lymphocytic leukemia, Hodgkin's and non-Hodgkin's lymphoma; breast and ovarian carcinoma; Waldenström's macroglobulinemia, testicular carcinoma, thrombocythemia, choriocarcinoma

Mechanism of Action Interferes with DNA replication and RNA transcription by alkylation and cross-linking the strands of DNA

Labeled Contraindications Hypersensitivity to chlorambucil or any component of the formulation; pregnancy

(Continued)

Chlorambucil *(Continued)*

Warnings/Precautions Hazardous agent - use appropriate precautions for handling and disposal. See Safe Handling of Hazardous Drugs *on page 1034* in the Appendix. Use with caution in patients with seizure disorder and bone marrow suppression. Reduce initial dosage if patient has received radiation therapy, myelosuppressive drugs, or has a depressed baseline leukocyte or platelet count within the previous 4 weeks. Can severely suppress bone marrow function; effects human fertility; is carcinogenic in humans and probably mutagenic and terato-genic as well. Chromosomal damage has been documented. Secondary AML may be associated with chronic therapy.

Adverse Reactions

>10%:
  Dermatologic: Skin rash
  Hematologic: Myelosuppression (common, dose-limiting)
    Onset: 7 days
    Nadir: 14 days
    Recovery: 28 days; may be prolonged to 6-8 weeks in some patients
  Hepatic: Transient elevations in liver enzymes
1% to 10%:
  Endocrine & metabolic: Hyperuricemia, menstrual cramps
  Gastrointestinal: Mild nausea or vomiting, diarrhea, stomatitis
<1%: Agitation, amenorrhea, angioneurotic edema, ataxia, chromosomal damage, confusion, fever, hallucination, hepatic necrosis, hepatotox-icity, infertility (may be irreversible in some patients), muscular twitching, myoclonia, neuropathy, primary AML, secondary malignan-cies, seizure (rare), skin hypersensitivity, tremor, weakness; interstitial pneumonitis or fibrosis including cough, dyspnea, fever, hypoxia, pulmonary dysplasia (related to long-term [>6 months] or high-dose [>2000 mg] therapy), rales, respiratory distress, urticaria

Emetic Potential Very low (<10%)

Overdosage/Toxicology Symptoms of overdose include vomiting, ataxia, coma, seizures, and pancytopenia. There are no known antidotes for chlorambucil intoxication. Treatment is mainly supportive and sympto-matic.

Drug Interactions

Decreased Effect: Patients may experience impaired immune response to vaccines; possible infection after administration of live vaccines in patients receiving immunosuppressants.

Ethanol/Nutrition/Herb Interactions Food: Avoid acidic foods and hot foods. Avoid spices.

Storage/Stability Store in refrigerator at 2°C to 8°C (36°F to 46°F). Protect from light.

Pharmacodynamics/Kinetics

Absorption: 70% to 80% with meals
Distribution: V_d: 0.14-0.24 L/kg
Protein binding: ~99%
Metabolism: Hepatic; active metabolite, phenylacetic acid mustard
Bioavailability: Reduced 10% to 20% with food
Half-life elimination: 1.5 hours; Phenylacetic acid mustard: 2.5 hours
Excretion: Urine (60% primarily as metabolites, <1% as unchanged drug)

Dosage Oral (refer to individual protocols):

Children:

General short courses: 0.1-0.2 mg/kg/day **OR** 4.5 mg/m^2/day for 3-6 weeks for remission induction (usual: 4-10 mg/day); maintenance therapy: 0.03-0.1 mg/kg/day (usual: 2-4 mg/day)

Nephrotic syndrome: 0.1-0.2 mg/kg/day every day for 5-15 weeks with low-dose prednisone

Chronic lymphocytic leukemia (CLL):

Biweekly regimen: Initial: 0.4 mg/kg/dose every 2 weeks; increase dose by 0.1 mg/kg every 2 weeks until a response occurs and/or myelosuppression occurs

Monthly regimen: Initial: 0.4 mg/kg, increase dose by 0.2 mg/kg every 4 weeks until a response occurs and/or myelosuppression occurs

Malignant lymphomas:

Non-Hodgkin's lymphoma: 0.1 mg/kg/day

Hodgkin's lymphoma: 0.2 mg/kg/day

Adults: 0.1-0.2 mg/kg/day **or**

3-6 mg/m^2/day for 3-6 weeks, then adjust dose on basis of blood counts **or**

0.4 mg/kg and increased by 0.1 mg/kg biweekly or monthly **or**

14 mg/m^2/day for 5 days, repeated every 21-28 days

Hemodialysis: Supplemental dosing is not necessary

Peritoneal dialysis: Supplemental dosing is not necessary

Combination Regimens

Leukemia, chronic lymphocytic:

CHL + PRED *on page 859*

CP (Leukemia) *on page 867*

Lymphoma, Hodgkin's:

ChlVPP *on page 859*

LOPP *on page 905*

Administration Usually administered as a single dose; preferably on an empty stomach

Dosage Forms Tablet [film coated]: 2 mg

Monitoring Parameters Liver function tests, CBC, platelets, serum uric acid

Patient Information Take as directed. Maintain adequate hydration (2-3 L/day of fluids unless instructed to restrict fluid intake). Avoid OTC medications unless approved by prescriber. Hair may be lost during treatment (reversible). You may experience menstrual irregularities and/or sterility. You will be more susceptible to infection; avoid crowds and exposure to infection. Frequent mouth care with a soft toothbrush or cotton swab may reduce occurrence of mouth sores. Report easy bruising or bleeding; fever or chills; numbness, pain, or tingling of extremities; muscle cramping or weakness; unusual swelling of extremities; menstrual irregularities; or any difficulty breathing. Contraceptive measures are recommended during therapy.

Special Geriatric Considerations Toxicity to immunosuppressives is increased in the elderly. Start with lowest recommended adult doses (Dosage). Signs of infection, such as fever and rise in WBCs, may not occur. Lethargy and confusion may be more prominent signs of infection.

Extemporaneous Preparations A 2 mg/mL oral suspension can be prepared by crushing sixty 2 mg tablets in a mortar and then mixing in (Continued)

Chlorambucil *(Continued)*

small amounts of methylcellulose (mix in a total of 30 mL of methylcellulose). Next, add a sufficient quantity of syrup to make 60 mL of final product. Transfer to amber container. Label "shake well," "refrigerate," and "protect from light." Refrigerated stability is 7 days.

> Nahata MC and Hipple TF, *Pediatric Drug Formulations*, 4th ed, Cincinnati, OH: Harvey Whitney Books Co, 2000.
>
> Dressman JB and Poust RI, "Stability of Allopurinol and of Five Antineoplastics in Suspension," *Am J Hosp Pharm*, 1983, 40(4):616-8.

Selected Readings

Begleiter A, Mowat M, Israels LG, et al, "Chlorambucil in Chronic Lymphocytic Leukemia: Mechanism of Action," *Leuk Lymphoma*, 1996, 23(3-4):187-201.

Brittinger G, Hellriegel KP, and Hiddemann W, "Chronic Lymphocytic Leukemia and Hairy-Cell Leukemia-Diagnosis and Treatment: Results of a Consensus Meeting of the German CLL Cooperative Group," *Ann Hematol*, 1997, 74(6):291-4.

Rozman C and Montserrat E, "Chronic Lymphocytic Leukemia," *N Engl J Med*, 1995, 333(16);1052-7.

Vandenberg SA, Kulig K, Spoerke DG, et al, "Chlorambucil Overdose: Accidental Ingestion of an Antineoplastic Drug," *J Emerg Med*, 1988, 6(6):495-8.

♦ **Chlorambucilum** *see* Chlorambucil *on page 175*

♦ **Chloraminophene** *see* Chlorambucil *on page 175*

♦ **Chlorbutinum** *see* Chlorambucil *on page 175*

♦ **Chlorethazine** *see* Mechlorethamine *on page 521*

♦ **Chlorethazine Mustard** *see* Mechlorethamine *on page 521*

♦ **Chlormeprazine** *see* Prochlorperazine *on page 691*

♦ **2-Chlorodeoxyadenosine** *see* Cladribine *on page 196*

ChlorproMAZINE *(klor PROE ma zeen)*

Medication Safety Issues

Sound-alike/look-alike issues:

ChlorproMAZINE may be confused with chlorproPAMIDE, clomiPRAMINE, prochlorperazine, promethazine

Thorazine® may be confused with thiamine, thioridazine

U.S. Brand Names Thorazine® [DSC]

Canadian Brand Names Apo-Chlorpromazine®; Largactil®; Novo-Chlorpromazine

Generic Available Yes: Tablet

Synonyms Chlorpromazine Hydrochloride; CPZ

Pharmacologic Category Antipsychotic Agent, Phenothiazine, Aliphatic

Pregnancy Risk Factor C

Lactation Enters breast milk/not recommended (AAP rates "of concern")

Use Control of mania; treatment of schizophrenia; control of nausea and vomiting; relief of restlessness and apprehension before surgery; acute intermittent porphyria; adjunct in the treatment of tetanus; intractable hiccups; combativeness and/or explosive hyperexcitable behavior in children 1-12 years of age and in short-term treatment of hyperactive children

Unlabeled/Investigational Use Management of psychotic disorders

Mechanism of Action Chlorpromazine is an aliphatic phenothiazine antipsychotic which blocks postsynaptic mesolimbic dopaminergic receptors in the brain; exhibits a strong alpha-adrenergic blocking effect and depresses the release of hypothalamic and hypophyseal hormones; believed to depress the reticular activating system, thus affecting basal metabolism, body temperature, wakefulness, vasomotor tone, and emesis

Labeled Contraindications Hypersensitivity to chlorpromazine or any component of the formulation (cross-reactivity between phenothiazines may occur); severe CNS depression; coma

Warnings/Precautions Highly sedating, use with caution in disorders where CNS depression is a feature and in patients with Parkinson's disease. Use with caution in patients with hemodynamic instability, bone marrow suppression, predisposition to seizures, subcortical brain damage, severe cardiac, hepatic, renal, or respiratory disease. Esophageal dysmotility and aspiration have been associated with antipsychotic use - use with caution in patients at risk of aspiration pneumonia (ie, Alzheimer's disease). Caution in breast cancer or other prolactin-dependent tumors (may elevate prolactin levels). May alter temperature regulation or mask toxicity of other drugs due to antiemetic effects. May alter cardiac conduction - life-threatening arrhythmias have occurred with therapeutic doses of neuroleptics.

Use with caution in patients at risk of hypotension (orthostasis is common) or those who would tolerate transient hypotensive episodes (cerebrovascular disease, cardiovascular disease, or other medications which may predispose). Significant hypotension may occur, particularly with parenteral administration. Injection contains sulfites and benzyl alcohol.

Use with caution in patients with decreased gastrointestinal motility, urinary retention, BPH, xerostomia, or visual problems (ie, narrow-angle glaucoma - screening is recommended) and myasthenia gravis. Relative to other neuroleptics, chlorpromazine has a moderate potency of cholinergic blockade.

May cause extrapyramidal symptoms, neuroleptic malignant syndrome (NMS) or pigmentary retinopathy.

Adverse Reactions

Cardiovascular: Postural hypotension, tachycardia, dizziness, nonspecific QT changes

Central nervous system: Drowsiness, dystonias, akathisia, pseudoparkinsonism, tardive dyskinesia, neuroleptic malignant syndrome, seizure

Dermatologic: Photosensitivity, dermatitis, skin pigmentation (slate gray)

Endocrine & metabolic: Lactation, breast engorgement, false-positive pregnancy test, amenorrhea, gynecomastia, hyper- or hypoglycemia

Gastrointestinal: Xerostomia, constipation, nausea

Genitourinary: Urinary retention, ejaculatory disorder, impotence

Hematologic: Agranulocytosis, eosinophilia, leukopenia, hemolytic anemia, aplastic anemia, thrombocytopenic purpura

Hepatic: Jaundice

Ocular: Blurred vision, corneal and lenticular changes, epithelial keratopathy, pigmentary retinopathy

Vesicant No

Emetic Potential Very low (<10%)

Overdosage/Toxicology Symptoms of overdose include deep sleep, coma, extrapyramidal symptoms, abnormal involuntary muscle movements, and hypotension. Following initiation of essential overdose management, toxic symptom treatment and supportive treatment should be initiated. Neuroleptics often cause extrapyramidal symptoms (Continued)

179

ChlorproMAZINE *(Continued)*

(eg, dystonic reactions) requiring management with anticholinergic agents such as benztropine mesylate 1-2 mg for adult patients (oral, I.M., I.V.) or diphenhydramine 25-50 mg (oral, I.M., I.V.) may be effective.

Drug Interactions

Cytochrome P450 Effect: Substrate of CYP1A2 (minor), 2D6 (major), 3A4 (minor); **Inhibits** CYP2D6 (strong), 2E1 (weak)

Increased Effect/Toxicity: The levels/effects of chlorpromazine may be increased by delavirdine, fluoxetine, miconazole, paroxetine, pergolide, quinidine, quinine, ritonavir, ropinirole, and other CYP2D6 inhibitors. Effects on CNS depression may be additive when chlorpromazine is combined with CNS depressants (narcotic analgesics, ethanol, barbiturates, cyclic antidepressants, antihistamines, or sedative-hypnotics). Chlorpromazine may increase the levels/effects of amphetamines, selected beta-blockers, dextromethorphan, fluoxetine, lidocaine, mirtazapine, nefazodone, paroxetine, risperidone, ritonavir, thioridazine, tricyclic antidepressants, and venlafaxine and other CYP2D6 substrates. Chlorpromazine may increase the effects/toxicity of anticholinergics, antihypertensives, lithium (rare neurotoxicity), trazodone, or valproic acid. Concurrent use with TCA may produce increased toxicity or altered therapeutic response. Chloroquine and propranolol may increase chlorpromazine concentrations. Hypotension may occur when chlorpromazine is combined with epinephrine. May increase the risk of arrhythmia when combined with antiarrhythmics, cisapride, pimozide, sparfloxacin, or other drugs which prolong QT interval. Metoclopramide may increase risk of extrapyramidal symptoms (EPS).

Decreased Effect: Chlorpromazine may decrease the levels/effects of CYP2D6 prodrug substrates; example prodrug substrates include codeine, hydrocodone, oxycodone, and tramadol. Phenothiazines inhibit the ability of bromocriptine to lower serum prolactin concentrations. Benztropine (and other anticholinergics) may inhibit the therapeutic response to chlorpromazine and excess anticholinergic effects may occur. Antihypertensive effects of guanethidine and guanadrel may be inhibited by chlorpromazine. Chlorpromazine may inhibit the antiparkinsonian effect of levodopa. Chlorpromazine and possibly other low potency antipsychotics may reverse the pressor effects of epinephrine.

Ethanol/Nutrition/Herb Interactions

Ethanol: Avoid ethanol (may increase CNS depression).

Herb/Nutraceutical: Avoid St John's wort (may decrease chlorpromazine levels, increase photosensitization, or enhance sedative effect). Avoid dong quai (may enhance photosensitization). Avoid kava kava, gotu kola, valerian (may increase CNS depression).

Storage/Stability Injection: Protect from light. A slightly yellowed solution does not indicate potency loss, but a markedly discolored solution should be discarded. Diluted injection (1 mg/mL) with NS and stored in 5 mL vials remains stable for 30 days.

Reconstitution Dilute injection (1 mg/mL) with NS for I.V. administration.

Compatibility Stable in dextran 6% in dextrose, dextran 6% in NS, D_5LR, $D_5^{1}/_4NS$, $D_5^{1}/_2NS$, D_5NS, D_5W, $D_{10}W$, LR, $^{1}/_2NS$, NS

Y-site administration: Compatible: Amsacrine, cisatracurium, cisplatin, cladribine, cyclophosphamide, cytarabine, docetaxel, doxorubicin,

doxorubicin liposome, famotidine, filgrastim, fluconazole, gatifloxacin, gemcitabine, granisetron, heparin, hydrocortisone sodium succinate, ondansetron, potassium chloride, propofol, teniposide, thiotepa, vinorelbine, vitamin B complex with C. **Incompatible:** Allopurinol, amifostine, amphotericin B cholesteryl sulfate complex, aztreonam, cefepime, etoposide phosphate, fludarabine, furosemide, linezolid, melphalan, methotrexate, paclitaxel, piperacillin/tazobactam, sargramostim. **Variable (consult detailed reference):** Remifentanil, TPN

Compatibility in syringe: Compatible: Atropine, benztropine, butorphanol, diphenhydramine, doxapram, droperidol, fentanyl, glycopyrrolate, hydromorphone, hydroxyzine, meperidine, metoclopramide, midazolam, morphine, pentazocine, perphenazine, prochlorperazine edisylate, promazine, promethazine, scopolamine. **Incompatible:** Cimetidine, dimenhydrinate, heparin, pentobarbital, thiopental. **Variable (consult detailed reference):** Ranitidine

Compatibility when admixed: Compatible: Ascorbic acid injection, ethacrynate, netilmicin, theophylline, vitamin B complex with C. **Incompatible:** Aminophylline, amphotericin B, ampicillin, chloramphenicol, chlorothiazide, floxacillin, furosemide, methohexital, penicillin G potassium, penicillin G sodium, phenobarbital. **Variable (consult detailed reference):** Pentobarbital

Pharmacodynamics/Kinetics

Onset of action: I.M.: 15 minutes; Oral: 30-60 minutes

Absorption: Rapid

Distribution: V_d: 20 L/kg; crosses the placenta; enters breast milk

Protein binding: 92% to 97%

Metabolism: Extensively hepatic to active and inactive metabolites

Bioavailability: 20%

Half-life, biphasic: Initial: 2 hours; Terminal: 30 hours

Excretion: Urine (<1% as unchanged drug) within 24 hours

Dosage

Children ≥6 months:

Schizophrenia/psychoses:

Oral: 0.5-1 mg/kg/dose every 4-6 hours; older children may require 200 mg/day or higher

I.M., I.V.: 0.5-1 mg/kg/dose every 6-8 hours

<5 years (22.7 kg): Maximum: 40 mg/day

5-12 years (22.7-45.5 kg): Maximum: 75 mg/day

Nausea and vomiting:

Oral: 0.5-1 mg/kg/dose every 4-6 hours as needed

I.M., I.V.: 0.5-1 mg/kg/dose every 6-8 hours

<5 years (22.7 kg): Maximum: 40 mg/day

5-12 years (22.7-45.5 kg): Maximum: 75 mg/day

Adults:

Schizophrenia/psychoses:

Oral: Range: 30-2000 mg/day in 1-4 divided doses, initiate at lower doses and titrate as needed; usual dose: 400-600 mg/day; some patients may require 1-2 g/day

I.M., I.V.: Initial: 25 mg, may repeat (25-50 mg) in 1-4 hours, gradually increase to a maximum of 400 mg/dose every 4-6 hours until patient is controlled; usual dose: 300-800 mg/day

Intractable hiccups: Oral, I.M.: 25-50 mg 3-4 times/day

(Continued)

ChlorproMAZINE *(Continued)*

Nausea and vomiting:
Oral: 10-25 mg every 4-6 hours
I.M., I.V.: 25-50 mg every 4-6 hours

Elderly: Behavioral symptoms associated with dementia: Initial: 10-25 mg 1-2 times/day; increase at 4- to 7-day intervals by 10-25 mg/day. Increase dose intervals (bid, tid, etc) as necessary to control behavior response or side effects; maximum daily dose: 800 mg; gradual increases (titration) may prevent some side effects or decrease their severity.

Dosing comments in renal impairment: Hemodialysis: Not dialyzable (0% to 5%)

Dosing adjustment/comments in hepatic impairment: Avoid use in severe hepatic dysfunction

Administration Note: Avoid skin contact with oral solution or injection solution; may cause contact dermatitis.

Oral: Dilute oral concentrate solution in juice before administration. Chlorpromazine concentrate is not compatible with carbamazepine suspension; schedule dosing at least 1-2 hours apart from each other.

I.V.: Direct of intermittent infusion: Infuse 1 mg or portion thereof over 1 minute.

Dosage Forms [DSC] = Discontinued product

Injection, solution, as hydrochloride (Thorazine® [DSC]): 25 mg/mL (10 mL) [contains benzyl alcohol, sodium bisulfite, and sodium sulfite]

Tablet, as hydrochloride: 10 mg, 25 mg, 50 mg, 100 mg, 200 mg

Monitoring Parameters Vital signs; lipid profile, fasting blood glucose/Hgb A_{1c}; BMI; mental status; abnormal involuntary movement scale (AIMS); extrapyramidal symptoms (EPS)

Patient Information Do not stop taking unless informed by your prescriber. Do not take antacid within 1 hour of taking drug. Avoid alcohol. Avoid excess sun exposure (use sun block). May cause drowsiness; rise slowly from recumbent position. Use of supportive stockings may help prevent orthostatic hypotension.

Special Geriatric Considerations See Warnings/Precautions, Adverse Reactions, and Overdose/Toxicology. Elderly patients have an increased risk of adverse response to side effects or adverse reactions to antipsychotics.

♦ **Chlorpromazine Hydrochloride** *see* ChlorproMAZINE *on page 178*

♦ **Ciloxan**® *see* Ciprofloxacin *on page 182*

♦ **Cipro**® *see* Ciprofloxacin *on page 182*

Ciprofloxacin *(sip roe FLOKS a sin)*

Medication Safety Issues

Sound-alike/look-alike issues:
Ciprofloxacin may be confused with cephalexin
Ciloxan® may be confused with cinoxacin, Cytoxan®
Cipro® may be confused with Ceftin®

U.S. Brand Names Ciloxan®; Cipro®; Cipro® XR

Canadian Brand Names Ciloxan®; Cipro®; Cipro® XL

Generic Available Yes: Suspension, tablet

Synonyms Ciprofloxacin Hydrochloride

Pharmacologic Category Antibiotic, Ophthalmic; Antibiotic, Quinolone

Pregnancy Risk Factor C

Lactation Enters breast milk/not recommended (AAP rates "compatible")

Use

Children: Complicated urinary tract infections and pyelonephritis due to *E. coli*. **Note:** Although effective, ciprofloxacin is not the drug of first choice in children.

Children and adults: To reduce incidence or progression of disease following exposure to aerolized *Bacillus anthracis*. Ophthalmologically, for superficial ocular infections (corneal ulcers, conjunctivitis) due to susceptible strains

Adults: Treatment of the following infections when caused by susceptible bacteria: Urinary tract infections; acute uncomplicated cystitis in females; chronic bacterial prostatitis; lower respiratory tract infections (including acute exacerbations of chronic bronchitis); acute sinusitis; skin and skin structure infections; bone and joint infections; complicated intra-abdominal infections (in combination with metronidazole); infectious diarrhea; typhoid fever due to *Salmonella typhi* (eradication of chronic typhoid carrier state has not been proven); uncomplicated cervical and urethra gonorrhea (due to *N. gonorrhoeae*); nosocomial pneumonia; empirical therapy for febrile neutropenic patients (in combination with piperacillin)

Unlabeled/Investigational Use Acute pulmonary exacerbations in cystic fibrosis (children); cutaneous/gastrointestinal/oropharyngeal anthrax (treatment, children and adults); disseminated gonococcal infection (adults); chancroid (adults); prophylaxis to *Neisseria meningitidis* following close contact with an infected person

Mechanism of Action Inhibits DNA-gyrase in susceptible organisms; inhibits relaxation of supercoiled DNA and promotes breakage of double-stranded DNA

Labeled Contraindications Hypersensitivity to ciprofloxacin, any component of the formulation, or other quinolones

Warnings/Precautions CNS stimulation may occur (tremor, restlessness, confusion, and very rarely hallucinations or seizures). Use with caution in patients with known or suspected CNS disorder. Prolonged use may result in superinfection. Tendon inflammation and/or rupture have been reported with ciprofloxacin and other quinolone antibiotics. Risk may be increased with concurrent corticosteroids, particularly in the elderly. Discontinue at first sign of tendon inflammation or pain. Adverse effects, including those related to joints and/or surrounding tissues, are increased in pediatric patients. Rare cases of peripheral neuropathy may occur.

Severe hypersensitivity reactions, including anaphylaxis, have occurred with quinolone therapy. Quinolones may exacerbate myasthenia gravis, use with caution (rare, potentially life-threatening weakness of respiratory muscles may occur). Use caution in renal impairment. Avoid excessive sunlight; may cause moderate-to-severe phototoxicity reactions.

Adverse Reactions

1% to 10%:

Central nervous system: Neurologic events (children 2%, includes dizziness, insomnia, nervousness, somnolence); fever (children 2%); headache (I.V. administration); restlessness (I.V. administration)

Dermatologic: Rash (children 2%, adults 1%)

(Continued)

Ciprofloxacin *(Continued)*

Gastrointestinal: Nausea (children/adults 3%); diarrhea (children 5%, adults 2%); vomiting (children 5%, adults 1%); abdominal pain (children 3%, adults <1%); dyspepsia (children 3%)

Hepatic: ALT/AST increased (adults 1%)

Local: Injection site reactions (I.V. administration)

Respiratory: Rhinitis (children 3%)

<1%: Abnormal gait, acute renal failure, agitation, allergic reactions, anaphylaxis, anemia, angina pectoris, angioedema, anorexia, arthralgia, ataxia, atrial flutter, breast pain, bronchospasm, candidiasis, cardiopulmonary arrest, cerebral thrombosis, chills, cholestatic jaundice, confusion, chromatopsia, crystalluria (particularly in alkaline urine), cylindruria, depersonalization, depression, dizziness, drowsiness, dyspnea, edema, eosinophilia, erythema nodosum, fever (adults), gastrointestinal bleeding, hallucinations, headache (oral), hematuria, hyperpigmentation, hyper-/hypotension, insomnia, interstitial nephritis, intestinal perforation, irritability, joint pain, laryngeal edema, lightheadedness, lymphadenopathy, malaise, manic reaction, migraine, MI, nephritis, nightmares, palpitation, paranoia, paresthesia, peripheral neuropathy, petechia, photosensitivity, pulmonary edema, seizure, syncope, tachycardia, thrombophlebitis, tinnitus, tremor, urethral bleeding, vaginitis, ventricular ectopy, visual disturbance, weakness

Postmarketing and/or case reports: Agranulocytosis, albuminuria, anosmia, bone marrow depression (life-threatening), candiduria, constipation, delirium, dyspepsia (adults), dysphagia, erythema multiforme, exfoliative dermatitis, fixed eruption, flatulence, hemolytic anemia, hepatic failure, hepatic necrosis, hyperesthesia, hyperglycemia, hypertonia, jaundice, methemoglobinemia, moniliasis, myalgia, myasthenia gravis, myoclonus, nystagmus, orthostatic hypotension, pancreatitis, pancytopenia (life-threatening or fatal), prolongation of PT/INR, pseudomembranous colitis, psychosis, renal calculi, serum cholesterol increased, serum glucose increased, serum sickness-like reactions, serum triglycerides increased, Stevens-Johnson syndrome, taste loss, tendon rupture, tendonitis, toxic epidermal necrolysis, torsade de pointes, twitching, vaginal candidiasis, vasculitis

Vesicant No

Emetic Potential Very low (<10%)

Overdosage/Toxicology Symptoms of overdose include acute renal failure and seizures. Treatment is supportive. The drug is not removed by peritoneal or hemodialysis.

Drug Interactions

Cytochrome P450 Effect: Inhibits CYP1A2 (strong), 3A4 (weak)

Increased Effect/Toxicity: Ciprofloxacin may increase the effects/toxicity of caffeine, CYP1A2 substrates (eg, aminophylline, fluvoxamine, mexiletine, mirtazapine, ropinirole, and trifluoperazine), glyburide, methotrexate, ropivacaine, theophylline, and warfarin. Concomitant use with corticosteroids may increase the risk of tendon rupture. Concomitant use with foscarnet may increase the risk of seizures. Probenecid may increase ciprofloxacin levels.

Decreased Effect: Concurrent administration of metal cations, including most antacids, oral electrolyte supplements, quinapril, sucralfate, and some didanosine formulations (chewable/buffered tablets and pediatric powder for oral suspension), may decrease quinolone levels; separate doses. Ciprofloxacin may decrease phenytoin levels.

Ethanol/Nutrition/Herb Interactions

Food: Food decreases rate, but not extent, of absorption. Ciprofloxacin serum levels may be decreased if taken with dairy products or calcium-fortified juices. Ciprofloxacin may increase serum caffeine levels if taken with caffeine.

Enteral feedings may decrease plasma concentrations of ciprofloxacin probably by >30% inhibition of absorption. Ciprofloxacin should not be administered with enteral feedings. The feeding would need to be discontinued for 1-2 hours prior to and after ciprofloxacin administration. Nasogastric administration produces a greater loss of ciprofloxacin bioavailability than does nasoduodenal administration.

Herb/Nutraceutical: Avoid dong quai, St John's wort (may also cause photosensitization).

Storage/Stability

Injection:

Premixed infusion: Store between 5°C to 25°C (41°F to 77°F). Protect from light. Avoid freezing.

Vial: Store between 5°C to 30°C (41°F to 86°F). Protect from light. Avoid freezing. Diluted solutions of 0.5-2 mg/mL are stable for up to 14 days refrigerated or at room temperature.

Ophthalmic solution/ointment: Store at 36°F to 77°F (2°C to 25°C). Protect from light.

Microcapsules for oral suspension: Prior to reconstitution, store below 25°C (77°F). Protect from freezing. Following reconstitution, store below 30°C (86°F) for up to 14 days. Protect from freezing.

Tablet:

Immediate release: Store below 30°C (86°F).

Extended release: Store at room temperature of 15°C to 30°C (59°F to 86°F).

Reconstitution Injection, vial: May be diluted with NS, D_5W, SWFI, $D_{10}W$, $D_5^{1}/_4NS$, $D_5^{1}/_2NS$, LR.

Compatibility Stable in $D_5^{1}/_4NS$, $D_5^{1}/_2NS$, D_5W, $D_{10}W$, LR, NS; **variable stability (consult detailed reference)** in peritoneal dialysis solution

Y-site administration: Compatible: Amifostine, amino acids (dextrose), aztreonam, calcium gluconate, ceftazidime, cisatracurium, clarithromycin, digoxin, diltiazem, diphenhydramine, dobutamine, docetaxel, dopamine, doxorubicin liposome, etoposide phosphate, gemcitabine, gentamicin, granisetron, hydroxyzine, lidocaine, linezolid, lorazepam, metoclopramide, midazolam, midodrine, piperacillin, potassium acetate, potassium chloride, potassium phosphates, promethazine, ranitidine, remifentanil, Ringer's injection (lactated), sodium chloride, tacrolimus, teniposide, thiotepa, tobramycin, verapamil. **Incompatible:** Aminophylline, ampicillin/sulbactam, cefepime, dexamethasone sodium phosphate, furosemide, heparin, hydrocortisone sodium succinate, methylprednisolone sodium succinate, phenytoin, propofol, sodium phosphates, warfarin. **Variable (consult detailed reference):** Magnesium sulfate, sodium bicarbonate, teicoplanin, TPN

Compatibility when admixed: Compatible: Amikacin, aztreonam, ceftazidime, cyclosporine, gentamicin, metronidazole, netilmicin, piperacillin, potassium chloride, ranitidine, tobramycin, vitamin B complex. **Incompatible:** Aminophylline, clindamycin, floxacillin, heparin

(Continued)

Ciprofloxacin *(Continued)*

Pharmacodynamics/Kinetics

Absorption: Oral: Immediate release tablet: Rapid (~50% to 85%)

Distribution: V_d: 2.1-2.7 L/kg; tissue concentrations often exceed serum concentrations especially in kidneys, gallbladder, liver, lungs, gynecological tissue, and prostatic tissue; CSF concentrations: 10% of serum concentrations (noninflamed meninges), 14% to 37% (inflamed meninges); crosses placenta; enters breast milk

Protein binding: 20% to 40%

Metabolism: Partially hepatic; forms 4 metabolites (limited activity)

Half-life elimination: Children: 2.5 hours; Adults: Normal renal function: 3-5 hours

Time to peak: Oral: Immediate release tablet: 0.5-2 hours; Extended release tablet: 1-2.5 hours

Excretion: Urine (30% to 50% as unchanged drug); feces (15% to 40%)

Dosage Note: Extended release tablets and immediate release formulations are not interchangeable. Unless otherwise specified, oral dosing reflects the use of immediate release formulations.

Children (see Warnings/Precautions):

Oral:

Complicated urinary tract infection or pyelonephritis: Children 1-17 years: 20-30 mg/kg/day in 2 divided doses (every 12 hours) for 10-21 days; maximum: 1.5 g/day

Cystic fibrosis (unlabeled use): Children 5-17 years: 40 mg/kg/day divided every 12 hours administered following 1 week of I.V. therapy has been reported in a clinical trial; total duration of therapy: 10-21 days

Anthrax:

Inhalational (postexposure prophylaxis): 15 mg/kg/dose every 12 hours for 60 days; maximum: 500 mg/dose

Cutaneous (treatment, CDC guidelines): 10-15 mg/kg every 12 hours for 60 days (maximum: 1 g/day); amoxicillin 80 mg/kg/day divided every 8 hours is an option for completion of treatment after clinical improvement. **Note:** In the presence of systemic involvement, extensive edema, lesions on head/neck, refer to I.V. dosing for treatment of inhalational/gastrointestinal/oropharyngeal anthrax

I.V.:

Complicated urinary tract infection or pyelonephritis: Children 1-17 years: 6-10 mg/kg every 8 hours for 10-21 days (maximum: 400 mg/dose)

Cystic fibrosis (unlabeled use): Children 5-17 years: 30 mg/kg/day divided every 8 hours for 1 week, followed by oral therapy, has been reported in a clinical trial

Anthrax:

Inhalational (postexposure prophylaxis): 10 mg/kg/dose every 12 hours for 60 days; do **not** exceed 400 mg/dose (800 mg/day)

Inhalational/gastrointestinal/oropharyngeal (treatment, CDC guidelines): Initial: 10-15 mg/kg every 12 hours for 60 days (maximum: 500 mg/dose); switch to oral therapy when clinically appropriate; refer to Adults dosing for notes on combined therapy and duration

Adults: Oral:

Urinary tract infection:

Acute uncomplicated: Immediate release formulation: 100 mg or 250 mg every 12 hours for 3 days

Acute uncomplicated pyelonephritis: Extended release formulation: 1000 mg every 24 hours for 7-14 days

Uncomplicated/acute cystitis: Extended release formulation: 500 mg every 24 hours for 3 days

Mild/moderate: Immediate release formulation: 250 mg every 12 hours for 7-14 days

Severe/complicated:

Immediate release formulation: 500 mg every 12 hours for 7-14 days

Extended release formulation: 1000 mg every 24 hours for 7-14 days

Lower respiratory tract, skin/skin structure infections: 500-750 mg twice daily for 7-14 days depending on severity and susceptibility

Bone/joint infections: 500-750 mg twice daily for 4-6 weeks, depending on severity and susceptibility

Infectious diarrhea: 500 mg every 12 hours for 5-7 days

Intra-abdominal (in combination with metronidazole): 500 mg every 12 hours for 7-14 days

Typhoid fever: 500 mg every 12 hours for 10 days

Urethral/cervical gonococcal infections: 250-500 mg as a single dose (CDC recommends concomitant doxycycline or azithromycin due to developing resistance; avoid use in Asian or Western Pacific travelers)

Disseminated gonococcal infection (CDC guidelines): 500 mg twice daily to complete 7 days of therapy (initial treatment with ceftriaxone 1 g I.M./I.V. daily for 24-48 hours after improvement begins)

Chancroid (CDC guidelines): 500 mg twice daily for 3 days

Sinusitis (acute): 500 mg every 12 hours for 10 days

Chronic bacterial prostatitis: 500 mg every 12 hours for 28 days

Anthrax:

Inhalational (postexposure prophylaxis): 500 mg every 12 hours for 60 days

Cutaneous (treatment, CDC guidelines): Immediate release formulation: 500 mg every 12 hours for 60 days. **Note:** In the presence of systemic involvement, extensive edema, lesions on head/neck, refer to I.V. dosing for treatment of inhalational/gastrointestinal/oropharyngeal anthrax

Adults: I.V.:

Bone/joint infections:

Mild to moderate: 400 mg every 12 hours for 4-6 weeks

Severe or complicated: 400 mg every 8 hours for 4-6 weeks

Lower respiratory tract, skin/skin structure infections:

Mild to moderate: 400 mg every 12 hours for 7-14 days

Severe or complicated: 400 mg every 8 hours for 7-14 days

Nosocomial pneumonia (mild to moderate to severe): 400 mg every 8 hours for 10-14 days

Prostatitis (chronic, bacterial): 400 mg every 12 hours for 28 days

Sinusitis (acute): 400 mg every 12 hours for 10 days

Urinary tract infection:

Mild to moderate: 200 mg every 12 hours for 7-14 days

(Continued)

Ciprofloxacin *(Continued)*

Severe or complicated: 400 mg every 12 hours for 7-14 days

Febrile neutropenia (with piperacillin): 400 mg every 8 hours for 7-14 days

Intra-abdominal infection (with metronidazole): 400 mg every 12 hours for 7-14 days

Anthrax:

Inhalational (postexposure prophylaxis): 400 mg every 12 hours for 60 days

Inhalational/gastrointestinal/oropharyngeal (treatment, CDC guidelines): 400 mg every 12 hours. **Note:** Initial treatment should include two or more agents predicted to be effective (per CDC recommendations). Agents suggested for use in conjunction with ciprofloxacin or doxycycline include rifampin, vancomycin, imipenem, penicillin, ampicillin, chloramphenicol, clindamycin, and clarithromycin. May switch to oral antimicrobial therapy when clinically appropriate. Continue combined therapy for 60 days.

Elderly: No adjustment needed in patients with normal renal function

Ophthalmic:

Solution: Children >1 year and Adults:

Bacterial conjunctivitis: Instill 1-2 drops in eye(s) every 2 hours while awake for 2 days and 1-2 drops every 4 hours while awake for the next 5 days

Corneal ulcer: Instill 2 drops into affected eye every 15 minutes for the first 6 hours, then 2 drops into the affected eye every 30 minutes for the remainder of the first day. On day 2, instill 2 drops into the affected eye hourly. On days 3-14, instill 2 drops into affected eye every 4 hours. Treatment may continue after day 14 if re-epithelialization has not occurred.

Ointment: Children >2 years and Adults: Bacterial conjunctivitis: Apply a $\frac{1}{2}$" ribbon into the conjunctival sac 3 times/day for the first 2 days, followed by a $\frac{1}{2}$" ribbon applied twice daily for the next 5 days

Dosing adjustment in renal impairment: Adults:

Cl_{cr} 30-50 mL/minute: Oral: 250-500 mg every 12 hours

Cl_{cr} <30 mL/minute: Acute uncomplicated pyelonephritis or complicated UTI: Oral: Extended release formulation: 500 mg every 24 hours

Cl_{cr} 5-29 mL/minute:

Oral: 250-500 mg every 18 hours

I.V.: 200-400 mg every 18-24 hours

Dialysis: Only small amounts of ciprofloxacin are removed by hemo- or peritoneal dialysis (<10%); usual dose: Oral: 250-500 mg every 24 hours following dialysis

Continuous arteriovenous or venovenous hemodiafiltration effects: Administer 200-400 mg I.V. every 12 hours

Administration

Oral: May administer with food to minimize GI upset; avoid antacid use; maintain proper hydration and urine output. Administer at least 2 hours before or 6 hours after antacids or other products containing calcium, iron, or zinc (including dairy products or calcium-fortified juices). Separate oral administration from drugs which may impair absorption (see Drug Interactions).

Oral suspension: Should not be administered through feeding tubes (due to its physical characteristics). Patients should avoid chewing on the microcapsules if the suspension is administered orally. Do not administer commercial 5% or 10% oral suspension via enteral feeding tubes (due to physical characteristics of the suspension).

Tablet, extended release: Do not crush, split, or chew. May be administered with meals containing dairy products (calcium content <800 mg), but not with dairy products alone.

Parenteral: Administer by slow I.V. infusion over 60 minutes to reduce the risk of venous irritation (burning, pain, erythema, and swelling); final concentration for administration should not exceed 2 mg/mL

Dosage Forms

Infusion, [premixed in D_5W] (Cipro®): 200 mg (100 mL); 400 mg (200 mL) [latex free]

Injection, solution (Cipro®): 10 mg/mL (20 mL, 40 mL, 120 mL)

Microcapsules for oral suspension (Cipro®): 250 mg/5 mL (100 mL); 500 mg/5 mL (100 mL) [strawberry flavor]

Ointment, ophthalmic, as hydrochloride (Ciloxan®): 3.33 mg/g [0.3% base] (3.5 g)

Solution, ophthalmic, as hydrochloride (Ciloxan®): 3.5 mg/mL [0.3% base] (2.5 mL, 5 mL, 10 mL) [contains benzalkonium chloride]

Tablet [film coated]: 250 mg, 500 mg, 750 mg

Cipro®: 100 mg, 250 mg, 500 mg, 750 mg

Tablet, extended release [film coated] (Cipro® XR): 500 mg [equivalent to ciprofloxacin hydrochloride 287.5 mg and ciprofloxacin base 212.6 mg]; 1000 mg [equivalent to ciprofloxacin hydrochloride 574.9 mg and ciprofloxacin base 425.2 mg]

Monitoring Parameters

Patients receiving concurrent ciprofloxacin, theophylline, or cyclosporine should have serum levels monitored; CBC, renal and hepatic function during prolonged therapy

Dietary Considerations

Food: Drug may cause GI upset; take without regard to meals (manufacturer prefers that immediate release tablet is taken 2 hours after meals). Extended release tablet may be taken with meals that contain dairy products (calcium content <800 mg), but not with dairy products alone.

Dairy products, calcium-fortified juices, oral multivitamins, and mineral supplements: Absorption of ciprofloxacin is decreased by divalent and trivalent cations. The manufacturer states that the usual dietary intake of calcium (including meals which include dairy products) has not been shown to interfere with ciprofloxacin absorption. Ciprofloxacin may be taken 2 hours before or 6 hours after any of these products.

Caffeine: Patients consuming regular large quantities of caffeinated beverages may need to restrict caffeine intake if excessive cardiac or CNS stimulation occurs.

Patient Information

Take as directed, preferably on an empty stomach, 2 hours after meals. Extended release tablet may be taken with meals containing dairy products, but not with dairy products alone; do not crush, split, or chew extended release tablet. Swallow oral suspension, do not chew microcapsules. Take entire prescription even if feeling better. Maintain adequate hydration (2-3 L/day of fluids unless instructed to restrict fluid intake) to avoid concentrated urine and crystal formation. You may experience nausea, vomiting, or anorexia (small frequent meals, frequent mouth care, sucking lozenges, or chewing gum may help). You may experience increased sensitivity to sunlight; use sunblock, wear protective clothing and dark glasses, or avoid direct exposure to sunlight. (Continued)

Ciprofloxacin *(Continued)*

Report immediately any signs of skin rash, joint or back pain, or difficulty breathing. Report unusual fever or chills; vaginal itching or foul-smelling vaginal discharge; easy bruising or bleeding. Report immediately any pain, inflammation, or rupture of tendon.

Special Geriatric Considerations Ciprofloxacin should not be used as first-line therapy unless the culture and sensitivity findings show resistance to usual therapy. The interactions with caffeine and theophylline can result in serious toxicity in the elderly. Adjust dose for renal function.

Selected Readings

Bayer A, Gajewska A, Stephens M, et al, "Pharmacokinetics of Ciprofloxacin in the Elderly," *Respiration*, 1987, 51(4):292-5.

Campoli-Richards DM, Monk JP, Price A, et al, "Ciprofloxacin: A Review of Its Antibacterial Activity, Pharmacokinetic Properties and Therapeutic Use," *Drugs*, 1988, 35(4):373-447.

Davis R, Markham A, and Balfour JA, "Ciprofloxacin. An Updated Review of Its Pharmacology, Therapeutic Efficacy and Tolerability," *Drugs*, 1996, 51(6):1019-74.

♦ **Ciprofloxacin Hydrochloride** *see* Ciprofloxacin *on page 182*

♦ **Cipro® XL (Can)** *see* Ciprofloxacin *on page 182*

♦ **Cipro® XR** *see* Ciprofloxacin *on page 182*

Cisplatin *(SIS pla tin)*

Medication Safety Issues

Sound-alike/look-alike issues:

Cisplatin may be confused with carboplatin

Platinol®-AQ may be confused with Paraplatin®, Patanol®, Plaquenil®

Related Information

Fertility and Cancer Therapy *on page 962*

Safe Handling of Hazardous Drugs *on page 1034*

Transplantation *on page 1019*

U.S. Brand Names Platinol®-AQ

Generic Available Yes

Synonyms CDDP

Pharmacologic Category Antineoplastic Agent, Alkylating Agent

Pregnancy Risk Factor D

Lactation Enters breast milk/contraindicated (AAP rates "compatible")

Use Treatment of head and neck, breast, testicular, and ovarian cancer; Hodgkin's and non-Hodgkin's lymphoma; neuroblastoma; sarcomas; bladder, gastric, lung, esophageal, cervical, and prostate cancer; myeloma, melanoma, mesothelioma, small cell lung cancer, and osteosarcoma

Mechanism of Action Inhibits DNA synthesis by the formation of DNA cross-links; denatures the double helix; covalently binds to DNA bases and disrupts DNA function; may also bind to proteins; the *cis*-isomer is 14 times more cytotoxic than the *trans*-isomer; both forms cross-link DNA but cis-platinum is less easily recognized by cell enzymes and, therefore, not repaired. Cisplatin can also bind two adjacent guanines on the same strand of DNA producing intrastrand cross-linking and breakage.

Labeled Contraindications Hypersensitivity to cisplatin, other platinum-containing compounds, or any component of the formulation (anaphylactic-like reactions have been reported); pre-existing renal insufficiency; myelosuppression; hearing impairment; pregnancy

Warnings/Precautions Hazardous agent - use appropriate precautions for handling and disposal. See Safe Handling of Hazardous Drugs *on*

page 1034 in the Appendix. All patients should receive adequate hydration, with or without diuretics, prior to and for 24 hours after cisplatin administration. Reduce dosage in renal impairment. Cumulative renal toxicity may be severe. Dose-related toxicities include myelosuppression, nausea, and vomiting. Ototoxicity, especially pronounced in children, is manifested by tinnitus or loss of high frequency hearing and occasionally, deafness. **Serum magnesium, as well as other electrolytes, should be monitored both before and within 48 hours after cisplatin therapy.** When administered as sequential infusions, taxane derivatives (docetaxel, paclitaxel) should be administered before platinum derivatives (carboplatin, cisplatin).

Adverse Reactions

>10%:

Central nervous system: Neurotoxicity: Peripheral neuropathy is dose- and duration-dependent.

Dermatologic: Mild alopecia

Gastrointestinal: Nausea and vomiting (76% to 100%)

Hematologic: Myelosuppressive: Mild with moderate doses, mild to moderate with high-dose therapy

WBC: Mild

Platelets: Mild

Onset: 10 days

Nadir: 14-23 days

Recovery: 21-39 days

Hepatic: Elevation of liver enzymes

Renal: Nephrotoxicity: Acute renal failure and chronic renal insufficiency

Otic: Ototoxicity (10% to 30%), manifested as high frequency hearing loss. Baseline audiography should be performed. Ototoxicity is especially pronounced in children.

1% to 10%: Local: Tissue irritation

<1%: Anaphylactic reaction, arrhythmias, blurred vision, bradycardia, hemolytic uremic syndrome, mild alopecia, mouth sores, optic neuritis, orthostatic hypotension, papilledema, phlebitis, SIADH, thrombophlebitis

Vesicant No

Emetic Potential

<50 mg/m^2: Moderately high (60% to 90%)

≥50 mg/m^2: High (>90%)

Overdosage/Toxicology Symptoms of overdose include severe myelosuppression, intractable nausea and vomiting, kidney and liver failure, deafness, ocular toxicity, and neuritis. There is no known antidote. Hemodialysis appears to have little effect. Treatment is supportive.

Drug Interactions

Increased Effect/Toxicity: Cisplatin and ethacrynic acid have resulted in severe ototoxicity in animals. Delayed bleomycin elimination with decreased glomerular filtration rate. When administered as sequential infusions, observational studies indicate a potential for increased toxicity when platinum derivatives (carboplatin, cisplatin) are administered before taxane derivatives (docetaxel, paclitaxel).

Decreased Effect: Sodium thiosulfate theoretically inactivates drug systemically; has been used clinically to reduce systemic toxicity with intraperitoneal administration of cisplatin.

(Continued)

Cisplatin *(Continued)*

Ethanol/Nutrition/Herb Interactions Herb/Nutraceutical: Avoid black cohosh, dong quai in estrogen-dependent tumors.

Storage/Stability Store intact vials at room temperature 15°C to 25°C (59°F to 77°F) and protect from light. Do not refrigerate solution as a precipitate may form. Further dilution stability is dependent on the chloride ion concentration and should be mixed in solutions of NS (at least 0.3% NaCl). After initial entry into the vial, solution is stable for 28 days protected from light or for at least 7 days under fluorescent room light at room temperature.

Standard I.V. dilution: Dose/250-1000 mL NS, D_5/NS or D_5/0.45% NaCl; stable for 72 hours at 4°C to 25°C.

Reconstitution Further dilutions in NS, D_5/0.45% NaCl or D_5/NS to a concentration of 0.05-2 mg/mL are stable for 72 hours at 4°C to 25°C. The infusion solution should have a final sodium chloride concentration of ≥0.2%.

Compatibility Stable in D_5¼NS, D_5½NS, D_5NS, ¼NS, ⅓NS, ½NS, NS, not stable in sodium bicarbonate 5%; **variable stability (consult detailed reference)** in D_5W

Y-site administration: Compatible: Allopurinol, aztreonam, bleomycin, chlorpromazine, cimetidine, cladribine, cyclophosphamide, dexamethasone sodium phosphate, diphenhydramine, doxorubicin, doxorubicin liposome, droperidol, etoposide phosphate, famotidine, filgrastim, fludarabine, fluorouracil, furosemide, ganciclovir, gatifloxacin, gemcitabine, granisetron, heparin, hydromorphone, leucovorin, linezolid, lorazepam, melphalan, methotrexate, methylprednisolone sodium succinate, metoclopramide, mitomycin, morphine, ondansetron, paclitaxel, prochlorperazine edisylate, promethazine, propofol, ranitidine, sargramostim, teniposide, topotecan, vinblastine, vincristine, vinorelbine. **Incompatible:** Amifostine, amphotericin B cholesteryl sulfate complex, cefepime, piperacillin/tazobactam, thiotepa

Compatibility in syringe: Compatible: Bleomycin, cyclophosphamide, doxapram, doxorubicin, droperidol, fluorouracil, furosemide, heparin, leucovorin, methotrexate, metoclopramide, mitomycin, vinblastine, vincristine

Compatibility when admixed: Compatible: Carboplatin, cyclophosphamide with etoposide, etoposide, etoposide with floxuridine, floxuridine, floxuridine with leucovorin, hydroxyzine, ifosfamide, ifosfamide with etoposide, leucovorin, magnesium sulfate, mannitol, ondansetron. **Incompatible:** Fluorouracil, mesna, thiotepa. **Variable (consult detailed reference):** Etoposide with mannitol and potassium chloride, paclitaxel

Pharmacodynamics/Kinetics

Distribution: I.V.: Rapidly into tissue; high concentrations in kidneys, liver, ovaries, uterus, and lungs

Protein binding: >90%

Metabolism: Nonenzymatic; inactivated (in both cell and bloodstream) by sulfhydryl groups; covalently binds to glutathione and thiosulfate

Half-life elimination: Initial: 20-30 minutes; Beta: 60 minutes; Terminal: ~24 hours; Secondary half-life: 44-73 hours

Excretion: Urine (>90%); feces (10%)

Dosage

Children: Various dosage schedules range from 30-100 mg/m^2 once every 2-3 weeks; may also dose similar to adult dosing

Recurrent brain tumors: 60 mg/m^2 once daily for 2 consecutive days every 3-4 weeks

Adults:

Advanced bladder cancer: 50-70 mg/m^2 every 3-4 weeks

Head and neck cancer: 100-120 mg/m^2 every 3-4 weeks

Malignant pleural mesothelioma (in combination with pemetrexed): 75 mg/m^2 on day 1 of each 21-day cycle; see Pemetrexed monograph for additional details

Metastatic ovarian cancer: 75-100 mg/m^2 every 3 weeks

Intraperitoneal: Cisplatin has been administered intraperitoneal with systemic sodium thiosulfate for ovarian cancer; doses up to 90-270 mg/m^2 have been administered and retained for 4 hours before draining

Testicular cancer: 10-20 mg/m^2/day for 5 days repeated every 3-4 weeks

Dosing adjustment in renal impairment:

Cl_{cr} 10-50 mL/minute: Administer 50% of normal dose

Cl_{cr} <10 mL/minute: Do not administer

Hemodialysis: Partially cleared by hemodialysis; administer dose posthemodialysis

CAPD effects: Unknown

CAVH effects: Unknown

Combination Regimens

Adenocarcinoma, unknown primary: EP (Adenocarcinoma) *on page 878*

Bladder cancer:

CAP *on page 851*

CISCA *on page 861*

Cisplatin-Docetaxel *on page 861*

CMV *on page 863*

Gemcitabine-Cisplatin *on page 896*

M-VAC (Bladder Cancer) *on page 917*

Breast Cancer: M-VAC (Breast Cancer) *on page 921*

Brain tumors:

8 in 1 (Brain Tumors) *on page 841*

CDDP/VP-16 *on page 856*

COPE *on page 866*

Cervical cancer:

Cisplatin-Fluorouracil *on page 861*

Cisplatin-Vinorelbine *on page 862*

M-VAC (Cervical Cancer) *on page 921*

Colorectal cancer: PFL (Colorectal Cancer) *on page 929*

Endometrial cancer:

AP *on page 845*

M-VAC (Endometrial Cancer) *on page 921*

Esophageal cancer:

TCF *on page 939*

TIP *on page 940*

Gastric cancer:

EAP *on page 875*

ECF *on page 875*

FUP *on page 894*

(Continued)

Cisplatin *(Continued)*

Administration Pretreatment hydration with 1-2 L of fluid is recommended prior to cisplatin administration; adequate hydration and urinary output (>100 mL/hour) should be maintained for 24 hours after administration.

I.V.: Rate of administration has varied from a 15- to 120-minute infusion, 1 mg/minute infusion, 6- to 8-hour infusion, 24-hour infusion, or per protocol; maximum rate of infusion of 1 mg/minute in patients with CHF

Dosage Forms
Injection, solution: 1 mg/mL (50 mL, 100 mL, 200 mL)
  Platinol®-AQ: 1 mg/mL (50 mL, 100 mL)

High Dose Considerations
High Dose: Continuous I.V.: 55 mg/m^2/24 hours for 72 hours; total dose: 165 mg/m^2; generally combined with other high-dose chemotherapy
Unique Toxicities:
Central nervous system: Autonomic neuropathy, ototoxicity
Gastrointestinal: Highly emetogenic
Hematologic: Myelosuppression
Endocrine & metabolic: Hypokalemia, hypomagnesemia
Neuromuscular & skeletal: Peripheral neuropathy
Ocular: Optic neuropathy, retinal vascular occlusion and myelopathy (concurrent administration of high-dose carmustine)
Renal: Acute renal failure, serum creatinine increased, azotemia
Miscellaneous: Transient pain at tumor, transient autoimmune disorders

Monitoring Parameters Renal function (serum creatinine, BUN, Cl$_{cr}$); electrolytes (particularly magnesium, calcium, potassium) before and within 48 hours after cisplatin therapy; hearing test, neurologic exam (with high dose); liver function tests periodically, CBC with differential and platelet count; urine output, urinalysis

Dietary Considerations Sodium content: 9 mg/mL (equivalent to 0.9% sodium chloride solution)

Patient Information This drug is usually given I.V. and numerous adverse side effects can occur. Maintaining adequate hydration is extremely important to help avoid kidney damage (2-3 L/day of fluids unless instructed to restrict fluid intake). Nausea and vomiting can be severe and can be delayed for up to 48 hours after infusion and last for 1 week; consult prescriber immediately for appropriate antiemetic medication. May cause hair loss (reversible). You will be susceptible to infection; avoid crowds or infectious situations (do not have any vaccinations
(Continued)

Cisplatin *(Continued)*

without consulting prescriber). Report all unusual symptoms promptly to prescriber. Contraceptive measures are recommended during therapy.

Additional Information
Sodium content: 9 mg/mL (equivalent to 0.9% sodium chloride solution)
Osmolality of Platinol®-AQ = 285-286 mOsm

Recommendations for minimizing nephrotoxicity include:
Prepare cisplatin in saline-containing vehicles
Infuse dose over 24 hours
Vigorous hydration (125-150 mL/hour) before, during, and after cisplatin administration
Simultaneous administration of either mannitol or furosemide
Pretreatment with amifostine
Avoid other nephrotoxic agents (aminoglycosides, amphotericin, etc)

Recommendations for minimizing nephrotoxicity include:
Prepare cisplatin in saline-containing vehicles
Infuse dose over 24 hours
Vigorous hydration (125-150 mL/hour) before, during, and after cisplatin administration
Simultaneous administration of either mannitol or furosemide
Pretreatment with amifostine
Avoid other nephrotoxic agents (aminoglycosides, amphotericin, etc)

Selected Readings
Farris FF, Dedrick RL, and King FG, "Cisplatin Pharmacokinetics: Applications of a Physiological Model," *Toxicol Lett*, 1988, 43(1-3):117-37.

Loehrer PJ and Einhorn LH, "Drugs Five Years Later. Cisplatin," *Ann Intern Med*, 1984, 100(5):704-13.

Long DF and Repta AJ, "Cisplatin: Chemistry, Distribution and Biotransformation," *Biopharm Drug Dispos*, 1981, 2(1):1-16.

Prestayko AW, D'Aoust JC, Isell BF, et al, "Cisplatin (cis-diamminedichloroplatinum II)," *Cancer Treat Rev*, 1979, 6(1):17-39.

Reed E, "Cisplatin," *Cancer Chemother Biol Response Modif*, 1999, 18:144-51.

Siddik ZH, "Cisplatin: Mode of Cytotoxic Action and Molecular Basis of Resistance," *Oncogene*, 2003, 22(47):7265-79.

Sleijfer DT, Meijer S, and Mulder NH, "Cisplatin: A Review of Clinical Applications and Renal Toxicity," *Pharm Weekbl Sci*, 1985, 7(6):237-44.

♦ **Citrovorum Factor** *see Leucovorin on page 497*
♦ **CL-118,532** *see Triptorelin on page 801*
♦ **CL-825** *see Pentostatin on page 661*
♦ **CL-184116** *see Porfimer on page 676*

Cladribine *(KLA dri been)*

Medication Safety Issues
Sound-alike/look-alike issues:
Leustatin® may be confused with lovastatin

Related Information
Safe Handling of Hazardous Drugs *on page 1034*

U.S. Brand Names Leustatin®

Canadian Brand Names Leustatin®

Generic Available Yes

Synonyms 2-CdA; 2-Chlorodeoxyadenosine

Pharmacologic Category Adjuvant, Radiosensitizing Agent; Antineoplastic Agent, Antimetabolite (Purine Antagonist); Antineoplastic Agent, Antimetabolite

Pregnancy Risk Factor D

Lactation Enters breast milk/contraindicated

Use Treatment of hairy cell leukemia, chronic lymphocytic leukemia (CLL), chronic myelogenous leukemia (CML)

Unlabeled/Investigational Use Non-Hodgkin's lymphomas, progressive multiple sclerosis

Mechanism of Action A purine nucleoside analogue; prodrug which is activated via phosphorylation by deoxycytidine kinase to a 5'-triphosphate derivative. This active form incorporates into DNA to result in the breakage of DNA strand and shutdown of DNA synthesis. This also results in a depletion of nicotinamide adenine dinucleotide and adenosine triphosphate (ATP). Cladribine is cell-cycle nonspecific.

Labeled Contraindications Hypersensitivity to cladribine or any component of the formulation; pregnancy

Warnings/Precautions Hazardous agent - use appropriate precautions for handling and disposal. See Safe Handling of Hazardous Drugs *on page 1034* in the Appendix. Because of its myelosuppressive properties, cladribine should be used with caution in patients with pre-existing hematologic or immunologic abnormalities.

Adverse Reactions

>10%:

Allergic: Fever (70%), chills (18%); skin reactions (erythema, itching) at the catheter site (18%)

Central nervous system: Fatigue (17%), headache (13%)

Dermatologic: Rash

Hematologic: Myelosuppression, common, dose-limiting; leukopenia (70%); anemia (37%); thrombocytopenia (12%)

Nadir: 5-10 days

Recovery: 4-8 weeks

1% to 10%:

Cardiovascular: Edema, tachycardia

Central nervous system: Dizziness; pains; chills; malaise; severe infection, possibly related to thrombocytopenia

Dermatologic: Pruritus, erythema

Gastrointestinal: Nausea, mild to moderate, usually not seen at doses <0.3 mg/kg/day; constipation; abdominal pain

Neuromuscular & skeletal: Myalgia, arthralgia, weakness

Renal: Renal failure at high (>0.3 mg/kg/day) doses

Miscellaneous: Diaphoresis, delayed herpes zoster infection, tumor lysis syndrome

<1%, postmarketing and/or case reports: Paraparesis, quadriplegia (reported at high doses); increased risk of opportunistic infection

Vesicant No

Emetic Potential Very low (<10%)

Ethanol/Nutrition/Herb Interactions Ethanol: Avoid ethanol (due to GI irritation).

Storage/Stability Store intact vials under refrigeration 2°C to 8°C (36°F to 46°F). Dilutions in 500 mL NS are stable for 72 hours. Stable in PVC containers for 24 hours at room temperature of 15°C to 30°C (59°F to 86°F) and 7 days in Pharmacia Deltec® cassettes.

Reconstitution Dilute in 250-1000 mL. Solutions for 7-day infusion should be prepared in bacteriostatic NS.

Compatibility Stable in NS; **incompatible** with D_5W

(Continued)

197

Cladribine *(Continued)*

Y-site administration: Compatible: Aminophylline, bumetanide, bupre-norphine, butorphanol, calcium gluconate, carboplatin, chlorpromazine, cimetidine, cisplatin, cyclophosphamide, cytarabine, dexamethasone sodium phosphate, diphenhydramine, dobutamine, dopamine, doxorubicin, droperidol, enalaprilat, etoposide, famotidine, furosemide, granisetron, haloperidol, heparin, hydrocortisone sodium phosphate, hydrocortisone sodium succinate, hydromorphone, hydroxyzine, idarubicin, leucovorin, lorazepam, mannitol, meperidine, mesna, methylprednisolone sodium succinate, metoclopramide, mitoxantrone, morphine, nalbuphine, ondansetron, paclitaxel, potassium chloride, prochlorperazine edisylate, promethazine, ranitidine, sodium bicarbonate, teniposide, vincristine

Pharmacodynamics/Kinetics

Absorption: Oral: 55%; SubQ: 100%; Rectal: 20%

Distribution: V_d: 4.52 ± 2.82 L/kg

Protein binding, plasma: 20%

Metabolism: Hepatic; 5′-triphosphate moiety-active

Half-life elimination: Biphasic: Alpha: 25 minutes; Beta: 6.7 hours; Terminal, mean: Normal renal function: 5.4 hours

Excretion: Urine (21% to 44%)

Clearance: Estimated systemic: 640 mL/hour/kg

Dosage I.V.: Refer to individual protocols.

Pediatrics: Acute leukemias: 6.2-7.5 mg/m^2/day continuous infusion for days 1-5; maximum tolerated dose was 8.9 mg/m^2/day.

Adults:

Hairy cell leukemia: Continuous infusion:

0.09-0.1 mg/kg/day days 1-7; may be repeated every 28-35 days **or** 3.4 mg/m^2/day SubQ days 1-7

Chronic lymphocytic leukemia: Continuous infusion:

0.1 mg/kg/day days 1-7 **or**

0.028-0.14 mg/kg/day as a 2-hour infusion days 1-5

Chronic myelogenous leukemia: 15 mg/m^2/day as a 1-hour infusion days 1-5; if no response increase dose to 20 mg/m^2/day in the second course.

Administration I.V.: Administer as a 1- to 2-hour infusion or by continuous infusion

Dosage Forms Injection, solution [preservative free]: 1 mg/mL (10 mL)

Monitoring Parameters Monitor periodic assessment of peripheral blood counts, particularly during the first 4-8 weeks post-treatment, is recommended to detect the development of anemia, neutropenia, and thrombocytopenia and for early detection of any potential sequelae (ie, infection or bleeding)

Selected Readings

Baltz JK and Montello MJ, "Cladribine for the Treatment of Hematologic Malignancies," *Clin Pharm*, 1993, 12(11):805-13.

Beutler E, "Cladribine (2-Chlorodeoxyadenosine)," *Lancet*, 1992, 340(8825):952-6.

Kearns CM, Biakley RL, Santane VM, et al, "Pharmacokinetics of Cladribine (2-Chlorodioxyadenosine) in Children with Acute Leukemia," *Cancer Res*, 1994, 54:1235-39.

Liliemark J, "The Clinical Pharmacokinetics of Cladribine," *Clin Pharmacokinet*, 1997, 32(2):120-31.

Saven A and Piro LD, "2-Chlorodeoxyadenosine: A Potent Antimetabolite With Major Activity in the Treatment of Indolent Lymphoproliferative Disorders," *Hematol Cell Ther*, 1996, 38(Suppl 2):93-101.

Tortorella C, Rovaris M, and Filippi M, "Cladribine. Ortho Biotech Inc," Curr Opin Investig Drugs, 2001, 2(12):1751-6.

Clodronate (KLOE droh nate)

Canadian Brand Names Bonefos®; Ostac®

Synonyms Clodronate Disodium

Pharmacologic Category Bisphosphonate Derivative

Pregnancy Risk Factor Not assigned; similar agents rated X

Lactation Excretion in breast milk unknown/contraindicated

Use Management of hypercalcemia of malignancy

Mechanism of Action A bisphosphonate which inhibits bone resorption via actions on osteoclasts or on osteoclast precursors.

Restrictions Not available in U.S.

Labeled Contraindications Hypersensitivity to clodronate, bisphosphonates, or any component of the formulation; severe GI inflammation; renal impairment (serum creatinine >5 mg/dL, SI 440 µmol/L); pregnancy or breast-feeding

Warnings/Precautions Use caution in patients with renal impairment. May cause irritation to upper gastrointestinal mucosa. Esophagitis, esophageal ulcers, esophageal erosions, and esophageal stricture (rare) have been reported with bisphosphonates (oral). Use with caution in patients with dysphagia, esophageal disease, gastritis, duodenitis, or ulcers (may worsen underlying condition). Safety and efficacy have not been established in pediatric patients.

For I.V. preparation: Dilute prior to use; adequate hydration should be ensured prior to infusion; avoid infiltration/extravasation. May cause venous irritation, hypocalcemia, or transient hypophosphatemia. Do not administer as bolus injection.

Adverse Reactions

1% to 10%:

Endocrine & metabolic: Hypocalcemia (2%)

Gastrointestinal: Incidence highest with oral administration: Vomiting (4%), nausea (3%), diarrhea (2%), anorexia (1%)

Renal: Serum creatinine increased (1%), BUN increased

<1%: Bronchospasm, hypersensitivity reactions (angioedema, pruritus, rash, urticaria), oliguria, proteinuria, transaminases increased

Postmarketing and/or case reports: Osteonecrosis

Overdosage/Toxicology Symptoms of overdose include hypocalcemia, ECG changes, seizures, bleeding, paresthesia, carpopedal spasm, and fever. Treat with I.V. calcium gluconate, and general supportive care; fever and hypotension can be treated with corticosteroids.

Drug Interactions

Increased Effect/Toxicity: I.V. ranitidine has been shown to double the bioavailability of an oral bisphosphonate (alendronate). An increased incidence of adverse renal or GI effects may occur when used concurrently with NSAIDs or aspirin-containing products. Loop diuretics may increase risk of hypocalcemia.

Decreased Effect: Oral medications (especially those containing multivalent cations, including aluminum, calcium, iron, or magnesium) may interfere with clodronate absorption; wait at least 30 minutes before taking any oral medications. Thiazide diuretics may alter hypocalcemic effects.

(Continued)

Clodronate *(Continued)*

Ethanol/Nutrition/Herb Interactions Food: All food and beverages may interfere with absorption. Coadministration with dairy products may decrease absorption. Beverages (especially orange juice and coffee), food, and medications (eg, antacids, calcium, iron, and multivalent cations) may reduce the absorption of bisphosphonates as much as 60%.

Storage/Stability Store capsules and undiluted ampuls at room temperature (15°C to 30°C).

Reconstitution Injection must be diluted in 500 mL of NS or D_5W.

Compatibility Stable in D_5W or 0.9% NS

Pharmacodynamics/Kinetics

Onset of effect: 24-48 hours

Peak effect: 5-7 days

Duration: 2-3 weeks

Distribution: V_d: 20 L

Bioavailability: Oral: 1% to 3%

Half-life (terminal): 13 hours (serum); prolonged in bone tissue

Elimination: Urine (as unchanged drug)

Dosage

I.V.:

Multiple infusions: 300 mg/day; should not be prolonged beyond 10 days.

Single infusion: 1500 mg as a single dose

Oral: Recommended daily maintenance dose following I.V. therapy: Range: 1600 mg (4 capsules) to 2400 mg (6 capsules) given in single or 2 divided doses; maximum recommended daily dose: 3200 mg (8 capsules). Should be taken at least 1 hour before or after food, because food may decrease the amount of clodronate absorbed by the body.

Dosage adjustment in renal impairment:

Cl_{cr} >5 mg/dL: Use is contraindicated

Cl_{cr} ≥2.5-5 mg/dL: Dosage reduction is recommended; no specific guidelines available

Administration

Capsules: Administer with copious fluids (not milk).

Injection: Do not administer as bolus injection; infuse over 2-6 hours

Dosage Forms

Injection, as disodium: 30 mg/mL (10 mL); 60 mg/mL (5 mL)

Capsule, as disodium: 400 mg

Monitoring Parameters Serum electrolytes, monitor for hypocalcemia for at least 2 weeks after therapy; serum calcium, phosphate, magnesium, potassium, serum creatinine, CBC with differential, hepatic function

Patient Information Take as directed, with a full glass of water first thing in the morning and at least 30 minutes before the first food or beverage of the day. Wait at least 30 minutes after taking clodronate before taking any supplement. Avoid NSAIDs, aspirin or aspirin-containing medications. You may experience GI upset (eg, flatulence, bloating, nausea, acid regurgitation); small, frequent meals may help. Report acute headache or gastric pain, unresolved GI upset, or acid stomach.

Selected Readings

Ostac® product monograph, Hoffman-La Roche Ltd/Ltee, Ontario, June 1998.

♦ **Clodronate Disodium** *see* Clodronate *on page 199*

Clofarabine (klo FARE a been)

U.S. Brand Names Clolar™

Generic Available No

Synonyms Clofarex, NSC606869

Pharmacologic Category Antineoplastic Agent, Antimetabolite (Purine Antagonist)

Pregnancy Risk Factor D

Lactation Excretion in breast milk unknown/not recommended

Use Treatment of relapsed or refractory acute lymphoblastic leukemia

Unlabeled/Investigational Use Adults: Relapsed and refractory acute myeloid leukemia (AML), chronic myeloid leukemia (CML) in blast phase, acute lymphocytic leukemia (ALL), myelodysplastic syndrome

Mechanism of Action Clofarabine, a purine (deoxyadenosine) nucleoside analog, is metabolized to clofarabine 5'-triphosphate. Clofarabine 5'-triphosphate decreases cell replication and repair as well as causing cell death. To decrease cell replication and repair, clofarabine 5'-triphosphate competes with deoxyadenosine triphosphate for the enzymes ribonucleotide reductase and DNA polymerase. Cell replication is decreased when clofarabine 5'-triphosphate inhibits ribonucleotide reductase from reacting with deoxyadenosine triphosphate to produce deoxynucleotide triphosphate which is needed for DNA synthesis. Cell replication is also decreased when clofarabine 5'-triphosphate competes with DNA polymerase for incorporation into the DNA chain; when done during the repair process, cell repair is affected. To cause cell death, clofarabine 5'-triphosphate alters the mitochondrial membrane by releasing proteins, an inducing factor and cytochrome C.

Labeled Contraindications Hypersensitivity to clofarabine or any component of the formulation

Warnings/Precautions Hazardous agent - use appropriate precautions for handling and disposal. See Safe Handling of Hazardous Drugs *on page 1034* in the Appendix. Tumor lysis syndrome and cytokine release may develop into systemic inflammatory response syndrome (SIRS)/ capillary leak syndrome, and organ dysfunction; discontinuation of clofarabine should be considered with the presentation of SIRS or capillary leak syndrome (see Tumor Lysis Syndrome *on page 1002* in the Appendix). Safety and efficacy have not been established with renal or hepatic dysfunction; use with caution. Safety and efficacy in pediatric patients <1 year of age or >21 years have not been established.

Adverse Reactions

>10%:

Cardiovascular: Pericardial effusion (35%), tachycardia (34%), hypotension (29%), left ventricular systolic dysfunction (27%), edema (20%), flushing (18%), hypertension (11%)

Central nervous system: Headache (46%), pyrexia (41%), fatigue (36%) anxiety (22%), pain (19%), dizziness (16%), depression (11%), irritability (11%), lethargy (1%)

Dermatologic: Pruritus (47%), dermatitis (41%), petechiae (29%), erythema (18%), palmar-plantar erythrodysesthesia syndrome (13%), oral candidiasis (13%), cellulitis (11%)

Gastrointestinal: Vomiting (83%), nausea (75%), diarrhea (53%), abdominal pain (36%), anorexia (30%), constipation (21%), mucosal inflammation (18%), gingival bleeding (15%), sore throat (14%), appetite decreased (11%)

(Continued)

Clofarabine *(Continued)*

Genitourinary: Hematuria (17%)

Hematologic: Febrile neutropenia (57%)

Hepatic: ALT increased (44%), AST increased (38%), bilirubin increased (15%), hepatomegaly (15%), jaundice (15%)

Neuromuscular & skeletal: Rigors (38%), pain in limb (29%), myalgia (14%), back pain (13%), arthralgia (11%)

Respiratory: Epistaxis (31%), cough (19%), respiratory distress (14%), dyspnea (13%)

Miscellaneous: Infection (85%), injection site pain (14%), staphylococcal infection (13%), herpes simplex (11%)

1% to 10%:

Central nervous system: Somnolence (10%)

Gastrointestinal: Weight gain (10%)

Genitourinary: Creatinine increased (6%)

Neuromuscular & skeletal: Tremor (10%)

Respiratory: Pleural effusion (10%), pneumonia (10%), systemic inflammatory response syndrome (SIRS)/capillary leak syndrome

Miscellaneous: Transfusion reaction (10%), bacteremia (10%)

Vesicant No

Emetic Potential High (60% to 90%)

Overdosage/Toxicology No known overdoses have been reported; treatment should be symptom directed and supportive.

Storage/Stability Store undiluted and diluted at room temperature of 15°C to 30°C (59°F to 86°F); diluted solution must be used within 24 hours.

Reconstitution Clofarabine should be filtered through a 0.2 micrometer filter then diluted with 100-500 mL D_5W or NS

Pharmacodynamics/Kinetics

Distribution: V_d: 172 L/m^2

Protein binding: 47%

Metabolism: Intracellular by deoxycytidine kinase and mono- and diphosphokinases to active metabolite clofarabine 5'-triphosphate

Half-life elimination: ~5.2 hours

Excretion: Urine (49% to 60% unchanged)

Dosage I.V.: Children and Adults 1-21 years: ALL: 52 mg/m^2 I.V. days 1 through 5; repeat every 2-6 weeks

Dosage adjustment in renal/hepatic impairment: Safety not established; use with caution

Administration I.V. infusion: Over 2 hours. Continuous I.V. fluids are encouraged to decrease adverse events and tumor lysis effects. Discontinue if the patient becomes hypotensive during administration; retreatment at a lower dose should only be considered if the hypotension was transient, not requiring pharmacological intervention.

Dosage Forms Injection, solution [preservative free]: 1 mg/mL (20 mL)

Monitoring Parameters Blood pressure, cardiac function, and respiratory status during infusion; periodic CBC with platelet count (increase frequency in patients who develop cytopenias); liver and kidney function during 5 days of clofarabine administration; signs and symptoms of tumor lysis syndrome and cytokine release syndrome (tachypnea, tachycardia, hypotension, pulmonary edema); hydration status

Additional Information The use of prophylactic steroids (hydrocortisone 100 mg/m^2 on days 1-3) may be of benefit in preventing signs of SIRS or capillary leak syndrome; allopurinol may be used if hyperuricemia is anticipated. Dosage should be based on BSA, calculated based upon the height and weight prior to each cycle.

Selected Readings
"Clofarabine," *Drugs R D*, 2004, 5(4):213-7.
Sternberg A, "Clofarabine. Bioenvision/ILEX," *Curr Opin Investig Drugs*, 2003, 4(12):1479-87.

♦ **Clofarex, NSC606869** *see* Clofarabine *on page 201*
♦ **Clolar**™ *see* Clofarabine *on page 201*
♦ **Clotrimaderm (Can)** *see* Clotrimazole *on page 203*

Clotrimazole (kloe TRIM a zole)

Medication Safety Issues
Sound-alike/look-alike issues:
Clotrimazole may be confused with co-trimoxazole
Lotrimin® may be confused with Lotrisone®, Otrivin®
Mycelex® may be confused with Myoflex®

Related Information
Management of Infections *on page 978*

U.S. Brand Names Cruex® Cream [OTC]; Gyne-Lotrimin® 3 [OTC]; Lotrimin® AF Athlete's Foot Cream [OTC]; Lotrimin® AF Athlete's Foot Solution [OTC]; Lotrimin® AF Jock Itch Cream [OTC]; Mycelex®; Mycelex®-7 [OTC]; Mycelex® Twin Pack [OTC]

Canadian Brand Names Canesten® Topical; Canesten® Vaginal; Clotrimaderm; Trivagizole-3®

Generic Available Yes: Cream, solution, troche

Pharmacologic Category Antifungal Agent, Oral Nonabsorbed; Antifungal Agent, Topical; Antifungal Agent, Vaginal

Pregnancy Risk Factor B (topical); C (troches)

Lactation Excretion in breast milk unknown

Use Treatment of susceptible fungal infections, including oropharyngeal candidiasis, dermatophytoses, superficial mycoses, and cutaneous candidiasis, as well as vulvovaginal candidiasis; limited data suggest that clotrimazole troches may be effective for prophylaxis against oropharyngeal candidiasis in neutropenic patients

Mechanism of Action Binds to phospholipids in the fungal cell membrane altering cell wall permeability resulting in loss of essential intracellular elements

Labeled Contraindications Hypersensitivity to clotrimazole or any component of the formulation

Warnings/Precautions Clotrimazole should not be used for treatment of ocular or systemic fungal infection. Use with caution with hepatic impairment. Safety and effectiveness of clotrimazole lozenges (troches) in children <3 years of age have not been established. When using topical formulation, avoid contact with eyes.

Adverse Reactions
Oral:
>10%: Hepatic: Abnormal liver function tests
1% to 10%:
Gastrointestinal: Nausea and vomiting may occur in patients on clotrimazole troches
(Continued)

Clotrimazole *(Continued)*

Local: Mild burning, irritation, stinging to skin or vaginal area

Vaginal:

1% to 10%: Genitourinary: Vulvar/vaginal burning

<1% (Limited to important or life-threatening): Vulvar itching, soreness, edema, or discharge; polyuria; burning or itching of penis of sexual partner

Emetic Potential Very low (<10%)

Drug Interactions

Cytochrome P450 Effect: Inhibits CYP1A2 (weak), 2A6 (weak), 2B6 (weak), 2C8/9 (weak), 2C19 (weak), 2D6 (weak), 2E1 (weak), 3A4 (moderate)

Increased Effect/Toxicity: Clotrimazole may increase the levels/ effects of selected benzodiazepines, calcium channel blockers, cisapride, cyclosporine, ergot derivatives, selected HMG-CoA reductase inhibitors, mesoridazine, mirtazapine, nateglinide, nefazodone, pimozide, quinidine, sildenafil (and other PDE-5 inhibitors), tacrolimus, thioridazine, venlafaxine, and other CYP3A4 substrates.

Pharmacodynamics/Kinetics

Absorption: Topical: Negligible through intact skin

Time to peak, serum:

Oral topical (troche): Salivary levels occur within 3 hours following 30 minutes of dissolution time

Vaginal cream: High vaginal levels: 8-24 hours

Vaginal tablet: High vaginal levels: 1-2 days

Excretion: Feces (as metabolites)

Dosage

Children >3 years and Adults:

Oral:

Prophylaxis: 10 mg troche dissolved 3 times/day for the duration of chemotherapy or until steroids are reduced to maintenance levels

Treatment: 10 mg troche dissolved slowly 5 times/day for 14 consecutive days

Topical (cream, solution): Apply twice daily; if no improvement occurs after 4 weeks of therapy, re-evaluate diagnosis

Children >12 years and Adults:

Vaginal:

Cream:

1%: Insert 1 applicatorful vaginal cream daily (preferably at bedtime) for 7 consecutive days

2%: Insert 1 applicatorful vaginal cream daily (preferably at bedtime) for 3 consecutive days

Tablet: Insert 100 mg/day for 7 days or 500 mg single dose

Topical (cream, solution): Apply to affected area twice daily (morning and evening) for 7 consecutive days

Administration

Oral: Allow to dissolve slowly over 15-30 minutes.

Topical: Avoid contact with eyes. For external use only. Apply sparingly. Protect hands with latex gloves. Do not use occlusive dressings.

Dosage Forms

Combination pack (Mycelex®-7): Vaginal tablet 100 mg (7s) and vaginal cream 1% (7 g)

Cream, topical: 1% (15 g, 30 g, 45 g)

Cruex®: 1% (15 g)
Lotrimin® AF Athlete's Foot: 1% (12 g, 24 g)
Lotrimin® AF Jock Itch: 1% (12 g)
Cream, vaginal: 2% (21 g)
Mycelex®-7: 1% (45 g)
Solution, topical: 1% (10 mL, 30 mL)
Lotrimin® AF Athlete's Foot: 1% (10 mL)
Tablet, vaginal (Gyne-Lotrimin® 3): 200 mg (3s)
Troche (Mycelex®): 10 mg

Monitoring Parameters Periodic liver function tests during oral therapy with clotrimazole troche

Patient Information Oral: Do not swallow oral medication whole; allow to dissolve slowly in mouth. You may experience nausea or vomiting (small frequent meals, frequent mouth care, chewing gum, or sucking lozenges may help). Report signs of opportunistic infection (eg, white plaques in mouth, fever, chills, perianal itching or vaginal discharge, fatigue, unhealed wounds or sores).

Topical: Wash hands before applying or wear gloves. Apply thin film to affected area. May apply porous dressing. Report persistent burning, swelling, itching, worsening of condition, or lack of response to therapy.

Vaginal: Wash hands before using. Insert full applicator into vagina gently and expel cream, or insert tablet into vagina, at bedtime. Wash applicator with soap and water following use. Remain lying down for 30 minutes following administration. Avoid intercourse during therapy (sexual partner may experience penile burning or itching). Report adverse reactions (eg, vulvar itching, frequent urination), worsening of condition, or lack of response to therapy. Contact prescriber if symptoms do not improve within 3 days or you do not feel well within 7 days. Do not use tampons until therapy is complete. Contact prescriber immediately if you experience abdominal pain, fever, or foul-smelling discharge.

Special Geriatric Considerations Localized fungal infections frequently follow broad spectrum antimicrobial therapy. Specifically, oral and vaginal infections due to *Candida*.

Selected Readings
Duhm B, Medenwald H, Puetter J, et al, "The Pharmacokinetics of Clotrimazole 14C," *Postgrad Med J*, 1974, 50(Suppl 1):13-6.

♦ **CMV-IGIV** *see* Cytomegalovirus Immune Globulin (Intravenous-Human) *on page 236*

♦ **Coagulation Factor VIIa** *see* Factor VIIa (Recombinant) *on page 326*

Codeine (KOE deen)

Medication Safety Issues

Sound-alike/look-alike issues:
Codeine may be confused with Cardene®, Cophene®, Cordran®, iodine, Lodine®

Canadian Brand Names Codeine Contin®

Generic Available Yes

Synonyms Codeine Phosphate; Codeine Sulfate; Methylmorphine

Pharmacologic Category Analgesic, Narcotic; Antitussive

Pregnancy Risk Factor C/D (prolonged use or high doses at term)

Lactation Enters breast milk/use caution (AAP rates "compatible")

(Continued)

Codeine *(Continued)*

Use Treatment of mild to moderate pain; antitussive in lower doses; dextromethorphan has equivalent antitussive activity but has much lower toxicity in accidental overdose

Mechanism of Action Binds to opiate receptors in the CNS, causing inhibition of ascending pain pathways, altering the perception of and response to pain; causes cough supression by direct central action in the medulla; produces generalized CNS depression

Restrictions C-II

Labeled Contraindications Hypersensitivity to codeine or any component of the formulation; pregnancy (prolonged use or high doses at term)

Warnings/Precautions An opioid-containing analgesic regimen should be tailored to each patient's needs and based upon the type of pain being treated (acute versus chronic), the route of administration, degree of tolerance for opioids (naive versus chronic user), age, weight, and medical condition. The optimal analgesic dose varies widely among patients. Doses should be titrated to pain relief/prevention.

Use with caution in patients with hypersensitivity reactions to other phenanthrene derivative opioid agonists (morphine, hydrocodone, hydromorphone, levorphanol, oxycodone, oxymorphone); respiratory diseases including asthma, emphysema, COPD, or severe liver or renal insufficiency; some preparations contain sulfites which may cause allergic reactions; tolerance or drug dependence may result from extended use

Not recommended for use for cough control in patients with a productive cough; not recommended as an antitussive for children <2 years of age; the elderly may be particularly susceptible to the CNS depressant and confusion as well as constipating effects of narcotics

Not approved for I.V. administration (although this route has been used clinically). If given intravenously, must be given slowly and the patient should be lying down. Rapid intravenous administration of narcotics may increase the incidence of serious adverse effects, in part due to limited opportunity to assess response prior to administration of the full dose. Access to respiratory support should be immediately available

Adverse Reactions

Frequency not defined: Increased AST, ALT

>10%:

Central nervous system: Drowsiness

Gastrointestinal: Constipation

1% to 10%:

Cardiovascular: Tachycardia or bradycardia, hypotension

Central nervous system: Dizziness, lightheadedness, false feeling of well being, malaise, headache, restlessness, paradoxical CNS stimulation, confusion

Dermatologic: Rash, urticaria

Gastrointestinal: Xerostomia, anorexia, nausea, vomiting

Genitourinary: Decreased urination, ureteral spasm

Hepatic: Increased LFTs

Local: Burning at injection site

Neuromuscular & skeletal: Weakness

Ocular: Blurred vision

Respiratory: Dyspnea

Miscellaneous: Histamine release

<1%: Convulsions, hallucinations, mental depression, nightmares, insomnia, paralytic ileus, biliary spasm, stomach cramps, muscle rigidity, trembling

Vesicant No

Overdosage/Toxicology Symptoms of overdose include CNS and respiratory depression, GI cramping, and constipation. Naloxone, 2 mg I.V. with repeat administration as necessary up to a total of 10 mg, can also be used to reverse toxic effects of the opiate.

Drug Interactions

Cytochrome P450 Effect: Substrate of CYP2D6 (major), 3A4 (minor); **Inhibits** CYP2D6 (weak)

Increased Effect/Toxicity: May cause severely increased toxicity of codeine when taken with CNS depressants, phenothiazines, tricyclic antidepressants, other narcotic analgesics, guanabenz, MAO inhibitors, and neuromuscular blockers.

Decreased Effect: CYP2D6 inhibitors may decrease the effects of codeine. Example inhibitors include chlorpromazine, delavirdine, fluoxetine, miconazole, paroxetine, pergolide, quinidine, quinine, ritonavir, and ropinirole. Decreased effect with cigarette smoking.

Ethanol/Nutrition/Herb Interactions

Ethanol: May increase CNS depression.

Herb/Nutraceutical: St John's wort may decrease codeine levels. Avoid valerian, St John's wort, kava kava, gotu kola (may increase CNS depression).

Storage/Stability Store injection between 15°C to 30°C, avoid freezing. Do not use if injection is discolored or contains a precipitate. Protect injection from light.

Compatibility Compatibility in syringe: Compatible: Glycopyrrolate, hydroxyzine

Pharmacodynamics/Kinetics

Onset of action: Oral: 0.5-1 hour; I.M.: 10-30 minutes

Peak effect: Oral: 1-1.5 hours; I.M.: 0.5-1 hour

Duration: 4-6 hours

Absorption: Oral: Adequate

Distribution: Crosses placenta; enters breast milk

Protein binding: 7%

Metabolism: Hepatic to morphine (active)

Half-life elimination: 2.5-3.5 hours

Excretion: Urine (3% to 16% as unchanged drug, norcodeine, and free and conjugated morphine)

Dosage Note: These are guidelines and do not represent the maximum doses that may be required in all patients. Doses should be titrated to pain relief/prevention. Doses >1.5 mg/kg body weight are not recommended.

Analgesic:

Children: Oral, I.M., SubQ: 0.5-1 mg/kg/dose every 4-6 hours as needed; maximum: 60 mg/dose

Adults:

Oral: 30 mg every 4-6 hours as needed; patients with prior opiate exposure may require higher initial doses. Usual range: 15-120 mg every 4-6 hours as needed

(Continued)

Codeine *(Continued)*

Oral, controlled release formulation (Codeine Contin®, not available in U.S.): 50-300 mg every 12 hours. **Note:** A patient's codeine requirement should be established using prompt release formulations; conversion to long acting products may be considered when chronic, continuous treatment is required. Higher dosages should be reserved for use only in opioid-tolerant patients.

I.M., SubQ: 30 mg every 4-6 hours as needed; patients with prior opiate exposure may require higher initial doses. Usual range: 15-120 mg every 4-6 hours as needed; more frequent dosing may be needed

Antitussive: Oral (for nonproductive cough):

Children: 1-1.5 mg/kg/day in divided doses every 4-6 hours as needed: Alternative dose according to age:

2-6 years: 2.5-5 mg every 4-6 hours as needed; maximum: 30 mg/day
6-12 years: 5-10 mg every 4-6 hours as needed; maximum: 60 mg/day

Adults: 10-20 mg/dose every 4-6 hours as needed; maximum: 120 mg/day

Dosing adjustment in renal impairment:

Cl_{cr} 10-50 mL/minute: Administer 75% of dose
Cl_{cr} <10 mL/minute: Administer 50% of dose

Dosing adjustment in hepatic impairment: Probably necessary in hepatic insufficiency

Administration I.M., Oral, SubQ: Not approved for I.V. administration (although this route has been used clinically). Rapid intravenous administration of narcotics may increase the incidence of serious adverse effects, in part due to limited opportunity to assess response prior to administration of the full dose. Access to respiratory support should be immediately available.

Dosage Forms

Injection, as phosphate: 15 mg/mL (2 mL); 30 mg/mL (2 mL) [contains sodium metabisulfite]

Solution, oral, as phosphate: 15 mg/5 mL (5 mL, 500 mL) [strawberry flavor]

Tablet, controlled release (Codeine Contin®) [not available in U.S.]: 50 mg, 100 mg, 150 mg, 200 mg

Tablet, as phosphate: 30 mg, 60 mg

Tablet, as sulfate: 15 mg, 30 mg, 60 mg

Monitoring Parameters Pain relief, respiratory and mental status, blood pressure, heart rate

Patient Information Avoid alcohol; may cause drowsiness, impaired judgment, or coordination; may cause physical and psychological dependence with prolonged use

Special Geriatric Considerations The elderly may be particularly susceptible to CNS depression and confusion as well as the constipating effects of narcotics.

- ◆ **Codeine Contin® (Can)** *see* Codeine *on page 205*
- ◆ **Codeine Phosphate** *see* Codeine *on page 205*
- ◆ **Codeine Sulfate** *see* Codeine *on page 205*
- ◆ **Colocort®** *see* Hydrocortisone *on page 419*
- ◆ **Compazine® [DSC]** *see* Prochlorperazine *on page 691*

- **Compound F** *see* Hydrocortisone *on page 419*
- **Compro**™ *see* Prochlorperazine *on page 691*
- **Correctol® Tablets [OTC]** *see* Bisacodyl *on page 133*
- **CortaGel® Maximum Strength [OTC] [DSC]** *see* Hydrocortisone *on page 419*
- **Cortaid® Intensive Therapy [OTC]** *see* Hydrocortisone *on page 419*
- **Cortaid® Maximum Strength [OTC]** *see* Hydrocortisone *on page 419*
- **Cortaid® Sensitive Skin [OTC]** *see* Hydrocortisone *on page 419*
- **Cortamed® (Can)** *see* Hydrocortisone *on page 419*
- **Cortate® (Can)** *see* Hydrocortisone *on page 419*
- **Cortef®** *see* Hydrocortisone *on page 419*
- **Cortenema® (Can)** *see* Hydrocortisone *on page 419*
- **Corticool® [OTC]** *see* Hydrocortisone *on page 419*
- **Cortifoam®** *see* Hydrocortisone *on page 419*
- **Cortisol** *see* Hydrocortisone *on page 419*
- **Cortizone®-10 Maximum Strength [OTC]** *see* Hydrocortisone *on page 419*
- **Cortizone®-10 Plus Maximum Strength [OTC]** *see* Hydrocortisone *on page 419*
- **Cortizone®-10 Quick Shot [OTC]** *see* Hydrocortisone *on page 419*
- **Cortoderm (Can)** *see* Hydrocortisone *on page 419*
- **Cosmegen®** *see* Dactinomycin *on page 245*
- **Co-Trimoxazole** *see* Sulfamethoxazole and Trimethoprim *on page 727*
- **Co-Vidarabine** *see* Pentostatin *on page 661*
- **CP358774** *see* Erlotinib *on page 308*
- **CPM** *see* Cyclophosphamide *on page 209*
- **CPT-11** *see* Irinotecan *on page 478*
- **CPZ** *see* ChlorproMAZINE *on page 178*
- **Creatinine Clearance Estimating Methods in Patients with Stable Renal Function** *see page 1048*
- **Cruex® Cream [OTC]** *see* Clotrimazole *on page 203*
- **CsA** *see* CycloSPORINE *on page 216*
- **CTX** *see* Cyclophosphamide *on page 209*
- **CyA** *see* CycloSPORINE *on page 216*

Cyclophosphamide (sye kloe FOS fa mide)

Medication Safety Issues

Sound-alike/look-alike issues:

Cyclophosphamide may be confused with cycloSPORINE

Cytoxan® may be confused with cefoxitin, Centoxin®, Ciloxan®, cytarabine, CytoGam®, Cytosar®, Cytosar-U®, Cytotec®

Related Information

Fertility and Cancer Therapy *on page 962*
Safe Handling of Hazardous Drugs *on page 1034*
Transplantation *on page 1019*

U.S. Brand Names Cytoxan®

Canadian Brand Names Cytoxan®; Procytox®

Generic Available Yes: Tablet

Synonyms CPM; CTX; CYT; NSC-26271

Pharmacologic Category Antineoplastic Agent, Alkylating Agent

(Continued)

Cyclophosphamide *(Continued)*

Pregnancy Risk Factor D

Lactation Enters breast milk/contraindicated

Use

> **Oncologic:** Treatment of Hodgkin's and non-Hodgkin's lymphoma, Burkitt's lymphoma, chronic lymphocytic leukemia (CLL), chronic myelocytic leukemia (CML), acute myelocytic leukemia (AML), acute lymphocytic leukemia (ALL), mycosis fungoides, multiple myeloma, neuroblastoma, retinoblastoma, rhabdomyosarcoma, Ewing's sarcoma; breast, testicular, endometrial, ovarian, and lung cancers, and in conditioning regimens for bone marrow transplantation

> **Nononcologic:** Prophylaxis of rejection for kidney, heart, liver, and bone marrow transplants, severe rheumatoid disorders, nephrotic syndrome, Wegener's granulomatosis, idiopathic pulmonary hemosideroses, myasthenia gravis, multiple sclerosis, systemic lupus erythematosus, lupus nephritis, autoimmune hemolytic anemia, idiopathic thrombocytic purpura (ITP), macroglobulinemia, and antibody-induced pure red cell aplasia

Mechanism of Action Cyclophosphamide is an alkylating agent that prevents cell division by cross-linking DNA strands and decreasing DNA synthesis. It is a cell cycle phase nonspecific agent. Cyclophosphamide also possesses potent immunosuppressive activity. Cyclophosphamide is a prodrug that must be metabolized to active metabolites in the liver.

Labeled Contraindications Hypersensitivity to cyclophosphamide or any component of the formulation; pregnancy

Warnings/Precautions Hazardous agent - use appropriate precautions for handling and disposal. See Safe Handling of Hazardous Drugs *on page 1034* in the Appendix. Dosage adjustment needed for renal or hepatic failure.

Adverse Reactions

> >10%:

>> Dermatologic: Alopecia (40% to 60%) but hair will usually regrow although it may be a different color and/or texture. Hair loss usually begins 3-6 weeks after the start of therapy.

>> Endocrine & metabolic: Fertility: May cause sterility; interferes with oogenesis and spermatogenesis; may be irreversible in some patients; gonadal suppression (amenorrhea)

>> Gastrointestinal: Nausea and vomiting, usually beginning 6-10 hours after administration; anorexia, diarrhea, mucositis, and stomatitis are also seen

>> Genitourinary: Severe, potentially fatal acute hemorrhagic cystitis or urinary fibrosis (7% to 40%)

>> Hematologic: Thrombocytopenia and anemia are less common than leukopenia

>>> Onset: 7 days

>>> Nadir: 10-14 days

>>> Recovery: 21 days

> 1% to 10%:

>> Cardiovascular: Facial flushing

>> Central nervous system: Headache

>> Dermatologic: Skin rash

Renal: SIADH may occur, usually with doses >50 mg/kg (or 1 g/m^2); renal tubular necrosis, which usually resolves with discontinuation of the drug, is also reported

Respiratory: Nasal congestion occurs when I.V. doses are administered too rapidly; patients experience runny eyes, rhinorrhea, sinus congestion, and sneezing during or immediately after the infusion.

<1%: High-dose therapy may cause cardiac dysfunction manifested as CHF; cardiac necrosis or hemorrhagic myocarditis has occurred rarely, but may be fatal. Cyclophosphamide may also potentiate the cardiac toxicity of anthracyclines. Other adverse reactions include anaphylactic reactions, dizziness, darkening of skin/fingernails, hypokalemia, hyperuricemia, hepatotoxicity, jaundice, neutrophilic eccrine hidradenitis, radiation recall, secondary malignancy (eg, bladder carcinoma), Stevens-Johnson syndrome, toxic epidermal necrolysis, hemorrhagic colitis, hemorrhagic ureteritis, renal tubular necrosis; interstitial pneumonitis and pulmonary fibrosis is occasionally seen with high doses.

Vesicant No

Emetic Potential

Very high (>90%): >1500 mg/m^2

High (60% to 90%): >750 mg/m^2, ≤1500 mg/m^2

Moderate (30% to 60%): ≤750 mg/m^2

Oral: Moderate (30% to 60%)

Overdosage/Toxicology Symptoms of overdose include myelosuppression, alopecia, nausea, and vomiting. Treatment is supportive.

Drug Interactions

Cytochrome P450 Effect: Substrate of CYP2A6 (minor), 2B6 (major), 2C8/9 (minor), 2C19 (minor), 3A4 (major); **Inhibits** CYP3A4 (weak); **Induces** CYP2B6 (weak), 2C8/9 (weak)

Increased Effect/Toxicity: Allopurinol may cause an increase in bone marrow depression and may result in significant elevations of cyclophosphamide cytotoxic metabolites.

Anesthetic agents: Cyclophosphamide reduces serum pseudocholinesterase concentrations and may prolong the neuromuscular blocking activity of succinylcholine. Use with caution with halothane, nitrous oxide, and succinylcholine.

Chloramphenicol causes prolonged cyclophosphamide half-life and increased toxicity.

CYP2B6 inducers: CYP2B6 inducers may increase the levels/effects of acrolein (the active metabolite of cyclophosphamide). Example inducers include carbamazepine, nevirapine, phenobarbital, phenytoin, and rifampin.

CYP3A4 inducers: CYP3A4 inducers may increase the levels/effects of acrolein (the active metabolite of cyclophosphamide). Example inducers include aminoglutethimide, carbamazepine, nafcillin, nevirapine, phenobarbital, phenytoin, and rifamycins.

Doxorubicin: Cyclophosphamide may enhance cardiac toxicity of anthracyclines.

Tetrahydrocannabinol results in enhanced immunosuppression in animal studies.

Thiazide diuretics: Leukopenia may be prolonged.

Decreased Effect: Cyclophosphamide may decrease digoxin serum levels. CYP2B6 inhibitors may decrease the levels/effects of acrolein (the active metabolite of cyclophosphamide); example inhibitors include

(Continued)

Cyclophosphamide *(Continued)*

desipramine, paroxetine, and sertraline. CYP3A4 inhibitors may decrease the levels/effects of acrolein (the active metabolite of cyclophosphamide); example inhibitors include azole antifungals, ciprofloxacin, clarithromycin, diclofenac, doxycycline, erythromycin, imatinib, isoniazid, nefazodone, nicardipine, propofol, protease inhibitors, quinidine, and verapamil.

Ethanol/Nutrition/Herb Interactions Herb/Nutraceutical: Avoid black cohosh, dong quai in estrogen-dependent tumors.

Storage/Stability Store intact vials of powder at room temperature of (25°C to 35°C). Reconstituted solutions are stable for 24 hours at room temperature (25°C) and 6 days under refrigeration (5°C). Further dilutions in D$_5$W or NS are stable for 24 hours at room temperature (25°C) and 6 days at refrigeration (5°C).

Reconstitution Reconstitute vials with SWI, NS, or D$_5$W to a concentration of 20 mg/mL.

Compatibility Stable in D$_5$LR, D$_5$NS, D$_5$W, LR, $\frac{1}{2}$NS, NS

Y-site administration: Compatible: Allopurinol, amifostine, amikacin, ampicillin, azlocillin, aztreonam, bleomycin, cefamandole, cefazolin, cefepime, cefoperazone, cefotaxime, cefoxitin, cefuroxime, chloramphenicol, chlorpromazine, cimetidine, cisplatin, cladribine, clindamycin, co-trimoxazole, dexamethasone sodium phosphate, diphenhydramine, doxorubicin, doxorubicin liposome, doxycycline, droperidol, erythromycin lactobionate, etoposide phosphate, famotidine, filgrastim, fludarabine, fluorouracil, furosemide, ganciclovir, gatifloxacin, gemcitabine, gentamicin, granisetron, heparin, hydromorphone, idarubicin, kanamycin, leucovorin, linezolid, lorazepam, melphalan, methotrexate, methylprednisolone sodium succinate, metoclopramide, metronidazole, minocycline, mitomycin, morphine, nafcillin, ondansetron, oxacillin, paclitaxel, penicillin G potassium, piperacillin, piperacillin/tazobactam, prochlorperazine edisylate, promethazine, propofol, ranitidine, sargramostim, sodium bicarbonate, teniposide, thiotepa, ticarcillin, ticarcillin/clavulanate, tobramycin, topotecan, vancomycin, vinblastine, vincristine, vinorelbine. **Incompatible:** Amphotericin B cholesteryl sulfate complex

Compatibility in syringe: Compatible: Bleomycin, cisplatin, doxapram, doxorubicin, droperidol, fluorouracil, furosemide, heparin, leucovorin, methotrexate, metoclopramide, mitomycin, vinblastine, vincristine

Compatibility when admixed: Compatible: Cisplatin with etoposide, dacarbazine, fluorouracil, hydroxyzine, mesna, methotrexate, methotrexate with fluorouracil, mitoxantrone, ondansetron

Pharmacodynamics/Kinetics

Absorption: Oral: Well absorbed

Distribution: V$_d$: 0.48-0.71 L/kg; crosses placenta; crosses into CSF (not in high enough concentrations to treat meningeal leukemia)

Protein binding: 10% to 56%

Metabolism: Hepatic to active metabolites acrolein, 4-aldophosphamide, 4-hydroperoxycyclophosphamide, and nor-nitrogen mustard

Bioavailability: >75%

Half-life elimination: 4-8 hours

Time to peak, serum: Oral: ~1 hour

Excretion: Urine (<30% as unchanged drug, 85% to 90% as metabolites)

Dosage Refer to individual protocols

Children:

SLE: I.V.: 500-750 mg/m^2 every month; maximum dose: 1 g/m^2

JRA/vasculitis: I.V.: 10 mg/kg every 2 weeks

Children and Adults:

Oral: 50-100 mg/m^2/day as continuous therapy or 400-1000 mg/m^2 in divided doses over 4-5 days as intermittent therapy

I.V.:

Single doses: 400-1800 mg/m^2 (30-50 mg/kg) per treatment course (1-5 days) which can be repeated at 2-4 week intervals

Continuous daily doses: 60-120 mg/m^2 (1-2.5 mg/kg) per day

Autologous BMT: IVPB: 50 mg/kg/dose x 4 days or 60 mg/kg/dose for 2 days; total dose is usually divided over 2-4 days

Nephrotic syndrome: Oral: 2-3 mg/kg/day every day for up to 12 weeks when corticosteroids are unsuccessful

Dosing adjustment in renal impairment: A large fraction of cyclophosphamide is eliminated by hepatic metabolism

Some authors recommend no dose adjustment unless severe renal insufficiency (Cl_{cr} <20 mL/minute)

Cl_{cr} >10 mL/minute: Administer 100% of normal dose

Cl_{cr} <10 mL/minute: Administer 75% of normal dose

Hemodialysis: Moderately dialyzable (20% to 50%); administer dose posthemodialysis

CAPD effects: Unknown

CAVH effects: Unknown

Dosing adjustment in hepatic impairment: The pharmacokinetics of cyclophosphamide are not significantly altered in the presence of hepatic insufficiency. No dosage adjustments are recommended.

Combination Regimens

Bladder cancer:

CAP *on page 851*

CISCA *on page 861*

Brain tumors:

8 in 1 (Brain Tumors) *on page 841*

COPE *on page 866*

Breast cancer:

AC *on page 843*

CAF *on page 850*

CEF *on page 857*

CMF *on page 862*

CMF-IV *on page 863*

CNF *on page 863*

FAC *on page 884*

FEC *on page 888*

TAC *on page 938*

Gestational trophoblastic tumor:

CHAMOCA *on page 858*

EMA/CO *on page 877*

Leukemia, acute lymphocytic:

Larson Regimen *on page 904*

VAD/CVAD *on page 944*

Leukemia, acute myeloid: Hyper-CVAD *on page 898*

Leukemia, chronic lymphocytic: CVP (Leukemia) *on page 869*

Lung cancer (small cell): CAVE *on page 853*

(Continued)

Cyclophosphamide *(Continued)*

VAC Pulse *on page 943*
Sarcoma: CYVADIC *on page 871*
Wilms' tumor: ACAV (J) *on page 844*

Administration Oral, I.P., intrapleurally, IVPB, or continuous I.V. infusion; may also be administered slow IVP in doses ≤1 g.

I.V. infusions may be administered over 1-24 hours

Doses >500 mg to approximately 2 g may be administered over 20-30 minutes

To minimize bladder toxicity, increase normal fluid intake during and for 1-2 days after cyclophosphamide dose. Most adult patients will require a fluid intake of at least 2 L/day. High-dose regimens should be accompanied by vigorous hydration with or without mesna therapy.

Tablets are not scored and should not be cut or crushed; should be administered during or after meals.

Dosage Forms

Injection, powder for reconstitution:
Cytoxan®: 500 mg, 1 g, 2 g [contains mannitol 75 mg per cyclophosphamide 100 mg]

Tablet (Cytoxan®): 25 mg, 50 mg

High Dose Considerations

High Dose:

I.V.:
60 mg/kg/day for 2 days (total dose: 120 mg/kg)
50 mg/kg/day for 4 days (total dose: 200 mg/kg)
1.8 g/m^2/day for 4 days (total dose: 7.2 g/m^2)
1875 mg/m^2/24 hours for 72 hours (total dose: 5625 mg/m^2)
Continuous I.V.: 1.5 g/m^2/24 hours for 96 hours (total dose: 6 g/m^2)
Duration of infusion is 1-24 hours; generally combined with other high-dose chemotherapeutic drugs, lymphocyte immune globulin, or total body irradiation (TBI).

Unique Toxicities:

Cardiovascular: Heart failure, cardiac necrosis, pericardial tamponade, heart block

Endocrine & metabolic: Hyponatremia, acquired pseudocholinesterase deficiency, transient diabetes insipidus

Hematologic: Methemoglobinemia

Neuromuscular & skeletal: Rhabdomyolysis

Respiratory: Pleural effusion, interstitial pneumonitis

Comments: Approaches to reduction of hemorrhagic cystitis include infusion of 0.9% NaCl 3 L/m^2/24 hours, infusion of 0.9% NaCl 3 L/m^2/24 hours with continuous 0.9% NaCl bladder irrigation 300-1000 mL/hour, and infusion of 0.9% NaCl 1.5-3 L/m^2/24 hours with intravenous mesna. Hydration should begin at least 4 hours before cyclophosphamide and continue at least 24 hours after completion of cyclophosphamide. The dose of daily mesna used should equal the daily dose of cyclophosphamide. Mesna can be administered as a continuous 24-hour intravenous infusion or be given in divided doses every 4 hours. Mesna should begin at the start of treatment, and continue at least 24 hours following the last dose of cyclophosphamide.

Enhanced bioactivation of cyclophosphamide may increase the risk of cardiotoxicity. A 30-minute infusion of thiotepa administered 1 hour before a 60-minute infusion of cyclophosphamide reduced bioactivation of cyclophosphamide to 4-hydroxycyclophosphamide in 20 patients.
(Continued)

Cyclophosphamide *(Continued)*

This effect did not occur with administration of thiotepa 1 hour following infusion of cyclophosphamide. Intravascular red blood cell hemolysis requiring transfusion support occurred during continuous flow plasmapheresis performed 12 hours following infusion of cyclophosphamide 60 mg/kg.

Monitoring Parameters CBC with differential and platelet count, BUN, UA, serum electrolytes, serum creatinine

Dietary Considerations Tablets should be administered during or after meals.

Patient Information Tablets may be taken during or after meals to reduce GI effects. Maintain adequate fluid balance (2-3 L/day of fluids unless instructed to restrict fluid intake). Void frequently and report any difficulty or pain with urination. May cause hair loss (reversible after treatment), sterility, or amenorrhea (sometimes reversible). If you are diabetic, you will need to monitor serum glucose closely to avoid hypoglycemia. You may be more susceptible to infection; avoid crowds and unnecessary exposure to infection. Report unusual bleeding or bruising; persistent fever or sore throat; blood in urine, stool (black stool), or vomitus; delayed healing of any wounds; skin rash; yellowing of skin or eyes; or changes in color of urine or stool. Contraceptive measures are recommended during therapy.

Special Geriatric Considerations Toxicity to immunosuppressives is increased in the elderly. Start with lowest recommended adult doses. Signs of infection, such as fever and WBC rise, may not occur. Lethargy and confusion may be more prominent signs of infection; adjust dose for renal function in the elderly.

Extemporaneous Preparations A 2 mg/mL oral elixir was stable for 14 days when refrigerated when made as follows: Reconstitute a 200 mg vial with aromatic elixir, withdraw the solution, and add sufficient aromatic elixir to make a final volume of 100 mL (store in amber glass container).

Brook D, Davis RE, and Bequette RJ, "Chemical Stability of Cyclophosphamide in Aromatic Elixir U.S.P.," *Am J Health Syst Pharm*, 1973, 30:618-20.

Selected Readings

Ahmed AR and Hombal SM, "Cyclophosphamide (Cytoxan®). A Review on Relevant Pharmacology and Clinical Uses," *J Am Acad Dermatol*, 1984, 11(6):1115-26.

Colvin OM, "An Overview of Cyclophosphamide Development and Clinical Applications," *Curr Pharm Des*, 1999, 5(8):555-60.

Fleming RA, "An Overview of Cyclophosphamide and Ifosfamide Pharmacology," *Pharmacotherapy*, 1997, 17(5 Pt 2):146S-154S.

Fraiser LH, Kanekal S, and Kehrer JP, "Cyclophosphamide Toxicity. Characterizing and Avoiding the Problem," *Drugs*, 1991, 42(5):781-95.

Langford CA, "Complications of Cyclophosphamide Therapy," *Eur Arch Otorhinolaryngol*, 1997, 254(2):65-72.

♦ **Cyclosporin A** see CycloSPORINE on page 216

CycloSPORINE *(SYE kloe spor een)*

Medication Safety Issues

Sound-alike/look-alike issues:

CycloSPORINE may be confused with cyclophosphamide, Cyklokapron®, cycloSERINE

Gengraf® may be confused with Prograf®

Neoral® may be confused with Neurontin®, Nizoral®

Sandimmune® may be confused with Sandostatin®

Related Information
Safe Handling of Hazardous Drugs *on page 1034*
Transplantation *on page 1019*

U.S. Brand Names Gengraf®; Neoral®; Restasis™; Sandimmune®

Canadian Brand Names Apo-Cyclosporine®; Neoral®; Rhoxal-cyclosporine; Sandimmune® I.V.

Generic Available Yes

Synonyms CsA; CyA; Cyclosporin A

Pharmacologic Category Immunosuppressant Agent

Pregnancy Risk Factor C

Lactation Enters breast milk/contraindicated

Use Prophylaxis of organ rejection in kidney, liver, and heart transplants, has been used with azathioprine and/or corticosteroids; severe, active rheumatoid arthritis (RA) not responsive to methotrexate alone; severe, recalcitrant plaque psoriasis in nonimmunocompromised adults unresponsive to or unable to tolerate other systemic therapy

Ophthalmic emulsion (Restasis™): Increase tear production when suppressed tear production is presumed to be due to keratoconjunctivitis sicca-associated ocular inflammation (in patients not already using topical anti-inflammatory drugs or punctal plugs)

Unlabeled/Investigational Use Short-term, high-dose cyclosporine as a modulator of multidrug resistance in cancer treatment; allogenic bone marrow transplants for prevention and treatment of graft-versus-host disease; also used in some cases of severe autoimmune disease (ie, SLE, myasthenia gravis) that are resistant to corticosteroids and other therapy; focal segmental glomerulosclerosis

Mechanism of Action Inhibition of production and release of interleukin II and inhibits interleukin II-induced activation of resting T-lymphocytes.

Labeled Contraindications Hypersensitivity to cyclosporine or any component of the formulation. Rheumatoid arthritis and psoriasis: Abnormal renal function, uncontrolled hypertension, malignancies. Concomitant treatment with PUVA or UVB therapy, methotrexate, other immunosuppressive agents, coal tar, or radiation therapy are also contraindications for use in patients with psoriasis. Ophthalmic emulsion is contraindicated in patients with active ocular infections.

Warnings/Precautions Use caution with other potentially nephrotoxic drugs. Increased risk of lymphomas and other malignancies. Increased risk of infection. May cause hypertension. Use caution when changing dosage forms. Monitor cyclosporine concentrations closely following the addition, modification, or deletion of other medications; live, attenuated vaccines may be less effective; use should be avoided.

Transplant patients: May cause significant hyperkalemia and hyperuricemia, seizures (particularly if used with high dose corticosteroids), and encephalopathy. Make dose adjustments based on cyclosporine blood concentrations. Anaphylaxis has been reported with I.V. use; reserve for patients who cannot take oral form.

Psoriasis: Patients should avoid excessive sun exposure. Safety and efficacy in children <18 have not been established.

Rheumatoid arthritis: Safety and efficacy for use in juvenile rheumatoid arthritis have not been established. If receiving other immunosuppressive
(Continued)

CycloSPORINE *(Continued)*

agents, radiation or UV therapy, concurrent use of cyclosporine is not recommended.

Ophthalmic emulsion: Safety and efficacy have not been established in patients <16 years of age.

Products may contain corn oil, castor oil, ethanol, or propylene glycol; injection also contains Cremophor® EL (polyoxyethylated castor oil).

Adverse Reactions Note: Adverse reactions reported with kidney, liver, and heart transplantation, unless otherwise noted. Although percentage is reported for specific condition, reaction may occur in anyone taking cyclosporine. [Reactions reported for rheumatoid arthritis (RA) are based on cyclosporine (modified) 2.5 mg/kg/day versus placebo.]

>10%:

Cardiovascular: Hypertension (13% to 53%; psoriasis 25% to 27%)

Central nervous system: Headache (2% to 15%; RA 17%, psoriasis 14% to 16%)

Dermatologic: Hirsutism (21% to 45%), hypertrichosis (RA 19%)

Endocrine & metabolic: Increased triglycerides (psoriasis 15%), female reproductive disorder (psoriasis 8% to 11%)

Gastrointestinal: Nausea (RA 23%), diarrhea (RA 12%), gum hyperplasia (4% to 16%), abdominal discomfort (RA 15%), dyspepsia (RA 12%)

Neuromuscular & skeletal: Tremor (12% to 55%)

Renal: Renal dysfunction/nephropathy (25% to 38%; RA 10%, psoriasis 21%), creatinine elevation ≥50% (RA 24%), increased creatinine (psoriasis 16% to 20%)

Respiratory: Upper respiratory infection (psoriasis 8% to 11%)

Miscellaneous: Infection (psoriasis 24% to 25%)

Kidney, liver, and heart transplant only (≤2% unless otherwise noted):

Cardiovascular: Flushes (<1% to 4%), MI

Central nervous system: Convulsions (1% to 5%), anxiety, confusion, fever, lethargy

Dermatologic: Acne (1% to 6%), brittle fingernails, hair breaking, pruritus

Endocrine & metabolic: Gynecomastia (<1% to 4%), hyperglycemia

Gastrointestinal: Nausea (2% to 10%), vomiting (2% to 10%), diarrhea (3% to 8%), abdominal discomfort (<1% to 7%), cramps (0% to 4%), anorexia, constipation, gastritis, mouth sores, pancreatitis, swallowing difficulty, upper GI bleed, weight loss

Hematologic: Leukopenia (<1% to 6%), anemia, thrombocytopenia

Hepatic: Hepatotoxicity (<1% to 7%)

Neuromuscular & skeletal: Paresthesia (1% to 3%), joint pain, muscle pain, tingling, weakness

Ocular: Conjunctivitis, visual disturbance

Otic: Hearing loss, tinnitus

Renal: Hematuria

Respiratory: Sinusitis (<1% to 7%)

Miscellaneous: Lymphoma (<1% to 6%), allergic reactions, hiccups, night sweats

Rheumatoid arthritis only (1% to <3% unless otherwise noted):

Cardiovascular: Hypertension (8%), edema (5%), chest pain (4%), arrhythmia (2%), abnormal heart sounds, cardiac failure, MI, peripheral ischemia

Central nervous system: Dizziness (8%), pain (6%), insomnia (4%), depression (3%), migraine (2%), anxiety, hypoesthesia, emotional lability, impaired concentration, malaise, nervousness, paranoia, somnolence, vertigo

Dermatologic: Purpura (3%), abnormal pigmentation, angioedema, cellulitis, dermatitis, dry skin, eczema, folliculitis, nail disorder, pruritus, skin disorder, urticaria

Endocrine & metabolic: Menstrual disorder (3%), breast fibroadenosis, breast pain, diabetes mellitus, goiter, hot flashes, hyperkalemia, hyperuricemia, hypoglycemia, libido increased/decreased

Gastrointestinal: Vomiting (9%), flatulence (5%), gingivitis (4%), gum hyperplasia (2%), constipation, dry mouth, dysphagia, enanthema, eructation, esophagitis, gastric ulcer, gastritis, gastroenteritis, gingival bleeding, glossitis, peptic ulcer, salivary gland enlargement, taste perversion, tongue disorder, tooth disorder, weight loss/gain

Genitourinary: Leukorrhea (1%), abnormal urine, micturition urgency, nocturia, polyuria, pyelonephritis, urinary incontinence, uterine hemorrhage

Hematologic: Anemia, leukopenia

Hepatic: Bilirubinemia

Neuromuscular & skeletal: Paresthesia (8%), tremor (8%), leg cramps/muscle contractions (2%), arthralgia, bone fracture, joint dislocation, myalgia, neuropathy, stiffness, synovial cyst, tendon disorder, weakness

Ocular: Abnormal vision, cataract, conjunctivitis, eye pain

Otic: Tinnitus, deafness, vestibular disorder

Renal: Increased BUN, hematuria, renal abscess

Respiratory: Cough (5%), dyspnea (5%), sinusitis (4%), abnormal chest sounds, bronchospasm, epistaxis

Miscellaneous: Infection (9%), abscess, allergy, bacterial infection, carcinoma, fungal infection, herpes simplex, herpes zoster, lymphadenopathy, moniliasis, diaphoresis increased, tonsillitis, viral infection

Psoriasis only (1% to <3% unless otherwise noted):

Cardiovascular: Chest pain, flushes

Central nervous system: Psychiatric events (4% to 5%), pain (3% to 4%), dizziness, fever, insomnia, nervousness, vertigo

Dermatologic: Hypertrichosis (5% to 7%), acne, dry skin, folliculitis, keratosis, pruritus, rash, skin malignancies

Endocrine & metabolic: Hot flashes

Gastrointestinal: Nausea (5% to 6%), diarrhea (5% to 6%), gum hyperplasia (4% to 6%), abdominal discomfort (3% to 6%), dyspepsia (2% to 3%), abdominal distention, appetite increased, constipation, gingival bleeding

Genitourinary: Micturition increased

Hematologic: Bleeding disorder, clotting disorder, platelet disorder, red blood cell disorder

Hepatic: Hyperbilirubinemia

Neuromuscular & skeletal: Paresthesia (5% to 7%), arthralgia (1% to 6%)

Ocular: Abnormal vision

(Continued)

CycloSPORINE *(Continued)*

Respiratory: Bronchospasm (5%), cough (5%), dyspnea (5%), rhinitis (5%), respiratory infection

Miscellaneous: Flu-like symptoms (8% to 10%)

Postmarketing and/or case reports (any indication): Death (due to renal deterioration), mild hypomagnesemia, hyperkalemia, increased uric acid, gout, hyperbilirubinemia, increased cholesterol, encephalopathy, impaired consciousness, neurotoxicity

Ophthalmic emulsion (Restasis™):

>10%: Ocular: Burning (17%)

1% to 10%: Ocular: Hyperemia (conjunctival 5%), eye pain, pruritus, stinging

Vesicant No

Emetic Potential Very low (<10%)

Overdosage/Toxicology Symptoms of overdose include hepatotoxicity, nephrotoxicity, nausea, vomiting, tremor. CNS secondary to direct action of the drug may not be reflected in serum concentrations, may be more predictable by renal magnesium loss. Forced emesis may be beneficial if done within 2 hours of ingestion of cyclosporine capsules (modified). Treatment is symptomatic and supportive. Cyclosporine is not dialyzable.

Drug Interactions

Cytochrome P450 Effect: Substrate of CYP3A4 (major); **Inhibits** CYP2C8/9 (weak), 3A4 (moderate)

Increased Effect/Toxicity: The levels/effects of cyclosporine may be increased by allopurinol, azole antifungals, ciprofloxacin, clarithromycin, diclofenac, doxycycline, erythromycin, imatinib, isoniazid, metoclopramide, nefazodone, nicardipine, octreotide, propofol, protease inhibitors, quinidine, telithromycin, verapamil, and other CYP3A4 inhibitors. Cyclosporine may increase the levels/effects of selected benzodiazepines, calcium channel blockers, cisapride, cyclosporine, ergot alkaloids, selected HMG-CoA reductase inhibitors, mesoridazine, mirtazapine, nateglinide, nefazodone, pimozide, prednisolone (dosage adjustment may be required), quinidine, sildenafil (and other PDE-5 inhibitors), tacrolimus, thioridazine, venlafaxine, and other CYP3A4 substrates. Drugs that enhance nephrotoxicity of cyclosporine include aminoglycosides, amphotericin B, acyclovir, cimetidine, ketoconazole, lovastatin, melphalan, NSAIDs, ranitidine, and trimethoprim and sulfamethoxazole, Cyclosporine increases toxicity of digoxin, diuretics, methotrexate, nifedipine.

Decreased Effect: Isoniazid and ticlopidine decrease cyclosporine concentrations. The levels/effects of cyclosporine may be decreased by aminoglutethimide, carbamazepine, nafcillin, nevirapine, phenobarbital, phenytoin, rifamycins, and other CYP3A4 inducers. Orlistat may decrease absorption of cyclosporine; avoid concomitant use. Vaccination may be less effective; avoid use of live vaccines during therapy.

Ethanol/Nutrition/Herb Interactions

Food: Grapefruit juice increases absorption; unsupervised use should be avoided.

Herb/Nutraceutical: Avoid St John's wort; as an enzyme inducer, it may increase the metabolism of and decrease plasma levels of cyclosporine; organ rejection and graft loss have been reported. Avoid cat's claw, echinacea (have immunostimulant properties).

Storage/Stability

Capsule: Store at controlled room temperature

Injection: Store at controlled room temperature; do not refrigerate. Ampuls should be protected from light. Stability of injection of parenteral admixture at room temperature (25°C) is 6 hours in PVC; 24 hours in Excel®, PAB® containers, or glass.

Ophthalmic emulsion: Store at 15°C to 25°C (59°F to 77°F). Vials are single-use; discard immediately following administration.

Oral solution: Store at controlled room temperature; do not refrigerate. Use within 2 months after opening; should be mixed in glass containers.

Reconstitution Sandimmune® injection: Injection should be further diluted [1 mL (50 mg) of concentrate in 20-100 mL of D_5W or NS] for administration by intravenous infusion.

Compatibility Stable in D_5W, fat emulsion 10%, fat emulsion 20%, NS

Y-site administration: Compatible: Alatrofloxacin, gatifloxacin, linezolid, propofol, sargramostim. **Incompatible:** Amphotericin B cholesteryl sulfate complex

Compatibility when admixed: Compatible: Ciprofloxacin. **Incompatible:** Magnesium sulfate

Pharmacodynamics/Kinetics

Absorption:

Ophthalmic emulsion: Serum concentrations not detectable.

Oral:

Cyclosporine (non-modified): Erratic and incomplete; dependent on presence of food, bile acids, and GI motility; larger oral doses are needed in pediatrics due to shorter bowel length and limited intestinal absorption

Cyclosporine (modified): Erratic and incomplete; increased absorption, up to 30% when compared to cyclosporine (non-modified); less dependent on food, bile acids, or GI motility when compared to cyclosporine (non-modified)

Distribution: Widely in tissues and body fluids including the liver, pancreas, and lungs; crosses placenta; enters breast milk

V_{dss}: 4-6 L/kg in renal, liver, and marrow transplant recipients (slightly lower values in cardiac transplant patients; children <10 years have higher values)

Protein binding: 90% to 98% to lipoproteins

Metabolism: Extensively hepatic via CYP; forms at least 25 metabolites; extensive first-pass effect following oral administration

Bioavailability: Oral:

Cyclosporine (non-modified): Dependent on patient population and transplant type (<10% in adult liver transplant patients and as high as 89% in renal transplant patients); bioavailability of Sandimmune® capsules and oral solution are equivalent; bioavailability of oral solution is ~30% of the I.V. solution

Children: 28% (range: 17% to 42%); gut dysfunction common in BMT patients and oral bioavailability is further reduced

Cyclosporine (modified): Bioavailability of Neoral® capsules and oral solution are equivalent:

Children: 43% (range: 30% to 68%)

Adults: 23% greater than with cyclosporine (non-modified) in renal transplant patients; 50% greater in liver transplant patients

(Continued)

CycloSPORINE *(Continued)*

Half-life elimination: Oral: May be prolonged in patients with hepatic impairment and shorter in pediatric patients due to the higher metabolism rate

Cyclosporine (non-modified): Biphasic: Alpha: 1.4 hours; Terminal: 19 hours (range: 10-27 hours)

Cyclosporine (modified): Biphasic: Terminal: 8.4 hours (range: 5-18 hours)

Time to peak, serum: Oral:

Cyclosporine (non-modified): 2-6 hours; some patients have a second peak at 5-6 hours

Cyclosporine (modified): Renal transplant: 1.5-2 hours

Excretion: Primarily feces; urine (6%, 0.1% as unchanged drug and metabolites)

Dosage Note: Neoral® and Sandimmune® are not bioequivalent and cannot be used interchangeably

Children: Transplant: Refer to adult dosing; children may require, and are able to tolerate, larger doses than adults.

Adults:

Newly-transplanted patients: Adjunct therapy with corticosteroids is recommended. Initial dose should be given 4-12 hours prior to transplant or may be given postoperatively; adjust initial dose to achieve desired plasma concentration

Oral: Dose is dependent upon type of transplant and formulation:

Cyclosporine (modified):

Renal: 9 ± 3 mg/kg/day, divided twice daily

Liver: 8 ± 4 mg/kg/day, divided twice daily

Heart: 7 ± 3 mg/kg/day, divided twice daily

Cyclosporine (non-modified): Initial dose: 15 mg/kg/day as a single dose (range 14-18 mg/kg); lower doses of 10-14 mg/kg/day have been used for renal transplants. Continue initial dose daily for 1-2 weeks; taper by 5% per week to a maintenance dose of 5-10 mg/kg/day; some renal transplant patients may be dosed as low as 3 mg/kg/day

Note: When using the non-modified formulation, cyclosporine levels may increase in liver transplant patients when the T-tube is closed; dose may need decreased

I.V.: Cyclosporine (non-modified): Initial dose: 5-6 mg/kg/day as a single dose (1/3 the oral dose), infused over 2-6 hours; use should be limited to patients unable to take capsules or oral solution; patients should be switched to an oral dosage form as soon as possible

Conversion to cyclosporine (modified) from cyclosporine (non-modified): Start with daily dose previously used and adjust to obtain preconversion cyclosporine trough concentration. Plasma concentrations should be monitored every 4-7 days and dose adjusted as necessary, until desired trough level is obtained. When transferring patients with previously poor absorption of cyclosporine (non-modified), monitor trough levels at least twice weekly (especially if initial dose exceeds 10 mg/kg/day); high plasma levels are likely to occur.

Rheumatoid arthritis: Oral: Cyclosporine (modified): Initial dose: 2.5 mg/kg/day, divided twice daily; salicylates, NSAIDs, and oral glucocorticoids may be continued (refer to Drug Interactions); dose may be increased by 0.5-0.75 mg/kg/day if insufficient response is seen after 8

weeks of treatment; additional dosage increases may be made again at 12 weeks (maximum dose: 4 mg/kg/day). Discontinue if no benefit is seen by 16 weeks of therapy.

Note: Increase the frequency of blood pressure monitoring after each alteration in dosage of cyclosporine. Cyclosporine dosage should be decreased by 25% to 50% in patients with no history of hypertension who develop sustained hypertension during therapy and, if hypertension persists, treatment with cyclosporine should be discontinued.

Psoriasis: Oral: Cyclosporine (modified): Initial dose: 2.5 mg/kg/day, divided twice daily; dose may be increased by 0.5 mg/kg/day if insufficient response is seen after 4 weeks of treatment. Additional dosage increases may be made every 2 weeks if needed (maximum dose: 4 mg/kg/day). Discontinue if no benefit is seen by 6 weeks of therapy. Once patients are adequately controlled, the dose should be decreased to the lowest effective dose. Doses lower than 2.5 mg/kg/day may be effective. Treatment longer than 1 year is not recommended.

Note: Increase the frequency of blood pressure monitoring after each alteration in dosage of cyclosporine. Cyclosporine dosage should be decreased by 25% to 50% in patients with no history of hypertension who develop sustained hypertension during therapy and, if hypertension persists, treatment with cyclosporine should be discontinued.

Focal segmental glomerulosclerosis: Initial: 3 mg/kg/day divided every 12 hours

Autoimmune diseases: 1-3 mg/kg/day

Keratoconjunctivitis sicca: Ophthalmic: Children ≥16 years and Adults: Instill 1 drop in each eye every 12 hours

Dosage adjustment in renal impairment: For severe psoriasis:

Serum creatinine levels ≥25% above pretreatment levels: Take another sample within 2 weeks; if the level remains ≥25% above pretreatment levels, decrease dosage of cyclosporine (modified) by 25% to 50%. If two dosage adjustments do not reverse the increase in serum creatinine levels, treatment should be discontinued.

Serum creatinine levels ≥50% above pretreatment levels: Decrease cyclosporine dosage by 25% to 50%. If two dosage adjustments do not reverse the increase in serum creatinine levels, treatment should be discontinued.

Hemodialysis: Supplemental dose is not necessary.

Peritoneal dialysis: Supplemental dose is not necessary.

Dosage adjustment in hepatic impairment: Probably necessary; monitor levels closely

Administration

Oral solution: Do not administer liquid from plastic or styrofoam cup. May dilute Neoral® oral solution with orange juice or apple juice. May dilute Sandimmune® oral solution with milk, chocolate milk, or orange juice. Avoid changing diluents frequently. Mix thoroughly and drink at once. Use syringe provided to measure dose. Mix in a glass container and rinse container with more diluent to ensure total dose is taken. Do not rinse syringe before or after use (may cause dose variation).

I.V.: Following dilution, intravenous admixture should be administered over 2-6 hours. Discard solution after 24 hours. Anaphylaxis has been reported with I.V. use; reserve for patients who cannot take oral form. Patients should be under continuous observation for at least the first 30 minutes of the infusion, and should be monitored frequently thereafter. (Continued)

CycloSPORINE *(Continued)*

Maintain patent airway; other supportive measures and agents for treating anaphylaxis should be present when I.V. drug is given.

Ophthalmic emulsion: Prior to use, invert vial several times to obtain a uniform emulsion. Remove contact lenses prior to instillation of drops; may be reinserted 15 minutes after administration. May be used with artificial tears; allow 15 minute interval between products.

Dosage Forms

Capsule, soft gel, modified: 25 mg, 100 mg [contains castor oil, ethanol]
Gengraf®: 25 mg, 100 mg [contains ethanol, castor oil, propylene glycol]
Neoral®: 25 mg, 100 mg [contains dehydrated ethanol, corn oil, castor oil, propylene glycol]

Capsule, soft gel, non-modified (Sandimmune®): 25 mg, 100 mg [contains dehydrated ethanol, corn oil]

Emulsion, ophthalmic [preservative free, single-use vial] (Restasis™): 0.05% (0.4 mL) [contains glycerin, castor oil, polysorbate 80, carbomer 1342; 32 vials/box]

Injection, solution, non-modified (Sandimmune®): 50 mg/mL (5 mL) [contains Cremophor® EL (polyoxyethylated castor oil), ethanol]

Solution, oral, modified:
Gengraf®: 100 mg/mL (50 mL) [contains castor oil, propylene glycol]
Neoral®: 100 mg/mL (50 mL) [contains dehydrated ethanol, corn oil, castor oil, propylene glycol]

Solution, oral, non-modified (Sandimmune®): 100 mg/mL (50 mL) [contains olive oil, ethanol]

Monitoring Parameters Monitor blood pressure and serum creatinine after any cyclosporine dosage changes or addition, modification, or deletion of other medications. Monitor plasma concentrations periodically.

Transplant patients: Cyclosporine trough levels, serum electrolytes, renal function, hepatic function, blood pressure, lipid profile

Psoriasis therapy: Baseline blood pressure, serum creatinine (2 levels each), BUN, CBC, serum magnesium, potassium, uric acid, lipid profile. Biweekly monitoring of blood pressure, complete blood count, and levels of BUN, uric acid, potassium, lipids, and magnesium during the first 3 months of treatment for psoriasis. Monthly monitoring is recommended after this initial period. Also evaluate any atypical skin lesions prior to therapy. Increase the frequency of blood pressure monitoring after each alteration in dosage of cyclosporine. Cyclosporine dosage should be decreased by 25% to 50% in patients with no history of hypertension who develop sustained hypertension during therapy and, if hypertension persists, treatment with cyclosporine should be discontinued.

Rheumatoid arthritis: Baseline blood pressure, and serum creatinine (2 levels each); serum creatinine every 2 weeks for first 3 months, then monthly if patient is stable. Increase the frequency of blood pressure monitoring after each alteration in dosage of cyclosporine. Cyclosporine dosage should be decreased by 25% to 50% in patients with no history of hypertension who develop sustained hypertension during therapy and, if hypertension persists, treatment with cyclosporine should be discontinued.

Dietary Considerations Administer this medication consistently with relation to time of day and meals.

Patient Information Use glass container for liquid solution (do not use plastic or styrofoam cup). Diluting oral solution improves flavor. May dilute Neoral® oral solution with orange juice or apple juice. May dilute Sandimmune® oral solution with milk, chocolate milk, or orange juice. Avoid changing what you mix with your cyclosporine. Mix thoroughly and drink at once. Use syringe provided to measure dose. Mix in a glass container and rinse container with more juice/milk to ensure total dose is taken. Do not rinse syringe before or after use (may cause dose variation). Take dose at the same time each day. You will be susceptible to infection; avoid crowds and exposure to any infectious diseases. Do not have any vaccinations without consulting prescriber. Practice good oral hygiene to reduce gum inflammation; see dentist regularly during treatment. Report severe headache; unusual hair growth or deepening of voice; mouth sores or swollen gums; persistent nausea, vomiting, or abdominal pain; muscle pain or cramping; unusual swelling of extremities, weight gain, or change in urination; or chest pain or rapid heartbeat. Increases in blood pressure or damage to the kidney are possible. Your prescriber will need to monitor closely. Do not change one brand of cyclosporine for another; any changes must be done by your prescriber. If you are taking this medication for psoriasis, your risk of cancer may be increased when taking additional medications.

Ophthalmic emulsion: Prior to use, invert vial several times to obtain a uniform emulsion. Remove contact lenses prior to instillation of drops; may be reinserted 15 minutes after administration. May be used with artificial tears; allow 15 minute interval between products.

Additional Information Cyclosporine (modified): Refers to the capsule dosage formulation of cyclosporine in an aqueous dispersion (previously referred to as "microemulsion"). Cyclosporine (modified) has increased bioavailability as compared to cyclosporine (non-modified) and cannot be used interchangeably without close monitoring.

Selected Readings

Andrews DJ and Cramb R, "Cyclosporin: Revisions in Monitoring Guidelines and Review of Current Analytical Methods," *Ann Clin Biochem*, 2002, 39(Pt 5):424-35.

Dunn CJ, Wagstaff AJ, Perry CM, et al, "Cyclosporin: An Updated Review of the Pharmacokinetic Properties, Clinical Efficacy and Tolerability of a Microemulsion-Based Formulation (Neoral)1 in Organ Transplantation," *Drugs*, 2001, 61(13):1957-2016.

Pollard S, Nashan B, Johnston A, et al, "A Pharmacokinetic and Clinical Review of the Potential Clinical Impact of Using Different Formulations of Cyclosporin A. Berlin, Germany, November 19, 2001," *Clin Ther*, 2003, 25(6):1654-69.

♦ **Cyklokapron**® *see* Tranexamic Acid *on page 788*

Cyproheptadine (si proe HEP ta deen)

Medication Safety Issues

Sound-alike/look-alike issues:

Cyproheptadine may be confused with cyclobenzaprine

Periactin may be confused with Perative®, Percodan®, Persantine®

Canadian Brand Names Periactin®

Generic Available Yes

Synonyms Cyproheptadine Hydrochloride; Periactin

Pharmacologic Category Antihistamine

Pregnancy Risk Factor B

Lactation Excretion in breast milk unknown/contraindicated

Use Perennial and seasonal allergic rhinitis and other allergic symptoms including urticaria

(Continued)

Cyproheptadine *(Continued)*

Unlabeled/Investigational Use Appetite stimulation, blepharospasm, cluster headaches, migraine headaches, Nelson's syndrome, pruritus, schizophrenia, spinal cord damage associated spasticity, and tardive dyskinesia

Mechanism of Action A potent antihistamine and serotonin antagonist, competes with histamine for H_1-receptor sites on effector cells in the gastrointestinal tract, blood vessels, and respiratory tract

Labeled Contraindications Hypersensitivity to cyproheptadine or any component of the formulation; narrow-angle glaucoma; bladder neck obstruction; acute asthmatic attack; stenosing peptic ulcer; GI tract obstruction; concurrent use of MAO inhibitors; avoid use in premature and term newborns due to potential association with SIDS

Warnings/Precautions Do not use in the presence of symptomatic prostate hypertrophy. Antihistamines are more likely to cause dizziness, excessive sedation, syncope, toxic confusion states, and hypotension in the elderly. In case reports, cyproheptadine has promoted weight gain in anorexic adults, though it has not been specifically studied in the elderly. All cases of weight loss or decreased appetite should be adequately assessed.

Adverse Reactions

>10%:
  Central nervous system: Slight to moderate drowsiness
  Respiratory: Thickening of bronchial secretions

1% to 10%:
  Central nervous system: Headache, fatigue, nervousness, dizziness
  Gastrointestinal: Appetite stimulation, nausea, diarrhea, abdominal pain, xerostomia
  Neuromuscular & skeletal: Arthralgia
  Respiratory: Pharyngitis

<1%: Tachycardia, palpitation, edema, sedation, CNS stimulation, seizure, depression, photosensitivity, rash, angioedema, hemolytic anemia, leukopenia, thrombocytopenia, hepatitis, myalgia, paresthesia, bronchospasm, epistaxis, allergic reactions

Emetic Potential Very low (<10%)

Overdosage/Toxicology Symptoms of overdose include CNS depression or stimulation, dry mouth, flushed skin, fixed and dilated pupils, and apnea. There is no specific treatment for antihistamine overdose. Clinical toxicity is due to blockade of cholinergic receptors. For anticholinergic overdose with severe life-threatening symptoms, physostigmine 1-2 mg I.V. slowly, may be given to reverse these effects.

Drug Interactions

Increased Effect/Toxicity: Cyproheptadine may potentiate the effect of CNS depressants. MAO inhibitors may cause hallucinations when taken with cyproheptadine.

Ethanol/Nutrition/Herb Interactions Ethanol: Avoid ethanol (may increase CNS sedation).

Pharmacodynamics/Kinetics

Absorption: Completely
Metabolism: Almost completely hepatic
Excretion: Urine (>50% primarily as metabolites); feces (~25%)

Dosage Oral:
Children:
Allergic conditions: 0.25 mg/kg/day or 8 mg/m^2/day in 2-3 divided doses
or
2-6 years: 2 mg every 8-12 hours (not to exceed 12 mg/day)
7-14 years: 4 mg every 8-12 hours (not to exceed 16 mg/day)
Migraine headaches: 4 mg 2-3 times/day
Children ≥12 years and Adults: Spasticity associated with spinal cord damage: 4 mg at bedtime; increase by a 4 mg dose every 3-4 days; average daily dose: 16 mg in divided doses; not to exceed 36 mg/day
Children >13 years and Adults: Appetite stimulation (anorexia nervosa): 2 mg 4 times/day; may be increased gradually over a 3-week period to 8 mg 4 times/day
Adults:
Allergic conditions: 4-20 mg/day divided every 8 hours (not to exceed 0.5 mg/kg/day)
Cluster headaches: 4 mg 4 times/day
Migraine headaches: 4-8 mg 3 times/day
Dosage adjustment in hepatic impairment: Reduce dosage in patients with significant hepatic dysfunction

Dosage Forms
Syrup, as hydrochloride: 2 mg/5 mL (473 mL) [contains alcohol 5%; mint flavor]
Tablet, as hydrochloride: 4 mg

Patient Information May cause drowsiness; may stimulate appetite; avoid alcohol and other CNS depressants; may impair judgment and coordination

Additional Information May stimulate appetite; in case reports, cyproheptadine has promoted weight gain in anorexic adults.

Special Geriatric Considerations Elderly may not tolerate anticholinergic effects.

Selected Readings
Carlton MC, Kunkel DB, and Curry SC, "Ergotism Treated With Cyproheptadine," *Clin Toxicol*, 1995, 33(5):552.
Craven JL and Rodin GM, "Cyproheptadine Dependence Associated With an Atypical Somatoform Disorder," *Can J Psychiatry*, 1987, 32(2):143-5.
Herzog DB and Copeland PM, "Eating Disorders," *N Engl J Med*, 1985, 313(5):295-303.
Lappin RI and Auchincloss EL, "Treatment of the Serotonin Syndrome With Cyproheptadine," *N Engl J Med*, 1994, 331(15):1021-2.
Wians FH, Norton JT, and Wirebaugh, "False-Positive Serum Tricyclic Antidepressant Screen With Cyproheptadine," *Clin Chem*, 1993, 39(6):1355-6.

♦ **Cyproheptadine Hydrochloride** *see* Cyproheptadine *on page 225*

Cyproterone (sye PROE ter one)

Canadian Brand Names Alti-CPA; Androcur®; Androcur® Depot; Gen-Cyproterone
Generic Available Yes (Canada)
Synonyms Cyproterone Acetate
Pharmacologic Category Antiandrogen
Pregnancy Risk Factor Not indicated for use in women
Use Palliative treatment of advanced prostate carcinoma
Mechanism of Action Cyproterone is a steroidal compound with antiandrogenic, antigonadotropic, and progestin-like activity.
Restrictions Not available in U.S.
(Continued)

Cyproterone *(Continued)*

Labeled Contraindications Hypersensitivity to cyproterone or any component of the formulation; active liver disease or hepatic dysfunction; renal impairment

Warnings/Precautions Cyproterone has been associated with hepatic toxicity (jaundice, hepatitis, hepatic failure); typically this toxicity develops after several months of therapy. Monitor hepatic function and consider discontinuation of therapy in patients with evidence of hepatic injury.

Use caution in patients with a history of depression. Cyproterone has been associated with an increased incidence of depression, particularly early in the course of therapy (initial 6-8 weeks). Use with caution in patients with diabetes or impaired glucose tolerance, may cause alterations in glucose metabolism. Use with caution in conditions that may be aggravated by fluid retention, or cardiovascular disease. May increase the risk of thromboembolism and/or alter lipid profiles.

Adverse Reactions Frequency not defined.

Cardiovascular: Heart failure, hemorrhage, hypotension, MI, stroke, shock, stroke, syncope, tachycardia, thrombosis (DVT, pulmonary embolism, retinal vein thrombosis)

Central nervous system: Libido increased, lassitude, fatigue, weakness, dizziness, encephalopathy, depression, headache

Dermatologic: Dry skin (sebum reduction), patchy loss of body hair, eczema, urticaria, erythema nodosum, rash, exfoliative dermatitis, photosensitivity, scleroderma, pruritus, hirsutism, skin discoloration

Endocrine & metabolic: Hyperglycemia, negative nitrogen balance, gynecomastia, hot flashes, benign nodular breast hyperplasia, galactorrhea, inhibition of spermatogenesis, impotence, adrenal suppression (dose related), hypercalcemia, diabetes mellitus, weight gain/loss

Gastrointestinal: Constipation, diarrhea, dyspepsia, nausea, anorexia, pancreatitis, glossitis, vomiting

Genitourinary: Hematuria, urinary frequency, bladder carcinoma

Hematologic: PT decreased, fibrinogen increased, thrombocytopenia, anemia, hemolytic anemia, leukopenia, leukocytosis

Hepatic: Hepatic dysfunction (dose related), hepatitis, transaminases increased, cholestatic jaundice, cirrhosis, hepatic failure, hepatic necrosis, ascites, hepatic coma, hepatomegaly, hepatoma, hepatic carcinoma

Local: Injection site reaction

Neuromuscular and skeletal: Weakness, myasthenia, osteoporosis

Ocular: Optic neuritis, optic atrophy, abnormal accommodation, abnormal vision, retinal disorder, blindness

Renal: Serum creatinine increased, renal failure

Respiratory: Asthma, bronchospasm, cough, dyspnea, pulmonary embolism, pulmonary fibrosis

Miscellaneous: Allergic reaction

Overdosage/Toxicology Toxicity is unlikely following single exposures of excessive doses. Any treatment following emesis and charcoal administration should be supportive and symptomatic.

Ethanol/Nutrition/Herb Interactions

Ethanol: May reduce the effect of cyproterone (not established in the treatment of prostatic carcinoma); avoid concurrent use.

Storage/Stability Store at controlled room temperature of 25°C (77°F).

Pharmacodynamics/Kinetics

Absorption: Oral: Rapid and complete

Metabolism: Hepatic, some metabolites have activity

Half-life elimination: Oral: 38 hours; Depot injection: 4 days

Time to peak, plasma: Oral: 3-4 hours; Depot injection: 3 days

Excretion: Urine (35%, as metabolites); feces (60%)

Dosage Adults: Males: Prostatic carcinoma (palliative treatment):

Oral: 200-300 mg/day in 2-3 divided doses; following orchiectomy, reduce dose to 100-200 mg/day; should be taken with meals

I.M. (depot): 300 mg (3 mL) once weekly; reduce dose in orchiectomized patients to 300 mg every 2 weeks

Dosage adjustment in renal impairment: Use is contraindicated

Dosage adjustment in hepatic impairment: Use is contraindicated with hepatic impairment or active liver disease

Administration Administer at the same time each day. Take with meals.

Dosage Forms

Injection, solution, as acetate (Androcur® Depot): 100 mg/mL (3 mL) [contains benzyl benzoate and castor oil]

Tablet, as acetate (Androcur®): 50 mg

Monitoring Parameters Liver function tests should be performed at baseline and periodically thereafter, or whenever signs or symptoms suggestive of hepatotoxicity are noted. Adrenal function should be monitored periodically.

Patient Information Immediately report pain or muscle soreness; warmth, swelling, pain, or redness in calves; shortness of breath; sudden loss of vision; unresolved leg/foot swelling; acute abdominal cramping; CNS changes (blurred vision, confusion, acute anxiety, or unresolved depression); or significant weight gain (>5 lb/week). Notify prescriber of changes in contact lens tolerance.

Selected Readings

Barradell LB and Faulds D, "Cyproterone. A Review of its Pharmacology and Therapeutic Efficacy in Prostate Cancer," *Drugs Aging*, 1994, 5(1):59-80.

Goldenberg SL and Bruchovsky N, "Use of Cyproterone Acetate in Prostate Cancer," *Urol Clin North Am*, 1991, 18(1):111-22.

Neumann F and Kalmus J, "Cyproterone Acetate in the Treatment of Sexual Disorders: Pharmacological Base and Clinical Experience," *Exp Clin Endocrinol*, 1991, 98(2):71-80.

Neumann F, "Pharmacology and Potential Use of Cyproterone Acetate," *Horm Metab Res*, 1977, 9(1):1-13.

Neumann F, "The Antiandrogen Cyproterone Acetate: Discovery, Chemistry, Basic Pharmacology, Clinical Use and Tool in Basic Research," *Exp Clin Endocrinol*, 1994, 102(1):1-32.

Schroder FH, "Cyproterone Acetate - Mechanism of Action and Clinical Effectiveness in Prostate Cancer Treatment," *Cancer*, 1993, 72(12 Suppl):3810-5.

♦ **Cyproterone Acetate** *see* Cyproterone *on page 227*

♦ **CYT** *see* Cyclophosphamide *on page 209*

♦ **Cytadren®** *see* Aminoglutethimide *on page 63*

Cytarabine (sye TARE a been)

Medication Safety Issues

Sound-alike/look-alike issues:

Cytarabine may be confused with Cytadren®, Cytosar®, Cytoxan®, vidarabine

Cytosar-U® may be confused with cytarabine, Cytovene®, Cytoxan®, Neosar®

(Continued)

Cytarabine *(Continued)*

Related Information
Fertility and Cancer Therapy *on page 962*
Safe Handling of Hazardous Drugs *on page 1034*
Transplantation *on page 1019*

U.S. Brand Names Cytosar-U®

Canadian Brand Names Cytosar®

Generic Available Yes

Synonyms Arabinosylcytosine; Ara-C; Cytarabine Hydrochloride; Cytosine Arabinosine Hydrochloride; NSC-63878

Pharmacologic Category Antineoplastic Agent, Antimetabolite (Purine Antagonist); Antineoplastic Agent, Antimetabolite

Pregnancy Risk Factor D

Lactation Excretion in breast milk unknown/not recommended

Use Treatment of acute myelogenous leukemia; lymphoma, meningeal leukemia, and meningeal lymphoma; has little use in the treatment of solid tumors

Mechanism of Action Inhibition of DNA synthesis. Cytosine gains entry into cells by a carrier process, and then must be converted to its active compound, aracytidine triphosphate. Cytosine is a purine analog and is incorporated into DNA; however, the primary action is inhibition of DNA polymerase resulting in decreased DNA synthesis and repair. The degree of cytotoxicity correlates linearly with incorporation into DNA; therefore, incorporation into the DNA is responsible for drug activity and toxicity. Cytarabine is specific for the S phase of the cell cycle.

Labeled Contraindications Hypersensitivity to cytarabine or any component of the formulation

Warnings/Precautions The U.S. Food and Drug Administration (FDA) currently recommends that procedures for proper handling and disposal of antineoplastic agents be considered. Use with caution in patients with impaired renal and hepatic function.

Adverse Reactions
>10%:
Central nervous system: Fever (>80%)
Dermatologic: Alopecia
Gastrointestinal: Nausea, vomiting, diarrhea, and mucositis which subside quickly after discontinuing the drug; GI effects may be more pronounced with divided I.V. bolus doses than with continuous infusion
Hematologic: Myelosuppression; neutropenia and thrombocytopenia are severe, anemia may also occur
Onset: 4-7 days
Nadir: 14-18 days
Recovery: 21-28 days
Hepatic: Hepatic dysfunction, mild jaundice, transaminases increased (acute)
Ocular: Tearing, ocular pain, foreign body sensation, photophobia, and blurred vision may occur with high-dose therapy; ophthalmic corticosteroids or 0.9% NaCl usually prevents or relieves the condition
1% to 10%:
Cardiovascular: Thrombophlebitis, cardiomegaly

Central nervous system: Dizziness, headache, somnolence, confusion, malaise; a severe cerebellar toxicity occurs in about 8% of patients receiving a high dose (>36-48 g/m²/cycle); it is irreversible or fatal in about 1%

Dermatologic: Skin freckling, itching, cellulitis at injection site; rash, pain, erythema, and skin sloughing of the palmar and plantar surfaces may occur with high-dose therapy. Prophylactic topical steroids and/or skin moisturizers may be useful.

Genitourinary: Urinary retention

Neuromuscular & skeletal: Myalgia, bone pain

Respiratory: Syndrome of sudden respiratory distress, including tachypnea, hypoxemia, interstitial and alveolar infiltrates progressing to pulmonary edema, pneumonia

<1%: Increases in amylase and lipase levels; isolated cases of pancreatitis have been reported; dysphagia (reported with intrathecal use); peripheral neuropathy, neuritis; accessory nerve paralysis (reported with intrathecal use); diplopia (reported with intrathecal use); cough, hoarseness (reported with intrathecal use); aphonia (reported with intrathecal use)

Vesicant No

Emetic Potential High (60% to 90%)

Overdosage/Toxicology Symptoms of overdose include myelosuppression, megaloblastosis, nausea, vomiting, respiratory distress, and pulmonary edema. A syndrome of sudden respiratory distress progressing to pulmonary edema and cardiomegaly has been reported following high doses. Treatment is symptomatic and supportive.

Drug Interactions

Increased Effect/Toxicity: Alkylating agents and radiation and purine analogs when coadministered with cytarabine may result in increased toxic effects. Methotrexate, when administered prior to cytarabine, may enhance the efficacy and toxicity of cytarabine; some combination treatment regimens (eg, hyper-CVAD) have been designed to take advantage of this interaction.

Decreased Effect: Decreased effect of gentamicin, flucytosine. Decreased digoxin oral tablet absorption.

Storage/Stability

Powder for reconstitution: Store intact vials of powder at room temperature 15°C to 30°C (59°F to 86°F). Reconstituted solutions are for up to 8 days at room temperature.

Solution: Prior to dilution, store at room temperature, 15°C to 30°C (59°F to 86°F); protect from light. Do not refrigerate solution; precipitate may form.

Reconstitution Reconstitute powder with bacteriostatic water for injection, bacteriostatic 0.9% sodium chloride, 0.9% sodium chloride, or D_5W; for I.T. use, reconstitute with preservative free diluents. Dilute in 250-1000 mL 0.9% sodium chloride or D_5W for I.V. infusion.

Note: Solutions containing bacteriostatic agents should not be used for the preparation of either high doses or intrathecal doses of cytarabine; may be used for I.M., SubQ, and low-dose (100-200 mg/m²) I.V. solution.

Compatibility Stable in D_5LR, $D_5^{1}/_4NS$, D_5NS, $D_{10}NS$, D_5W, LR, NS

Y-site administration: Compatible: Amifostine, amsacrine, aztreonam, cefepime, chlorpromazine, cimetidine, cladribine, dexamethasone

(Continued)

Cytarabine *(Continued)*

sodium phosphate, diphenhydramine, doxorubicin liposome, droperidol, etoposide phosphate, famotidine, filgrastim, fludarabine, furosemide, gatifloxacin, gemcitabine, gentamicin, granisetron, heparin, hydrocortisone sodium succinate, hydromorphone, idarubicin, linezolid, lorazepam, melphalan, methotrexate, methylprednisolone sodium succinate, metoclopramide, morphine, ondansetron, paclitaxel, piperacillin/tazobactam, prochlorperazine edisylate, promethazine, propofol, ranitidine, sargramostim, sodium bicarbonate, teniposide, thiotepa, vinorelbine. **Incompatible:** Allopurinol, amphotericin B cholesteryl sulfate complex, ganciclovir

Compatibility in syringe: Compatible: Metoclopramide

Compatibility when admixed: Compatible: Corticotropin, dacarbazine, daunorubicin with etoposide, etoposide, hydroxyzine, lincomycin, methotrexate, mitoxantrone, ondansetron, potassium chloride, sodium bicarbonate, vincristine. **Incompatible:** Fluorouracil, heparin, insulin (regular), nafcillin, oxacillin, penicillin G sodium. **Variable (consult detailed reference):** Gentamicin, hydrocortisone sodium succinate, methylprednisolone sodium succinate

Pharmacodynamics/Kinetics

Distribution: V_d: Total body water; widely and rapidly since it enters the cells readily; crosses blood-brain barrier with CSF levels of 40% to 50% of plasma level

Metabolism: Primarily hepatic; aracytidine triphosphate is the active moiety; about 86% to 96% of dose is metabolized to inactive uracil arabinoside

Half-life elimination: Initial: 7-20 minutes; Terminal: 0.5-2.6 hours

Excretion: Urine (~80% as metabolites) within 24-36 hours

Dosage I.V. bolus: Refer to individual protocols. Children and Adults:

Remission induction:

I.V.: 100-200 mg/m²/day for 5-10 days; a second course, beginning 2-4 weeks after the initial therapy, may be required in some patients.

I.T.: 5-75 mg/m² every 2-7 days until CNS findings normalize; or age-based dosing:

<1 year: 20 mg

1-2 years: 30 mg

2-3 years: 50 mg

>3 years: 75 mg

Remission maintenance:

I.V.: 70-200 mg/m²/day for 2-5 days at monthly intervals

I.M., SubQ: 1-1.5 mg/kg single dose for maintenance at 1- to 4-week intervals

High-dose therapies:

Doses as high as 1-3 g/m² have been used for refractory or secondary leukemias or refractory non-Hodgkin's lymphoma.

Doses of 1-3 g/m² every 12 hours for up to 12 doses have been used

Bone marrow transplant: 1.5 g/m² continuous infusion over 48 hours

Hemodialysis: Supplemental dose is not necessary.

Peritoneal dialysis: Supplemental dose is not necessary.

Dosage adjustment in hepatic impairment: Dose may need to be adjusted since cytarabine is partially detoxified in the liver.

Combination Regimens

Brain tumors: 8 in 1 (Brain Tumors) *on page 841*

Leukemia, acute lymphocytic:
  FIS-HAM *on page 889*
  Linker Protocol *on page 904*
  PVA (POG 8602) *on page 932*
Leukemia, acute myeloid:
  5 + 2 *on page 840*
  7 + 3 (Daunorubicin) *on page 840*
  7 + 3 (Idarubicin) *on page 840*
  7 + 3 (Mitoxantrone) *on page 841*
  7 + 3 + 7 *on page 841*
  CA *on page 849*
  DA *on page 871*
  DAT *on page 872*
  DAV *on page 872*
  EMA 86 *on page 877*
  FIS-HAM *on page 889*
  FLAG *on page 889*
  Hyper-CVAD *on page 898*
  Idarubicin, Cytarabine, Etoposide (ICE Protocol) *on page 900*
  Idarubicin, Cytarabine, Etoposide (IDA-Based BF12) *on page 901*
  TAD *on page 938*
  V-TAD *on page 949*
Lymphoma, Hodgkin's: mini-BEAM *on page 910*
Lymphoma, non-Hodgkin's:
  CODOX-M *on page 865*
  COMLA *on page 865*
  DHAP *on page 872*
  ESHAP *on page 880*
  IVAC *on page 904*
  Pro-MACE-CytaBOM *on page 931*
Neuroblastoma: N4SE Protocol *on page 922*
Retinoblastoma: 8 in 1 (Retinoblastoma) *on page 842*

Administration Can be administered I.M., I.V. infusion, I.T., or SubQ at a
concentration not to exceed 100 mg/mL

I.V. may be administered either as a bolus, IVPB (high doses of >500 mg/
m^2), or continuous intravenous infusion (doses of 100-200 mg/m^2)

I.V. doses of ≥1.5 g/m^2 may produce conjunctivitis which can be ameliorated with prophylactic use of corticosteroid (0.1% dexamethasone) eye
drops. Dexamethasone eye drops should be administered at 1-2 drops
every 6 hours during and for 2-7 days after cytarabine is done.

Dosage Forms
Injection, powder for reconstitution: 100 mg, 500 mg, 1 g, 2 g
Injection, solution: 20 mg/mL (5 mL, 25 mL, 50 mL); 100 mg/mL (20 mL)

High Dose Considerations
High Dose: I.V.: 2-3 g/m^2/dose every 12-24 hours for 4-12 doses; duration of infusion is 1-3 hours; maximum single-agent dose: 36 g/m^2;
generally combined with other high-dose chemotherapeutic drugs or
total body irradiation (TBI).

Unique Toxicities:
Central nervous system: Cerebellar toxicity which includes nystagmus,
dysarthria, disdiadochokinesis, slurred speech; cerebral toxicity which
includes somnolence, confusion
Dermatologic: Rash, desquamation may occur
(Continued)

Cytarabine *(Continued)*

Gastrointestinal: Severe nausea and vomiting, mucositis, diarrhea, ageusia

Ocular: Photophobia, excessive tearing, blurred vision, local discomfort, chemical conjunctivitis, optic neuropathy, visual loss

Respiratory: Noncardiogenic pulmonary edema (onset 22-27 days following completion of therapy)

Miscellaneous: Anosmia

Comments: Risk of cerebellar toxicity increases with creatinine clearance <60 mL/minute, age older than 50 years, pre-existing CNS lesion, and alkaline phosphatase levels exceeding 3 times the upper limit of normal. Conjunctivitis is prevented and treated with saline or corticosteroid eye drops. As prophylaxis, eye drops should be started 6-12 hours before initiation of cytarabine and continued 24 hours following the last dose.

Monitoring Parameters Liver function tests, CBC with differential and platelet count, serum creatinine, BUN, serum uric acid

Patient Information This drug can only be given by injection. You will be more susceptible to infection; avoid crowds and exposure to infection. Do not have any vaccinations without consulting prescriber. Small frequent meals, frequent mouth care, sucking lozenges, or chewing gum may reduce incidence of nausea or vomiting or loss of appetite. If these measures are ineffective, consult prescriber for antiemetic medication. Report immediately any signs of CNS changes or change in gait, easy bruising or bleeding, yellowing of eyes or skin, change in color of urine or blackened stool, respiratory difficulty, or palpitations. Contraceptive measures are recommended during therapy.

Additional Information Latex-free products: 100 mg, 500 mg, 1 g, 2 g vials (Cytosar-U®) by Pharmacia-Upjohn

Pyridoxine has been administered on days of high-dose Ara-C therapy for prophylaxis of CNS toxicity.

Selected Readings

Capizzi RL, "Curative Chemotherapy for Acute Myeloid Leukemia: The Development of High-Dose Ara-C From the Laboratory to Bedside," *Invest New Drugs*, 1996, 14(3):249-56.

Capizzi RL, White JC, Powell BL, et al, "Effect of Dose on the Pharmacokinetic and Pharmacodynamic Effects of Cytarabine," *Semin Hematol*, 1991, 28(3 Suppl 4):54-69.

Hamada A, Kawaguchi T, and Nakano M, "Clinical Pharmacokinetics of Cytarabine Formulations," *Clin Pharmacokinet*, 2002, 41(10):705-18.

Hiddemann W, "Cytosine Arabinoside in the Treatment of Acute Myeloid Leukemia: The Role and Place of High-Dose Regimens," *Ann Hematol*, 1991, 62(4):119-28.

Stasi R, Venditti A, Del Poeta G, et al, "High-Dose Chemotherapy in Adult Acute Myeloid Leukemia: Rationale and Results," *Leuk Res*, 1996, 20(7):535-49.

Stentoft J, "The Toxicity of Cytarabine," *Drug Saf*, 1990, 5(1):7-27.

♦ **Cytarabine Hydrochloride** *see* Cytarabine *on page 229*

Cytarabine (Liposomal) *(sye TARE a been lip po SOE mal)*

Medication Safety Issues

Sound-alike/look-alike issues:

Cytarabine may be confused with Cytadren®, Cytosar®, Cytoxan®, vidarabine

DepoCyt™ may be confused with Depoject®

Related Information

Safe Handling of Hazardous Drugs *on page 1034*

U.S. Brand Names DepoCyt™

Canadian Brand Names DepoCyt™

Generic Available No

Pharmacologic Category Antineoplastic Agent, Antimetabolite

Pregnancy Risk Factor D

Lactation Excretion in breast milk unknown/not recommended

Use Treatment of neoplastic (lymphomatous) meningitis

Mechanism of Action This is a sustained-release formulation of the active ingredient cytarabine, which acts through inhibition of DNA synthesis; cell cycle-specific for the S phase of cell division; cytosine gains entry into cells by a carrier process, and then must be converted to its active compound; cytosine acts as an analog and is incorporated into DNA; however, the primary action is inhibition of DNA polymerase resulting in decreased DNA synthesis and repair; degree of its cytotoxicity correlates linearly with its incorporation into DNA; therefore, incorporation into the DNA is responsible for drug activity and toxicity

Labeled Contraindications Hypersensitivity to cytarabine or any component of the formulation; active meningeal infection; pregnancy

Warnings/Precautions The U.S. Food and Drug Administration (FDA) currently recommends that procedures for proper handling and disposal of antineoplastic agents be considered. The incidence and severity of chemical arachnoiditis is reduced by coadministration with dexamethasone. May cause neurotoxicity. Blockage to CSF flow may increase the risk of neurotoxicity.

Adverse Reactions

>10%:

Central nervous system: Headache (28%), confusion (14%), somnolence (12%), fever (11%), pain (11%); chemical arachnoiditis is commonly observed, and may include neck pain, neck rigidity, headache, fever, nausea, vomiting, and back pain; may occur in up to 100% of cycles without dexamethasone prophylaxis; incidence is reduced to 33% when dexamethasone is used concurrently

Gastrointestinal: Vomiting (12%), nausea (11%)

1% to 10%:

Cardiovascular: Peripheral edema (7%)

Gastrointestinal: Constipation (7%)

Genitourinary: Incontinence (3%)

Hematologic: Neutropenia (9%), thrombocytopenia (8%), anemia (1%)

Neuromuscular & skeletal: Back pain (7%), weakness (19%), abnormal gait (4%)

<1% Anaphylaxis, neck pain

Vesicant No

Emetic Potential Low (10% to 30%)

Overdosage/Toxicology No overdosage with liposomal cytarabine has been reported. See Cytarabine *on page 229* for toxicology related to systemic administration.

Drug Interactions

Increased Effect/Toxicity: No formal studies of interactions with other medications have been conducted. The limited systemic exposure minimizes the potential for interaction between liposomal cytarabine and other medications.

(Continued)

Cytarabine (Liposomal) *(Continued)*

Decreased Effect: No formal studies of interactions with other medications have been conducted. The limited systemic exposure minimizes the potential for interaction between liposomal cytarabine and other medications.

Storage/Stability Store under refrigeration (2°C to 8°C); protect from freezing and avoid aggressive agitation. Solutions should be used within 4 hours of withdrawal from the vial. Particles may settle in diluent over time, and may be resuspended by gentle agitation or inversion of the vial.

Pharmacodynamics/Kinetics

Absorption: Systemic exposure following intrathecal administration is negligible since transfer rate from CSF to plasma is slow

Metabolism: In plasma to ara-U (inactive)

Half-life elimination, CSF: 100-263 hours

Time to peak, CSF: Intrathecal: ~5 hours

Excretion: Primarily urine (as metabolites - ara-U)

Dosage Note: Patients should be started on dexamethasone 4 mg twice daily (oral or I.V.) for 5 days, beginning on the day of liposomal cytarabine injection

Adults:

Induction: 50 mg intrathecally every 14 days for a total of 2 doses (weeks 1 and 3)

Consolidation: 50 mg intrathecally every 14 days for 3 doses (weeks 5, 7, and 9), followed by an additional dose at week 13

Maintenance: 50 mg intrathecally every 28 days for 4 doses (weeks 17, 21, 25, and 29)

If drug-related neurotoxicity develops, the dose should be reduced to 25 mg. If toxicity persists, treatment with liposomal cytarabine should be discontinued.

Administration For intrathecal use only. Dose should be removed from vial immediately before administration (must be administered within 4 hours of removal). An in-line filter should **not** be used. Administer directly into the CSF via an intraventricular reservoir or by direct injection into the lumbar sac. Injection should be made slowly (over 1-5 minutes). Patients should lie flat for 1 hour after lumbar puncture.

Dosage Forms Injection, suspension: 10 mg/mL (5 mL) [preservative free]

Monitoring Parameters Monitor closely for signs of an immediate reaction

Patient Information Report fever, sore throat, bleeding, or bruising. Contraceptive measures are recommended during therapy.

♦ **CytoGam®** *see* Cytomegalovirus Immune Globulin (Intravenous-Human) *on page 236*

Cytomegalovirus Immune Globulin (Intravenous-Human)

(sye toe meg a low VYE rus i MYUN GLOB yoo lin in tra VEE nus HYU man)

Medication Safety Issues

Sound-alike/look-alike issues:

CytoGam® may be confused with Cytoxan®, Gamimune® N

Related Information
Management of Infections *on page 978*

U.S. Brand Names CytoGam®

Generic Available No

Synonyms CMV-IGIV

Pharmacologic Category Immune Globulin

Pregnancy Risk Factor C

Lactation Excretion in breast milk unknown

Use Prophylaxis of cytomegalovirus (CMV) disease associated with kidney, lung, liver, pancreas, and heart transplants; concomitant use with ganciclovir should be considered in organ transplants (other than kidney) from CMV seropositive donors to CMV seronegative recipients

Unlabeled/Investigational Use Adjunct therapy in the treatment of CMV disease in immunocompromised patients

Mechanism of Action CMV-IGIV is a preparation of immunoglobulin G derived from pooled healthy blood donors with a high titer of CMV antibodies; administration provides a passive source of antibodies against cytomegalovirus

Labeled Contraindications Hypersensitivity to CMV-IGIV, other immunoglobulins, or any component of the formulation; immunoglobulin A deficiency

Warnings/Precautions Monitor for anaphylactic reactions during infusion. May theoretically transmit blood-borne viruses. Use with caution in patients with renal insufficiency, diabetes mellitus, patients >65 years of age, volume depletion, sepsis, paraproteinemia, or patients on concomitant nephrotoxic drugs. Stabilized with sucrose and albumin, contains no preservative.

Adverse Reactions

<6%:

Cardiovascular: Flushing

Central nervous system: Fever, chills

Gastrointestinal: Nausea, vomiting

Neuromuscular & skeletal: Arthralgia, back pain, muscle cramps

Respiratory: Wheezing

<1%: Blood pressure decreased

Postmarketing and/or case reports: Acute renal failure, acute tubular necrosis, anaphylactic shock, angioneurotic edema, anuria, aseptic meningitis syndrome (AMS), BUN increased, serum creatinine increased, oliguria, osmotic nephrosis, proximal tubular nephropathy

Vesicant No

Emetic Potential Very low (<10%)

Overdosage/Toxicology Symptoms related to volume overload would be expected to occur with overdose; treatment is symptom-directed and supportive.

Drug Interactions

Decreased Effect: Decreased effect of live vaccines may be seen if given within 3 months of IGIV administration. Defer vaccination or revaccinate.

Storage/Stability Store between 2°C and 8°C (35.6°F and 46.4°F)

Reconstitution Dilution is not recommended. Do not shake vials. Do not use if turbid.

(Continued)

Cytomegalovirus Immune Globulin (Intravenous-Human) *(Continued)*

Compatibility Infusion with other products is not recommended. If unavoidable, may be piggybacked into an I.V. line of sodium chloride, 2.5% dextrose in water, 5% dextrose in water, 10% dextrose in water, or 20% dextrose in water. Do not dilute more than 1:2.

Dosage I.V.: Adults:

Kidney transplant:

Initial dose (within 72 hours of transplant): 150 mg/kg/dose

2-, 4-, 6-, and 8 weeks after transplant: 100 mg/kg/dose

12 and 16 weeks after transplant: 50 mg/kg/dose

Liver, lung, pancreas, or heart transplant:

Initial dose (within 72 hours of transplant): 150 mg/kg/dose

2-, 4-, 6-, and 8 weeks after transplant: 150 mg/kg/dose

12 and 16 weeks after transplant: 100 mg/kg/dose

Severe CMV pneumonia: Various regimens have been used, including 400 mg/kg CMV-IGIV in combination with ganciclovir on days 1, 2, 7, or 8, followed by 200 mg/kg CMV-IGIV on days 14 and 21

Elderly: Use with caution in patients >65 years of age, may be at increased risk of renal insufficiency

Dosage adjustment in renal impairment: Use with caution; specific dosing adjustments are not available. Infusion rate should be the minimum practical; do not exceed 180 mg/kg/hour

Administration Administer through an I.V. line containing an in-line filter (pore size 15 micron) using an infusion pump. Do not mix with other infusions; do not use if turbid. Begin infusion within 6 hours of entering vial, complete infusion within 12 hours.

Infuse at 15 mg/kg/hour. If no adverse reactions occur within 30 minutes, may increase rate to 30 mg/kg/hour. If no adverse reactions occur within the second 30 minutes, may increase rate to 60 mg/kg/hour; maximum rate of infusion: 75 mL/hour. When infusing subsequent doses, may decrease titration interval from 30 minutes to 15 minutes. If patient develops nausea, back pain, or flushing during infusion, slow the rate or temporarily stop the infusion. Discontinue if blood pressure drops or in case of anaphylactic reaction.

Dosage Forms Injection, solution [preservative free]: 50 mg ± 10 mg/mL (50 mL) [contains human albumin and sucrose]

Monitoring Parameters Vital signs (throughout infusion), flushing, chills, muscle cramps, back pain, fever, nausea, vomiting, wheezing, decreased blood pressure, or anaphylaxis; renal function and urine output

Selected Readings

Levinson ML and Jacobson PA, "Treatment and Prophylaxis of Cytomegalovirus Disease," *Pharmacotherapy*, 1992, 12(4):300-18.

Reed EC, Bowden RA, Dandliker PS, et al, "Efficacy of Cytomegalovirus Immunoglobulin in Marrow Transplant Recipients With Cytomegalovirus Pneumonia," *J Infect Dis*, 1987, 156:641-5.

Reed EC, Bowden RA, Dandliker PS, et al, "Treatment of Cytomegalovirus Pneumonia With Ganciclovir and Intravenous Cytomegalovirus Immunoglobulin in Patients With Bone Marrow Transplants," *Ann Intern Med*, 1988, 109:783-8.

"Renal Insufficiency and Failure Associated With Immune Globulin Intravenous Therapy - United States, 1985-1998." *MMWR*, 1999, 48(24):518-21.

Snydman DR, "Cytomegalovirus Immunoglobulins in the Prevention and Treatment of Cytomegalovirus Disease," *Rev Infect Dis*, 1990, 12(Suppl 7):839-48.

♦ **Cytosar® (Can)** *see* Cytarabine *on page 229*

♦ **Cytosar-U**® *see Cytarabine on page 229*
♦ **Cytosine Arabinoside Hydrochloride** *see Cytarabine on page 229*
♦ **Cytovene**® *see Ganciclovir on page 382*
♦ **Cytoxan**® *see Cyclophosphamide on page 209*

Dacarbazine (da KAR ba zeen)

Medication Safety Issues
Sound-alike/look-alike issues:
Dacarbazine may be confused with Dicarbosil®, procarbazine

Related Information
Management of Drug Extravasations *on page 965*
Safe Handling of Hazardous Drugs *on page 1034*

U.S. Brand Names DTIC-Dome®

Canadian Brand Names DTIC®

Generic Available Yes

Synonyms DIC; Dimethyl Triazeno Imidazole Carboxamide; DTIC; Imidazole Carboxamide; Imidazole Carboxamide Dimethyltriazenene; WR-139007

Pharmacologic Category Antineoplastic Agent, Alkylating Agent (Triazene)

Pregnancy Risk Factor C

Lactation Excretion in breast milk unknown/not recommended

Use Treatment of malignant melanoma, Hodgkin's disease, soft-tissue sarcomas, fibrosarcomas, rhabdomyosarcoma, islet cell carcinoma, medullary carcinoma of the thyroid, and neuroblastoma

Mechanism of Action Alkylating agent which appears to form methylcarbonium ions that attack nucleophilic groups in DNA; cross-links strands of DNA resulting in the inhibition of DNA, RNA, and protein synthesis, the exact mechanism of action is still unclear.

Labeled Contraindications Hypersensitivity to dacarbazine or any component of the formulation

Warnings/Precautions Hazardous agent - use appropriate precautions for handling and disposal. See Safe Handling of Hazardous Drugs *on page 1034* in the Appendix. Use with caution in patients with bone marrow depression. In patients with renal and/or hepatic impairment, dosage reduction may be necessary.

Adverse Reactions
>10%:
Gastrointestinal: Nausea and vomiting (>90%), can be severe and dose-limiting; nausea and vomiting decrease on successive days when dacarbazine is given daily for 5 days; diarrhea
Hematologic: Myelosuppression, leukopenia, thrombocytopenia - dose-limiting
Onset: 5-7 days
Nadir: 7-10 days
Recovery: 21-28 days
Local: Pain on infusion, may be minimized by administration through a central line, or by administration as a short infusion (eg, 1-2 hours as opposed to bolus injection)
1% to 10%:
Dermatologic: Alopecia, rash, photosensitivity
Gastrointestinal: Anorexia, metallic taste
Miscellaneous: Flu-like syndrome (fever, myalgia, malaise)

(Continued)

Dacarbazine *(Continued)*

<1%: Anaphylactic reactions, diarrhea (following high-dose bolus injection), eosinophilia, headache, hepatic necrosis, hepatic vein occlusion, liver enzymes increased (transient), paresthesia

Vesicant No; irritant

Emetic Potential High (>90%)

Overdosage/Toxicology Symptoms of overdose include myelosuppression and diarrhea. There are no known antidotes and treatment is symptomatic and supportive.

Drug Interactions

Cytochrome P450 Effect: Substrate (major) of CYP1A2, 2E1

Increased Effect/Toxicity: CYP1A2 inhibitors may increase the levels/ effects of dacarbazine; example inhibitors include amiodarone, ciprofloxacin, fluvoxamine, ketoconazole, norfloxacin, ofloxacin, and rofecoxib. CYP2E1 inhibitors may increase the levels/effects of dacarbazine; example inhibitors include disulfiram, isoniazid, and miconazole.

Decreased Effect: CYP1A2 inducers may decrease the levels/effects of dacarbazine; example inducers include aminoglutethimide, carbamazepine, phenobarbital, and rifampin. Patients may experience impaired immune response to vaccines; possible infection after administration of live vaccines in patients receiving immunosuppressants.

Ethanol/Nutrition/Herb Interactions

Ethanol: Avoid ethanol (due to GI irritation).

Herb/Nutraceutical: Avoid dong quai, St John's wort (may also cause photosensitization).

Storage/Stability Store intact vials under refrigeration (2°C to 8°C) and protect from light. Vials are stable for 4 weeks at room temperature. Reconstituted solution is stable for 24 hours at room temperature (20°C) and 96 hours under refrigeration (4°C). Solutions for infusion (in D_5W or NS) are stable for 24 hours at room temperature and protected from light. Decomposed drug turns pink.

Reconstitution Reconstitute to a concentration of 10-20 mg/mL with SWI, D_5W, or NS.

Standard I.V. dilution: Dilute in 250-1000 mL D_5W or NS

Compatibility Stable in NS, sterile water for injection; **variable stability (consult detailed reference)** in D_5W

Y-site administration: Compatible: Amifostine, aztreonam, etoposide phosphate, filgrastim, fludarabine, granisetron, melphalan, ondansetron, paclitaxel, sargramostim, teniposide, thiotepa, vinorelbine. **Incompatible:** Allopurinol, cefepime, piperacillin/tazobactam. **Variable (consult detailed reference):** Heparin

Compatibility when admixed: Compatible: Bleomycin, carmustine, cyclophosphamide, cytarabine, dactinomycin, doxorubicin, fluorouracil, hydrocortisone sodium phosphate, lidocaine, mercaptopurine, methotrexate, ondansetron, vinblastine. **Incompatible:** Hydrocortisone sodium succinate. **Variable (consult detailed reference):** Ondansetron with doxorubicin

Pharmacodynamics/Kinetics

Onset of action: I.V.: 18-24 days

Distribution: V_d: 0.6 L/kg, exceeding total body water; suggesting binding to some tissue (probably liver)

Protein binding: 5%

Metabolism: Extensively hepatic; hepatobiliary excretion is probably of some importance; metabolites may also have an antineoplastic effect

Half-life elimination: Biphasic: Initial: 20-40 minutes; Terminal: 5 hours

Excretion: Urine (~30% to 50% as unchanged drug)

Dosage Refer to individual protocols. Some dosage regimens include:

Intra-arterial: 50-400 mg/m^2 for 5-10 days

I.V.:

Hodgkin's disease, ABVD: 375 mg/m^2 days 1 and 15 every 4 weeks **or** 100 mg/m^2/day for 5 days

Metastatic melanoma (alone or in combination with other agents): 150-250 mg/m^2 days 1-5 every 3-4 weeks

Metastatic melanoma: 850 mg/m^2 every 3 weeks

High dose: Bone marrow/blood cell transplantation: I.V.: 1-3 g/m^2; maximum dose as a single agent: 3.38 g/m^2; generally combined with other high-dose chemotherapeutic drugs

Dosage adjustment in renal/hepatic impairment: No guidelines exist for adjustment

Combination Regimens

Brain tumors: 8 in 1 (Brain Tumors) *on page 841*

Lymphoma, Hodgkin's:

ABVD *on page 843*

MOPP/ABVD *on page 913*

Melanoma:

BOLD *on page 849*

CCDT *on page 855*

CVD *on page 868*

Dacarbazine/Tamoxifen *on page 871*

Dacarbazine- Carboplatin-Aldesleukin-Interferon *on page 871*

Dartmouth Regimen *on page 872*

IL-2 + IFN *on page 902*

Neuroblastoma: CCDDT (Neuroblastomas) *on page 855*

Sarcoma: CYVADIC *on page 871*

Sarcoma, soft tissue:

AD *on page 844*

MAID *on page 908*

Administration Infuse over 30-60 minutes; rapid infusion may cause severe venous irritation.

Dosage Forms Injection, powder for reconstitution: 100 mg, 200 mg, 500 mg

DTIC-Dome®: 200 mg

High Dose Considerations

High Dose: I.V.: 1-3 g/m^2; maximum dose as a single agent: 3.38 g/m^2; generally combined with other high-dose chemotherapeutic drugs.

Unique Toxicities:

Cardiovascular: Hypotension (infusion-related)

Gastrointestinal: Severe nausea and vomiting

Comments: Doses of 6591 mg/m^2 have been administered, although hypotension is considered the nonhematologic dose-limiting side effect for doses >3380 mg/m^2. Infusion-related hypotension may be secondary to calcium chelation by citric acid in formulation.

Monitoring Parameters CBC with differential, liver function

(Continued)

Dacarbazine *(Continued)*

Patient Information Limit oral intake for 4-6 hours before therapy. Do not use alcohol, aspirin-containing products, and/or OTC medications without consulting prescriber. It is important to maintain adequate nutrition and hydration (2-3 L/day of fluids unless instructed to restrict fluid intake) during therapy; frequent small meals may help. You may experience nausea or vomiting (frequent small meals, frequent mouth care, sucking lozenges, or chewing gum may help). If this is ineffective, consult prescriber for antiemetic medication. You may experience loss of hair (reversible); you will be more susceptible to infection (avoid crowds and exposure to infection as much as possible); you will be more sensitive to sunlight; use sunblock, wear protective clothing and dark glasses, or avoid direct exposure to sunlight. Flu-like symptoms (eg, malaise, fever, myalgia) may occur 1 week after infusion and persist for 1-3 weeks; consult prescriber for severe symptoms. Report fever, chills, unusual bruising or bleeding, signs of infection, excessive fatigue, yellowing of eyes or skin, or change in color of urine or stool. Contraceptive measures are recommended during therapy.

Selected Readings

Buesa JM and Urrechaga E, "Clinical Pharmacokinetics of High-Dose DTIC," *Cancer Chemother Pharmacol*, 1991, 28(6):475-9.

Eggermont AM and Kirkwood JM, "Re-Evaluating the Role of Dacarbazine in Metastatic Melanoma: What Have We Learned in 30 Years?" *Eur J Cancer*, 2004, 40(12):1825-36.

Finklestein JZ, Albo V, Ertel I, et al, "5-(3,3-Dimethyl-l-triazeno) imidazole-4-carboxamide (NSC-45388) in the Treatment of Solid Tumors in Children," *Cancer Chemother Rep*, 1975, 59(2 Pt 1):351-7.

Daclizumab *(dac KLYE zue mab)*

Related Information

Investigational Drug Service *on page 1031*

U.S. Brand Names Zenapax®

Canadian Brand Names Zenapax®

Generic Available No

Pharmacologic Category Immunosuppressant Agent

Pregnancy Risk Factor C

Lactation Excretion in breast milk unknown/use caution

Use Part of an immunosuppressive regimen (including cyclosporine and corticosteroids) for the prophylaxis of acute organ rejection in patients receiving renal transplant

Unlabeled/Investigational Use Graft-versus-host disease

Mechanism of Action Daclizumab is a chimeric (90% human, 10% murine) monoclonal IgG antibody produced by recombinant DNA technology. Daclizumab inhibits immune reactions by binding and blocking the alpha-chain of the interleukin-2 receptor (CD25) located on the surface of activated lymphocytes.

Labeled Contraindications Hypersensitivity to daclizumab or any component of the formulation

Warnings/Precautions Patients on immunosuppressive therapy are at increased risk for infectious complications and secondary malignancies. Long-term effects of daclizumab on immune function are unknown. Severe hypersensitivity reactions have been rarely reported; anaphylaxis has been observed on initial exposure and following re-exposure; medications for the management of severe allergic reaction should be available for immediate use. Anti-idiotype antibodies have been measured in patients that have received daclizumab (adults 14%; children 34%); detection of antibodies may be influenced by multiple factors and may therefore be misleading.

In cardiac transplant patients, the combined use of daclizumab, cyclo-sporine, mycophenolate mofetil, and corticosteroids has been associated with an increased mortality. Higher mortality may be associated with the use of antilymphocyte globulin and a higher incidence of severe infections.

Adverse Reactions Although reported adverse events are frequent, when daclizumab is compared with placebo the incidence of adverse effects is similar between the two groups. Many of the adverse effects reported during clinical trial use of daclizumab may be related to the patient population, transplant procedure, and concurrent transplant medications. Diarrhea, fever, postoperative pain, pruritus, respiratory tract infection, urinary tract infection, and vomiting occurred more often in children than adults.

≥5%:

Cardiovascular: Chest pain, edema, hyper-/hypotension, tachycardia, thrombosis

Central nervous system: Dizziness, fatigue, fever, headache, insomnia, pain, post-traumatic pain, tremor

Dermatologic: Acne, cellulitis, wound healing impaired

Gastrointestinal: Abdominal distention, abdominal pain, constipation, diarrhea, dyspepsia, epigastric pain, nausea, pyrosis, vomiting

Genitourinary: Dysuria

Hematologic: Bleeding

Neuromuscular & skeletal: Back pain, musculoskeletal pain

Renal: Oliguria, renal tubular necrosis

Respiratory: Cough, dyspnea, pulmonary edema,

Miscellaneous: Lymphocele, wound infection

≥2% to <5%:

Central nervous system: Anxiety, depression, shivering

Dermatologic: Hirsutism, pruritus, rash

Endocrine & metabolic: Dehydration, diabetes mellitus, fluid overload

Gastrointestinal: Flatulence, gastritis, hemorrhoids

Genitourinary: Urinary retention, urinary tract bleeding

Local: Application site reaction

Neuromuscular & skeletal: Arthralgia, leg cramps, myalgia, weakness

Ocular: Vision blurred

Renal: Hydronephrosis, renal damage, renal insufficiency

Respiratory: Atelectasis, congestion, hypoxia, pharyngitis, pleural effusion, rales, rhinitis

Miscellaneous: Night sweats, prickly sensation, diaphoresis

<1%, postmarketing, and/or case reports: Severe hypersensitivity reactions (rare): Anaphylaxis, bronchospasm, cardiac arrest, cytokine release syndrome, hypotension, laryngeal edema, pulmonary edema, pruritus, urticaria

Vesicant No

Emetic Potential Very low (<10%)

Overdosage/Toxicology Overdose has not been reported.

(Continued)

Daclizumab *(Continued)*

Drug Interactions

Increased Effect/Toxicity: The combined use of daclizumab, cyclosporine, mycophenolate mofetil, and corticosteroids has been associated with an increased mortality in a population of cardiac transplant recipients, particularly in patients who received antilymphocyte globulin and in patients with severe infections.

Storage/Stability Refrigerate vials at 2°C to 8°C (36°F to 46°F). Do not shake or freeze; protect undiluted solution against direct sunlight. Diluted solution is stable for 24 hours at 4°C or for 4 hours at room temperature.

Reconstitution Dose should be further diluted in 50 mL 0.9% sodium chloride solution. When mixing, gently invert bag to avoid foaming; do not shake. Do not use if solution is discolored.

Compatibility Do not mix with other medications or infuse other medications through same I.V. line.

Pharmacodynamics/Kinetics

Distribution: V_d:

Adults: Central compartment: 0.031 L/kg; Peripheral compartment: 0.043 L/kg

Children: Central compartment: 0.067 L/kg; Peripheral compartment: 0.047 L/kg

Half-life elimination (estimated): Adults: Terminal: 20 days; Children: 13 days

Dosage Daclizumab is used adjunctively with other immunosuppressants (eg, cyclosporine, corticosteroids, mycophenolate mofetil, and azathioprine): I.V.:

Children: Use same weight-based dose as adults

Adults:

Immunoprophylaxis against acute renal allograft rejection: 1 mg/kg infused over 15 minutes within 24 hours before transplantation (day 0), then every 14 days for 4 additional doses

Treatment of graft-versus-host disease (unlabeled use, limited data): 0.5-1.5 mg/kg, repeat same dosage for transient response. Repeat doses have been administered 11-48 days following the initial dose.

Dosage adjustment in renal impairment: No adjustment needed.

Dosage adjustment in hepatic impairment: No data available for patients with severe impairment.

Administration For I.V. administration following dilution. Daclizumab solution should be administered within 4 hours of preparation if stored at room temperature; infuse over a 15-minute period via a peripheral or central vein.

Dosage Forms Injection, solution [preservative free]: 5 mg/mL (5 mL)

Patient Information This medication can only be given by I.V. infusion by a healthcare professional. May cause side effects similar to those caused by surgery as well as other medications that you may be taking.

Selected Readings

Carswell CI, Plosker GL, and Wagstaff AJ, "Daclizumab: A Review of its Use in the Management of Organ Transplantation," *BioDrugs*, 2001, 15(11):745-73.

Vincenti F, Kirkman R, Light S, et al, "Interleukin-2-Receptor Blockade With Daclizumab to Prevent Acute Rejection in Renal Transplantation. Daclizumab Triple Therapy Study Group," *N Engl J Med*, 1998, 338(3):161-5.

Wiseman LR and Faulds D, "Daclizumab: A Review of its Use in the Prevention of Acute Rejection in Renal Transplant Recipients," *Drugs*, 1999, 58(6):1029-42.

♦ **DACT** *see* Dactinomycin *on page 245*

Dactinomycin (dak ti noe MYE sin)

Medication Safety Issues
Sound-alike/look-alike issues:
Dactinomycin may be confused with DAUNOrubicin
Actinomycin may be confused with Achromycin

Related Information
Safe Handling of Hazardous Drugs *on page 1034*

U.S. Brand Names Cosmegen®

Canadian Brand Names Cosmegen®

Generic Available No

Synonyms ACT; Act-D; Actinomycin; Actinomycin Cl; Actinomycin D; DACT; NSC-3053

Pharmacologic Category Antineoplastic Agent, Antibiotic

Pregnancy Risk Factor C

Lactation Excretion in breast milk unknown/contraindicated

Use Treatment of testicular tumors, melanoma, choriocarcinoma, Wilms' tumor, neuroblastoma, retinoblastoma, rhabdomyosarcoma, uterine sarcomas, Ewing's sarcoma, Kaposi's sarcoma, sarcoma botryoides, and soft tissue sarcoma

Mechanism of Action Binds to the guanine portion of DNA intercalating between guanine and cytosine base pairs inhibiting DNA and RNA synthesis and protein synthesis

Labeled Contraindications Hypersensitivity to dactinomycin or any component of the formulation; patients with concurrent or recent chickenpox or herpes zoster; avoid in infants <6 months of age

Warnings/Precautions Hazardous agent - use appropriate precautions for handling and disposal. See Safe Handling of Hazardous Drugs *on page 1034* in the Appendix. Drug is extremely irritating to tissues and must be administered I.V. If extravasation occurs during I.V. use, severe damage to soft tissues will occur. Use with caution in patients who have received radiation therapy or in the presence of hepatobiliary dysfunction. Reduce dosage in patients who are receiving radiation therapy simultaneously. Toxic effects may be delayed in onset (2-4 days following a course of treatment). Effects may require 1-2 weeks to reach maximum severity.

Adverse Reactions
>10%:
Central nervous system: Fatigue, malaise, fever, lethargy
Dermatologic: Alopecia (reversible), skin eruptions, acne, increased pigmentation or sloughing of previously irradiated skin, maculopapular rash
Endocrine & metabolic: Hypocalcemia
Gastrointestinal: Severe nausea, vomiting, anorexia
Hematologic: Myelosuppression, anemia
Onset: 7 days
Nadir: 14-21 days
Recovery: 21-28 days
Local: Tissue necrosis, pain, and ulceration (following extravasation)
1% to 10%: Gastrointestinal: Mucositis, stomatitis, diarrhea, abdominal pain

(Continued)

Dactinomycin *(Continued)*

<1%: Anaphylactoid reaction, hepatitis, hyperuricemia, LFT abnormalities, liver toxicity, ascites, hepatomegaly

Vesicant Yes; see Management of Drug Extravasations *on page 965*.

Emetic Potential High (60% to 90%)

Overdosage/Toxicology Symptoms of overdose include myelosuppression, nausea, vomiting, glossitis, and oral ulceration. There are no known antidotes and treatment is symptomatic and supportive. Toxic effects may not be apparent until 2-4 days after a treatment course (peak after 1-2 weeks).

Drug Interactions

Increased Effect/Toxicity: Dactinomycin potentiates the effects of radiation therapy.

Storage/Stability Store intact vials at controlled room temperature 15°C to 30°C (59°F to 86°F) and protect from light, humidity, and heat. Reconstituted solutions are chemically stable under refrigeration for up to 60 days. Solutions in 50 mL D_5W or NS are stable for 24 hours at room temperature.

Reconstitution Dilute with 1.1 mL of preservative-free SWI to yield a final concentration of 500 mcg/mL; do not use preservative diluent as precipitation may occur.

Compatibility Stable in D_5W, NS, SWFI

Y-site administration: Compatible: Allopurinol, amifostine, aztreonam, cefepime, etoposide phosphate, fludarabine, gemcitabine, granisetron, melphalan, ondansetron, sargramostim, teniposide, thiotepa, vinorelbine. **Incompatible:** Filgrastim

Compatibility when admixed: Compatible: Dacarbazine

Pharmacodynamics/Kinetics

Distribution: High concentrations found in bone marrow and tumor cells, submaxillary gland, liver, and kidney; crosses placenta; poor CSF penetration

Metabolism: Hepatic, minimal

Half-life elimination: 36 hours

Time to peak, serum: I.V.: 2-5 minutes

Excretion: Bile (50%); feces (14%); urine (~10% as unchanged drug)

Dosage Refer to individual protocols: I.V.:

Note: Medication orders for dactinomycin are commonly written in MICROgrams (eg, 150 mcg) although many regimens list the dose in MILLIgrams (eg, mg/kg or mg/m². One-time doses for >1000 mcg, or multiple-day doses for >500 mcg/day are not common. Some practitioners recommend calculation of the dosage for obese or edematous patients on the basis of body surface area in an effort to relate dosage to lean body mass.

Children >6 months: 15 mcg/kg/day **or** 400-600 mcg/m²/day for 5 days every 3-6 weeks

Adults: 2.5 mg/m² in divided doses over 1 week, repeated every 2 weeks **or**

0.75-2 mg/m² every 1-4 weeks **or**

400-600 mcg/m²/day for 5 days, repeated every 3-6 weeks

Dosing in renal impairment: No adjustment necessary

Combination Regimens
  Gestational trophoblastic tumor:

Administration Avoid extravasation. Extremely damaging to soft tissue and will cause a severe local reaction if extravasation occurs. Administer slow I.V. push over 10-15 minutes. Do not give I.M. or SubQ

Dosage Forms Injection, powder for reconstitution: 0.5 mg [contains mannitol 20 mg]

Monitoring Parameters CBC with differential and platelet count, liver function tests, and renal function tests

Patient Information Limit oral intake for 4-6 hours before therapy. It is important to maintain adequate nutrition and hydration (2-3 L/day of fluids unless instructed to restrict fluid intake) during therapy; frequent small meals may help. You may experience nausea or vomiting (frequent small meals, frequent mouth care, sucking lozenges, or chewing gum may help). If this is ineffective, consult prescriber for antiemetic medication. You may experience loss of hair (reversible); you will be more susceptible to infection (avoid crowds and exposure to infection as much as possible); you will be more sensitive to sunlight; use sunblock, wear protective clothing and dark glasses, or avoid direct exposure to sunlight. Flu-like symptoms (eg, malaise, fever, myalgia) may occur 1 week after infusion and persist for 1-3 weeks; consult prescriber for severe symptoms. Report fever, chills, unusual bruising or bleeding, signs of infection, excessive fatigue, yellowing of eyes or skin, or change in color of urine or stool. Contraceptive measures are recommended during therapy.

Selected Readings
Berkowitz RS and Goldstein DP, "Gestational Trophoblastic Disease," *Cancer*, 1995, 76(10 Suppl):2079-85.
Blatt J, Trigg ME, Pizzo PA, et al, "Tolerance to Single-Dose Dactinomycin in Combination Chemotherapy for Solid Tumors," *Cancer Treat Rep*, 1981, 65(1-2):145-7.
Carli M, Pastore G, Perilongo G, et al, "Tumor Response and Toxicity After Single High-Dose Versus Standard Five-Day Divided Dose Dactinomycin in Childhood Rhabdomyosarcoma," *J Clin Oncol*, 1988, 6(4):654-8.
Horowitz ME, "Ewing's Sarcoma: Current Status of Diagnosis and Treatment," *Oncology*, 1989, 3(3):101-6.
Mehta MP, Bastin KT, and Wiersma SR, "Treatment of Wilms' Tumor. Current Recommendations," *Drugs*, 1991, 42(5):766-80.

♦ **DAD** *see* Mitoxantrone *on page 584*

♦ **Daunomycin** *see* DAUNOrubicin Hydrochloride *on page 250*

DAUNOrubicin Citrate (Liposomal)
(daw noe ROO bi sin SI trate lip po SOE mal)

Medication Safety Issues
Sound-alike/look-alike issues:

DAUNOrubicin may be confused with dactinomycin, DOXOrubicin

Liposomal formulations (DaunoXome®) may be confused with conventional formulations (Adriamycin PFS®, Adriamycin RDF®, Cerubidine®, Rubex®)

Related Information
Safe Handling of Hazardous Drugs *on page 1034*

U.S. Brand Names DaunoXome®

Generic Available No

Pharmacologic Category Antineoplastic Agent, Anthracycline

Pregnancy Risk Factor D

Lactation Excretion in breast milk unknown/not recommended

Use First-line cytotoxic therapy for advanced HIV-associated Kaposi's sarcoma

Mechanism of Action Liposomes have been shown to penetrate solid tumors more effectively, possibly because of their small size and longer circulation time. Once in tissues, daunorubicin is released. Daunorubicin inhibits DNA and RNA synthesis by intercalation between DNA base pairs and by steric obstruction; and intercalates at points of local uncoiling of the double helix. Although the exact mechanism is unclear, it appears that direct binding to DNA (intercalation) and inhibition of DNA repair (topoisomerase II inhibition) result in blockade of DNA and RNA synthesis and fragmentation of DNA.

Labeled Contraindications Hypersensitivity to daunorubicin or any component of the formulation; pregnancy

Warnings/Precautions Hazardous agent - use appropriate precautions for handling and disposal. See Safe Handling of Hazardous Drugs *on page 1034* in the Appendix. Daunorubicin is associated with a dose-related cardiac toxicity. The risk of similar toxicity with liposome-encapsulated daunorubicin is not certain. Use caution in patients with previous therapy with high cumulative doses of anthracyclines, cyclophosphamide, or thoracic radiation, or who have pre-existing cardiac disease.

Adverse Reactions
>10%:

Central nervous system: Fatigue (51%), headache (28%), neuropathy (13%)

Hematologic: Myelosuppression, neutropenia (51%), thrombocytopenia, anemia

Onset: 7 days

Nadir: 14 days

Recovery: 21 days

Gastrointestinal: Abdominal pain, vomiting, anorexia (23%); diarrhea (38%); nausea (55%)

Respiratory: Cough (28%), dyspnea (26%), rhinitis

Miscellaneous: Allergic reactions (24%)

1% to 10%:
  Cardiovascular: CHF (incidence unknown), hypertension, palpitation, syncope, tachycardia, chest pain, edema
  Dermatologic: Alopecia (8%), pruritus (7%)
  Endocrine & metabolic: Hot flashes
  Gastrointestinal: Constipation (7%), stomatitis (10%)
  Neuromuscular & skeletal: Arthralgia (7%), myalgia (7%)
  Ocular: Conjunctivitis, eye pain (5%)
  Respiratory: Sinusitis

Vesicant No; may be an irritant

Emetic Potential Moderate (30% to 60%)

Overdosage/Toxicology Symptoms of acute overdose are increased severity of the observed dose-limiting toxicities of therapeutic doses, myelosuppression (especially granulocytopenia), fatigue, nausea, and vomiting. Treatment is symptomatic.

Drug Interactions
  Decreased Effect: Patients may experience impaired immune response to vaccines; possible infection after administration of live vaccines in patients receiving immunosuppressants.

Storage/Stability Store in refrigerator 2°C to 8°C (37°F to 45°F); do not freeze. Protect from light.

Reconstitution Only fluid which may be mixed with DaunoXome® is D_5W. Must not be mixed with saline, bacteriostatic agents such as benzyl alcohol, or any other solution.

Compatibility Incompatible with sodium bicarbonate and fluorouracil, heparin, and dexamethasone.

Pharmacodynamics/Kinetics
  Distribution: V_d: 3-6.4 L
  Metabolism: Similar to daunorubicin, but metabolite plasma levels are low
  Half-life elimination: Distribution: 4.4 hours; Terminal: 3-5 hours
  Excretion: Primarily feces; some urine
    Clearance, plasma: 17.3 mL/minute

Dosage Refer to individual protocols. Adults: I.V.:
  20-40 mg/m² every 2 weeks
  100 mg/m² every 3 weeks
  Dosing adjustment in renal impairment: Serum creatinine >3 mg/dL: Administer 50% of normal dose
  Dosing adjustment in hepatic impairment:
    Bilirubin 1.2-3 mg/dL: Administer 75% of normal dose
    Bilirubin >3 mg/dL: Administer 50% of normal dose

Administration Infuse over 1 hour; do not mix with other drugs.

Dosage Forms Injection, solution [preservative free]: 2 mg/mL (25 mL) [contains sucrose 2125 mg/25 mL]

Monitoring Parameters Observe patient closely and monitor chemical and laboratory tests extensively. Evaluate cardiac, renal, and hepatic function. Repeat blood counts prior to each dose and withhold if the absolute granulocyte count is <750 cells/mm³. Monitor serum uric acid levels.

Selected Readings
Eckardt JR, Campbell E, Burris HA, et al, "A Phase II Trial of DaunoXome®, Liposome-Encapsulated Daunorubicin, in Patients With Metastatic Adenocarcinoma of the Colon," *Am J Clin Oncol*, 1994, 17(6):498-501.

Gill PS, Espina BM, Muggia F, et al, "Phase I/II Clinical and Pharmacokinetic Evaluation of Liposomal Daunorubicin," *J Clin Oncol*, 1995, 13(4):996-1003.

(Continued)

DAUNOrubicin Citrate (Liposomal) *(Continued)*

Gill PS, Wernz J, Scadden DT, et al, "Randomized Phase III Trial of Liposomal Daunoru-bicin Versus Doxorubicin, Bleomycin, and Vincristine in AIDS-Related Kaposi's Sarcoma," *J Clin Oncol*, 1996, 14(8):2353-64.

Guaglianone P, Chan K, Dela Flor-Weiss E, et al, "Phase I and Pharmacologic Study of Liposomal Daunorubicin (DaunoXome®)," *Invest New Drugs*, 1994, 12(2):103-10.

Schurmann D, Dormann A, Grunewald T, et al, "Successful Treatment of AIDS-Related Pulmonary Kaposi's Sarcoma With Liposomal Daunorubicin," *Eur Respir J*, 1994, 7(4):824-5.

DAUNOrubicin Hydrochloride

(daw noe ROO bi sin hye droe KLOR ide)

Medication Safety Issues

Sound-alike/look-alike issues:

DAUNOrubicin may be confused with dactinomycin, DOXOrubicin

Conventional formulations (Cerubidine®) may be confused with liposomal formulations (DaunoXome®, Doxil®)

Related Information

Safe Handling of Hazardous Drugs *on page 1034*

U.S. Brand Names Cerubidine®

Canadian Brand Names Cerubidine®

Generic Available Yes

Synonyms Daunomycin; DNR; NSC-82151; Rubidomycin Hydrochloride

Pharmacologic Category Antineoplastic Agent, Anthracycline

Pregnancy Risk Factor D

Lactation Excretion in breast milk unknown/not recommended

Use Treatment of acute lymphocytic (ALL) and nonlymphocytic (ANLL) leukemias

Mechanism of Action Inhibition of DNA and RNA synthesis by intercalation between DNA base pairs and by steric obstruction. Daunomycin intercalates at points of local uncoiling of the double helix. Although the exact mechanism is unclear, it appears that direct binding to DNA (inter-calation) and inhibition of DNA repair (topoisomerase II inhibition) result in blockade of DNA and RNA synthesis and fragmentation of DNA.

Labeled Contraindications Hypersensitivity to daunorubicin or any component of the formulation; congestive heart failure or arrhythmias; previous therapy with high cumulative doses of daunorubicin and/or doxorubicin; pre-existing bone marrow suppression; pregnancy

Warnings/Precautions Hazardous agent - use appropriate precautions for handling and disposal. See Safe Handling of Hazardous Drugs *on page 1034* in the Appendix. I.V. use only, severe local tissue necrosis will result if extravasation occurs. Reduce dose in patients with impaired hepatic, renal, or biliary function. Severe myelosuppression is possible when used in therapeutic doses. Total cumulative dose should take into account previous or concomitant treatment with cardiotoxic agents or irradiation of chest. Use with caution in patients with previous therapy with anthracyclines, cyclophosphamide, thoracic radiation, or pre-existing cardiac disease.

Irreversible myocardial toxicity may occur as total dosage approaches:

550 mg/m^2 in adults

400 mg/m^2 in patients receiving chest radiation

300 mg/m^2 in children >2 years of age

If daunorubicin contacts the skin, wash and flush thoroughly with water.

Adverse Reactions

>10%:

Cardiovascular: Transient ECG abnormalities (supraventricular tachycardia, S-T wave changes, atrial or ventricular extrasystoles); generally asymptomatic and self-limiting. CHF, dose related, may be delayed for 7-8 years after treatment. Cumulative dose, radiation therapy, age, and use of cyclophosphamide all increase the risk. Recommended maximum cumulative doses:

No risk factors: 550-600 mg/m^2

Concurrent radiation: 450 mg/m^2

Regardless of cumulative dose, if the left ventricular ejection fraction is <30% to 40%, the drug is usually not given

Dermatologic: Alopecia, radiation recall

Gastrointestinal: Mild nausea or vomiting, stomatitis

Genitourinary: Discoloration of urine (red)

Hematologic: Myelosuppression, primarily leukopenia; thrombocytopenia and anemia

Onset: 7 days

Nadir: 10-14 days

Recovery: 21-28 days

1% to 10%:

Dermatologic: Skin "flare" at injection site; discoloration of saliva, sweat, or tears

Endocrine & metabolic: Hyperuricemia

Gastrointestinal: GI ulceration, diarrhea

<1%: Systemic hypersensitivity (including urticaria, pruritus, angioedema, dysphagia, dyspnea), pericarditis, myocarditis, MI, skin rash, pigmentation of nail beds, nail banding, onycholysis, infertility, sterility, elevated bilirubin and transaminases, hepatitis

Vesicant Yes; see Management of Drug Extravasations *on page 965*.

Emetic Potential Moderate (30% to 60%)

Overdosage/Toxicology Symptoms of overdose include myelosuppression, nausea, vomiting, and stomatitis. There are no known antidotes. Treatment is symptomatic and supportive.

Drug Interactions

Decreased Effect: Patients may experience impaired immune response to vaccines; possible infection after administration of live vaccines in patients receiving immunosuppressants.

Ethanol/Nutrition/Herb Interactions Ethanol: Avoid ethanol (due to GI irritation).

Storage/Stability Store intact vials at room temperature and protect from light. Reconstituted solution is stable for 4 days at 15°C to 25°C. Further dilution in D_5W, LR, or NS is stable at room temperature (25°C) for up to 4 weeks if protected from light.

Reconstitution Dilute vials with 4 mL SWFI for a final concentration of 5 mg/mL.

Compatibility Incompatible with heparin, sodium bicarbonate, fluorouracil, and dexamethasone.

Stable in D_5W, LR, NS, sterile water for injection

(Continued)

DAUNOrubicin Hydrochloride *(Continued)*

Y-site administration: Compatible: Amifostine, etoposide phosphate, filgrastim, gemcitabine, granisetron, melphalan, methotrexate, ondansetron, sodium bicarbonate, teniposide, thiotepa, vinorelbine. **Incompatible:** Allopurinol, aztreonam, cefepime, fludarabine, piperacillin/tazobactam

Compatibility when admixed: Compatible: Cytarabine with etoposide, hydrocortisone sodium succinate. **Incompatible:** Dexamethasone sodium phosphate, heparin

Pharmacodynamics/Kinetics

Distribution: Many body tissues, particularly the liver, kidneys, lung, spleen, and heart; not into CNS; crosses placenta; V_d: 40 L/kg

Metabolism: Primarily hepatic to daunorubicinol (active), then to inactive aglycones, conjugated sulfates, and glucuronides

Half-life elimination: Distribution: 2 minutes; Elimination: 14-20 hours; Terminal: 18.5 hours; Daunorubicinol plasma half-life: 24-48 hours

Excretion: Feces (40%); urine (~25% as unchanged drug and metabolites)

Dosage I.V. (refer to individual protocols):

Children:

ALL combination therapy: Remission induction: 25-45 mg/m^2 on day 1 every week for 4 cycles **or** 30-45 mg/m^2/day for 3 days

AML combination therapy: Induction: I.V. continuous infusion: 30-60 mg/m^2/day on days 1-3 of cycle

Note: In children <2 years or <0.5 m^2, daunorubicin should be based on weight - mg/kg: 1 mg/kg per protocol with frequency dependent on regimen employed

Cumulative dose should not exceed 300 mg/m^2 in children >2 years; maximum cumulative doses for younger children are unknown.

Adults:

Range: 30-60 mg/m^2/day for 3-5 days, repeat dose in 3-4 weeks

AML: Single agent induction: 60 mg/m^2/day for 3 days; repeat every 3-4 weeks

AML: Combination therapy induction: 45 mg/m^2/day for 3 days of the first course of induction therapy; subsequent courses: Every day for 2 days

ALL combination therapy: 45 mg/m^2/day for 3 days

Cumulative dose should not exceed 600-800 mg/m^2

Dosing adjustment in renal impairment:

Cl_{cr} <10 mL/minute: Administer 75% of normal dose

S_{cr} >3 mg/dL: Administer 50% of normal dose

Dosing adjustment in hepatic impairment:

Serum bilirubin 1.2-3 mg/dL or AST 60-180 int. units: Reduce dose to 75%

Serum bilirubin 3.1-5 mg/dL or AST >180 int. units: Reduce dose to 50%

Serum bilirubin >5 mg/dL: Omit use

Combination Regimens

Leukemia, acute lymphocytic:

DVP *on page 875*

Larson Regimen *on page 904*

Linker Protocol *on page 904*

PVDA *on page 936*

Leukemia, acute myeloid:

5 + 2 *on page 840*
7 + 3 (Daunorubicin) *on page 840*
7 + 3 + 7 *on page 841*
DA *on page 871*
DAT *on page 872*
DAV *on page 872*
TAD *on page 938*
V-TAD *on page 949*

Administration Not for I.M. or SubQ administration. Administer IVP over 1-5 minutes into the tubing of a rapidly infusing I.V. solution of D_5W or NS; or diluted in 100 mL of D_5W or NS and infused over 15-30 minutes.

Dosage Forms

Injection, powder for reconstitution: 20 mg, 50 mg
Cerubidine®: 20 mg
Injection, solution: 5 mg/mL (4 mL, 10 mL)

Monitoring Parameters CBC with differential and platelet count, liver function test, ECG, ventricular ejection fraction, renal function test

Patient Information This medication can only be administered I.V. During therapy, do not use alcohol, aspirin-containing products, and/or OTC medications without consulting prescriber. It is important to maintain adequate nutrition and hydration (2-3 L/day of fluids unless instructed to restrict fluid intake) during therapy; frequent small meals may help. You may experience nausea or vomiting (frequent small meals, frequent mouth care, sucking lozenges, or chewing gum may help). You may experience loss of hair (reversible); you will be more susceptible to infection (avoid crowds and exposure to infection as much as possible). Urine may turn red (normal). Yogurt or buttermilk may help reduce diarrhea (if unresolved, contact prescriber). Report fever, chills, unusual bruising or bleeding, signs of infection, abdominal pain or blood in stools, excessive fatigue, yellowing of eyes or skin, swelling of extremities, difficulty breathing, or unresolved diarrhea. Contraceptive measures are recommended during therapy.

Selected Readings

Aubel-Sadron G and Londos-Gagliardi D, "Daunorubicin and Doxorubicin, Anthracycline Antibiotics, A Physicochemical and Biological Review," *Biochimie*, 1984, 66(5):333-52.

Davis HL and Davis TE, "Daunorubicin and Adriamycin in Cancer Treatment: An Analysis of Their Roles and Limitations," *Cancer Treat Rep*, 1979, 63(5):809-15.

Maral RJ and Jouanne M, "Toxicology of Daunorubicin in Animals and Man," *Cancer Treat Rep*, 1981, 65 Suppl 4:9-18.

Riggs CE Jr, "Clinical Pharmacology of Daunorubicin in Patients With Acute Leukemia," *Semin Oncol*, 1984, 11(4 Suppl 3):2-11.

Speth PA, Minderman H, and Haanen C, "Idarubicin v Daunorubicin: Preclinical and Clinical Pharmacokinetic Studies," *Semin Oncol*, 1989, 16(1 Suppl 2):2-9.

Weiss RB and Bruno S, "Daunorubicin Treatment of Adult Solid Tumors," *Cancer Treat Rep*, 1981, 65 Suppl 4:25-8.

♦ **DaunoXome®** *see* DAUNOrubicin Citrate (Liposomal) *on page 248*

♦ **DAVA** *see* Vindesine *on page 825*

♦ **dCF** *see* Pentostatin *on page 661*

♦ **DDAVP®** *see* Desmopressin *on page 259*

♦ **Deacetyl Vinblastine Carboxamide** *see* Vindesine *on page 825*

♦ **1-Deamino-8-D-Arginine Vasopressin** *see* Desmopressin *on page 259*

♦ **Decadron®** *see* Dexamethasone *on page 263*

♦ **Decadron® Phosphate [DSC]**   *see* Dexamethasone *on page 263*

Deferoxamine (de fer OKS a meen)

Medication Safety Issues
Sound-alike/look-alike issues:
Deferoxamine may be confused with cefuroxime
Desferal® may be confused with desflurane, Dexferrum®, Disophrol®

U.S. Brand Names Desferal®

Canadian Brand Names Desferal®; PMS-Deferoxamine

Generic Available Yes

Synonyms Deferoxamine Mesylate

Pharmacologic Category Antidote

Pregnancy Risk Factor C

Lactation Excretion in breast milk unknown/contraindicated

Use Acute iron intoxication when serum iron is >450-500 mcg/dL or when clinical signs of significant iron toxicity exist; chronic iron overload secondary to multiple transfusions; iron overload secondary to congenital anemias; hemochromatosis

Unlabeled/Investigational Use Removal of corneal rust rings following surgical removal of foreign bodies; diagnostic test for iron and aluminum overload
Investigational: Treatment of aluminum accumulation in renal failure; treatment of aluminum-induced bone disease

Mechanism of Action Complexes with trivalent ions (ferric ions) to form ferrioxamine, which are removed by the kidneys

Labeled Contraindications Hypersensitivity to deferoxamine or any component of the formulation; patients with anuria, primary hemochromatosis

Warnings/Precautions Use with caution in patients with severe renal disease, pyelonephritis. May increase susceptibility to *Yersinia enterocolitica*. Ocular and auditory disturbances, as well as growth retardation (children only), have been reported following prolonged administration. Has been associated with adult respiratory distress syndrome (ARDS) following excessively high-dose treatment of acute intoxication.

Adverse Reactions Frequency not defined.
Cardiovascular: Flushing, hypotension, tachycardia, shock, edema
Central nervous system: Convulsions, fever, dizziness, neuropathy, paresthesia, seizure, exacerbation of aluminum-related encephalopathy (dialysis), headache, CNS depression, coma, aphasia, agitation
Dermatologic: Erythema, urticaria, pruritus, rash, cutaneous wheal formation
Endocrine & metabolic: Hypocalcemia
Gastrointestinal: Abdominal discomfort, diarrhea, nausea
Genitourinary: Dysuria
Hematologic: Thrombocytopenia, leukopenia
Local: Pain and induration at injection site
Neuromuscular & skeletal: Leg cramps
Ocular: Blurred vision, visual loss, scotoma, visual field defects, impaired vision, optic neuritis, cataracts, retinal pigmentary abnormalities
Otic: Hearing loss, tinnitus
Renal: Renal impairment, acute renal failure
Respiratory: Acute respiratory distress syndrome (with dyspnea, cyanosis)

Miscellaneous: Anaphylaxis

Overdosage/Toxicology Symptoms of overdose include hypotension, blurring of vision, diarrhea, leg cramps, and tachycardia. Treatment is symptomatic and supportive.

Drug Interactions

Increased Effect/Toxicity: May cause loss of consciousness when administered with prochlorperazine. Concomitant treatment with vitamin C (>500 mg/day) has been associated with cardiac impairment.

Storage/Stability Protect from light.

Reconstitution Reconstituted solutions (sterile water) may be stored at room temperature for 7 days.

Compatibility Stable in D_5W, LR, NS, sterile water for injection

Pharmacodynamics/Kinetics

Absorption: Oral: <15%

Metabolism: Hepatic to ferrioxamine

Half-life elimination: Parent drug: 6.1 hours; Ferrioxamine: 5.8 hours

Excretion: Urine (as unchanged drug and metabolites)

Dosage

Children and Adults:

Acute iron toxicity: I.V. route is used when severe toxicity is evidenced by systemic symptoms (coma, shock, metabolic acidosis, or severe gastrointestinal bleeding) or potentially severe intoxications (serum iron level >500 mcg/dL). When severe symptoms are not present, the I.M. route may be preferred; however, the use of deferoxamine in situations where the serum iron concentration is <500 mcg/dL or when severe toxicity is not evident is a subject of some clinical debate.

Dose: For the first 1000 mg, infuse at 15 mg/kg/hour (although rates up to 40-50 mg/kg/hour have been given in patients with massive iron intoxication); may be followed by 500 mg every 4 hours for up to 2 doses; subsequent doses of 500 mg have been administered every 4-12 hours

Maximum recommended dose: 6 g/day (however, doses as high as 16-37 g have been administered)

Children:

Chronic iron overload: SubQ: 20-40 mg/kg/day over 8-12 hours (via a portable, controlled infusion device)

Aluminum-induced bone disease (unlabeled use): 20-40 mg/kg every hemodialysis treatment, frequency dependent on clinical status of the patient

Adults: Chronic iron overload:

I.M.: 500-1000 mg/day; in addition, 2000 mg should be given with each unit of blood transfused (administer separately from blood)

I.V.: 2 g after each unit of blood infusion at 15 mg/kg/hour

SubQ: 1-2 g every day over 8-24 hours

Dosing adjustment in renal impairment: Cl_{cr} <10 mL/minute: Administer 50% of dose

Has been used investigationally as a single 40 mg/kg I.V. dose over 2 hours, to promote mobilization of aluminum from tissue stores as an aid in the diagnosis of aluminum-associated osteodystrophy

Administration Administer I.M., slow SubQ, or I.V. infusion

(Continued)

Deferoxamine *(Continued)*

I.M.: I.M. administration is preferred in patients not in shock. Add 2 mL sterile water to 500 mg vial. For I.M. or SubQ administration, no further dilution is required.

I.V.: The manufacturer states that the I.M. route is preferred; however, the I.V. route is generally preferred in patients with severe toxicity (ie, patients in shock). Urticaria, hypotension, and shock have occurred following rapid I.V. administration; maximum I.V. rate: 15 mg/kg/hour for first 1000 mg; subsequent dosing, if needed, should not exceed 125 mg/hour

Dosage Forms Injection, powder for reconstitution, as mesylate: 500 mg, 2 g

Monitoring Parameters Serum iron, total iron-binding capacity; ophthalmologic exam (fundoscopy, slit-lamp exam) and audiometry with chronic therapy

Patient Information May turn urine pink; blood and urine tests are necessary to follow therapy

Selected Readings

Allain P, Mauras Y, Chaleil D, et al, "Pharmacokinetics and Renal Elimination of Desferrioxamine and Ferrioxamine in Healthy Subjects and Patients With Haemochromatosis," *Br J Clin Pharmacol*, 1987, 24(2):207-12.

Bentur Y, McGuigan M, and Koren G, "Deferoxamine (Desferrioxamine): New Toxicities for an Old Drug," *Drug Saf*, 1991, 6(1):37-46.

Cheney K, Gumbiner C, Benson B, et al, "Survival After a Severe Iron Poisoning Treated With Intermittent Infusions of Deferoxamine," *J Toxicol Clin Toxicol*, 1995, 33(1):61-6.

Cohen AR, Mizanin J, and Schwartz E, "Rapid Removal of Excessive Iron With Daily, High-Dose Intravenous Chelation Therapy," *J Pediatr*, 1989, 115(1):151-5.

Douglas D and Smilkstein M, "Deferoxamine-Iron Induced Pulmonary Injury and N-Acetylcysteine," *Clin Toxicol*, 1995, 33(5):495.

Fouad AA, Eldin NAS, and Eweda MH, "Protective Effects of Desferrioxamine on Cadmium Induced Testicular Toxicity in Rats," *Clin Toxicol*, 1995, 33(5):539-40.

Freedman MH, Olivieri N, Benson L, et al, "Clinical Studies on Iron Chelation in Patients With Thalassemia Major," *Haematologica*, 1990, 75(Suppl 5):74-83.

Giardina PJ, Grady RW, Ehlers KH, et al, "Current Therapy of Cooley's Anemia: A Decade of Experience With Subcutaneous Desferrioxamine," *Ann N Y Acad Sci*, 1990, 612:275-85.

Gomez HF, McClafferty H, Flory D, et al, "Prevention of GI Iron Absorption by an Orally Administered Deferoxamine/Charcoal Mixture," *Clin Toxicol*, 1995, 33(5):556.

Hershko C, Konijn AM, and Link G, "Iron Chelators for Thalassaemia," *Br J Haematol*, 1998, 101(3):399-406.

Jackson TW, Ling LJ, and Washington V, "The Effect of Oral Deferoxamine on Iron Absorption in Humans," *J Toxicol Clin Toxicol*, 1995, 33(4):325-9.

Kirking MH, "Treatment of Chronic Iron Overload," *Clin Pharm*, 1991, 10(10):775-83.

Krishnan K, Trobe JD, and Adams PT, "Myasthenia Gravis Following Iron Chelation Therapy With Intravenous Desferrioxamine," *Eur J Haematol*, 1995, 55(2):138-9.

Metwalley HE and Melies AE, "Protective Effects of Desferroxamine on Cadmium Induced Liver and Kidney Toxicity in Rats," *Clin Toxicol*, 1995, 33(5):541.

Pippard MJ, "Iron Metabolism and Iron Chelation in the Thalassemia Disorders," *Haematologica*, 1990, 75(Suppl 5):66-71.

Shannon M, "Desferrioxamine in Acute Iron Poisoning," *Lancet*, 1992, 339(8809):1601.

Voest EE, Vreugdenhil G, and Marx JJ, "Iron-Chelating Agents in Noniron Overload Conditions," *Ann Intern Med*, 1994, 120(6):490-9.

Winship KA, "Toxicity of Aluminum: A Historical Review, Part 2," *Adverse Drug React Toxicol Rev*, 1993, 12(3):177-211.

Yatscoff RW, Wayne EA, and Tenenbein M, "An Objective Criterion for the Cessation of Deferoxamine Therapy in the Acutely Iron Poisoned Patient," *J Toxicol Clin Toxicol*, 1991, 29(1):1-10.

♦ **Deferoxamine Mesylate** *see Deferoxamine on page 254*

♦ **Dehydrobenzperidol** *see Droperidol on page 294*

♦ **Delta-9-Tetrahydro-Cannabinol** *see Dronabinol on page 292*

♦ **Delta-9 THC** *see Dronabinol on page 292*

♦ **Deltacortisone** *see PredniSONE on page 683*

♦ **Deltadehydrocortisone** *see PredniSONE on page 683*

♦ **Deltahydrocortisone** *see PrednisoLONE on page 679*

♦ **Demerol®** *see Meperidine on page 535*

♦ **4-Demethoxydaunorubicin** *see Idarubicin on page 443*

Denileukin Diftitox (de ni LOO kin DIF ti toks)

Related Information
  Safe Handling of Hazardous Drugs *on page 1034*
U.S. Brand Names ONTAK®
Generic Available No
Pharmacologic Category Antineoplastic Agent, Miscellaneous
Pregnancy Risk Factor C
Lactation Excretion in breast milk unknown/contraindicated
Use Treatment of persistent or recurrent cutaneous T-cell lymphoma whose malignant cells express the CD25 component of the IL-2 receptor
Mechanism of Action Denileukin diftitox is a fusion protein (a combination of amino acid sequences from diphtheria toxin and interleukin-2) which selectively delivers the cytotoxic activity of diphtheria toxin to targeted cells. It interacts with the high-affinity IL-2 receptor on the surface of malignant cells to inhibit intracellular protein synthesis, rapidly leading to cell death.
Labeled Contraindications Hypersensitivity to denileukin diftitox, diphtheria toxin, interleukin-2, or any component of the formulation
Warnings/Precautions Hazardous agent - use appropriate precautions for handling and disposal. See Safe Handling of Hazardous Drugs *on page 1034* in the Appendix. Acute hypersensitivity reactions, including anaphylaxis, may occur; most events occur during or within 24 hours of the first dose of a treatment cycle. Has been associated with a delayed-onset vascular leak syndrome, which may be severe. Denileukin diftitox may impair immune function. Use with caution in patients with pre-existing cardiovascular disease and in patients >65 years of age.
Adverse Reactions
  The following list of symptoms reported during treatment includes all levels of severity:
  >10%:
  Cardiovascular: Edema (47%; Grade 3 and 4, 15%), hypotension (36%), chest pain (24%), vasodilation (22%), tachycardia (12%)
  Central nervous system: Fever/chills (81%; Grade 3 and 4, 22%), headache (26%), pain (48%; Grade 3 and 4, 13%), dizziness (22%), nervousness (11%)
  Dermatologic: Rash (34%; Grade 3 and 4, 13%), pruritus (20%)
  Endocrine & metabolic: Hypoalbuminemia (83%; Grade 3 and 4, 14%), hypocalcemia (17%), weight loss (14%)
  Gastrointestinal: Nausea/vomiting (64%; Grade 3 and 4, 14%), anorexia (36%), diarrhea (29%)
  Hematologic: Decreased lymphocyte count (34%), anemia (18%)
  Hepatic: Transaminases increased (61%; Grade 3 and 4, 15%)
  Neuromuscular & skeletal: Asthenia (66%; Grade 3 and 4, 22%), myalgia (17%), paresthesia (13%)
(Continued)

Denileukin Diftitox *(Continued)*

Respiratory: Dyspnea (29%; Grade 3 and 4, 14%), increased cough (26%), pharyngitis (17%), rhinitis (13%)

Miscellaneous: Flu-like syndrome (91%; beginning several hours to days following infusion), hypersensitivity (69%; reactions are variable, but may include hypotension, back pain, dyspnea, vasodilation, rash, chest pain, tachycardia, dysphagia, syncope, or anaphylaxis), infection (48%; Grade 3 and 4, 24%), vascular leak syndrome (27%; characterized by hypotension, edema, or hypoalbuminemia; the syndrome usually developed within the first 2 weeks of infusion; 6% of patients who developed this syndrome required hospitalization; the symptoms may persist or even worsen despite cessation of denileukin diftitox)

1% to 10%:

Cardiovascular: Hypertension (6%), arrhythmia (6%), MI (1%)

Central nervous system: Insomnia (9%), confusion (8%)

Endocrine & metabolic: Dehydration (9%), hypokalemia (6%), hyperthyroidism (<5%), hypothyroidism (<5%)

Gastrointestinal: Constipation (9%), dyspepsia (7%), dysphagia (6%), pancreatitis (<5%)

Hematologic: Thrombotic events (7%), thrombocytopenia (8%), leukopenia (6%)

Local: Injection site reaction (8%), anaphylaxis (1%)

Neuromuscular & skeletal: Arthralgia (8%)

Renal: Hematuria (10%), albuminuria (10%), pyuria (10%), creatinine increased (7%), acute renal insufficiency (<5%)

Respiratory: Lung disorder (8%)

Miscellaneous: Anaphylaxis (1%), decreased diaphoresis (10%)

Vesicant No

Emetic Potential High (60% to 90%)

Overdosage/Toxicology Although there is no human experience in overdose, dose-limiting toxicities include nausea, vomiting, fever, chills and persistent asthenia. Treatment is supportive and symptom-directed. Fluid balance, as well as hepatic and renal function, should be closely monitored.

Storage/Stability Store frozen at or -10°C; cannot be refrozen. Solutions ≥15 mcg/mL in NS should be used within 6 hours. DO NOT use glass syringes or containers.

Reconstitution Must be brought to room temperature (25°C or 77°F) before preparing the dose. Do **not** heat vials. Thaw in refrigerator for not more than 24 hours or at room temperature for 1-2 hours. Avoid vigorous agitation. Solution may be mixed by gentle swirling. Dilute with NS to a concentration of ≥15 mcg/mL.

Compatibility Do **not** use glass syringes or containers.

Pharmacodynamics/Kinetics

Distribution: V_d: 0.06-0.08 L/kg

Metabolism: Hepatic via proteolytic degradation (animal studies)

Half-life elimination: Distribution: 2-5 minutes; Terminal: 70-80 minutes

Dosage Adults: I.V.: 9 or 18 mcg/kg/day days 1 through 5 every 21 days.

Administration For I.V. use only. Should be infused over at least 15 minutes. Should not be given as an I.V. bolus.

Dosage Forms Injection, solution [frozen]: 150 mcg/mL (2 mL)

Monitoring Parameters CBC, blood chemistry panel, renal and hepatic function tests as well as a serum albumin level; these tests should be repeated at weekly intervals during therapy. During the infusion, the patient should be monitored for symptoms of an acute hypersensitivity reaction. After infusion, the patient should be monitored for the development of a delayed vascular leak syndrome (usually in the first 2 weeks), including careful monitoring of weight, blood pressure, and serum albumin.

Additional Information Formulation includes EDTA and polysorbate 20, and has a pH of 6.9-7.2.

Selected Readings

Duvic M, "Bexarotene and DAB(389)IL-2 (denileukin diftitox, ONTAK) in Treatment of Cutaneous T-cell Lymphomas: Algorithms," *Clin Lymphoma*, 2000, 1(Suppl 1):51-5.

Figgitt DP, Lamb HM, and Goa KL "Denileukin Diftitox," *Am J Clin Dermatol*, 2000, 1(1):67-72.

Foss FM, "DAB(389)IL-2 (denileukin diftitox, ONTAK): A New Fusion Protein Technology," *Clin Lymphoma*, 2000, 1(Suppl 1):27-31.

Kuzel TM, "DAB(389)IL-2 (denileukin diftitox, ONTAK): Review of Clinical Trials to Date," *Clin Lymphoma*, 2000, 1(Suppl 1):33-6.

LeMaistre CF, "DAB(389)IL-2 (denileukin diftitox, ONTAK): Other Potential Applications," *Clin Lymphoma*, 2000, 1(Suppl 1):37-40.

Nichols J, Foss F, Kuzel TM, et al, "Interleukin-2 Fusion Protein: An Investigational Therapy for Interleukin-2 Receptor Expressing Malignancies, *Eur J Cancer*, 1997, 33(Suppl 1):34-6.

- **Deoxycoformycin** *see Pentostatin on page 661*
- **2'-Deoxycoformycin** *see Pentostatin on page 661*
- **DepoCyt™** *see Cytarabine (Liposomal) on page 234*
- **DepoDur™** *see Morphine Sulfate on page 588*
- **Depo-Medrol®** *see MethylPREDNISolone on page 558*
- **Depo-Prevera® (Can)** *see MedroxyPROGESTERone on page 524*
- **Depo-Provera®** *see MedroxyPROGESTERone on page 524*
- **Depo-Provera® Contraceptive** *see MedroxyPROGESTERone on page 524*
- **depo-subQ provera 104™** *see MedroxyPROGESTERone on page 524*
- **Dermarest Dricort® [OTC]** *see Hydrocortisone on page 419*
- **Dermtex® HC [OTC]** *see Hydrocortisone on page 419*
- **Desacetyl Vinblastine Amide Sulfate** *see Vindesine on page 825*
- **Desferal®** *see Deferoxamine on page 254*

Desmopressin (des moe PRES in)

U.S. Brand Names DDAVP®; Stimate™

Canadian Brand Names Apo-Desmopressin®; DDAVP®; Minirin®; Octostim®

Generic Available Yes: Excludes tablet

Synonyms 1-Deamino-8-D-Arginine Vasopressin; Desmopressin Acetate

Pharmacologic Category Antihemophilic Agent; Hemostatic Agent; Vasopressin Analog, Synthetic

Pregnancy Risk Factor B

Lactation Excretion in breast milk unknown/use caution

Use Treatment of diabetes insipidus; control of bleeding in hemophilia A, and mild-to-moderate classic von Willebrand disease (type I); primary nocturnal enuresis

(Continued)

Desmopressin *(Continued)*

Mechanism of Action Enhances reabsorption of water in the kidneys by increasing cellular permeability of the collecting ducts; possibly causes smooth muscle constriction with resultant vasoconstriction; raises plasma levels of von Willebrand factor and factor VIII

Labeled Contraindications Hypersensitivity to desmopressin or any component of the formulation; hemophilia B, severe classic von Willebrand disease (type IIB); patients with ≤5% factor VIII activity level; factor VIII antibodies

Warnings/Precautions Fluid intake should be adjusted downward in the elderly and very young patients to decrease the possibility of water intoxication and hyponatremia. Avoid overhydration especially when drug is used for its hemostatic effect. Use caution with cystic fibrosis or other conditions associated with fluid and electrolyte imbalance due to potential hyponatremia. Use caution with coronary artery insufficiency or hypertensive cardiovascular disease; may increase or decrease blood pressure leading to changes in heart rate. Consider switching from nasal to intravenous solution if changes in the nasal mucosa (scarring, edema) occur leading to unreliable absorption. Use caution in patients predisposed to thrombus formation; thrombotic events (acute cerebrovascular thrombosis, acute myocardial infarction) have occurred (rare). Use may rarely lead to extreme decreases in plasma osmolality, resulting in seizures and coma.

Adverse Reactions Frequency not defined (may be dose or route related).

  Cardiovascular: Acute cerebrovascular thrombosis, acute MI, blood pressure increased/decreased, chest pain, edema, facial flushing, palpitation

  Central nervous system: Agitation, chills, coma, dizziness, headache, insomnia, somnolence

  Endocrine & metabolic: Hyponatremia, water intoxication

  Gastrointestinal: Abdominal cramps, dyspepsia, nausea, sore throat, vomiting

  Genitourinary: Balanitis, vulval pain

  Local: Injection: Burning pain, erythema, and swelling at the injection site

  Respiratory: Cough, nasal congestion, epistaxis

  Miscellaneous: Allergic reactions (rare), anaphylaxis (rare)

Vesicant No

Emetic Potential Very low (<10%)

Overdosage/Toxicology Symptoms of overdose include drowsiness, headache, confusion, anuria, and water intoxication. In case of overdose, decrease or discontinue desmopressin.

Drug Interactions

  Increased Effect/Toxicity: Chlorpropamide, fludrocortisone may increase ADH response.

  Decreased Effect: Demeclocycline and lithium may decrease ADH response.

Ethanol/Nutrition/Herb Interactions Ethanol: Avoid ethanol (may decrease antidiuretic effect).

Storage/Stability

DDAVP®:

Tablet, nasal spray: Store at controlled room temperature of 20°C to 25°C (68°F to 77°F). Keep nasal spray in upright position.

Rhinal tube: Store refrigerated at 2°C to 8°C (36°F to 46°F). May store at room temperature for up to 3 weeks.

Injection: Store refrigerated at 2°C to 8°C (36°F to 46°F).

Stimate™: Store refrigerated at 2°C to 8°C (36°F to 46°F). May store at room temperature for up to 3 weeks.

Reconstitution Dilute in 10-50 mL NS for I.V. infusion (10 mL for children ≤10 kg; 50 mL for adults and children >10 kg)

Compatibility Compatible: Stable in NS

Pharmacodynamics/Kinetics

Intranasal administration: Onset of increased factor VIII activity: 30 minutes (dose related)

Peak effect 1.5 hours

I.V. infusion:

Onset of increased factor VIII activity: 30 minutes (dose related)

Peak effect: 1.5-2 hours

Half-life elimination: Terminal: 75 minutes

Oral tablets:

Onset of action: ADH: ~1 hour

Peak effect: 4-7 hours

Half-life elimination: 1.5-2.5 hours

Bioavailability: 5% compared to intranasal; 0.16% compared to I.V.

Dosage

Children:

Diabetes insipidus:

Intranasal (using 100 mcg/mL nasal solution): 3 months to 12 years: Initial: 5 mcg/day (0.05 mL/day) divided 1-2 times/day; range: 5-30 mcg/day (0.05-0.3 mL/day) divided 1-2 times/day; adjust morning and evening doses separately for an adequate diurnal rhythm of water turnover; doses <10 mcg should be administered using the rhinal tube system

Oral: ≥4 years: Initial: 0.05 mg twice daily; total daily dose should be increased or decreased as needed to obtain adequate antidiuresis (range: 0.1-1.2 mg divided 2-3 times/day)

Hemophilia A and von Willebrand disease (type I):

I.V.: >3 months: 0.3 mcg/kg by slow infusion; may repeat dose if needed; begin 30 minutes before procedure

Intranasal: ≥11 months: Refer to adult dosing.

Nocturnal enuresis:

Intranasal (using 100 mcg/mL nasal solution): ≥6 years: Initial: 20 mcg (0.2 mL) at bedtime; range: 10-40 mcg; it is recommended that ¹/₂ of the dose be given in each nostril

Oral: 0.2 mg at bedtime; dose may be titrated up to 0.6 mg to achieve desired response. Patients previously on intranasal therapy can begin oral tablets 24 hours after the last intranasal dose.

Children ≥12 years and Adults:

Diabetes insipidus:

I.V., SubQ: 2-4 mcg/day (0.5-1 mL) in 2 divided doses or ¹/₁₀ of the maintenance intranasal dose

(Continued)

Desmopressin *(Continued)*

Intranasal (using 100 mcg/mL nasal solution): 10-40 mcg/day (0.1-0.4 mL) divided 1-3 times/day; adjust morning and evening doses separately for an adequate diurnal rhythm of water turnover. **Note:** The nasal spray pump can only deliver doses of 10 mcg (0.1 mL) or multiples of 10 mcg (0.1 mL); if doses other than this are needed, the rhinal tube delivery system is preferred.

Oral: Initial: 0.05 mg twice daily; total daily dose should be increased or decreased as needed to obtain adequate antidiuresis (range: 0.1-1.2 mg divided 2-3 times/day)

Hemophilia A and mild to moderate von Willebrand disease (type I):

I.V.: 0.3 mcg/kg by slow infusion, begin 30 minutes before procedure

Intranasal: Using high concentration spray (1.5 mg/mL): <50 kg: 150 mcg (1 spray); >50 kg: 300 mcg (1 spray each nostril); repeat use is determined by the patient's clinical condition and laboratory work; if using preoperatively, administer 2 hours before surgery

Administration

I.V.: Infuse over 15-30 minutes

Intranasal: DDAVP®: Nasal pump spray delivers 0.1 mL (10 mcg); for other doses which are not multiples, use rhinal tube. DDAVP® Nasal spray delivers fifty 10 mcg doses. Any solution remaining after 50 doses should be discarded. Pump must be primed prior to first use.

Dosage Forms

Injection, solution, as acetate (DDAVP®): 4 mcg/mL (1 mL, 10 mL)

Solution, intranasal, as acetate (DDAVP®): 100 mcg/mL (2.5 mL) [with rhinal tube]

Solution, intranasal spray, as acetate: 100 mcg/mL (5 mL) [delivers 10 mcg/spray]

DDAVP®: 100 mcg/mL (5 mL) [delivers 10 mcg/spray]

Stimate™: 1.5 mg/mL (2.5 mL) [delivers 150 mcg/spray]

Tablet, as acetate (DDAVP®): 0.1 mg, 0.2 mg

Monitoring Parameters Blood pressure and pulse should be monitored during I.V. infusion

Diabetes insipidus: Fluid intake, urine volume, specific gravity, plasma and urine osmolality, serum electrolytes

Hemophilia: Factor VIII antigen levels, aPTT, bleeding time (for von Willebrand disease and thrombocytopathies)

Patient Information Avoid overhydration. Report headache, shortness of breath, heartburn, nausea, abdominal cramps, or vulval pain.

Additional Information 10 mcg of desmopressin acetate is equivalent to 40 int. units

Special Geriatric Considerations Elderly patients should be cautioned not to increase their fluid intake beyond that sufficient to satisfy their thirst in order to avoid water intoxication and hyponatremia.

Selected Readings

Cattaneo M, "Review of Clinical Experience of Desmopressin in Patients With Congenital and Acquired Bleeding Disorder," *Eur J Anesthesiol Suppl*, 1997, 14:10-4.

Chistolini A, Dragoni F, Ferrari A, et al, "Intranasal DDAVP®: Biological and Clinical Evaluation in Mild Factor VIII Deficiency," *Haemostasis*, 1991, 21(5):273-7.

Lindeman RD, Lee TD Jr, Yiengst MJ, et al, "Influence of Age, Renal Disease, Hypertension, Diuretics, and Calcium on the Antidiuretic Responses to Suboptimal Infusions of Vasopressin," *J Lab Clin Med*, 1966, 68(2):206-23.

Lusher JM, "Response to 1-Deamino-8-D-Arginine Vasopressin in von Willebrand Disease," *Haemostasis*, 1994, 24(5):276-84.

Mannucci PM and Cattaneo M, "Desmopressin: A Nontransfusional Treatment of Hemophilia and von Willebrand Disease," *Haemostasis*, 1992, 22(5)276-80.

Richardson DW and Robinson AG, "Desmopressin," *Ann Intern Med*, 1985, 103(2):228-39.

♦ **Desmopressin Acetate** *see* Desmopressin *on page 259*

Dexamethasone (deks a METH a sone)

Medication Safety Issues

Sound-alike/look-alike issues:

Dexamethasone may be confused with desoximetasone

Decadron® may be confused with Percodan®

Maxidex® may be confused with Maxzide®

Related Information

Management of Nausea and Vomiting *on page 982*

U.S. Brand Names Decadron®; Decadron® Phosphate [DSC]; Dexamethasone Intensol®; DexPak® TaperPak®; Maxidex®

Canadian Brand Names Decadron®; Dexasone®; Diodex®; Maxidex®; PMS-Dexamethasone

Generic Available Yes

Synonyms Dexamethasone Sodium Phosphate

Pharmacologic Category Antiemetic; Anti-inflammatory Agent; Anti-inflammatory Agent, Ophthalmic; Corticosteroid, Ophthalmic; Corticosteroid, Systemic; Corticosteroid, Topical

Pregnancy Risk Factor C

Lactation Excretion in breast milk unknown

Use Systemically and locally for chronic swelling; allergic, hematologic, neoplastic, and autoimmune diseases; may be used in management of cerebral edema, septic shock, as a diagnostic agent, antiemetic

Unlabeled/Investigational Use General indicator consistent with depression; diagnosis of Cushing's syndrome

Mechanism of Action Decreases inflammation by suppression of neutrophil migration, decreased production of inflammatory mediators, and reversal of increased capillary permeability; suppresses normal immune response. Dexamethasone's mechanism of antiemetic activity is unknown.

Labeled Contraindications Hypersensitivity to dexamethasone or any component of the formulation; active untreated infections; ophthalmic use in viral, fungal, or tuberculosis diseases of the eye

Warnings/Precautions Use with caution in patients with hypothyroidism, cirrhosis, hypertension, CHF, ulcerative colitis, or thromboembolic disorders. Corticosteroids should be used with caution in patients with diabetes, osteoporosis, peptic ulcer, glaucoma, cataracts, or tuberculosis. Use caution following acute MI (corticosteroids have been associated with myocardial rupture). Use caution in hepatic impairment. Because of the risk of adverse effects, systemic corticosteroids should be used cautiously in the elderly in the smallest possible effective dose for the shortest duration.

May cause suppression of hypothalamic-pituitary-adrenal (HPA) axis, particularly in younger children or in patients receiving high doses for prolonged periods. Symptoms of adrenocortical insufficiency in suppressed patients may result from rapid discontinuation/withdrawal; deficits in HPA response may persist for months following discontinuation and require supplementation during metabolic stress. Patients receiving 20 mg/day of prednisone (or equivalent) may be most susceptible. (Continued)

Dexamethasone *(Continued)*

Particular care is required when patients are transferred from systemic corticosteroids to inhaled products due to possible adrenal insufficiency or exacerbation of underlying disease, including an increase in allergic symptoms. Fatalities have occurred due to adrenal insufficiency in asthmatic patients during and after transfer from systemic corticosteroids to aerosol steroids; aerosol steroids do **not** provide the systemic steroid needed to treat patients having trauma, surgery, or infections. Dexamethasone does not provide adequate mineralocorticoid activity in adrenal insufficiency (may be employed as a single dose while cortisol assays are performed).

To minimize the systemic effects of orally-inhaled and intranasal corticosteroids, each patient should be titrated to the lowest effective dose.

May suppress the immune system; patients may be more susceptible to infection. Use with caution in patients with systemic infections or ocular herpes simplex. Avoid exposure to chickenpox and measles.

Adverse Reactions Frequency not defined.

Cardiovascular: Edema, hypertension, arrhythmia, cardiomyopathy, myocardial rupture (post-MI), syncope, thromboembolism, thrombophlebitis, vasculitis

Central nervous system: Insomnia, nervousness, vertigo, seizure, psychosis, pseudotumor cerebri (usually following discontinuation), headache, mood swings, delirium, hallucinations, euphoria

Dermatologic: Hirsutism, acne, skin atrophy, bruising, hyperpigmentation, pruritus (generalized), perianal pruritus (following I.V. injection), urticaria

Endocrine & metabolic: Diabetes mellitus, adrenal suppression, hyperlipidemia, Cushing's syndrome, pituitary-adrenal axis suppression, growth suppression, glucose intolerance, gynecomastia, hypokalemia, alkalosis, amenorrhea, sodium and water retention, hyperglycemia, hypercalciuria, weight gain

Gastrointestinal: Appetite increased, indigestion, peptic ulcer, nausea, vomiting, abdominal distention, ulcerative esophagitis, pancreatitis, intestinal perforation

Genitourinary: Altered (increased or decreased) spermatogenesis

Hematologic: Transient leukocytosis

Hepatic: Transaminases increased, hepatomegaly

Neuromuscular & skeletal: Arthralgia, muscle weakness, osteoporosis, fractures, myopathy (particularly in conjunction with neuromuscular disease or neuromuscular blocking agents), tendon rupture, vertebral compression fractures, neuropathy, neuritis, parasthesia

Ocular: Cataracts, glaucoma, exophthalmos, intraocular pressure increased

Miscellaneous: Infections, anaphylactoid reaction, anaphylaxis, angioedema, avascular necrosis, secondary malignancy, Kaposi's sarcoma, intractable hiccups, impaired wound healing, abnormal fat deposition, moon face

Topical: <1%: Itching, dryness, folliculitis, hypertrichosis, acneiform eruptions, hypopigmentation, perioral dermatitis, allergic contact dermatitis, skin maceration, skin atrophy, striae, miliaria, local burning, irritation. secondary infection

Vesicant No

Emetic Potential Very low (<10%); may cause nausea/indigestion if taken orally on an empty stomach

Overdosage/Toxicology When consumed in high doses over prolonged periods, systemic hypercorticism and adrenal suppression may occur. In these cases, discontinuation of the corticosteroid should be done judiciously.

Drug Interactions

Cytochrome P450 Effect: Substrate of CYP3A4 (minor); **Induces** CYP2A6 (weak), 2B6 (weak), 2C8/9 (weak), 3A4 (weak)

Increased Effect/Toxicity: Aprepitant, azole antifungals, calcium channel blockers (nondihydropyridine), cyclosporine, and estrogens may increase the serum levels of corticosteroids. Antacids may increase the absorption of corticosteroids, separate administration by 2 hours. Corticosteroids may increase the serum levels of cyclosporine.

Concurrent use of nonsteroidal anti-inflammatory drugs (NSAIDs) and salicylates with corticosteroids may lead to an increased incidence of gastrointestinal adverse effects. Concurrent use with anticholinergic agents may lead to severe weakness in patients with myasthenia gravis. Concurrent use of fluoroquinolone antibiotics may increase the risk of tendon rupture, particularly in elderly patients (overall incidence rare). Concurrent use of neuromuscular blocking agents with corticosteroids may increase the risk of myopathy. The concurrent use of thalidomide with corticosteroids may increase the risk of selected adverse effects (toxic epidermal necrolysis and DVT).

Decreased Effect: Bile acid sequestrants may reduce the absorption of corticosteroids; separate administration by 2 hours. Aminoglutethimide may reduce the serum levels/effects of dexamethasone.

Serum concentrations of isoniazid and phenytoin may be decreased by corticosteroids. Corticosteroids may lead to a reduction in warfarin effect. Corticosteroids may suppress the response to vaccinations. The use of live vaccines is contraindicated in immunosuppressed patients. In patients receiving high doses of systemic corticosteroids for ≥14 days, wait at least 1 month between discontinuing steroid therapy and administering immunization.

Ethanol/Nutrition/Herb Interactions

Ethanol: Avoid ethanol (may enhance gastric mucosal irritation).

Food: Dexamethasone interferes with calcium absorption. Limit caffeine.

Herb/Nutraceutical: Avoid cat's claw, echinacea (have immunostimulant properties).

Storage/Stability Injection solution: Store at room temperature; protect from light and freezing.

Stability of injection of parenteral admixture at room temperature (25°C): 24 hours

Stability of injection of parenteral admixture at refrigeration temperature (4°C): 2 days; protect from light and freezing

Reconstitution Injection should be diluted in 50-100 mL NS or D_5W.

Compatibility Stable in D_5W, NS

Y-site administration: Compatible: Acyclovir, allopurinol, amifostine, amikacin, amphotericin B cholesteryl sulfate complex, amsacrine, aztreonam, cefepime, cefpirome, cisatracurium, cisplatin, cladribine, cyclophosphamide, cytarabine, docetaxel, doxorubicin, doxorubicin liposome, etoposide phosphate, famotidine, filgrastim, fluconazole, (Continued)

Dexamethasone *(Continued)*

fludarabine, foscarnet, gatifloxacin, gemcitabine, granisetron, heparin, heparin with hydrocortisone sodium succinate, levofloxacin, linezolid, lorazepam, melphalan, meperidine, meropenem, morphine, ondansetron, paclitaxel, piperacillin/tazobactam, potassium chloride, propofol, remifentanil, sargramostim, sodium bicarbonate, sufentanil, tacrolimus, teniposide, theophylline, thiotepa, vinorelbine, vitamin B complex with C, zidovudine. **Incompatible:** Ciprofloxacin, idarubicin, midazolam, topotecan. **Variable (consult detailed reference):** Methotrexate

Compatibility in syringe: Compatible: Granisetron, metoclopramide, ranitidine, sufentanil. **Incompatible:** Doxapram, glycopyrrolate. **Variable (consult detailed reference):** Diphenhydramine, hydromorphone, ondansetron

Compatibility when admixed: Compatible: Aminophylline, bleomycin, cimetidine, floxacillin, furosemide, granisetron, lidocaine, meropenem, mitomycin, nafcillin, netilmicin, ondansetron, prochlorperazine edisylate, ranitidine, verapamil. **Incompatible:** Daunorubicin, diphenhydramine with lorazepam and metoclopramide, metaraminol, vancomycin. **Variable (consult detailed reference):** Amikacin

Pharmacodynamics/Kinetics

Onset of action: Acetate: Prompt

Duration of metabolic effect: 72 hours; acetate is a long-acting repository preparation

Metabolism: Hepatic

Half-life elimination: Normal renal function: 1.8-3.5 hours; Biological half-life: 36-54 hours

Time to peak, serum: Oral: 1-2 hours; I.M.: ~8 hours

Excretion: Urine and feces

Dosage

Children:

Antiemetic (prior to chemotherapy): I.V. (should be given as sodium phosphate): 5-20 mg given 15-30 minutes before treatment

Anti-inflammatory immunosuppressant: Oral, I.M., I.V. (injections should be given as sodium phosphate): 0.08-0.3 mg/kg/day **or** 2.5-10 mg/m^2/day in divided doses every 6-12 hours

Extubation or airway edema: Oral, I.M., I.V. (injections should be given as sodium phosphate): 0.5-2 mg/kg/day in divided doses every 6 hours beginning 24 hours prior to extubation and continuing for 4-6 doses afterwards

Cerebral edema: I.V. (should be given as sodium phosphate): Loading dose: 1-2 mg/kg/dose as a single dose; maintenance: 1-1.5 mg/kg/day (maximum: 16 mg/day) in divided doses every 4-6 hours for 5 days then taper for 5 days, then discontinue

Bacterial meningitis in infants and children >2 months: I.V. (should be given as sodium phosphate): 0.6 mg/kg/day in 4 divided doses every 6 hours for the first 4 days of antibiotic treatment; start dexamethasone at the time of the first dose of antibiotic

Physiologic replacement: Oral, I.M., I.V.: 0.03-0.15 mg/kg/day **or** 0.6-0.75 mg/m^2/day in divided doses every 6-12 hours

Adults:

Antiemetic:

Prophylaxis: Oral, I.V.: 10-20 mg 15-30 minutes before treatment on each treatment day

Continuous infusion regimen: Oral or I.V.: 10 mg every 12 hours on each treatment day

Mildly emetogenic therapy: Oral, I.M., I.V.: 4 mg every 4-6 hours

Delayed nausea/vomiting: Oral: 4-10 mg 1-2 times/day for 2-4 days **or**

8 mg every 12 hours for 2 days; then

4 mg every 12 hours for 2 days **or**

20 mg 1 hour before chemotherapy; then

10 mg 12 hours after chemotherapy; then

8 mg every 12 hours for 4 doses; then

4 mg every 12 hours for 4 doses

Anti-inflammatory:

Oral, I.M., I.V. (injections should be given as sodium phosphate): 0.75-9 mg/day in divided doses every 6-12 hours

Intra-articular, intralesional, or soft tissue (as sodium phosphate): 0.4-6 mg/day

Ophthalmic:

Ointment: Apply thin coating into conjunctival sac 3-4 times/day; gradually taper dose to discontinue

Suspension: Instill 2 drops into conjunctival sac every hour during the day and every other hour during the night; gradually reduce dose to every 3-4 hours, then to 3-4 times/day

Topical: Apply 1-4 times/day. Therapy should be discontinued when control is achieved; if no improvement is seen, reassessment of diagnosis may be necessary.

Chemotherapy: Oral, I.V.: 40 mg every day for 4 days, repeated every 4 weeks (VAD regimen)

Cerebral edema: I.V. 10 mg stat, 4 mg I.M./I.V. (should be given as sodium phosphate) every 6 hours until response is maximized, then switch to oral regimen, then taper off if appropriate; dosage may be reduced after 24 days and gradually discontinued over 5-7 days

Dexamethasone suppression test (depression indicator) (unlabeled use): Oral: 1 mg at 11 PM, draw blood at 8 AM the following day for plasma cortisol determination

Cushing's syndrome, diagnostic: Oral: 1 mg at 11 PM, draw blood at 8 AM; greater accuracy for Cushing's syndrome may be achieved by the following:

Dexamethasone 0.5 mg by mouth every 6 hours for 48 hours (with 24-hour urine collection for 17-hydroxycorticosteroid excretion)

Differentiation of Cushing's syndrome due to ACTH excess from Cushing's due to other causes: Oral: Dexamethasone 2 mg every 6 hours for 48 hours (with 24-hour urine collection for 17-hydroxycorticosteroid excretion)

Multiple sclerosis (acute exacerbation): 30 mg/day for 1 week, followed by 4-12 mg/day for 1 month

Physiological replacement: Oral, I.M., I.V. (should be given as sodium phosphate): 0.03-0.15 mg/kg/day **or** 0.6-0.75 mg/m²/day in divided doses every 6-12 hours

Treatment of shock:

Addisonian crisis/shock (ie, adrenal insufficiency/responsive to steroid therapy): I.V. (given as sodium phosphate): 4-10 mg as a single dose, which may be repeated if necessary

(Continued)

Dexamethasone *(Continued)*

Unresponsive shock (ie, unresponsive to steroid therapy): I.V. (given as sodium phosphate): 1-6 mg/kg as a single I.V. dose or up to 40 mg initially followed by repeat doses every 2-6 hours while shock persists

Hemodialysis: Supplemental dose is not necessary

Peritoneal dialysis: Supplemental dose is not necessary

Combination Regimens

Leukemia, acute lymphocytic:
TVTG *on page 942*
VAD/CVAD *on page 944*
Leukemia, acute myeloid:
Hyper-CVAD *on page 898*
TVTG *on page 942*
Lymphoma, non-Hodgkin's:
DHAP *on page 872*
m-BACOD *on page 908*
Multiple myeloma:
DTPACE *on page 874*
DVD *on page 874*
Thalidomide + Dexamethasone *on page 939*
VAD *on page 943*
Prostate cancer: Cyclophosphamide + Vincristine + Dexamethasone *on page 870*

Administration

Oral: Administer with meals to decrease GI upset.

I.M.: Acetate injection is **not** for I.V. use.

I.V.: Administer as a 5-10 minute bolus; rapid injection is associated with a high incidence of perianal discomfort.

Topical: For external use. Do not use on open wounds. Apply sparingly to occlusive dressings. Should not be used in the presence of open or weeping lesions.

Dosage Forms [DSC] = Discontinued product

Elixir, as base: 0.5 mg/5 mL (240 mL) [contains alcohol 5%; raspberry flavor]

Injection, solution, as sodium phosphate: 4 mg/mL (1 mL, 5 mL, 10 mL, 25 mL, 30 mL); 10 mg/mL (1 mL, 10 mL)

Decadron® Phosphate: 4 mg/mL (5 mL, 25 mL); 24 mg/mL (5 mL) [contains sodium bisulfite] [DSC]

Ointment, ophthalmic, as sodium phosphate: 0.05% (3.5 g)

Solution, ophthalmic, as sodium phosphate: 0.1% (5 mL)

Solution, oral: 0.5 mg/5 mL (500 mL) [cherry flavor]

Solution, oral concentrate (Dexamethasone Intensol®): 1 mg/mL (30 mL) [contains alcohol 30%]

Suspension, ophthalmic (Maxidex®): 0.1% (5 mL, 15 mL)

Tablet: 0.25 mg, 0.5 mg, 0.75 mg, 1 mg, 1.5 mg, 2 mg, 4 mg, 6 mg [some 0.5 mg tablets may contain tartrazine]

Decadron®: 0.5 mg, 0.75 mg, 4 mg

DexPak® TaperPak®: 1.5 mg [51 tablets on taper dose card]

Monitoring Parameters Hemoglobin, occult blood loss, serum potassium, and glucose

Dietary Considerations May be taken with meals to decrease GI upset. May need diet with increased potassium, pyridoxine, vitamin C, vitamin D, folate, calcium, and phosphorus.

Patient Information Notify prescriber of any signs of infection or injuries during therapy; inform physician or dentist before surgery if you are taking a corticosteroid; may cause GI upset, take with food; do not overuse; use only as prescribed and for no longer than the period prescribed; notify prescriber if condition being treated persists or worsens

Ophthalmic: For ophthalmic use only. Wash hands before using. Tilt head back and look upward. Put drops of suspension or apply thin ribbon of ointment inside lower eyelid. Close eye and roll eyeball in all directions. Do not blink for $1/2$ minute. Apply gentle pressure to inner corner of eye for 30 seconds. Do not use any other eye preparation for at least 10 minutes. Do not let tip of applicator touch eye; do not contaminate tip of applicator (may cause eye infection, eye damage, or vision loss). Do not share medication with anyone else. Wear sunglasses when in sunlight; you may be more sensitive to bright light. Inform prescriber if condition worsens or fails to improve or if you experience eye pain, disturbances of vision, or other adverse eye response.

Topical: Thin film of cream or ointment is effective, do not overuse; do not use tight-fitting diapers or plastic pants on children being treated in the diaper area; use only as prescribed, and for no longer than the period prescribed; rub in lightly; avoid contact with eyes

Additional Information Effects of inhaled/intranasal steroids on growth have been observed in the absence of laboratory evidence of HPA axis suppression, suggesting that growth velocity is a more sensitive indicator of systemic corticosteroid exposure in pediatric patients than some commonly used tests of HPA axis function. The long-term effects of this reduction in growth velocity associated with orally-inhaled and intranasal corticosteroids, including the impact on final adult height, are unknown. The potential for "catch up" growth following discontinuation of treatment with inhaled corticosteroids has not been adequately studied.

Withdrawal/tapering of therapy: Corticosteroid tapering following short-term use is limited primarily by the need to control the underlying disease state; tapering may be accomplished over a period of days. Following longer-term use, tapering over weeks to months may be necessary to avoid signs and symptoms of adrenal insufficiency and to allow recovery of the HPA axis. Testing of HPA axis responsiveness may be of value in selected patients. Subtle deficits in HPA response may persist for months after discontinuation of therapy, and may require supplemental dosing during periods of acute illness or surgical stress.

Special Geriatric Considerations Because of the risk of adverse effects, systemic corticosteroids should be used cautiously in the elderly in the smallest possible dose, and for the shortest possible time.

♦ **Dexamethasone Intensol®** *see* Dexamethasone *on page 263*

♦ **Dexamethasone Sodium Phosphate** *see* Dexamethasone *on page 263*

♦ **Dexasone® (Can)** *see* Dexamethasone *on page 263*

♦ **Dexferrum®** *see* Iron Dextran Complex *on page 484*

♦ **Dexiron™ (Can)** *see* Iron Dextran Complex *on page 484*

♦ **DexPak® TaperPak®** *see* Dexamethasone *on page 263*

Dexrazoxane (deks ray ZOKS ane)

Medication Safety Issues
Sound-alike/look-alike issues:
Zinecard® may be confused with Gemzar®

Related Information
Safe Handling of Hazardous Drugs *on page 1034*

U.S. Brand Names Zinecard®

Canadian Brand Names Zinecard®

Generic Available No

Synonyms ICRF-187

Pharmacologic Category Cardioprotectant

Pregnancy Risk Factor C

Lactation Excretion in breast milk unknown/not recommended

Use Reduction of the incidence and severity of cardiomyopathy associated with doxorubicin administration in women with metastatic breast cancer who have received a cumulative doxorubicin dose of 300 mg/m^2 and who would benefit from continuing therapy with doxorubicin. It is not recommended for use with the initiation of doxorubicin therapy.

Mechanism of Action Derivative of EDTA; potent intracellular chelating agent. The mechanism of cardioprotectant activity is not fully understood. Appears to be converted intracellularly to a ring-opened chelating agent that interferes with iron-mediated oxygen free radical generation thought to be responsible, in part, for anthracycline-induced cardiomyopathy.

Labeled Contraindications Do not use with chemotherapy regimens that do not contain an anthracycline

Warnings/Precautions Hazardous agent - use appropriate precautions for handling and disposal. See Safe Handling of Hazardous Drugs *on page 1034* in the Appendix. Dexrazoxane may add to the myelosuppression caused by chemotherapeutic agents. Dexrazoxane does not eliminate the potential for anthracycline-induced cardiac toxicity. Carefully monitor cardiac function.

Adverse Reactions Unless specified, frequency not defined.
Dermatologic: Alopecia, urticaria, recall skin reaction, extravasation
Endocrine & metabolic: Serum amylase increased, serum calcium decreased, serum triglycerides increased
Gastrointestinal: Nausea, vomiting (mild)
Hematologic: Myelosuppression, neutropenia (~12%), thrombocytopenia (~4%)
Hepatic: AST/ALT increased, bilirubin increased

Vesicant No

Emetic Potential Low (high incidence of mild nausea)

Overdosage/Toxicology Management includes supportive care until resolution of myelosuppression and related conditions is complete. Retention of a significant dose fraction of unchanged drug in the plasma pool, minimal tissue partitioning or binding, and availability of >90% of systemic drug levels in the unbound form suggest that dexrazoxane could be removed using conventional peritoneal or hemodialysis.

Storage/Stability Store intact vials at controlled room temperature (15°C to 30°C/59°F to 86°F). Reconstituted and diluted solutions are stable for 6 hours at controlled room temperature or under refrigeration (2°C to 8°C/ 36°F to 46°F).

Reconstitution Must be reconstituted with 0.167 Molar (M/6) sodium lactate injection to a concentration of 10 mg dexrazoxane/mL sodium lactate. Reconstituted dexrazoxane solution may be diluted with either 0.9% sodium chloride injection or 5% dextrose injection to a concentration of 1.3-5 mg/mL in intravenous infusion bags.

Compatibility Compatible: Stable in NS, D_5W

Pharmacodynamics/Kinetics

Distribution: V_d: 22-22.4 L/m^2

Protein binding: None

Half-life elimination: 2.1-2.5 hours

Excretion: Urine (42%)

Clearance, renal: 3.35 L/hour/m^2; Plasma: 6.25-7.88 L/hour/m^2

Dosage Adults: I.V.: A 10:1 ratio of dexrazoxane:doxorubicin (500 mg/m^2 dexrazoxane: 50 mg/m^2 doxorubicin)

Dosage adjustment in hepatic impairment: Since doxorubicin dosage is reduced in hyperbilirubinemia, a proportional reduction in dexrazoxane dosage is recommended (maintain ratio of 10:1).

Administration Administer by slow I.V. push or rapid (5-15 minutes) I.V. infusion from a bag. Administer doxorubicin within 30 minutes after beginning the infusion with dexrazoxane.

Dosage Forms Injection, powder for reconstitution: 250 mg, 500 mg [10 mg/mL when reconstituted]

Monitoring Parameters Since dexrazoxane will always be used with cytotoxic drugs, and since it may add to the myelosuppressive effects of cytotoxic drugs, frequent complete blood counts are recommended

Additional Information Reimbursement Guarantee Program: 1-800-808-9111

Selected Readings

Hellmann K, "Overview and Historical Development of Dexrazoxane," *Semin Oncol*, 1998, 25(4 Suppl 10):48-54.

Hochster HS, "Clinical Pharmacology of Dexrazoxane," *Semin Oncol*, 1998, 25(4 Suppl 10):37-42.

Kwok JC and Richardson DR, "The Cardioprotective Effect of the Iron Chelator Dexrazoxane (ICRF-187) on Anthracycline-Mediated Cardiotoxicity," *Redox Rep*, 2000, 5(6):317-24.

Lopez M and Vici P, "European Trials With Dexrazoxane in Amelioration of Doxorubicin and Epirubicin-Induced Cardiotoxicity," *Semin Oncol*, 1998, 25(4 Suppl 10):55-60.

Sehested M, et al, "Dexrazoxane for Protection Against Cardiotoxic Effects of Anthracyclines," *J Clin Oncol*, 1996, 14:2884.

Weiss G, Loyevsky M, and Gordeuk VR, "Dexrazoxane (ICRF-187)," *Gen Pharmacol*, 1999, 32(1):155-8.

Wiseman LR and Spencer CM, "Dexrazoxane. A Review of Its Use as a Cardioprotective Agent in Patients Receiving Anthracycline-Based Chemotherapy," *Drugs*, 1998, 56(3):385-403.

- **Dihydrohydroxycodeinone** *see* Oxycodone *on page 633*
- **Dihydromorphinone** *see* Hydromorphone *on page 426*
- **Dihydroxyanthracenedione Dihydrochloride** *see* Mitoxantrone *on page 584*
- **Dihydroxydeoxynorvinkaleukoblastine** *see* Vinorelbine *on page 826*
- **Dilaudid®** *see* Hydromorphone *on page 426*
- **Dilaudid-HP®** *see* Hydromorphone *on page 426*
- **Dilaudid-HP-Plus® (Can)** *see* Hydromorphone *on page 426*
- **Dilaudid® Sterile Powder (Can)** *see* Hydromorphone *on page 426*
- **Dilaudid-XP® (Can)** *see* Hydromorphone *on page 426*
- **Dimethyl Triazeno Imidazole Carboxamide** *see* Dacarbazine *on page 239*
- **Diocarpine (Can)** *see* Pilocarpine *on page 666*
- **Diodex® (Can)** *see* Dexamethasone *on page 263*
- **Diogent® (Can)** *see* Gentamicin *on page 398*
- **Diopred® (Can)** *see* PrednisoLONE *on page 679*
- **Disodium Thiosulfate Pentahydrate** *see* Sodium Thiosulfate *on page 722*
- **5071-1DL(6)** *see* Megestrol *on page 528*
- **4-DMDR** *see* Idarubicin *on page 443*
- **DNA-Derived Humanized Monoclonal Antibody** *see* Alemtuzumab *on page 37*
- **DNR** *see* DAUNOrubicin Hydrochloride *on page 250*

Docetaxel (doe se TAKS el)

Medication Safety Issues
Sound-alike/look-alike issues:
Taxotere® may be confused with Taxol®

Related Information
Safe Handling of Hazardous Drugs *on page 1034*

U.S. Brand Names Taxotere®

Canadian Brand Names Taxotere®

Generic Available No

Synonyms NSC-628503; RP-6976

Pharmacologic Category Antineoplastic Agent, Natural Source (Plant) Derivative

Pregnancy Risk Factor D

Lactation Excretion in breast milk unknown/contraindicated

Use Treatment of locally-advanced or metastatic breast cancer; adjuvant treatment of operable node-positive breast cancer (in combination with doxorubicin and cyclophosphamide); treatment of locally-advanced or metastatic nonsmall cell lung cancer (NSCLC) in combination with cisplatin in treatment of patients who have not previously received chemotherapy for unresected NSCLC; treatment of prostate cancer (hormone refractory, metastatic)

Unlabeled/Investigational Use Investigational: Treatment of gastric, pancreatic, head and neck, and ovarian cancers, soft tissue sarcoma, and melanoma

Mechanism of Action Docetaxel promotes the assembly of microtubules from tubulin dimers, and inhibits the depolymerization of tubulin which stabilizes microtubules in the cell. This results in inhibition of DNA, RNA, and protein synthesis. Most activity occurs during the M phase of the cell cycle.

Labeled Contraindications Hypersensitivity to docetaxel or any component of the formulation; pre-existing bone marrow suppression (neutrophils <1500 cells/mm³); pregnancy

Warnings/Precautions Hazardous agent - use appropriate precautions for handling and disposal. See Safe Handling of Hazardous Drugs *on page 1034* in the Appendix. Patients should be premedicated with a steroid to prevent hypersensitivity reactions and fluid retention. A common regimen is dexamethasone 4-8 mg orally twice daily for 3-5 days, starting the day before docetaxel administration.

Fluid retention syndrome (pleural effusions, ascites, edema, and 2-15 kg weight gain) may occur. The incidence and severity of the syndrome increase sharply at cumulative doses ≥400 mg/m².

Neutropenia was the dose-limiting toxicity. Patients with an absolute neutrophil count <1500 cells/mm³ should not receive docetaxel. Hepatic dysfunction increases risk of neutropenia and severe infections. Should generally not be given to patients with bilirubin greater than the upper limit of normal or to patients with AST (SGOT) and/or ALT (SGPT) greater than 1.5x the upper limit of normal concomitantly with alkaline phosphatase greater than 2.5x the upper limit of normal. Obtain baseline levels prior to administration. If docetaxel contacts the skin, wash and flush thoroughly with water. Contains Polysorbate 80®; diluent contains ethanol.

When administered as sequential infusions, taxane derivatives (docetaxel, paclitaxel) should be administered before platinum derivatives (carboplatin, cisplatin) to limit myelosuppression and to enhance efficacy.

Adverse Reactions Note: Frequencies cited for nonsmall cell lung cancer and breast cancer treatment. Exact frequency may vary based on tumor type, prior and/or current treatment, premedication, and dosage of docetaxel.

>10%:

Cardiovascular: Fluid retention, including peripheral edema, pleural effusion, and ascites (33% to 47%); may be more common at cumulative doses ≥400 mg/m². Up to 64% in breast cancer patients with dexamethasone premedication.

Dermatologic: Alopecia (56% to 76%); nail disorder (11% to 31%, banding, onycholysis, hypo- or hyperpigmentation)

Gastrointestinal: Mucositis/stomatitis (26% to 42%, severe in 6% to 7%), may be dose-limiting (premedication may reduce frequency and severity); nausea and vomiting (40% to 80%, severe in 1% to 5%); diarrhea (33% to 43%)

Hematologic: Myelosuppression, neutropenia (75% to 85%), thrombocytopenia, anemia

Onset: 4-7 days

Nadir: 5-9 days

Recovery: 21 days

Hepatic: Transaminases increased (18%)

Neuromuscular & skeletal: Myalgia (3% to 21%); neurosensory changes (paresthesia, dysesthesia, pain) noted in 23% to 49% (severe in up to 6%). Motor neuropathy (including weakness) noted in
(Continued)

Docetaxel *(Continued)*

as many as 16% of lung cancer patients (severe in up to 5%). Neuropathy may be more common at higher cumulative docetaxel dosages or with prior cisplatin therapy.

Ocular: Epiphora associated with canalicular stenosis (up to 77% with weekly administration; up to 1% with every-3-week administration)

Miscellaneous: Hypersensitivity reactions (6% to 13%; angioedema, rash, flushing, fever, hypotension); frequency substantially reduced by premedication with dexamethasone starting one day prior to docetaxel administration.

1% to 10%:

Cardiovascular: Hypotension (3%)

Dermatologic: Rash and skin eruptions (6%)

Gastrointestinal: Taste perversion (6%)

Hepatic: Bilirubin increased (9%)

Neuromuscular & skeletal: Arthralgia (3% to 9%)

Miscellaneous: Infusion site reactions (up to 4%)

<1%, postmarketing and/or case reports (Limited to important or life-threatening): Arrhythmias, atrial fibrillation, acute respiratory distress syndrome (ARDS), confusion, dehydration, erythema multiforme, gastrointestinal hemorrhage, gastrointestinal obstruction, gastrointestinal perforation, hepatitis, ileus, interstitial pneumonia, ischemic colitis, loss of consciousness (transient), MI, neutropenic enterocolitis, pulmonary edema, pulmonary embolism, pulmonary fibrosis, radiation recall, seizure, Stevens-Johnson syndrome, visual disturbances

Vesicant No; may be an irritant

Emetic Potential Moderate (30% to 60%)

Drug Interactions

Cytochrome P450 Effect: Substrate of CYP3A4 (major); **Inhibits** CYP3A4 (weak)

Increased Effect/Toxicity: CYP3A4 inhibitors may increase the levels/effects of docetaxel; example inhibitors include azole antifungals, ciprofloxacin, clarithromycin, diclofenac, doxycycline, erythromycin, imatinib, isoniazid, nefazodone, nicardipine, propofol, protease inhibitors, quinidine, and verapamil. When administered as sequential infusions, observational studies indicate a potential for increased toxicity when platinum derivatives (carboplatin, cisplatin) are administered before taxane derivatives (docetaxel, paclitaxel).

Decreased Effect: CYP3A4 inducers may decrease the levels/effects of docetaxel; example inducers include aminoglutethimide, carbamazepine, nafcillin, nevirapine, phenobarbital, phenytoin, and rifamycins.

Ethanol/Nutrition/Herb Interactions

Ethanol: Avoid ethanol (due to GI irritation).

Herb/Nutraceutical: St John's wort may decrease docetaxel levels.

Storage/Stability Intact vials should be stored at 2°C to 25°C (36°F to 77°F) and protected from light. Freezing does not adversely affect the product. Vials should be stored at room temperature for approximately 5 minutes before using. Following dilution, vials are stable for 8 hours at room temperature or under refrigeration. Following dilution for infusion, solutions are stable for up to 4 weeks at room temperature 15°C to 25°C (59°F to 77°F) in polyolefin containers.

Reconstitution Intact vials of solution should be diluted with 13% (w/w) ethanol/water to a final concentration of 10 mg/mL. Do not shake. Docetaxel dose should then be further diluted with NS or D_5W to a final concentration of 0.3-0.74 mg/mL and dispensed in a glass bottle, polypropylene, or polyolefin plastic bag.

Compatibility Stable in D_5W, NS

Y-site administration: Compatible: Acyclovir, amifostine, amikacin, aminophylline, ampicillin, ampicillin/sulbactam, aztreonam, bumetanide, buprenorphine, butorphanol, calcium gluconate, cefazolin, cefepime, cefoperazone, cefotaxime, cefotetan, cefoxitin, ceftazidime, ceftizoxime, ceftriaxone, cefuroxime, chlorpromazine, cimetidine, ciprofloxacin, clindamycin, co-trimoxazole, dexamethasone sodium phosphate, diphenhydramine, dobutamine, dopamine, doxycycline, droperidol, enalaprilat, famotidine, fluconazole, furosemide, ganciclovir, gemcitabine, gentamicin, granisetron, haloperidol, heparin, hydrocortisone sodium phosphate, hydrocortisone sodium succinate, hydromorphone, hydroxyzine, imipenem/cilastatin, leucovorin, lorazepam, magnesium sulfate, mannitol, meperidine, meropenem, mesna, metoclopramide, metronidazole, minocycline, morphine, netilmicin, ofloxacin, ondansetron, piperacillin, piperacillin/tazobactam, potassium chloride, prochlorperazine edisylate, promethazine, ranitidine, Ringer's injection (lactated), sodium bicarbonate, ticarcillin, ticarcillin/clavulanate, tobramycin, vancomycin, zidovudine. **Incompatible:** Amphotericin B, doxorubicin liposome, methylprednisolone sodium succinate, nalbuphine

Pharmacodynamics/Kinetics Exhibits linear pharmacokinetics at the recommended dosage range

Distribution: Extensive extravascular distribution and/or tissue binding; V_d: 80-90 L/m^2, V_{dss}: 113 L (mean steady state)

Protein binding: 94%, primarily to alpha$_1$-acid glycoprotein, albumin, and lipoproteins

Metabolism: Hepatic; oxidation via CYP3A4 to metabolites

Half-life elimination: Alpha, beta, gamma: 4 minutes, 36 minutes, and 10-18 hours, respectively

Excretion: Feces (75%); urine (6%); ~80% within 48 hours

Clearance: Total body: Mean: 21 L/hour/m^2

Dosage Children ≥16 years and Adults: I.V. infusion: Refer to individual protocols:

Breast cancer:

Locally-advanced or metastatic: 60-100 mg/m^2 every 3 weeks; patients initially started at 60 mg/m^2 who do not develop toxicity may tolerate higher doses

Operable, node-positive (adjuvant treatment): 75 mg/m^2 every 3 weeks for 6 courses

Nonsmall-cell lung cancer: I.V.: 75 mg/m^2 every 3 weeks

Prostate cancer: 75 mg/m^2 every 3 weeks; prednisone (5 mg twice daily) is administered continuously

Dosing adjustment for toxicity:

Note: Toxicity includes febrile neutropenia, neutrophils ≤500/mm^3 for >1 week, severe or cumulative cutaneous reactions; in nonsmall cell lung cancer, this may also include other grade 3/4 nonhematologic toxicities.

(Continued)

Docetaxel *(Continued)*

Breast cancer: Patients dosed initially at 100 mg/m²; reduce dose to 75 mg/m²; **Note:** If the patient continues to experience these adverse reactions, the dosage should be reduced to 55 mg/m² or therapy should be discontinued

Breast cancer, adjuvant treatment: TAC regimen should be administered when neutrophils are ≥1500 cells/mm³. Patients experiencing febrile neutropenia should receive G-CSF in all subsequent cycles. Patients continuing to experience febrile neutropenia or patients experiencing severe/cumulative cutaneous reactions or moderate neurosensory effects (signs/symptoms) should receive a reduced dose (60 mg/m²) of docetaxel. Discontinue therapy in patients continuing to experience these reactions after dosage reduction.

Nonsmall cell lung cancer:

Monotherapy: Patients dosed initially at 75 mg/m² should have dose held until toxicity is resolved, then resume at 55 mg/m²; discontinue patients who develop ≥ grade 3 peripheral neuropathy.

Combination therapy: Patients dosed initially at 75 mg/m², in combination with cisplatin, should have the docetaxel dosage reduced to 65 mg/m² in subsequent cycles; if further adjustment is required, dosage may be reduced to 50 mg/m²

Prostate cancer: Reduce dose to 60 mg/m²; discontinue therapy if adverse reactions persist at lower dose.

Dosing adjustment in hepatic impairment: Total bilirubin ≥ the upper limit of normal (ULN), or AST/ALT >1.5 times ULN concomitant with alkaline phosphatase >2.5 times ULN: Docetaxel **should not be administered**.

Combination Regimens

Bladder cancer: Cisplatin-Docetaxel *on page 861*

Breast cancer: TAC *on page 938*

Lung cancer (nonsmall cell): Docetaxel-Cisplatin *on page 873*

Osteosarcoma: Gemcitabine-Docetaxel *on page 896*

Prostate cancer:

Estramustine + Docetaxel *on page 881*

Estramustine + Docetaxel + Carboplatin *on page 882*

Estramustine + Docetaxel + Hydrocortisone *on page 882*

Sarcoma, soft tissue: Gemcitabine-Docetaxel *on page 896*

Administration

Prevention of fluid retention/anaphylactoid-like reactions: Premedication with dexamethasone (4-8 mg orally twice daily for 3 or 5 days starting 1 day prior to administration of docetaxel).

Administer I.V. infusion over 1-hour through nonsorbing (nonpolyvinylchloride) tubing. When administered as sequential infusions, taxane derivatives should be administered before platinum derivatives (cisplatin, carboplatin) to limit myelosuppression and to enhance efficacy.

Dosage Forms Injection, solution [concentrate]: 20 mg/0.5 mL (0.5 mL, 2 mL) [contains Polysorbate 80®; diluent contains ethanol 13%]

Monitoring Parameters Monitor for hypersensitivity reactions, fluid retention, epiphora, and canalicular stenosis

Patient Information This medication can only be administered intravenously. You may experience nausea or vomiting (frequent small meals, frequent mouth care, sucking lozenges, or chewing gum may help); you may experience loss of hair (reversible); you will be more susceptible to infection (avoid crowds and exposure to infection as much as possible). Yogurt or buttermilk may help reduce diarrhea (if unresolved, contact prescriber for medication relief). Report swelling of extremities, difficulty breathing, unusual weight gain, abdominal distention, fever, chills, unusual bruising or bleeding, signs of infection, excessive fatigue, or unresolved diarrhea. Contraceptive measures are recommended during therapy.

Additional Information Premedication with oral corticosteroids is recommended for all patients to decrease the incidence and severity of fluid retention and severity of hypersensitivity reactions. Suggested regimen: Dexamethasone: Oral: 4-10 mg twice daily, beginning the day before docetaxel infusion.

Selected Readings

Bruno R and Sanderink GJ, "Pharmacokinetics and Metabolism of Taxotere® (Docetaxel)," *Cancer Surv*, 1993, 17:305-13.

Cortes JE and Pazdur R, "Docetaxel," *J Clin Oncol*, 1995, 13(10):2643-55.

Fulton B and Spencer CM, "Docetaxel. A Review of Its Pharmacodynamic and Pharmacokinetic Properties and Therapeutic Efficacy in the Management of Metastatic Breast Cancer," *Drugs*, 1996, 51(6):1075-92.

Ravdin PM, "The International Experience With Docetaxel in the Treatment of Breast Cancer," *Oncology*, 1997, 11(3 Suppl 2):38-42.

Trudeau ME, "Docetaxel: A Review of Its Pharmacology and Clinical Activity," *Can J Oncol*, 1996, 6(1):443-57.

Dolasetron (dol A se tron)

Medication Safety Issues

Sound-alike/look-alike issues:
Anzemet® may be confused with Aldomet®

Related Information

Management of Nausea and Vomiting *on page 982*

U.S. Brand Names Anzemet®

Canadian Brand Names Anzemet®

Generic Available No

Synonyms Dolasetron Mesylate; MDL 73,147EF

Pharmacologic Category Antiemetic; Selective 5-HT$_3$ Receptor Antagonist

Pregnancy Risk Factor B

Lactation Excretion in breast milk unknown

Use Prevention of nausea and vomiting associated with emetogenic cancer chemotherapy; prevention of postoperative nausea and vomiting and treatment of postoperative nausea and vomiting (injectable form only)

Not recommended for treatment of existing chemotherapy-induced emesis (CIE).

Mechanism of Action Selective serotonin receptor (5-HT$_3$) antagonist, blocking serotonin both peripherally (primary site of action) and centrally at the chemoreceptor trigger zone

Labeled Contraindications Hypersensitivity to dolasetron or any component of the formulation

Warnings/Precautions Administer with caution in patients who have or may develop prolongation of cardiac conduction intervals, particularly QT$_c$ intervals. These include patients with hypokalemia, hypomagnesemia, patients taking diuretics which may cause electrolyte disturbances, (Continued)

Dolasetron *(Continued)*

patients with congenital QT syndrome, patients taking antiarrhythmic drugs or drug which prolong QT interval, and cumulative high-dose anthracycline therapy.

Adverse Reactions

>10%:

Central nervous system: Headache (31%), dizziness, lightheadedness (23%)

Gastrointestinal: Loose stools/diarrhea (50%); increased appetite (27%); taste alterations (12%)

1% to 10%:

Cardiovascular: Hypertension, hypotension (6%), ECG abnormalities, prolonged P-R, QRS, and QT_c intervals

Central nervous system: Sedation (8%), slow movement (3%), nervousness (3%), fatigue (2%), listlessness, grogginess

Gastrointestinal: Nausea (6%), constipation (3%), diarrhea, abdominal pain, flatulence

Hepatic: Mild elevations of serum aminotransferases (7%)

Local: Pain at injection site (1%)

Neuromuscular & skeletal: Paresthesia

Ocular: Visual disturbances (mostly blurred vision) (9%); photosensitivity (2%)

Vesicant No

Emetic Potential Very low (<10%)

Overdosage/Toxicology Prolongation of QT, AV block, severe hypotension, and dizziness have been reported. Treatment is supportive, and continuous ECG monitoring (telemetry) is recommended.

Drug Interactions

Cytochrome P450 Effect: Substrate (minor) of CYP2C8/9, 3A4; **Inhibits** CYP2D6 (weak)

Increased Effect/Toxicity: Increased blood levels of active metabolite may occur during concurrent administration of cimetidine and atenolol. Inhibitors of this isoenzyme may increase blood levels of active metabolite. Due to the potential to potentiate QT_c prolongation, drugs which may prolong QT interval directly (eg, antiarrhythmics) or by causing alterations in electrolytes (eg, diuretics) should be used with caution.

Decreased Effect: Blood levels of active metabolite are decreased during coadministration of rifampin.

Ethanol/Nutrition/Herb Interactions Herb/Nutraceutical: St John's wort may decrease dolasetron levels.

Storage/Stability Store intact vials at room temperature. Protect from light. After dilution, I.V. dolasetron is stable under normal lighting conditions at room temperature for 24 hours or under refrigeration for 48 hours with the following **compatible** intravenous fluids: 0.9% sodium chloride injection, 5% dextrose injection, 5% dextrose and 0.45% sodium chloride injection, 5% dextrose and lactated Ringer's injection, lactated Ringer's injection, and 10% mannitol injection

Reconstitution Dilute in 50-100 mL of a compatible solution.

Compatibility Compatible: Stable in D_5W, $D_5W^{1/2}NS$, D_5WLR, LR, NS, $^{1/2}NS$, and 10% mannitol injection

Pharmacodynamics/Kinetics

Distribution: V_d: 5.8-10 L/kg

Metabolism: Hepatic to a reduced alcohol (active metabolite MDL 74,156)

Bioavailability: 59% to 80%

Half-life elimination: Dolasetron: 10 minutes; MDL 74,156: 8 hours

Time to peak concentration:

I.V.: 0.6 hours

Oral: 1-1.5 hours

Excretion:

Urine: 45% to 68% as metabolites

Feces: 25% to 33%

Dosage

Children <2 years: Not recommended for use

Nausea and vomiting prophylaxis, chemotherapy-induced (including initial and repeat courses):

Children 2-16 years:

Oral: 1.8 mg/kg within 1 hour before chemotherapy; maximum: 100 mg/dose

I.V.: 1.8 mg/kg ~30 minutes before chemotherapy; maximum: 100 mg/dose

Adults:

Oral: 200 mg single dose

I.V.:

0.6-5 mg/kg as a single dose

50 mg 1-2 minute bolus

2.4-3 mg/kg 20-minute infusion

Prevention of postoperative nausea and vomiting:

Children 2-16 years:

Oral: 1.2 mg/kg within 2 hours before surgery; maximum: 100 mg/dose

I.V.: 0.35 mg/kg (maximum: 12.5 mg) ~15 minutes before stopping anesthesia

Adults:

Oral: 100 mg within 2 hours before surgery

I.V.: 12.5 mg ~15 minutes before stopping anesthesia

Treatment of postoperative nausea and vomiting: I.V. (only):

Children: 0.35 mg/kg (maximum: 12.5 mg) as soon as needed

Adults: 12.5 mg as soon as needed

Dosing adjustment for elderly, renal/hepatic impairment: No dosage adjustment is recommended

Administration I.V. injection may be given either undiluted IVP over 30 seconds or infused over 15 minutes. Dolasetron injection may be diluted in apple or apple-grape juice and taken orally.

Dosage Forms

Injection, solution, as mesylate: 20 mg/mL (0.625 mL, 5 mL) [single-use ampuls and vial]; 20 mg/mL (25 mL) [multidose vial]

Tablet, as mesylate: 50 mg, 100 mg

Monitoring Parameters Liver function tests, blood pressure and pulse, and ECG in patients with cardiovascular disease

Additional Information Efficacy of dolasetron, for chemotherapy treatment, is enhanced with concomitant administration of dexamethasone 20 mg (increases complete response by 10% to 20%). Oral administration of the intravenous solution is equivalent to tablets. A single I.V. dose of (Continued)

Dolasetron *(Continued)*

dolasetron mesylate (1.8 or 2.4 mg/kg) has comparable safety and efficacy to a single 32 mg I.V. dose of ondansetron in patients receiving cisplatin chemotherapy.

Selected Readings

Balfour JA and Goa KL, "Dolasetron. A Review of its Pharmacology and Therapeutic Potential in the Management of Nausea and Vomiting Induced by Chemotherapy, Radiotherapy or Surgery," *Drugs*, 1997, 54(2):273-98.

Hui YF and Ignoffo RJ, "Dolasetron. A New 5-Hydroxytryptamine3 Receptor Antagonist," *Cancer Pract*, 1997, 5(5):324-8.

♦ **Dolasetron Mesylate** *see* Dolasetron *on page 277*

♦ **Dolophine®** *see* Methadone *on page 545*

♦ **Dom-Benzydamine (Can)** *see* Benzydamine *on page 123*

♦ **Doxidan® *(reformulation)* [OTC]** *see* Bisacodyl *on page 133*

♦ **Doxil®** *see* DOXOrubicin (Liposomal) *on page 286*

DOXOrubicin (doks oh ROO bi sin)

Medication Safety Issues

Sound-alike/look-alike issues:

DOXOrubicin may be confused with dactinomycin, DAUNOrubicin, doxacurium, doxapram, doxazosin, idarubicin

Adriamycin PFS® may be confused with achromycin, Aredia®, Idamycin®

Rubex® may be confused with Robaxin®

Conventional formulations (Adriamycin PFS®, Adriamycin RDF®, Rubex®) may be confused with liposomal formulations (DaunoXome®, Doxil®)

Related Information

Fertility and Cancer Therapy *on page 962*

Safe Handling of Hazardous Drugs *on page 1034*

Transplantation *on page 1019*

U.S. Brand Names Adriamycin PFS®; Adriamycin RDF®; Rubex®

Canadian Brand Names Adriamycin®

Generic Available Yes

Synonyms ADR; Adria; Doxorubicin Hydrochloride; Hydroxydaunomycin Hydrochloride; Hydroxyldaunorubicin Hydrochloride; NSC-123127

Pharmacologic Category Antineoplastic Agent, Anthracycline

Pregnancy Risk Factor D

Lactation Enters breast milk/contraindicated

Use Treatment of leukemias, lymphomas, multiple myeloma, osseous and nonosseous sarcomas, mesotheliomas, germ cell tumors of the ovary or testis, and carcinomas of the head and neck, thyroid, lung, breast, stomach, pancreas, liver, ovary, bladder, prostate, uterus, and neuroblastoma

Mechanism of Action Inhibition of DNA and RNA synthesis by intercalation between DNA base pairs by inhibition of topoisomerase II and by steric obstruction. Doxorubicin intercalates at points of local uncoiling of the double helix. Although the exact mechanism is unclear, it appears that direct binding to DNA (intercalation) and inhibition of DNA repair (topoisomerase II inhibition) result in blockade of DNA and RNA synthesis and fragmentation of DNA. Doxorubicin is also a powerful iron chelator; the iron-doxorubicin complex can bind DNA and cell membranes and produce free radicals that immediately cleave the DNA and cell membranes.

Labeled Contraindications Hypersensitivity to doxorubicin or any component of the formulation; congestive heart failure or arrhythmias; previous therapy with high cumulative doses of doxorubicin and/or daunorubicin; pre-existing bone marrow suppression; pregnancy

Warnings/Precautions Hazardous agent - use appropriate precautions for handling and disposal. See Safe Handling of Hazardous Drugs *on page 1034* in the Appendix. Total dose should not exceed 550 mg/m² or 450 mg/m² in patients with previous or concomitant treatment with daunorubicin, cyclophosphamide, or irradiation of the cardiac region. Irreversible myocardial toxicity may occur as total dosage approaches 550 mg/m². I.V. use only, severe local tissue necrosis will result if extravasation occurs. Elderly and pediatric patients are at higher risk of cardiotoxicity (delayed). Reduce dose in patients with impaired hepatic function. Severe myelosuppression is also possible. Administration of live vaccines to immunosuppressed patients may be hazardous. Heart failure may occur during therapy or months to years after therapy. Treatment may increase the risk of other neoplasms. Secondary acute myelogenous leukemia may occur following treatment.

Adverse Reactions
>10%:

Dermatologic: Alopecia, radiation recall

Gastrointestinal: Nausea, vomiting, stomatitis, GI ulceration, anorexia, diarrhea

Genitourinary: Discoloration of urine, mild dysuria, urinary frequency, hematuria, bladder spasms, cystitis following bladder instillation

Hematologic: Myelosuppression, primarily leukopenia (75%); thrombocytopenia and anemia

Onset: 7 days

Nadir: 10-14 days

Recovery: 21-28 days

1% to 10%:

Cardiovascular: Transient ECG abnormalities (supraventricular tachycardia, S-T wave changes, atrial or ventricular extrasystoles); generally asymptomatic and self-limiting. CHF, dose related, may be delayed for 7-8 years after treatment. Cumulative dose, mediastinal/pericardial radiation therapy, cardiovascular disease, age, and use of cyclophosphamide (or other cardiotoxic agents) all increase the risk.

Recommended maximum cumulative doses:

No risk factors: 550 mg/m²

Concurrent radiation: 450 mg/m²

Note: Regardless of cumulative dose, if the left ventricular ejection fraction is <30% to 40%, the drug is usually not given.

Dermatologic: Skin "flare" at injection site; discoloration of saliva, sweat, or tears

Endocrine & metabolic: Hyperuricemia

<1%: Pericarditis, myocarditis, myocardial infection, skin rash, pigmentation of nail beds, nail banding, onycholysis, urticaria, infertility, sterility, elevations of bilirubin and transaminases, hepatitis, systemic hypersensitivity (including urticaria, pruritus, angioedema, dysphagia, and dyspnea)

Vesicant Yes; see Management of Drug Extravasations *on page 965*. (Continued)

DOXOrubicin *(Continued)*

Emetic Potential
≤20 mg: Moderately low (10% to 30%)
>20 mg or <60 mg: Moderate (30% to 60%)
≥60 mg: Moderately high (60% to 90%)

Overdosage/Toxicology Symptoms of overdose include myelosuppression, nausea, vomiting, and myocardial toxicity. Treatment of acute overdose consists of treatment of the severely myelosuppressed patient with hospitalization, antibiotics, platelet and granulocyte transfusions, and symptomatic treatment of mucositis.

Drug Interactions
Cytochrome P450 Effect: Substrate (major) of CYP2D6, 3A4; **Inhibits** CYP2B6 (moderate), 2D6 (weak), 3A4 (weak)

Increased Effect/Toxicity: Allopurinol may enhance the antitumor activity of doxorubicin (animal data only). Cyclosporine may increase doxorubicin levels, enhancing hematologic toxicity or may induce coma or seizures. Cyclophosphamide enhances the cardiac toxicity of doxorubicin by producing additional myocardial cell damage. Mercaptopurine increases doxorubicin toxicities. Streptozocin greatly enhances leukopenia and thrombocytopenia. Verapamil alters the cellular distribution of doxorubicin and may result in increased cell toxicity by inhibition of the P-glycoprotein pump. Paclitaxel reduces doxorubicin clearance and increases toxicity if administered prior to doxorubicin. High doses of progesterone enhance toxicity (neutropenia and thrombocytopenia).

Doxorubicin may increase the levels/effects of bupropion, promethazine, propofol, selegiline, sertraline, and other CYP2B6 substrates. The levels/effects of doxorubicin may be increased by azole antifungals, chlorpromazine, ciprofloxacin, clarithromycin, delavirdine, diclofenac, doxycycline, erythromycin, fluoxetine, imatinib, isoniazid, miconazole, nefazodone, nicardipine, paroxetine, pergolide, propofol, protease inhibitors, quinidine, quinine, ritonavir, ropinirole, telithromycin, verapamil and other inhibitors of CYP2D6 or 3A4. Based on mouse studies, cardiotoxicity may be enhanced by verapamil. Concurrent therapy with actinomycin-D may result in recall pneumonitis following radiation.

Decreased Effect: The levels/effects of doxorubicin may be decreased by aminoglutethimide, carbamazepine, nafcillin, nevirapine, phenobarbital, phenytoin, rifamycins, and other CYP3A4 inducers. Doxorubicin may decrease plasma levels and effectiveness of digoxin. Doxorubicin may decrease the antiviral activity of zidovudine.

Ethanol/Nutrition/Herb Interactions Herb/Nutraceutical: St John's wort may decrease doxorubicin levels. Avoid black cohosh, dong quai in estrogen-dependent tumors.

Storage/Stability Store intact vials of solution under refrigeration at 2°C to 8°C and protected from light. Store intact vials of lyophilized powder at room temperature (15°C to 30°C). Reconstituted vials are stable for 7 days at room temperature (25°C) and 15 days under refrigeration (5°C) when protected from light. Infusions are stable for 48 hours at room temperature (25°C) when protected from light.

Reconstitution Reconstitute lyophilized powder with NS to a final concentration of 2 mg/mL.
Further dilution in 50-1000 mL D_5W or NS

Unstable in solutions with a pH <3 or >7.

Compatibility Stable in D_5W, LR, NS

> **Y-site administration: Compatible:** Amifostine, aztreonam, bleomycin, chlorpromazine, cimetidine, cisplatin, cladribine, cyclophosphamide, dexamethasone sodium phosphate, diphenhydramine, droperidol, etoposide phosphate, famotidine, filgrastim, fludarabine, fluorouracil, gatifloxacin, gemcitabine, granisetron, hydromorphone, leucovorin, linezolid, lorazepam, melphalan, methotrexate, methylprednisolone sodium succinate, metoclopramide, mitomycin, morphine, ondansetron, paclitaxel, prochlorperazine edisylate, promethazine, ranitidine, sargramostim, sodium bicarbonate, teniposide, thiotepa, topotecan, vinblastine, vincristine, vinorelbine. **Incompatible:** Allopurinol, amphotericin B cholesteryl sulfate complex, cefepime, ganciclovir, piperacillin/tazobactam, propofol. **Variable (consult detailed reference):** Furosemide, heparin
>
> **Compatibility in syringe: Compatible:** Bleomycin, cisplatin, cyclophosphamide, droperidol, leucovorin, methotrexate, metoclopramide, mitomycin, vinblastine, vincristine. **Incompatible:** Furosemide, heparin. **Variable (consult detailed reference):** Fluorouracil
>
> **Compatibility when admixed: Compatible:** Dacarbazine, ondansetron, ondansetron with vincristine, paclitaxel, vinblastine. **Incompatible:** Aminophylline, diazepam, fluorouracil. **Variable (consult detailed reference):** Dacarbazine with ondansetron, etoposide with vincristine

Pharmacodynamics/Kinetics

Absorption: Oral: Poor (<50%)

Distribution: V_d: 25 L/kg; to many body tissues, particularly liver, spleen, kidney, lung, heart; does not distribute into the CNS; crosses placenta

Protein binding, plasma: 70%

Metabolism: Primarily hepatic to doxorubicinol (active), then to inactive aglycones, conjugated sulfates, and glucuronides

Half-life elimination:
  Distribution: 10 minutes
  Elimination: Doxorubicin: 1-3 hours; Metabolites: 3-3.5 hours
  Terminal: 17-30 hours
  Male: 54 hours; Female: 35 hours

Excretion: Feces (~40% to 50% as unchanged drug); urine (~3% to 10% as metabolites, 1% doxorubicinol, <1% Adriamycin aglycones, and unchanged drug)

Clearance: Male: 113 L/hour; Female: 44 L/hour

Dosage Refer to individual protocols. I.V.:

Children:
  35-75 mg/m^2 as a single dose, repeat every 21 days **or**
  20-30 mg/m^2 once weekly **or**
  60-90 mg/m^2 given as a continuous infusion over 96 hours every 3-4 weeks

Adults: Usual or typical dose: 60-75 mg/m^2 as a single dose, repeat every 21 days **or** other dosage regimens like 20-30 mg/m^2/day for 2-3 days, repeat in 4 weeks **or** 20 mg/m^2 once weekly

Dosing adjustment in renal impairment:
  Mild to moderate renal failure: Adjustment is not required
  Cl_{cr} <10 mL/minute: Administer 75% of normal dose

Hemodialysis: Supplemental dose is not necessary

Dosing adjustment in hepatic impairment:
  ALT/AST 2-3 times ULN: Administer 75% of dose

(Continued)

DOXOrubicin *(Continued)*

ALT/AST >3 times ULN **or** bilirubin 1.2-3 mg/dL (20-51 µmol/L): Administer 50% of dose

Bilirubin 3.1-5 mg/dL (51-85 µmol/L): Administer 25% of dose

Bilirubin >5 mg/dL (85 µmol/L): Do not administer

Combination Regimens

Bladder cancer:

Breast cancer:

Cervical cancer:

Endometrial cancer:

Gastric cancer:

Gestational trophoblastic tumor:

Head and neck cancer:

Hepatoblastoma:

Leukemia, acute lymphocytic:

Leukemia, acute myeloid:

Lung cancer (small cell):

Lymphoma, Hodgkin's:

Lymphoma, non-Hodgkin's:

Multiple myeloma:
Neuroblastoma:
Prostate cancer:
Sarcoma, soft tissue:
Wilms' tumor:
Administration I.V. push over 1-2 minutes, IVPB over 15-60 minutes, or continuous infusion.

Dosage Forms
Injection, powder for reconstitution, as hydrochloride: 10 mg, 20 mg, 50 mg [contains lactose]
  Adriamycin RDF®: 10 mg, 20 mg, 50 mg, 150 mg [contains lactose; rapid dissolution formula]
  Rubex®: 50 mg, 100 mg [contains lactose]
Injection, solution, as hydrochloride [preservative free]: 2 mg/mL (5 mL, 10 mL, 25 mL, 100 mL)
  Adriamycin PFS® [preservative free]: 2 mg/mL (5 mL, 10 mL, 25 mL, 37.5 mL, 100 mL)

Monitoring Parameters CBC with differential and platelet count, cardiac and liver function tests

Patient Information This medication can only be administered intravenously. During therapy, do not use aspirin-containing products, and/or OTC medications without consulting prescriber. It is important to maintain adequate nutrition during therapy; frequent small meals may help. You may experience nausea or vomiting (frequent small meals, frequent mouth care, sucking lozenges, or chewing gum may help). You may (Continued)

DOXOrubicin *(Continued)*

experience loss of hair (reversible); you will be more susceptible to infection (avoid crowds and exposure to infection as much as possible). Urine may turn darker yellow. Yogurt or buttermilk may help reduce diarrhea (if unresolved, contact prescriber for medication relief). Frequent mouth care and use of a soft toothbrush or cotton swabs may reduce mouth sores. Report fever, chills, unusual bruising or bleeding, signs of infection, abdominal pain or blood in stools, excessive fatigue, yellowing of eyes or skin, swelling of extremities, difficulty breathing, or unresolved diarrhea. Contraceptive measures are recommended during therapy.

Selected Readings

Brown JR and Iman SH, "Recent Studies on Doxorubicin and Its Analogues," *Prog Med Chem*, 1984, 21:169-236.

Cummings J and Smyth JF, "Pharmacology of Adriamycin: The Message to the Clinician," *Eur J Cancer Clin Oncol*, 1988, 24(4):579-82.

Speth PA, van Hoesel QG, and Haanen C, "Clinical Pharmacokinetics of Doxorubicin," *Clin Pharmacokinet*, 1988, 15(1):15-31.

◆ **Doxorubicin Hydrochloride** *see* DOXOrubicin *on page 280*

◆ **Doxorubicin Hydrochloride (Liposomal)** *see* DOXOrubicin (Liposomal) *on page 286*

DOXOrubicin (Liposomal)

(doks oh ROO bi sin lip pah SOW mal)

Medication Safety Issues

Sound-alike/look-alike issues:

DOXOrubicin may be confused with dactinomycin, DAUNOrubicin, doxacurium, doxapram, doxazosin, idarubicin

Doxil® may be confused with Doxy®, Paxil®

Liposomal formulations (Doxil®) may be confused with conventional formulations (Adriamycin PFS®, Adriamycin RDF®, Cerubidine®, Rubex®).

Related Information

Safe Handling of Hazardous Drugs *on page 1034*

U.S. Brand Names Doxil®

Canadian Brand Names Caelyx®

Generic Available No

Synonyms Doxorubicin Hydrochloride (Liposomal)

Pharmacologic Category Antineoplastic Agent, Anthracycline

Pregnancy Risk Factor D

Lactation Excretion in breast milk unknown/contraindicated

Use Treatment of AIDS-related Kaposi's sarcoma, breast cancer, ovarian cancer, solid tumors

Mechanism of Action Doxorubicin inhibits DNA and RNA synthesis by intercalating between DNA base pairs causing steric obstruction and inhibits topoisomerase-II at the point of DNA cleavage. Doxorubicin is also a powerful iron chelator. The iron-doxorubicin complex can bind DNA and cell membranes, producing free hydroxyl (OH) radicals that cleave DNA and cell membranes. Active throughout entire cell cycle.

Labeled Contraindications Hypersensitivity to doxorubicin, other anthracyclines, or any component of the formulation; breast-feeding, pregnancy

Warnings/Precautions Hazardous agent - use appropriate precautions for handling and disposal. See Safe Handling of Hazardous Drugs *on page 1034* in the Appendix.

Doxorubicin is associated with dose-related myocardial damage leading to congestive heart failure. Doxorubicin and liposomal doxorubicin should be used cautiously in patients with high cumulative doses of anthracyclines, anthracenediones, and cyclophosphamide. Caution should also be used in patients with previous thoracic radiation or who have pre-existing cardiac disease. Total cumulative doses of anthracyclines, including liposomal doxorubicin and anthracenediones should not exceed 550 mg/m^2 or 400 mg/m^2 in patients with previous or concomitant treatment (with daunorubicin, cyclophosphamide, or irradiation of the cardiac region); irreversible myocardial toxicity may occur at these doses. Symptoms of anthracycline-induced CHF and/or cardiomyopathy may be delayed in onset (up to 7-8 years in some cases). For I.V. use only; reduce dose in patients with impaired hepatic function; severe myelosuppression is also possible. Acute infusion reactions may occur, some may be serious/life-threatening. **Liposomal formulations of doxorubicin should not be substituted for doxorubicin hydrochloride on a mg-per-mg basis.**

Hand-foot syndrome (palmar-plantar erythrodysesthesia) has been reported in up to 51% of patients with ovarian cancer (and significantly lower frequency in patients with Kaposi's sarcoma). May occur early in treatment, but is usually seen after 2-3 treatment cycles. Dosage modification may be required. In severe cases, treatment discontinuation may be required.

Adverse Reactions

>10%:

Cardiovascular: Peripheral edema (up to 11%)

Central nervous system: Fever (8% to 12%), headache (up to 11%), pain (up to 21%)

Dermatologic: Alopecia (9% to 19%); palmar-plantar erythrodysesthesia/hand-foot syndrome (up to 51% in ovarian cancer, 4% in Kaposi's sarcoma), rash (up to 29% in ovarian cancer, up to 5% in Kaposi's sarcoma)

Gastrointestinal: Stomatitis (5% to 41%), vomiting (8% to 33%), nausea (18% to 46%), mucositis (up to 14%), constipation (up to 30%), anorexia (up to 20%), diarrhea (5% to 21%), dyspepsia (up to 12%), intestinal obstruction (up to 11%)

Hematologic: Myelosuppression, neutropenia (12% to 62%), leukopenia (36%), thrombocytopenia (13% to 65%), anemia (6% to 74%)

Onset: 7 days

Nadir: 10-14 days

Recovery: 21-28 days

Neuromuscular & skeletal: Weakness (7% to 40%), back pain (up to 12%)

Respiratory: Pharyngitis (up to 16%), dyspnea (up to 15%)

1% to 10%:

Cardiovascular: Cardiac arrest, chest pain, edema, hypotension, pallor, tachycardia, vasodilation

Central nervous system: Agitation, anxiety, chills, confusion, depression, dizziness, emotional lability, insomnia, somnolence, vertigo

(Continued)

DOXOrubicin (Liposomal) *(Continued)*

Dermatologic: Acne, dry skin (6%), dermatitis, furunculosis, herpes simplex/zoster, maculopapular rash, pruritus, skin discoloration, vesiculobullous rash

Endocrine & metabolic: Dehydration, hyperbilirubinemia, hyperglycemia, hypocalcemia, hypokalemia, hyponatremia

Gastrointestinal: Abdomen enlarged, ascites, cachexia, dyspepsia, dysphagia, esophagitis, flatulence, gingivitis, glossitis, ileus, mouth ulceration, rectal bleeding, taste perversion, weight loss, xerostomia

Genitourinary: Cystitis, dysuria, leukorrhea, pelvic pain, polyuria, urinary incontinence, urinary tract infection, urinary urgency, vaginal bleeding

Hematologic: Ecchymosis, hemolysis, prothrombin time increased

Hepatic: ALT increased

Local: Thrombophlebitis

Neuromuscular & skeletal: Arthralgia, hypertonia, myalgia, neuralgia, neuritis (peripheral), neuropathy, paresthesia (up to 10%), pathological fracture,

Ocular: Conjunctivitis, dry eyes, retinitis

Otic: Ear pain

Renal: Albuminuria, hematuria

Respiratory: Apnea, cough increased (up to 10%), epistaxis, pleural effusion, pneumonia, rhinitis, sinusitis

Miscellaneous: Allergic reaction; infusion-related reactions (bronchospasm, chest tightness, chills, dyspnea, facial edema, flushing, headache, hypotension, pruritus); moniliasis, diaphoresis

<1%: Abscess, acute brain syndrome, abnormal vision, anaphylactic or anaphylactoid reaction, appetite increased, asthma, balanitis, blindness, bone pain, bronchitis, BUN increased, bundle branch block, cardiomegaly, cellulitis, colitis, creatinine increased, cryptococcosis, diabetes mellitus, erythema multiforme, erythema nodosum, eosinophilia, eye pain, fecal impaction, flu-like syndrome, gastritis, glucosuria, heart arrest, hematuria, hemiplegia, hemorrhage, hepatic failure, hepatitis, hepatosplenomegaly, hypercalcemia, hyperkalemia, hypernatremia, hyper-/hypotonia, hyperuricemia, hyperventilation, hypoglycemia, hypokinesia, hypolipidemia, hypomagnesemia, hyponatremia, hypophosphatemia, hypoproteinemia, hypothermia, injection site hemorrhage, injection site pain, jaundice, ketosis, lactic dehydrogenase increased, kidney failure, lymphadenopathy, lymphangitis, migraine, myositis, optic neuritis, otitis media, palpitation, pancreatitis, pericardial effusion, petechia, pleural effusion, pneumothorax, radiation injury, sclerosing cholangitis, seizure, sepsis, skin necrosis, skin ulcer, syncope, tenesmus, thrombophlebitis, thromboplastin decreased, thrombosis, tinnitus, urticaria, visual field defect, ventricular arrhythmia, weight gain

Vesicant No; may be an irritant

Emetic Potential Low (10% to 30%)

Overdosage/Toxicology Symptoms of overdose include increases in mucositis, leukopenia, and thrombocytopenia. For acute overdose, treatment of the severely myelosuppressed patient consists of hospitalization, antibiotics, hematopoietic growth factors, platelet and granulocyte transfusion, and symptomatic treatment of mucositis.

Drug Interactions

Cytochrome P450 Effect: Substrate (major) of CYP2D6, 3A4; **Inhibits** CYP2B6 (moderate), 2D6 (weak), 3A4 (weak)

Increased Effect/Toxicity: Allopurinol may enhance the antitumor activity of doxorubicin (animal data only). Cyclosporine may increase doxorubicin levels, enhancing hematologic toxicity or may induce coma or seizures. Cyclophosphamide enhances the cardiac toxicity of doxorubicin by producing additional myocardial cell damage. Mercaptopurine increases doxorubicin toxicities. Streptozocin greatly enhances leukopenia and thrombocytopenia. Verapamil alters the cellular distribution of doxorubicin and may result in increased cell toxicity by inhibition of the P-glycoprotein pump. Paclitaxel reduces doxorubicin clearance and increases toxicity if administered prior to doxorubicin. High doses of progesterone enhance toxicity (neutropenia and thrombocytopenia).

Doxorubicin may increase the levels/effects of bupropion, promethazine, propofol, selegiline, sertraline, and other CYP2B6 substrates. The levels/effects of doxorubicin may be increased by azole antifungals, chlorpromazine, ciprofloxacin, clarithromycin, delavirdine, diclofenac, doxycycline, erythromycin, fluoxetine, imatinib, isoniazid, miconazole, nefazodone, nicardipine, paroxetine, pergolide, propofol, protease inhibitors, quinidine, quinine, ritonavir, ropinirole, telithromycin, verapamil and other inhibitors of CYP2D6 or 3A4. Based on mouse studies, cardiotoxicity may be enhanced by verapamil. Concurrent therapy with actinomycin-D may result in recall pneumonitis following radiation.

Decreased Effect: The levels/effects of doxorubicin may be decreased by aminoglutethimide, carbamazepine, nafcillin, nevirapine, phenobarbital, phenytoin, rifamycins, and other CYP3A4 inducers. Doxorubicin may decrease plasma levels and effectiveness of digoxin. Doxorubicin may decrease the antiviral activity of zidovudine.

Ethanol/Nutrition/Herb Interactions

Ethanol: Avoid ethanol (due to GI irritation).

Herb/Nutraceutical: St John's wort may decrease doxorubicin levels. Avoid black cohosh, dong quai in estrogen-dependent tumors.

Storage/Stability Store intact vials of solution under refrigeration (2°C to 8°C); avoid freezing. Prolonged freezing may adversely affect liposomal drug products, however, short-term freezing (<1 month) does not appear to have a deleterious effect. Diluted doxorubicin hydrochloride liposome injection may be refrigerated at 2°C to 8°C or at room temperature; administer within 24 hours. **Do not use with in-line filters.**

Reconstitution Doses Doxil® ≤90 mg must be diluted in 250 mL of D_5W prior to administration. Doses >90 mg should be diluted in 500 mL D_5W.

Compatibility Stable in D_5W

Y-site administration: Compatible: Acyclovir, allopurinol, aminophylline, ampicillin, aztreonam, bleomycin, butorphanol, calcium gluconate, carboplatin, cefazolin, cefepime, cefoxitin, ceftizoxime, ceftriaxone, chlorpromazine, cimetidine, ciprofloxacin, cisplatin, clindamycin, co-trimoxazole, cyclophosphamide, cytarabine, dexamethasone sodium phosphate, diphenhydramine, dobutamine, dopamine, droperidol, enalaprilat, etoposide, famotidine, fluconazole, ganciclovir, gentamicin, granisetron, haloperidol, hydrocortisone sodium succinate, hydromorphone, ifosfamide, leucovorin, lorazepam, magnesium sulfate, mesna, methotrexate, methylprednisolone sodium succinate, (Continued)

DOXOrubicin (Liposomal) *(Continued)*

metronidazole, netilmicin, ondansetron, piperacillin, potassium chloride, prochlorperazine edisylate, ranitidine, ticarcillin, ticarcillin/clavulanate, tobramycin, vancomycin, vinblastine, vincristine, vinorelbine, zidovudine. **Incompatible:** Amphotericin B, amphotericin B cholesteryl sulfate complex, buprenorphine, cefoperazone, ceftazidime, docetaxel, fluorouracil, furosemide, heparin, hydroxyzine, mannitol, meperidine, metoclopramide, mitoxantrone, morphine, ofloxacin, paclitaxel, piperacillin/tazobactam, promethazine, sodium bicarbonate

Recommended Dose Modification Guidelines

Toxicity Grade	Dose Adjustment
HAND FOOT SYNDROME (HFS)	
1 (Mild erythema, swelling, or desquamation not interfering with daily activities)	Redose unless patient has experienced previous Grade 3 or 4 toxicity. If so, delay up to 2 weeks and decrease dose by 25%; return to original dosing interval.
2 (Erythema, desquamation, or swelling interfering with, but not precluding, normal physical activities; small blisters or ulcerations <2 cm in diameter)	Delay dosing up to 2 weeks or until resolved to Grade 0-1. If after 2 weeks there is no resolution, liposomal doxorubicin should be discontinued. Otherwise, if no prior Grade 3-4 HFS, continue treatment at previous dose and dosage interval. If a prior Grade 3-4 HFS has occurred, continue prior dosage interval, but decrease dose by 25%.
3 (Blistering, ulceration, or swelling interfering with walking or normal daily activities; cannot wear regular clothing)	Delay dosing up to 2 weeks or until resolved to Grade 0-1. Decrease dose by 25% and return to original dosing interval; if after 2 weeks there is no resolution, liposomal doxorubicin should be discontinued.
4 (Diffuse or local process causing infectious complications, or a bedridden state or hospitalization)	Delay dosing up to 2 weeks or until resolved to Grade 0-1. Decrease dose by 25% and return to original dosing interval. If after 2 weeks there is no resolution, liposomal doxorubicin should be discontinued.
STOMATITIS	
1 (Painless ulcers, erythema, or mild soreness)	Redose unless patient has experienced previous Grade 3 or 4 toxicity. If so, delay up to 2 weeks and decrease by 25%. Return to original dosing interval.
2 (Painful erythema, edema, or ulcers, but can eat)	Delay dosing up to 2 weeks or until resolved to Grade 0-1. If after 2 weeks there is no resolution, liposomal doxorubicin should be discontinued. Otherwise, if not prior Grade 3-4 stomatitis, continue treatment at previous dose and dosage interval. If prior Grade 3-4 toxicity, continue treatment with previous dosage interval, but decrease dose by 25%.
3 (Painful erythema, edema, or ulcers, but cannot eat)	Delay dosing up to 2 weeks or until resolved to Grade 0-1. Decrease dose by 25% and return to original dosing interval. If after 2 weeks there is no resolution, liposomal doxorubicin should be discontinued.
4 (Requires parenteral or enteral support)	Delay dosing up to 2 weeks or until resolved to Grade 0-1. Decrease dose by 25% and return to original dosing interval. If after 2 weeks there is no resolution, liposomal doxorubicin should be discontinued.

Pharmacodynamics/Kinetics

Distribution: V_{dss}: 2.8 L/m^2

Protein binding, plasma: Unknown; nonliposomal doxorubicin 70%

Half-life elimination: Terminal: Distribution: 4.7-5.2 hours, Elimination: 44-55 hours

Metabolism: Hepatic and in plasma to doxorubicinol and the sulfate and glucuronide conjugates of 4-demethyl,7-deoxyaglycones

Excretion: Urine (5% as doxorubicin or doxorubicinol)

Clearance: Mean: 0.041 L/hour/m^2

Dosage Note: Liposomal formulations of doxorubicin should not be substituted for doxorubicin hydrochloride on a mg-per-mg basis. Refer to individual protocols.

AIDS-KS patients: I.V.: 20 mg/m^2/dose once every 3 weeks

Breast cancer: I.V.: 20-80 mg/m^2/dose every 8 weeks has been studied in a limited number of phase I/II trials

Ovarian cancer: I.V.: 50 mg/m^2/dose every 4 weeks

Solid tumors: I.V.: 50-60 mg/m^2/dose every 3-4 weeks

See table: "Recommended Dose Modification Guidelines" on previous page.

Dosing adjustment in hepatic impairment:

ALT/AST 2-3 times ULN: Administer 75% of dose

ALT/AST >3 times ULN **or** bilirubin 1.2-3 mg/dL (20-51 µmol/L): Administer 50% of dose

Bilirubin 3.1-5 mg/dL (51-85 µmol/L): Administer 25% of dose

Bilirubin >5 mg/dL (85 µmol/L): Do not administer

See table "Hematological Toxicity" on next page.

Administration Administer IVPB over 30 minutes; administer at initial rate of 1 mg/minute to minimize risk of infusion reactions; do not administer as a bolus injection or undiluted solution. **Do not administer I.M. or SubQ. Do not use with in-line filters.** Avoid extravasation associated with severe ulceration and soft tissue necrosis. Flush with 5-10 mL of D$_5$W solution before and after drug administration. Incompatible with heparin. Monitor for local erythematous streaking along vein and/or facial flushing (may indicate rapid infusion rate).

Dosage Forms Injection, solution, as hydrochloride: 2 mg/mL (10 mL, 25 mL)

Monitoring Parameters CBC with differential and platelet count, liver function tests

Cardiac function should be carefully monitored; echocardiography, MUGA scan may be used during therapy. Endomyocardial biopsy is the most definitive test for anthracycline myocardial injury.

Patient Information This medication can only be administered I.V. During therapy, do not use alcohol, aspirin-containing products, and/or OTC medications without consulting prescriber. It is important to maintain adequate nutrition and hydration (2-3 L/day of fluids unless instructed to restrict fluid intake) during therapy; frequent small meals may help. You may experience nausea or vomiting (frequent small meals, frequent mouth care, sucking lozenges, or chewing gum may help). You may experience loss of hair (reversible); you will be more susceptible to infection (avoid crowds and exposure to infection as much as possible). Urine may turn red-brown (normal). Yogurt or buttermilk may help reduce diarrhea (if unresolved, contact prescriber for medication relief). Frequent mouth care and use of a soft toothbrush or cotton swabs may reduce mouth sores. Report fever, chills, unusual bruising or bleeding, signs of infection, abdominal pain or blood in stools, excessive fatigue, yellowing of eyes or skin, darkening in color of urine or pale colored stools, swelling of extremities, difficulty breathing, or unresolved diarrhea. Contraceptive measures are recommended during therapy

(Continued)

DOXOrubicin (Liposomal) *(Continued)*

Hematological Toxicity

Grade	ANC	Platelets	Modification
1	1500-1900	75,000-150,000	Resume treatment with no dose reduction.
2	1000-<1500	50,000-<75,000	Wait until ANC ≥1500 and platelets ≥75,000; redose with no dose reduction.
3	500-999	25,000-<50,000	Wait until ANC ≥1500 and platelets ≥75,000; redose with no dose reduction.
4	<500	<25,000	Wait until ANC ≥1500 and platelets ≥75,000; redose at 25% dose reduction or continue full dose with cytokine support.

Selected Readings
Forbes C, Wilby J, Richardson G, et al, "A Systematic Review and Economic Evaluation of Pegylated Liposomal Doxorubicin Hydrochloride for Ovarian Cancer," *Health Technol Assess*, 2002, 6(23):1-119.

Gabizon A, Shmeeda H, and Barenholz Y, "Pharmacokinetics of Pegylated Liposomal Doxorubicin: Review of Animal and Human Studies," *Clin Pharmacokinet*, 2003, 42(5):419-36.

King PD and Perry MC, "Hepatotoxicity of Chemotherapy," *Oncologist*, 2001, 6(2):162-76.

Orditura M, Quaglia F, Morgillo F, et al, "Pegylated Liposomal Doxorubicin: Pharmacologic and Clinical Evidence of Potent Antitumor Activity With Reduced Anthracycline-induced Cardiotoxicity (Review)," *Oncol Rep*, 2004, 12(3):549-56.

O'Shaughnessy JA, "Pegylated Liposomal Doxorubicin in the Treatment of Breast Cancer," *Clin Breast Cancer*, 2003, 4(5):318-28.

Sharpe M, Easthope SE, Keating GM, et al, "Polyethylene Glycol-Liposomal Doxorubicin: A Review of Its Use in the Management of Solid and Haematological Malignancies and AIDS-Related Kaposi's Sarcoma," *Drugs*, 2002, 62(14):2089-126.

Stebbing J and Gaya A, "Pegylated Liposomal Doxorubicin (Caelyx) in Recurrent Ovarian Cancer," *Cancer Treat Rev*, 2002, 28(2):121-5.

Waterhouse DN, Tardi PG, Mayer LD, et al, "A Comparison of Liposomal Formulations of Doxorubicin With Drug Administered in Free Form: Changing Toxicity Profiles," *Drug Saf*, 2001, 24(12):903-20.

Dronabinol *(droe NAB i nol)*

Medication Safety Issues
Sound-alike/look-alike issues:
Dronabinol may be confused with droperidol

Related Information
Management of Nausea and Vomiting *on page 982*

U.S. Brand Names Marinol®

Canadian Brand Names Marinol®

Generic Available No

Synonyms Delta-9-Tetrahydro-Cannabinol; Delta-9 THC; Tetrahydrocannabinol; THC

Pharmacologic Category Antiemetic; Appetite Stimulant

Pregnancy Risk Factor C

Lactation Enters breast milk/contraindicated

Use Chemotherapy-associated nausea and vomiting refractory to other antiemetic; AIDS- and cancer-related anorexia

Mechanism of Action Unknown, may inhibit endorphins in the emetic center, suppress prostaglandin synthesis, and/or inhibit medullary activity through an unspecified cortical action

Restrictions C-III

Labeled Contraindications Hypersensitivity to dronabinol or any component of the formulation, or marijuana; should be avoided in patients with a history of schizophrenia

Warnings/Precautions Use with caution in patients with heart disease, hepatic disease, or seizure disorders. Reduce dosage in patients with severe hepatic impairment. May have potential for abuse; drug is psycho-active substance in marijuana. Monitor for possible psychotic reaction with first dose.

Adverse Reactions

>10%:

Central nervous system: Drowsiness (48%), sedation (53%), confusion (30%), dizziness (21%), detachment, anxiety, difficulty concentrating, mood change

Gastrointestinal: Appetite increased (when used as an antiemetic), xerostomia (38% to 50%)

1% to 10%:

Cardiovascular: Orthostatic hypotension, tachycardia

Central nervous system: Ataxia (4%), depression (7%), headache, vertigo, hallucinations (5%), memory lapse (4%)

Neuromuscular & skeletal: Paresthesia, weakness

<1%: Syncope, nightmares, diarrhea, myalgia, tinnitus, diaphoresis

Emetic Potential Very low (<10%)

Overdosage/Toxicology Symptoms of overdose include tachycardia, hyper- and hypotension. Treatment is symptomatic.

Drug Interactions

Increased Effect/Toxicity: Increased toxicity (drowsiness) with alcohol, barbiturates, and benzodiazepines.

Ethanol/Nutrition/Herb Interactions

Ethanol: Avoid ethanol (may increase CNS depression).

Food: Administration with high-lipid meals may increase absorption.

Herb/Nutraceutical: St John's wort may decrease dronabinol levels.

Storage/Stability Store in a cool place.

Pharmacodynamics/Kinetics

Onset of action: Within 1 hour

Absorption: Oral: 90% to 95%; ~5% to 10% of dose gets into systemic circulation

Distribution: V_d: 2.5-6.4 L; tetrahydrocannabinol is highly lipophilic and distributes to adipose tissue

Protein binding: 97% to 99%

Metabolism: Hepatic to at least 50 metabolites, some of which are active; 11-hydroxytetrahydrocannabinol (11-OH-THC) is the major metabolite; extensive first-pass effect

Half-life elimination: THC: 19-24 hours; THC metabolites: 49-53 hours

Time to peak, serum: 2-3 hours

Excretion: Feces (35% as unconjugated metabolites); urine (10% to 15% as acid metabolites and conjugates)

Dosage Refer to individual protocols. Oral:

Antiemetic:

Children: 5 mg/m² starting 6-8 hours before chemotherapy and every 4-6 hours after to be continued for 12 hours after chemotherapy is discontinued

Adults: 5 mg/m² 1-3 hours before chemotherapy, then 5 mg/m²/dose every 2-4 hours after chemotherapy for a total of 4-6 doses/day;

(Continued)

Dronabinol *(Continued)*

increase doses in increments of 2.5 mg/m^2 to a maximum of 15 mg/ m^2/dose.

Appetite stimulant: Initial: 2.5 mg twice daily (before lunch and dinner); titrate up to a maximum of 20 mg/day.

Administration Oral; administration with high lipid meals may increase absorption.

Dosage Forms Capsule, gelatin: 2.5 mg, 5 mg, 10 mg [contains sesame oil]

Monitoring Parameters CNS effects, heart rate, blood pressure

Patient Information Avoid activities such as driving which require motor coordination, avoid alcohol and other CNS depressants; may impair coordination and judgment

Selected Readings

Anderson PO and Muire GG, "Delta-9-Tetrahydrocannabinol as an Antiemetic," *Am J Hosp Pharm*, 1981, 38:639-46.

Cat LK and Coleman RL, "Treatment for HIV Wasting Syndrome," *Ann Pharmacother*, 1994, 28(5):595-7.

Plasse TF, Gorter RW, Krasnow SH, et al, "Recent Clinical Experience With Dronabinol," *Pharmacol Biochem Behav*, 1991, 40(3):695-700.

Struwe M, Kaempfer SH, Geiger CJ, et al, "Effect of Dronabinol on Nutritional Status in HIV Infection," *Ann Pharmacother*, 1993, 27(7-8):827-31.

Voth EA and Schwartz RH, "Medicinal Applications of Delta-9-Tetrahydrocannabinol and Marijuana," *Ann Intern Med*, 1979, 126(10):791-8.

Droperidol *(droe PER i dole)*

Medication Safety Issues

Sound-alike/look-alike issues:

Droperidol may be confused with dronabinol

Inapsine® may be confused with Nebcin®

Related Information

Management of Nausea and Vomiting *on page 982*

U.S. Brand Names Inapsine®

Generic Available Yes

Synonyms Dehydrobenzperidol

Pharmacologic Category Antiemetic; Antipsychotic Agent, Butyrophenone

Pregnancy Risk Factor C

Lactation Excretion in breast milk unknown

Use Antiemetic in surgical and diagnostic procedures; preoperative medication in patients when other treatments are ineffective or inappropriate

Mechanism of Action Droperidol is a butyrophenone antipsychotic; antiemetic effect is a result of blockade of dopamine stimulation of the chemoreceptor trigger zone. Other effects include alpha-adrenergic blockade, peripheral vascular dilation, and reduction of the pressor effect of epinephrine resulting in hypotension and decreased peripheral vascular resistance; may also reduce pulmonary artery pressure

Labeled Contraindications Hypersensitivity to droperidol or any component of the formulation; known or suspected QT prolongation, including congenital long QT syndrome (prolonged QT$_c$ is defined as >440 msec in males or >450 msec in females)

Warnings/Precautions May alter cardiac conduction. Cases of QT prolongation and torsade de pointes, including some fatal cases, have been reported. Use extreme caution in patients with bradycardia (<50

bpm), cardiac disease, concurrent MAOI therapy, Class I and Class III antiarrhythmics or other drugs known to prolong QT interval, and electrolyte disturbances (hypokalemia or hypomagnesemia), including concomitant drugs which may alter electrolytes (diuretics).

Use with caution in patients with seizures, bone marrow suppression, or severe liver disease. May be sedating, use with caution in disorders where CNS depression is a feature. Caution in patients with hemodynamic instability, predisposition to seizures, subcortical brain damage, renal or respiratory disease. Esophageal dysmotility and aspiration have been associated with antipsychotic use. Caution in breast cancer or other prolactin-dependent tumors. May cause orthostatic hypotension - use with caution in patients at risk of this effect. Significant hypotension may occur; injection contains benzyl alcohol; injection also contains sulfites which may cause allergic reaction.

Relative to other neuroleptics, droperidol has a low potency of cholinergic blockade. Use with caution in patients with decreased gastrointestinal motility, urinary retention, BPH, xerostomia, or visual problems. May worsen myasthenia gravis.

May cause extrapyramidal symptoms, including tardive dyskinesia. May be associated with neuroleptic malignant syndrome (NMS) or pigmentary retinopathy. Safety in children <6 months of age has not been established.

Adverse Reactions

>10%:

Cardiovascular: QT_c prolongation (dose dependent)

Central nervous system: Restlessness, anxiety, extrapyramidal symptoms, dystonic reactions, pseudoparkinsonian signs and symptoms, tardive dyskinesia, seizure, altered central temperature regulation, sedation, drowsiness

Endocrine & metabolic: Swelling of breasts

Gastrointestinal: Weight gain, constipation

1% to 10%:

Cardiovascular: Hypotension (especially orthostatic), tachycardia, abnormal T waves with prolonged ventricular repolarization, hypertension

Central nervous system: Hallucinations, persistent tardive dyskinesia, akathisia

Gastrointestinal: Nausea, vomiting

Genitourinary: Dysuria

<1%: Adynamic ileus, agranulocytosis, alopecia, amenorrhea, arrhythmia, blurred vision, cholestatic jaundice, contact dermatitis, galactorrhea, gynecomastia, heat stroke, hyperpigmentation, laryngospasm, leukopenia (usually with large doses for prolonged periods), neuroleptic malignant syndrome (NMS), obstructive jaundice, overflow incontinence, photosensitivity (rare), priapism, pruritus, rash, respiratory depression, retinal pigmentation, sexual dysfunction, tardive dystonia, torsade de pointes, urinary retention, ventricular tachycardia, visual acuity decreased (may be irreversible), xerostomia

Vesicant No

Emetic Potential Very low (<10%)

(Continued)

Droperidol *(Continued)*

Overdosage/Toxicology Symptoms of overdose include hypotension, tachycardia, hallucinations, and extrapyramidal symptoms. Following initiation of essential overdose management, toxic symptom treatment and supportive treatment should be initiated. Prolonged QT interval, seizures, and arrhythmias have been reported.

Drug Interactions

Increased Effect/Toxicity: Droperidol in combination with certain forms of conduction anesthesia may produce peripheral vasodilitation and hypotension. Droperidol and CNS depressants will likely have additive CNS effects. Droperidol and cyclobenzaprine may have an additive effect on prolonging the QT interval. Use caution with other agents known to prolong QT interval (Class I or Class III antiarrhythmics, some quinolone antibiotics, cisapride, some phenothiazines, pimozide, tricyclic antidepressants). Potassium- or magnesium-depleting agents (diuretics, aminoglycosides, amphotericin B, cyclosporine) may increase risk of arrhythmias. Metoclopramide may increase risk of extrapyramidal symptoms (EPS).

Storage/Stability Droperidol ampuls/vials should be stored at room temperature and protected from light. Solutions diluted in NS or D_5W are stable at room temperature for up to 7 days.

Compatibility Stable in D_5W, LR, NS

Y-site administration: Compatible: Alatrofloxacin, amifostine, aztreonam, bleomycin, cisatracurium, cisplatin, cladribine, cyclophosphamide, cytarabine, docetaxel, doxorubicin, doxorubicin liposome, etoposide phosphate, famotidine, filgrastim, fluconazole, fludarabine, gatifloxacin, gemcitabine, granisetron, hydrocortisone sodium succinate, idarubicin, linezolid, melphalan, meperidine, metoclopramide, mitomycin, ondansetron, paclitaxel, potassium chloride, propofol, remifentanil, sargramostim, teniposide, thiotepa, vinblastine, vincristine, vinorelbine, vitamin B complex with C. **Incompatible:** Allopurinol, amphotericin B cholesteryl sulfate complex, cefepime, fluorouracil, foscarnet, furosemide, leucovorin, nafcillin, piperacillin/tazobactam. **Variable (consult detailed reference):** Heparin, methotrexate

Compatibility in syringe: Compatible: Atropine, bleomycin, butorphanol, chlorpromazine, cimetidine, cisplatin, cyclophosphamide, dimenhydrinate, diphenhydramine, doxorubicin, fentanyl, glycopyrrolate, hydroxyzine, meperidine, metoclopramide, midazolam, mitomycin, morphine, nalbuphine, pentazocine, perphenazine, prochlorperazine edisylate, promazine, promethazine, scopolamine, vinblastine, vincristine. **Incompatible:** Fluorouracil, furosemide, heparin, leucovorin, methotrexate, ondansetron, pentobarbital

Pharmacodynamics/Kinetics

Onset of action: Peak effect: Parenteral: ~30 minutes

Duration: Parenteral: 2-4 hours, may extend to 12 hours

Absorption: I.M.: Rapid

Distribution: Crosses blood-brain barrier and placenta

V_d: Children: ~0.25-0.9 L/kg; Adults: ~2 L/kg

Protein binding: Extensive

Metabolism: Hepatic, to *p*-fluorophenylacetic acid, benzimidazolone, *p*-hydroxypiperidine

Half-life elimination: Adults: 2.3 hours

Excretion: Urine (75%, <1% as unchanged drug); feces (22%, 11% to 50% as unchanged drug)

Dosage Titrate carefully to desired effect

Children 2-12 years: Nausea and vomiting: I.M., I.V.: 0.05-0.06 mg/kg (maximum initial dose: 0.1 mg/kg); additional doses may be repeated to achieve effect; administer additional doses with caution

Adults: Nausea and vomiting: I.M., I.V.: Initial: 2.5 mg; additional doses of 1.25 mg may be administered to achieve desired effect; administer additional doses with caution

Administration Administer I.M. or I.V.; I.V. should be administered as a rapid IVP (over 30-60 seconds); for I.V. infusion, dilute in 50-100 mL NS or D$_5$W. ECG monitoring for 2-3 hours after administration is recommended.

Dosage Forms Injection, solution: 2.5 mg/mL (1 mL, 2 mL)

Monitoring Parameters To identify QT prolongation, a 12-lead ECG prior to use is recommended; continued ECG monitoring for 2-3 hours following administration is recommended. Vital signs; lipid profile, fasting blood glucose/Hgb A$_{1c}$, serum magnesium and potassium; BMI; mental status, abnormal involuntary movement scale (AIMS); observe for dystonias, extrapyramidal side effects, and temperature changes

Additional Information Does not possess analgesic effects; has little or no amnesic properties.

Special Geriatric Considerations Use of droperidol in the elderly may result in severe and often irreversible undesirable effects. Before initiating antipsychotic therapy, the clinician should investigate possible reversible causes.

Selected Readings

Cersosimo RJ, Bromer R, Hoffer S, et al, "The Antiemetic Activity of Droperidol Administered by Intramuscular Injection During Cisplatin Chemotherapy: A Pilot Study," *Drug Intell Clin Pharm*, 1985, 19(2):118-21.

Foster PN, Stickle BR, Dale M, et al, "Akathisia After Low-Dose Droperidol," *Br J Anaesth*, 1995, 74:477P.

Ghoneim MM and Korttila K, "Pharmacokinetics of Intravenous Anaesthetics: Implications for Clinical Use," *Clin Pharmacokinet*, 1977, 2(5):344-72.

Grunberg SM and Hesketh PJ, "Control of Chemotherapy-Induced Emesis," *N Engl J Med*, 1993, 329(24):1790-6.

Kao LW, Kirk MA, Evers SJ, et al, "Droperidol, QT Prolongation, and Sudden Death: What Is the Evidence," *Ann Emerg Med*, 2003, 41(4):546-58.

Peabody CA, Warner MD, Whiteford HA, et al, "Neuroleptics and the Elderly," *J Am Geriatr Soc*, 1987, 35(3):233-8.

Risse SC and Barnes R, "Pharmacologic Treatment of Agitation Associated With Dementia," *J Am Geriatr Soc*, 1986, 34(5):368-76.

Rosen C, Ratliff AF, Wolfe RW, et al, "The Efficacy of Droperidol in the Prehospital Setting," *Acad Emerg Med*, 1995, 2:446.

Saltz BL, Woerner MG, Kane JM, et al, "Prospective Study of Tardive Dyskinesia Incidence in the Elderly," *JAMA*, 1991, 266(17):2402-6.

Seifert RD, "Therapeutic Drug Monitoring: Psychotropic Drugs," *J Pharm Pract*, 1984, 6:403-16.

Sridhar KS and Donnelly E, "Combination Antiemetics for Cisplatin Chemotherapy," *Cancer*, 1988, 61(8):1508-17.

Tortorice PV and O'Connell MB, "Management of Chemotherapy-Induced Nausea and Vomiting," *Pharmacotherapy*, 1990, 10(2):129-45.

Wilson J, Weltz M, Solimando D, et al, "Continuous Infusion Droperidol: Antiemetic Therapy for Cis-Platinum (DDP) Toxicity," *Proc Am Soc Clin Oncol*, 1981, C-351.

Yaster M, Sola JE, Pegoli W Jr, et al, "The Night After Surgery: Postoperative Management of the Pediatric Outpatient - Surgical and Anesthetic Aspects," *Pediatr Clin North Am*, 1994, 41(1):199-220.

♦ **Droxia**™ *see* Hydroxyurea *on page 432*

Epirubicin (ep i ROO bi sin)

Medication Safety Issues
Sound-alike/look-alike issues:
Ellence® may be confused with Elase®

Related Information
Safe Handling of Hazardous Drugs *on page 1034*

U.S. Brand Names Ellence®

Canadian Brand Names Ellence®; Pharmorubicin®

Generic Available No

Synonyms Pidorubicin; Pidorubicin Hydrochloride

Pharmacologic Category Antineoplastic Agent, Anthracycline

Pregnancy Risk Factor D

Lactation Excretion in breast milk unknown/contraindicated

Use Adjuvant therapy for primary breast cancer

Mechanism of Action Epirubicin is an anthracycline antibiotic. Epirubicin is known to inhibit DNA and RNA synthesis by steric obstruction after intercalating between DNA base pairs; active throughout entire cell cycle. Intercalation triggers DNA cleavage by topoisomerase II, resulting in cytocidal activity. Epirubicin also inhibits DNA helicase, and generates cytotoxic free radicals.

Labeled Contraindications Hypersensitivity to epirubicin, other anthracyclines, or anthracenediones; severe myocardial insufficiency, severe arrhythmias; recent myocardial infarction; severe hepatic dysfunction; baseline neutrophil count 1500 cells/mm^3; previous anthracycline treatment up to maximum cumulative dose; pregnancy

Warnings/Precautions Hazardous agent - use appropriate precautions for handling and disposal. See Safe Handling of Hazardous Drugs *on page 1034* in the Appendix. The primary toxicity is myelosuppression; severe thrombocytopenia or anemia may occur. Thrombophlebitis and thromboembolic phenomena (including pulmonary embolism) have occurred.

Potential cardiotoxicity, particularly in patients who have received prior anthracyclines, prior radiotherapy to the mediastinal/pericardial area, or who have pre-existing cardiac disease, may occur. Acute toxicity (primarily arrhythmias) and delayed toxicity (CHF) have been described. Delayed toxicity usually develops late in the course of therapy or within 2-3 months after completion, however, events with an onset of several months to years after termination of treatment have been described. The risk of delayed cardiotoxicity increases more steeply at dosages above 900 mg/m^2, and this dose should be exceeded only with extreme caution. Toxicity may be additive with other anthracyclines or anthracenediones, and may be increased in pediatric patients. Regular monitoring of LVEF and discontinuation at the first sign of impairment is recommended especially in patients with risk factors or impaired cardiac function.

Reduce dosage and use with caution in mild to moderate hepatic impairment or in severe renal dysfunction (serum creatinine >5 mg/dL). May cause tumor lysis syndrome or radiation recall. Treatment with anthracyclines may increase the risk of secondary leukemias. For I.V. administration only, severe local tissue necrosis will result if extravasation occurs. Epirubicin is emetogenic. Women ≥70 years of age should be especially monitored for toxicity; women of childbearing age should be advised to avoid becoming pregnant.

Adverse Reactions

>10%:

Central nervous system: Lethargy (1% to 46%)

Dermatologic: Alopecia (69% to 95%)

Endocrine & metabolic: Amenorrhea (69% to 72%), hot flashes (5% to 39%)

Gastrointestinal: Nausea, vomiting (83% to 92%), mucositis (9% to 59%), diarrhea (7% to 25%)

Hematologic: Leukopenia (49% to 80%; Grade 3 and 4: 1.5% to 58.6%), neutropenia (54% to 80%), anemia (13% to 72%), thrombocytopenia (5% to 49%)

Local: Injection site reactions (3% to 20%)

Ocular: Conjunctivitis (1% to 15%)

Miscellaneous: Infection (15% to 21%)

1% to 10%:

Cardiovascular: CHF (0.4% to 1.5%), decreased LVEF (asymptomatic) (1.4% to 1.8%); recommended maximum cumulative dose: 900 mg/m^2

Central nervous system: Fever (1% to 5%)

(Continued)

Epirubicin *(Continued)*

Dermatologic: Rash (1% to 9%), skin changes (0.7% to 5%)

Gastrointestinal: Anorexia (2% to 3%)

Other reactions (percentage not specified): Acute lymphoid leukemia, acute myelogenous leukemia (0.2% at 3 years), anaphylaxis, hypersensitivity, photosensitivity reaction, premature menopause in women, pulmonary embolism, radiation recall, skin and nail hyperpigmentation, thromboembolic phenomena, thrombophlebitis, transaminases increased, urticaria

Vesicant Yes

Emetic Potential High (60% to 90%)

Overdosage/Toxicology Symptoms of overdose are generally extensions of known cytotoxic effects, including myelosuppression, mucositis, gastrointestinal bleeding, lactic acidosis, multiple organ failure, and death. Treatment is supportive.

Drug Interactions

Increased Effect/Toxicity: Cimetidine increased the blood levels of epirubicin (AUC increased by 50%).

Ethanol/Nutrition/Herb Interactions

Ethanol: Avoid ethanol (due to GI irritation).

Herb/Nutraceutical: St John's wort may decrease doxorubicin levels. Avoid black cohosh, dong quai in estrogen-dependent tumors.

Storage/Stability Store refrigerated (2°C to 8°C/36°F to 46°F). Protect from light. Solution should be used within 24 hours.

Reconstitution May administer undiluted for IVP or dilute in 50-250 mL NS or D_5W for infusion.

Compatibility Stable in D_5W, LR, NS; **incompatible** with heparin, fluorouracil, or any solution of alkaline pH

Compatibility in syringe: Compatible: Ifosfamide. **Incompatible:** Fluorouracil, ifosfamide with mesna, any solution of alkaline pH

Pharmacodynamics/Kinetics

Distribution: V_{ss} 21-27 L/kg

Protein binding: 77% to albumin

Metabolism: Extensively via hepatic and extrahepatic (including RBCs) routes

Half-life elimination: Triphasic; Mean terminal: 33 hours

Excretion: Feces; urine (lesser extent)

Dosage Adults: I.V.: 100-120 mg/m² once every 3-4 weeks **or** 50-60 mg/m² days 1 and 8 every 3-4 weeks

Breast cancer:

CEF-120: 60 mg/m² on days 1 and 8 every 28 days for 6 cycles

FEC-100: 100 mg/m² on day 1 every 21 days for 6 cycles

Note: Note: Patients receiving 120 mg/m²/cycle as part of combination therapy should also receive prophylactic therapy with sulfamethoxazole/trimethoprim or a fluoroquinolone.

Dosage modifications:

Delay day 1 dose until platelets are ≥100,000/mm³, ANC ≥1500/mm³, and nonhematologic toxicities have recovered to ≤grade 1

Reduce day 1 dose in subsequent cycles to 75% of previous day 1 dose if patient experiences nadir platelet counts <50,000/mm³, ANC <250/mm³, neutropenic fever, or grade 3/4 nonhematologic toxicity during the previous cycle

For divided doses (day 1 and day 8), reduce day 8 dose to 75% of day 1 dose if platelet counts are 75,000-100,000/mm^3 and ANC is 1000-1499/mm^3; omit day 8 dose if platelets are <75,000/mm^3, ANC <1000/mm^3, or grade 3/4 nonhematologic toxicity

Dosage adjustment in bone marrow dysfunction: Heavily-treated patients, patients with pre-existing bone marrow depression or neoplastic bone marrow infiltration: Lower starting doses (75-90 mg/mm^2) should be considered.

Elderly: Plasma clearance of epirubicin in elderly female patients was noted to be reduced by 35%. Although no initial dosage reduction is specifically recommended, particular care should be exercised in monitoring toxicity and adjusting subsequent dosage in elderly patients (particularly females >70 years of age).

Dosage adjustment in renal impairment: Severe renal impairment (serum creatinine >5 mg/dL): Lower doses should be considered

Dosage adjustment in hepatic impairment:
Bilirubin 1.2-3 mg/dL or AST 2-4 times the upper limit of normal: 50% of recommended starting dose
Bilirubin >3 mg/dL or AST >4 times the upper limit of normal: 25% of recommended starting dose

Combination Regimens
Breast cancer:
CEF *on page 857*
FEC *on page 888*
Tamoxifen-Epirubicin *on page 939*
Gastric cancer: ECF *on page 875*
Rhabdomyosarcoma: CEV *on page 857*

Administration I.V.: The manufacturer recommends that starting doses of 100-120 mg/m^2 should be infused over 15-20 minutes; lower doses may be pushed into the tubing of a free flowing intravenous infusion (NS or D$_5$W) over 3-10 minutes.

Dosage Forms Injection, solution [preservative free]: 2 mg/mL (25 mL, 100 mL)

Monitoring Parameters Monitor injection site during infusion for possible extravasation or local reactions; CBC with differential and platelet count, liver function tests, renal function, ECG, and left ventricular ejection fraction

Patient Information Report any stinging or change in sensation during the infusion. This medication can only be administered I.V. During therapy, do not use alcohol, aspirin-containing products, and OTC medications without consulting prescriber. It is important to maintain adequate nutrition and hydration (2-3 L/day of fluids unless instructed to restrict fluid intake) during therapy; frequent small meals may help. You may experience nausea or vomiting (frequent small meals, frequent mouth care, sucking lozenges, or chewing gum may help). You may experience loss of hair (reversible); you will be more susceptible to infection (avoid crowds and exposure to infection as much as possible). Yogurt or buttermilk may help reduce diarrhea (if unresolved, contact prescriber for medication relief). Frequent mouth care and use of a soft toothbrush or cotton swabs may reduce mouth sores. May discolor urine (red/pink). Report fever, chills, unusual bruising or bleeding, signs of infection, abdominal pain or blood in stools, excessive fatigue, yellowing of eyes or skin, (Continued)

Epirubicin *(Continued)*

swelling of extremities, difficulty breathing, or unresolved diarrhea. Barrier contraceptive measures are recommended for both males and females while receiving this drug and for at least one month following administration. Risks of treatment include irreversible heart damage, treatment-related leukemia, and premature menopause in women.

Selected Readings

Coukell AJ and Faulds D, "Epirubicin. An Updated Review of Its Pharmacodynamic and Pharmacokinetic Properties and Therapeutic Efficacy in the Management of Breast Cancer," *Drugs*, 1997, 53(3):453-82.

Gluck S, "The Expanding Role of Epirubicin in the Treatment of Breast Cancer," *Cancer Control*, 2002, 9(2 Suppl):16-27.

Onrust SV, Wiseman LR, and Goa KL, "Epirubicin: A Review of Its Intravesical Use in Superficial Bladder Cancer," *Drugs Aging*, 1999, 15(4):307-33.

Trudeau M and Pagani O, "Epirubicin in Combination With the Taxanes," *Semin Oncol*, 2001, 28(4 Suppl 12):41-50.

♦ **EPO** *see Epoetin Alfa on page 302*

Epoetin Alfa (e POE e tin AL fa)

Medication Safety Issues

Sound-alike/look-alike issues:

Epogen® may be confused with Neupogen®

U.S. Brand Names Epogen®; Procrit®

Canadian Brand Names Eprex®

Generic Available No

Synonyms EPO; Erythropoietin; rHuEPO-α

Pharmacologic Category Colony Stimulating Factor

Pregnancy Risk Factor C

Lactation Excretion in breast milk unknown/use caution

Use Treatment of anemia related to HIV therapy, chronic renal failure, and antineoplastic therapy; reduction of allogeneic blood transfusion for elective, noncardiac, nonvascular surgery

Unlabeled/Investigational Use Anemia associated with rheumatic disease; hypogenerative anemia of Rh hemolytic disease; sickle cell anemia; acute renal failure; Gaucher's disease; Castleman's disease; paroxysmal nocturnal hemoglobinuria; anemia of critical illness (limited documentation); anemia of prematurity

Mechanism of Action Induces erythropoiesis by stimulating the division and differentiation of committed erythroid progenitor cells; induces the release of reticulocytes from the bone marrow into the bloodstream, where they mature to erythrocytes. There is a dose response relationship with this effect. This results in an increase in reticulocyte counts followed by a rise in hematocrit and hemoglobin levels.

Labeled Contraindications Hypersensitivity to albumin (human) or mammalian cell-derived products; uncontrolled hypertension

Warnings/Precautions Use caution with history of seizures or hypertension; blood pressure should be controlled prior to start of therapy and monitored closely throughout treatment. Excessive rate of rise of hematocrit may be possibly associated with the exacerbation of hypertension or seizures; decrease the epoetin dose if the hemoglobin increase exceeds 1 g/dL in any 2-week period. Use caution in patients at risk for thrombosis or with history of cardiovascular disease. Increased mortality has occurred when aggressive dosing is used in CHF or anginal patients undergoing hemodialysis.

Pure red cell aplasia (PRCA) with neutralizing antibodies to erythropoietin has been reported in limited patients treated with recombinant products; may occur more in patients with CRF.

Prior to and during therapy iron stores must be evaluated. Iron supplementation should be given during therapy.

Use caution with porphyria. Not recommended for acute correction of severe anemia or as a substitute for transfusion.

Adverse Reactions
>10%:
   Cardiovascular: Hypertension
   Central nervous system: Headache, fever
   Gastrointestinal: Nausea
   Neuromuscular & skeletal: Arthralgias
1% to 10%:
   Cardiovascular: Edema, chest pain
   Central nervous system: Fatigue, seizure
   Gastrointestinal: Vomiting, diarrhea
   Hematologic: Clotted access
   Neuromuscular & skeletal: Asthenia
<1%: CVA, flu-like syndrome, hyperkalemia, hypersensitivity reactions, MI, rash, thrombosis, TIA

Vesicant No

Emetic Potential Very low (<10%)

Overdosage/Toxicology Symptoms of overdose include erythrocytosis. Maintain adequate airway and provide other supportive measures and agents for treating anaphylaxis when the I.V. drug is given.

Storage/Stability Vials should be stored at 2°C to 8°C (36°F to 46°F); **do not freeze or shake**.

Single-dose 1 mL vial contains no preservative: Use one dose per vial; do not re-enter vial; discard unused portions.

   Single-use vials (except 40,000 units/mL vial) are stable for 2 weeks at room temperature; single-dose 40,000 units/mL vial is stable for 1 week at room temperature.

Multidose 1 mL or 2 mL vial contains preservative; store at 2°C to 8°C after initial entry and between doses; discard 21 days after initial entry. Multidose vials (with preservative) are stable for 1 week at room temperature.

   Dilutions of 1:10 and 1:20 (1 part epoetin:19 parts sodium chloride) are stable for 18 hours at room temperature.

Reconstitution Mix with 20 mL bacteriostatic 0.9% sodium chloride.

Compatibility Stable in $D_{10}W$ with albumin 0.05%, $D_{10}W$ with albumin 0.1%; not stable in $D_{10}W$ with albumin 0.01%, $D_{10}W$, NS; **variable stability (consult detailed reference)** in TPN

Pharmacodynamics/Kinetics
Onset of action: Several days
   Peak effect: 2-3 weeks
Distribution: V_d: 9 L; rapid in the plasma compartment; concentrated in liver, kidneys, and bone marrow
Metabolism: Some degradation does occur
(Continued)

Epoetin Alfa *(Continued)*

Bioavailability: SubQ: ~21% to 31%; intraperitoneal epoetin: 3% (a few patients)

Half-life elimination: Circulating: Chronic renal failure: 4-13 hours; Healthy volunteers: 20% shorter

Time to peak, serum: SubQ: Chronic renal failure: 5-24 hours

Excretion: Feces (majority); urine (small amounts, 10% unchanged in normal volunteers)

Dosage

Chronic renal failure patients: I.V., SubQ:

Children: Initial dose: 50 units/kg 3 times/week

Adults: Initial dose: 50-100 units/kg 3 times/week

Dose adjustment: Children and Adults: Reduce dose by 25% when hemoglobin approaches 12 g/dL **or** hemoglobin increases 1 g/dL in any 2-week period. Increase dose by 25% if hemoglobin does not increase by 2 g/dL after 8 weeks of therapy and hemoglobin is below suggested target range. Suggested target hemoglobin range: 10-12 g/dL.

Maintenance dose: Individualize to target range; limit additional dosage increases to every 4 weeks (or longer)

Dialysis patients: Median dose:

Children: 167 units/kg/week **or** 76 units/kg 2-3 times/week

Adults: 75 units/kg 3 times/week

Nondialysis patients:

Children: Dosing range: 50-250 units/kg 1-3 times/week

Adults: Median dose: 75-150 units/kg

Zidovudine-treated, HIV-infected patients (patients with erythropoietin levels >500 mU/mL are **unlikely** to respond): I.V., SubQ:

Children: Initial dose: Reported dosing range: 50-400 units/kg 2-3 times/week

Adults: 100 units/kg 3 times/week for 8 weeks. **Dose adjustment:** Increase dose by 50-100 units/kg 3 times/week if response is not satisfactory in terms of reducing transfusion requirements or increasing hemoglobin after 8 weeks of therapy. Evaluate response every 4-8 weeks thereafter and adjust the dose accordingly by 50-100 units/kg increments 3 times/week. If patient has not responded satisfactorily to a 300 unit/kg dose 3 times/week, a response to higher doses is unlikely. Stop dose if hemoglobin exceeds 13 g/dL and resume treatment at a 25% dose reduction when hemoglobin drops to 12 g/dL.

Cancer patient on chemotherapy: Treatment of patients with erythropoietin levels >200 mU/mL is **not recommended**

Children: I.V., SubQ: Dosing range: 25-300 units/kg 3-7 times/week; commonly reported initial dose: 150 units/kg

Adults: SubQ: Initial dose: 150 units/kg 3 times/week or 40,000 units once weekly; commonly used doses range from 10,000 units 3 times/week to 40,000-60,000 units once weekly.

Dose adjustment: Children and Adults: If response is not satisfactory after a sufficient period of evaluation (8 weeks of 3 times/week and 4 weeks of once-weekly therapy), the dose may be increased every 4 weeks (or longer) up to 300 units/kg 3 times/week, **or** when dosed weekly, increased all at once to 60,000 units weekly. If patient does not respond, a response to higher doses is unlikely. Stop dose if hemoglobin exceeds 13 g/dL and resume treatment at a 25% dose reduction when hemoglobin drops to 12 g/dL; reduce dose by 25% if hemoglobin increases by 1 g/dL in any 2-week period, or if hemoglobin approaches 12 g/dL.

Alternative dose (unlabeled dosing): Adults: SubQ: Initial dose: 60,000 units once weekly for 8 weeks. **Dose adjustment:** If patient does not respond, a response to higher doses is unlikely. If response is adequate (hemoglobin increases >2 g/dL after 8 weeks), begin maintenance dose of 120,000 units, to be given once every 3 weeks. During any point of initial or maintenance therapy, if the hemoglobin increases 1.3 g/dL in a 2-week period, decrease dose to 40,000 units once weekly. Stop dose if hemoglobin exceeds 15 g/dL and resume treatment at 20,000 units once-weekly when hemoglobin drops to 13 g/dL (Patton, 2003).

Surgery patients: Prior to initiating treatment, obtain a hemoglobin to establish that is >10 mg/dL or ≤13 mg/dL: Adults: SubQ: Initial dose: 300 units/kg/day for 10 days before surgery, on the day of surgery, and for 4 days after surgery

Alternative dose: 600 units/kg in once weekly doses (21, 14, and 7 days before surgery) plus a fourth dose on the day of surgery

Anemia of critical illness (unlabeled use): Adults: SubQ: 40,000 units once weekly

Anemia of prematurity (unlabeled use): Infants: I.V., SubQ: Dosing range: 500-1250 units/kg/week; commonly used dose: 250 units/kg 3 times/ week; supplement with oral iron therapy 3-8 mg/kg/day

Dosage adjustment in renal impairment:

Dialysis patient: Usually administered as I.V. bolus 3 times/week. While administration is independent of the dialysis procedure, it may be administered into the venous line at the end of the dialysis procedure to obviate the need for additional venous access.

Chronic renal failure patients not on dialysis: May be given either as an I.V. or SubQ injection.

Hemodialysis: Supplemental dose is not necessary.

Peritoneal dialysis: Supplemental dose is not necessary.

Administration SubQ, I.M., I.V. (not recommended; I.V. administration may require up to 40% more drug as SubQ/I.M. administration to achieve the same therapeutic result)

Patients with CRF on dialysis: May be administered I.V. bolus into the venous line after dialysis.

Patients with CRF not on dialysis: May be administered I.V. or SubQ

Dosage Forms

Injection, solution [preservative free]: 2000 units/mL (1 mL); 3000 units/ mL (1 mL); 4000 units/mL (1 mL); 10,000 units/mL (1 mL); 40,000 units/ mL (1 mL) [contains human albumin]

Injection, solution [with preservative]: 10,000 units/mL (2 mL); 20,000 units/mL (1 mL) [contains human albumin and benzyl alcohol]

Monitoring Parameters Blood pressure; hemoglobin/hematocrit

Hematocrit should be determined twice weekly until stabilization within the target range (30% to 36%), and twice weekly for at least 2-6 weeks after a dose increase.

Patient Information You will require blood tests to determine appropriate dosage. Do not take other medications, vitamin or iron supplements, or make significant changes in your diet without consulting prescriber. (Continued)

Epoetin Alfa *(Continued)*

Report signs or symptoms of edema (eg, swollen extremities, difficulty breathing, rapid weight gain), onset of severe headache, acute back pain, chest pain, muscular tremors, or seizure activity.

Additional Information Due to the delayed onset of erythropoiesis (7-10 days to increase reticulocyte count; 2-6 weeks to increase hemoglobin), erythropoietin is of no value in the acute treatment of anemia. Emergency/stat orders for erythropoietin are inappropriate.

Factors Limiting Response to Epoetin Alfa

Factor	Mechanism
Iron deficiency	Limits hemoglobin synthesis
Blood loss/hemolysis	Counteracts epoetin alfa-stimulated erythropoiesis
Infection/inflammation	Inhibits iron transfer from storage to bone marrow
	Suppresses erythropoiesis through activated macrophages
Aluminum overload	Inhibits iron incorporation into heme protein
Bone marrow replacement Hyperparathyroidism Metastatic, neoplastic	Limits bone marrow volume
Folic acid/vitamin B_{12} deficiency	Limits hemoglobin synthesis
Patient compliance	Self-administered epoetin alfa or iron therapy

Professional Services:
Amgen (Epogen®): 1-800-772-6436
Ortho Biotech (Procrit®): 1-800-325-7504
Reimbursement Assistance:
Amgen: 1-800-272-9376
Ortho Biotech: 1-800-553-3851

Special Geriatric Considerations There is limited information about the use of epoetin alfa in the elderly. Endogenous erythropoietin secretion has been reported to be decreased in older adults with normocytic or iron-deficiency anemias or those with a serum hemoglobin concentration <12 g/dL; one study did not find such a relationship in the elderly with chronic anemia. A blunted erythropoietin response to anemia has been reported in patients with cancer, rheumatoid arthritis, and AIDS.

Selected Readings

Blanche S, Caniglia M, Fischer A, et al, "Zidovudine Therapy in Children With Acquired Immunodeficiency Syndrome," *Am J Med*, 1988, 85(2A):203-7.

Brown KR, Carter W Jr, and Lombardi GE, "Recombinant Erythropoietin Overdose," *Am J Emerg Med*, 1993, 11(6):619-21.

Brown MS and Keith JF 3rd, "Comparison Between Two and Five Doses a Week of Recombinant Human Erythropoietin for Anemia of Prematurity: A Randomized Trial," *Pediatrics*, 1999, 104(2 Pt 1):210-5.

Carpenter MA, Kendall RG, O'Brien AE, et al, "Reduced Erythropoietin Response to Anaemia in Elderly Patients With Normocytic Anaemia," *Eur J Haematol*, 1992, 49(3):119-21.

Corwin HL, Gettinger A, Pearl RG, et al, "Efficacy of Recombinant Human Erythropoietin in Critically Ill Patients: A Randomized Controlled Trial," *JAMA*, 2002, 288(22):2827-35.

Donato H, Vain N, Rendo P, et al, "Effect of Early Versus Late Administration of Human Recombinant Erythropoietin on Transfusion Requirements in Premature Infants: Results of a Randomized, Placebo-Controlled, Multicenter Trial," *Pediatrics*, 2000, 105(5):1066-72.

Erslev AJ, "Erythropoietin," *N Engl J Med*, 1991, 324(19):1339-44.

Feusner J and Hastings C, "Recombinant Human Erythropoietin in Pediatric Oncology: A Review," *Med Pediatr Oncol*, 2002, 39(4):463-8.

Gareau R, Gagnon MG, Thellend C, et al, "Transferrin Soluble Receptor: A Possible Probe for Detection of Erythropoietin Abuse by Athletes," *Horm Metab Res*, 1994, 26(6):311-2.

Goodnough LT, Price TH, Parvin CA, "The Indigenous Erythropoietin Response and the Erythropoietic Response to Blood Loss Anemia: The Effects of Age and Gender," *J Lab Clin Med*, 1995, 126(1):57-64.

Halperin DS, Wacker P, Lacourt G, et al, "Effects of Recombinant Human Erythropoietin in Infants With the Anemia of Prematurity: A Pilot Study," *J Pediatr*, 1990, 116(5):779-86.

Hebert PC, Wells G, Blajchman MA, et al, "A Multicenter, Randomized, Controlled Clinical Trial of Transfusion Requirements in Critical Care. Transfusion Requirements in Critical Care Investigators, Canadian Critical Care Trials Group," *N Engl J Med*, 1999, 340(6):409-17.

Henry DH, "Recombinant Human Erythropoietin Treatment of Anemic Cancer Patients," *Cancer Pract*, 1996, 4(4):180-4.

Henry DH and Spivak JL, "Clinical Use of Erythropoietin," *Curr Opin Hematol*, 1995, 2(2):118-24.

Henry DH and Thatcher N, "Patient Selection and Predicting Response to Recombinant Human Erythropoietin in Anemic Cancer Patients," *Semin Hematol*, 1996, 33(1 Suppl 1):2-5.

Joosten E, Van Hove L, Lesaffre E, et al, "Serum Erythropoietin Levels in Elderly Inpatients With Anemia of Chronic Disorders and Iron Deficiency Anemia," *J Am Geriatr Soc*, 1993, 41(12):1301-4.

Juul SE and Christensen RD, "Absorption of Enteral Recombinant Human Erythropoietin By Neonates," *Ann Pharmacother*, 2003, 37(6):782-6.

Kario K, Matsuo T, and Nakao K, "Serum Erythropoietin Levels in the Elderly," *Gerontology*, 1991, 37(6):345-8.

MacDougall IC, "Adverse Reactions Profile: Erythropoietin in Chronic Renal Failure," *Prescribers J*, 1992, 32:40-4.

Maier RF, Obladen M, Muller-Hansen I, et al, "Early Treatment With Erythropoietin Beta Ameliorates Anemia and Reduces Transfusion Requirements in Infants With Birth Weights Below 1000 g," *J Pediatr*, 2002, 141(1):8-15.

Means RT Jr, "Erythropoietin in the Treatment of Anemia in Chronic Infectious, Inflammatory, and Malignant Diseases," *Curr Opin Hematol*, 1995, 2(3):210-3.

Nafziger J, Pailla K, Luciani L, et al, "Decreased Erythropoietin Responsiveness to Iron Deficiency Anemia in the Elderly," *Am J Hematol*, 1993, 43(3):172-6.

Ohls RK and Christensen, RD, "Stability of Human Recombinant Epoetin Alfa in Commonly Used Neonatal Intravenous Solutions," *Ann Pharmacother*, 1996, 30(5):466-468.

Ohls RK, Ehrenkranz RA, Wright LL, et al, "Effects of Early Erythropoietin Therapy on the Transfusion Requirements of Preterm Infants Below 1250 Grams Birth Weight: A Multicenter, Randomized, Controlled Trial," *Pediatrics*, 2001, 108(4):934-42.

Ohls RK, Veerman MW, and Christensen RD, "Pharmacokinetics and Effectiveness of Recombinant Erythropoietin Administered to Preterm Infants by Continuous Infusion in Total Parenteral Nutrition Solution," *J Pediatr*, 1996, 128(4):518-23.

Patton J, Kuzur M, Liggett W, et al, "Epoetin Alfa 60,000 U Once Weekly Followed by 120,000 U Every 3 Weeks Increases and Maintains Hemoglobin Levels in Anemic Cancer Patients Undergoing Chemotherapy," *Oncologist*, 2004, 9(1):90-6.

Powers JS, Krantz SB, Collins JC, et al, "Erythropoietin Response to Anemia as a Function of Age," *J Am Geriatr Soc*, 1991, 39(1):30-2.

Rhondeau SM, Christensen RD, Ross MP, et al, "Responsiveness to Recombinant Human Erythropoietin of Marrow Erythroid Progenitors From Infants With the Anemia of Prematurity," *J Pediatr*, 1988, 112(6):935-40.

Rubins J, "Metastatic Renal Cell Carcinoma: Response to Treatment With Human Recombinant Erythropoietin," *Ann Intern Med*, 1995, 122(9):676-7.

Schwenk MH and Halstenson CE, "Recombinant Human Erythropoietin," *DICP*, 1989, 23(7-8):528-36.

Shannon KM, Keith JF 3rd, Mentzer WC, et al, "Recombinant Human Erythropoietin Stimulates Erythropoiesis and Reduces Erythrocyte Transfusions in Very Low Birth Weight Preterm Infants," *Pediatrics*, 1995, 95(1):1-8.

(Continued)

Epoetin Alfa *(Continued)*

Sinai-Trieman L, Salusky IB, and Fine RN, "Use of Subcutaneous Recombinant Human Erythropoietin in Children Undergoing Continuous Cycling Peritoneal Dialysis," *J Pediatr*, 1989, 114(4 Pt 1):550-4.

Steinberg H, "Erythropoietin and Visual Hallucinations," *N Engl J Med*, 1991, 325(4):285.

Weinthal JA, "The Role of Cytokines Following Bone Marrow Transplantation: Indications and Controversies," *Bone Marrow Transplant*, 1996, 18(Suppl 3):10-4.

Erslev AJ, "Erythropoietin," *N Engl J Med*, 1991, 324(19):1339-44.

Feusner J and Hastings C, "Recombinant Human Erythropoietin in Pediatric Oncology: A Review," *Med Pediatr Oncol*, 2002, 39(4):463-8.

Henry DH, "Recombinant Human Erythropoietin Treatment of Anemic Cancer Patients," *Cancer Pract*, 1996, 4(4):180-4.

Henry DH and Spivak JL, "Clinical Use of Erythropoietin," *Curr Opin Hematol*, 1995, 2(2):118-24.

MacDougall IC, "Adverse Reactions Profile: Erythropoietin in Chronic Renal Failure," *Prescribers J*, 1992, 32:40-4.

♦ **Epogen®** *see Epoetin Alfa on page 302*

♦ **Eprex® (Can)** *see Epoetin Alfa on page 302*

♦ **Epsilon Aminocaproic Acid** *see Aminocaproic Acid on page 61*

♦ **EPT** *see Teniposide on page 754*

♦ **Eptacog Alfa (Activated)** *see Factor VIIa (Recombinant) on page 326*

♦ **Erbitux™** *see Cetuximab on page 172*

Erlotinib (er LOE tye nib)

U.S. Brand Names Tarceva™

Generic Available No

Synonyms CP358774; Erlotinib Hydrochloride; NSC-718781; OSI-774; R 14-15

Pharmacologic Category Antineoplastic Agent, Tyrosine Kinase Inhibitor; Epidermal Growth Factor Receptor (EGFR) Inhibitor

Pregnancy Risk Factor D

Lactation Excretion in breast milk unknown/not recommended

Use Salvage therapy of advanced or metastatic nonsmall-cell lung cancer

Unlabeled/Investigational Use Salvage therapy of advanced or metastatic breast, colorectal, and head and neck tumors

Mechanism of Action The mechanism of erlotinib's antitumor action is not fully characterized. The drug is known to inhibit overall epidermal growth factor receptor (HER1/EGFR)- tyrosine kinase. Active competitive inhibition of adenosine triphosphate inhibits downstream signal transduction of ligand dependent HER1/EGFR activation.

Labeled Contraindications Hypersensitivity to erlotinib or any component of the formulation; pregnancy

Warnings/Precautions Hazardous agent - use appropriate precautions for handling and disposal. See Safe Handling of Hazardous Drugs *on page 1034* in the Appendix. Rare, sometimes fatal, pulmonary toxicity (interstitial pneumonia, interstitial lung disease, obliterative bronchiolitis, pulmonary fibrosis) has occurred; an interruption of therapy should occur with unexplained pulmonary symptoms (dyspnea, cough, and fever); use caution in hepatic or severe renal impairment. Safety and efficacy in pediatric patients have not been established.

Adverse Reactions

>10%:

Central nervous system: Fatigue (14% to 55%), anxiety (21%), headache (17%), depression (16%), insomnia (12%)

Dermatologic: Acneiform rash (50% to 88%), pruritus (13% to 55%), dry skin (12% to 35%), erythema (18%)

Gastrointestinal: Diarrhea (30% to 56%), anorexia (23% to 52%), nausea (11% to 33%), vomiting (23%), mucositis (17% to 18%), glossodynia (18%), xerostomia (17%), pain (14%), constipation (12%), dyspepsia (12%), dysphagia (12%), weight loss (12%), abnormal taste (11%), abdominal pain (11%)

Hepatic: Hyperbilirubinemia (20%)

Neuromuscular & Skeletal: Arthralgia (14%), paresthesia (11%)

Ocular: Conjunctivitis (12%), keratoconjunctivitis sicca (12%)

Respiratory: Dyspnea (21% to 41%), cough (16% to 33%)

Miscellaneous: Infection (24%)

1% to 10%:

Hepatic: Liver function test abnormalities (4%)

Ocular: Keratitis (6%)

Respiratory: Pneumonitis (6%)

<1%: Corneal ulcerations, gastrointestinal bleeding, interstitial lung disease-related events

Overdosage/Toxicology Specific overdose-related toxicities include diarrhea, rash, and liver transaminase elevation. Overdose management should include withdrawal of erlotinib, and symptom-based and supportive treatment.

Drug Interactions

Cytochrome P450 Effect: Substrate of CYP1A2 (minor), 3A4 (major)

Increased Effect/Toxicity: Ketoconazole and CYP3A4 inhibitors may increase erlotinib levels/effects; example inhibitors include azole antifungals, ciprofloxacin, clarithromycin, diclofenac, doxycycline, erythromycin, imatinib, isoniazid, nefazodone, nicardipine, propofol, protease inhibitors, quinidine, and verapamil.

Decreased Effect: Rifamycins and CYP3A4 inducers may decrease erlotinib levels/effects; example inducers include aminoglutethimide, carbamazepine, nafcillin, nevirapine, phenobarbital, and phenytoin.

Ethanol/Nutrition/Herb Interactions

Herb/Nutraceutical: Avoid St John's wort (may increase metabolism and decrease erlotinib concentrations).

Storage/Stability Store at room temperature between 15°C and 30°C (59°F and 86°F).

Pharmacodynamics/Kinetics

Absorption: Oral: 60% on an empty stomach; ~100% on a full stomach

Distribution: 94-232 L

Protein binding: 92% to 95%, albumin and α_1-acid glycoprotein

Metabolism: Hepatic, CYP3A4 (major), CYP1A1 (minor), CYP1A2 (minor), and CYP1C (minor)

Bioavailability: 100% when given with food

Half-life elimination: 24-36 hours

Time to peak, plasma: 1-7 hours

Excretion: Primarily as metabolites: Feces (83%); urine (8%)

Dosage Oral: Adults: 150 mg/day until disease progression or unacceptable toxicity occurs; dose reduction (if required) should be done in increments of 50 mg

Note: Dose reductions are more likely to be needed when erlotinib is administered concomitantly with strong CYP3A4 inhibitors. Likewise, the CYP3A4 inducers may require increased doses; doses of >150

(Continued)

Erlotinib *(Continued)*

mg/day should be considered with rifampin. (Note: See Drug Interactions for examples of CYP3A4 inhibitors and inducers).

Dosage adjustment for toxicity: Patients experiencing poorly-tolerated diarrhea or a severe skin reaction may benefit from a brief therapy interruption. Patients experiencing acute onset (or worsening) of pulmonary symptoms should have therapy interrupted and be evaluated for drug-induced interstitial lung disease.

Dosage adjustment in hepatic impairment: Dose reduction or interruption should be considered if liver function changes are severe.

Administration The manufacturer recommends administration on an empty stomach (at least 1 hour before or 2 hours after the ingestion of food) even though this reduces drug absorption by approximately 40%. Administration after a meal results in nearly 100% absorption.

Dosage Forms Tablet: 25 mg, 100 mg, 150 mg

Monitoring Parameters Periodic liver function tests (asymptomatic increases in liver enzymes have occurred)

Special Geriatric Considerations In clinical trials, there was no significant difference between older and younger adults in survival benefit, safety, or pharmacokinetics. No dosage adjustment necessary in elderly patients.

Selected Readings

Bonomi P, "Erlotinib: A New Therapeutic Approach for Non-Small Cell Lung Cancer," *Expert Opin Investig Drugs*, 2003, 12(8):1395-401.

Bulgaru AM, Mani S, Goel S, et al, "Erlotinib (Tarceva): A Promising Drug Targeting Epidermal Growth Factor Receptor Tyrosine Kinase," *Expert Rev Anticancer Ther*, 2003, 3(3):269-79.

Hidalgo M and Bloedow D, "Pharmacokinetics and Pharmacodynamics: Maximizing the Clinical Potential of Erlotinib (Tarceva)," *Semin Oncol*, 2003, 30(3 Suppl 7):25-33.

♦ **Erlotinib Hydrochloride** *see Erlotinib on page 308*

♦ *Erwinia* **Asparaginase** *see Asparaginase on page 106*

♦ **Erythropoietin** *see Epoetin Alfa on page 302*

Estramustine *(es tra MUS teen)*

Medication Safety Issues

Sound-alike/look-alike issues:

Emcyt® may be confused with Eryc®

Related Information

Safe Handling of Hazardous Drugs *on page 1034*

U.S. Brand Names Emcyt®

Canadian Brand Names Emcyt®

Generic Available No

Synonyms Estramustine Phosphate Sodium; NSC-89199

Pharmacologic Category Antineoplastic Agent, Alkylating Agent; Antineoplastic Agent, Hormone; Antineoplastic Agent, Hormone (Estrogen/ Nitrogen Mustard)

Pregnancy Risk Factor C

Lactation Excretion in breast milk unknown/contraindicated

Use Palliative treatment of prostatic carcinoma (progressive or metastatic)

Mechanism of Action Mechanism is not completely clear. It appears to bind to microtubule proteins, preventing normal tubulin function. The antitumor effect may be due solely to an estrogenic effect. Estramustine causes a marked decrease in plasma testosterone and an increase in estrogen levels.

Labeled Contraindications Hypersensitivity to estramustine or any component, estradiol or nitrogen mustard; active thrombophlebitis or thromboembolic disorders

Warnings/Precautions Hazardous agent - use appropriate precautions for handling and disposal. See Safe Handling of Hazardous Drugs *on page 1034* in the Appendix. Glucose tolerance may be decreased; elevated blood pressure may occur. Exacerbation of peripheral edema or congestive heart disease may occur. Use with caution in patients with impaired liver function, renal insufficiency, metabolic bone diseases, or history of cardiovascular disease (eg, thrombophlebitis, thrombosis, or thromboembolic disease). Patients with prostate cancer and osteoblastic metastases should have their calcium monitored regularly.

Adverse Reactions
>10%:
  Cardiovascular: Impaired arterial circulation; ischemic heart disease; venous thromboembolism; cardiac decompensation (58%), about 50% of complications occur within the first 2 months of therapy, 85% occur within the first year; edema
  Endocrine & metabolic: Sodium and water retention, gynecomastia, breast tenderness, libido decreased
  Gastrointestinal: Nausea, vomiting, may be dose-limiting
  Hematologic: Thrombocytopenia
  Local: Thrombophlebitis (nearly 100% with I.V. administration)
  Respiratory: Dyspnea
1% to 10%:
  Cardiovascular: Myocardial infarction
  Central nervous system: Insomnia, lethargy
  Gastrointestinal: Diarrhea, anorexia, flatulence
  Hematologic: Leukopenia
  Hepatic: Serum transaminases increased, jaundice
  Neuromuscular & skeletal: Leg cramps
  Respiratory: Pulmonary embolism
<1%: Allergic reactions, angioedema, cardiac arrest, depression, gynecomastia, hypercalcemia, hyperpigmentation, hot flashes, impotence, rash, urticaria

Emetic Potential Moderate (10% to 60%)

Overdosage/Toxicology Symptoms of overdose include nausea, vomiting, and myelosuppression. There are no known antidotes; treatment is symptomatic and supportive.

Drug Interactions
  Decreased Effect: Milk products and calcium-rich foods/drugs may impair the oral absorption of estramustine phosphate sodium.

Ethanol/Nutrition/Herb Interactions Food: Estramustine serum levels may be decreased if taken with dairy products.

Storage/Stability Refrigerate at 2°C to 8°C (36°F to 46°F). Capsules may be stored outside of refrigerator for up to 24-48 hours without affecting potency.

Pharmacodynamics/Kinetics
  Absorption: Oral: 75%
  Metabolism:
  GI tract: Initial dephosphorylation

(Continued)

311

Estramustine *(Continued)*

Hepatic: Oxidation and hydrolysis; metabolites include estramustine, estrone, estradiol, nitrogen mustard

Half-life elimination: Terminal: 20-24 hours

Time to peak, serum: 2-3 hours

Excretion: Feces (2.9% to 4.8% as unchanged drug)

Dosage Refer to individual protocols.

Oral: 10-16 mg/kg/day (14 mg/kg/day is most common) or 140 mg 4 times/day (some patients have been maintained for >3 years on therapy)

Combination Regimens

Prostate cancer:

Cyclophosphamide + Estramustine *on page 870*

Doxorubicin + Ketoconazole/Estramustine + Vinblastine *on page 874*

Estramustine + Docetaxel *on page 881*

Estramustine + Docetaxel + Carboplatin *on page 882*

Estramustine + Docetaxel + Hydrocortisone *on page 882*

Estramustine + Etoposide *on page 882*

Estramustine + Vinorelbine *on page 883*

EV *on page 883*

Paclitaxel + Estramustine + Carboplatin *on page 926*

Paclitaxel + Estramustine + Etoposide *on page 926*

PE *on page 928*

Administration Oral: Administer on an empty stomach, at least 1 hour before or 2 hours after eating.

Dosage Forms Capsule, as phosphate sodium: 140 mg

Monitoring Parameters Serum calcium, liver function tests

Dietary Considerations Should be taken at least 1 hour before or 2 hours after eating.

Patient Information It may take several weeks to manifest effects of this medication. Store capsules in refrigerator. Do not take with milk or milk products. Preferable to take on empty stomach (1 hour before or 2 hours after meals). Small frequent meals and frequent mouth care may reduce incidence of nausea or vomiting. You may experience flatulence, diarrhea, decreased libido (reversible), breast tenderness or enlargement. Report sudden acute pain or cramping in legs or calves, chest pain, shortness of breath, weakness or numbness of arms or legs, difficulty breathing, or edema (increased weight, swelling of legs or feet); contraceptive measures are recommended during therapy.

Selected Readings

Benson R and Hartley-Asp B, "Mechanisms of Action and Clinical Uses of Estramustine," *Cancer Invest*, 1990, 8(3-4):375-80.

Bergenheim AT and Henriksson R, "Pharmacokinetics and Pharmacodynamics of Estramustine Phosphate," *Clin Pharmacokinet*, 1998, 34(2):163-72.

Hudes GR, "Estramustine-Based Chemotherapy," *Semin Urol Oncol*, 1997, 15(1):13-9.

Kreis W, "Estramustine Revisited," *Cancer Treat Res*, 1995, 78:163-84.

Perry CM and McTavish D, "Estramustine Phosphate Sodium. A Review of Its Pharmacodynamic and Pharmacokinetic Properties, and Therapeutic Efficacy in Prostate Cancer," *Drugs Aging*, 1995, 7(1):49-74.

♦ **Estramustine Phosphate Sodium** *see* Estramustine *on page 310*

♦ **ETAF** *see* Aldesleukin *on page 32*

♦ **Ethiofos** *see* Amifostine *on page 53*

♦ **Ethoxynaphthamido Penicillin Sodium** *see* Nafcillin *on page 605*

♦ **Ethyol**® *see* Amifostine *on page 53*

Etidronate Disodium (e ti DROE nate dye SOW dee um)

Medication Safety Issues

Sound-alike/look-alike issues:

Etidronate may be confused with etidocaine, etomidate, etretinate

U.S. Brand Names Didronel®

Canadian Brand Names Didronel®; Gen-Etidronate

Generic Available No

Synonyms EHDP; Sodium Etidronate

Pharmacologic Category Bisphosphonate Derivative

Pregnancy Risk Factor C

Lactation Excretion in breast milk unknown/use caution

Use Symptomatic treatment of Paget's disease and heterotopic ossification due to spinal cord injury or after total hip replacement, hypercalcemia associated with malignancy

Mechanism of Action Decreases bone resorption by inhibiting osteocystic osteolysis; decreases mineral release and matrix or collagen breakdown in bone

Labeled Contraindications Hypersensitivity to bisphosphonates or any component of the formulation; serum creatinine >5 mg/dL

Warnings/Precautions Use with caution in patients with restricted calcium and vitamin D intake; dosage modification required in renal impairment; I.V. form may be nephrotoxic and should be used with caution, if at all, in patients with impaired renal function (serum creatinine: 2.5-4.9 mg/dL).

Adverse Reactions

>10%: Neuromuscular & skeletal: Bone pain (10% to 20%, Paget's)

1% to 10%:

Central nervous system: Fever (9%), convulsions (3%)

Endocrine & metabolic: Hypophosphatemia (3%), hypomagnesemia (3%), fluid overload (6%), hypercalcemia of malignancy

Gastrointestinal: Diarrhea and nausea (7% to 30%, dose related), constipation (3%), abnormal taste (3%)

Hepatic: LFT changes (3%)

Respiratory: Dyspnea (3%)

Renal: Increased serum creatinine (10%)

<1%: Pain, angioedema, rash, occult blood in stools, increased risk of fractures, nephrotoxicity, hypersensitivity reactions, urticaria

Postmarketing and/or case reports: Osteonecrosis

Vesicant No

Emetic Potential Low (10% to 30%)

Overdosage/Toxicology Symptoms of overdose include diarrhea, nausea, vomiting, paresthesias, tetany, and coma. Antidote is calcium.

Drug Interactions

Increased Effect/Toxicity: Foscarnet and plicamycin may have additive hypocalcemic effect.

Ethanol/Nutrition/Herb Interactions Food: Food decreases the absorption and bioavailability of the drug.

Storage/Stability Store ampuls at room temperature and avoid excess heat (>40°C/104°F); intravenous solution diluted in ≥250 mL normal saline is stable for 48 hours at room temperature or refrigerated

(Continued)

Etidronate Disodium *(Continued)*

Reconstitution I.V. doses should be diluted in at least 250 mL normal saline.

Pharmacodynamics/Kinetics

Onset of action: 1-3 months

Duration: Can persist for 12 months without continuous therapy

Absorption: Dose dependent

Metabolism: None

Excretion: Primarily urine (as unchanged drug); feces (as unabsorbed drug)

Dosage Adults: Oral formulation should be taken on an empty stomach 2 hours before any meal.

Paget's disease: Oral

Initial: 5-10 mg/kg/day (not to exceed 6 months) or 11-20 mg/kg/day (not to exceed 3 months). Doses >10 mg/kg/day are **not** recommended.

Retreatment: Initiate only after etidronate-free period ≥90 days. Monitor patients every 3-6 months. Retreatment regimens are the same as for initial treatment.

Heterotopic ossification: Oral:

Caused by spinal cord injury: 20 mg/kg/day for 2 weeks, then 10 mg/kg/day for 10 weeks; total treatment period: 12 weeks

Complicating total hip replacement: 20 mg/kg/day for 1 month preoperatively then 20 mg/kg/day for 3 months postoperatively; total treatment period is 4 months

Hypercalcemia associated with malignancy:

I.V. (dilute dose in at least 250 mL NS): 7.5 mg/kg/day for 3 days; there should be at least 7 days between courses of treatment

Oral: Start 20 mg/kg/day on the last day of infusion and continue for 30-90 days

Dosing adjustment in renal impairment:

S_{cr} 2.5-5 mg/dL: Use with caution

S_{cr} >5 mg/dL: **Not recommended**

Administration Administer intravenous dose over at least 2 hours; tablet should be administered on an empty stomach 2 hours before meals

Dosage Forms

Injection, solution: 50 mg/mL (6 mL)

Tablet: 200 mg, 400 mg

Monitoring Parameters Serum calcium and phosphorous; serum creatinine and BUN

Dietary Considerations Administer tablet with water, black coffee, tea, or fruit juice on an empty stomach; avoid administering foods/supplements with calcium, iron, or magnesium within 2 hours of drug; maintain adequate intake of calcium and vitamin D.

Selected Readings

Beauchesne MF and Miller PF, "Etidronate and Alendronate in the Treatment of Postmenopausal Osteoporosis," *Ann Pharmacother*, 1999, 33(5):587-99.

Horowitz E, Miller JL, and Rose LI, "Etidronate for Hypercalcemia of Malignancy and Osteoporosis," *Am Fam Physician*, 1991, 43(6):2155-9.

Krane SM, "Etidronate Disodium in the Treatment of Paget's Disease of Bone," *Ann Intern Med*, 1982, 96(5):619-25.

♦ **Etopophos**® *see* Etoposide Phosphate *on page 320*

Etoposide (e toe POE side)

Medication Safety Issues

Sound-alike/look-alike issues:

VePesid® may be confused with Versed

Related Information

Safe Handling of Hazardous Drugs *on page 1034*

Transplantation *on page 1019*

U.S. Brand Names Toposar®; VePesid®

Canadian Brand Names VePesid®

Generic Available Yes

Synonyms Epipodophyllotoxin; VP-16; VP-16-213

Pharmacologic Category Antineoplastic Agent, Podophyllotoxin Derivative

Pregnancy Risk Factor D

Lactation Enters breast milk/contraindicated

Use Treatment of lymphomas, ANLL, lung, testicular, bladder, and prostate carcinoma, hepatoma, rhabdomyosarcoma, uterine carcinoma, neuroblastoma, mycosis fungoides, Kaposi's sarcoma, histiocytosis, gestational trophoblastic disease, Ewing's sarcoma, Wilms' tumor, and brain tumors

Mechanism of Action Etoposide does not inhibit microtubular assembly. It has been shown to delay transit of cells through the S phase and arrest cells in late S or early G_2 phase. The drug may inhibit mitochondrial transport at the NADH dehydrogenase level or inhibit uptake of nucleosides into HeLa cells. Etoposide is a topoisomerase II inhibitor and appears to cause DNA strand breaks.

Labeled Contraindications Hypersensitivity to etoposide or any component of the formulation; pregnancy

Warnings/Precautions Hazardous agent - use appropriate precautions for handling and disposal. See Safe Handling of Hazardous Drugs *on page 1034* in the Appendix. Severe myelosuppression with resulting infection or bleeding may occur. **Must be diluted - do not give IVP**. Dosage should be adjusted in patients with hepatic or renal impairment.

Adverse Reactions

>10%:

Cardiovascular: Hypotension if the drug is infused too fast

Dermatologic: Alopecia (22% to 93%)

Endocrine & metabolic: Ovarian failure (38%), amenorrhea

Gastrointestinal: Mild to moderate nausea and vomiting; mucositis, especially at high doses; anorexia (10% to 13%)

Hematologic: Myelosuppression, leukopenia (91%), thrombocytopenia (41%), anemia

Onset: 5-7 days

Nadir: 7-14 days

Recovery: 21-28 days

1% to 10%:

Gastrointestinal: Stomatitis (1% to 6%), diarrhea (1% to 13%), abdominal pain

Neuromuscular & skeletal: Peripheral neuropathies (0.7% to 2%)

<1%: Tachycardia, CHF, MI, somnolence, fatigue, headache, anovulatory cycles, hypomenorrhea, hepatitis, thrombophlebitis, anaphylactoid

(Continued)

Etoposide (Continued)

reactions (chills, fever, bronchospasm, dyspnea, hypotension); possibly related to rapid infusion (0.7% to 2%)

Vesicant No; an irritant

Emetic Potential Mild (10% to 30%)

Overdosage/Toxicology Symptoms of overdose include bone marrow suppression, leukopenia, thrombocytopenia, nausea, and vomiting. Treatment is supportive.

Drug Interactions

Cytochrome P450 Effect: Substrate of CYP1A2 (minor), 2E1 (minor), 3A4 (major); **Inhibits** CYP2C8/9 (weak), 3A4 (weak)

Increased Effect/Toxicity: The effects of etoposide may be increased by calcium antagonists (increased effects noted *in vitro*). Cyclosporine may increase the levels of etoposide. Etoposide may increase the effects/toxicity of methotrexate and warfarin. There have been reports of frequent hepatic dysfunction with hyperbilirubinemia, ascites, and thrombocytopenia when etoposide is combined with carmustine. CYP3A4 inhibitors may increase the levels/effects of etoposide; example inhibitors include azole antifungals, ciprofloxacin, clarithromycin, diclofenac, doxycycline, erythromycin, imatinib, isoniazid, nefazodone, nicardipine, propofol, protease inhibitors, quinidine, and verapamil.

Decreased Effect: CYP3A4 inducers may decrease the levels/effects of etoposide; example inducers include aminoglutethimide, carbamazepine, nafcillin, nevirapine, phenobarbital, phenytoin, and rifamycins.

Ethanol/Nutrition/Herb Interactions

Ethanol: Avoid ethanol (may increase GI irritation).

Food: Administration of food does not affect GI absorption with doses ≤200 mg of injection.

Herb/Nutraceutical: St John's wort may decrease etoposide levels.

Storage/Stability Store intact vials of injection at room temperature and protected from light. Store oral capsules under refrigeration. Capsules are stable for 3 months at room temperature.

Reconstitution Etoposide should be further diluted in 250-1000 mL D_5W or NS for administration. Diluted solutions have concentration-dependent stability: More concentrated solutions have shorter stability times.

At room temperature in D_5W or NS in polyvinyl chloride, the concentration is stable as follows:

0.2 mg/mL: 96 hours

0.4 mg/mL: 48 hours

Standard I.V. dilution: Dilute in 250-1000 mL NS or D_5W

High-dose regimens (>1g/dose): Total dose should be drawn into an empty Viaflex® container.

Compatibility Variable stability (consult detailed reference) in NS, D_5W, LR (see Storage/Stability)

Y-site administration: Compatible: Allopurinol, amifostine, aztreonam, cladribine, doxorubicin liposome, fludarabine, gemcitabine, granisetron, melphalan, ondansetron, paclitaxel, piperacillin/tazobactam, sargramostim, sodium bicarbonate, teniposide, thiotepa, topotecan, vinorelbine. **Incompatible:** Cefepime, filgrastim, idarubicin

Compatibility when admixed: Compatible: Carboplatin, cisplatin, cisplatin with cyclophosphamide, cisplatin with floxuridine, cytarabine,

cytarabine with daunorubicin, floxuridine, fluorouracil, hydroxyzine, ifosfamide, ifosfamide, ifosfamide with carboplatin, ifosfamide with cisplatin, ondansetron. **Variable (consult detailed reference):** Cisplatin with mannitol and potassium chloride, doxorubicin with vincristine

Pharmacodynamics/Kinetics

Absorption: Oral: 25% to 75%; significant inter- and intrapatient variation

Distribution: Average V_d: 3-36 L/m²; poor penetration across the blood-brain barrier; CSF concentrations <10% of plasma concentrations

Protein binding: 94% to 97%

Metabolism: Hepatic to hydroxy acid and cislactone metabolites

Half-life elimination: Terminal: 4-15 hours; Children: Normal renal/hepatic function: 6-8 hours

Time to peak, serum: Oral: 1-1.5 hours

Excretion:

Children: Urine (≤55% as unchanged drug)

Adults: Urine (42% to 67%; 8% to 35% as unchanged drug) within 24 hours; feces (up to 16%)

Dosage Refer to individual protocols:

Children: I.V.: 60-120 mg/m²/day for 3-5 days every 3-6 weeks

AML:

Remission induction: 150 mg/m²/day for 2-3 days for 2-3 cycles

Intensification or consolidation: 250 mg/m²/day for 3 days, courses 2-5

Brain tumor: 150 mg/m²/day on days 2 and 3 of treatment course

Neuroblastoma: 100 mg/m²/day over 1 hour on days 1-5 of cycle; repeat cycle every 4 weeks

BMT conditioning regimen used in patients with rhabdomyosarcoma or neuroblastoma: I.V. continuous infusion: 160 mg/m²/day for 4 days

Conditioning regimen for allogenic BMT: 60 mg/kg/dose as a single dose

Adults:

Small cell lung cancer:

Oral: Twice the I.V. dose rounded to the nearest 50 mg given once daily if total dose ≤400 mg or in divided doses if >400 mg

I.V.: 35 mg/m²/day for 4 days or 50 mg/m²/day for 5 days every 3-4 weeks total dose ≤400 mg/day or in divided doses if >400 mg/day

IVPB: 60-100 mg/m²/day for 3 days (with cisplatin)

CIV: 500 mg/m² over 24 hours every 3 weeks

Testicular cancer:

IVPB: 50-100 mg/m²/day for 5 days repeated every 3-4 weeks

I.V.: 100 mg/m² every other day for 3 doses repeated every 3-4 weeks

BMT/relapsed leukemia: I.V.: 2.4-3.5 g/m² or 25-70 mg/kg administered over 4-36 hours

Dosing adjustment in renal impairment:

Cl_{cr} 10-50 mL/minute: Administer 75% of normal dose

Cl_{cr} <10 mL minute: Administer 50% of normal dose

Hemodialysis: Supplemental dose is not necessary

Peritoneal dialysis: Supplemental dose is not necessary

CAPD effects: Unknown

CAVH effects: Unknown

Dosing adjustment in hepatic impairment:

Bilirubin 1.5-3 mg/dL or AST 60-180 units: Reduce dose by 50%

(Continued)

Etoposide *(Continued)*

Bilirubin 3-5 mg/dL or AST >180 units: Reduce by 75%
Bilirubin >5 mg/dL: Do not administer

Combination Regimens

Adenocarcinoma, unknown primary:
EP (Adenocarcinoma) *on page 878*
Paclitaxel, Carboplatin, Etoposide *on page 926*

Brain tumors:
CDDP/VP-16 *on page 856*
COPE *on page 866*

Gastric cancer:
EAP *on page 875*
ELF *on page 877*

Gestational trophoblastic tumor:
EMA/CO *on page 877*
EP/EMA *on page 879*

Leukemia, acute myeloid:
7 + 3 + 7 *on page 841*
DAV *on page 872*
EMA 86 *on page 877*
Idarubicin, Cytarabine, Etoposide (ICE Protocol) *on page 900*
Idarubicin, Cytarabine, Etoposide (IDA-Based BF12) *on page 901*
MV *on page 917*
V-TAD *on page 949*

Lung cancer (small cell):
CAVE *on page 853*
EC (Small Cell Lung Cancer) *on page 876*
EP (Small Cell Lung Cancer) *on page 878*
VIP (Small Cell Lung Cancer) *on page 947*
VP (Small Cell Lung Cancer) *on page 948*

Lung cancer (nonsmall cell):
EC (Nonsmall Cell Lung Cancer) *on page 876*
EP (Nonsmall Cell Lung Cancer) *on page 878*
EP/PE *on page 880*

Lymphoma, Hodgkin's:
BEACOPP *on page 846*
EVA *on page 884*
mini-BEAM *on page 910*
Stanford V *on page 937*

Lymphoma, non-Hodgkin's:
CEPP(B) *on page 857*
EPOCH *on page 880*
ESHAP *on page 880*
ICE (Lymphoma, non-Hodgkin's) *on page 899*
IMVP-16 *on page 902*
IVAC *on page 904*
MINE *on page 909*
MINE-ESHAP *on page 909*
Pro-MACE-CytaBOM *on page 931*

Multiple myeloma: DTPACE *on page 874*

Neuroblastoma:
CAV-P/VP *on page 853*
CDDP/VP-16 *on page 856*

Administration

Oral: Doses should be rounded to the nearest 50 mg; doses ≤400 mg/day should be given as a single daily dose. Doses ≥400 mg/day should be given in 2-4 divided doses.

I.V.: As a bolus over 45-60 minutes or 24-hour continuous infusion. **Infusion of doses in <45 minutes greatly increases the risk of hypotension.**

Dosage Forms

Capsule, softgel (VePesid®): 50 mg

Injection, solution: 20 mg/mL (5 mL, 25 mL, 50 mL) [may contain benzyl alcohol or alcohol]

Toposar®: 20 mg/mL (5 mL, 10 mL, 25 mL) [contains benzyl alcohol]

VePesid®: 20 mg/mL (5 mL, 7.5 mL, 25 mL, 50 mL) [contains benzyl alcohol and alcohol 30%]

High Dose Considerations

High Dose: I.V.: 750-2400 mg/m^2; 10-60 mg/kg; duration of infusion is 1-4 hours to 24 hours; generally combined with other high-dose chemotherapeutic drugs or total body irradiation (TBI).

Unique Toxicities:

Cardiovascular: Hypotension (infusion-related)

Central nervous system: Confusion, somnolence, seizure activity increased

Dermatologic: Skin lesions resembling Stevens-Johnson syndrome, alopecia

Endocrine & metabolic: Metabolic acidosis, parotitis

Gastrointestinal: Severe nausea and vomiting, mucositis

Hepatic: Hepatitis

(Continued)

Etoposide *(Continued)*

Neuromuscular & skeletal: Peripheral neuropathy, motor deficits exacerbated

Miscellaneous: Secondary malignancy, ethanol intoxication

Comments: The etoposide formulation contains ethanol 30.3% (v/v). Etoposide 2.4 mg/m^2 delivers ethanol 45 g/m^2 I.V. Adverse effects may be increased with administration of etoposide to patients with decreased creatinine clearance. Etoposide 400-1600 mg/m^2 has been drawn into plastic syringes undiluted (20 mg/mL) for administration over 3-4 hours. Etoposide 800 mg/m^2 was pharmacokinetically equivalent to etoposide phosphate 910 mg/m^2 in patients with refractory hematologic malignancies.

Monitoring Parameters CBC with differential, platelet count, and hemoglobin, vital signs (blood pressure), bilirubin, and renal function tests

Patient Information During therapy, do not use alcohol, aspirin-containing products, and/or OTC medications without consulting prescriber. It is important to maintain adequate nutrition and hydration (2-3 L/day of fluids unless instructed to restrict fluid intake) during therapy; frequent small meals may help. You may experience mild nausea or vomiting (frequent small meals, frequent mouth care, sucking lozenges, or chewing gum may help). You may experience loss of hair (reversible); you will be more susceptible to infection (avoid crowds and exposure to infection as much as possible). Yogurt or buttermilk may help reduce diarrhea. Frequent mouth care and use of a soft toothbrush or cotton swabs may help prevent mouth sores. This drug may cause sterility or birth defects. Report extreme fatigue, pain or numbness in extremities, severe GI upset or diarrhea, bleeding or bruising, fever, chills, sore throat, vaginal discharge, difficulty breathing, yellowing of eyes or skin, and any changes in color of urine or stool. Contraceptive measures are recommended during therapy. The drug may be excreted in breast milk, therefore, an alternative form of feeding your baby should be used.

Selected Readings

Clark PL and Slevin ML, "The Clinical Pharmacology of Etoposide and Teniposide," *Clin Pharmacokinet*, 1987, 12(4):223-52.

Hainsworth JD and Greco FA, "Etoposide: Twenty Years Later," *Ann Oncol*, 1995, 6(4):325-41.

Joel SP, Shah R, and Slevin ML, "Etoposide Dosage and Pharmacodynamics," *Cancer Chemother Pharmacol*, 1994, 34(Suppl):69-75.

Meresse P, Dechaux E, Monneret C, et al, "Etoposide: Discovery and Medicinal Chemistry," *Curr Med Chem*, 2004, 11(18):2443-66.

Toffoli G, Corona G, Basso B, et al, "Pharmacokinetic Optimisation of Treatment With Oral Etoposide," *Clin Pharmacokinet*, 2004, 43(7):441-66.

Etoposide Phosphate *(e toe POE side FOS fate)*

Related Information

Safe Handling of Hazardous Drugs *on page 1034*

U.S. Brand Names Etopophos®

Generic Available No

Pharmacologic Category Antineoplastic Agent, Podophyllotoxin Derivative

Pregnancy Risk Factor D

Lactation Enters breast milk/contraindicated

Use Treatment of refractory testicular tumors and small cell lung cancer

Mechanism of Action Etoposide phosphate is converted *in vivo* to the active moiety, etoposide, by dephosphorylation. Etoposide inhibits mitotic activity; inhibits cells from entering prophase; inhibits DNA synthesis. Initially thought to be mitotic inhibitors similar to podophyllotoxin, but actually have no effect on microtubule assembly. However, later shown to induce DNA strand breakage and inhibition of topoisomerase II (an enzyme which breaks and repairs DNA); etoposide acts in late S or early G2 phases.

Labeled Contraindications Hypersensitivity to etoposide, etoposide phosphate, or any component of the formulation; pregnancy

Warnings/Precautions Hazardous agent - use appropriate precautions for handling and disposal. See Safe Handling of Hazardous Drugs *on page 1034* in the Appendix. Severe myelosuppression with resulting infection or bleeding may occur. Dosage should be adjusted in patients with hepatic or renal impairment. Use caution in elderly patients (may be more likely to develop severe myelosuppression, GI effects, and/or alopecia).

Adverse Reactions Based on **etoposide**:

>10%:

Cardiovascular: Hypotension if the drug is infused too fast

Dermatologic: Alopecia (22% to 93%)

Endocrine & metabolic: Ovarian failure (38%), amenorrhea

Gastrointestinal: Mild to moderate nausea and vomiting; mucositis, especially at high doses; anorexia (10% to 13%)

Hematologic: Myelosuppression, leukopenia (91%), thrombocytopenia (41%), anemia

Onset: 5-7 days

Nadir: 7-14 days

Recovery: 21-28 days

1% to 10%:

Gastrointestinal: Stomatitis (1% to 6%), diarrhea (1% to 13%), abdominal pain

Neuromuscular & skeletal: Peripheral neuropathies (0.7% to 2%)

<1%: Tachycardia, CHF, MI, somnolence, fatigue, headache, anovulatory cycles, hypomenorrhea, hepatitis, thrombophlebitis, anaphylactoid reactions (chills, fever, bronchospasm, dyspnea, hypotension); possibly related to rapid infusion (0.7% to 2%)

Vesicant No

Emetic Potential Mild (10% to 30%)

Overdosage/Toxicology Symptoms of overdose include bone marrow suppression, leukopenia, thrombocytopenia, nausea, and vomiting. Treatment is supportive.

Drug Interactions

Cytochrome P450 Effect: Substrate of CYP1A2 (minor), 2E1 (minor), 3A4 (major); **Inhibits** CYP2C8/9 (weak), 3A4 (weak)

Increased Effect/Toxicity: Etoposide taken with warfarin may result in prolongation of bleeding times. Alteration of methotrexate transport has been found as a slow efflux of methotrexate and its polyglutamated form out of the cell, leading to intercellular accumulation of methotrexate. Calcium antagonists increase the rate of VP-16-induced DNA damage and cytotoxicity *in vitro*. Use with carmustine has shown reports of frequent hepatic dysfunction with hyperbilirubinemia, ascites, and thrombocytopenia. Cyclosporine may cause additive cytotoxic (Continued)

Etoposide Phosphate *(Continued)*

effects on tumor cells. CYP3A4 inhibitors may increase the levels/effects of etoposide; example inhibitors include azole antifungals, ciprofloxacin, clarithromycin, diclofenac, doxycycline, erythromycin, imatinib, isoniazid, nefazodone, nicardipine, propofol, protease inhibitors, quinidine, and verapamil.

Decreased Effect: CYP3A4 inducers may decrease the levels/effects of etoposide; example inducers include aminoglutethimide, carbamazepine, nafcillin, nevirapine, phenobarbital, phenytoin, and rifamycins.

Ethanol/Nutrition/Herb Interactions

Ethanol: Avoid ethanol (may increase GI irritation).

Food: Administration of food does not affect GI absorption with doses ≤200 mg of injection.

Herb/Nutraceutical: St John's wort may decrease etoposide levels.

Storage/Stability Store intact vials of injection and capsules under refrigeration 2°C to 8°C (36°F to 46°F). Protect vials from light. Solutions are stable in glass or plastic containers at room temperature 20°C to 25°C (68°F to 77°F) or under refrigeration 2°C to 8°C (36°F to 47°F) for up to 24 hours.

Reconstitution Reconstitute vials with SWI, D_5W, NS, bacteriostatic SWI, or bacteriostatic NS to a concentration of 20 mg/mL or 10 mg/mL etoposide (22.7 mg/mL or 11.4 mg/mL etoposide phosphate). These solutions may be administered without further dilution or may be further diluted in 50-500 mL D_5W or NS.

Compatibility Stable in D_5W, NS, sterile water for injection

Y-site administration: Compatible: Acyclovir, amikacin, aminophylline, ampicillin, ampicillin/sulbactam, aztreonam, bleomycin, bumetanide, buprenorphine, butorphanol, calcium gluconate, carboplatin, carmustine, cefazolin, cefoperazone, cefotaxime, cefotetan, cefoxitin, ceftazidime, ceftizoxime, ceftriaxone, cefuroxime, cimetidine, ciprofloxacin, cisplatin, clindamycin, co-trimoxazole, cyclophosphamide, cytarabine, dacarbazine, dactinomycin, daunorubicin, dexamethasone sodium phosphate, diphenhydramine, dobutamine, dopamine, doxorubicin, doxycycline, droperidol, enalaprilat, famotidine, floxuridine, fluconazole, fludarabine, fluorouracil, furosemide, ganciclovir, gatifloxacin, gemcitabine, gentamicin, granisetron, haloperidol, heparin, hydrocortisone sodium phosphate, hydrocortisone sodium succinate, hydromorphone, hydroxyzine, idarubicin, ifosfamide, leucovorin, linezolid, lorazepam, magnesium sulfate, mannitol, meperidine, mesna, methotrexate, metoclopramide, metronidazole, minocycline, mitoxantrone, morphine, nalbuphine, netilmicin, ofloxacin, ondansetron, paclitaxel, piperacillin, piperacillin/tazobactam, plicamycin, potassium chloride, promethazine, ranitidine, sodium bicarbonate, streptozocin, teniposide, thiotepa, ticarcillin, ticarcillin/clavulanate, tobramycin, vancomycin, vinblastine, vincristine, zidovudine. **Incompatible:** Amphotericin B, cefepime, chlorpromazine, imipenem/cilastatin, methylprednisolone sodium succinate, mitomycin, prochlorperazine edisylate

Pharmacodynamics/Kinetics

Distribution: Average V_d: 3-36 L/m^2; poor penetration across blood-brain barrier; concentrations in CSF being <10% that of plasma

Protein binding: 94% to 97%

Metabolism: Hepatic (with a biphasic decay)

Half-life elimination: Terminal: 4-15 hours; Children: Normal renal/hepatic function: 6-8 hours

Excretion: Urine (as unchanged drug and metabolites), feces (2% to 16%); Children: I.V.: Urine (≤55% as unchanged drug)

Dosage Refer to individual protocols. **Note**: Etoposide phosphate may be substituted for etoposide, using the desired etoposide dose. Dosage should be expressed as the desired etoposide dose; **not** as the etoposide phosphate dose (eg, etoposide phosphate equivalent to ___ mg etoposide). See Etoposide *on page 315* for recommended doses.

Adults:

Dosage adjustment in renal impairment:

Cl_{cr} 15-50 mL/minute: Administer 75% of normal dose

Cl_{cr} <15 mL minute: Data are not available and further dose reduction should be considered in these patients.

Hemodialysis: Supplemental dose is not necessary

Peritoneal dialysis: Supplemental dose is not necessary

CAPD effects: Unknown

CAVH effects: Unknown

Dosage adjustment in hepatic impairment:

Bilirubin 1.5-3 mg/dL or AST 60-180 units: Reduce dose by 50%

Bilirubin 3-5 mg/dL or AST >180 units: Reduce by 75%

Bilirubin >5 mg/dL: Do not administer

Administration I.V. infusion, usually over 5-210 minutes, infusions over 10-12 hours are reported.

Dosage Forms Injection, powder for reconstitution, as base: 100 mg

High Dose Considerations

High Dose: I.V.: 0.5-2 g/m^2 divided into 2 daily doses; maximum single-dose agent: 3.2 g/m^2; generally combined with other high-dose chemotherapeutic drugs.

Unique Toxicities: Gastrointestinal: Nausea, vomiting, mucositis

Comments: In contrast to etoposide, metabolic acidosis is not a frequent adverse effect of high-dose etoposide phosphate. Etoposide 800 mg/m^2 was pharmacokinetically equivalent to etoposide phosphate 910 mg/m^2 in patients with refractory hematologic malignancies.

Monitoring Parameters CBC with differential, platelet count, and hemoglobin, vital signs (blood pressure), bilirubin, and renal function tests

Patient Information This drug can only be administered by infusion. During therapy, do not use alcohol, aspirin-containing products, and/or OTC medications without consulting prescriber. It is important to maintain adequate nutrition and hydration (2-3 L/day of fluids unless instructed to restrict fluid intake) during therapy; frequent small meals may help. You may experience mild nausea or vomiting (frequent small meals, frequent mouth care, sucking lozenges, or chewing gum may help). You may experience loss of hair (reversible); you will be more susceptible to infection (avoid crowds and exposure to infection as much as possible). Yogurt or buttermilk may help reduce diarrhea. Frequent mouth care and use of a soft toothbrush or cotton swabs may help prevent mouth sores. This drug may cause sterility or birth defects. Report extreme fatigue, pain or numbness in extremities, severe GI upset or diarrhea, bleeding or bruising, fever, chills, sore throat, vaginal discharge, difficulty breathing, yellowing of eyes or skin, and any changes in color of urine or stool. Contraceptive measures should be used during therapy. The drug may cause permanent sterility and may cause birth defects. The drug may be (Continued)

Etoposide Phosphate *(Continued)*

excreted in breast milk, therefore, an alternative form of feeding your baby should be used.

Special Geriatric Considerations Elderly patients may be more susceptible to severe myelosuppression. Other adverse effects including GI toxicity, infectious complications, weakness, and alopecia may occur more frequently in elderly.

Selected Readings

Budman DR, "Early Studies of Etoposide Phosphate, a Water-Soluble Prodrug," *Semin Oncol*, 1996, 23(6 Suppl 13):8-14.

Dorr RT, Briggs A, Kintzel P, et al, "Comparative Pharmacokinetic Study of High-Dose Etoposide and Etoposide Phosphate in Patients With Lymphoid Malignancy Receiving Autologous Stem Cell Transplantation," *Bone Marrow Transplant*, 2003, 31(8):643-9.

Greco FA and Hainsworth JD, "Clinical Studies With Etoposide Phosphate," *Semin Oncol*, 1996, 23(6 Suppl 13):45-50.

Mummaneni V, Kaul S, Igwemezie LN, et al, "Bioequivalence Assessment of Etoposide Phosphate and Etoposide Using Pharmacodynamic and Traditional Pharmacokinetic Parameters," *J Pharmacokinet Biopharm*, 1996, 24(4):313-25.

Schacter LP, Igwemezie LN, Seyedsadr M, et al, "Clinical and Pharmacokinetic Overview of Parenteral Etoposide Phosphate," *Cancer Chemother Pharmacol*, 1994, 34(Suppl):58-63.

Witterland AH, Koks CH, and Beijnen JH, "Etoposide Phosphate, the Water Soluble Prodrug of Etoposide," *Pharm World Sci*, 1996, 18(5):163-70.

♦ **Euflex® (Can)** *see* Flutamide *on page 366*

♦ **Eulexin®** *see* Flutamide *on page 366*

Exemestane *(ex e MES tane)*

Related Information

Safe Handling of Hazardous Drugs *on page 1034*

U.S. Brand Names Aromasin®

Canadian Brand Names Aromasin®

Generic Available No

Pharmacologic Category Antineoplastic Agent, Aromatase Inactivator

Pregnancy Risk Factor D

Lactation Excretion in breast milk unknown/use caution

Use Treatment of advanced breast cancer in postmenopausal women whose disease has progressed following tamoxifen therapy

Mechanism of Action Exemestane is an irreversible, steroidal aromatase inactivator. It prevents conversion of androgens to estrogens by tying up the enzyme aromatase. In breast cancers where growth is estrogen-dependent, this medicine will lower circulating estrogens.

Labeled Contraindications Hypersensitivity to exemestane or any component of the formulation; pregnancy

Warnings/Precautions Not indicated for premenopausal women; not to be given with estrogen-containing agents. Use with caution in hepatic impairment or renal insufficiency.

Adverse Reactions

>10%:

Central nervous system: Fatigue (22%), pain (13%), depression (13%), insomnia (11%), anxiety (10%)

Endocrine & metabolic: Hot flashes (13%)

Gastrointestinal: Nausea (18%)

1% to 10%:

Cardiovascular: Edema (7%), hypertension (5%), chest pain

Central nervous system: Dizziness (8%), headache (8%), fever (5%), hypoesthesia, confusion

Dermatologic: Rash, itching, alopecia

Gastrointestinal: Vomiting (7%), abdominal pain (6%), anorexia (6%), constipation (5%), diarrhea (4%), increased appetite (3%), dyspepsia

Genitourinary: Urinary tract infection

Neuromuscular & skeletal: Weakness, paresthesia, pathological fracture, arthralgia

Respiratory: Dyspnea (10%), cough (6%), bronchitis, sinusitis, pharyngitis, rhinitis

Miscellaneous: Influenza-like symptoms (6%), diaphoresis (6%), lymphedema, infection

<1%: GGT increased, transaminases increased

A dose-dependent decrease in sex hormone-binding globulin has been observed with daily doses of 25 mg or more. Serum luteinizing hormone and follicle-stimulating hormone levels have increased with this medicine.

Emetic Potential Low (10% to 30%)

Overdosage/Toxicology If an overdose should occur, general supportive care would be indicated.

Drug Interactions

Cytochrome P450 Effect: Substrate of CYP3A4 (major)

Decreased Effect: CYP3A4 inducers may decrease the levels/effects of exemestane (example inducers include aminoglutethimide, carbamazepine, nafcillin, nevirapine, phenobarbital, phenytoin, and rifamycins). Rifampin may decrease exemestane levels; increased dosage recommended.

Ethanol/Nutrition/Herb Interactions

Food: Plasma levels increased by 40% when exemestane was taken with a fatty meal.

Herb/Nutraceutical: St John's wort may decrease exemestane levels. Avoid black cohosh, dong quai in estrogen-dependent tumors.

Storage/Stability Store at 25°C (77°F)

Pharmacodynamics/Kinetics

Absorption: Rapid and moderate (~42%) following oral administration; absorption increases ~40% following high-fat meal

Distribution: Extensive

Protein binding: 90%, primarily to albumin and α_1-acid glycoprotein

Metabolism: Extensively hepatic; oxidation (CYP3A4) of methylene group, reduction of 17-keto group with formation of many secondary metabolites; metabolites are inactive

Half-life elimination: 24 hours

Time to peak: Women with breast cancer: 1.2 hours

Excretion: Urine (<1% as unchanged drug, 39% to 45% as metabolites); feces (36% to 48%)

Dosage Adults: Oral: 25 mg once daily

Dosage adjustment with CYP3A4 inducers: 50 mg once daily when used with potent inducers (eg, rifampin, phenytoin)

Dosing adjustment in renal/hepatic impairment: Safety of chronic doses has not been studied

Administration Oral, preferably after a meal.

Dosage Forms Tablet: 25 mg

(Continued)

Exemestane *(Continued)*

Patient Information Take after a meal; use caution if you have uncontrolled high blood pressure. Avoid driving or doing other tasks or hobbies that require alertness until you know how this medicine affects you. Take at approximately the same time every day.

Selected Readings

Boeddinghaus IM and Dowsett M, "Comparative Clinical Pharmacology and Pharmacokinetic Interactions of Aromatase Inhibitors," *J Steroid Biochem Mol Biol*, 2001, 79(1-5):85-91.

Buzdar AU, Robertson JF, Eiermann W, et al, "An Overview of the Pharmacology and Pharmacokinetics of the Newer Generation Aromatase Inhibitors Anastrozole, Letrozole, and Exemestane," *Cancer*, 2002, 95(9):2006-16.

Lonning PE, "Pharmacological Profiles of Exemestane and Fromestane, Steroidal Aromatase Inhibitors Used for Treatment of Postmenopausal Breast Cancer," *Breast Cancer Res Treat*, 1998, 49(Suppl 1):45-52.

Njar VC and Brodie AM, "Comprehensive Pharmacology and Clinical Efficacy of Aromatase Inhibitors," *Drugs*, 1999, 58(2):233-55.

Scott LJ and Wiseman LR, "Exemestane," *Drugs*, 1999, 58(4):675-80.

♦ **309F** *see* Suramin *on page 733*

♦ **Factive**® *see* Gemifloxacin *on page 392*

Factor VIIa (Recombinant)

(FAK ter SEV en ree KOM be nant)

Medication Safety Issues

Sound-alike/look-alike issues:

NovoSeven® may be confused with Novacet®

U.S. Brand Names NovoSeven®

Canadian Brand Names Niastase®

Generic Available No

Synonyms Coagulation Factor VIIa; Eptacog Alfa (Activated); rFVIIa

Pharmacologic Category Antihemophilic Agent; Blood Product Derivative

Pregnancy Risk Factor C

Lactation Excretion in breast milk unknown/compatible

Use Treatment of bleeding episodes in patients with hemophilia A or B when inhibitors to factor VIII or factor IX are present

Mechanism of Action Recombinant factor VIIa, a vitamin K-dependent glycoprotein, promotes hemostasis by activating the extrinsic pathway of the coagulation cascade. It replaces deficient activated coagulation factor VII, which complexes with tissue factor and may activate coagulation factor X to Xa and factor IX to IXa. When complexed with other factors, coagulation factor Xa converts prothrombin to thrombin, a key step in the formation of a fibrin-platelet hemostatic plug.

Labeled Contraindications Hypersensitivity to factor VII or any component of the formulation; hypersensitivity to mouse, hamster, or bovine proteins

Warnings/Precautions Patients should be monitored for signs and symptoms of activation of the coagulation system or thrombosis. Thrombotic events may be increased in patients with disseminated intravascular coagulation (DIC), advanced atherosclerotic disease, sepsis or crush injury. Decreased dosage or discontinuation is warranted in confirmed DIC. Efficacy with prolonged infusions and data evaluating this agent's long-term adverse effects are limited.

Adverse Reactions

1% to 10%:

Cardiovascular: Hypertension

Hematologic: Hemorrhage, decreased plasma fibrinogen

Musculoskeletal: Hemarthrosis

<1%: Abnormal renal function, allergic reactions, arthrosis, bradycardia, coagulation disorder, disseminated intravascular coagulation (DIC), edema, fibrinolysis increased, headache, hypotension, injection-site reactions, prothrombin decreased, pneumonia, prothrombin decreased, pruritus, purpura, rash, vomiting

Overdosage/Toxicology Experience with overdose in humans is limited; an increased risk of thrombotic events may occur in overdosage. Treatment is symptomatic and supportive.

Storage/Stability Store under refrigeration (2°C to 8°C/36°F to 46°F). Reconstituted solutions may be stored at room temperature or under refrigeration, but must be infused within 3 hours of reconstitution.

Pharmacodynamics/Kinetics

Distribution: V_d: 103 mL/kg (78-139)

Half-life elimination: 2.3 hours (1.7-2.7)

Excretion: Clearance: 33 mL/kg/hour (27-49)

Dosage Children and Adults: I.V. administration only: 90 mcg/kg every 2 hours until hemostasis is achieved or until the treatment is judged ineffective. The dose and interval may be adjusted based upon the severity of bleeding and the degree of hemostasis achieved. The duration of therapy following hemostasis has not been fully established; for patients experiencing severe bleeds, dosing should be continued at 3-6 hour intervals after hemostasis has been achieved and the duration of dosing should be minimized.

Note: In clinical trials, dosages have ranged from 35-120 mcg/kg

Administration I.V. administration only

Dosage Forms Injection, powder for reconstitution [preservative free]: 1.2 mg, 2.4 mg, 4.8 mg [latex free; contains sodium 0.44 mEq/mg rFVIIa, polysorbate 80]

Monitoring Parameters Monitor for evidence of hemostasis; although the prothrombin time, aPTT, and factor VII clotting activity have no correlation with achieving hemostasis, these parameters may be useful as adjunct tests to evaluate efficacy and guide dose or interval adjustments

Dietary Considerations Contains sodium 0.44 mEq/mg rFVIIa

Factor IX (FAK ter nyne)

U.S. Brand Names AlphaNine® SD; BeneFix®; Mononine®

Canadian Brand Names BeneFix®; Immunine® VH; Mononine®

Generic Available No

Pharmacologic Category Antihemophilic Agent; Blood Product Derivative

Pregnancy Risk Factor C

Use Control bleeding in patients with factor IX deficiency (hemophilia B or Christmas disease)

Mechanism of Action Replaces deficient clotting factor IX; concentrate of factor IX; hemophilia B, or Christmas disease, is an X-linked inherited disorder of blood coagulation characterized by insufficient or abnormal synthesis of the clotting protein factor IX. Factor IX is a vitamin (Continued)

Factor IX *(Continued)*

K-dependent coagulation factor which is synthesized in the liver. Factor IX is activated by factor XIa in the intrinsic coagulation pathway. Activated factor IX (IXa), in combination with factor VII:C activates factor X to Xa, resulting ultimately in the conversion of prothrombin to thrombin and the formation of a fibrin clot. The infusion of exogenous factor IX to replace the deficiency present in hemophilia B temporarily restores hemostasis.

Labeled Contraindications Hypersensitivity to mouse protein (Mononine®), hamster protein (BeneFix®), or any component of the formulation

Warnings/Precautions Use with caution in patients with liver dysfunction; some products prepared from pooled human plasma - the risk of viral transmission is not totally eradicated; monitor patients who receive repeated doses twice daily with PTT and level of factor being replaced (eg, IX). Observe closely for signs or symptoms of intravascular coagulation or thrombosis. Caution should be exercised when administering to patients with liver disease, postoperatively, neonates, or patients at risk of thromboembolic phenomena or disseminated intravascular coagulation because of the potential risk of thromboembolic complications.

AlphaNine® SD, Mononine® contain **nondetectable levels of factors II, VII, and X** (<0.0025 units per factor IX unit using standard coagulation assays) and are, therefore, **NOT INDICATED** for replacement therapy of any of these clotting factors.

BeneFix®, Mononine® are **NOT INDICATED** in the treatment or reversal of coumarin-induced anticoagulation or in a hemorrhagic state caused by hepatitis-induced lack of production of liver dependent coagulation factors.

Adverse Reactions Frequency not defined.

Cardiovascular: Angioedema, cyanosis, flushing, hypotension, tightness in chest, tightness in neck, thrombosis (following high dosages because of presence of activated clotting factors)

Central nervous system: Fever, headache, chills, somnolence, dizziness, drowsiness, lightheadedness

Dermatologic: Urticaria, rash

Gastrointestinal: Nausea, vomiting, abnormal taste

Hematologic: Disseminated intravascular coagulation (DIC)

Local: Injection site discomfort

Neuromuscular & skeletal: Tingling

Respiratory: Dyspnea, laryngeal edema, allergic rhinitis

Miscellaneous: Transient fever (following rapid administration), anaphylaxis, burning sensation in jaw/skull

Overdosage/Toxicology Symptoms of overdose include disseminated intravascular coagulation (DIC).

Drug Interactions

Increased Effect/Toxicity: Do not coadminister with aminocaproic acid; may increase risk for thrombosis.

Storage/Stability When stored at refrigerator temperature, 2°C to 8°C (36°F to 46°F), coagulation factor IX is stable for the period indicated by the expiration date on its label. Avoid freezing which may damage container for the diluent.

AlphaNine® SD: May also be stored at ≤30°C (≤86°F) for up to 3 months.

BeneFix®: May also be stored at ≤25°C (≤77°F) for up to 6 months.

Mononine®: May also be stored at ≤30°C (≤86°F) for up to 1 month.

Stability of parenteral admixture at room temperature (25°C): 3 hours

Reconstitution Mononine®: When reconstituted to ~100 int. units/mL, infusion rate should be up to 225 units/minute (2 mL/minute).

Pharmacodynamics/Kinetics Half-life elimination: IX component: 23-31 hours

Dosage Dosage is expressed in units of factor IX activity and must be individualized. I.V. only:

Formula for units required to raise blood level %:

AlphaNine® SD, Mononine®: Children and Adults:

Number of Factor IX Units Required = body weight (in kg) x desired Factor IX level increase (% normal) x 1 unit/kg

For example, for a 100% level a patient who has an actual level of 20%: Number of Factor IX Units needed = 70 kg x 80% x 1 Unit/kg = 5600 Units

BeneFix®:

Children <15 years:

Number of Factor IX Units Required = body weight (in kg) x desired Factor IX level increase (% normal) x 1.4 units/kg

Adults:

Number of Factor IX Units Required = body weight (in kg) x desired Factor IX level increase (% normal) x 1.2 units/kg

Guidelines: As a general rule, the level of factor IX required for treatment of different conditions is listed below:

Minor spontaneous hemorrhage, prophylaxis:

Desired levels of factor IX for hemostasis: 15% to 25%

Initial loading dose to achieve desired level: 20-30 units/kg

Frequency of dosing: Every 12-24 hours if necessary

Duration of treatment: 1-2 days

Moderate hemorrhage:

Desired levels of factor IX for hemostasis: 25% to 50%

Initial loading dose to achieve desired level: 25-50 units/kg

Frequency of dosing: Every 12-24 hours

Duration of treatment: 2-7 days

Major hemorrhage:

Desired levels of factor IX for hemostasis: >50%

Initial loading dose to achieve desired level: 30-50 units/kg

Frequency of dosing: Every 12-24 hours, depending on half-life and measured factor IX levels (after 3-5 days, maintain at least 20% activity)

Duration of treatment: 7-10 days, depending upon nature of insult

Surgery:

Desired levels of factor IX for hemostasis: 50% to 100%

Initial loading dose to achieve desired level: 50-100 units/kg

Frequency of dosing: Every 12-24 hours, depending on half-life and measured factor IX levels

Duration of treatment: 7-10 days, depending upon nature of insult

Administration Solution should be infused at room temperature

I.V. administration only: Should be infused **slowly**: The rate of administration should be determined by the response and comfort of the patient. (Continued)

Factor IX *(Continued)*

Mononine®: Intravenous dosage administration rates of up to 225 units/minute (~2 mL/minute) have been regularly tolerated without incident. **Infuse at a rate not exceeding 2 mL/minute**.

Dosage Forms Injection, powder for reconstitution (**Note:** Exact potency labeled on each vial):

AlphaNine® SD [human derived; solvent detergent treated; virus filtered; contains nondetectable levels of factors II, VII, X; supplied with diluent]

BeneFix® [recombinant formulation; supplied with diluent]

Mononine® [human derived; monoclonal antibody purified; contains nondetectable levels of factors II, VII, X; supplied with diluent]

Monitoring Parameters Levels of factors IX, PTT

Patient Information Early signs of hypersensitivity reactions including hives, generalized urticaria, tightness of the chest, wheezing, hypotension, and anaphylaxis indicate discontinuation of use of the concentrate and prescriber should be contacted if these symptoms occur

Factor IX Complex (Human)

(FAK ter nyne KOM pleks HYU man)

U.S. Brand Names Bebulin® VH; Profilnine® SD; Proplex® T

Generic Available No

Synonyms Prothrombin Complex Concentrate

Pharmacologic Category Antihemophilic Agent; Blood Product Derivative

Pregnancy Risk Factor C

Use

Control bleeding in patients with factor IX deficiency (hemophilia B or Christmas disease) **Note:** Factor IX concentrate containing **only** factor IX is also available and preferable for this indication.

Prevention/control of bleeding in hemophilia A patients with inhibitors to factor VIII

Prevention/control of bleeding in patients with factor VII deficiency

Emergency correction of the coagulopathy of warfarin excess in critical situations.

Mechanism of Action Replaces deficient clotting factor including factor X; hemophilia B, or Christmas disease, is an X-linked recessively inherited disorder of blood coagulation characterized by insufficient or abnormal synthesis of the clotting protein factor IX. Factor IX is a vitamin K-dependent coagulation factor which is synthesized in the liver. Factor IX is activated by factor XIa in the intrinsic coagulation pathway. Activated factor IX (IXa), in combination with factor VII:C activates factor X to Xa, resulting ultimately in the conversion of prothrombin to thrombin and the formation of a fibrin clot. The infusion of exogenous factor IX to replace the deficiency present in hemophilia B temporarily restores hemostasis.

Labeled Contraindications Liver disease with signs of intravascular coagulation or fibrinolysis, not for use in factor VII deficiencies, patients undergoing elective surgery

Warnings/Precautions Use with caution in patients with liver dysfunction. Prepared from pooled human plasma - the risk of viral transmission is not totally eradicated. Thromboembolic complications (more likely to occur during postoperative period or in patients with risk factors) rarely occurs. Treatment should stop if respiratory distress or any changes in blood pressure or pulse rate occur.

Adverse Reactions

1% to 10%:

Central nervous system: Fever, headache, chills

Neuromuscular & skeletal: Tingling

Miscellaneous: Following rapid administration: Transient fever

<1%: Disseminated intravascular coagulation (DIC), flushing, nausea, somnolence, thrombosis following high dosages because of presence of activated clotting factors, tightness in chest, tightness in neck, urticaria, vomiting

Overdosage/Toxicology Symptoms of overdose include disseminated intravascular coagulation (DIC).

Drug Interactions

Increased Effect/Toxicity: Do not coadminister with aminocaproic acid; may increase risk for thrombosis.

Storage/Stability When stored at refrigerator temperature, 2°C to 8°C (36°F to 46°F), coagulation factor IX is stable for the period indicated by the expiration date on its label. Avoid freezing which may damage container for the diluent. Once diluted should be used promptly; stable for up to 3 hours.

Reconstitution Refer to instructions for individual products. Diluent and Factor IX complex should come to room temperature before combining. Diluent vial should be inverted over concentrate vial. After diluent is pulled, disconnect. The provided filter needle should be used to withdraw concentrate. Remove needle and attach to infusion set or replace needle for infusion.

Pharmacodynamics/Kinetics

Half-life elimination:

VII component: Initial: 4-6 hours; Terminal: 22.5 hours

IX component: 24 hours

Dosage Children and Adults: Dosage is expressed in units of factor IX activity and must be individualized. I.V. only:

Formula for units required to raise blood level %:

Total blood volume (mL blood/kg) = 70 mL/kg (adults), 80 mL/kg (children)

Plasma volume = total blood volume (mL) x [1 - Hct (in decimals)]

For example, for a 70 kg adult with a Hct = 40%: Plasma volume = [70 kg x 70 mL/kg] x [1 - 0.4] = 2940 mL

To calculate number of units needed to increase level to desired range (highly individualized and dependent on patient's condition): Number of units = desired level increase [desired level - actual level] x plasma volume (in mL)

For example, for a 100% level in the above patient who has an actual level of 20%: Number of units needed = [1 (for a 100% level) - 0.2] x 2940 mL = 2352 units

As a general rule, the level of factor IX required for treatment of different conditions is listed below:

Minor Spontaneous Hemorrhage, Prophylaxis:

Desired levels of factor IX for hemostasis: 15% to 25%

Initial loading dose to achieve desired level: <20-30 units/kg

Frequency of dosing: Once; repeated in 24 hours if necessary

Duration of treatment: Once; repeated if necessary

(Continued)

Factor IX Complex (Human) *(Continued)*

Major Trauma or Surgery:
  Desired levels of factor IX for hemostasis: 25% to 50%
  Initial loading dose to achieve desired level: <75 units/kg
  Frequency of dosing: Every 18-30 hours, depending on half-life and measured factor IX levels
  Duration of treatment: Up to 10 days, depending upon nature of insult

Factor VIII inhibitor patients: 75 units/kg/dose; may be given every 6-12 hours

Anticoagulant overdosage: I.V.: 15 units/kg

Administration I.V. administration only: Should be infused **slowly**. Rate should not exceed 2 mL/minute for Bebulin® VH, 3 mL/minute for Proplex® T, or 10 mL/minute for Profilnine® SD.

Dosage Forms Injection, powder for reconstitution (**Note:** Exact potency labeled on each vial):
  Bebulin® VH [single-dose vial; vapor heated; supplied with sterile water for injection]
  Profilnine® SD [single-dose vial; solvent detergent treated]
  Proplex® T [single-dose vial; heat treated; supplied with sterile water for injection]

Monitoring Parameters Levels of factors being replaced (eg, VII or IX), PT, PTT

Patient Information Early signs of hypersensitivity reactions including hives, generalized urticaria, tightness of the chest, wheezing, hypotension, and anaphylaxis indicate discontinuation of use of the concentrate and prescriber should be contacted if these symptoms occur

♦ **Factor VIII (Human)** *see* Antihemophilic Factor (Human) *on page 87*
♦ **Factor VIII (Porcine)** *see* Antihemophilic Factor (Porcine) *on page 90*
♦ **Factor VIII (Recombinant)** *see* Antihemophilic Factor (Recombinant) *on page 92*

Famciclovir *(fam SYE kloe veer)*

U.S. Brand Names Famvir®
Canadian Brand Names Famvir®
Generic Available No
Pharmacologic Category Antiviral Agent
Pregnancy Risk Factor B
Lactation Excretion in breast milk unknown/contraindicated
Use Management of acute herpes zoster (shingles) and recurrent episodes of genital herpes; treatment of recurrent herpes simplex in immunocompetent patients
Mechanism of Action After undergoing rapid biotransformation to the active compound, penciclovir, famciclovir is phosphorylated by viral thymidine kinase in HSV-1, HSV-2, and VZV-infected cells to a monophosphate form; this is then converted to penciclovir triphosphate and competes with deoxyguanosine triphosphate to inhibit HSV-2 polymerase (ie, herpes viral DNA synthesis/replication is selectively inhibited)
Labeled Contraindications Hypersensitivity to famciclovir or any component of the formulation
Warnings/Precautions Hazardous agent - use appropriate precautions for handling and disposal. See Safe Handling of Hazardous Drugs *on*

page 1034 in the Appendix. Has not been studied in immunocompromised patients or patients with ophthalmic or disseminated zoster. Dosage adjustment is required in patients with renal insufficiency (Cl_{cr} <60 mL/minute) and in patients with noncompensated hepatic disease. Safety and efficacy have not been established in children <18 years of age. May be carcinogenic/mutagenic.

Adverse Reactions
1% to 10%:
  Central nervous system: Fatigue (4% to 6%), fever (1% to 3%), dizziness (3% to 5%), somnolence (1% to 2%), headache
  Dermatologic: Pruritus (1% to 4%)
  Gastrointestinal: Diarrhea (4% to 8%), vomiting (1% to 5%), constipation (1% to 5%), anorexia (1% to 3%), abdominal pain (1% to 4%), nausea
  Neuromuscular & skeletal: Paresthesia (1% to 3%)
  Respiratory: Sinusitis/pharyngitis (2%)
<1%: Rigors, arthralgia, upper respiratory infection

Emetic Potential Low (10% to 30%)

Overdosage/Toxicology Supportive and symptomatic care is recommended. Hemodialysis may enhance elimination.

Drug Interactions
Increased Effect/Toxicity:
  Cimetidine: Penciclovir AUC may increase due to impaired metabolism.
  Digoxin: C_{max} of digoxin increases by ~19%.
  Probenecid: Penciclovir serum levels significantly increase.
  Theophylline: Penciclovir AUC/C_{max} may increase and renal clearance decrease, although not clinically significant.

Ethanol/Nutrition/Herb Interactions Food: Rate of absorption and/or conversion to penciclovir and peak concentration are reduced with food, but bioavailability is not affected.

Pharmacodynamics/Kinetics
Absorption: Food decreases maximum peak concentration and delays time to peak; AUC remains the same
Distribution: V_{dss}: 0.98-1.08 L/kg
Protein binding: 20%
Metabolism: Rapidly deacetylated and oxidized to penciclovir; not via CYP
Bioavailability: 77%
Half-life elimination: Penciclovir: 2-3 hours (10, 20, and 7 hours in HSV-1, HSV-2, and VZV-infected cells, respectively); prolonged with renal impairment
Time to peak: 0.9 hours; C_{max} and T_{max} are decreased and prolonged with noncompensated hepatic impairment
Excretion: Urine (>90% as unchanged drug)

Dosage Initiate therapy as soon as herpes zoster is diagnosed:
Adults: Oral:
Acute herpes zoster: 500 mg every 8 hours for 7 days
Recurrent herpes simplex in immunocompetent patients: 125 mg twice daily for 5 days
Genital herpes:
  First episode: 250 mg 3 times/day for 7-10 days
  Recurrent episodes: 125 mg twice daily for 5 days
  Prophylaxis: 250 mg twice daily
  Severe (hospitalized patients): 250 mg twice daily
(Continued)

Famciclovir *(Continued)*

Dosing interval in renal impairment:
Herpes zoster:
Cl_{cr} ≥60 mL/minute: Administer 500 mg every 8 hours
Cl_{cr} 40-59 mL/minute: Administer 500 mg every 12 hours
Cl_{cr} 20-39 mL/minute: Administer 500 mg every 24 hours
Cl_{cr} <20 mL/minute: Administer 250 mg every 24 hours
Recurrent genital herpes:
Cl_{cr} ≥40 mL/minute: Administer 125 mg every 12 hours
Cl_{cr} 20-39 mL/minute: Administer 125 mg every 24 hours
Cl_{cr} <20 mL/minute: Administer 125 mg every 48 hours
Suppression of recurrent genital herpes:
Cl_{cr} ≥40 mL/minute: Administer 250 mg every 12 hours
Cl_{cr} 20-39 mL/minute: Administer 125 mg every 12 hours
Cl_{cr} <20 mL/minute: Administer 125 mg every 24 hours
Recurrent orolabial or genital herpes in HIV-infected patients:
Cl_{cr} ≥40 mL/minute: Administer 500 mg every 12 hours
Cl_{cr} 20-39 mL/minute: Administer 500 mg every 24 hours
Cl_{cr} <20 mL/minute: Administer 250 mg every 24 hours

Administration Initiate therapy as soon as herpes zoster is diagnosed.

Dosage Forms Tablet: 125 mg, 250 mg, 500 mg

Monitoring Parameters Periodic CBC during long-term therapy

Dietary Considerations May be taken with food or on an empty stomach.

Patient Information Initiate therapy as soon as herpes zoster is diagnosed; may take medication with food or on an empty stomach

Additional Information Most effective if therapy is initiated within 72 hours of initial lesion.

Special Geriatric Considerations For herpes zoster (shingles) infections, famciclovir should be started within 72 hours of the appearance of the rash to be effective. Famciclovir has been shown to accelerate healing, reduce the duration of viral shedding, and resolve posthepatic neuralgia faster than placebo. Comparison trials to acyclovir or valacyclovir are not available. Adjust dose for estimated renal function.

Selected Readings
Boike SC, Pue MA, and Freed MI, "Pharmacokinetics of Famciclovir in Subjects With Varying Degrees of Renal Impairment," *Clin Pharmacol Ther*, 1994, 55(4):418-26.
Gill KS and Wood MJ, "The Clinical Pharmacokinetics of Famciclovir," *Clin Pharmacokinet*, 1996, 31(1):1-8.
Hodge RA, "Famciclovir and Penciclovir: The Mode of Action of Famciclovir Including Its Conversion to Penciclovir," *Antivir Chem Chemother*, 1993, 4:67-84.
Perry CM and Wagstaff AJ, "Famciclovir. A Review of Its Pharmacological Properties and Therapeutic Efficacy in Herpesvirus Infections," *Drugs*, 1995, 50(2):396-415.
Pue MA and Benet LZ, "Pharmacokinetics of Famciclovir in Man," *Antivir Chem Chemother*, 1993, 4(Suppl 1):47-55.

♦ **Famvir®** *see* Famciclovir *on page 332*
♦ **Fareston®** *see* Toremifene *on page 779*
♦ **Faslodex®** *see* Fulvestrant *on page 372*
♦ **5-FC** *see* Flucytosine *on page 354*
♦ **FC1157a** *see* Toremifene *on page 779*
♦ **FDA Pregnancy Categories** *see page 18*
♦ **Femara®** *see* Letrozole *on page 494*

♦ **Femilax**™ **[OTC]** *see* Bisacodyl *on page 133*

Fentanyl (FEN ta nil)
Medication Safety Issues
Sound-alike/look-alike issues:
Fentanyl may be confused with alfentanil, sufentanil

Transdermal patch may contain conducting metal (eg, aluminum); remove patch prior to MRI.

U.S. Brand Names Actiq®; Duragesic®; Sublimaze®

Canadian Brand Names Actiq®; Duragesic®

Generic Available Yes: Excludes lozenge

Synonyms Fentanyl Citrate

Pharmacologic Category Analgesic, Narcotic; General Anesthetic

Pregnancy Risk Factor C/D (prolonged use or high doses at term)

Lactation Enters breast milk/not recommended (AAP rates "compatible")

Use
Injection: Sedation, relief of pain, preoperative medication, adjunct to general or regional anesthesia

Transdermal: Management of moderate-to-severe chronic pain

Transmucosal (Actiq®): Management of breakthrough cancer pain

Mechanism of Action Binds with stereospecific receptors at many sites within the CNS, increases pain threshold, alters pain reception, inhibits ascending pain pathways

Restrictions C-II

Labeled Contraindications Hypersensitivity to fentanyl or any component of the formulation; increased intracranial pressure; severe respiratory disease or depression including acute asthma (unless patient is mechanically ventilated); paralytic ileus; severe liver or renal insufficiency; pregnancy (prolonged use or high doses near term)

Transmucosal lozenges (Actiq®) or transdermal patches must not be used in patients who are intolerant to opioids. Patients are considered opioid-tolerant if they are taking at least 60 mg morphine/day, 30 mg oral oxycodone/day, 8 mg oral hydromorphone/day, 50 mcg transdermal fentanyl/hour, or an equivalent dose of another opioid for ≥1 week. Transdermal patches are not for use in acute pain, mild pain, or postoperative pain management.

Warnings/Precautions An opioid-containing analgesic regimen should be tailored to each patient's needs and based upon the type of pain being treated (acute versus chronic), the route of administration, degree of tolerance for opioids (naive versus chronic user), age, weight, and medical condition. The optimal analgesic dose varies widely among patients. Doses should be titrated to pain relief/prevention. Fentanyl shares the toxic potentials of opiate agonists, and precautions of opiate agonist therapy should be observed. Use with caution in patients with bradycardia. Rapid I.V. infusion may result in skeletal muscle and chest wall rigidity leading to respiratory distress and/or apnea, bronchoconstriction, laryngospasm. Inject slowly over 3-5 minutes. Nondepolarizing skeletal muscle relaxant may be required. Tolerance or drug dependence may result from extended use. Use caution in patients with a history of drug dependence or abuse. The elderly may be particularly susceptible to the CNS depressant and constipating effects of narcotics.
(Continued)

Fentanyl *(Continued)*

Topical patches: Serious or life-threatening hypoventilation may occur, even in opioid-tolerant patients. Serum fentanyl concentrations may increase approximately 33% for patients with a body temperature of 40°C secondary to a temperature-dependent increase in fentanyl release from the system and increased skin permeability. Patients who experience adverse reactions should be monitored for at least 24 hours after removal of the patch. Transdermal patch may contain conducting metal (eg, aluminum); remove patch prior to MRI. Safety and efficacy of transdermal system have been limited to children >2 years of age who are opioid tolerant.

Adverse Reactions

>10%:

Cardiovascular: Hypotension, bradycardia

Central nervous system: CNS depression, confusion, drowsiness, sedation

Gastrointestinal: Nausea, vomiting, constipation, xerostomia

Neuromuscular & skeletal: Chest wall rigidity (high dose I.V.), weakness

Ocular: Miosis

Respiratory: Respiratory depression

Miscellaneous: Diaphoresis

1% to 10%:

Cardiovascular: Cardiac arrhythmia, edema, orthostatic hypotension, hypertension, syncope

Central nervous system: Abnormal dreams, abnormal thinking, agitation, amnesia, dizziness, euphoria, fatigue, fever, hallucinations, headache, insomnia, nervousness, paranoid reaction

Dermatologic: Erythema, papules, pruritus, rash

Gastrointestinal: Abdominal pain, anorexia, biliary tract spasm, diarrhea, dyspepsia, flatulence

Local: Application site reaction

Neuromuscular & skeletal: Abnormal coordination, abnormal gait, back pain, paresthesia, rigors, tremor

Respiratory: Apnea, bronchitis, dyspnea, hemoptysis, pharyngitis, rhinitis, sinusitis, upper respiratory infection

Miscellaneous: Hiccups, flu-like syndrome, speech disorder

<1%: Abdominal distention, ADH release, amblyopia, aphasia, bladder pain, bradycardia, bronchospasm, circulatory depression, CNS excitation or delirium, cold/clammy skin, convulsions, depersonalization, dysesthesia, exfoliative dermatitis, hyper-/hypotonia, hostility, laryngospasm, oliguria, paradoxical dizziness, physical and psychological dependence with prolonged use, polyuria, pustules, stertorous breathing, stupor, urinary tract spasm, urticaria, vertigo

Postmarketing and/or case reports: Anorgasmia, blurred vision, dental caries (Actiq®), ejaculatory difficulty, gum line erosion (Actiq®), libido decreased, tachycardia, tooth loss (Actiq®), weight loss

Vesicant No

Overdosage/Toxicology

Symptoms of overdose include CNS depression, respiratory depression, and miosis. Treatment is supportive. Naloxone, 2 mg I.V. with repeat administration as necessary up to a total of 10 mg, can also be used to reverse toxic effects of the opiate. Patients who experience adverse reactions during use of transdermal fentanyl should be monitored for at least 24 hours after removal of the patch.

Drug Interactions

Cytochrome P450 Effect: Substrate of CYP3A4 (major); **Inhibits** CYP3A4 (weak)

Increased Effect/Toxicity: Increased sedation with CNS depressants, phenothiazines. Tricyclic antidepressants may potentiate fentanyl's adverse effects. Potential for serotonin syndrome if combined with other serotonergic drugs. CYP3A4 inhibitors may increase the levels/effects of fentanyl; potentially fatal respiratory depression may occur when a potent inhibitor is used in a patient receiving chronic fentanyl (eg, transdermal); example inhibitors include azole antifungals, ciprofloxacin, clarithromycin, diclofenac, doxycycline, erythromycin, imatinib, isoniazid, nefazodone, nicardipine, propofol, protease inhibitors, quinidine, and verapamil.

Decreased Effect: CYP3A4 inducers (including carbamazepine, phenytoin, phenobarbital, rifampin) may decrease serum levels of fentanyl by increasing metabolism.

Ethanol/Nutrition/Herb Interactions

Ethanol: Avoid ethanol (may increase CNS depression).

Food: Glucose may cause hyperglycemia.

Herb/Nutraceutical: St John's wort may decrease fentanyl levels. Avoid valerian, St John's wort, kava kava, gotu kola (may increase CNS depression).

Storage/Stability

Injection formulation: Store at controlled room temperature of 15°C to 25°C (59°F to 86°F). Protect from light.

Transdermal: Do not store above 25°C (77°F).

Transmucosal: Store at controlled room temperature of 15°C to 30°C (59°F to 86°F).

Compatibility Stable in D_5W, NS

Y-site administration: Compatible: Alatrofloxacin, amphotericin B cholesteryl sulfate complex, atracurium, cisatracurium, diltiazem, dobutamine, dopamine, enalaprilat, epinephrine, esmolol, etomidate, furosemide, gatifloxacin, heparin, hydrocortisone sodium succinate, hydromorphone, labetalol, levofloxacin, linezolid, lorazepam, midazolam, milrinone, morphine, nafcillin, nicardipine, nitroglycerin, norepinephrine, pancuronium, potassium chloride, propofol, ranitidine, remifentanil, sargramostim, thiopental, vecuronium, vitamin B complex with C

Compatibility in syringe: Compatible: Atracurium, atropine, bupivacaine with ketamine, butorphanol, chlorpromazine, cimetidine, clonidine with lidocaine, dimenhydrinate, diphenhydramine, droperidol, heparin, hydromorphone, hydroxyzine, meperidine, metoclopramide, midazolam, morphine, ondansetron, pentazocine, perphenazine, prochlorperazine edisylate, promazine, promethazine, ranitidine, scopolamine. **Incompatible:** Pentobarbital

Compatibility when admixed: Compatible: Bupivacaine. **Incompatible:** Fluorouracil, methohexital, pentobarbital, thiopental

Pharmacodynamics/Kinetics

Onset of action: Analgesic: I.M.: 7-15 minutes; I.V.: Almost immediate; Transmucosal: 5-15 minutes

Peak effect: Transmucosal: Analgesic: 20-30 minutes

(Continued)

Fentanyl *(Continued)*

Duration: I.M.: 1-2 hours; I.V.: 0.5-1 hour; Transmucosal: Related to blood level; respiratory depressant effect may last longer than analgesic effect

Absorption: Transmucosal: Rapid, ~25% from the buccal mucosa; 75% swallowed with saliva and slowly absorbed from GI tract

Distribution: Highly lipophilic, redistributes into muscle and fat

Metabolism: Hepatic, primarily via CYP3A4

Bioavailability: Transmucosal: ~50% (range: 36% to 71%)

Half-life elimination: 2-4 hours; Transmucosal: 6.6 hours (range: 5-15 hours); Transdermal: 17 hours (half-life is influenced by absorption rate)

Excretion: Urine (primarily as metabolites, 10% as unchanged drug)

Dosage Note: These are guidelines and do not represent the maximum doses that may be required in all patients. Doses should be titrated to pain relief/prevention. Monitor vital signs routinely. Single I.M. doses have a duration of 1-2 hours, single I.V. doses last 0.5-1 hour.

Children 1-12 years:

Sedation for minor procedures/analgesia: I.M., I.V.: 1-2 mcg/kg/dose; may repeat at 30- to 60-minute intervals. **Note:** Children 18-36 months of age may require 2-3 mcg/kg/dose

Continuous sedation/analgesia: Initial I.V. bolus: 1-2 mcg/kg then 1 mcg/kg/hour; titrate upward; usual: 1-3 mcg/kg/hour

Pain management: Transdermal (limited to children >2 years who are opioid tolerant): Initial dose: 25 mcg/hour system (higher doses have been used based on equianalgesic conversion); change patch every 72 hours

Children >12 years and Adults:

Sedation for minor procedures/analgesia: I.M., I.V.: 0.5-1 mcg/kg/dose; higher doses are used for major procedures

Pain management: Transdermal:

Initial: To convert patients from oral or parenteral opioids to transdermal formulation, a 24-hour analgesic requirement should be calculated (based on prior opiate use). This analgesic requirement should be converted to the equianalgesic oral morphine dose. The initial fentanyl dosage may be approximated from the 24-hour morphine dosage and titrated to minimize adverse effects and provide analgesia. Change patch every 72 hours.

Titration: Short-acting agents may be required until analgesic efficacy is established and/or as supplements for "breakthrough" pain. The amount of supplemental doses should be closely monitored. Appropriate dosage increases may be based on daily supplemental dosage using the ratio of 45 mg/24 hours of oral morphine to a 12.5 mcg/hour increase in fentanyl dosage.

Frequency of adjustment: The dosage should not be titrated more frequently than every 3 days after the initial dose or every 6 days thereafter. Patients should wear a consistent fentanyl dosage through two applications (6 days) before dosage increase based on supplemental opiate dosages can be estimated.

Frequency of application: The majority of patients may be controlled on every 72-hour administration; however, a small number of patients require every 48-hour administration.

Adults:

Premedication: I.M., slow I.V.: 50-100 mcg/dose 30-60 minutes prior to surgery

Adjunct to regional anesthesia: I.M., slow I.V.: 50-100 mcg/dose; if I.V. used, give over 1-2 minutes

Severe pain: I.M.: 50-100 mcg/dose every 1-2 hours as needed; patients with prior opiate exposure may tolerate higher initial doses

Adjunct to general anesthesia: Slow I.V.:

Low dose: Initial: 2 mcg/kg/dose; Maintenance: Additional doses infrequently needed

Moderate dose: Initial: 2-20 mcg/kg/dose; Maintenance: 25-100 mcg/dose may be given slow I.V. or I.M. as needed

High dose: Initial: 20-50 mcg/kg/dose; Maintenance: 25 mcg to one-half the initial loading dose may be given as needed

General anesthesia without additional anesthetic agents: Slow I.V.: 50-100 mcg/kg with O_2 and skeletal muscle relaxant

Mechanically-ventilated patients (based on 70 kg patient): Slow I.V.: 0.35-1.5 mcg/kg every 30-60 minutes as needed; infusion: 0.7-10 mcg/kg/hour

Patient-controlled analgesia (PCA): I.V.: Usual concentration: 50 mcg/mL

Demand dose: Usual: 10 mcg; range: 10-50 mcg

Lockout interval: 5-8 minutes

Breakthrough cancer pain: Adults: Transmucosal: Initial starting dose: 200 mcg; second dose may be started 15 minutes after completion of the first dose. Consumption should be limited to 4 units/day or less. Patients needing more than 4 units/day should have the dose of their long-term opioid re-evaluated.

The majority of patients are controlled on every 72-hour administration, however, a small number of patients require every 48-hour administration.

Elderly >65 years: Transmucosal: Actiq®: Dose should be reduced to 2.5-5 mcg/kg

Dosing adjustment in hepatic impairment: Fentanyl kinetics may be altered in hepatic disease

Administration

I.V.: Muscular rigidity may occur with rapid I.V. administration.

Transdermal: Apply to nonirritated and nonirradiated skin, such as chest, back, flank, or upper arm. Do not shave skin; hair at application site should be clipped. Prior to application, clean site with clear water and allow to dry completely. Do not cut patch. Firmly press in place and hold for 30 seconds. Change patch every 72 hours. Do **not** use soap, alcohol, or other solvents to remove transdermal gel if it accidentally touches skin; use copious amounts of water. Avoid exposing application site to external heat sources (eg, heating pad, electric blanket, heat lamp, hot tub).

Transmucosal: Foil overwrap should be removed just prior to administration. Place the unit in mouth and allow it to dissolve. Do **not** chew. Actiq® units may be moved from one side of the mouth to the other. The unit should be consumed over a period of 15 minutes. Unit should be removed after it is consumed or if patient has achieved an adequate response and/or shows signs of respiratory depression. For patients

(Continued)

Fentanyl (Continued)

who have received transmucosal product within 6-12 hours, it is recommended that if other narcotics are required, they should be used at starting doses $1/4$ to $1/3$ those usually recommended.

Dosage Forms

Infusion [premixed in NS]: 0.05 mg (10 mL); 1 mg (100 mL); 1.25 mg (250 mL); 2 mg (100 mL); 2.5 mg (250 mL)

Injection, solution, as citrate [preservative free]: 0.05 mg/mL (2 mL, 5 mL, 10 mL, 20 mL, 30 mL, 50 mL)

Sublimaze®: 0.05 mg/mL (2 mL, 5 mL, 10 mL, 20 mL)

Lozenge, oral transmucosal, as citrate (Actiq®): 200 mcg, 400 mcg, 600 mcg, 800 mcg, 1200 mcg, 1600 mcg [mounted on a plastic radiopaque handle; raspberry flavor]

Transdermal system: 25 mcg/hour [6.25 cm^2] (5s); 50 mcg/hour [12.5 cm^2] (5s); 75 mcg/hour [18.75 cm^2]; 100 mcg/hour [25 cm^2] (5s)

Duragesic®: 12 mcg/hour [5 cm^2] (5s); 25 mcg/hour [10 cm^2] (5s); 50 mcg/hour [20 cm^2] (5s); 75 mcg/hour [30 cm^2] (5s); 100 mcg/hour [40 cm^2] (5s)

Monitoring Parameters Respiratory and cardiovascular status, blood pressure, heart rate

Transdermal: Monitor for 24 hours after application of first dose

Dietary Considerations Actiq® contains 2 g sugar per unit.

Patient Information Actiq® preparations contain an amount of medication that can be fatal to children. Keep all units out of the reach of children and discard any open units properly. Actiq® Welcome Kits are available which contain educational materials, safe storage and disposal instructions.

Additional Information Fentanyl is 50-100 times as potent as morphine; morphine 10 mg I.M. is equivalent to fentanyl 0.1-0.2 mg I.M.; fentanyl has less hypotensive effects than morphine due to lack of histamine release. However, fentanyl may cause rigidity with high doses. If the patient has required high-dose analgesia or has used for a prolonged period (~7 days), taper dose to prevent withdrawal; monitor for signs and symptoms of withdrawal.

Transmucosal (oral lozenge): Disposal of Actiq® units: After consumption of a complete unit, the handle may be disposed of in a trash container that is out of the reach of children. For a partially-consumed unit, or a unit that still has any drug matrix remaining on the handle, the handle should be placed under hot running tap water until the drug matrix has dissolved. Special child-resistant containers are available to temporarily store partially consumed units that cannot be disposed of immediately.

Transdermal system (Duragesic®): Upon removal of the patch, ~17 hours are required before serum concentrations fall to 50% of their original values. Opioid withdrawal symptoms are possible. Gradual downward titration (potentially by the sequential use of lower-dose patches) is recommended. Keep transdermal product (both used and unused) out of the reach of children. Do **not** use soap, alcohol, or other solvents to remove transdermal gel if it accidentally touches skin as they may increase transdermal absorption, use copious amounts of water.

Special Geriatric Considerations The elderly may be particularly susceptible to the CNS depressant and constipating effects of narcotics; therefore, use with caution.

Selected Readings

Clotz MA and Nahata MC, "Clinical Uses of Fentanyl, Sufentanil, and Alfentanil," *Clin Pharm*, 1991, 10(8):581-93.

Fine PG, "Fentanyl in the Treatment of Cancer Pain," *Semin Oncol*, 1997, 24(5 Suppl 16):16-20-7.

Grond S, Radbruch L, and Lehmann KA, "Clinical Pharmacokinetics of Transdermal Opioids: Focus on Transdermal Fentanyl," *Clin Pharmacokinet*, 2000, 38(1):59-89.

Jeal W and Benfield P, "Transdermal Fentanyl. A Review of Its Pharmacological Properties and Therapeutic Efficacy in Pain Control," *Drugs*, 1997, 53(1):109-38.

Peng PW and Sandler AN, "Review of the Use of Fentanyl Analgesia in the Management of Acute Pain in Adults," *Anesthesiology*, 1999, 90(2):576-99.

Poklis A, "Fentanyl: A Review for Clinical and Analytical Toxicologists," *J Toxicol Clin Toxicol*, 1995, 33(5):439-47.

Scholz J, Steinfath M, and Schulz M, "Clinical Pharmacokinetics of Alfentanil, Fentanyl, and Sufentanil. An Update," *Clin Pharmacokinet*, 1996, 31(4):275-92.

Wedell D and Hersh EV, "A Review of the Opioid Analgesics Fentanyl, Alfentanil, and Sufentanil," *Compendium*, 1991, 12(3):184-7.

Willens JS and Myslinski NR, "Pharmacodynamics, Pharmacokinetics, and Clinical Uses of Fentanyl, Sufentanil, and Alfentanil," *Heart Lung*, 1993, 22(3):239-51.

♦ **Fentanyl Citrate** *see* Fentanyl *on page 335*

♦ **Fertility and Cancer Therapy** *see page 962*

Filgrastim (fil GRA stim)

Medication Safety Issues

Sound-alike/look-alike issues:

Neupogen® may be confused with Epogen®, Neumega®, Nutramigen®

Related Information

Management of Infections *on page 978*

Transplantation *on page 1019*

U.S. Brand Names Neupogen®

Canadian Brand Names Neupogen®

Generic Available No

Synonyms G-CSF; Granulocyte Colony Stimulating Factor

Pharmacologic Category Colony Stimulating Factor

Pregnancy Risk Factor C

Lactation Excretion in breast milk unknown/use caution

Use Stimulation of granulocyte production in patients with malignancies, including myeloid malignancies; receiving myelosuppressive therapy associated with a significant risk of neutropenia; severe chronic neutropenia (SCN); receiving bone marrow transplantation (BMT); undergoing peripheral blood progenitor cell (PBPC) collection

Mechanism of Action Stimulates the production, maturation, and activation of neutrophils; filgrastim activates neutrophils to increase both their migration and cytotoxicity. See table.

Comparative Effects — G-CSF vs GM-CSF

Proliferation/Differentiation	G-CSF (Filgrastim)	GM-CSF (Sargramostim)
Neutrophils	Yes	Yes
Eosinophils	No	Yes
Macrophages	No	Yes
Neutrophil migration	Enhanced	Inhibited

(Continued)

Filgrastim *(Continued)*

Labeled Contraindications Hypersensitivity to filgrastim, *E. coli*-derived proteins, or any component of the formulation; concurrent myelosuppressive chemotherapy or radiation therapy

Warnings/Precautions Do not use filgrastim in the period 24 hours before to 24 hours after administration of cytotoxic chemotherapy because of the potential sensitivity of rapidly dividing myeloid cells to cytotoxic chemotherapy. Precaution should be exercised in the usage of filgrastim in any malignancy with myeloid characteristics. Filgrastim can potentially act as a growth factor for any tumor type, particularly myeloid malignancies. Tumors of nonhematopoietic origin may have surface receptors for filgrastim.

Allergic-type reactions have occurred in patients receiving the parent compound, filgrastim with first or later doses. Reactions tended to occur more frequently with intravenous administration and within 30 minutes of infusion. Rare cases of splenic rupture or adult respiratory distress syndrome have been reported in association with filgrastim; patients must be instructed to report left upper quadrant pain or shoulder tip pain or respiratory distress. Use caution in patients with sickle cell diseases; sickle cell crises have been reported following filgrastim therapy.

Adverse Reactions

>10%:

Cardiovascular: Chest pain

Central nervous system: Fever

Dermatologic: Alopecia

Endocrine & metabolic: Fluid retention

Gastrointestinal: Nausea, vomiting, diarrhea, mucositis; splenomegaly - up to 33% of patients with cyclic neutropenia/congenital agranulocytosis receiving filgrastim for ≥14 days; rare in other patients

Neuromuscular & skeletal: Bone pain (24%), commonly in the lower back, posterior iliac crest, and sternum

1% to 10%:

Cardiovascular: S-T segment depression (3%)

Central nervous system: Headache

Dermatologic: Rash

Gastrointestinal: Anorexia, constipation, sore throat

Hematologic: Leukocytosis

Local: Pain at injection site

Neuromuscular & skeletal: Weakness

Respiratory: Dyspnea, cough

<1%: Transient supraventricular arrhythmia, pericarditis, hypotension, thrombophlebitis, hypersensitivity reactions

Vesicant No

Emetic Potential Low (10% to 30%)

Overdosage/Toxicology No clinical adverse effects have been seen with high doses producing ANC >10,000/mm^3.

Storage/Stability Intact vials and prefilled syringes should be stored under refrigeration at 2°C to 8°C (36°F to 46°F) and protected from direct sunlight. Filgrastim should be protected from freezing and temperatures

>30°C to avoid aggregation. If inadvertently frozen, thaw in a refrigerator and use within 24 hours; do not use if frozen >24 hours or frozen more than once. The solution should not be shaken since bubbles and/or foam may form. If foaming occurs, the solution should be left undisturbed for a few minutes until bubbles dissipate.

Filgrastim vials and prefilled syringes are stable for 7 days at 9°C to 30°C (47°F to 86°F), however, the manufacturer recommends discarding after 24 hours because of microbiological concerns. The product is packaged without a preservative.

Undiluted filgrastim is stable for 24 hours at 15°C to 30°C and for 2 weeks at 2°C to 8°C (36°F to 46°F) in tuberculin syringes. However, the manufacturer recommends to use immediately because of concern for bacterial contamination.

Filgrastim diluted for I.V. infusion ($\geq$15 mcg/mL) is stable for 7 days at 2°C to 8°C (36°F to 46°F).

Reconstitution Filgrastim may be diluted in dextrose 5% in water to a concentration $\geq$15 mcg/mL for I.V. infusion administration. Minimum concentration is 15 mcg/mL. Concentrations <15 mcg/mL require addition of albumin (1 mL of 5%) to the bag to prevent absorption to plastics/PVC.

Compatibility Stable in D_5W; **not stable** in NS

Y-site administration: Compatible: Acyclovir, allopurinol, amikacin, aminophylline, ampicillin, ampicillin/sulbactam, aztreonam, bleomycin, bumetanide, buprenorphine, butorphanol, calcium gluconate, carboplatin, carmustine, cefazolin, cefotetan, ceftazidime, chlorpromazine, cimetidine, cisplatin, co-trimoxazole, cyclophosphamide, cytarabine, dacarbazine, daunorubicin, dexamethasone sodium phosphate, diphenhydramine, doxorubicin, doxycycline, droperidol, enalaprilat, famotidine, floxuridine, fluconazole, fludarabine, ganciclovir, granisetron, haloperidol, hydrocortisone sodium phosphate, hydrocortisone sodium succinate, hydromorphone, hydroxyzine, idarubicin, ifosfamide, leucovorin, lorazepam, mechlorethamine, melphalan, meperidine, mesna, methotrexate, metoclopramide, minocycline, mitoxantrone, morphine, nalbuphine, netilmicin, ondansetron, plicamycin, potassium chloride, promethazine, ranitidine, sodium bicarbonate, streptozocin, ticarcillin, ticarcillin/clavulanate, tobramycin, vancomycin, vinblastine, vincristine, vinorelbine, zidovudine. **Incompatible:** Amphotericin B, cefepime, cefoperazone, cefotaxime, cefoxitin, ceftizoxime, ceftriaxone, cefuroxime, clindamycin, dactinomycin, etoposide, fluorouracil, furosemide, heparin, mannitol, methylprednisolone sodium succinate, metronidazole, mitomycin, piperacillin, prochlorperazine edisylate, thiotepa. **Variable (consult detailed reference):** Gentamicin, imipenem/cilastatin

Pharmacodynamics/Kinetics

Onset of action: ~24 hours; plateaus in 3-5 days

Duration: ANC decreases by 50% within 2 days after discontinuing filgrastim; white counts return to the normal range in 4-7 days; peak plasma levels can be maintained for up to 12 hours

Absorption: SubQ: 100%

Distribution: V_d: 150 mL/kg; no evidence of drug accumulation over a 11- to 20-day period

Metabolism: Systemically degraded

Half-life elimination: 1.8-3.5 hours

(Continued)

Filgrastim *(Continued)*

Time to peak, serum: SubQ: 2-6 hours

Dosage Refer to individual protocols.

Dosing, even in morbidly obese patients, should be based on actual body weight. Rounding doses to the nearest vial size enhances patient convenience and reduces costs without compromising clinical response.

Myelosuppressive therapy: 5 mcg/kg/day - doses may be increased by 5 mcg/kg according to the duration and severity of the neutropenia.

Bone marrow transplantation: 5-10 mcg/kg/day - doses may be increased by 5 mcg/kg according to the duration and severity of neutropenia; recommended steps based on neutrophil response:

When ANC >1000/mm^3 for 3 consecutive days: Reduce filgrastim dose to 5 mcg/kg/day

If ANC remains >1000/mm^3 for 3 more consecutive days: Discontinue filgrastim

If ANC decreases to <1000/mm^3: Resume at 5 mcg/kg/day

If ANC decreases <1000/mm^3 during the 5 mcg/kg/day dose, increase filgrastim to 10 mcg/kg/day and follow the above steps

Peripheral blood progenitor cell (PBPC) collection: 10 mcg/kg/day **or** 5-8 mcg/kg twice daily in donors. The optimal timing and duration of growth factor stimulation has not been determined.

Severe chronic neutropenia:

Congenital: 6 mcg/kg twice daily

Idiopathic/cyclic: 5 mcg/kg/day

Not removed by hemodialysis

Combination Regimens

Breast cancer: AC - dose dense *on page 843*

Leukemia, acute myeloid: FLAG *on page 889*

Lymphoma, non-Hodgkin's: ICE (Lymphoma, non-Hodgkin's) *on page 899*

Prostate cancer: Cyclophosphamide + Doxorubicin *on page 869*

Administration May be administered undiluted by SubQ or by I.V. infusion over 15-60 minutes in D$_5$W; **incompatible** with sodium chloride solutions

Dosage Forms

Injection, solution [preservative free]: 300 mcg/mL (1 mL, 1.6 mL) [vial; contains sodium 0.035 mg/mL and sorbitol]

Injection, solution [preservative free]: 600 mcg/mL (0.5 mL, 0.8 mL) [prefilled Singleject® syringe; contains sodium 0.035 mg/mL and sorbitol]

High Dose Considerations

High Dose: 5-10 mcg/kg/day

Monitoring Parameters WBC should be monitored 7-10 days after beginning filgrastim, then every 7-10 days until WBC recovers. Leukocytosis (white blood cell counts ≥100,000/mm^3) has been observed in ~2% of patients receiving filgrastim at doses >5 mcg/kg/day.

Dietary Considerations Injection solution contains sodium 0.035 mg/mL and sorbitol.

Patient Information Follow directions for proper storage and administration of SubQ medication. Never reuse syringes or needles. You may experience bone pain (request analgesic); nausea or vomiting (small frequent meals may help); hair loss (reversible); or sore mouth (frequent mouth care with a soft toothbrush or cotton swab may help). Report unusual fever or chills; unhealed sores; severe bone pain; pain, redness, or swelling at injection site; unusual swelling of extremities or difficulty breathing; or chest pain and palpitations.

Additional Information
Reimbursement Hotline: 1-800-272-9376
Professional Services [Amgen]: 1-800-77-AMGEN

Selected Readings
"1997 Update of Recommendations for the Use of Hematopoietic Colony-Stimulating Factors: Evidence-Based, Clinical Practice Guidelines. American Society of Clinical Oncology," *J Clin Oncol*, 1997, 15(10):3288.

Frampton JE, Lee CR, and Faulds D, "Filgrastim. A Review of Its Pharmacological Properties and Therapeutic Efficacy in Neutropenia," *Drugs*, 1994, 48(5):731-60.

Hollingshead LM, Goa KL, "Recombinant Granulocyte Colony-Stimulating Factor (rG-CSF). A Review of Its Pharmacological Properties and Prospective Role in Neutropenic Conditions," *Drugs*, 1991, 42(2):300-30.

Kuwabara T, Kobayashi S, and Sugiyama Y, "Pharmacokinetics and Pharmacodynamics of a Recombinant Human Granulocyte Colony-Stimulating Factor," *Drug Metab Rev*, 1996, 28(4):625-58.

Lieschke GJ and Burgess AW, "Granulocyte Colony-Stimulating Factor and Granulocyte-Macrophage Colony-Stimulating Factor," *N Engl J Med*, 1992, 327(1):28-35.

Nemunaitis J, "A Comparative Review of Colony-Stimulating Factors," *Drugs*, 1997, 54(5):709-29.

Finasteride (fi NAS teer ide)

Medication Safety Issues
Sound-alike/look-alike issues:
Proscar® may be confused with ProSom®, Prozac®, Psorcon®

Related Information
Safe Handling of Hazardous Drugs *on page 1034*

U.S. Brand Names Propecia®; Proscar®

Canadian Brand Names Propecia®; Proscar®

Generic Available No

Pharmacologic Category 5 Alpha-Reductase Inhibitor

Pregnancy Risk Factor X

Lactation Excretion in breast milk unknown/contraindicated

Use
Propecia®: Treatment of male pattern hair loss in **men only**. Safety and efficacy were demonstrated in men between 18-41 years of age.
Proscar®: Treatment of symptomatic benign prostatic hyperplasia (BPH); can be used in combination with an alpha blocker, doxazosin

Unlabeled/Investigational Use Adjuvant monotherapy after radical prostatectomy in the treatment of prostatic cancer; female hirsutism

Mechanism of Action Finasteride is a competitive inhibitor of both tissue and hepatic 5-alpha reductase. This results in inhibition of the conversion of testosterone to dihydrotestosterone and markedly suppresses serum dihydrotestosterone levels

Labeled Contraindications Hypersensitivity to finasteride or any component of the formulation; pregnancy; not for use in children

Warnings/Precautions Hazardous agent - use appropriate precautions for handling and disposal. See Safe Handling of Hazardous Drugs *on page 1034* in the Appendix. A minimum of 6 months of treatment may be necessary to determine whether an individual will respond to finasteride. Use with caution in those patients with hepatic dysfunction. Carefully (Continued)

Finasteride *(Continued)*

monitor patients with a large residual urinary volume or severely diminished urinary flow for obstructive uropathy. These patients may not be candidates for finasteride therapy.

Adverse Reactions Note: "Combination therapy" refers to finasteride and doxazosin.

>10%:

Endocrine & metabolic: Impotence (19%; combination therapy 23%), libido decreased (10%; combination therapy 12%)

Genitourinary: Neuromuscular & skeletal: Weakness (5%; combination therapy 17%)

1% to 10%:

Cardiovascular: Postural hypotension (9%; combination therapy 18%), edema (1%, combination therapy 3%)

Central nervous system: Dizziness (7%; combination therapy 23%), somnolence (2%; combination therapy 3%)

Genitourinary: Ejaculation disturbances (7%; combination therapy 14%), decreased volume of ejaculate

Endocrine & metabolic: Gynecomastia (2%)

Respiratory: Dyspnea (1%; combination therapy 2%), rhinitis (1%; combination therapy 2%)

<1%, postmarketing and/or case reports: Hypersensitivity (pruritus, rash, urticaria, swelling of face/lips); breast tenderness, breast enlargement, breast cancer (males), prostate cancer (high grade), testicular pain

Emetic Potential Very low (<10%)

Drug Interactions

Cytochrome P450 Effect: Substrate of CYP3A4 (minor)

Ethanol/Nutrition/Herb Interactions

Herb/Nutraceutical: St John's wort may decrease finasteride levels. Avoid saw palmetto (concurrent use has not been adequately studied).

Storage/Stability Store below 30°C (86°F). Protect from light.

Pharmacodynamics/Kinetics

Onset of action: 3-6 months of ongoing therapy

Duration:

After a single oral dose as small as 0.5 mg: 65% depression of plasma dihydrotestosterone levels persists 5-7 days

After 6 months of treatment with 5 mg/day: Circulating dihydrotestosterone levels are reduced to castrate levels without significant effects on circulating testosterone; levels return to normal within 14 days of discontinuation of treatment

Distribution: V_{dss}: 76 L

Protein binding: 90%

Metabolism: Hepatic via CYP3A4; two active metabolites (<20% activity of finasteride)

Bioavailability: Mean: 63%

Half-life elimination, serum: Elderly: 8 hours; Adults: 6 hours (3-16)

Time to peak, serum: 2-6 hours

Excretion: Feces (57%) and urine (39%) as metabolites

Dosage Oral: Adults:

Male:

Benign prostatic hyperplasia (Proscar®): 5 mg/day as a single dose; clinical responses occur within 12 weeks to 6 months of initiation of therapy; long-term administration is recommended for maximal response

Male pattern baldness (Propecia®): 1 mg daily

Female hirsutism (unlabeled use): 5 mg/day

Dosing adjustment in renal impairment: No dosage adjustment is necessary

Dosing adjustment in hepatic impairment: Use with caution in patients with liver function abnormalities because finasteride is metabolized extensively in the liver

Administration Administration with food may delay the rate and reduce the extent of oral absorption. Women of childbearing age should not touch or handle broken tablets.

Dosage Forms

Tablet [film coated]:
Propecia®: 1 mg
Proscar®: 5 mg

Monitoring Parameters Objective and subjective signs of relief of benign prostatic hyperplasia, including improvement in urinary flow, reduction in symptoms of urgency, and relief of difficulty in micturition

Special Geriatric Considerations Clearance of finasteride is decreased in the elderly, but no dosage reductions are necessary.

♦ **FK506** *see* Tacrolimus *on page 734*

♦ **Flagyl®** *see* Metronidazole *on page 568*

♦ **Flagyl ER®** *see* Metronidazole *on page 568*

♦ **Flagyl® I.V. RTU™** *see* Metronidazole *on page 568*

♦ **Flebogamma®** *see* Immune Globulin (Intravenous) *on page 458*

♦ **Fleet® Bisacodyl Enema [OTC]** *see* Bisacodyl *on page 133*

♦ **Fleet® Stimulant Laxative [OTC]** *see* Bisacodyl *on page 133*

♦ **Florazole® ER (Can)** *see* Metronidazole *on page 568*

♦ **Floxin®** *see* Ofloxacin *on page 618*

♦ **Floxin Otic Singles** *see* Ofloxacin *on page 618*

Floxuridine (floks YOOR i deen)

Medication Safety Issues

Sound-alike/look-alike issues:
FUDR® may be confused with Fludara®

Related Information

Safe Handling of Hazardous Drugs *on page 1034*

U.S. Brand Names FUDR®

Canadian Brand Names FUDR®

Generic Available Yes

Synonyms Fluorodeoxyuridine; FUDR; 5-FUDR; NSC-27640

Pharmacologic Category Antineoplastic Agent, Antimetabolite (Pyrimidine Antagonist)

Pregnancy Risk Factor D

Lactation Excretion in breast milk unknown/contraindicated

Use Management of hepatic metastases of colorectal and gastric cancers

Mechanism of Action Mechanism of action and pharmacokinetics are very similar to fluorouracil; floxuridine is the deoxyribonucleotide of fluorouracil. Floxuridine is a fluorinated pyrimidine antagonist which inhibits
(Continued)

Floxuridine *(Continued)*

DNA and RNA synthesis and methylation of deoxyuridylic acid to thymidylic acid.

Labeled Contraindications Hypersensitivity to floxuridine, fluorouracil, or any component of the formulation; pregnancy

Warnings/Precautions Hazardous agent - use appropriate precautions for handling and disposal. See Safe Handling of Hazardous Drugs *on page 1034* in the Appendix.

Use caution in impaired kidney or liver function. Discontinue if intractable vomiting or diarrhea, precipitous fall in leukocyte or platelet counts, or myocardial ischemia occur. Use with caution in patients who have had high-dose pelvic radiation or previous use of alkylating agents. Use of floxuridine with pentostatin has been associated with a high incidence of fatal pulmonary toxicity; this combination is not recommended.

If floxuridine contacts the skin, wash and flush thoroughly with water.

Adverse Reactions

>10%:

Gastrointestinal: Stomatitis, diarrhea; may be dose-limiting

Hematologic: Myelosuppression, may be dose-limiting; leukopenia, thrombocytopenia, anemia

Onset: 4-7 days

Nadir: 5-9 days

Recovery: 21 days

1% to 10%:

Dermatologic: Alopecia, photosensitivity, hyperpigmentation of the skin, localized erythema, dermatitis

Gastrointestinal: Anorexia

Hepatic: Biliary sclerosis, cholecystitis, jaundice

<1%: Nausea, vomiting, intrahepatic abscess

Vesicant No

Emetic Potential Very low (<10%)

Drug Interactions

Increased Effect/Toxicity: Any form of therapy which adds to the stress of the patient, interferes with nutrition, or depresses bone marrow function will increase the toxicity of floxuridine. Pentostatin and floxuridine administered together has resulted in fatal pulmonary toxicity.

Decreased Effect: Patients may experience impaired immune response to vaccines; possible infection after administration of live vaccines in patients receiving immunosuppressants.

Ethanol/Nutrition/Herb Interactions Ethanol: Avoid ethanol (due to GI irritation).

Storage/Stability Store intact vials at room temperature of 15°C to 30°C (59°F to 86°F). Reconstituted vials are stable for up to 2 weeks under refrigeration at 2°C to 8°C (36°C to 46°C). Further dilution in 500-1000 mL D_5W or NS is stable for 2 weeks at room temperature. Solutions in 0.9% sodium chloride are stable in some ambulatory infusion pumps for up to 21 days.

Reconstitution Reconstitute with 5 mL SWI for a final concentration of 100 mg/mL; further dilute in 500-1000 mL D_5W or NS for I.V. infusion.

Compatibility Stable in D_5W, NS, sterile water for injection

Y-site administration: Compatible: Amifostine, aztreonam, etoposide phosphate, filgrastim, fludarabine, gemcitabine, granisetron, melphalan, ondansetron, paclitaxel, piperacillin/tazobactam, sargramostim, teniposide, thiotepa, vinorelbine. **Incompatible:** Allopurinol, cefepime

Compatibility when admixed: Compatible: Carboplatin, cisplatin, cisplatin with etoposide, cisplatin with leucovorin, etoposide, fluorouracil, leucovorin

Pharmacodynamics/Kinetics

Metabolism: Hepatic; Active metabolites: Floxuridine monophosphate (FUDR-MP) and fluorouracil; Inactive metabolites: Urea, CO_2, α-fluoro-β-alanine, α-fluoro-β-guanidopropionic acid, α-fluoro-β-ureidopropionic acid, and dihydrofluorouracil

Excretion: Urine: Fluorouracil, urea, α-fluoro-β-alanine, α-fluoro-β-guanidopropionic acid, α-fluoro-β-ureidopropionic acid, and dihydrofluorouracil; exhaled gases (CO_2)

Dosage Refer to individual protocols.

Intra-arterial:

0.1-0.6 mg/kg/day

4-20 mg/day

I.V.:

0.15 mg/kg/day for 7-14 days

0.5-1 mg/kg/day for 6-15 days

30 mg/kg/day for 5 days, then 15 mg/kg/day every other day, up to 11 days

Administration Continuous intra-arterial or I.V. infusion

Dosage Forms Injection, powder for reconstitution: 500 mg

Selected Readings

Davidson BS, Izzo F, Chase JL, et al, "Alternating Floxuridine and 5-Fluorouracil Hepatic Arterial Chemotherapy for Colorectal Liver Metastases Minimizes Biliary Toxicity," *Am J Surg*, 1996, 172(3):244-7.

DeConti RC, Kaplan SR, Papac RJ, et al, "Continuous Infusions of 5-Fluoro-2-Deoxyuridine in the Treatment of Solid Tumors," *Cancer*, 1973, 31(4):894-8.

de Takats PG, Kerr DJ, Poole CJ, et al, "Hepatic Arterial Chemotherapy for Metastatic Colorectal Carcinoma," *Br J Cancer*, 1994, 69(2):372-8.

Hrushesky WJ, von Roemeling R, Lanning RM, et al, "Circadian-Shaped Infusions of Floxuridine for Progressive Metastatic Renal Cell Carcinoma," *J Clin Oncol*, 1990, 8(9):1504-13.

Kemeny N, Seiter K, Conti JA, et al, Hepatic Arterial Floxuridine and Leucovorin for Unresectable Liver Metastases From Colorectal Carcinoma. New Dose Schedules and Survival Update," *Cancer*, 1994, 73(4):1134-42.

Fluconazole (floo KOE na zole)

Medication Safety Issues

Sound-alike/look-alike issues:

Fluconazole may be confused with flecainide

Diflucan® may be confused with diclofenac, Diprivan®, disulfiram

Related Information

Management of Infections *on page 978*

U.S. Brand Names Diflucan®

Canadian Brand Names Apo-Fluconazole®; Diflucan®; Gen-Fluconazole; Novo-Fluconazole

Generic Available Yes

Pharmacologic Category Antifungal Agent, Oral; Antifungal Agent, Parenteral

Pregnancy Risk Factor C

Lactation Enters breast/not recommended (AAP rates "compatible")

(Continued)

Fluconazole *(Continued)*

Use Treatment of candidiasis (vaginal, oropharyngeal, esophageal, urinary tract infections, peritonitis, pneumonia, and systemic infections); cryptococcal meningitis; antifungal prophylaxis in allogeneic bone marrow transplant recipients

Mechanism of Action Interferes with cytochrome P450 activity, decreasing ergosterol synthesis (principal sterol in fungal cell membrane) and inhibiting cell membrane formation

Labeled Contraindications Hypersensitivity to fluconazole, other azoles, or any component of the formulation; concomitant administration with cisapride

Warnings/Precautions Should be used with caution in patients with renal and hepatic dysfunction or previous hepatotoxicity from other azole derivatives. Patients who develop abnormal liver function tests during fluconazole therapy should be monitored closely and discontinued if symptoms consistent with liver disease develop. Use caution in patients at risk of proarrhythmias.

Adverse Reactions Frequency not always defined.

Cardiovascular: Angioedema, pallor, QT prolongation, torsade de pointes

Central nervous system: Headache (2% to 13%), seizure, dizziness

Dermatologic: Rash (2%), alopecia, toxic epidermal necrolysis, Stevens-Johnson syndrome

Endocrine & metabolic: Hypercholesterolemia, hypertriglyceridemia, hypokalemia

Gastrointestinal: Nausea (4% to 7%), vomiting (2%), abdominal pain (2% to 6%), diarrhea (2% to 3%), taste perversion, dyspepsia

Hematologic: Agranulocytosis, leukopenia, neutropenia, thrombocytopenia

Hepatic: Hepatic failure (rare), hepatitis, cholestasis, jaundice, increased ALT/AST, increased alkaline phosphatase

Respiratory: Dyspnea

Miscellaneous: Anaphylactic reactions (rare)

Vesicant No

Emetic Potential Very low (<10%)

Overdosage/Toxicology Symptoms of overdose include decreased lacrimation, salivation, respiration and motility, urinary incontinence, and cyanosis. Treatment includes supportive measures. A 3-hour hemodialysis will remove 50%.

Drug Interactions

Cytochrome P450 Effect: Inhibits CYP1A2 (weak), 2C8/9 (strong), 2C19 (strong), 3A4 (moderate)

Increased Effect/Toxicity: Concurrent use of fluconazole with cisapride is contraindicated due to the potential for malignant arrhythmias. Fluconazole may increase the levels/effects of amiodarone, selected benzodiazepines, calcium channel blockers, cisapride, citalopram, cyclosporine, diazepam, ergot derivatives, fluoxetine, glimepiride, glipizide, HMG-CoA reductase inhibitors, methsuximide, mirtazapine, nateglinide, nefazodone, phenytoin, pioglitazone, propranolol, rosiglitazone, sertraline, sildenafil (and other PDE-5 inhibitors), tacrolimus, venlafaxine, warfarin, and other substrates of CYP2C8/9, 2C19, and 3A4.

Decreased Effect: Rifampin decreases concentrations of fluconazole.

Storage/Stability

Powder for oral suspension: Store dry powder at ≤30°C (86°F). Following reconstitution, store at 5°C to 30°C (41°F to 86°F). Discard unused portion after 2 weeks. Do not freeze.

Injection: Store injection in glass at 5°C to 30°C (41°F to 86°F). Store injection in Viaflex® at 5°C to 25°C (41°F to 77°F). Protect from freezing. Do not unwrap unit until ready for use.

Compatibility Stable in D_5W, LR, NS

Y-site administration: Compatible: Acyclovir, aldesleukin, allopurinol, amifostine, amikacin, aminophylline, ampicillin/sulbactam, aztreonam, benztropine, cefazolin, cefepime, cefotetan, cefoxitin, cefpirome, chlorpromazine, cimetidine, cisatracurium, dexamethasone sodium phosphate, diltiazem, diphenhydramine, dobutamine, docetaxel, dopamine, doxorubicin liposome, droperidol, etoposide phosphate, famotidine, filgrastim, fludarabine, foscarnet, ganciclovir, gatifloxacin, gemcitabine, gentamicin, granisetron, heparin, hydrocortisone sodium phosphate, immune globulin intravenous, leucovorin, linezolid, lorazepam, melphalan, meperidine, meropenem, metoclopramide, metronidazole, midazolam, morphine, nafcillin, nitroglycerin, ondansetron, oxacillin, paclitaxel, pancuronium, penicillin G potassium, phenytoin, piperacillin/tazobactam, prochlorperazine edisylate, promethazine, propofol, ranitidine, remifentanil, sargramostim, tacrolimus, teniposide, theophylline, thiotepa, ticarcillin/clavulanate, tobramycin, vancomycin, vecuronium, vinorelbine, zidovudine. **Incompatible:** Amphotericin B, amphotericin B cholesteryl sulfate complex, ampicillin, calcium gluconate, cefotaxime, ceftazidime, ceftriaxone, cefuroxime, chloramphenicol, clindamycin, co-trimoxazole, diazepam, digoxin, erythromycin lactobionate, furosemide, haloperidol, hydroxyzine, imipenem/cilastatin, pentamidine, piperacillin, ticarcillin

Compatibility when admixed: Compatible: Acyclovir, amikacin, amphotericin B, cefazolin, ceftazidime, clindamycin, gentamicin, heparin, meropenem, metronidazole, morphine, piperacillin, potassium chloride, ranitidine with ondansetron, theophylline. **Incompatible:** Co-trimoxazole

Pharmacodynamics/Kinetics

Distribution: Widely throughout body with good penetration into CSF, eye, peritoneal fluid, sputum, skin, and urine

Relative diffusion blood into CSF: Adequate with or without inflammation (exceeds usual MICs)

CSF:blood level ratio: Normal meninges: 70% to 80%; Inflamed meninges: >70% to 80%

Protein binding, plasma: 11% to 12%

Bioavailability: Oral: >90%

Half-life elimination: Normal renal function: ~30 hours

Time to peak, serum: Oral: 1-2 hours

Excretion: Urine (80% as unchanged drug)

Dosage The daily dose of fluconazole is the same for oral and I.V. administration

Neonates: First 2 weeks of life, especially premature neonates: Same dose as older children every 72 hours

Children: Once-daily dosing by indication: See table on page 353. (Continued)

Fluconazole *(Continued)*

Adults: Oral, I.V.: **Note:** Susceptibility for *Candida* is divided into susceptible, susceptible-dose dependent (SDD), and resistant. Increased dose (up to 400 mg/day) may be used to treat SDD strains, especially when there has been treatment failure at lower doses.

Once-daily dosing by indication: See table below.

Dosing adjustment/interval in renal impairment:

No adjustment for vaginal candidiasis single-dose therapy

For multiple dosing, administer usual load then adjust daily doses

$Cl_{cr} \leq 50$ mL/minute (no dialysis): Administer 50% of recommended dose or administer every 48 hours.

Fluconazole Once-Daily Dosing – Adults

Indication	Day 1	Daily Therapy	Minimum Duration of Therapy
Oropharyngeal candidiasis (OPC) (long-term suppression)	200 mg	200 mg	Chronic therapy in AIDS patients with history of OPC
Esophageal candidiasis	200 mg	100-200 mg	14-21 d after clinical improvement
Prevention of candidiasis in bone marrow transplant	400 mg	400 mg	3 d before neutropenia, 7 d after neutrophils >1000 cells/mm^3
Urinary candidiasis	--	200 mg	14 d
Candidemia, primary therapy, non-neutropenic	--	400-800 mg	14 d after last positive blood culture and resolution of signs/ symptoms
Candidemia, alternative therapy, non-neutropenic	--	800 mg with AmB for 4-7 d, followed by 800 mg/ day	14 d after last positive blood culture and resolution of signs/ symptoms
Candidemia, secondary, neutropenic	--	6-12 mg/ kg/day	14 d after last positive blood culture and resolution of signs/ symptoms
Cryptococcal meningitis consolidation (after induction with amphotericin plus flucytosine)	--	400 mg	10 wk
relapse suppression (maintenance)	--	200-400 mg	N/A
Vaginal candidiasis	150 mg	Single dose	N/A

N/A = not applicable. AmB = conventional deoxycholate amphotericin B.

Fluconazole Once-Daily Dosing – Children

Indication	Day 1	Daily Therapy	Minimum Duration of Therapy
Oropharyngeal candidiasis	6 mg/kg	3 mg/kg	14 d
Esophageal candidiasis	6 mg/kg	3-12 mg/kg	21 d and for at least 2 wk following resolution of symptoms
Systemic candidiasis	—	6 mg/kg every 12 hours	28 d
Cryptococcal meningitis acute	12 mg/kg	6-12 mg/kg	10-12 wk after CSF culture becomes negative
relapse suppression	6 mg/kg	6 mg/kg	N/A

N/A = Not applicable.

Hemodialysis: 50% is removed by hemodialysis; administer 100% of daily dose (according to indication) after each dialysis treatment.

Continuous arteriovenous or venovenous hemofiltration: Dose as for Cl_{cr} 10-50 mL/minute.

Administration

I.V.: I.V. infusion over approximately 1-2 hours; do not exceed 200 mg/hour

Oral: May be taken with or without food

Dosage Forms

Infusion [premixed in sodium chloride]: 2 mg/mL (100 mL, 200 mL)
   Diflucan® [premixed in sodium chloride or dextrose] 2 mg/mL (100 mL, 200 mL)

Powder for oral suspension (Diflucan®): 10 mg/mL (35 mL); 40 mg/mL (35 mL) [contains sodium benzoate; orange flavor]

Tablet (Diflucan®): 50 mg, 100 mg, 150 mg, 200 mg

Monitoring Parameters Periodic liver function tests (AST, ALT, alkaline phosphatase) and renal function tests, potassium

Dietary Considerations Take with or without regard to food.

Patient Information May take with food; complete full course of therapy; report if side effects develop

Special Geriatric Considerations Dose may need adjustment based on changes of renal function.

Selected Readings

Goa KL and Barradell LB, "Fluconazole. An Update of Its Pharmacodynamic and Pharmacokinetic Properties and Therapeutic Use in Major Superficial and Systemic Mycoses in Immunocompromised Patients," *Drugs*, 1995, 50(4):658-90.

Grant SM and Clissold SP, "Fluconazole: A Review of Its Pharmacodynamic and Pharmacokinetic Properties and Therapeutic Potential in Superficial and Systemic Mycoses," *Drugs*, 1990, 39(6):877-916.

Kowalsky SF and Dixon DM, "Fluconazole: A New Antifungal Agent," *Clin Pharm*, 1991, 10(3):179-94.

Lee JW, Seibel NL, Amantea M, et al, "Safety and Pharmacokinetics of Fluconazole in Children With Neoplastic Diseases," *J Pediatr*, 1992, 120(6):987-93.

Perry CM, Whittington R, and McTavish D, "Fluconazole. An Update of Its Antimicrobial Activity, Pharmacokinetic Properties, and Therapeutic Use in Vaginal Candidiasis," *Drugs*, 1995, 49(6):984-1006.

Flucytosine (floo SYE toe seen)
Medication Safety Issues
Sound-alike/look-alike issues:
Flucytosine may be confused with fluorouracil
Ancobon® may be confused with Oncovin®

U.S. Brand Names Ancobon®

Canadian Brand Names Ancobon®

Generic Available No

Synonyms 5-FC; 5-Flurocytosine

Pharmacologic Category Antifungal Agent, Oral

Pregnancy Risk Factor C

Lactation Excretion in breast milk unknown/not recommended

Use Adjunctive treatment of susceptible fungal infections (usually *Candida* or *Cryptococcus*); synergy with amphotericin B for certain fungal infections (*Cryptococcus* spp., *Candida* spp.)

Mechanism of Action Penetrates fungal cells and is converted to fluorouracil which competes with uracil interfering with fungal RNA and protein synthesis

Labeled Contraindications Hypersensitivity to flucytosine or any component of the formulation

Warnings/Precautions Use with extreme caution in patients with renal dysfunction; dosage adjustment required. Avoid use as monotherapy; resistance rapidly develops. Use with caution in patients with bone marrow depression; patients with hematologic disease or who have been treated with radiation or drugs that suppress the bone marrow may be at greatest risk. Bone marrow toxicity can be irreversible.

Adverse Reactions Frequency not defined.
Cardiovascular: Cardiac arrest, myocardial toxicity, ventricular dysfunction, chest pain
Central nervous system: Confusion, headache, hallucinations, dizziness, drowsiness, psychosis, parkinsonism, ataxia, sedation, pyrexia, seizure, fatigue
Dermatologic: Rash, photosensitivity, pruritus, urticaria, Lyell's syndrome
Endocrine & metabolic: Temporary growth failure, hypoglycemia, hypokalemia
Gastrointestinal: Nausea, vomiting, diarrhea, abdominal pain, loss of appetite, dry mouth, hemorrhage, ulcerative colitis
Hematologic: Bone marrow suppression, anemia, leukopenia, thrombocytopenia, agranulocytosis, aplastic anemia, eosinophilia, pancytopenia
Hepatic: Liver enzymes increased, hepatitis, jaundice, azotemia, bilirubin increased
Neuromuscular & skeletal: Peripheral neuropathy, paresthesia, weakness
Otic: Hearing loss
Renal: BUN and serum creatinine increased, renal failure, azotemia, crystalluria
Respiratory: Respiratory arrest, dyspnea
Miscellaneous: Anaphylaxis, allergic reaction

Emetic Potential Very low (<10%)

Overdosage/Toxicology Symptoms of overdose include nausea, vomiting, diarrhea, hepatitis, and bone marrow suppression. Treatment is supportive. Removed by hemodialysis.

Drug Interactions

Increased Effect/Toxicity: Increased effect with amphotericin B. Amphotericin B-induced renal dysfunction may predispose patient to flucytosine accumulation and myelosuppression.

Decreased Effect: Cytarabine may inactivate flucytosine activity.

Ethanol/Nutrition/Herb Interactions Food: Food decreases the rate, but not the extent of absorption.

Storage/Stability Store at 25°C (77°F). Protect from light.

Pharmacodynamics/Kinetics

Absorption: 75% to 90%

Distribution: Into CSF, aqueous humor, joints, peritoneal fluid, and bronchial secretions; V_d: 0.6 L/kg

Protein binding: 2% to 4%

Metabolism: Minimally hepatic; deaminated, possibly via gut bacteria, to 5-fluorouracil

Half-life elimination:

Normal renal function: 2-5 hours

Anuria: 85 hours (range: 30-250)

End stage renal disease: 75-200 hours

Time to peak, serum: ~2-6 hours

Excretion: Urine (>90% as unchanged drug)

Dosage Children and Adults: Oral: 50-150 mg/kg/day in divided doses every 6 hours

Dosing interval in renal impairment: Use lower initial dose:

Cl_{cr} 20-40 mL/minute: Administer every 12 hours

Cl_{cr} 10-20 mL/minute: Administer every 24 hours

Cl_{cr} <10 mL/minute: Administer every 24-48 hours

Hemodialysis: Dialyzable (50% to 100%); administer dose posthemodialysis

Peritoneal dialysis: Adults: Administer 0.5-1 g every 24 hours

Continuous arteriovenous or venovenous hemodiafiltration effects: Dose as for Cl_{cr} 10-50 mL/minute

Administration To avoid nausea and vomiting, administer a few capsules at a time over 15 minutes until full dose is taken.

Dosage Forms Capsule: 250 mg, 500 mg

Monitoring Parameters

Pretreatment: Electrolytes, CBC, BUN, renal function, blood culture

During treatment: CBC and LFTs frequently, serum flucytosine concentration, renal function

Patient Information Take capsules a few at a time with food over a 15-minute period to avoid nausea

Special Geriatric Considerations Adjust for renal function.

Extemporaneous Preparations Flucytosine oral liquid has been prepared by using the contents of ten 500 mg capsules triturated in a mortar and pestle with a small amount of distilled water; the mixture was transferred to a 500 mL volumetric flask; the mortar was rinsed several times with a small amount of distilled water and the fluid added to the flask; sufficient distilled water was added to make a total volume of 500 mL of a 10 mg/mL liquid; oral liquid was stable for 70 days when stored in glass or plastic prescription bottles at 4°C or for up to 14 days at room temperature.

(Continued)

Flucytosine *(Continued)*

Wintermeyer SM and Nahata MC, "Stability of Flucytosine in an Extemporaneously Compounded Oral Liquid," *Am J Health Syst Pharm*, 1996, 53:407-9.

Selected Readings

Baley JE, Meyers C, Kliegman RM, et al, "Pharmacokinetics, Outcome of Treatment, and Toxic Effects of Amphotericin B and 5-Fluorocytosine in Neonates," *J Pediatr*, 1990, 116(5):791-7.

Lau AH and Kronfol NO, "Elimination of Flucytosine by Continuous Hemofiltration," *Am J Nephrol*, 1995, 15(4):327-31.

Lyman CA and Walsh TJ, "Systemically Administered Antifungal Agents. A Review of Their Clinical Pharmacology and Therapeutic Applications," *Drugs*, 1992, 44(1):9-35.

Patel R, "Antifungal Agents. Part I. Amphotericin B Preparations and Flucytosine," *Mayo Clin Proc*, 1998, 73(12):1205-25.

◆ **Fludara**® *see Fludarabine on page 356*

Fludarabine *(floo DARE a been)*

Medication Safety Issues

Sound-alike/look-alike issues:

Fludarabine may be confused with Flumadine®

Fludara® may be confused with FUDR®

Related Information

Safe Handling of Hazardous Drugs *on page 1034*

Transplantation *on page 1019*

U.S. Brand Names Fludara®

Canadian Brand Names Fludara®

Generic Available Yes

Synonyms Fludarabine Phosphate

Pharmacologic Category Antineoplastic Agent, Antimetabolite (Purine Antagonist)

Pregnancy Risk Factor D

Lactation Excretion in breast milk unknown/contraindicated

Use Treatment of chronic lymphocytic leukemia (CLL) (including refractory CLL); non-Hodgkin's lymphoma in adults

Unlabeled/Investigational Use Treatment of non-Hodgkin's lymphoma and acute leukemias in pediatric patients; reduced-intensity conditioning regimens prior to allogeneic hematopoietic stem cell transplantation (generally administered in combination with busulfan and antithymocyte globulin or lymphocyte immune globulin, or in combination with melphalan and alemtuzumab)

Mechanism of Action Fludarabine inhibits DNA synthesis by inhibition of DNA polymerase and ribonucleotide reductase.

Labeled Contraindications Hypersensitivity of fludarabine or any component of the formulation; pregnancy

Warnings/Precautions Hazardous agent - use appropriate precautions for handling and disposal. See Safe Handling of Hazardous Drugs *on page 1034* in the Appendix. Use with caution with renal insufficiency, patients with a fever, documented infection, or pre-existing hematological disorders (particularly granulocytopenia) or in patients with pre-existing central nervous system disorder (epilepsy), spasticity, or peripheral neuropathy. Life-threatening and sometimes fatal autoimmune hemolytic anemia have occurred. Severe myelosuppression (trilineage bone marrow hypoplasia/aplasia) has been reported (rare); the duration of significant cytopenias in these cases may be prolonged (up to 1 year).

Adverse Reactions
>10%:
  Cardiovascular: Edema
  Central nervous system: Fatigue, somnolence (30%), chills, pain
  Dermatologic: Rash
  Hematologic: Myelosuppression, common, dose-limiting toxicity, primarily leukopenia and thrombocytopenia
    Nadir: 10-14 days
    Recovery: 5-7 weeks
  Neuromuscular & skeletal: Paresthesia, myalgia, weakness
1% to 10%:
  Cardiovascular: CHF
  Central nervous system: Malaise, headache
  Dermatologic: Alopecia
  Endocrine & metabolic: Hyperglycemia
  Gastrointestinal: Anorexia, stomatitis (1.5%), diarrhea (1.8%), mild nausea/vomiting (3% to 10%)
  Hematologic: Eosinophilia, hemolytic anemia, may be dose-limiting, possibly fatal in some patients
<1%: Blurred vision, diplopia, increased risk for opportunistic infection due to decreased CD4 counts, metabolic acidosis, metallic taste, muscle weakness, paresthesia, photophobia (primarily in patients receiving high doses)
  A syndrome characterized by cortical blindness, coma, and paralysis - 36% at doses >96 mg/m^2 for 5-7 days; <0.2% at doses <125 mg/m^2/cycle (onset of neurologic symptoms may be delayed for 3-4 weeks)
Postmarketing and/or case reports: Acute renal failure; pulmonary toxicity (including interstitial pneumonitis, pulmonary fibrosis, pulmonary hemorrhage, respiratory failure, or ARDS) has been reported (may improve with steroid administration). Trilineage (bone marrow hypoplasia or bone marrow aplasia) has been reported; may require several months for recovery.

Vesicant No

Emetic Potential Very low (<10%)

Overdosage/Toxicology High doses of fludarabine are associated with bone marrow depression including severe neutropenia and thrombocytopenia; irreversible central nervous system toxicity with delayed blindness, coma, and death has occurred. Discontinuation of drug and supportive therapy are recommended.

Drug Interactions
  Increased Effect/Toxicity: Combined use with pentostatin may lead to severe, even fatal, pulmonary toxicity.

Ethanol/Nutrition/Herb Interactions Ethanol: Avoid ethanol (due to GI irritation).

Storage/Stability Store intact vials under refrigeration (2°C to 8°C). Reconstituted solution is stable for 16 days at room temperature (22°C to 25°C) and under refrigeration (2°C to 8°C). Further dilution in 100 mL D$_5$W or NS is stable for 48 hours at room temperature or refrigeration.

Reconstitution Reconstitute vials with SWI, NS, or D$_5$W to a concentration of 10-25 mg/mL. Standard I.V. dilution: 50-100 mL D$_5$W or NS.

Compatibility Stable in D$_5$W, NS, sterile water for injection
(Continued)

Fludarabine *(Continued)*

Y-site administration: Compatible: Allopurinol, amifostine, amikacin, aminophylline, ampicillin, ampicillin/sulbactam, amsacrine, aztreonam, bleomycin, butorphanol, carboplatin, carmustine, cefazolin, cefepime, cefoperazone, cefotaxime, cefotetan, ceftazidime, ceftizoxime, ceftriaxone, cefuroxime, cimetidine, cisplatin, clindamycin, co-trimoxazole, cyclophosphamide, cytarabine, dacarbazine, dactinomycin, dexamethasone sodium phosphate, diphenhydramine, doxorubicin, doxycycline, droperidol, etoposide, etoposide phosphate, famotidine, filgrastim, floxuridine, fluconazole, fluorouracil, furosemide, gemcitabine, gentamicin, granisetron, haloperidol, heparin, hydrocortisone sodium phosphate, hydrocortisone sodium succinate, hydromorphone, ifosfamide, imipenem/cilastatin, lorazepam, magnesium sulfate, mannitol, mechlorethamine, melphalan, meperidine, mesna, methotrexate, methylprednisolone sodium succinate, metoclopramide, minocycline, mitoxantrone, morphine, multivitamins, nalbuphine, netilmicin, ondansetron, pentostatin, piperacillin, piperacillin/tazobactam, potassium chloride, promethazine, ranitidine, sodium bicarbonate, teniposide, thiotepa, ticarcillin, ticarcillin/clavulanate, tobramycin, vancomycin, vinblastine, vincristine, vinorelbine, zidovudine. **Incompatible:** Acyclovir, amphotericin B, chlorpromazine, daunorubicin, ganciclovir, hydroxyzine, prochlorperazine edisylate

Pharmacodynamics/Kinetics

Distribution: V_d: 38-96 L/m^2; widely with extensive tissue binding

Metabolism: I.V.: Fludarabine phosphate is rapidly dephosphorylated to 2-fluoro-vidarabine, which subsequently enters tumor cells and is phosphorylated to the active triphosphate derivative; rapidly dephosphorylated in the serum

Bioavailability: 75%

Half-life elimination: 2-fluoro-vidarabine: 9 hours

Excretion: Urine (60%, 23% as 2-fluoro-vidarabine) within 24 hours

Dosage I.V.:

Children (unlabeled use):

Acute leukemia: 10 mg/m^2 bolus over 15 minutes followed by continuous infusion of 30.5 mg/m^2/day for 5 days **or** 10.5 mg/m^2 bolus over 15 minutes followed by 30.5 mg/m^2/day for 48 hours

Solid tumors: 9 mg/m^2 bolus followed by 27 mg/m^2/day continuous infusion for 5 days

Adults:

Chronic lymphocytic leukemia: 25 mg/m^2/day for 5 days every 28 days

Non-Hodgkin's lymphoma: Loading dose: 20 mg/m^2 followed by 30 mg/m^2/day for 48 hours

Reduced-intensity conditioning regimens prior to allogeneic hematopoietic stem cell transplantation (unlabeled use): 120-150 mg/m^2 administered in divided doses over 4-5 days

Dosing in renal impairment:

Cl_{cr} 30-70 mL/minute: Reduce dose by 20%

Cl_{cr} <30 mL/minute: Not recommended

Combination Regimens

Leukemia, acute lymphocytic: FIS-HAM *on page 889*

Leukemia, acute myeloid:

FIS-HAM *on page 889*

FLAG *on page 889*

Leukemia, chronic lymphocytic: Fludarabine-Rituximab *on page 890*

Administration Fludarabine is administered intravenously, usually as a 15- to 30-minute infusion; continuous infusions are occasionally used

Dosage Forms Injection, powder for reconstitution, as phosphate: 50 mg

Monitoring Parameters CBC with differential, platelet count, AST, ALT, creatinine, serum albumin, uric acid

Selected Readings

Adkins JC, Peters DH, and Markham A, "Fludarabine. An Update of its Pharmacology and Use in the Treatment of Haematological Malignancies," *Drugs*, 1997, 53(6):1005-37.

Gandhi V and Plunkett W, "Cellular and Clinical Pharmacology of Fludarabine," *Clin Pharmacokinet*, 2002, 41(2):93-103.

Hood MA and Finley RS, "Fludarabine: A Review," *DICP*, 1991, 25(5):518-24.

Plosker GL and Figgitt DP, "Oral fludarabine," *Drugs*, 2003, 63(21):2317-23.

Rodriguez G, "Fludarabine Phosphate. A New Anticancer Drug With Significant Activity in Patients With Chronic Lymphocytic Leukemia and in Patients With Lymphoma," *Invest New Drugs*, 1994, 12(2):75-92.

Ross SR, McTavish D, and Faulds D, "Fludarabine. A Review of Its Pharmacological Properties and Therapeutic Potential in Malignancy," *Drugs*, 1993, 45(5):737-59.

♦ **Fludarabine Phosphate** *see* Fludarabine *on page 356*

♦ **Fluorodeoxyuridine** *see* Floxuridine *on page 347*

♦ **Fluoroplex**® *see* Fluorouracil *on page 359*

Fluorouracil (flure oh YOOR a sil)

Medication Safety Issues

Sound-alike/look-alike issues:

Fluorouracil may be confused with flucytosine

Efudex® may be confused with Efidac (Efidac 24®), Eurax®

Related Information

Fertility and Cancer Therapy *on page 962*

Safe Handling of Hazardous Drugs *on page 1034*

U.S. Brand Names Adrucil®; Carac™; Efudex®; Fluoroplex®

Canadian Brand Names Adrucil®; Efudex®

Generic Available Yes: Injection, topical solution

Synonyms 5-Fluorouracil; FU; 5-FU

Pharmacologic Category Antineoplastic Agent, Antimetabolite (Pyrimidine Antagonist)

Pregnancy Risk Factor D (injection); X (topical)

Lactation Excretion in breast milk unknown/not recommended

Use Treatment of carcinomas of the breast, colon, head and neck, pancreas, rectum, or stomach; topically for the management of actinic or solar keratoses and superficial basal cell carcinomas

Mechanism of Action A pyrimidine antimetabolite that interferes with DNA synthesis by blocking the methylation of deoxyuridylic acid; fluorouracil inhibits thymidylate synthetase (TS), or is incorporated into RNA. The reduced folate cofactor is required for tight binding to occur between the 5-FdUMP and TS.

Labeled Contraindications Hypersensitivity to fluorouracil or any component of the formulation; dihydropyrimidine dehydrogenase (DPD) enzyme deficiency; pregnancy

Warnings/Precautions Hazardous agent - use appropriate precautions for handling and disposal. See Safe Handling of Hazardous Drugs *on page 1034* in the Appendix. Use with caution in patients who have had high-dose pelvic radiation or previous use of alkylating agents. Use with (Continued)

Fluorouracil *(Continued)*

caution in patients with impaired kidney or liver function. The drug should be discontinued if intractable vomiting or diarrhea, precipitous fall in leukocyte or platelet counts or myocardial ischemia occurs. Systemic toxicity normally associated with parenteral administration (including neutropenia, neurotoxicity, and gastrointestinal toxicity) has been associated with topical use particularly in patients with a genetic deficiency of dihydropyrimidine dehydrogenase (DPD).

Adverse Reactions Toxicity depends on route and duration of treatment

I.V.:

Cardiovascular: Angina, myocardial ischemia, nail changes

Central nervous system: Acute cerebellar syndrome, confusion, disorientation, euphoria, headache, nystagmus

Dermatologic: Alopecia, dermatitis, dry skin, fissuring, palmar-plantar erythrodysesthesia syndrome, pruritic maculopapular rash, photosensitivity, vein pigmentations

Gastrointestinal: Anorexia, bleeding, diarrhea, esophagopharyngitis, nausea, sloughing, stomatitis, ulceration, vomiting

Hematologic: Agranulocytosis, anemia, leukopenia, pancytopenia, thrombocytopenia

Myelosuppression:
  Onset: 7-10 days
  Nadir: 9-14 days
  Recovery: 21-28 days

Local: Thrombophlebitis

Ocular: Lacrimation, lacrimal duct stenosis, photophobia, visual changes

Respiratory: Epistaxis

Miscellaneous: Anaphylaxis, generalized allergic reactions, loss of nails

Topical: Note: Systemic toxicity normally associated with parenteral administration (including neutropenia, neurotoxicity, and gastrointestinal toxicity) has been associated with topical use particularly in patients with a genetic deficiency of dihydropyrimidine dehydrogenase (DPD).

Central nervous system: Headache, telangiectasia

Dermatologic: Photosensitivity, pruritus, rash, scarring

Hematologic: Leukocytosis

Local: Allergic contact dermatitis, burning, crusting, dryness, edema, erosion, erythema, hyperpigmentation, irritation, pain, soreness, ulceration

Ocular: Eye irritation (burning, watering, sensitivity, stinging, itching)

Miscellaneous: Birth defects, miscarriage

Vesicant No

Emetic Potential Very low (<10%)

Overdosage/Toxicology Symptoms of overdose include myelosuppression, nausea, vomiting, diarrhea, and alopecia. No specific antidote exists. Monitor hematologically for at least 4 weeks. Treatment is supportive.

Drug Interactions

Increased Effect/Toxicity: Fluorouracil may increase effects of warfarin.

Ethanol/Nutrition/Herb Interactions

Ethanol: Avoid ethanol (due to GI irritation).

Herb/Nutraceutical: Avoid black cohosh, dong quai in estrogen-dependent tumors.

Storage/Stability

Injection: Store intact vials at room temperature and protect from light; slight discoloration does not usually denote decomposition. If exposed to cold, a precipitate may form; **gentle** heating to 60°C will dissolve the precipitate without impairing the potency; solutions in 50-1000 mL NS or D_5W, or undiluted solutions in syringes are stable for 72 hours at room temperature.

Topical: Store at controlled room temperature.

Reconstitution Dilute in 50-1000 mL NS, D_5W, or bacteriostatic NS for infusion.

Compatibility Stable in D_5LR, D_5W, NS, bacteriostatic NS; concentrations >25 mg/mL of fluorouracil and >2 mg/mL of leucovorin are incompatible (precipitation occurs).

Y-site administration: Compatible: Allopurinol, amifostine, aztreonam, bleomycin, cefepime, cisplatin, cyclophosphamide, doxorubicin, doxorubicin liposome, etoposide phosphate, fludarabine, furosemide, gatifloxacin, gemcitabine, granisetron, heparin, hydrocortisone sodium succinate, leucovorin, linezolid, mannitol, melphalan, methotrexate, metoclopramide, mitomycin, paclitaxel, piperacillin/tazobactam, potassium chloride, propofol, sargramostim, teniposide, thiotepa, vinblastine, vincristine, vitamin B complex with C. **Incompatible:** Amphotericin B cholesteryl sulfate complex, droperidol, filgrastim, ondansetron, topotecan, vinorelbine

Compatibility in syringe: Compatible: Bleomycin, cisplatin, cyclophosphamide, furosemide, heparin, leucovorin, methotrexate, metoclopramide, mitomycin, vinblastine, vincristine. **Incompatible:** Droperidol, epirubicin. **Variable (consult detailed reference):** Doxorubicin

Compatibility when admixed: Compatible: Bleomycin, cyclophosphamide, cyclophosphamide with methotrexate, etoposide, floxuridine, hydromorphone, ifosfamide, methotrexate, mitoxantrone, vincristine. **Incompatible:** Carboplatin, cisplatin, cytarabine, diazepam, doxorubicin, fentanyl, leucovorin, morphine

Pharmacodynamics/Kinetics

Duration: ~3 weeks

Distribution: V_d: ~22% of total body water; penetrates extracellular fluid, CSF, and third space fluids (eg, pleural effusions and ascitic fluid)

Metabolism: Hepatic (90%); via a dehydrogenase enzyme; FU must be metabolized to be active

Bioavailability: <75%, erratic and undependable

Half-life elimination: Biphasic: Initial: 6-20 minutes; two metabolites, FdUMP and FUTP, have prolonged half-lives depending on the type of tissue

Excretion: Lung (large amounts as CO_2); urine (5% as unchanged drug) in 6 hours

Dosage Adults:

Refer to individual protocols:

I.V. bolus: 500-600 mg/m^2 every 3-4 weeks **or** 425 mg/m^2 on days 1-5 every 4 weeks

(Continued)

Fluorouracil *(Continued)*

Continuous I.V. infusion: 1000 mg/m^2/day for 4-5 days every 3-4 weeks **or**

2300-2600 mg/m^2 on day 1 every week **or**

300-400 mg/m^2/day **or**

225 mg/m^2/day for 5-8 weeks (with radiation therapy)

Actinic keratoses: Topical:

Carac™: Apply thin film to lesions once daily for up to 4 weeks, as tolerated

Efudex®: Apply to lesions twice daily for 2-4 weeks; complete healing may not be evident for 1-2 months following treatment

Fluoroplex®: Apply to lesions twice daily for 2-6 weeks

Basal cell carcinoma: Topical: Efudex®: Apply to affected lesions twice daily for 3-6 weeks; treatment may be continued for up to 10-12 weeks

Dosage adjustment for renal impairment: Hemodialysis: Administer dose following hemodialysis.

Dosage adjustment for hepatic impairment: Bilirubin >5 mg/dL: Omit use.

Combination Regimens

Breast cancer:

CAF *on page 850*

CEF *on page 857*

CMF *on page 862*

CMF-IV *on page 863*

CNF *on page 863*

FAC *on page 884*

FEC *on page 888*

NFL *on page 923*

Cervical cancer: Cisplatin-Fluorouracil *on page 861*

Colorectal cancer:

F-CL *on page 886*

FLe *on page 890*

FOIL *on page 890*

FOLFOX 1 *on page 891*

FOLFOX 2 *on page 891*

FOLFOX 3 *on page 891*

FOLFOX 4 *on page 892*

FOLFOX 6 *on page 892*

FOLFOX 7 *on page 892*

FU/LV/CPT-11 *on page 893*

FU/LV/CPT-11 (Saltz Regimen) *on page 894*

PFL (Colorectal Cancer) *on page 929*

Esophageal cancer: TCF *on page 939*

Gastric cancer:

ECF *on page 875*

ELF *on page 877*

FAM *on page 885*

FAMTX *on page 886*

FUP *on page 894*

Head and neck cancer:

CF *on page 858*

FU HURT *on page 893*

PFL (Head and Neck Cancer) *on page 930*

PFL + IFN *on page 930*
Neuroblastoma: N4SE Protocol *on page 922*
Pancreatic cancer: FAM *on page 885*
Renal cell cancer: Interleukin 2-Interferon Alfa 2-Fluorouracil *on page 903*

Administration
I.V.: I.V. bolus as a slow push or short (5-15 minutes) bolus infusion, or as a continuous infusion. Warm to body temperature before using. I.V. formulation may be given orally mixed in water, grape juice, or carbonated beverage. It is generally best to drink undiluted solution, then rinse the mouth. CocaCola® has been recommended as the "best chaser" for oral fluorouracil.

Topical: Apply 10 minutes after washing, rinsing, and drying the affected area. Apply using fingertip (wash hands immediately after application) or nonmetal applicator. Avoid eyes, nostrils, and mouth. Do not cover area with an occlusive dressing.

Dosage Forms
Cream, topical:
Carac™: 0.5% (30 g)
Efudex®: 5% (25 g, 40 g)
Fluoroplex®: 1% (30 g) [contains benzyl alcohol]
Injection, solution: 50 mg/mL (10 mL, 20 mL, 50 mL, 100 mL)
Adrucil®: 50 mg/mL (10 mL, 50 mL, 100 mL)
Solution, topical (Efudex®): 2% (10 mL); 5% (10 mL)

Monitoring Parameters
CBC with differential and platelet count, renal function tests, liver function tests

Dietary Considerations
Increase dietary intake of thiamine.

Patient Information
Avoid alcohol and all OTC drugs unless approved by your prescriber. Maintain adequate hydration (2-3 L/day of fluids unless instructed to restrict fluid intake) and nutrition (small frequent meals may help). You may experience sensitivity to sunlight (use sunblock, wear protective clothing, or avoid direct sunlight); susceptibility to infection (avoid crowds or infected persons or persons with contagious diseases); nausea, vomiting, diarrhea, or loss of appetite (frequent small meals may help - request medication); weakness, lethargy, dizziness, decreased vision (use caution when driving or engaging in tasks requiring alertness until response to drug is known); headache (request medication). Report signs and symptoms of infection (eg, fever, chills, sore throat, burning urination, vaginal itching or discharge, fatigue, mouth sores); bleeding (eg, black or tarry stools, easy bruising, unusual bleeding); vision changes; unremitting nausea, vomiting, or abdominal pain; CNS changes; respiratory difficulty; chest pain or palpitations; severe skin reactions to topical application; or any other adverse reactions. Contraceptive measures are recommended during therapy. The drug may be excreted in breast milk, therefore, an alternative form of feeding your baby should be used.

Topical: Use as directed; do not overuse. Wash hands thoroughly before and after applying medication; avoid contact with eyes and mouth; avoid occlusive dressings; use a porous dressing. May cause local reaction (pain, burning, or swelling); if severe, contact prescriber.

Selected Readings
Diasio RB and Harris BE, "Clinical Pharmacology of 5-Fluorouracil," *Clin Pharmacokinet*, 1989, 16(4):215-37.
(Continued)

Fluorouracil (Continued)

Diasio RB and Johnson MR, "The Role of Pharmacogenetics and Pharmacogenomics in Cancer Chemotherapy With 5-Fluorouracil," *Pharmacology*, 2000, 61(3):199-203.

Grem JL, "5-Fluorouracil: Forty-Plus and Still Ticking. A Review of its Preclinical and Clinical Development," *Invest New Drugs*, 2000, 18(4):299-313.

Iyer L and Ratain MJ, "5-Fluorouracil Pharmacokinetics: Causes for Variability and Strategies for Modulation in Cancer Chemotherapy," *Cancer Invest*, 1999, 17(7):494-506.

Kuhn JG, "Fluorouracil and the New Oral Fluorinated Pyrimidines," *Ann Pharmacother*, 2001, 35(2):217-27.

Milano G and Chamorey AL, "Clinical Pharmacokinetics of 5-Fluorouracil With Consideration of Chronopharmacokinetics," *Chronobiol Int*, 2002, 19(1):177-89.

Parker WB and Cheng YC, "Metabolism and Mechanism of Action of 5-Fluorouracil," *Pharmacol Ther*, 1990, 48(3):381-95.

Schilsky RL, "Biochemical and Clinical Pharmacology of 5-Fluorouracil," *Oncology*, 1998, 12(10 Suppl 7):13-8.

♦ **5-Fluorouracil** *see* Fluorouracil *on page 359*

Fluoxymesterone (floo oks i MES te rone)

Medication Safety Issues

Sound-alike/look-alike issues:

Halotestin® may be confused with Haldol®, haloperidol, halothane, Halotussin®

U.S. Brand Names Halotestin®

Canadian Brand Names Halotestin®

Generic Available Yes

Pharmacologic Category Androgen

Pregnancy Risk Factor X

Lactation Excretion in breast milk unknown/contraindicated

Use Replacement of endogenous testicular hormone; in females, palliative treatment of breast cancer

Unlabeled/Investigational Use Stimulation of erythropoiesis, angioneurotic edema

Mechanism of Action Synthetic androgenic anabolic hormone responsible for the normal growth and development of male sex hormones and development of male sex organs and maintenance of secondary sex characteristics; synthetic testosterone derivative with significant androgen activity; stimulates RNA polymerase activity resulting in an increase in protein production; increases bone development; halogenated derivative of testosterone with up to 5 times the activity of methyltestosterone

Restrictions C-III

Labeled Contraindications Hypersensitivity to fluoxymesterone or any component of the formulation; serious cardiac disease, liver or kidney disease; pregnancy

Warnings/Precautions May accelerate bone maturation without producing compensatory gain in linear growth in children; in prepubertal children perform radiographic examination of the hand and wrist every 6 months to determine the rate of bone maturation and to assess the effect of treatment on the epiphyseal centers.

Adverse Reactions

>10%:

Male: Priapism

Female: Menstrual problems (amenorrhea), virilism, breast soreness

Cardiovascular: Edema

Dermatologic: Acne

1% to 10%:
  Male: Prostatic carcinoma, hirsutism (increase in pubic hair growth), impotence, testicular atrophy
  Cardiovascular: Edema
  Gastrointestinal: GI irritation, nausea, vomiting
  Genitourinary: Prostatic hyperplasia
  Hepatic: Hepatic dysfunction
<1%:
  Male: Gynecomastia
  Female: Amenorrhea
  Hypercalcemia, leukopenia, polycythemia, hepatic necrosis, cholestatic hepatitis, hypersensitivity reactions

Emetic Potential Very low (<10%)

Overdosage/Toxicology Symptoms of overdose include water retention. Abnormal liver function tests have been observed.

Drug Interactions
  Increased Effect/Toxicity: Fluoxymesterone may suppress clotting factors II, V, VII, and X; therefore, bleeding may occur in patients on anticoagulant therapy May elevate cyclosporine serum levels. May enhance hypoglycemic effect of insulin therapy; may decrease blood glucose concentrations and insulin requirements in patients with diabetes. Lithium may potentiate EPS and other CNS effect. May potentiate the effects of narcotics including respiratory depression
  Decreased Effect: May decrease barbiturate levels and fluphenazine effectiveness.

Storage/Stability Protect from light.

Pharmacodynamics/Kinetics
  Absorption: Rapid
  Protein binding: 98%
  Metabolism: Hepatic; enterohepatic recirculation
  Half-life elimination: 10-100 minutes
  Excretion: Urine (90%)

Dosage Adults: Oral:
  Male:
    Hypogonadism: 5-20 mg/day
    Delayed puberty: 2.5-20 mg/day for 4-6 months
  Female: Inoperable breast carcinoma: 10-40 mg/day in divided doses for 1-3 months

Combination Regimens
  Breast cancer: VATH *on page 944*

Dosage Forms [DSC] = Discontinued product
  Tablet: 10 mg
    Halotestin®: 2 mg, 5 mg, 10 mg [contains tartrazine; 10 mg tablet DSC]

Monitoring Parameters In prepubertal children, perform radiographic examination of the hand and wrist every 6 months

Patient Information Take as directed; do not discontinue without consulting prescriber. Diabetics should monitor serum glucose closely and notify prescriber of changes; this medication can alter hypoglycemic requirements. You may experience acne, growth of body hair, loss of libido, impotence, or menstrual irregularity (usually reversible); nausea or vomiting (small frequent meals, frequent mouth care, sucking lozenges, or chewing gum may help). Report changes in menstrual pattern; deepening of voice or unusual growth of body hair; fluid retention (swelling of (Continued)

Fluoxymesterone *(Continued)*

ankles, feet, or hands, difficulty breathing, or sudden weight gain); change in color of urine or stool; yellowing of eyes or skin; unusual bruising or bleeding; or other adverse reactions.

♦ **5-Flurocytosine** *see* Flucytosine *on page 354*

Flutamide *(FLOO ta mide)*

Medication Safety Issues
Sound-alike/look-alike issues:
Flutamide may be confused with Flumadine®, thalidomide
Eulexin® may be confused with Edecrin®, Eurax®

Related Information
Safe Handling of Hazardous Drugs *on page 1034*

U.S. Brand Names Eulexin®

Canadian Brand Names Apo-Flutamide®; Euflex®; Eulexin®; Novo-Flutamide; PMS-Flutamide

Generic Available Yes

Synonyms Niftolid; 4'-Nitro-3'-Trifluoromethylisobutyrantide; NSC-147834; SCH 13521

Pharmacologic Category Antineoplastic Agent, Antiandrogen

Pregnancy Risk Factor D

Lactation Excretion in breast milk unknown/not recommended

Use Treatment of metastatic prostatic carcinoma in combination therapy with LHRH agonist analogues

Unlabeled/Investigational Use Female hirsutism

Mechanism of Action Nonsteroidal antiandrogen that inhibits androgen uptake or inhibits binding of androgen in target tissues

Labeled Contraindications Hypersensitivity to flutamide or any component of the formulation; severe hepatic impairment; pregnancy

Warnings/Precautions Patients with glucose-6 phosphate dehydrogenase deficiency or hemoglobin M disease or smokers are at risk of toxicities associated with aniline exposure, including methemoglobinemia, hemolytic anemia, and cholestatic jaundice. Monitor methemoglobin levels. Severe and potentially fatal hepatic injury may occur (50% of cases within first 3 months of therapy). Serum transaminases should be monitored at baseline and monthly for the first four months of therapy, and periodically thereafter. These should also be repeated at the first sign and symptom of liver dysfunction. Use of flutamide is not recommended in patients with baseline elevation of transaminase levels (>2 times the upper limit of normal). Flutamide should be discontinued immediately at any time if the patient develops jaundice or elevation in serum transaminase levels (>2 times upper limit of normal).

Adverse Reactions
>10%:
Endocrine & metabolic: Gynecomastia, hot flashes, breast tenderness, galactorrhea (9% to 42%); impotence; decreased libido; tumor flare
Gastrointestinal: Nausea, vomiting (11% to 12%)
Hepatic: Increased AST (SGOT) and LDH levels, transient, mild
1% to 10%:
Cardiovascular: Hypertension (1%), edema
Central nervous system: Drowsiness, confusion, depression, anxiety, nervousness, headache, dizziness, insomnia

Dermatologic: Pruritus, ecchymosis, photosensitivity, herpes zoster
Gastrointestinal: Anorexia, increased appetite, constipation, indigestion, upset stomach (4% to 6%); diarrhea
Hematologic: Anemia (6%), leukopenia (3%), thrombocytopenia (1%)
Neuromuscular & skeletal: Weakness (1%)
<1%: Discoloration of urine (yellow), hepatitis, hepatic failure, jaundice, sulfhemoglobinemia, thrombophlebitis, malignant breast neoplasm (male), MI, pulmonary embolism

Emetic Potential Low (10% to 30%)

Overdosage/Toxicology Symptoms of overdose include hypoactivity, ataxia, anorexia, vomiting, slow respiration, and lacrimation. Induce vomiting. Management is supportive. Dialysis is of no benefit.

Drug Interactions
Cytochrome P450 Effect: Substrate (major) of CYP1A2, 3A4; **Inhibits** CYP1A2 (weak)
Increased Effect/Toxicity: CYP1A2 inhibitors may increase the levels/effects of flutamide; example inhibitors include amiodarone, ciprofloxacin, fluvoxamine, ketoconazole, lomefloxacin, ofloxacin, and rofecoxib. CYP3A4 inhibitors may increase the levels/effects of flutamide; example inhibitors include azole antifungals, ciprofloxacin, clarithromycin, diclofenac, doxycycline, erythromycin, imatinib, isoniazid, nefazodone, nicardipine, propofol, protease inhibitors, quinidine, and verapamil. Warfarin effects may be increased.
Decreased Effect: CYP1A2 inducers may decrease the levels/effects of flutamide; example inducers include aminoglutethimide, carbamazepine, phenobarbital, and rifampin. CYP3A4 inducers may decrease the levels/effects of flutamide; example inducers include aminoglutethimide, carbamazepine, nafcillin, nevirapine, phenobarbital, phenytoin, and rifamycins.

Ethanol/Nutrition/Herb Interactions
Food: No effect on bioavailability of flutamide.
Herb/Nutraceutical: St John's wort may decrease flutamide levels.

Storage/Stability Store at room temperature.

Pharmacodynamics/Kinetics
Absorption: Oral: Rapid and complete
Protein binding: Parent drug: 94% to 96%; 2-hydroxyflutamide: 92% to 94%
Metabolism: Extensively hepatic to more than 10 metabolites, primarily 2-hydroxyflutamide (active)
Half-life elimination: 5-6 hours (2-hydroxyflutamide)
Excretion: Primarily urine (as metabolites)

Dosage Oral: Adults:
Prostatic carcinoma: 250 mg 3 times/day; alternatively, once-daily doses of 0.5-1.5 g have been used (unlabeled dosing)
Female hirsutism (unlabeled use): 250 mg daily

Combination Regimens
Prostate cancer:
FL *on page 889*
FZ *on page 895*

Administration Oral: Usually in 3 divided doses; contents of capsule may be opened and mixed with applesauce, pudding, or other soft foods; mixing with a beverage is not recommended

Dosage Forms Capsule: 125 mg
(Continued)

Flutamide *(Continued)*

Monitoring Parameters Serum transaminase levels should be measured prior to starting treatment and monthly for the first 4 months of therapy, and periodically thereafter. LFTs should be checked at the first sign or symptom of liver dysfunction (eg, nausea, vomiting, abdominal pain, fatigue, anorexia, flu-like symptoms, hyperbilirubinuria, jaundice, or right upper quadrant tenderness). Other parameters include tumor reduction, testosterone/estrogen, and phosphatase serum levels.

Patient Information Take as directed; do not discontinue without consulting prescriber. You may experience decreased libido, impotence, swelling of breasts, or decreased appetite (small frequent meals may help). Report chest pain or palpitation; acute abdominal pain; pain, tingling, or numbness of extremities; swelling of extremities or unusual weight gain; difficulty breathing; or other persistent adverse effects.

Special Geriatric Considerations A study has shown that the addition of flutamide to leuprolide therapy in patients with advanced prostatic cancer increased median actuarial survival time to 34.9 months versus 27.9 months with leuprolide alone. No specific dose alterations are necessary in the elderly.

Selected Readings

Brogden RN and Chrisp P, "Flutamide. A Review of Its Pharmacodynamic and Pharmacokinetic Properties, and Therapeutic Use in Advanced Prostatic Cancer," *Drugs Aging*, 1991, 1(2):104-15.

Brogden RN and Clissold SP, "Flutamide. A Preliminary Review of Its Pharmacodynamic and Pharmacokinetic Properties, and Therapeutic Efficacy in Advanced Prostate Cancer," *Drugs*, 1989, 38(2):185-203.

Goldspiel BR and Kohler DR, "Flutamide: An Antiandrogen for Advanced Prostate Cancer," *DICP Ann Pharmacother*, 1990, 24(6):616-23.

Labrie F, "Mechanism of Action and Pure Antiandrogenic Properties of Flutamide," *Cancer*, 1993, 72(12 Suppl):3816-27.

♦ **Folinic Acid** *see* Leucovorin *on page 497*

♦ **5-Formyl Tetrahydrofolate** *see* Leucovorin *on page 497*

♦ **Forneau-309** *see* Suramin *on page 733*

♦ **Fortaz®** *see* Ceftazidime *on page 165*

Foscarnet *(fos KAR net)*

U.S. Brand Names Foscavir®

Canadian Brand Names Foscavir®

Generic Available No

Synonyms PFA; Phosphonoformate; Phosphonoformic Acid

Pharmacologic Category Antiviral Agent

Pregnancy Risk Factor C

Lactation Excretion in breast milk unknown/contraindicated

Use

Treatment of herpes virus infections suspected to be caused by acyclovir-resistant (HSV, VZV) or ganciclovir-resistant (CMV) strains; this occurs almost exclusively in immunocompromised persons (eg, with advanced AIDS) who have received prolonged treatment for a herpes virus infection

Treatment of CMV retinitis in persons with AIDS

Unlabeled/Investigational Use Other CMV infections in persons unable to tolerate ganciclovir; may be given in combination with ganciclovir in patients who relapse after monotherapy with either drug

Mechanism of Action Pyrophosphate analogue which acts as a noncompetitive inhibitor of many viral RNA and DNA polymerases as well as HIV reverse transcriptase. Similar to ganciclovir, foscarnet is a virostatic agent. Foscarnet does not require activation by thymidine kinase.

Labeled Contraindications Hypersensitivity to foscarnet or any component of the formulation; Cl_{cr} <0.4 mL/minute/kg during therapy

Warnings/Precautions Hazardous agent - use appropriate precautions for handling and disposal. See Safe Handling of Hazardous Drugs *on page 1034* in the Appendix. Renal impairment occurs to some degree in the majority of patients treated with foscarnet. Renal impairment may occur at any time (usually reversible within 1 week following dose adjustment or discontinuation, but some severe cases). Renal function should be closely monitored. Foscarnet may cause tooth disorders. Safety and effectiveness in children have not been studied. Monitor electrolytes carefully, particularly calcium, magnesium, phosphate, and potassium. Seizures have been experienced by up to 10% of AIDS patients. Risk factors for seizures include a low baseline absolute neutrophil count (ANC), impaired baseline renal function and low total serum calcium. Some patients who have experienced seizures have died, while others have been able to continue or resume foscarnet treatment after their mineral or electrolyte abnormality has been corrected, their underlying disease state treated, or their dose decreased. Foscarnet has been shown to be mutagenic *in vitro* and in mice at very high doses.

Adverse Reactions

>10%:

Central nervous system: Fever (65%), headache (26%), seizure (10%)

Gastrointestinal: Nausea (47%), diarrhea (30%), vomiting

Hematologic: Anemia (33%)

Renal: Abnormal renal function/decreased creatinine clearance (27%)

1% to 10%:

Central nervous system: Fatigue, malaise, dizziness, hypoesthesia, depression/confusion/anxiety (≥5%)

Dermatologic: Rash

Endocrine & metabolic: Electrolyte imbalance (especially potassium, calcium, magnesium, and phosphorus)

Gastrointestinal: Anorexia

Hematologic: Granulocytopenia, leukopenia (≥5%), thrombocytopenia, thrombosis

Local: Injection site pain

Neuromuscular & skeletal: Paresthesia, involuntary muscle contractions, rigors, neuropathy (peripheral), weakness

Ocular: Vision abnormalities

Respiratory: Coughing, dyspnea (≥5%)

Miscellaneous: Sepsis, diaphoresis (increased)

<1%: Cardiac failure, bradycardia, arrhythmia, cerebral edema, leg edema, peripheral edema, syncope, substernal chest pain, hypothermia, abnormal crying, malignant hyperpyrexia, vertigo, coma, speech disorders, gynecomastia, decreased gonadotropins, cholecystitis, cholelithiasis, hepatitis, hepatosplenomegaly, ascites, abnormal gait, dyskinesia, hypertonia, nystagmus, vocal cord paralysis

Vesicant No

Emetic Potential Moderate (30% to 60%)

(Continued)

Foscarnet *(Continued)*

Overdosage/Toxicology Symptoms of overdose include seizures, renal dysfunction, perioral or limb paresthesia, and hypocalcemia. Treatment is supportive.

Drug Interactions

Increased Effect/Toxicity: Concurrent use with ciprofloxacin (or other fluoroquinolone) increases seizure potential. Acute renal failure (reversible) has been reported with cyclosporine due most likely to a synergistic toxic effect. Nephrotoxic drugs (amphotericin B, I.V. pentamidine, aminoglycosides, etc) should be avoided, if possible, to minimize additive renal risk with foscarnet. Concurrent use of pentamidine also increases the potential for hypocalcemia. Protease inhibitors (ritonavir, saquinavir) have been associated with an increased risk of renal impairment during concurrent use of foscarnet

Storage/Stability Foscarnet injection is a clear, colorless solution. It should be stored at room temperature and protected from temperatures >40°C and from freezing. Diluted solution is stable for 24 hours at room temperature or refrigeration.

Reconstitution Foscarnet should be diluted in D_5W or NS. For peripheral line administration, foscarnet **must** be diluted to ≤12 mg/mL with D_5W or NS. For central line administration, foscarnet may be administered undiluted.

Compatibility Stable in D_5W, NS; not stable in LR; **incompatible** with dextrose 30%, TPN, and I.V. solutions containing calcium, magnesium, vancomycin

Y-site administration: Compatible: Aldesleukin, amikacin, aminophylline, ampicillin, aztreonam, cefazolin, cefoperazone, cefoxitin, ceftazidime, ceftizoxime, ceftriaxone, cefuroxime, chloramphenicol, cimetidine, clindamycin, dexamethasone sodium phosphate, dopamine, erythromycin lactobionate, fluconazole, flucytosine, furosemide, gentamicin, heparin, hydrocortisone sodium succinate, hydromorphone, hydroxyzine, imipenem/cilastatin, metoclopramide, metronidazole, morphine, nafcillin, oxacillin, penicillin G potassium, phenytoin, piperacillin, ranitidine, ticarcillin/clavulanate, tobramycin. **Incompatible:** Acyclovir, amphotericin B, diazepam, digoxin, diphenhydramine, dobutamine, droperidol, ganciclovir, haloperidol, leucovorin, midazolam, pentamidine, prochlorperazine edisylate, promethazine, trimetrexate. **Variable (consult detailed reference):** Co-trimoxazole, lorazepam, vancomycin

Compatibility when admixed: Compatible: Potassium chloride

Pharmacodynamics/Kinetics

Distribution: Up to 28% of cumulative I.V. dose may be deposited in bone

Metabolism: Biotransformation does not occur

Half-life elimination: ~3 hours

Excretion: Urine (≤28% as unchanged drug)

Dosage

CMV retinitis: I.V.:

Induction treatment: 60 mg/kg/dose every 8 hours **or** 100 mg/kg every 12 hours for 14-21 days

Maintenance therapy: 90-120 mg/kg/day as a single infusion

Acyclovir-resistant HSV induction treatment: I.V.: 40 mg/kg/dose every 8-12 hours for 14-21 days

Dosage adjustment in renal impairment:

Induction and maintenance dosing schedules based on creatinine clearance (mL/minute/kg): See tables.

Induction Dosing of Foscarnet in Patients With Abnormal Renal Function

Cl_{cr} (mL/min/kg)	HSV Equivalent to 40 mg/kg q12h	HSV Equivalent to 40 mg/kg q8h	CMV Equivalent to 60 mg/kg q8h	CMV Equivalent to 90 mg/kg q12h
<0.4	Not recommended	Not recommended	Not recommended	Not recommended
≥0.4-0.5	20 mg/kg every 24 hours	35 mg/kg every 24 hours	50 mg/kg every 24 hours	50 mg/kg every 24 hours
>0.5-0.6	25 mg/kg every 24 hours	40 mg/kg every 24 hours	60 mg/kg every 24 hours	60 mg/kg every 24 hours
>0.6-0.8	35 mg/kg every 24 hours	25 mg/kg every 12 hours	40 mg/kg every 12 hours	80 mg/kg every 24 hours
>0.8-1.0	20 mg/kg every 12 hours	35 mg/kg every 12 hours	50 mg/kg every 12 hours	50 mg/kg every 12 hours
>1.0-1.4	30 mg/kg every 12 hours	30 mg/kg every 8 hours	45 mg/kg every 8 hours	70 mg/kg every 12 hours
>1.4	40 mg/kg every 12 hours	40 mg/kg every 8 hours	60 mg/kg every 8 hours	90 mg/kg every 12 hours

Maintenance Dosing of Foscarnet in Patients With Abnormal Renal Function

Cl_{cr} (mL/min/kg)	CMV Equivalent to 90 mg/kg q24h	CMV Equivalent to 120 mg/kg q24h
<0.4	Not recommended	Not recommended
≥0.4-0.5	50 mg/kg every 48 hours	65 mg/kg every 48 hours
>0.5-0.6	60 mg/kg every 48 hours	80 mg/kg every 48 hours
>0.6-0.8	80 mg/kg every 48 hours	105 mg/kg every 48 hours
>0.8-1.0	50 mg/kg every 24 hours	65 mg/kg every 24 hours
>1.0-1.4	70 mg/kg every 24 hours	90 mg/kg every 24 hours
>1.4	90 mg/kg every 24 hours	120 mg/kg every 24 hours

Hemodialysis:

Foscarnet is highly removed by hemodialysis (30% in 4 hours HD)

Doses of 50 mg/kg/dose posthemodialysis have been found to produce similar serum concentrations as doses of 90 mg/kg twice daily in patients with normal renal function

Doses of 60-90 mg/kg/dose loading dose (posthemodialysis) followed by 45 mg/kg/dose posthemodialysis (3 times/week) with the monitoring of weekly plasma concentrations to maintain peak plasma concentrations in the range of 400-800 μMolar has been recommended by some clinicians

Continuous arteriovenous or venovenous hemodiafiltration effects: Dose as for Cl_{cr} 10-50 mL/minute

Administration Foscarnet is administered by intravenous infusion, using an infusion pump, at a rate not exceeding 1 mg/kg/minute. Undiluted (24 (Continued)

Foscarnet *(Continued)*

mg/mL) solution can be administered without further dilution when using a central venous catheter for infusion. For peripheral vein administration, the solution **must** be diluted to a final concentration **not to exceed** 12 mg/mL. The recommended dosage, frequency, and rate of infusion should not be exceeded.

Dosage Forms Injection, solution: 24 mg/mL (250 mL, 500 mL)

Patient Information Close monitoring is important and any symptom of electrolyte abnormalities should be reported immediately; maintain adequate fluid intake and hydration; regular ophthalmic examinations are necessary. Foscarnet is not a cure; disease progression may occur during or following treatment. Report any numbness in the extremities, paresthesias, or perioral tingling.

Additional Information Sodium loading with 500 mL of 0.9% sodium chloride solution before and after foscarnet infusion helps to minimize the risk of nephrotoxicity.

Special Geriatric Considerations Information on the use of foscarnet is lacking in the elderly. Dose adjustments and proper monitoring must be performed because of the decreased renal function common in older patients.

Selected Readings

Chrisp P and Clissold SP, "Foscarnet. A Review of Its Antiviral Activity, Pharmacokinetic Properties and Therapeutic Use in Immunocompromised Patients With Cytomegalovirus Retinitis," *Drugs*, 1991, 41(1):104-29.

Jacobson MA, "Review of the Toxicities of Foscarnet," *J Acquir Immune Defic Syndr*, 1992, 5(Suppl 1):11-7.

♦ **Foscavir**® *see* Foscarnet *on page 368*

♦ **Frusemide** *see* Furosemide *on page 374*

♦ **FU** *see* Fluorouracil *on page 359*

♦ **5-FU** *see* Fluorouracil *on page 359*

♦ **Fucidin**® **(Can)** *see* Fusidic Acid *on page 378*

♦ **Fucithalmic**® **(Can)** *see* Fusidic Acid *on page 378*

♦ **FUDR**® *see* Floxuridine *on page 347*

♦ **5-FUDR** *see* Floxuridine *on page 347*

Fulvestrant *(fool VES trant)*

U.S. Brand Names Faslodex®

Generic Available No

Synonyms ICI-182,780; Zeneca 182,780; ZM-182,780

Pharmacologic Category Antineoplastic Agent, Estrogen Receptor Antagonist

Pregnancy Risk Factor D

Lactation Excretion in breast milk unknown/contraindicated

Use Treatment of hormone receptor positive metastatic breast cancer in postmenopausal women with disease progression following antiestrogen therapy.

Unlabeled/Investigational Use Endometriosis; uterine bleeding

Mechanism of Action Steroidal compound which competitively binds to estrogen receptors on tumors and other tissue targets, producing a nuclear complex that decreases DNA synthesis and inhibits estrogen effects. Fulvestrant has no estrogen-receptor agonist activity. Causes down-regulation of estrogen receptors and inhibits tumor growth.

Labeled Contraindications Hypersensitivity to fulvestrant or any component of the formulation; contraindications to I.M. injections (bleeding diatheses, thrombocytopenia, or therapeutic anticoagulation); pregnancy

Warnings/Precautions Use caution in hepatic impairment.

Adverse Reactions

>10%:

Cardiovascular: Vasodilation (18%)

Central nervous system: Pain (19%), headache (15%)

Endocrine & metabolic: Hot flushes (19% to 24%)

Gastrointestinal: Nausea (26%), vomiting (13%), constipation (13%), diarrhea (12%), abdominal pain (12%)

Local: Injection site reaction (11%)

Neuromuscular & skeletal: Weakness (23%), bone pain (16%), back pain (14%)

Respiratory: Pharyngitis (16%), dyspnea (15%)

1% to 10%:

Cardiovascular: Edema (9%), chest pain (7%)

Central nervous system: Dizziness (7%), insomnia (7%), paresthesia (6%), fever (6%), depression (6%), anxiety (5%)

Dermatologic: Rash (7%)

Gastrointestinal: Anorexia (9%), weight gain (1% to 2%)

Genitourinary: Pelvic pain (10%), urinary tract infection (6%), vaginitis (2% to 3%)

Hematologic: Anemia (5%)

Neuromuscular and skeletal: Arthritis (3%)

Respiratory: Cough (10%)

Miscellaneous: Diaphoresis increased (5%)

<1%: Leukopenia, myalgia, thrombosis, vaginal bleeding, vertigo

Overdosage/Toxicology No specific experience in overdose. Treatment is supportive.

Drug Interactions

Cytochrome P450 Effect: Substrate of CYP3A4 (minor)

Storage/Stability Store under refrigeration at 2°C to 8°C (36°F to 46°F).

Pharmacodynamics/Kinetics

Duration: I.M.: Plasma levels maintained for at least 1 month

Distribution: V_d: 3-5 L/kg

Protein binding: 99%

Metabolism: Hepatic via multiple pathways (CYP3A4 substrate, relative contribution to metabolism unknown)

Bioavailability: Oral: Poor

Half-life elimination: ~40 days

Time to peak, plasma: I.M.: 7-9 days

Excretion: Feces (>90%); urine (<1%)

Dosage I.M.: Adults (postmenopausal women): 250 mg at 1-month intervals

Dosage adjustment in renal impairment: No adjustment required.

Dosage adjustment in hepatic impairment: Use in moderate to severe hepatic impairment has not been evaluated; use caution.

Administration I.M. injection into a relatively large muscle (ie, buttock); do not administer I.V., SubQ, or intra-arterially. May be administered as a single 5 mL injection or two concurrent 2.5 mL injections.

(Continued)

Fulvestrant *(Continued)*

Dosage Forms Injection, solution: 50 mg/mL (2.5 mL, 5 mL) [[prefilled syringe; contains alcohol, benzyl alcohol, benzyl stearate, castor oil]

Selected Readings

Bundred N and Howell A, "Fulvestrant (Faslodex): Current Status in the Therapy of Breast Cancer," *Expert Rev Anticancer Ther,* 2002, 2(2):151-60.

Curran M and Wiseman L, "Fulvestrant," *Drugs,* 2001, 61(6):807-13.

Wardley AM, "Fulvestrant: A Review of Its Development, Pre-clinical and Clinical Data," *Int J Clin Pract* 2002, 56(4):305-9.

♦ **Fungizone®** *see* Amphotericin B (Conventional) *on page 69*

Furosemide *(fyoor OH se mide)*

Medication Safety Issues

Sound-alike/look-alike issues:

Furosemide may be confused with torsemide

Lasix® may be confused with Esidrix®, Lanoxin®, Lidex®, Lomotil®, Luvox®, Luxiq®

U.S. Brand Names Lasix®

Canadian Brand Names Apo-Furosemide®; Lasix®; Lasix® Special

Generic Available Yes

Synonyms Frusemide

Pharmacologic Category Diuretic, Loop

Pregnancy Risk Factor C

Lactation Enters breast milk/use caution

Use Management of edema associated with congestive heart failure and hepatic or renal disease; alone or in combination with antihypertensives in treatment of hypertension

Mechanism of Action Inhibits reabsorption of sodium and chloride in the ascending loop of Henle and distal renal tubule, interfering with the chloride-binding cotransport system, thus causing increased excretion of water, sodium, chloride, magnesium, and calcium

Labeled Contraindications Hypersensitivity to furosemide, any component, or sulfonylureas; anuria; patients with hepatic coma or in states of severe electrolyte depletion until the condition improves or is corrected

Warnings/Precautions In cirrhosis, avoid electrolyte and acid/base imbalances that might lead to hepatic encephalopathy. Ototoxicity is associated with rapid I.V. administration, renal impairment, excessive doses, and concurrent use of other ototoxins. Hypersensitivity reactions can rarely occur. Monitor fluid status and renal function in an attempt to prevent oliguria, azotemia, electrolyte disturbances, dehydration, and reversible increases in BUN and creatinine. Coadministration of antihypertensives may increase the risk of hypotension. Avoid use of medications in which the toxicity is enhanced by hypokalemia (including quinolones with QT prolongation).

Chemical similarities are present among sulfonamides, sulfonylureas, carbonic anhydrase inhibitors, thiazides, and loop diuretics (except ethacrynic acid). Use in patients with sulfonylurea allergy is specifically contraindicated in product labeling, however, a risk of cross-reaction exists in patients with allergy to any of these compounds; avoid use when previous reaction has been severe.

Adverse Reactions Frequency not defined.

Cardiovascular: Orthostatic hypotension, necrotizing angiitis, thrombophlebitis, chronic aortitis, acute hypotension, sudden death from cardiac arrest (with I.V. or I.M. administration)

Central nervous system: Paresthesias, vertigo, dizziness, lightheadedness, headache, blurred vision, xanthopsia , fever, restlessness

Dermatologic: Exfoliative dermatitis, erythema multiforme, purpura, photosensitivity, urticaria, rash, pruritus, cutaneous vasculitis

Endocrine & metabolic: Gout, hyperglycemia, hyperuricemia, hypocalcemia, hypochloremia, hypokalemia, hypomagnesemia, hyponatremia, metabolic alkalosis

Gastrointestinal: Nausea, vomiting, anorexia, oral and gastric irritation, cramping, diarrhea, constipation, pancreatitis, intrahepatic cholestatic jaundice, ischemia hepatitis

Genitourinary: Urinary bladder spasm, urinary frequency

Hematological: Aplastic anemia (rare), thrombocytopenia, agranulocytosis (rare), hemolytic anemia, leukopenia, anemia, purpura

Neuromuscular & skeletal: Muscle spasm, weakness

Otic: Hearing impairment (reversible or permanent with rapid I.V. or I.M. administration), tinnitus, reversible deafness (with rapid I.V. or I.M. administration)

Renal: Vasculitis, allergic interstitial nephritis, glycosuria, fall in glomerular filtration rate and renal blood flow (due to overdiuresis), transient rise in BUN

Miscellaneous: Anaphylaxis (rare), exacerbate or activate systemic lupus erythematosus

Vesicant No

Emetic Potential Very low (<10%)

Overdosage/Toxicology Symptoms of overdose include electrolyte depletion, volume depletion, hypotension, dehydration, and circulatory collapse. Treatment is supportive.

Drug Interactions

Increased Effect/Toxicity: Furosemide-induced hypokalemia may predispose to digoxin toxicity and may increase the risk of arrhythmia with drugs which may prolong QT interval, including type Ia and type III antiarrhythmic agents, cisapride, and some quinolones (sparfloxacin, gatifloxacin, and moxifloxacin). The risk of toxicity from lithium and salicylates (high dose) may be increased by loop diuretics. Hypotensive effects and/or adverse renal effects of ACE inhibitors and NSAIDs are potentiated by furosemide-induced hypovolemia. The effects of peripheral adrenergic-blocking drugs or ganglionic blockers may be increased by furosemide.

Furosemide may increase the risk of ototoxicity with other ototoxic agents (aminoglycosides, cis-platinum), especially in patients with renal dysfunction. Synergistic diuretic effects occur with thiazide-type diuretics. Diuretics tend to be synergistic with other antihypertensive agents, and hypotension may occur.

Decreased Effect: Indomethacin, aspirin, phenobarbital, phenytoin, and NSAIDs may reduce natriuretic and hypotensive effects of furosemide. Colestipol, cholestyramine, and sucralfate may reduce the effect of furosemide; separate administration by 2 hours. Furosemide may antagonize the effect of skeletal muscle relaxants (tubocurarine). Glucose tolerance may be decreased by furosemide, requiring an

(Continued)

Furosemide *(Continued)*

adjustment in the dose of hypoglycemic agents. Metformin may decrease furosemide concentrations.

Ethanol/Nutrition/Herb Interactions

Food: Furosemide serum levels may be decreased if taken with food.

Herb/Nutraceutical: Avoid dong quai if using for hypertension (has estrogenic activity). Avoid ephedra, yohimbe, ginseng (may worsen hypertension). Limit intake of natural licorice. Avoid garlic (may have increased antihypertensive effect).

Storage/Stability Furosemide injection should be stored at controlled room temperature and protected from light. Exposure to light may cause discoloration. Do not use furosemide solutions if they have a yellow color. Refrigeration may result in precipitation or crystallization, however, resolubilization at room temperature or warming may be performed without affecting the drugs stability.

Reconstitution I.V. infusion solution mixed in NS or D_5W solution is stable for 24 hours at room temperature. May also be diluted for infusion 1-2 mg/mL (maximum: 10 mg/mL) over 10-15 minutes (following infusion rate parameters).

Compatibility Stable in D_5LR, D_5NS, D_5W, $D_{10}W$, $D_{20}W$, mannitol 20%, LR, NS

Y-site administration: Compatible: Allopurinol, amifostine, amikacin, amphotericin B cholesteryl sulfate complex, aztreonam, bleomycin, cefepime, cisplatin, cladribine, cyclophosphamide, cytarabine, docetaxel, doxorubicin liposome, epinephrine, etoposide phosphate, fentanyl, fludarabine, fluorouracil, foscarnet, granisetron, heparin, hydrocortisone sodium succinate, hydromorphone, indomethacin, kanamycin, leucovorin, linezolid, lorazepam, melphalan, meropenem, methotrexate, mitomycin, nitroglycerin, norepinephrine, paclitaxel, piperacillin/tazobactam, potassium chloride, propofol, ranitidine, remifentanil, sargramostim, tacrolimus, teniposide, thiotepa, tobramycin, tolazoline, vitamin B complex with C. **Incompatible:** Alatrofloxacin, amsacrine, chlorpromazine, ciprofloxacin, clarithromycin, diltiazem, droperidol, esmolol, filgrastim, fluconazole, gatifloxacin, gemcitabine, gentamicin, hydralazine, idarubicin, levofloxacin, metoclopramide, midazolam, milrinone, netilmicin, nicardipine, ondansetron, quinidine gluconate, thiopental, vecuronium, vinblastine, vincristine, vinorelbine. **Variable (consult detailed reference):** Cisatracurium, dobutamine, dopamine, doxorubicin, famotidine, labetalol, meperidine, morphine

Compatibility in syringe: Compatible: Bleomycin, cisplatin, cyclophosphamide, fluorouracil, heparin, leucovorin, methotrexate, mitomycin. **Incompatible:** Doxapram, doxorubicin, droperidol, metoclopramide, milrinone, vinblastine, vincristine

Compatibility when admixed: Compatible: Amikacin, aminophylline, ampicillin, atropine, bumetanide, calcium gluconate, cefamandole, cefoperazone, cefuroxime, cimetidine, dexamethasone sodium phosphate, diamorphine, digoxin, epinephrine, heparin, isosorbide, kanamycin, lidocaine, meropenem, morphine, nitroglycerin, penicillin G, potassium chloride, ranitidine, scopolamine, sodium bicarbonate, sulfadimidine, theophylline, tobramycin. **Incompatible:** Buprenorphine, chlorpromazine, diazepam, dobutamine, erythromycin lactobionate, isoproterenol, meperidine, metoclopramide, netilmicin, prochlorperazine edisylate, promethazine. **Variable (consult detailed reference):** Amiodarone, gentamicin, hydrocortisone sodium succinate, verapamil

Pharmacodynamics/Kinetics

Onset of action: Diuresis: Oral: 30-60 minutes; I.M.: 30 minutes; I.V.: ~5 minutes

Peak effect: Oral: 1-2 hours

Duration: Oral: 6-8 hours; I.V.: 2 hours

Absorption: Oral: 60% to 67%

Protein binding: >98%

Metabolism: Minimally hepatic

Half-life elimination: Normal renal function: 0.5-1.1 hours; End-stage renal disease: 9 hours

Excretion: Urine (Oral: 50%, I.V.: 80%) within 24 hours; feces (as unchanged drug); nonrenal clearance prolonged in renal impairment

Dosage

Infants and Children:

Oral: 1-2 mg/kg/dose increased in increments of 1 mg/kg/dose with each succeeding dose until a satisfactory effect is achieved to a maximum of 6 mg/kg/dose no more frequently than 6 hours.

I.M., I.V.: 1 mg/kg/dose, increasing by each succeeding dose at 1 mg/kg/dose at intervals of 6-12 hours until a satisfactory response up to 6 mg/kg/dose.

Adults:

Oral: 20-80 mg/dose initially increased in increments of 20-40 mg/dose at intervals of 6-8 hours; usual maintenance dose interval is twice daily or every day; may be titrated up to 600 mg/day with severe edematous states.

Hypertension (JNC 7): 20-80 mg/day in 2 divided doses

I.M., I.V.: 20-40 mg/dose, may be repeated in 1-2 hours as needed and increased by 20 mg/dose until the desired effect has been obtained. Usual dosing interval: 6-12 hours; for acute pulmonary edema, the usual dose is 40 mg I.V. over 1-2 minutes. If not adequate, may increase dose to 80 mg.

Continuous I.V. infusion: Initial I.V. bolus dose of 0.1 mg/kg followed by continuous I.V. infusion doses of 0.1 mg/kg/hour doubled every 2 hours to a maximum of 0.4 mg/kg/hour if urine output is <1 mL/kg/hour have been found to be effective and result in a lower daily requirement of furosemide than with intermittent dosing. Other studies have used a rate of ≤4 mg/minute as a continuous I.V. infusion.

Refractory heart failure: Oral, I.V.: Doses up to 8 g/day have been used.

Elderly: Oral, I.M., I.V.: Initial: 20 mg/day; increase slowly to desired response.

Dosing adjustment/comments in renal impairment: Acute renal failure: High doses (up to 1-3 g/day - oral/I.V.) have been used to initiate desired response; avoid use in oliguric states.

Dialysis: Not removed by hemo- or peritoneal dialysis; supplemental dose is not necessary.

Dosing adjustment/comments in hepatic disease: Diminished natriuretic effect with increased sensitivity to hypokalemia and volume depletion in cirrhosis; monitor effects, particularly with high doses.

Administration

I.V.: I.V. injections should be given slowly may be administered undiluted direct I.V. at a maximum rate of 0.5 mg/kg/minute for doses <120 mg and 4 mg/minute for doses >120 mg; maximum rate of administration (Continued)

Furosemide *(Continued)*

for IVPB or infusion: 4 mg/minute. For continuous infusion furosemide in patients with severely-impaired renal function, do not exceed 4 mg/minute.

Oral: May be taken with or without food.

Dosage Forms

Injection, solution: 10 mg/mL (2 mL, 4 mL, 8 mL, 10 mL)

Solution, oral: 10 mg/mL (60 mL, 120 mL) [orange flavor]; 40 mg/5 mL (5 mL, 500 mL) [pineapple-peach flavor]

Tablet (Lasix®): 20 mg, 40 mg, 80 mg

Monitoring Parameters Monitor weight and I & O daily; blood pressure, orthostasis, serum electrolytes, renal function; in high doses, monitor hearing

Dietary Considerations This product may cause a potassium loss; your healthcare provider may prescribe a potassium supplement, another medication to help prevent the potassium loss, or recommend that you eat foods high in potassium, especially citrus fruits; do not change your diet on your own while taking this medication, especially if you are taking potassium supplements or medications to reduce potassium loss; too much potassium can be as harmful as too little; ideally, should be administered on an empty stomach; however, may be administered with food or milk if GI distress; do not mix with acidic solutions. Sodium content of 1 mL (injection): 0.162 mEq

Patient Information May be taken with food or milk; rise slowly from a lying or sitting position to minimize dizziness, lightheadedness, or fainting; also use extra care when exercising, standing for long periods of time, and during hot weather; take last dose of day early in the evening to prevent nocturia

Special Geriatric Considerations Severe loss of sodium and/or increase in BUN can cause confusion. For any change in mental status in patients on furosemide, monitor electrolytes and renal function.

Fusidic Acid *(fyoo SI dik AS id)*

Canadian Brand Names Fucidin®; Fucithalmic®

Generic Available No

Synonyms Sodium Fusidate

Pharmacologic Category Antibiotic, Miscellaneous

Lactation Enters breast milk/use caution

Use

Systemic: Treatment of skin and soft tissue infections, or osteomyelitis, caused by susceptible organisms, including *Staphylococcus aureus* (penicillinase-producing or nonpenicillinase strains); may be used in the treatment of pneumonia, septicemia, endocarditis, burns, and cystic fibrosis caused by susceptible organisms when other antibiotics have failed

Topical: Treatment of primary and secondary skin infections caused by susceptible organisms

Ophthalmic: Treatment of superficial infections of the eye and conjunctiva caused by susceptible organisms

Mechanism of Action Inhibits protein synthesis by blocking aminoacyl-sRNA transfer to protein in susceptible bacteria.

Restrictions Not available in U.S.

Labeled Contraindications Hypersensitivity to fusidic acid or any component of the formulation

Warnings/Precautions Use with extreme caution in hepatic impairment; monitor liver function regularly during treatment. Intravenous formulation contains phosphate/citrate buffer; excessive amounts may lead to hypocalcemia. Use with extreme caution in patients with pre-existing hypocalcemia. Should not be administered I.M. or SubQ; local tissue injury may occur.

Adverse Reactions

Cardiovascular: Edema (leg), thrombophlebitis, venospasm

Central nervous system: Dizziness, headache, psychic disturbance

Dermatologic: Pruritus, rash

Gastrointestinal: Anorexia, dyspepsia, diarrhea, epigastric distress, nausea, vomiting

Hepatic: Jaundice

Local: Injection site reaction (redness, irritation)

Ocular: Blurred vision

Ophthalmic suspension: Ocular: Transient stinging, tearing, eyelid edema, temporary blurred vision

Overdosage/Toxicology Limited experience in overdose. Symptoms may include gastrointestinal distress, diarrhea, jaundice, and hepatic injury. Large amounts of intravenous solution may lead to hypophosphatemia (due to phosphate/citrate buffer). Not significantly removed by dialysis.

Drug Interactions

Increased Effect/Toxicity: Concurrent administration of rifampin (or other drugs with extensive biliary secretion) may increase the risk of jaundice.

Storage/Stability

Cream: Store below 25°C.

Injection, powder for reconstitution: Store below 25°C. Reconstituted solution may be further diluted with NS or D₅W; should be used within 24 hours.

Ointment: Store below 30°C.

Ophthalmic suspension: Store at 2°C to 25°C. Discard multidose vials 1 month after opening.

Reconstitution Injection, powder for reconstitution: Reconstitute 500 mg vial of powder for injection by adding 10 mL of supplied diluent containing phosphate/citrate buffer. Add to NS or D₅W to produce a final concentration of 1-2 mg/mL. For patients weighing <50 kg, reconstituted drug should be diluted at least 10-fold in a compatible solution. Discard solution if opalescence is observed.

Compatibility Stable in NS, D₅W, or LR; **incompatible** with calcium solutions, carbenicillin, gentamicin, or kanamycin

Incompatible with whole blood or amino acid solutions

Pharmacodynamics/Kinetics

Protein binding: 97%

Metabolism: Hepatic, to multiple metabolites

Half-life elimination: 5-6 hours

Time to peak, serum: Oral: 2-4 hours

Excretion: Feces (~100%, via bile)

(Continued)

Fusidic Acid *(Continued)*

Dosage

I.V.:

Children ≤12 years: 20 mg/kg/day in 3 divided doses

Children >12 years and Adults: 500 mg sodium fusidate 3 times/day

Ophthalmic: Children ≥2 years and Adults: Instill 1 drop in each eye every 12 hours for 7 days

Topical: Children and Adults: Apply to affected area 3-4 times/day until favorable results are achieved. If a gauze dressing is used, frequency of application may be reduced to 1-2 times/day.

Oral: Adults: 500 mg sodium fusidate 3 times/day. (**Note:** Oral dosage may be increased to 1000 mg 3 times/day in fulminating infections.)

Dosage adjustment in renal impairment: No dosage adjustment required

Dosage adjustment in hepatic impairment: Oral, I.V.: Use with extreme caution in patients with hepatic impairment; monitor liver function periodically during therapy

Administration I.V.: Should not be administered I.M. or SubQ. Intravenous administration should be via a large bore vein with good blood flow. Administer over 2 hours or more. Do not administer with whole blood or amino acid solutions.

Dosage Forms

Cream, as fusidic acid (Fucidin®): 2% (15 g, 30 g)

Injection, powder for reconstitution, as sodium fusidate (Fucidin®): 500 mg [packaged with 10 mL diluent/buffer solution]

Ointment, topical, as sodium fusidate (Fucidin®): 2% (15 g, 30 g) [contains lanolin]

Suspension, ophthalmic, as fusidic acid (Fucithalmic®): 10 mg/g [1%] (0.2 g) [unit-dose, without preservative]; (3 g, 5 g) [multidose, contains benzalkonium chloride]

Tablet [film coated], as sodium fusidate (Fucidin®): 250 mg

Monitoring Parameters Monitor liver function tests, including bilirubin periodically during systemic therapy

Dietary Considerations May take tablets with food to minimize gastrointestinal upset.

Gallium Nitrate *(GAL ee um NYE trate)*

Related Information

Safe Handling of Hazardous Drugs *on page 1034*

U.S. Brand Names Ganite™

Generic Available No

Synonyms NSC-15200

Pharmacologic Category Calcium-Lowering Agent

Pregnancy Risk Factor C

Lactation Excretion in breast milk unknown/not recommended

Use Treatment of hypercalcemia

Mechanism of Action Inhibits bone resorption by inhibiting osteoclast function

Labeled Contraindications Hypersensitivity to gallium nitrate or any component of the formulation; severe renal dysfunction (creatinine >2.5 mg/dL)

Warnings/Precautions Hazardous agent - use appropriate precautions for handling and disposal. See Safe Handling of Hazardous Drugs *on page 1034* in the Appendix. Use caution with renal impairment or when administering other nephrotoxic drugs (eg, aminoglycosides, amphotericin B); consider discontinuing gallium nitrate during treatment with nephrotoxic drugs. Maintain adequate hydration. Safety and efficacy in pediatric patients have not been established.

Adverse Reactions Not all frequencies defined.

Cardiovascular: Hypotension, tachycardia, edema of lower extremities

Central nervous system: Lethargy, confusion, dreams, hallucinations, hypothermia, fever

Dermatologic: Rash

Endocrine & metabolic: Hypophosphatemia (>50%, usually asymptomatic); hypocalcemia; mild respiratory alkalosis with hyperchloremia

Hematologic: Anemia, leukopenia

Gastrointestinal: Nausea (14%, generally mild), vomiting, diarrhea, constipation

Neuromuscular & skeletal: Paresthesia

Renal: Nephrotoxicity (>10%, generally reversible and reported to be minimized with adequate hydration and urine output)

Respiratory: Dyspnea, rales, rhonchi, pleural effusion, pulmonary infiltrates

Note: Toxicities reported with doses higher than those used to treat hypercalcemia (ie, in trials evaluating anticancer effect): Optic neuritis, tinnitus, hearing acuity decreased, metallic taste, hypomagnesemia, encephalopathy

Vesicant No

Emetic Potential Moderate (reported in 14% in one comparative trial, but reported as mild)

Overdosage/Toxicology Symptoms of overdose include nausea, vomiting, and increased risk of nephrotoxicity.

Drug Interactions

Increased Effect/Toxicity: Concurrent use of low-dose gallium nitrate with cyclophosphamide has been associated with dyspnea, stomatitis, asthenia, and rarely interstitial pneumonitis. Concurrent use nephrotoxic drugs (eg, aminoglycosides, amphotericin B) with gallium nitrate may increase nephrotoxic effects.

Storage/Stability Store unopened vials (25 mg/mL) at room temperature of 15°C to 30°C (59°F to 86°F); not light sensitive. Solutions in 0.9% NaCl or D$_5$W are stable for 48 hours at room temperature or for 7 days under refrigeration at 2°C to 8°C (36°F to 46°F).

Reconstitution Dilute in 250-1000 mL NS or D$_5$W for infusion

Compatibility Compatible: Stable in NS, D$_5$W

Pharmacodynamics/Kinetics

Onset of calcium lowering: Seen within 24-48 hours of beginning therapy, with normocalcemia achieved within 4-7 days of beginning therapy

Bioavailability: Oral: 5%

Distribution: Tissue concentrations were determined postmortem in one patient and concentrations were higher in liver and kidney than in lung, skin, muscle, heart, and cervix tumor; in dogs, tissue gallium concentrations were higher in renal cortex, bone, bone marrow, small intestine, and liver than in skeletal muscle and brain

Half-life elimination: Alpha: 1.25 hours; Beta: ~24 hours

(Continued)

Gallium Nitrate *(Continued)*

Elimination half-life varies with method of administration (72-115 hours with prolonged intravenous infusion versus 24 hours with bolus administration); long elimination half-life may be related to slow release from tissue such as bone

Excretion: Primarily renal with no prior metabolism in the liver or kidney

Dosage I.V.: Adults: 200 mg/m^2/day for 5 days; duration may be shortened during a course if normocalcemia is achieved. If hypercalcemia is mild and with very few symptoms, 100 mg/m^2/day may be used.

Dosage adjustment in renal impairment:

Serum creatinine >2.5 mg/dL: Contraindicated

Serum creatinine 2 to <2.5 mg/dL: No guidelines exist; frequent monitoring is recommended

Administration I.V. infusion; 30 minutes to 24 hours

Dosage Forms Injection, solution [preservative free]: 25 mg/mL (20 mL)

Monitoring Parameters Renal function, serum calcium (daily), serum phosphorus (twice weekly)

Selected Readings

Apseloff G, "Therapeutic Uses of Gallium Nitrate: Past, Present, and Future," *Am J Ther*, 1999, 6(6):327-39.

Chitambar CR, "Gallium Nitrate Revisited," *Semin Oncol*, 2003, 30(2 Suppl 5):1-4.

Hughes TE and Hansen LA, "Gallium Nitrate," *Ann Pharmacother*, 1992, 26(3):354-62.

Leyland-Jones B, "Pharmacokinetics and Therapeutic Index of Gallium Nitrate," *Semin Oncol*, 1991, 18(4 Suppl 5):16-20.

Todd PA and Fitton A, "Gallium Nitrate. A Review of its Pharmacological Properties and Therapeutic Potential in Cancer Related Hypercalcaemia," *Drugs*, 1991, 42(2):261-73.

♦ **Gamimune® N** *see* Immune Globulin (Intravenous) *on page 458*

♦ **Gammagard® S/D** *see* Immune Globulin (Intravenous) *on page 458*

♦ **Gammaphos** *see* Amifostine *on page 53*

♦ **Gammar®-P I.V.** *see* Immune Globulin (Intravenous) *on page 458*

♦ **Gamunex®** *see* Immune Globulin (Intravenous) *on page 458*

Ganciclovir *(gan SYE kloe veer)*

Medication Safety Issues

Sound-alike/look-alike issues:

Cytovene® may be confused with Cytosar®, Cytosar-U®

Related Information

Safe Handling of Hazardous Drugs *on page 1034*

U.S. Brand Names Cytovene®; Vitrasert®

Canadian Brand Names Cytovene®; Vitrasert®

Generic Available Yes: Capsule

Synonyms DHPG Sodium; GCV Sodium; Nordeoxyguanosine

Pharmacologic Category Antiviral Agent

Pregnancy Risk Factor C

Lactation Excretion in breast milk unknown/contraindicated

Use

Parenteral: Treatment of CMV retinitis in immunocompromised individuals, including patients with acquired immunodeficiency syndrome; prophylaxis of CMV infection in transplant patients

Oral: Alternative to the I.V. formulation for maintenance treatment of CMV retinitis in immunocompromised patients, including patients with AIDS, in whom retinitis is stable following appropriate induction therapy and for whom the risk of more rapid progression is balanced by the benefit associated with avoiding daily I.V. infusions.

Implant: Treatment of CMV retinitis

Unlabeled/Investigational Use May be given in combination with foscarnet in patients who relapse after monotherapy with either drug

Mechanism of Action Ganciclovir is phosphorylated to a substrate which competitively inhibits the binding of deoxyguanosine triphosphate to DNA polymerase resulting in inhibition of viral DNA synthesis

Labeled Contraindications Hypersensitivity to ganciclovir, acyclovir, or any component of the formulation; absolute neutrophil count <500/mm^3; platelet count <25,000/mm^3

Warnings/Precautions Hazardous agent - use appropriate precautions for handling and disposal. See Safe Handling of Hazardous Drugs *on page 1034* in the Appendix. Dosage adjustment or interruption of ganciclovir therapy may be necessary in patients with neutropenia and/or thrombocytopenia and patients with impaired renal function. Use with extreme caution in children since long-term safety has not been determined and due to ganciclovir's potential for long-term carcinogenic and adverse reproductive effects. Ganciclovir may adversely affect spermatogenesis and fertility. Due to its mutagenic potential, contraceptive precautions for female and male patients need to be followed during and for at least 90 days after therapy with the drug. Take care to administer only into veins with good blood flow.

Adverse Reactions

>10%:

Central nervous system: Fever (38% to 48%)

Dermatologic: Rash (15% oral, 10% I.V.)

Gastrointestinal: Abdominal pain (17% to 19%), diarrhea (40%), nausea (25%), anorexia (15%), vomiting (13%)

Hematologic: Anemia (20% to 25%), leukopenia (30% to 40%)

1% to 10%:

Central nervous system: Confusion, neuropathy (8% to 9%), headache (4%)

Dermatologic: Pruritus (5%)

Hematologic: Thrombocytopenia (6%), neutropenia with ANC <500/mm^3 (5% oral, 14% I.V.)

Neuromuscular & skeletal: Paresthesia (6% to 10%), weakness (6%)

Ocular: Retinal detachment (8% oral, 11% I.V.; relationship to ganciclovir not established)

Miscellaneous: Sepsis (4% oral, 15% I.V.)

<1% (Limited to important or life-threatening): Alopecia, arrhythmia, ataxia, bronchospasm, coma, dyspnea, encephalopathy, exfoliative dermatitis, extrapyramidal symptoms, nervousness, pancytopenia, psychosis, seizure, alopecia, urticaria, eosinophilia, hemorrhage, Stevens-Johnson syndrome, torsade de pointes, renal failure, SIADH, visual loss

Vesicant No

Overdosage/Toxicology Symptoms of overdose include neutropenia, vomiting, hypersalivation, bloody diarrhea, cytopenia, and testicular atrophy. Treatment is supportive. Hemodialysis removes 50% of the drug. Hydration may be of some benefit.

(Continued)

Ganciclovir *(Continued)*

Drug Interactions

Increased Effect/Toxicity: Immunosuppressive agents may increase hematologic toxicity of ganciclovir. Imipenem/cilastatin may increase seizure potential. Oral ganciclovir increases blood levels of zidovudine, although zidovudine decreases steady-state levels of ganciclovir. Since both drugs have the potential to cause neutropenia and anemia, some patients may not tolerate concomitant therapy with these drugs at full dosage. Didanosine levels are increased with concurrent ganciclovir. Other nephrotoxic drugs (eg, amphotericin and cyclosporine) may have additive nephrotoxicity with ganciclovir.

Decreased Effect: A decrease in blood levels of ganciclovir AUC may occur when used with didanosine.

Storage/Stability Reconstituted solution is stable for 12 hours at room temperature, however, conflicting data indicates that reconstituted solution is stable for 60 days under refrigeration (4°C). Stability of parenteral admixture at room temperature (25°C) and at refrigeration temperature (4°C) is 5 days.

Reconstitution Reconstitute powder with unpreserved, sterile water **not** bacteriostatic water because parabens may cause precipitation. Dilute in 250-1000 mL D_5W or NS to a concentration ≤10 mg/mL for infusion.

Compatibility Stable in D_5W, LR, NS; **incompatible** with paraben preserved bacteriostatic water for injection (may cause precipitation)

Y-site administration: Compatible: Allopurinol, amphotericin B cholesteryl sulfate complex, cisplatin, cyclophosphamide, docetaxel, doxorubicin liposome, enalaprilat, etoposide phosphate, filgrastim, fluconazole, gatifloxacin, granisetron, linezolid, melphalan, methotrexate, paclitaxel, propofol, remifentanil, tacrolimus, teniposide, thiotepa. **Incompatible:** Aldesleukin, amifostine, amsacrine, aztreonam, cefepime, cytarabine, doxorubicin, fludarabine, foscarnet, gemcitabine, ondansetron, piperacillin/tazobactam, sargramostim, vinorelbine. **Variable (consult detailed reference):** Cisatracurium

Pharmacodynamics/Kinetics

Distribution: V_d: 15.26 L/1.73 m²; widely to all tissues including CSF and ocular tissue

Protein binding: 1% to 2%

Bioavailability: Oral: Fasting: 5%; Following food: 6% to 9%; Following fatty meal: 28% to 31%

Half-life elimination: 1.7-5.8 hours; prolonged with renal impairment; End-stage renal disease: 5-28 hours

Excretion: Urine (80% to 99% as unchanged drug)

Dosage

CMV retinitis: Slow I.V. infusion (dosing is based on total body weight): Children >3 months and Adults:

Induction therapy: 5 mg/kg/dose every 12 hours for 14-21 days followed by maintenance therapy

Maintenance therapy: 5 mg/kg/day as a single daily dose for 7 days/week or 6 mg/kg/day for 5 days/week

CMV retinitis: Oral: 1000 mg 3 times/day with food **or** 500 mg 6 times/day with food

Prevention of CMV disease in patients with advanced HIV infection and normal renal function: Oral: 1000 mg 3 times/day with food

Prevention of CMV disease in transplant patients: Same initial and maintenance dose as CMV retinitis except duration of initial course is 7-14 days, duration of maintenance therapy is dependent on clinical condition and degree of immunosuppression

Intravitreal implant: One implant for 5- to 8-month period; following depletion of ganciclovir, as evidenced by progression of retinitis, implant may be removed and replaced

Elderly: Refer to adult dosing; in general, dose selection should be cautious, reflecting greater frequency of organ impairment

Dosing adjustment in renal impairment:

I.V. (Induction):

Cl_{cr} 50-69 mL/minute: Administer 2.5 mg/kg/dose every 12 hours

Cl_{cr} 25-49 mL/minute: Administer 2.5 mg/kg/dose every 24 hours

Cl_{cr} 10-24 mL/minute: Administer 1.25 mg/kg/dose every 24 hours

Cl_{cr} <10 mL/minute: Administer 1.25 mg/kg/dose 3 times/week following hemodialysis

I.V. (Maintenance):

Cl_{cr} 50-69 mL/minute: Administer 2.5 mg/kg/dose every 24 hours

Cl_{cr} 25-49 mL/minute: Administer 1.25 mg/kg/dose every 24 hours

Cl_{cr} 10-24 mL/minute: Administer 0.625 mg/kg/dose every 24 hours

Cl_{cr} <10 mL/minute: Administer 0.625 mg/kg/dose 3 times/week following hemodialysis

Oral:

Cl_{cr} 50-69 mL/minute: Administer 1500 mg/day or 500 mg 3 times/day

Cl_{cr} 25-49 mL/minute: Administer 1000 mg/day or 500 mg twice daily

Cl_{cr} 10-24 mL/minute: Administer 500 mg/day

Cl_{cr} <10 mL/minute: Administer 500 mg 3 times/week following hemodialysis

Hemodialysis effects: Dialyzable (50%) following hemodialysis; administer dose postdialysis. During peritoneal dialysis, dose as for Cl_{cr} <10 mL/minute. During continuous arteriovenous or venovenous hemofiltration, administer 2.5 mg/kg/dose every 24 hours.

Administration

Oral: Ganciclovir should be administered with food.

I.V.: Ganciclovir should not be administered by I.M., SubQ, or rapid IVP administration; administer by slow I.V. infusion over at least 1 hour

Dosage Forms

Capsule (Cytovene®): 250 mg, 500 mg

Implant, intravitreal (Vitrasert®): 4.5 mg [released gradually over 5-8 months]

Injection, powder for reconstitution, as sodium (Cytovene®): 500 mg

Monitoring Parameters CBC with differential and platelet count, serum creatinine, ophthalmologic exams

Dietary Considerations Sodium content of 500 mg vial: 46 mg

Patient Information Ganciclovir is not a cure for CMV retinitis; regular ophthalmologic examinations should be done; close monitoring of blood counts should be done while on therapy and dosage adjustments may need to be made; take with food to increase absorption

Special Geriatric Considerations Adjust dose based upon renal function.

Selected Readings

Gando S, Kameue T, Nanzaki S, et al, "Pharmacokinetics and Clearance of Ganciclovir During Continuous Hemodiafiltration," *Crit Care Med*, 1998, 26(1):184-7.

(Continued)

Ganciclovir *(Continued)*

Lake KD, Fletcher CV, Love KR, et al, "Ganciclovir Pharmacokinetics During Renal Impairment," *Antimicrob Agents Chemother*, 1988, 32(12):1899-900.

Matthews T and Boehme R, "Antiviral Activity and Mechanism of Action of Ganciclovir," *Rev Infect Dis*, 1988, 10(Suppl 3):490-4.

Paul S and Dummer S, "Topics in Clinical Pharmacology, Ganciclovir," *Am J Med Sci*, 1992, 304(4):272-7.

Sommadossi JP, Bevan R, Ling T, et al, "Clinical Pharmacokinetics of Ganciclovir in Patients With Normal and Impaired Renal Function," *Rev Infect Dis*, 1988, 10(Suppl 3):507-14.

♦ **Ganite**™ *see Gallium Nitrate on page 380*
♦ **Garamycin® (Can)** *see Gentamicin on page 398*
♦ **G-CSF** *see Filgrastim on page 341*
♦ **GCV Sodium** *see Ganciclovir on page 382*

Gefitinib *(ge FI tye nib)*

U.S. Brand Names Iressa™
Generic Available No
Synonyms NSC-715055; ZD1839
Pharmacologic Category Antineoplastic Agent, Tyrosine Kinase Inhibitor
Pregnancy Risk Factor D
Lactation Excretion in breast milk unknown/not recommended
Use Second-line treatment of nonsmall cell lung cancer (**Note:** In response to the lack of improved survival data from the ISEL trial, AstraZeneca has temporarily suspended promotion of this drug.)
Unlabeled/Investigational Use Brain cancer, breast cancer, colon cancer, head and neck cancer, ovarian cancer
Mechanism of Action The mechanism of antineoplastic action is not fully understood. Gefitinib inhibits tyrosine kinases (TK) associated with transmembrane cell surface receptors found on both normal and cancer cells. One such receptor is epidermal growth factor receptor. TK activity appears to be vitally important to cell proliferation and survival.
Labeled Contraindications Hypersensitivity to gefitinib or any component of the formulation; pregnancy
Warnings/Precautions Hazardous agent - use appropriate precautions for handling and disposal. See Safe Handling of Hazardous Drugs *on page 1034* in the Appendix. Rare, sometimes fatal, pulmonary toxicity (alveolitis, interstitial pneumonia, pneumonitis) has occurred; use caution in hepatic or severe renal impairment; safety and efficacy in pediatric patients have not been established
Adverse Reactions Based on 250 mg/day:
>10%:
  Dermatologic: Rash (43%), acne (25%), dry skin (13%)
  Gastrointestinal: Diarrhea (48%), nausea (13%), vomiting (12%)
1% to 10%:
  Cardiovascular: Peripheral edema (2%)
  Dermatologic: Pruritus (8%)
  Gastrointestinal: Anorexia (7%), weight loss (3%), mouth ulceration (1%)
  Neuromuscular & skeletal: Weakness (6%)
  Ocular: Amblyopia (2%), conjunctivitis (1%)
  Respiratory: Dyspnea (2%), interstitial lung disease (1%)

<1%: Aberrant eyelash growth, angioedema, corneal erosion and membrane sloughing, epistaxis, erythema multiforme, eye pain, hematuria, hemorrhage, ocular hemorrhaging, ocular ischemia, pancreatitis, toxic epidermal necrolysis, urticaria

Postmarketing and/or case reports: CNS hemorrhage and death were reported in clinical trials of pediatric patients with primary CNS tumors

Overdosage/Toxicology No specific overdose-related toxicities reported; Overdose management should be symptom-based and supportive.

Drug Interactions

Cytochrome P450 Effect: Substrate of CYP3A4 (major); **Inhibits** CYP2C19 (weak), 2D6 (weak)

Increased Effect/Toxicity: Gefitinib may increase the effects of warfarin. CYP3A4 inhibitors may increase the levels/effects of gefitinib; example inhibitors include azole antifungals, ciprofloxacin, clarithromycin, diclofenac, doxycycline, erythromycin, imatinib, isoniazid, nefazodone, nicardipine, propofol, protease inhibitors, quinidine, and verapamil.

Decreased Effect: Gefitinib effects may be decreased by H$_2$-receptor blockers and sodium bicarbonate. CYP3A4 inducers may decrease the levels/effects of gefitinib; example inducers include aminoglutethimide, carbamazepine, nafcillin, nevirapine, phenobarbital, phenytoin, and rifamycins.

Ethanol/Nutrition/Herb Interactions Food: Grapefruit juice may increase serum gefitinib concentrations; St John's wort may decrease serum gefitinib concentrations.

Storage/Stability Store tablets at controlled room temperature of 20°C to 25°C (68°F to 77°F).

Pharmacodynamics/Kinetics

Absorption: Oral: slow

Distribution: I.V.: 1400 L

Protein binding: 90%, albumin and alpha$_1$-acid glycoprotein

Metabolism: Hepatic, primarily via CYP3A4; forms metabolites

Bioavailability: 60%

Half-life elimination: I.V.: 48 hours

Time to peak, plasma: Oral: 3-7 hours

Excretion: Feces (86%); urine (<4%)

Dosage Note: In response to the lack of improved survival data from the ISEL trial, AstraZeneca has temporarily suspended promotion of this drug.

Oral: Adults: 250 mg/day; consider 500 mg/day in patients receiving effective CYP3A4 inducers (eg, rifampin, phenytoin)

Dosage adjustment in renal/hepatic impairment: No adjustment necessary

Dosage adjustment for toxicity: Patients experiencing poorly-tolerated diarrhea may benefit from a brief (up to 14 days) therapy interruption. Patients experiencing acute onset (or worsening) of pulmonary symptoms should have therapy interrupted and be evaluated for drug-induced interstitial lung disease. Patients experiencing new eye symptoms should consider therapy interruption until situation resolved.

Administration May administer with or without food.

Dosage Forms Tablet: 250 mg

(Continued)

Gefitinib (Continued)

Monitoring Parameters Periodic liver function tests (asymptomatic increases in liver enzymes have occurred)

Dietary Considerations Food does not affect gefitinib absorption.

Patient Information Contact prescriber if any of the following symptoms occur: Severe, persistent diarrhea; nausea or vomiting; breathing difficulties (shortness of breath, painful breathing, cough); eye irritation. Avoid becoming pregnant while on this medication.

Selected Readings

Cersosimo RJ, "Gefitinib: A New Antineoplastic for Advanced Non-Small-Cell Lung Cancer," *Am J Health Syst Pharm*, 2004, 61(9):889-98.

Culy CR and Faulds D, "Gefitinib," *Drugs*, 2002, 62(15):2237-48.

Hammond LA, "Pharmacokinetic Evaluation of Gefitinib When Administered With Chemotherapy," *Clin Lung Cancer*, 2003, 5 Suppl 1:S18-21.

Herbst RS, Fukuoka M, and Baselga J, "Gefitinib - A Novel Targeted Approach to Treating Cancer," *Nat Rev Cancer*, 2004, 4(12):956-65.

Ranson M and Wardell S, "Gefitinib, A Novel, Orally Administered Agent for the Treatment of Cancer," *J Clin Pharm Ther*, 2004, 29(2):95-103.

Gemcitabine (jem SITE a been)

Medication Safety Issues

Sound-alike/look-alike issues:

Gemzar® may be confused with Zinecard®

Related Information

Safe Handling of Hazardous Drugs *on page 1034*

U.S. Brand Names Gemzar®

Canadian Brand Names Gemzar®

Generic Available No

Synonyms Gemcitabine Hydrochloride

Pharmacologic Category Antineoplastic Agent, Antimetabolite (Pyrimidine Antagonist)

Pregnancy Risk Factor D

Lactation Excretion in breast milk unknown/contraindicated

Use

Adenocarcinoma of the pancreas; first-line therapy in locally-advanced (nonresectable stage II or stage III) or metastatic (stage IV) adenocarcinoma of the pancreas

Breast cancer: First-line therapy in metastatic breast cancer

Nonsmall-cell lung cancer: First-line therapy in locally-advanced (stage IIIA or IIIB) or metastatic (stage IV) nonsmall-cell lung cancer

Unlabeled/Investigational Use Bladder cancer, ovarian cancer

Mechanism of Action A pyrimidine antimetabolite that inhibits DNA synthesis by inhibition of DNA polymerase and ribonucleotide reductase, specific for the S-phase of the cycle.

Labeled Contraindications Hypersensitivity to gemcitabine or any component of the formulation; pregnancy

Warnings/Precautions Hazardous agent - use appropriate precautions for handling and disposal. See Safe Handling of Hazardous Drugs *on page 1034* in the Appendix. Prolongation of the infusion time >60 minutes and more frequent than weekly dosing have been shown to increase toxicity. Gemcitabine can suppress bone marrow function manifested by leukopenia, thrombocytopenia and anemia, and myelosuppression is usually the dose-limiting toxicity. Gemcitabine may cause fever in the absence of clinical infection. Gemcitabine should be used with caution in patients with pre-existing renal impairment and hepatic impairment. Safety and efficacy have not been established with radiation therapy or in pediatric patients.

Adverse Reactions Percentages reported with single-agent therapy for pancreatic cancer and other malignancies.

>10%:

Central nervous system: Pain (42% to 48%; grades 3 and 4: <1% to 9%), fever (38% to 41%; grades 3 and 4: ≤2%), somnolence (11%; grades 3 and 4: <1%). Fever was reported to occur in the absence of infection in pancreatic cancer treatment.

Dermatologic: Rash (28% to 30%; grades 3 and 4: <1%), alopecia (15% to 16%; grades 3 and 4: <1%). Rash in pancreatic cancer treatment was typically a macular or finely-granular maculopapular pruritic eruption of mild-to-moderate severity involving the trunk and extremities.

Gastrointestinal: Nausea and vomiting (69% to 71%; grades 3 and 4: 1% to 13%), constipation (23% to 31%; grades 3 and 4: <1% to 3%), diarrhea (19% to 30%; grades 3 and 4: ≤3%), stomatitis (10% to 11%; grades 3 and 4: <1%)

Hematologic: Anemia (73% to 68%; grades 3 and 4: 1% to 8%), leukopenia (62% to 64%; grades 3 and 4: <1% to 9%), neutropenia (61% to 63%; grades 3 and 4: 6% to 19%), thrombocytopenia (24% to 36%; grades 3 and 4: <1% to 7%), hemorrhage (4% to 17%; grades 3 or 4: <1%). Myelosuppression may be the dose-limiting toxicity with pancreatic cancer

Hepatic: Transaminases increased (68% to 78%; grades 3 and 4: 1% to 12%), alkaline phosphatase increased (55% to 77%; grades 3 and 4: 2% to 16%), bilirubin increased (13% to 26%; grades 3 or 4: <1% to 6%). Serious hepatotoxicity was reported rarely in pancreatic cancer treatment.

Renal: Proteinuria (32% to 45%; grades 3 and 4: <1%), hematuria (23% to 35%; grades 3 and 4: <1%), BUN increased (15% to 16%; grades 3 and 4: 0%)

Respiratory: Dyspnea (10% to 23%; grades 3 and 4: <1% to 3%)

Miscellaneous: Infection (10% to 16%; grades 3 or 4: <1% to 2%)

1% to 10%:

Local: Injection site reactions (4%)

Neuromuscular & skeletal: Paresthesias (10%)

Renal: Creatinine increased (6% to 8%)

Respiratory: Bronchospasm (<2%)

<1%: Anaphylactoid reaction, hemolytic uremic syndrome

Postmarketing and/or case reports (reported with single-agent use or with combination therapy, all reported rarely): Arrhythmias, cellulitis, CHF, gangrene, liver failure, MI, parenchymal toxicity, vascular toxicity

Vesicant No

Emetic Potential High (60% to 90%); usually mild, not requiring serotonin antagonists

Overdosage/Toxicology Symptoms of overdose include myelosuppression, paresthesia, and severe rash. The principle toxicities were seen when a single dose as high as 5700 mg/m^2 was administered by I.V. infusion over 30 minutes every 2 weeks. Monitor blood counts and administer supportive therapy as needed.

(Continued)

Gemcitabine *(Continued)*

Drug Interactions
Decreased Effect: No confirmed interactions have been reported. No specific drug interaction studies have been conducted.

Ethanol/Nutrition/Herb Interactions Ethanol: Avoid ethanol (due to GI irritation).

Storage/Stability Store intact vials at room temperature (20°C to 25°C/ 68°F to 77°F). Reconstituted vials and infusion solutions diluted in 0.9% sodium chloride are stable up to 24 hours. Do not refrigerate.

Reconstitution Reconstitute the 200 mg vial with preservative free 0.9% NaCl 5 mL or the 1000 mg vial with preservative free 25 mL 0.9% NaCl 25 mL.

Resulting solution is approximately 38 mg/mL, but is variable. Dilute with 50-500 mL 0.9% sodium chloride injection or D_5W to concentrations as low as 0.1 mg/mL.

Compatibility Stable in D_5W, NS

Y-site administration: Compatible: Amifostine, amikacin, aminophylline, ampicillin, ampicillin/sulbactam, aztreonam, bleomycin, bumetanide, buprenorphine, butorphanol, calcium gluconate, carboplatin, carmustine, cefazolin, cefotetan, cefoxitin, ceftazidime, ceftizoxime, ceftriaxone, cefuroxime, chlorpromazine, cimetidine, ciprofloxacin, cisplatin, clindamycin, co-trimoxazole, cyclophosphamide, cytarabine, dactinomycin, daunorubicin, dexamethasone sodium phosphate, dexrazoxane, diphenhydramine, dobutamine, docetaxel, dopamine, doxorubicin, doxycycline, droperidol, enalaprilat, etoposide, etoposide phosphate, famotidine, floxuridine, fluconazole, fludarabine, fluorouracil, gatifloxacin, gentamicin, granisetron, haloperidol, heparin, hydrocortisone sodium phosphate, hydrocortisone sodium succinate, hydromorphone, hydroxyzine, idarubicin, ifosfamide, leucovorin, linezolid, lorazepam, mannitol, meperidine, mesna, metoclopramide, metronidazole, minocycline, mitoxantrone, morphine, nalbuphine, netilmicin, ofloxacin, ondansetron, paclitaxel, plicamycin, potassium chloride, promethazine, ranitidine, sodium bicarbonate, streptozocin, teniposide, thiotepa, ticarcillin, ticarcillin/clavulanate, tobramycin, topotecan, vancomycin, vinblastine, vincristine, vinorelbine, zidovudine. **Incompatible:** Acyclovir, amphotericin B, cefoperazone, cefotaxime, furosemide, ganciclovir, imipenem/cilastatin, irinotecan, methotrexate, methylprednisolone sodium succinate, mitomycin, piperacillin, piperacillin/tazobactam, prochlorperazine edisylate

Pharmacodynamics/Kinetics
Distribution: V_d: Male: 15.6 mL mL/m²; Female: 11.3 L/m²

Protein binding: Low

Metabolism: Hepatic, metabolites: di- and triphosphates (active); uridine derivative (inactive)

Half-life elimination: Infusion time: ≤1 hour: 32-94 minutes; Infusion time: 3-4 hours: 4-10.5 hours

Time to peak: 30 minutes

Excretion: Urine (99%, 92% to 98% as intact drug or inactive uridine metabolite); feces (<1%)

Dosage Refer to individual protocols. **Note:** Prolongation of the infusion time >60 minutes has been shown to increase toxicity. I.V.:

Pancreatic cancer: Initial: 1000 mg/m² over 30 minutes once weekly for up to 7 weeks followed by 1 week rest; subsequent cycles once weekly for 3 consecutive weeks out of every 4 weeks. Dose adjustment: Patients who complete an entire cycle of therapy may have the dose in subsequent cycles increased by 25% as long as the absolute granulocyte count (AGC) nadir is >1500 x 10⁶/L, platelet nadir is >100,000 x 10⁶/L, and nonhematologic toxicity is less than WHO Grade 1. If the increased dose is tolerated (with the same parameters) the dose in subsequent cycles may again be increased by 20%.

Nonsmall cell lung cancer:
  28-day cycle: 1000 mg/m² over 30 minutes on days 1, 8, 15; repeat every 28 days

  or

  21-day cycle: 1250 mg/m² over 30 minutes on days 1, 8; repeat every 21 days

Breast cancer: 1250 mg/m² over 30 minutes on days 1 and 8 of each 21-day cycle

Bladder cancer (unlabeled use): 1000 mg/m² once weekly for 3 weeks; repeat cycle every 4 weeks

Ovarian cancer (unlabeled use): 1000 mg/m² once weekly for 3 weeks; repeat cycle every 4 weeks

Dosing adjustment for toxicity:
  Pancreatic cancer: Hematologic toxicity:
    AGC ≥1000 x 10⁶/L and platelet count ≥100,000 x 10⁶/L: Administer 100% of full dose
    AGC 500-999 x 10⁶/L or platelet count 50,000-90,000 x 10⁶/L: Administer 75% of full dose
    AGC <500 x 10⁶/L or platelet count <50,000 x 10⁶/L: Hold dose
  Nonsmall-cell lung cancer:
    Hematologic toxicity: Refer to guidelines for pancreatic cancer. Cisplatin dosage may also need adjusted.
    Severe (grades 3 or 4) nonhematologic toxicity (except alopecia, nausea, and vomiting): Hold or decrease dose by 50%.
  Breast cancer:
    Hematologic toxicity: Adjustments based on granulocyte and platelet counts on day 8:
      AGC ≥1200 x 10⁶/L and platelet count ≥75,000 x 10⁶/L: Administer 100% of full dose
      AGC 1000-1199 x 10⁶/L or platelet count ≥50,000-75,000 x 10⁶/L: Administer 75% of full dose
      AGC 700-999 x 10⁶/L and platelet count ≥ 50,000 x 10⁶/L: Administer 50% of full dose
      AGC <700 x 10⁶/L or platelet count <50,000 x 10⁶/L: Hold dose
    Severe (grades 3 or 4) nonhematologic toxicity (except alopecia, nausea, and vomiting): Hold or decrease dose by 50%. Paclitaxel dose may also need adjusted.

Dosing adjustment in renal/hepatic impairment: Use with caution; gemcitabine has not been studied in patients with significant renal or hepatic dysfunction

Combination Regimens

Bladder cancer: Gemcitabine-Cisplatin *on page 896*
Leukemia, acute lymphocytic: TVTG *on page 942*
Leukemia, acute myeloid: TVTG *on page 942*

(Continued)

Gemcitabine *(Continued)*

Lung cancer (nonsmall cell):

GC *on page 895*

Gemcitabine-Carboplatin *on page 896*

Gemcitabine-Cis *on page 896*

Gemcitabine-Vinorelbine *on page 897*

Vinorelbine-Gemcitabine *on page 946*

Osteosarcoma: Gemcitabine-Docetaxel *on page 896*

Ovarian cancer: Gemcitabine-Paclitaxel *on page 897*

Pancreatic cancer:

Gemcitabine/Capecitabine *on page 895*

Gemcitabine/Irinotecan *on page 897*

Sarcoma, soft tissue: Gemcitabine-Docetaxel *on page 896*

Administration Administer over 30 minutes. **Note**: Prolongation of the infusion time >60 minutes has been shown to increase toxicity.

Dosage Forms Injection, powder for reconstitution, as hydrochloride: 200 mg, 1 g

Monitoring Parameters Patients should be monitored prior to each dose with a complete blood count (CBC), including differential and platelet count. The diagnosis of hemolytic-uremic syndrome (HUS) should be considered if evidence of microangiopathic hemolysis is noted (elevation of bilirubin or LDH, reticulocytosis, severe thrombocytopenia, and/or renal failure).

Hepatic and renal function should be performed prior to initiation of therapy and periodically, thereafter

Special Geriatric Considerations Clearance is affected by age. There is no evidence; however, that unusual dose adjustment is necessary in patients older than 65 years of age. In general, adverse reaction rates were similar to patients older and younger than 65 years. Grade 3/4 thrombocytopenia was more common in the elderly.

Selected Readings

Aapro MS, Martin C, and Hatty S, "Gemcitabine - A Safety Review," *Anticancer Drugs*, 1998, 9(3):191-201.

Guchelaar HJ, Richel DJ, and van Knapen A, "Clinical, Toxicological and Pharmacological Aspects of Gemcitabine," *Cancer Treat Rev*, 1996, 22(1):15-31.

Hui YF and Reitz J, "Gemcitabine: A Cytidine Analogue Active Against Solid Tumors," *Am J Health Syst Pharm*, 1997, 54(2):162-70.

Noble S and Goa KL, "Gemcitabine. A Review of its Pharmacology and Clinical Potential in Nonsmall Cell Lung Cancer and Pancreatic Cancer, *Drugs*, 1997, 54(3):447-72.

Plunkett W, Huang P, Xu YZ, et al, "Gemcitabine: Metabolism, Mechanisms of Action, and Self-Potentiation," *Semin Oncol*, 1995, 22(4 Suppl 11):3-10.

Storniolo AM, Allerheiligen SR, and Pearce HL, "Preclinical, Pharmacologic, and Phase I Studies of Gemcitabine," *Semin Oncol* 1997, 24(2 Suppl 7):7-12.

♦ **Gemcitabine Hydrochloride** *see* Gemcitabine *on page 388*

Gemifloxacin *(je mi FLOKS a sin)*

U.S. Brand Names Factive®

Generic Available No

Synonyms DW286; Gemifloxacin Mesylate; LA 20304a; SB-265805

Pharmacologic Category Antibiotic, Quinolone

Pregnancy Risk Factor C

Lactation Excretion in breast milk unknown/not recommended

Use Treatment of acute exacerbation of chronic bronchitis; treatment of community-acquired pneumonia, including pneumonia caused by multi-drug-resistant strains of *S. pneumoniae* (MDRSP)

Unlabeled/Investigational Use Acute sinusitis, uncomplicated urinary tract infection

Mechanism of Action Gemifloxacin is a DNA gyrase inhibitor and also inhibits topoisomerase IV. DNA gyrase (topoisomerase IV) is an essential bacterial enzyme that maintains the superhelical structure of DNA. DNA gyrase is required for DNA replication and transcription, DNA repair, recombination, and transposition; bactericidal

Labeled Contraindications Hypersensitivity to gemifloxacin, other fluoroquinolones, or any component of the formulation

Warnings/Precautions Fluoroquinolones may prolong QT_c interval; avoid use of gemifloxacin in patients with uncorrected hypokalemia, hypomagnesemia, or concurrent administration of other medications known to prolong the QT interval (including class Ia and class III antiarrhythmics, cisapride, erythromycin, antipsychotics, and tricyclic antidepressants). Use with caution in patients with significant bradycardia or acute myocardial ischemia. Use with caution in individuals at risk of seizures (CNS disorders or concurrent therapy with medications which may lower seizure threshold). Discontinue in patients who experience significant CNS adverse effects (dizziness, hallucinations, suicidal ideation or actions). Use caution in renal dysfunction (dosage adjustment required).

Severe hypersensitivity reactions, including anaphylaxis, have occurred with quinolone therapy. If an allergic reaction occurs (itching, urticaria, dyspnea or facial edema, loss of consciousness, tingling, cardiovascular collapse), discontinue drug immediately. Prolonged use may result in superinfection; pseudomembranous colitis may occur and should be considered in all patients who present with diarrhea. Tendon inflammation and/or rupture has been reported with other quinolone antibiotics; risk may increase with concurrent corticosteroids, particularly in the elderly. Discontinue at first sign of tendon inflammation or pain. Peripheral neuropathy has been linked to the use of quinolones; these cases were rare. Experience with quinolones in immature animals has resulted in permanent arthropathy. Safety and effectiveness in pediatric patients (<18 years of age) have not been established.

Adverse Reactions

1% to 10%:

Central nervous system: Headache (1%), dizziness (1%)

Dermatologic: Rash (3%)

Gastrointestinal: Diarrhea (4%), nausea (3%), abdominal pain (1%), vomiting (1%)

Hepatic: Transaminases increased (1% to 2%)

<1%: Abnormal vision, anemia, anorexia, arthralgia, asthenia, back pain, bilirubin increased, constipation, CPK increased, cramps (leg), dermatitis, dry mouth, dyspepsia, dyspnea, eczema, eosinophilia, fatigue, flatulence, fungal infection, gastritis, genital moniliasis, GGT increased, granulocytopenia, hyperglycemia, insomnia, leukopenia, moniliasis, myalgia, nervousness, pharyngitis, photosensitivity, pruritus, somnolence, taste perversion, thrombocythemia, thrombocytopenia, tremor, urticaria, vaginitis, vertigo

(Continued)

393

Gemifloxacin *(Continued)*

Important adverse effects reported with other agents in this drug class include (not reported for gemifloxacin): Allergic reactions, CNS stimulation, hepatitis, jaundice, peripheral neuropathy, pneumonitis (eosinophilic), seizure; sensorimotor-axonal neuropathy (paresthesia, hypoesthesias, dysesthesias, weakness); severe dermatologic reactions (toxic epidermal necrolysis, Stevens-Johnson syndrome); tendon rupture, torsade de pointes, vasculitis

Overdosage/Toxicology Treatment should be symptom-directed and supportive; 20% to 30% removed by hemodialysis.

Drug Interactions

Increased Effect/Toxicity: Gemifloxacin may increase the effects/toxicity of glyburide and warfarin. Concomitant use with corticosteroids may increase the risk of tendon rupture. Concomitant use with other QT_c-prolonging agents (eg, Class Ia and Class III antiarrhythmics, erythromycin, cisapride, antipsychotics, and cyclic antidepressants) may result in arrhythmias, such as torsade de pointes. Probenecid may increase gemifloxacin levels.

Decreased Effect: Concurrent administration of metal cations, including most antacids, oral electrolyte supplements, quinapril, sucralfate, and some didanosine formulations (chewable/buffered tablets and pediatric powder for oral suspension), may decrease quinolone levels; separate doses.

Ethanol/Nutrition/Herb Interactions Herb/Nutraceutical: Avoid dong quai, St John's wort (may also cause photosensitization).

Storage/Stability Store at 25°C (77°F); excursions permitted to 15°C to 30°C (59°F to 86°F). Protect from light.

Pharmacodynamics/Kinetics

Absorption: Well absorbed from the GI tract

Bioavailability: 71%

Metabolism: Hepatic (minor); forms metabolites (CYP isoenzymes are not involved)

Time to peak, plasma: 1-2 hours

Protein binding: 60% to 70%

Half-life elimination: 7 hours (range 4-12 hours)

Excretion: Urine (30% to 40%); feces (60%)

Dosage Oral: Adults: 320 mg once daily

Duration of therapy:

Acute exacerbations of chronic bronchitis: 5 days

Community-acquired pneumonia (mild to moderate severity): 7 days

Dosage adjustment in renal impairment: Cl_{cr} ≤40 mL/minute (or patients on hemodialysis/CAPD): 160 mg once daily (administer dose following hemodialysis)

Dosage adjustment in hepatic impairment: No adjustment required.

Administration May be administered with or without food, milk, or calcium supplements. Gemifloxacin should be taken 3 hours before or 2 hours after supplements (including multivitamins) containing iron, zinc, or magnesium.

Dosage Forms Tablet, as mesylate: 320 mg

Monitoring Parameters WBC, signs/symptoms of infection

Dietary Considerations May take tablets with or without food, milk, or calcium supplements. Gemifloxacin should be taken 3 hours before or 2

hours after supplements (including multivitamins) containing iron, zinc, or magnesium.

Special Geriatric Considerations The risk of torsade de pointes and tendon inflammation and/or rupture associated with the concomitant use of corticosteroids and quinolones is increased in the elderly population. Adjust dose for renal function.

♦ **Gemifloxacin Mesylate** *see* Gemifloxacin *on page 392*

Gemtuzumab Ozogamicin

(gem TOO zoo mab oh zog a MY sin)

U.S. Brand Names Mylotarg®

Canadian Brand Names Mylotarg®

Generic Available No

Pharmacologic Category Antineoplastic Agent, Monoclonal Antibody

Pregnancy Risk Factor D

Lactation Excretion in breast milk unknown/not recommended

Use Treatment of relapsed acute myeloid leukemia (CD33 positive)

Mechanism of Action Antibody to CD33 antigen. Binding results in internalization of the antibody-antigen complex. Following internalization, the calicheamicin derivative is released inside the myeloid cell. The calicheamicin derivative binds to DNA resulting in double strand breaks and cell death. Pluripotent stem cells and nonhematopoietic cells are not affected.

Labeled Contraindications Hypersensitivity to gemtuzumab ozogamicin, calicheamicin derivatives, or any component of the formulation; patients with anti-CD33 antibody; pregnancy

Warnings/Precautions Hazardous agent - use appropriate precautions for handling and disposal. See Safe Handling of Hazardous Drugs *on page 1034* in the Appendix. Gemtuzumab has been associated with severe veno-occlusive disease or hepatotoxicity. Risk may be increased by combination chemotherapy, previous hepatic disease, or hematopoietic stem cell transplant.

Infusion-related events are common, generally reported to occur with the first dose at the end of the 2-hour intravenous infusion. These symptoms usually resolved after 2-4 hours with a supportive therapy of acetaminophen, diphenhydramine, and intravenous fluids. Fewer infusion-related events were observed after the second dose. **Infusion-related reactions may be severe (including anaphylaxis, pulmonary edema, or ARDS).** Symptomatic intrinsic lung disease or high peripheral blast counts may increase the risk of severe reactions. Consider discontinuation in patients who develop severe infusion-related reactions.

Severe myelosuppression occurs in all patients at recommended dosages. Use caution in patients with renal impairment (no clinical experience) and hepatic impairment (no clinical experience in patients with bilirubin >2 mg/dL). Tumor lysis syndrome may occur as a consequence of leukemia treatment, adequate hydration and prophylactic allopurinol must be instituted prior to use. Other methods to lower WBC <30,000 cells/mm^3 may be considered (hydroxyurea or leukapheresis) to minimize the risk of tumor lysis syndrome, and/or severe infusion reactions. Postinfusion reactions, which may include fever, chills, hypotension, or dyspnea, may occur during the first 24 hours after administration. Safety and efficacy have not been established in pediatric patients or in patients (Continued)

Gemtuzumab Ozogamicin *(Continued)*

with poor performance status and organ dysfunction have not been established.

Adverse Reactions Percentages established in adults >60 years of age.
Note: A postinfusion symptom complex (fever, chills, less commonly hypertension, and/or dyspnea) may occur within 24 hours of administration.

>10%:

Cardiovascular: Peripheral edema (21%), hypertension (16%), hypotension (20%)

Central nervous system: Chills (66%), fever (82%), headache (37%), pain (25%), dizziness (11%), insomnia (18%)

Dermatologic: Rash (23%), petechiae (21%), ecchymosis (15%), cutaneous herpes simplex (21%)

Endocrine & metabolic: Hypokalemia (30%)

Gastrointestinal: Nausea (68%), vomiting (58%), diarrhea (38%), anorexia (31%), abdominal pain (29%), constipation (28%), stomatitis/mucositis (25%), abdominal distention (11%), dyspepsia (11%)

Hematologic: Neutropenia (98%; median recovery 40.5 days), thrombocytopenia (99%; median recovery 39 days); anemia (52%), bleeding (15%), lymphopenia

Hepatic: Hyperbilirubinemia (29%), LDH increased (18%), transaminases increased (9% to 18%)

Local: Local reaction (25%)

Neuromuscular & skeletal: Weakness (45%), back pain (18%)

Respiratory: Dyspnea (26%), epistaxis (29%; severe 3%), cough (19%), pharyngitis (14%)

Miscellaneous: Infection (30%), sepsis (24%), neutropenic fever (20%)

1% to 10%:

Cardiovascular: Tachycardia (10%)

Central nervous system: Depression (10%), cerebral hemorrhage (2%), intracranial hemorrhage (2%)

Dermatologic: Pruritus (6%)

Endocrine & metabolic: Hypomagnesemia (4%), hyperglycemia (10%)

Genitourinary: Hematuria (10%; severe 1%), vaginal hemorrhage (7%)

Hematologic: Hemorrhage (8%), disseminated intravascular coagulation (DIC) (2%)

Hepatic: PT increased, veno-occlusive disease (range: 1% to 20% in relapsed patients; higher frequency in patients with prior history of subsequent hematopoietic stem cell transplant)

Neuromuscular & skeletal: Arthralgia (10%)

Respiratory: Rhinitis (10%), hypoxia (6%), pneumonia (10%)

<1% (Limited to important or life-threatening symptoms): Hepatic failure, jaundice, hepatosplenomegaly

Postmarketing and/or case reports: Acute respiratory distress syndrome, anaphylaxis, gastrointestinal hemorrhage, hypersensitivity reactions, noncardiogenic pulmonary edema, renal failure (secondary to tumor lysis syndrome)

Overdosage/Toxicology Symptoms are unknown. General supportive measures should be instituted. Gemtuzumab ozogamicin is not dialyzable.

Drug Interactions

Increased Effect/Toxicity: No formal drug interaction studies have been conducted.

Decreased Effect: No formal drug interaction studies have been conducted.

Ethanol/Nutrition/Herb Interactions Ethanol: Avoid ethanol (due to GI irritation).

Storage/Stability Light sensitive; protect from light. Store vials under refrigeration 2°C to 8°C or 36°F to 46°F.

Reconstitution Prepare in biologic safety hood with the fluorescent light turned **off**. Allow to warm to room temperature prior to reconstitution. Reconstitute vial with 5 mL sterile water for injection, USP. Final concentration in vial is 1 mg/mL. Dilute desired dose in 100 mL of 0.9% sodium chloride injection. The resulting I.V. bag should be placed in a UV protectant bag and infused immediately. Reconstituted vials may be stored under refrigeration for up to 8 hours.

Compatibility No information; infuse via separate line

Pharmacodynamics/Kinetics Half-life elimination: Calicheamicin: Total: Initial: 45 hours, Repeat dose: 60 hours; Unconjugated: 100 hours (no change noted in repeat dosing)

Dosage I.V.: Adults ≥60 years: 9 mg/m^2, infused over 2 hours. A full treatment course is a total of two doses administered with 14 days between doses. Full hematologic recovery is not necessary for administration of the second dose. There has been only limited experience with repeat courses of gemtuzumab ozogamicin.

Note: The patient should receive diphenhydramine 50 mg orally and acetaminophen 650-1000 mg orally 1 hour prior to administration of each dose. Acetaminophen dosage should be repeated as needed every 4 hours for two additional doses. Pretreatment with methylprednisolone may ameliorate infusion-related symptoms.

Dosage adjustment in renal impairment: No recommendation (not studied)

Dosage adjustment in hepatic impairment: No recommendation (not studied)

Administration I.V.: Over at least 2 hours. Use of a low protein binding 1.2 micron in-line filter is recommended. Premedication with acetaminophen and diphenhydramine should be administered prior to each infusion.

Dosage Forms Injection, powder for reconstitution: 5 mg

Monitoring Parameters Monitor vital signs during the infusion and for 4 hours following the infusion. Monitor for signs/symptoms of postinfusion reaction. Monitor electrolytes, LFTs, CBC with differential, and platelet counts frequently. Monitor for signs and symptoms of hepatitis reaction (weight gain, right upper quadrant abdominal pain, hepatomegaly, ascites).

Patient Information This medication can only be administered I.V. During therapy do not use ethanol, aspirin-containing products, antiplatelet medications (ticlopidine, clopidogrel, or dipyridamole), OTC medications, or supplements/herbal products without consulting prescriber. It is important to maintain adequate nutrition and hydration. You may experience nausea and vomiting (small frequent meals, frequent mouth care, sucking lozenges or chewing gum may help). Frequent mouth care and use of a soft toothbrush or cotton swabs may reduce mouth sores. You will be susceptible to infection (avoid crowds and exposure to infection). (Continued)

Gemtuzumab Ozogamicin *(Continued)*

Report fever, chills, unusual bruising or bleeding, signs of infection, dizziness, lightheadedness, difficulty breathing, or yellowing of the eyes or skin to prescriber. Keep all appointments and get required blood work done.

Selected Readings

Giles F, Estey E, and O'Brien S, "Gemtuzumab Ozogamicin in the Treatment of Acute Myeloid Leukemia," *Cancer*, 2003, 98(10):2095-104.

Giles FJ, "Gemtuzumab Ozogamicin: Promise and Challenge in Patients With Acute Myeloid Leukemia," *Expert Rev Anticancer Ther*, 2002, 2(6):630-40.

Larson RA, "Current Use and Future Development of Gemtuzumab Ozogamicin," *Semin Hematol*, 2001, 38(3 Suppl 6):24-31.

McGavin JK and Spencer CM, "Gemtuzumab Ozogamicin," *Drugs*, 2001, 61(9):1317-22.

Stadtmauer EA, "Gemtuzumab Ozogamicin in the Treatment of Acute Myeloid Leukemia," *Curr Oncol Rep*, 2002, 4(5):375-80.

♦ **Gemzar®** *see* Gemcitabine *on page 388*

♦ **Gen-Acyclovir (Can)** *see* Acyclovir *on page 26*

♦ **Gen-Cyproterone (Can)** *see* Cyproterone *on page 227*

♦ **Gen-Etidronate (Can)** *see* Etidronate Disodium *on page 313*

♦ **Gen-Fluconazole (Can)** *see* Fluconazole *on page 349*

♦ **Gengraf®** *see* CycloSPORINE *on page 216*

♦ **Gen-Hydroxyurea (Can)** *see* Hydroxyurea *on page 432*

♦ **Gen-Medroxy (Can)** *see* MedroxyPROGESTERone *on page 524*

♦ **Genoptic®** *see* Gentamicin *on page 398*

♦ **Gentacidin® [DSC]** *see* Gentamicin *on page 398*

♦ **Gentak®** *see* Gentamicin *on page 398*

Gentamicin *(jen ta MYE sin)*

Medication Safety Issues

Sound-alike/look-alike issues:

Gentamicin may be confused with kanamycin

Garamycin® may be confused with kanamycin, Terramycin®

Related Information

Management of Infections *on page 978*

U.S. Brand Names Genoptic®; Gentacidin® [DSC]; Gentak®

Canadian Brand Names Alcomicin®; Diogent®; Garamycin®; Minim's Gentamicin 0.3%; SAB-Gentamicin

Generic Available Yes

Synonyms Gentamicin Sulfate

Pharmacologic Category Antibiotic, Aminoglycoside; Antibiotic, Ophthalmic; Antibiotic, Topical

Pregnancy Risk Factor C

Lactation Enters breast milk (small amounts)/use caution (AAP rates "compatible")

Use Treatment of susceptible bacterial infections, normally gram-negative organisms including *Pseudomonas*, *Proteus*, *Serratia*, and gram-positive *Staphylococcus*; treatment of bone infections, respiratory tract infections, skin and soft tissue infections, as well as abdominal and urinary tract infections, endocarditis, and septicemia; used topically to treat superficial infections of the skin or ophthalmic infections caused by susceptible bacteria; prevention of bacterial endocarditis prior to dental or surgical procedures

Mechanism of Action Interferes with bacterial protein synthesis by binding to 30S and 50S ribosomal subunits resulting in a defective bacterial cell membrane

Labeled Contraindications Hypersensitivity to gentamicin or other aminoglycosides

Warnings/Precautions Not intended for long-term therapy due to toxic hazards associated with extended administration. Pre-existing renal insufficiency, vestibular or cochlear impairment, myasthenia gravis, hypocalcemia, conditions which depress neuromuscular transmission.

Parenteral aminoglycosides have been associated with significant nephrotoxicity or ototoxicity. Ototoxicity may be directly proportional to the amount of drug given and the duration of treatment and may not be reversible. Tinnitus or vertigo are indications of vestibular injury and impending hearing loss. Renal damage is usually reversible.

Adverse Reactions

>10%:

Central nervous system: Neurotoxicity (vertigo, ataxia)

Neuromuscular & skeletal: Gait instability

Otic: Ototoxicity (auditory), ototoxicity (vestibular)

Renal: Nephrotoxicity, decreased creatinine clearance

1% to 10%:

Cardiovascular: Edema

Dermatologic: Skin itching, reddening of skin, rash

<1%: Drowsiness, headache, pseudomotor cerebri, photosensitivity, allergic reaction, erythema, anorexia, nausea, vomiting, weight loss, increased salivation, enterocolitis, granulocytopenia, agranulocytosis, thrombocytopenia, elevated LFTs, burning, stinging, tremor, muscle cramps, weakness, dyspnea

Vesicant No

Emetic Potential Very low (<10%)

Overdosage/Toxicology Symptoms of overdose include ototoxicity, nephrotoxicity, and neuromuscular toxicity. Serum level monitoring is recommended. The treatment of choice, following a single acute overdose, appears to be maintenance of urine output of at least 3 mL/kg/hour during the acute treatment phase. Dialysis is of questionable value in enhancing aminoglycoside elimination.

Drug Interactions

Increased Effect/Toxicity: Penicillins, cephalosporins, amphotericin B, loop diuretics may increase nephrotoxic potential. Aminoglycosides may potentiate the effects of neuromuscular blocking agents.

Storage/Stability Gentamicin is a colorless to slightly yellow solution which should be stored between 2°C to 30°C, but refrigeration is not recommended.

Reconstitution I.V. infusion solutions mixed in NS or D_5W solution are stable for 24 hours at room temperature and refrigeration.

Premixed bag: Manufacturer expiration date; remove from overwrap stability: 30 days

Compatibility Stable in dextran 40, D_5W, $D_{10}W$, mannitol 20%, LR, NS; **not stable** in fat emulsion 10%; **variable stability (consult detailed reference)** in peritoneal dialysis solution

(Continued)

Gentamicin *(Continued)*

Y-site administration: Compatible: Acyclovir, alatrofloxacin, amifostine, amiodarone, amsacrine, atracurium, aztreonam, cefpirome, ciprofloxacin, cisatracurium, clarithromycin, cyclophosphamide, cytarabine, diltiazem, docetaxel, doxorubicin liposome, enalaprilat, esmolol, etoposide phosphate, famotidine, fluconazole, fludarabine, foscarnet, gatifloxacin, gemcitabine, granisetron, hydromorphone, IL-2, insulin (regular), labetalol, levofloxacin, linezolid, lorazepam, magnesium sulfate, melphalan, meperidine, meropenem, midazolam, morphine, multivitamins, ondansetron, paclitaxel, pancuronium, perphenazine, remifentanil, sargramostim, tacrolimus, teniposide, theophylline, thiotepa, tolazoline, vecuronium, vinorelbine, vitamin B complex with C, zidovudine. **Incompatible:** Allopurinol, amphotericin B cholesteryl sulfate complex, cefamandole, furosemide, heparin, hetastarch, idarubicin, indomethacin, iodipamide meglumine, phenytoin, propofol, warfarin. **Variable (consult detailed reference):** Filgrastim

Compatibility in syringe: Compatible: Clindamycin, diatrizoate meglumine 52% and diatrizoate sodium 8%, diatrizoate sodium 60%, iohexol, iopamidol, iothalamate meglumine 60%, penicillin G sodium. **Incompatible:** Ampicillin, cefamandole, heparin. **Variable (consult detailed reference):** Ioxaglate meglumine 39.3% and ioxaglate sodium 19.6%

Compatibility when admixed: Compatible: Atracurium, aztreonam, bleomycin, cefoxitin, cimetidine, chloroprocaine, ciprofloxacin, fluconazole, hexylcaine, lidocaine, lidocaine with epinephrine, mepivacaine, meropenem, metronidazole, metronidazole with sodium bicarbonate, ofloxacin, penicillin G sodium, piperocaine, procaine, ranitidine, verapamil. **Incompatible:** Amphotericin B, ampicillin, cefamandole, cefazolin with clindamycin, cefepime, heparin, nafcillin, ticarcillin. **Variable (consult detailed reference):** Cefotaxime, cefotetan, cefuroxime, clindamycin, cytarabine, dopamine, floxacillin, furosemide

Pharmacodynamics/Kinetics

Absorption: Oral: None

Distribution: Crosses placenta

V_d: Increased by edema, ascites, fluid overload; decreased with dehydration

Neonates: 0.4-0.6 L/kg

Children: 0.3-0.35 L/kg

Adults: 0.2-0.3 L/kg

Relative diffusion from blood into CSF: Minimal even with inflammation

CSF:blood level ratio: Normal meninges: Nil; Inflamed meninges: 10% to 30%

Protein binding: <30%

Half-life elimination:

Infants: <1 week old: 3-11.5 hours; 1 week to 6 months old: 3-3.5 hours

Adults: 1.5-3 hours; End-stage renal disease: 36-70 hours

Time to peak, serum: I.M.: 30-90 minutes; I.V.: 30 minutes after 30-minute infusion

Excretion: Urine (as unchanged drug)

Clearance: Directly related to renal function

Dosage Individualization is **critical** because of the low therapeutic index. **Use of ideal body weight (IBW) for determining the mg/kg/dose appears to be more accurate than dosing on the basis of total**

body weight (TBW). In morbid obesity, dosage requirement may best be estimated using a dosing weight of IBW + 0.4 (TBW - IBW).

Initial and periodic plasma drug levels (eg, peak and trough with conventional dosing) should be determined, particularly in critically-ill patients with serious infections or in disease states known to significantly alter aminoglycoside pharmacokinetics (eg, cystic fibrosis, burns, or major surgery).

Infants and Children <5 years: I.M., I.V.: 2.5 mg/kg/dose every 8 hours*

Children ≥5 years: I.M., I.V.: 2-2.5 mg/kg/dose every 8 hours*

Prevention of bacterial endocarditis: Dental, oral, upper respiratory procedures, GI/GU procedures: 1.5 mg/kg with ampicillin (50 mg/kg) 30 minutes prior to procedure

*Note: Higher individual doses and/or more frequent intervals (eg, every 6 hours) may be required in selected clinical situations (cystic fibrosis) or serum levels document the need

Children and Adults:

Intrathecal: 4-8 mg/day

Ophthalmic:

Ointment: Instill 1/2" (1.25 cm) 2-3 times/day to every 3-4 hours

Solution: Instill 1-2 drops every 2-4 hours, up to 2 drops every hour for severe infections

Topical: Apply 3-4 times/day to affected area

Adults: I.M., I.V.: Systemic infections:

Severe, life-threatening infections:

Conventional dosing: 2-2.5 mg/kg/dose every 8-12 hours; to ensure adequate peak concentrations early in therapy, higher initial dosages may be considered in selected patients when extracellular water is increased (edema, septic shock, postsurgical, or trauma)

Once-daily dosing: Some clinicians suggest a daily dose of 4-7 mg/kg once daily for all patients with normal renal function; this dose is at least as efficacious with similar, if not less, toxicity than conventional dosing.

Urinary tract infections: 1.5 mg/kg/dose every 8 hours

Synergy (for gram-positive infections): 1 mg/kg/dose

Prevention of bacterial endocarditis:

Dental, oral, or upper respiratory procedures: 1.5 mg/kg (not to exceed 80 mg) with ampicillin (1-2 g) 30 minutes prior to procedure

GI/GU surgery: 1.5 mg/kg (not to exceed 80 mg) with ampicillin (2 g) 30 minutes prior to procedure

Dosing interval in renal impairment:

Conventional dosing:

Cl_{cr} ≥60 mL/minute: Administer every 8 hours

Cl_{cr} 40-60 mL/minute: Administer every 12 hours

Cl_{cr} 20-40 mL/minute: Administer every 24 hours

Cl_{cr} <20 mL/minute: Loading dose, then monitor levels

High-dose therapy: Interval may be extended (eg, every 48 hours) in patients with moderate renal impairment (Cl_{cr} 30-59 mL/minute) and/or adjusted based on serum level determinations.

Hemodialysis: Dialyzable; removal by hemodialysis: 30% removal of aminoglycosides occurs during 4 hours of HD; administer dose after dialysis and follow levels

(Continued)

Gentamicin *(Continued)*

Removal by continuous ambulatory peritoneal dialysis (CAPD):

Administration via CAPD fluid:

Gram-negative infection: 4-8 mg/L (4-8 mcg/mL) of CAPD fluid

Gram-positive infection (eg, synergy): 3-4 mg/L (3-4 mcg/mL) of CAPD fluid

Administration via I.V., I.M. route during CAPD: Dose as for Cl_{cr} <10 mL/minute and follow levels

Removal via continuous arteriovenous or venovenous hemofiltration: Dose as for Cl_{cr} 10-40 mL/minute and follow levels

Dosing adjustment/comments in hepatic disease: Monitor plasma concentrations

Administration Administer other antibiotics at least 1 hour before or 1 hour after gentamicin.

Dosage Forms [DSC] = Discontinued product

Cream, topical, as sulfate: 0.1% (15 g, 30 g)

Infusion, as sulfate [premixed in NS]: 40 mg (50 mL); 60 mg (50 mL, 100 mL); 70 mg (50 mL); 80 mg (50 mL, 100 mL); 90 mg (100 mL); 100 mg (50 mL, 100 mL); 120 mg (100 mL)

Injection, solution, as sulfate [ADD-Vantage® vial]: 10 mg/mL (6 mL, 8 mL, 10 mL)

Injection, solution, as sulfate: 40 mg/mL (2 mL, 20 mL) [may contain sodium metabisulfite]

Injection, solution, pediatric, as sulfate: 10 mg/mL (2 mL) [may contain sodium metabisulfite]

Injection, solution, pediatric, as sulfate [preservative free]: 10 mg/mL (2 mL)

Ointment, ophthalmic, as sulfate (Gentak®): 0.3% [3 mg/g] (3.5 g)

Ointment, topical, as sulfate: 0.1% (15 g, 30 g)

Solution, ophthalmic, as sulfate: 0.3% (5 mL, 15 mL) [contains benzalkonium chloride]

Genoptic®: 0.3% (1 mL) [contains benzalkonium chloride]

Gentacidin®: 0.3% (5 mL) [contains benzalkonium chloride] [DSC]

Gentak®: 0.3% (5 mL, 15 mL) [contains benzalkonium chloride]

Monitoring Parameters Urinalysis, urine output, BUN, serum creatinine; hearing should be tested before, during, and after treatment; particularly in those at risk for ototoxicity or who will be receiving prolonged therapy (>2 weeks)

Dietary Considerations Calcium, magnesium, potassium: Renal wasting may cause hypocalcemia, hypomagnesemia, and/or hypokalemia.

Patient Information Report any dizziness or sensations of ringing or fullness in ears; do not touch ophthalmics to eye; use no other eye drops within 5-10 minutes of instilling ophthalmic

Special Geriatric Considerations Aminoglycosides are important therapeutic interventions for susceptible organisms and as empiric therapy in seriously ill patients. Their use is not without risk of toxicity, however. Additional studies comparing high-dose, once-daily aminoglycosides to traditional dosing regimens in the elderly are needed before once-daily aminoglycoside dosing can be routinely adopted to this patient population.

Selected Readings

Begg EJ and Barclay ML, "Aminoglycosides - 50 Years On," *Br J Clin Pharmacol*, 1995, 39(6):597-603.

Cunha BA, "Aminoglycosides: Current Role in Antimicrobial Therapy," *Pharmacotherapy*, 1988, 8(6):334-50.

♦ **Gentamicin Sulfate** *see* Gentamicin *on page 398*
♦ **Gen-Tamoxifen (Can)** *see* Tamoxifen *on page 743*
♦ **Gentlax® [OTC]** *see* Bisacodyl *on page 133*
♦ **Gleevec®** *see* Imatinib *on page 449*
♦ **Gliadel®** *see* Carmustine *on page 154*
♦ **Glivec** *see* Imatinib *on page 449*
♦ **GM-CSF** *see* Sargramostim *on page 713*
♦ **GnRH Agonist** *see* Histrelin *on page 415*

Goserelin (GOE se rel in)

Related Information

Safe Handling of Hazardous Drugs *on page 1034*

U.S. Brand Names Zoladex®

Canadian Brand Names Zoladex®; Zoladex® LA

Generic Available No

Synonyms D-Ser(Bu^t)^6,Azgly^{10}-LHRH; Goserelin Acetate; ICI-118630; NSC-606864

Pharmacologic Category Gonadotropin Releasing Hormone Agonist

Pregnancy Risk Factor X (endometriosis, endometrial thinning); D (advanced breast cancer)

Lactation Enters breast milk/contraindicated

Use Palliative treatment of advanced breast cancer and carcinoma of the prostate; treatment of endometriosis, including pain relief and reduction of endometriotic lesions; endometrial thinning agent as part of treatment for dysfunctional uterine bleeding

Mechanism of Action Goserelin is a synthetic analog of luteinizing-hormone-releasing hormone (LHRH). Following an initial increase in luteinizing hormone (LH) and follicle stimulating hormone (FSH), chronic administration of goserelin results in a sustained suppression of pituitary gonadotropins. Serum testosterone falls to levels comparable to surgical castration. The exact mechanism of this effect is unknown, but may be related to changes in the control of LH or down-regulation of LH receptors.

Labeled Contraindications Hypersensitivity to goserelin or any component of the formulation; pregnancy (or potential to become pregnant); breast-feeding

Warnings/Precautions Transient worsening of signs and symptoms (tumor flare) may develop during the first few weeks of treatment. Urinary tract obstruction or spinal cord compression have been reported when used for prostate cancer; closely observe patients for weakness, paresthesias, and urinary tract obstruction in first few weeks of therapy. Decreased bone density has been reported in women and may be irreversible; use caution if other risk factors are present; evaluate and institute preventative treatment if necessary. Safety and efficacy have not been established in pediatric patients.

Adverse Reactions Percentages reported in males with prostatic carcinoma and females with endometriosis using the 1-month implant: (Continued)

Goserelin *(Continued)*

>10%:

Central nervous system: Headache (female 75%, male 1% to 5%), emotional lability (female 60%), depression (female 54%, male 1% to 5%), pain (female 17%, male 8%), insomnia (female 11%, male 5%)

Endocrine & metabolic: Hot flashes (female 96%, male 62%), sexual dysfunction (21%), erections decreased (18%), libido decreased (female 61%), breast enlargement (female 18%)

Genitourinary: Lower urinary symptoms (male 13%), vaginitis (75%), dyspareunia (female 14%)

Miscellaneous: Diaphoresis (female 45%, male 6%); infection (female 13%)

1% to 10%:

Cardiovascular: CHF (male 5%), arrhythmia, cerebrovascular accident, hypertension, MI, peripheral vascular disorder, chest pain, palpitation, tachycardia, edema

Central nervous system: Lethargy (male 8%), dizziness (female 6%, male 5%), abnormal thinking, anxiety, chills, fever, malaise, migraine, somnolence

Dermatologic: Rash (female >1%, male 6%), alopecia, bruising, dry skin, skin discoloration

Endocrine & metabolic: Breast pain (female 7%), breast swelling/tenderness (male 1% to 5%), dysmenorrhea, gout, hyperglycemia

Gastrointestinal: Anorexia (female >1%, male 5%), nausea (male 5%), constipation, diarrhea, flatulence, dyspepsia, ulcer, vomiting, weight increased, xerostomia

Genitourinary: Renal insufficiency, urinary frequency, urinary obstruction, urinary tract infection, vaginal hemorrhage

Hematologic: Anemia, hemorrhage

Neuromuscular & skeletal: Arthralgia, bone mineral density decreased (female; ~4% decrease in 6 months), joint disorder, paresthesia

Ocular: Amblyopia, dry eyes

Respiratory: Upper respiratory tract infection (male 7%), COPD (male 5%), pharyngitis (female 5%), bronchitis, cough, epistaxis, rhinitis, sinusitis

Miscellaneous: Allergic reaction

Vesicant No

Emetic Potential Low (10% to 30%)

Overdosage/Toxicology Symptomatic management

Storage/Stability Zoladex® should be stored at room temperature not to exceed 25°C (77°F). Protect from light. Should be dispensed in a light-proof bag.

Pharmacodynamics/Kinetics Note: Data reported using the 1-month implant.

Absorption: SubQ: Rapid and can be detected in serum in 10 minutes

Distribution: V_d: Male: 44.1 L; Female: 20.3 L

Time to peak, serum: SubQ: Male: 12-15 days, Female: 8-22 days

Half-life elimination: SubQ: Male: ~4 hours, Female: ~2 hours; Renal impairment: Male: 12 hours

Excretion: Urine (90%)

Dosage SubQ: Adults:

Prostate cancer:

Monthly implant: 3.6 mg injected into upper abdomen every 28 days

3-month implant: 10.8 mg injected into the upper abdominal wall every 12 weeks

Breast cancer, endometriosis, endometrial thinning: Monthly implant: 3.6 mg injected into upper abdomen every 28 days

Note: For breast cancer, treatment may continue indefinitely; for endometriosis, it is recommended that duration of treatment not exceed 6 months. Only 1-2 doses are recommended for endometrial thinning.

Dosing adjustment in renal/hepatic impairment: No adjustment is necessary

Combination Regimens

Prostate cancer:

Bicalutamide + LHRH-A *on page 848*

FZ *on page 895*

Administration Subcutaneous implant: Insert the hypodermic needle into the subcutaneous fat. Do not try to aspirate with the goserelin syringe. If the needle is in a large vessel, blood will immediately appear in the syringe chamber. Change the direction of the needle so it parallels the abdominal wall. Push the needle in until the barrel hub touches the patient's skin. Fully depress the plunger to discharge. Withdraw needle and bandage the site. Confirm discharge by ensuring tip of the plunger is visible within the tip of the needle.

Dosage Forms

Injection, solution, 1-month implant [disposable syringe; single-dose]: 3.6 mg [with 16-gauge hypodermic needle]

Injection, solution, 3-month implant [disposable syringe; single-dose]: 10.8 mg [with 14-gauge hypodermic needle]

Patient Information This drug must be implanted under the skin of your abdomen every 28 days; it is important to maintain appointment schedule. You may experience systemic hot flashes (cool clothes and temperatures may help), headache (analgesic may help), constipation (increased bulk and water in diet or stool softener may help), sexual dysfunction (decreased libido, decreased erection). Symptoms may worsen temporarily during first weeks of therapy. Report unusual nausea or vomiting, any chest pain, respiratory difficulty, unresolved dizziness, or constipation. Females must use reliable contraception during therapy.

Selected Readings

Ahmann FR, Citrin DL, deHaan HA, et al, "Zoladex: A Sustained-Release, Monthly Luteinizing Hormone-Releasing Hormone Analog for the Treatment of Advanced Prostate Cancer," *J Clin Oncol*, 1987, 5(6):912-7.

Brogden RN and Faulds D, "Goserelin. A Review of Its Pharmacodynamic and Pharmacokinetic Properties and Therapeutic Efficacy in Prostate Cancer," *Drugs Aging*, 1995, 6(4);324-43.

Goldspiel BR and Kohler DR, "Goserelin Acetate Implant: A Depot Luteinizing Hormone-Releasing Hormone Analog for Advanced Prostate Cancer," *DICP*, 1991, 25(7-8):796-804.

♦ **Goserelin Acetate** *see* Goserelin *on page 403*

♦ **GR38032R** *see* Ondansetron *on page 622*

Granisetron (gra NI se tron)

Related Information

Management of Nausea and Vomiting *on page 982*

U.S. Brand Names Kytril®

Canadian Brand Names Kytril®

Generic Available No

(Continued)

Granisetron *(Continued)*

Synonyms BRL 43694

Pharmacologic Category Antiemetic; Selective 5-HT$_3$ Receptor Antagonist

Pregnancy Risk Factor B

Lactation Excretion in breast milk unknown/use caution

Use Prophylaxis of chemotherapy-related emesis; prophylaxis of nausea and vomiting associated with radiation therapy, including total body irradiation and fractionated abdominal radiation; prophylaxis of postoperative nausea and vomiting (PONV)

Generally **not** recommended for treatment of existing chemotherapy-induced emesis (CIE) or for prophylaxis of nausea from agents with a low emetogenic potential.

Mechanism of Action Selective 5-HT$_3$-receptor antagonist, blocking serotonin, both peripherally on vagal nerve terminals and centrally in the chemoreceptor trigger zone

Labeled Contraindications Previous hypersensitivity to granisetron, other 5-HT$_3$ receptor antagonists, or any component of the formulation

Warnings/Precautions Chemotherapy-related emesis: **Granisetron should be used on a scheduled basis, not on an "as needed" (PRN) basis**, since data support the use of this drug in the prevention of nausea and vomiting and not in the rescue of nausea and vomiting. Granisetron should be used only in the first 24-48 hours of receiving chemotherapy or radiation. Data do not support any increased efficacy of granisetron in delayed nausea and vomiting. May be prescribed for patients who are refractory to or have severe adverse reactions to standard antiemetic therapy or young patients (ie, <45 years of age who are more likely to develop extrapyramidal symptoms to high-dose metoclopramide) who are to receive highly emetogenic chemotherapeutic agents. Should not be prescribed for chemotherapeutic agents with a low emetogenic potential (eg, bleomycin, busulfan, etoposide, 5-fluorouracil, vinblastine, vincristine).

Routine prophylaxis for PONV is not recommended. In patients where nausea and vomiting must be avoided postoperatively, administer to all patients even when expected incidence of nausea and vomiting is low. Use caution following abdominal surgery or in chemotherapy-induced nausea and vomiting; may mask progressive ileus or gastric distention. Use caution in patients with liver disease or in pregnancy. Safety and efficacy in children <2 years of age have not been established. Injection contains benzyl alcohol and should not be used in neonates.

Adverse Reactions

>10%:

Central nervous system: Headache (8% to 21%)

Gastrointestinal: Constipation (3% to 18%)

1% to 10%:

Cardiovascular: Hypertension (1% to 2%)

Central nervous system: Dizziness, insomnia, anxiety, somnolence, fever (3% to 8%), pain (10%)

Gastrointestinal: Abdominal pain, diarrhea (1% to 9%), dyspepsia

Hepatic: Elevated liver enzymes (5% to 6%)

Neuromuscular & skeletal: Weakness (5% to 18%)

<1%: Arrhythmias, agitation, hot flashes, angina, atrial fibrillation, syncope, hypotension, anaphylaxis, allergic reactions

Vesicant No

Overdosage/Toxicology Treatment should be symptomatic and supportive.

Drug Interactions

Cytochrome P450 Effect: Substrate of CYP3A4 (minor)

Ethanol/Nutrition/Herb Interactions Herb/Nutraceutical: St John's wort may decrease granisetron levels.

Storage/Stability

I.V.: Store at 25°C (77°F); excursions permitted to 15°C to 30°C (59°F to 86°F). Protect from light. Do not freeze vials. Stable when mixed in NS or D_5W for 7 days under refrigeration and for 3 days at room temperature.

Oral: Store tablet or oral solution at 15°C to 30°C (59°F to 86°F). Protect from light.

Compatibility Stable in $D_5^{1/2}NS$, D_5NS, D_5W, NS, bacteriostatic water

Y-site administration: Compatible: Acyclovir, allopurinol, amifostine, amikacin, aminophylline, amphotericin B cholesteryl sulfate complex, ampicillin, ampicillin/sulbactam, amsacrine, aztreonam, bleomycin, bumetanide, buprenorphine, butorphanol, calcium gluconate, carboplatin, carmustine, cefazolin, cefepime, cefoperazone, cefotaxime, cefotetan, cefoxitin, ceftazidime, ceftizoxime, ceftriaxone, cefuroxime, chlorpromazine, cimetidine, ciprofloxacin, cisplatin, cladribine, clindamycin, co-trimoxazole, cyclophosphamide, cytarabine, dacarbazine, dactinomycin, daunorubicin, dexamethasone sodium phosphate, diphenhydramine, dobutamine, docetaxel, dopamine, doxorubicin, doxorubicin liposome, doxycycline, droperidol, enalaprilat, etoposide, etoposide phosphate, famotidine, filgrastim, floxuridine, fluconazole, fludarabine, fluorouracil, furosemide, ganciclovir, gatifloxacin, gemcitabine, gentamicin, haloperidol, heparin, hydrocortisone sodium phosphate, hydrocortisone sodium succinate, hydromorphone, hydroxyzine, idarubicin, ifosfamide, imipenem/cilastatin, leucovorin, levoleucovorin, linezolid, lorazepam, magnesium sulfate, mechlorethamine, melphalan, meperidine, mesna, methotrexate, methylprednisolone sodium succinate, metoclopramide, metronidazole, minocycline, mitomycin, mitoxantrone, morphine, nalbuphine, netilmicin, ofloxacin, paclitaxel, piperacillin, piperacillin/tazobactam, plicamycin, potassium chloride, prochlorperazine edisylate, promethazine, propofol, ranitidine, sargramostim, sodium bicarbonate, streptozocin, teniposide, thiotepa, ticarcillin, ticarcillin/clavulanate, tobramycin, topotecan, vancomycin, vinblastine, vincristine, vinorelbine, zidovudine. **Incompatible:** Amphotericin B

Compatibility in syringe: Compatible: Dexamethasone sodium phosphate, methylprednisolone sodium succinate

Compatibility when admixed: Compatible: Dexamethasone sodium phosphate, methylprednisolone sodium succinate

Pharmacodynamics/Kinetics

Duration: Generally up to 24 hours

Distribution: V_d: 2-4 L/kg; widely throughout body

Protein binding: 65%

Metabolism: Hepatic via N-demethylation, oxidation, and conjugation; some metabolites may have 5-HT_3 antagonist activity

(Continued)

Granisetron *(Continued)*

Half-life elimination: Cancer patients: 10-12 hours; Healthy volunteers: 4-5 hours; PONV: 9 hours

Excretion: Urine (12% as unchanged drug, 49% as metabolites); feces (34% as metabolites)

Dosage

Oral: Adults:

Prophylaxis of chemotherapy-related emesis: 2 mg once daily up to 1 hour before chemotherapy or 1 mg twice daily; the first 1 mg dose should be given up to 1 hour before chemotherapy.

Prophylaxis of radiation therapy-associated emesis: 2 mg once daily given 1 hour before radiation therapy.

I.V.:

Children ≥2 years and Adults: Prophylaxis of chemotherapy-related emesis:

Within U.S.: 10 mcg/kg/dose (or 1 mg/dose) administered IVPB over 5 minutes given within 30 minutes of chemotherapy: for some drugs (eg, carboplatin, cyclophosphamide) with a later onset of emetic action, 10 mcg/kg every 12 hours may be necessary.

Outside U.S.: 40 mcg/kg/dose (or 3 mg/dose); maximum: 9 mg/24 hours

Breakthrough: Repeat the dose 2-3 times within the first 24 hours as necessary **(not based on controlled trials, or generally recommended)**

Adults: PONV:

Prevention: 1 mg given undiluted over 30 seconds; administer before induction of anesthesia or before reversal of anesthesia

Treatment: 1 mg given undiluted over 30 seconds

Dosing interval in renal impairment: No dosage adjustment required.

Dosing interval in hepatic impairment: Kinetic studies in patients with hepatic impairment showed that total clearance was approximately halved, however, standard doses were very well tolerated

Administration

Oral: Doses should be given up to 1 hour prior to initiation of chemotherapy/radiation

I.V.: Administer as rapid (30 second) I.V. push or a short (5-10 minutes) infusion

For prevention of PONV, administer before induction of anesthesia or before reversal of anesthesia.

For PONV, administer undiluted over 30 seconds.

Dosage Forms

Injection, solution: 1 mg/mL (4 mL) [contains benzyl alcohol]

Injection, solution [preservative free]: 0.1 mg/mL (1 mL); 1 mg/mL (1 mL)

Solution, oral: 2 mg/10 mL (30 mL) [contains sodium benzoate; orange flavor]

Tablet: 1 mg

Special Geriatric Considerations Clinical trials with patients older than 65 years of age are limited; however, the data indicates that safety and efficacy are similar to that observed in younger adults. No adjustment in dose necessary for elderly.

Extemporaneous Preparations A 0.2 mg/mL oral suspension may be prepared by crushing twelve (12) 1 mg tablets and mixing with 30 mL water and enough cherry syrup to provide a final volume of 60 mL; this preparation is stable for 14 days at room temperature or when refrigerated

Quercia RA, Zhang JH, Fan C, et al, "Stability of Granisetron (Kytril®) in an Extemporaneously Prepared Oral Liquid," *International Pharmaceutical Abstracts*, 1996, May 15, Vol 33.

Selected Readings

Andrews PL, "The Pharmacologic Profile of Granisetron (Kytril®)," *Semin Oncol*, 1994, 21(3 Suppl 5):3-9.

Blower P, "A Pharmacologic Profile of Oral Granisetron (Kytril® Tablets)," *Semin Oncol*, 1995, 22(4 Suppl 10):3-5.

Morrow GR, Hickok JT, and Rosenthal SN, "Progress in Reducing Nausea and Emesis. Comparisons of Ondansetron (Zofran®), Granisetron (Kytril®), and Tropisetron (Navoban®)," *Cancer*, 1995, 76(3):343-57.

Palmer R, "Efficacy and Safety of Granisetron (Kytril®) in Two Special Populations: Children and Adults With Impaired Hepatic Function," *Semin Oncol*, 1994, 21(3 Suppl 5):22-5.

Plosker GL and Goa KL, "Granisetron: A Review of Its Pharmacological Properties and Therapeutic Use as an Antiemetic," *Drugs*, 1991, 42(5):805-24.

Yarker YE and McTavish D, "Granisetron. An Update of Its Therapeutic Use in Nausea and Vomiting Induced by Antineoplastic Therapy," *Drugs*, 1994, 48(5):761-93.

♦ **Granulocyte Colony Stimulating Factor** *see Filgrastim on page 341*

♦ **Granulocyte-Macrophage Colony Stimulating Factor** *see Sargramostim on page 713*

♦ **Gyne-Lotrimin® 3 [OTC]** *see Clotrimazole on page 203*

♦ **Haldol®** *see Haloperidol on page 409*

♦ **Haldol® Decanoate** *see Haloperidol on page 409*

Haloperidol (ha loe PER i dole)

Medication Safety Issues

Sound-alike/look-alike issues:

Haloperidol may be confused Halotestin®

Haldol® may be confused with Halcion®, Halenol®, Halog®, Halotestin®, Stadol®

Related Information

Management of Nausea and Vomiting *on page 982*

U.S. Brand Names Haldol®; Haldol® Decanoate

Canadian Brand Names Apo-Haloperidol®; Apo-Haloperidol LA®; Halo-peridol-LA Omega; Haloperidol Long Acting; Novo-Peridol; Peridol; PMS-Haloperidol LA

Generic Available Yes

Synonyms Haloperidol Decanoate; Haloperidol Lactate

Pharmacologic Category Antipsychotic Agent, Butyrophenone

Pregnancy Risk Factor C

Lactation Enters breast milk/not recommended (AAP rates "of concern")

Use Management of schizophrenia; control of tics and vocal utterances of Tourette's disorder in children and adults; severe behavioral problems in children

Unlabeled/Investigational Use Treatment of psychosis; may be used for the emergency sedation of severely-agitated or delirious patients; adjunctive treatment of ethanol dependence; antiemetic

Mechanism of Action Haloperidol is a butyrophenone antipsychotic which blocks postsynaptic mesolimbic dopaminergic D_1 and D_2 receptors in the brain; depresses the release of hypothalamic and hypophyseal hormones; believed to depress the reticular activating system thus (Continued)

Haloperidol *(Continued)*

affecting basal metabolism, body temperature, wakefulness, vasomotor tone, and emesis

Labeled Contraindications Hypersensitivity to haloperidol or any component of the formulation; Parkinson's disease; severe CNS depression; bone marrow suppression; severe cardiac or hepatic disease; coma

Warnings/Precautions May be sedating, use with caution in disorders where CNS depression is a feature. Caution in patients with hemodynamic instability, predisposition to seizures, subcortical brain damage, renal or respiratory disease. Esophageal dysmotility and aspiration have been associated with antipsychotic use - use with caution in patients at risk of pneumonia (ie, Alzheimer's disease). Caution in breast cancer or other prolactin-dependent tumors (may elevate prolactin levels). May alter temperature regulation or mask toxicity of other drugs due to antiemetic effects. Hypotension may occur, particularly with parenteral administration. Decanoate form should never be administered I.V. Adverse effects of decanoate may be prolonged. Avoid in thyrotoxicosis.

May alter cardiac conduction - life-threatening arrhythmias have occurred with therapeutic doses of antipsychotics. Use with caution in patients at risk of hypotension (orthostasis) or those who would tolerate transient hypotensive episodes (cerebrovascular disease, cardiovascular disease, or other medications which may predispose).

Use with caution in patients with decreased gastrointestinal motility, urinary retention, BPH, xerostomia, or visual problems. May exacerbate narrow-angle glaucoma (screening is recommended) or worsen myasthenia gravis. Relative to other neuroleptics, haloperidol has a low potency of cholinergic blockade.

May cause extrapyramidal symptoms, including pseudoparkinsonism, acute dystonic reactions, akathisia, and tardive dyskinesia (risk of these reactions is high relative to other neuroleptics). May be associated with neuroleptic malignant syndrome (NMS) or pigmentary retinopathy. Some tablets contain tartrazine.

Adverse Reactions Frequency not defined.

Cardiovascular: Hyper-/hypotension, tachycardia, arrhythmia, abnormal T waves with prolonged ventricular repolarization, torsade de pointes (case-control study ~4%)

Central nervous system: Restlessness, anxiety, extrapyramidal symptoms, dystonic reactions, pseudoparkinsonian signs and symptoms, tardive dyskinesia, neuroleptic malignant syndrome (NMS), altered central temperature regulation, akathisia, tardive dystonia, insomnia, euphoria, agitation, drowsiness, depression, lethargy, headache, confusion, vertigo, seizure

Dermatologic: Hyperpigmentation, pruritus, rash, contact dermatitis, alopecia, photosensitivity (rare)

Endocrine & metabolic: Amenorrhea, galactorrhea, gynecomastia, sexual dysfunction, lactation, breast engorgement, mastalgia, menstrual irregularities, hyperglycemia, hypoglycemia, hyponatremia

Gastrointestinal: Nausea, vomiting, anorexia, constipation, diarrhea, hypersalivation, dyspepsia, xerostomia

Genitourinary: Urinary retention, priapism

Hematologic: Cholestatic jaundice, obstructive jaundice

Ocular: Blurred vision

Respiratory: Laryngospasm, bronchospasm

Miscellaneous: Heat stroke, diaphoresis

Vesicant No

Emetic Potential Very low (<10%)

Overdosage/Toxicology Symptoms of overdose include deep sleep, dystonia, agitation, dysrhythmias, and extrapyramidal symptoms. Treatment is supportive and symptomatic.

Drug Interactions

Cytochrome P450 Effect: Substrate of CYP1A2 (minor), 2D6 (major), 3A4 (major); **Inhibits** CYP2D6 (moderate), 3A4 (moderate)

Increased Effect/Toxicity: Haloperidol concentrations/effects may be increased by chloroquine, propranolol, and sulfadoxine-pyridoxine. The levels/effects of haloperidol may be increased by azole antifungals, chlorpromazine, ciprofloxacin, clarithromycin, delavirdine, diclofenac, doxycycline, erythromycin, fluoxetine, imatinib, isoniazid, miconazole, nefazodone, nicardipine, paroxetine, pergolide, propofol, protease inhibitors, quinidine, quinine, ritonavir, ropinirole, telithromycin, verapamil, and other CYP2D6 or 3A4 inhibitors.

Haloperidol may increase the levels/effects of amphetamines, selected beta-blockers, selected benzodiazepines, calcium channel blockers, cisapride, cyclosporine, dextromethorphan, ergot alkaloids, fluoxetine, selected HMG-CoA reductase inhibitors, lidocaine, mesoridazine, mirtazapine, nateglinide, nefazodone, paroxetine, risperidone, ritonavir, sildenafil (and other PDE-5 inhibitors), tacrolimus, thioridazine, tricyclic antidepressants, venlafaxine, and other substrates of CYP2D6 or 3A4.

Haloperidol may increase the effects of antihypertensives, CNS depressants (ethanol, narcotics, sedative-hypnotics), lithium, trazodone, and TCAs. Haloperidol in combination with indomethacin may result in drowsiness, tiredness, and confusion. Metoclopramide may increase risk of extrapyramidal symptoms (EPS).

Decreased Effect: Haloperidol may inhibit the ability of bromocriptine to lower serum prolactin concentrations. Benztropine (and other anticholinergics) may inhibit the therapeutic response to haloperidol and excess anticholinergic effects may occur. Barbiturates, carbamazepine, and cigarette smoking may enhance the hepatic metabolism of haloperidol. Haloperidol may inhibit the antiparkinsonian effect of levodopa; avoid this combination. The levels/effects of haloperidol may be decreased by aminoglutethimide, carbamazepine, nafcillin, nevirapine, phenobarbital, phenytoin, rifamycins, and other CYP3A4 inducers. Haloperidol may decrease the levels/effects of CYP2D6 prodrug substrates (eg, codeine, hydrocodone, oxycodone, tramadol).

Ethanol/Nutrition/Herb Interactions

Ethanol: Avoid ethanol (may increase CNS depression).

Herb/Nutraceutical: Avoid valerian, St John's wort, kava kava, gotu kola (may increase CNS depression).

Storage/Stability Protect oral dosage forms from light. Haloperidol lactate injection should be stored at controlled room temperature and protected from light, freezing, and temperatures >40°C. Exposure to light may cause discoloration and the development of a grayish-red precipitate over several weeks.

(Continued)

Haloperidol *(Continued)*

Reconstitution Haloperidol lactate may be administered IVPB or I.V. infusion in D_5W solutions. NS solutions should not be used due to reports of decreased stability and incompatibility.

Standardized dose: 0.5-100 mg/50-100 mL D_5W

Stability of standardized solutions is 38 days at room temperature (24°C).

Compatibility Stable in D_5W; **variable stability (consult detailed reference)** in $D_5^1/_4NS$, LR, $^1/_2NS$, NS

Y-site administration: Compatible: Amifostine, amsacrine, aztreonam, cimetidine, cisatracurium, cladribine, dobutamine, docetaxel, dopamine, doxorubicin liposome, etoposide phosphate, famotidine, filgrastim, fludarabine, gatifloxacin, gemcitabine, granisetron, lidocaine, linezolid, lorazepam, melphalan, midazolam, nitroglycerin, norepinephrine ondansetron, paclitaxel, phenylephrine, propofol, remifentanil, sufentanil, tacrolimus, teniposide, theophylline, thiotepa, vinorelbine. **Incompatible:** Allopurinol, amphotericin B cholesteryl sulfate complex, cefepime, fluconazole, foscarnet, heparin, piperacillin/tazobactam, sargramostim. **Variable (consult detailed reference):** Sodium nitroprusside

Compatibility in syringe: Compatible: Hydromorphone, sufentanil. **Incompatible:** Diphenhydramine, heparin, hydroxyzine, ketorolac. **Variable (consult detailed reference):** Benztropine, cyclizine, diamorphine, morphine

Pharmacodynamics/Kinetics

Onset of action: Sedation: I.V.: ~1 hour

Duration: Decanoate: ~3 weeks

Distribution: Crosses placenta; enters breast milk

Protein binding: 90%

Metabolism: Hepatic to inactive compounds

Bioavailability: Oral: 60%

Half-life elimination: 20 hours

Time to peak, serum: 20 minutes

Excretion: Urine (33% to 40% as metabolites) within 5 days; feces (15%)

Dosage

Children: 3-12 years (15-40 kg): Oral:

Initial: 0.05 mg/kg/day or 0.25-0.5 mg/day given in 2-3 divided doses; increase by 0.25-0.5 mg every 5-7 days; maximum: 0.15 mg/kg/day

Usual maintenance:

Agitation or hyperkinesia: 0.01-0.03 mg/kg/day once daily

Nonpsychotic disorders: 0.05-0.075 mg/kg/day in 2-3 divided doses

Psychotic disorders: 0.05-0.15 mg/kg/day in 2-3 divided doses

Children 6-12 years: Sedation/psychotic disorders: I.M. (as lactate): 1-3 mg/dose every 4-8 hours to a maximum of 0.15 mg/kg/day; change over to oral therapy as soon as able

Adults:

Psychosis:

Oral: 0.5-5 mg 2-3 times/day; usual maximum: 30 mg/day

I.M. (as lactate): 2-5 mg every 4-8 hours as needed

I.M. (as decanoate): Initial: 10-20 times the daily oral dose administered at 4-week intervals

Maintenance dose: 10-15 times initial oral dose; used to stabilize psychiatric symptoms

Delirium in the intensive care unit (unlabeled use, unlabeled route):

I.V.: 2-10 mg; may repeat bolus doses every 20-30 minutes until calm achieved then administer 25% of the maximum dose every 6 hours; monitor ECG and QT_c interval

Intermittent I.V.: 0.03-0.15 mg/kg every 30 minutes to 6 hours

Oral: Agitation: 5-10 mg

Continuous intravenous infusion (100 mg/100 mL D_5W): Rates of 3-25 mg/hour have been used

Rapid tranquilization of severely-agitated patient (unlabeled use): Administer every 30-60 minutes:

Oral: 5-10 mg

I.M.: 5 mg

Average total dose (oral or I.M.) for tranquilization: 10-20 mg

Elderly: Initial: Oral: 0.25-0.5 mg 1-2 times/day; increase dose at 4- to 7-day intervals by 0.25-0.5 mg/day; increase dosing intervals (twice daily, 3 times/day, etc) as necessary to control response or side effects

Hemodialysis/peritoneal dialysis: Supplemental dose is not necessary

Administration The decanoate injectable formulation should be administered I.M. only, **do not administer decanoate I.V.** Dilute the oral concentrate with water or juice before administration. Avoid skin contact with oral suspension or solution; may cause contact dermatitis.

Dosage Forms Note: Strength expressed as base:

Injection, oil, as decanoate (Haldol®️ Decanoate): 50 mg/mL (1 mL, 5 mL); 100 mg/mL (1 mL, 5 mL) [contains benzyl alcohol, sesame oil]

Injection, solution, as lactate (Haldol®️): 5 mg/mL (1 mL, 10 mL)

Solution, oral concentrate, as lactate: 2 mg/mL (15 mL, 120 mL)

Tablet: 0.5 mg, 1 mg, 2 mg, 5 mg, 10 mg, 20 mg

Monitoring Parameters Vital signs; lipid profile, fasting blood glucose/ Hgb A_{1c}; BMI; mental status, abnormal involuntary movement scale (AIMS), extrapyramidal symptoms (EPS)

Patient Information May cause drowsiness, restlessness; avoid alcohol and other CNS depressants; rise slowly from recumbent position; use of supportive stockings may help prevent orthostatic hypotension; do not alter dosage or discontinue without consulting prescriber; oral concentrate must be diluted in 2-4 oz of liquid (water, fruit juice, carbonated drinks, milk, or pudding)

Special Geriatric Considerations (See Warnings/Precautions, Adverse Reactions, and Overdose/Toxicology.) Elderly patients have an increased risk of adverse response to side effects or adverse reactions to antipsychotics.

Selected Readings

"American Academy of Pediatrics Committee on Drugs. The Transfer of Drugs and Other Chemicals Into Human Milk," *Pediatrics*, 2001, 108(3):776-89.

Aunsholt NA, "Prolonged QT Interval and Hypokalemia Caused by Haloperidol," *Acta Psychiatr Scand*, 1989, 79(4):411-2.

Barton MD, Libonati M, and Cohen PJ, "The Use of Haloperidol for Treatment of Postoperative Nausea and Vomiting - A Double-Blind Placebo-Controlled Trial," *Anesthesiology*, 1975, 42(4):508-12.

Bauer M, "Concurrent Agranulocytosis and Acute Hepatitis Resulting From Combination of Classic Neuroleptics and Subsequent Successful Clozapine Treatment," *Pharmacopsychiatry*, 1995, 28(1):29-31.

Cole RM, Robinson F, Harvey L, et al, "Successful Control of Intractable Nausea and Vomiting Requiring Combined Ondansetron and Haloperidol in a Patient With Advanced Cancer," *J Pain Symptom Manage*, 1994, 9(1):48-50.

Di Salvo TG and O'Gara PT, "Torsade de Pointes Caused by High-Dose Intravenous Haloperidol in Cardiac Patients," *Clin Cardiol*, 1995, 18(5):285-90.

(Continued)

Haloperidol *(Continued)*

Doenecke AL and Heuermann RC, "Treatment of Haloperidol Abuse With Diphenhydramine," *Am J Psychiatry*, 1980, 137(4):487-8.

Fisher H, "A New Approach to Emergency Department Therapy of Migraine Headache With Intravenous Haloperidol: A Case Series," *J Emerg Med*, 1995, 13(1):119-22.

Harada H, Igarashi M, Sugae S, et al, "A Schizophrenic Patient Who Developed Extreme Hypothermia After an Increase in the Dose of Haloperidol: A Case Report," *Jpn J Psychiatry Neurol*, 1994, 48(3):595-8.

Jacobi J, Fraser GL, Coursin DB, et al, "Clinical Practice Guidelines for the Sustained Use of Sedatives and Analgesics in the Critically Ill Adult," *Crit Care Med*, 2002, 30(1):119-41. Available at: http://www.sccm.org/pdf/sedatives.pdf. Accessed August 2, 2003.

Kubota T, Ishikura T, and Jibiki I, "Alopecia Areata Associated With Haloperidol," *Jpn J Psychiatry Neurol*, 1994, 48(3):579-81.

Mahutte CK, Nakasato SK, and Light RW, "Haloperidol and Sudden Death Due to Pulmonary Edema," *Arch Intern Med*, 1982, 142(10):1951-2.

Medlin R, Ransom M, and Kline J, "Ethanol Potentiates Electromechanical Depression Induced by Haloperidol," *Clin Toxicol*, 1995, 33(5):499.

Neidhart JA, Gagen MM, Wilson HE, et al, "Comparative Trial of the Antiemetic Effects of THC and Haloperidol," *J Clin Pharmacol*, 1981, 21(8-9 Suppl):38-42.

Peabody CA, Warner MD, Whiteford HA, et al, "Neuroleptics and the Elderly," *J Am Geriatr Soc*, 1987, 35(3):233-8.

Plotkin DA, Plotkin D, and Okun R, "Haloperidol in the Treatment of Nausea and Vomiting Due to Cytotoxic Drug Administration," *Curr Ther Res Clin Exp*,1973, 15(9):599-602.

Riker RR, Fraser GL, and Cox PM, "Continuous Infusion of Haloperidol Controls Agitation in Critically Ill Patients," *Crit Care Med*, 1994, 22(3):433-40.

Risse SC and Barnes R, "Pharmacologic Treatment of Agitation Associated With Dementia," *J Am Geriatr Soc*, 1986, 34(5):368-76.

Saltz BL, Woerner MG, Kane JM, et al, "Prospective Study of Tardive Dyskinesia Incidence in the Elderly," *JAMA*, 1991, 266(17):2402-6.

Schwartz M, Weller B, Erdreich M, et al, "Rabbit Syndrome and Tardive Dyskinesia: Two Complications of Chronic Neuroleptic Treatment," *J Clin Psychiatry*, 1995, 56(5):212.

Seifert RD, "Therapeutic Drug Monitoring: Psychotropic Drugs," *J Pharm Pract*, 1984, 6:403-16.

Serrano AC, "Haloperidol - Its Use in Children," *J Clin Psychiatry*, 1981, 42(4):154-6.

Sharma ND, Rosman HS, Padhi ID, et al, "Torsades de Pointes Associated With Intravenous Haloperidol in Critically Ill Patients," *Am J Cardiol*, 1998, 81(2):238-40.

Silvey L, Carpenter JT Jr, Wheeler RH, et al, "A Randomized Comparison of Haloperidol Plus Dexamethasone Versus Prochlorperazine Plus Dexamethasone in Preventing Nausea and Vomiting in Patients Receiving Chemotherapy for Breast Cancer," *J Clin Oncol*, 1988, 6(9):1397-400.

Spencer EK, Kafantaris V, Padron-Gayol MV, et al, "Haloperidol in Schizophrenic Children: Early Findings From a Study in Progress," *Psychopharmacol Bull*, 1992, 28(2):183-6.

Wilt JL, Minnema AM, Johnson RF, et al, "Torsade de Pointes Associated With the Use of Intravenous Haloperidol," *Ann Intern Med*, 1993, 119(5):391-4.

Histrelin (his TREL in)

U.S. Brand Names Vantas™

Generic Available No

Synonyms GnRH Agonist; Histrelin Acetate; LH-RH Agonist

Pharmacologic Category Gonadotropin Releasing Hormone Agonist

Pregnancy Risk Factor X

Lactation Excretion in breast milk unknown/contraindicated

Use Palliative treatment of advanced prostate cancer

Mechanism of Action Potent inhibitor of gonadotropin secretion; continuous administration results in, after an initiation phase, the suppression of luteinizing hormone (LH), follicle-stimulating hormone (FSH), and a subsequent decrease in testosterone.

Labeled Contraindications Hypersensitivity to histrelin acetate, GnRH, GnRH-agonist analogs, or any component of the formulation; children; females

Warnings/Precautions Transient increases in testosterone serum levels occur during the first week of use. Worsening symptoms such as bone pain, neuropathy, ureteral or bladder outlet obstruction, and spinal cord compression have been reported. Spinal cord compression and ureteral obstruction may contribute to paralysis; close attention should be given during the first few weeks of therapy to both patients having metastatic vertebral lesions and/or urinary tract obstructions, and to any patients reporting weakness, paresthesias or poor urine output. Safety and efficacy have not been established in patients with hepatic dysfunction.

Adverse Reactions

>10%: Endocrine & metabolic: Expected pharmacological consequence of testosterone suppression: Hot flashes (66%)

2% to 10%:

Central nervous system: Fatigue (10%), headache (3%), insomnia (3%)

Endocrine & metabolic: Expected pharmacological consequences of testosterone suppression: Gynecomastia (4%), sexual dysfunction (4%), libido decreased (2%)

Gastrointestinal: Constipation (4%), weight gain (2%)

Genitourinary: Expected pharmacological consequence of testosterone suppression: Testicular atrophy (5%)

Local: Implant site reaction (6%)

Renal: Renal impairment (5%)

<2%: Abdominal discomfort, alopecia, anemia, appetite increased, arthralgia, AST increased, back pain, bone density decreased, bone pain, breast pain, breast tenderness, contusion, craving food, creatinine increased, depression, diaphoresis, dizziness, dyspnea (exertional), dysuria, feeling cold, fluid retention, genital pruritus, hematuria, hypercalcemia, hypercholesterolemia, hyperglycemia, irritability, LDH increased, lethargy, liver disorder, malaise, muscle twitching, nausea, neck pain, palpitation, peripheral edema, prostatic acid phosphatase increased, renal calculi, renal failure, stent occlusion, testosterone increased, tremor, urinary frequency, urinary retention, ventricular asystoles, weight loss

Drug Interactions

Increased Effect/Toxicity: Not studied

Storage/Stability Vantas™: Upon delivery, separate contents of implant carton. Store implant under refrigeration at 2°C to 8°C (36°F to 46°F), (Continued)

Histrelin *(Continued)*

wrapped in the amber pouch for protection from light. Do not freeze. The implantation kit does not require refrigeration.

Pharmacodynamics/Kinetics

Onset: Chemical castration: 14 days

Duration: 1 year

Distribution: V_d: ~58 L

Protein binding: 70% ± 9%

Metabolism: Hepatic via C-terminal dealkylation and hydrolysis

Bioavailability: 92%

Half-life elimination: Terminal: ~4 hours

Time to peak, serum: 12 hours

Dosage SubQ:

Adults: 50 mg implant surgically inserted every 12 months

Elderly: See Adults dosing

Dosage adjustment in renal impairment: Cl_{cr}: 15-60 mL/minute: Adjustment not needed

Administration SubQ: The implant must be removed from within the glass vial prior to implantation. Surgical implantation into the inner portion of the upper arm requires the use of the implantation device provided. Use the patient's nondominant arm for placement. Removal must occur after 12 months; a replacement implant may be required.

Dosage Forms Implant: 50 mg [released over 12 months; packaged with implantation kit]

Monitoring Parameters LH and FSH levels, serum testosterone levels, prostate specific antigen (PSA), bone mineral density; weakness, paresthesias, and urinary tract obstruction (especially during first few weeks of therapy)

Patient Information May experience disease flare (increased bone pain) and urinary retention during early treatment (usually resolves). Until response to drug is known use caution when driving or engaging in tasks that require alertness; dizziness, headache, lethargy or faintness may occur. Wait at least 24 hours before allowing moisture or water to touch the arm and 7 days before participating in strenuous exertion or heavy lifting. Wear lighter clothing or seek a cooler environment if hot flashes or flushing occur. May develop swelling or tenderness of the breast or a decrease in libido. Notify prescriber if any of the following occur: rapid heartbeat, palpitations, chest pain, inability to void or changes in urinary pattern; continual nausea or vomiting, numbness of extremities, or pain or swelling at implantation site.

- **Histrelin Acetate** *see* Histrelin *on page 415*
- **HMM** *see* Altretamine *on page 51*
- **HMR 3647** *see* Telithromycin *on page 747*
- **HN₂** *see* Mechlorethamine *on page 521*
- **Horse Antihuman Thymocyte Gamma Globulin** *see* Antithymocyte Globulin (Equine) *on page 96*
- **Humanized IgG1 Anti-CD52 Monoclonal Antibody** *see* Alemtuzumab *on page 37*
- **Humate-P**® *see* Antihemophilic Factor (Human) *on page 87*
- **HXM** *see* Altretamine *on page 51*

Hyaluronidase (hye al yoor ON i dase)

Medication Safety Issues

Sound-alike/look-alike issues:

Wydase may be confused with Lidex®, Wyamine®

U.S. Brand Names Amphadase™; Vitrase®

Generic Available No

Pharmacologic Category Enzyme

Pregnancy Risk Factor C

Lactation Excretion in breast milk unknown/use caution

Use Increase the dispersion and absorption of other drugs; increase rate of absorption of parenteral fluids given by hypodermoclysis; adjunct in subcutaneous urography for improving resorption of radiopaque agents

Unlabeled/Investigational Use Management of drug extravasations

Mechanism of Action Modifies the permeability of connective tissue through hydrolysis of hyaluronic acid, one of the chief ingredients of tissue cement which offers resistance to diffusion of liquids through tissues; hyaluronidase increases both the distribution and absorption of locally injected substances.

Labeled Contraindications Hypersensitivity to hyaluronidase or any component of the formulation

Warnings/Precautions Do not inject in or around infected or inflamed areas; may spread localized infection. Should not be used for extravasation management of dopamine or alpha agonists or to reduce swelling of bites or stings. Do not administer intravenously. Do not apply directly to the cornea.

Adverse Reactions

Frequency not defined: Local: Injection site reactions

<1%: Allergic reactions, anaphylactic-like reactions (retrobulbar block or I.V. injections), angioedema, urticaria

Overdosage/Toxicology Treatment is symptom-directed and supportive.

Drug Interactions

Increased Effect/Toxicity: Absorption and toxicity of local anesthetics may be increased.

Storage/Stability

Amphadase™: Store in refrigerator at 2°C to 8°C (35°F to 46°F). Do not freeze.

Vitrase®: Store unopened vial in refrigerator at 2°C to 8°C (35°F to 46°F). After reconstitution, store at 20°C to 25°C (68°F to 77°F) and use within 6 hours.

Reconstitution Vitrase®: Add 6.2 mL of NaCl to vial (1000 units/mL). Further dilute with NaCl before administration.

For 50 units/mL, draw up 0.05 mL of hyaluronidase reconstituted solution (1000 units/mL) and add 0.95 mL of NaCl.

For 75 units/mL, draw up 0.075 mL of hyaluronidase reconstituted solution and add 0.925 mL of NaCl.

For 150 units/mL, draw up 0.15 mL of hyaluronidase reconstituted solution and add 0.85 mL of NaCl.

For 300 units/mL, draw up 0.3 mL of hyaluronidase reconstituted solution and add 0.7 mL of NaCl.

Compatibility Stable in dextran 6% in dextrose, dextran 6% in NS, D_5LR, $D_5^{1}/_4NS$, $D_5^{1}/_2NS$, D_5NS, D_5W, $D_{10}W$, LR, $^{1}/_2NS$, NS

(Continued)

417

Hyaluronidase *(Continued)*

Compatibility in syringe: Compatible: Diatrizoate meglumine 34.3%, diatrizoate sodium 35%, iothalamate meglumine 60%, iothalamate sodium 80%, pentobarbital, thiopental. **Incompatible:** Hydromorphone. **Variable (consult detailed reference):** Diatrizoate meglumine 52%, diatrizoate sodium 8%, diatrizoate sodium 75%, iodipamide meglumine 52%

Compatibility when admixed: Compatible: Amikacin, sodium bicarbonate. **Incompatible:** Epinephrine, heparin

Pharmacodynamics/Kinetics

Onset of action: SubQ: Immediate

Duration: 24-48 hours

Dosage Note: A preliminary skin test for hypersensitivity can be performed. ACTH, antihistamines, corticosteroids, estrogens, and salicylates, when used in large doses, may cause tissues to be partly resistant to hyaluronidase. May require larger doses of hyaluronidase for the same effect.

Skin test: Intradermal: 0.02 mL (3 units) of a 150 units/mL solution. Positive reaction consists of a wheal with pseudopods appearing within 5 minutes and persisting for 20-30 minutes with localized itching.

Hypodermoclysis: SubQ: 15 units is added to each 100 mL of I.V. fluid to be administered

Premature Infants and Neonates: Volume of a single clysis should not exceed 25 mL/kg and the rate of administration should not exceed 2 mL/minute

Children <3 years: Volume of a single clysis should not exceed 200 mL

Children ≥3 years and Adults: Rate and volume of a single clysis should not exceed those used for infusion of I.V. fluids

Extravasation (unlabeled use): Adults: SubQ: Inject 1 mL of a 150 unit/mL solution (as 5-10 injections of 0.1-0.2 mL) into affected area; doses of 15-250 units have been reported.

Elderly: See Adults dosing. Adjust dose carefully to individual patient.

Administration Do **not** administer I.V.

Dosage Forms

Injection, powder for reconstitution (Vitrase®): 6200 units [ovine derived; contains lactose]

Injection, solution (Amphadase™): 150 units/mL (2 mL) [bovine derived; contains edetate disodium 1 mg, thimerosal ≤0.1 mg]

Injection, solution [preservative free] (Vitrase®): 200 units/mL (2 mL) [ovine derived; contains lactulose]

Special Geriatric Considerations The most common use of hyaluronidase in the elderly is in hypodermoclysis. Hypodermoclysis is very useful in dehydrated patients in whom oral intake is minimal and I.V. access is a problem.

Selected Readings

Berger EY, "Nutrition by Hypodermoclysis," *J Am Geriatr Soc*, 1984, 32(3):199-203.

Bertelli G, "Prevention and Management of Extravasation of Cytotoxic Drugs," *Drug Saf*, 1995, 12(4):245-55.

Bertelli G, Dini D, Forno GB, et al, "Hyaluronidase as an Antidote to Extravasation of Vinca Alkaloids: Clinical Results," *J Cancer Res Clin Oncol*, 1994, 120(8):505-6.

Cochran ST, Bomyea K, and Kahn M, "Treatment of Iodinated Contrast Material Extravasation With Hyaluronidase," *Acad Radiol*, 2002, 9(Suppl 2):544-6.

Dorr RT, "Vinca Alkaloid Ulceration: Experimental Mouse Model and Effects of Local Antidotes," *Proc Am Soc Clin Oncol*, 1982, 1:428.

Elam EA, Dorr RT, Lagel KE, et al, "Cutaneous Ulceration Due to Contrast Extravasation. Experimental Assessment of Injury and Potential Antidotes," *Invest Radiol*, 1991, 26(1):13-6.

Kumar MM and Sprung J, "The Use of Hyaluronidase to Treat Mannitol Extravasation," *Anesth Analg*, 2003, 97(4):1199-200.

Lipschitz S, Campbell AJ, Roberts MS, et al, "Subcutaneous Fluid Administration in Elderly Subjects: Validation of an Underused Technique," *J Am Geriatr Soc*, 1991, 39(1):6-9.

Raszka WV Jr, Kueser TK, Smith FR, et al, "The Use of Hyaluronidase in the Treatment of Intravenous Extravasation Injuries," *J Perinatol*, 19909, 10(2):146-9.

Sokol DK, Dahlmann A, and Dunn DW, "Hyaluronidase Treatment for Intravenous Phenytoin Extravasation," *J Child Neurol*, 1998, 13(5):246-7.

Zenk KE, "Hyaluronidase: An Antidote for Intravenous Extravasations," *CSHP Voice*, 1981, 66-8.

Zenk KE, "Management of Intravenous Extravasations," *Infusion*, 1981, 5:77-9.

Zenk KE, "Treating I.V. Extravasations With Hyaluronidase," *ASHP Signal*, 1986, 10:25,29.

Zenk KE, Dungy CI, and Greene GR, "Nafcillin Extravasation Injury: Use of Hyaluronidase as an Antidote," *Am J Dis Child*, 1981, 135(12):1113-4.

♦ **Hyate:C®** *see* Antihemophilic Factor (Porcine) *on page 90*

♦ **Hycamptamine** *see* Topotecan *on page 776*

♦ **Hycamtin®** *see* Topotecan *on page 776*

♦ **Hycort™ (Can)** *see* Hydrocortisone *on page 419*

♦ **Hydeltra T.B.A.® (Can)** *see* PrednisoLONE *on page 679*

♦ **Hyderm (Can)** *see* Hydrocortisone *on page 419*

♦ **Hydrea®** *see* Hydroxyurea *on page 432*

Hydrocortisone (hye droe KOR ti sone)

Medication Safety Issues

Sound-alike/look-alike issues:

Hydrocortisone may be confused with hydrocodone, hydroxychloroquine, hydrochlorothiazide

Anusol® may be confused with Anusol-HC®, Aplisol®, Aquasol®

Anusol-HC® may be confused with Anusol®

Cortef® may be confused with Lortab®

Cortizone® may be confused with cortisone

Hytone® may be confused with Vytone®

Proctocort® may be confused with ProctoCream®

ProctoCream® may be confused with Proctocort®

U.S. Brand Names Anucort-HC®; Anusol-HC®; Anusol® HC-1 [OTC]; Aquanil™ HC [OTC]; Beta-HC®; Caldecort® [OTC]; Cetacort®; Colocort®; CortaGel® Maximum Strength [OTC] [DSC]; Cortaid® Intensive Therapy [OTC]; Cortaid® Maximum Strength [OTC]; Cortaid® Sensitive Skin [OTC]; Cortef®; Corticool® [OTC]; Cortifoam®; Cortizone®-10 Maximum Strength [OTC]; Cortizone®-10 Plus Maximum Strength [OTC]; Cortizone®-10 Quick Shot [OTC]; Dermarest Dricort® [OTC]; Dermtex® HC [OTC]; EarSol® HC; Hemril®-30; Hydrocortone® [OTC]; HydroZone Plus [OTC]; Hytone®; IvySoothe® [OTC]; LactiCare-HC® [DSC]; Locoid®; Locoid Lipocream®; Nupercainal® Hydrocortisone Cream [OTC]; Nutracort®; Pandel®; Post Peel Healing Balm [OTC]; Preparation H® Hydrocortisone [OTC]; Proctocort®; ProctoCream® HC; Procto-Kit™; Procto-Pak™; Proctosert; Proctosol-HC®; Proctozone-HC™; Sarnol®-HC [OTC]; Solu-Cortef®; Summer's Eve® SpecialCare™ Medicated Anti-Itch Cream [OTC]; Texacort®; Westcort®

Canadian Brand Names Aquacort®; Cortamed®; Cortate®; Cortef®; Cortenema®; Cortifoam™; Cortoderm; Emo-Cort®; Hycort™; Hyderm; HydroVal®; Locoid®; Prevex® HC; Sarna® HC; Solu-Cortef®; Westcort® (Continued)

Hydrocortisone *(Continued)*

Generic Available Yes: Excludes acetate foam, butyrate cream and ointment, gel as base, otic drops as base, probutate cream, sodium succinate injection

Synonyms A-hydroCort; Compound F; Cortisol; Hemorrhoidal HC; Hydrocortisone Acetate; Hydrocortisone Butyrate; Hydrocortisone Probutate; Hydrocortisone Sodium Succinate; Hydrocortisone Valerate

Pharmacologic Category Corticosteroid, Rectal; Corticosteroid, Systemic; Corticosteroid, Topical

Pregnancy Risk Factor C

Lactation Excretion in breast milk unknown/use caution

Use Management of adrenocortical insufficiency; relief of inflammation of corticosteroid-responsive dermatoses (low and medium potency topical corticosteroid); adjunctive treatment of ulcerative colitis

Mechanism of Action Decreases inflammation by suppression of migration of polymorphonuclear leukocytes and reversal of increased capillary permeability

Labeled Contraindications Hypersensitivity to hydrocortisone or any component of the formulation; serious infections, except septic shock or tuberculous meningitis; viral, fungal, or tubercular skin lesions

Warnings/Precautions Use with caution in patients with hyperthyroidism, cirrhosis, nonspecific ulcerative colitis, hypertension, osteoporosis, thromboembolic tendencies, CHF, convulsive disorders, myasthenia gravis, thrombophlebitis, peptic ulcer, diabetes, glaucoma, cataracts, or tuberculosis. Use caution in hepatic impairment. May cause HPA axis suppression. Acute adrenal insufficiency may occur with abrupt withdrawal after long-term therapy or with stress. Young pediatric patients may be more susceptible to adrenal axis suppression from topical therapy. Avoid use of topical preparations with occlusive dressings or on weeping or exudative lesions. Because of the risk of adverse effects, systemic corticosteroids should be used cautiously in the elderly, in the smallest possible dose, and for the shortest possible time.

Adverse Reactions

Systemic:

>10%:

Central nervous system: Insomnia, nervousness

Gastrointestinal: Increased appetite, indigestion

1% to 10%:

Dermatologic: Hirsutism

Endocrine & metabolic: Diabetes mellitus

Neuromuscular & skeletal: Arthralgia

Ocular: Cataracts

Respiratory: Epistaxis

<1%: Hypertension, edema, euphoria, headache, delirium, hallucinations, seizure, mood swings, acne, dermatitis, skin atrophy, bruising, hyperpigmentation, hypokalemia, hyperglycemia, Cushing's syndrome, sodium and water retention, bone growth suppression, amenorrhea, peptic ulcer, abdominal distention, ulcerative esophagitis, pancreatitis, muscle wasting, hypersensitivity reactions, immunosuppression

Topical:

>10%: Dermatologic: Eczema (12.5%)

1% to 10%: Dermatologic: Pruritus (6%), stinging (2%), dry skin (2%)

<1%: Allergic contact dermatitis, burning, dermal atrophy, folliculitis, HPA axis suppression, hypopigmentation; metabolic effects (hyperglycemia, hypokalemia); striae

Overdosage/Toxicology When consumed in high doses for prolonged periods, systemic hypercorticism and adrenal suppression may occur. In those cases, discontinuation of the corticosteroid should be done judiciously.

Drug Interactions

Cytochrome P450 Effect: Substrate of CYP3A4 (minor); **Induces** CYP3A4 (weak)

Increased Effect/Toxicity: Hydrocortisone in combination with oral anticoagulants may increase prothrombin time. Potassium-depleting diuretics increase risk of hypokalemia. Cardiac glycosides increase risk of arrhythmias or digitalis toxicity secondary to hypokalemia.

Decreased Effect: Hydrocortisone may decrease the hypoglycemic effect of insulin. Phenytoin, phenobarbital, ephedrine, and rifampin increase metabolism of hydrocortisone resulting in a decreased steroid blood level.

Ethanol/Nutrition/Herb Interactions

Ethanol: Avoid ethanol (may enhance gastric mucosal irritation).

Food: Hydrocortisone interferes with calcium absorption.

Herb/Nutraceutical: St John's wort may decrease hydrocortisone levels. Avoid cat's claw, echinacea (have immunostimulant properties).

Storage/Stability Store at controlled room temperature 20°C to 25°C (59°F to 86°F). Hydrocortisone sodium phosphate and hydrocortisone sodium succinate are clear, light yellow solutions which are heat labile.

Sodium succinate: After initial reconstitution, hydrocortisone sodium succinate solutions are stable for 3 days at room temperature or under refrigeration when protected from light. Stability of parenteral admixture (Solu-Cortef®) at room temperature (25°C) and at refrigeration temperature (4°C) is concentration-dependent:

Stability of concentration 1 mg/mL: 24 hours

Stability of concentration 2 mg/mL to 60 mg/mL: At least 4 hours

Solutions for I.V. infusion: Reconstituted solutions may be added to an appropriate volume of compatible solution for infusion. Concentration should generally not exceed 1 mg/mL. However, in cases where administration of a small volume of fluid is desirable, 100-3000 mg may be added to 50 mL of D_5W or NS (stability limited to 4 hours).

Reconstitution

Sodium succinate: Reconstitute 100 mg vials with bacteriostatic water (not >2 mL). Act-O-Vial (self-contained powder for injection plus diluent) may be reconstituted by pressing the activator to force diluent into the powder compartment. Following gentle agitation, solution may be withdrawn via syringe through a needle inserted into the center of the stopper. May be administered (I.V. or I.M.) without further dilution.

Solutions for I.V. infusion: Reconstituted solutions may be added to an appropriate volume of compatible solution for infusion. Concentration should generally not exceed 1 mg/mL. However, in cases where administration of a small volume of fluid is desirable, 100-3000 mg may be added to 50 mL of D_5W or NS (stability limited to 4 hours).

Compatibility

Hydrocortisone sodium phosphate: Stable in D_5W, NS, fat emulsion 10%

(Continued)

Hydrocortisone *(Continued)*

Y-site administration: Compatible: Allopurinol, amifostine, aztreonam, cefepime, cladribine, clarithromycin, docetaxel, etoposide, famotidine, filgrastim, fluconazole, fludarabine, gemcitabine, granisetron, melphalan, ondansetron, paclitaxel, piperacillin/tazobactam, teniposide, thiotepa, vinorelbine. **Incompatible:** Sargramostim

Compatibility in syringe: Compatible: Metoclopramide. **Incompatible:** Doxapram

Compatibility when admixed: Compatible: Amikacin, amphotericin B, amphotericin B with heparin, bleomycin, dacarbazine, metaraminol, sodium bicarbonate, verapamil. **Variable (consult detailed reference):** Mitoxantrone

Hydrocortisone sodium succinate: Stable in dextran 6% in dextrose, dextran 6% in NS, D_5LR, $D_5^{1}/_4NS$, $D_5^{1}/_2NS$, D_5NS, D_5W, $D_{10}W$, $D_{20}W$, LR, $^{1}/_2NS$, NS, fat emulsion 10%

Y-site administration: Compatible: Acyclovir, allopurinol, amifostine, aminophylline, amphotericin B cholesteryl sulfate complex, ampicillin, amsacrine, atracurium, atropine, aztreonam, betamethasone sodium phosphate, calcium gluconate, cefepime, chlordiazepoxide, chlorpromazine, cisatracurium, cladribine, cyanocobalamin, cytarabine, dexamethasone sodium phosphate, digoxin, diphenhydramine, docetaxel, dopamine, doxorubicin liposome, droperidol, droperidol and fentanyl, edrophonium, enalaprilat, epinephrine, esmolol, estrogens (conjugated), ethacrynate sodium, etoposide, famotidine, fentanyl, filgrastim, fludarabine, fluorouracil, foscarnet, furosemide, gatifloxacin, gemcitabine, granisetron, heparin, hydralazine, inamrinone, insulin (regular), isoproterenol, kanamycin, lidocaine, linezolid, lorazepam, magnesium sulfate, melphalan, menadiol sodium diphosphate, meperidine, methoxamine, methylergonovine, minocycline, morphine, neostigmine, norepinephrine, ondansetron, oxacillin, oxytocin, paclitaxel, pancuronium, penicillin G potassium, pentazocine, phytonadione, piperacillin/tazobactam, procainamide, prochlorperazine edisylate, propofol, propranolol, pyridostigmine, remifentanil, scopolamine, sodium bicarbonate, succinylcholine, tacrolimus, teniposide, theophylline, thiotepa, trimethaphan camsylate, trimethobenzamide, vecuronium, vinorelbine. **Incompatible:** Ciprofloxacin, diazepam, ergotamine, idarubicin, midazolam, phenytoin, sargramostim. **Variable (consult detailed reference):** Diltiazem, methylprednisolone sodium succinate, promethazine

Compatibility in syringe: Compatible: Diatrizoate meglumine 52%, diatrizoate sodium 8%, diatrizoate sodium 60%, iohexol, iopamidol, iothalamate meglumine 60%, ioxaglate meglumine 39.3%, ioxaglate sodium 19.6%, metoclopramide, thiopental. **Incompatible:** Doxapram

Compatibility when admixed: Compatible: Amikacin, aminophylline, amphotericin B, calcium chloride, calcium gluconate, chloramphenicol, clindamycin, corticotropin, daunorubicin, diphenhydramine, dopamine, erythromycin lactobionate, floxacillin, lidocaine, magnesium sulfate, mephentermine, metronidazole, metronidazole with sodium bicarbonate, mitomycin, mitoxantrone, norepinephrine, penicillin G potassium, penicillin G sodium, piperacillin, polymyxin B sulfate, potassium chloride, procaine, sodium bicarbonate, theophylline, thiopental, vancomycin, verapamil, vitamin B complex with C. **Incompatible:** Aminophylline with cephalothin, bleomycin, colistimethate, ephedrine, hydralazine, nafcillin, pentobarbital, phenobarbital, prochlorperazine edisylate, promethazine. **Variable (consult detailed reference):** Amobarbital, ampicillin, cytarabine, dimenhydrinate, furosemide, heparin, kanamycin, metaraminol

Pharmacodynamics/Kinetics

Onset of action:

Hydrocortisone acetate: Slow

Hydrocortisone sodium succinate (water soluble): Rapid

Duration: Hydrocortisone acetate: Long

Absorption: Rapid by all routes, except rectally

Metabolism: Hepatic

Half-life elimination: Biologic: 8-12 hours

Excretion: Urine (primarily as 17-hydroxysteroids and 17-ketosteroids)

Dosage Dose should be based on severity of disease and patient response

Acute adrenal insufficiency: I.M., I.V.:

Infants and young Children: Succinate: 1-2 mg/kg/dose bolus, then 25-150 mg/day in divided doses every 6-8 hours

Older Children: Succinate: 1-2 mg/kg bolus then 150-250 mg/day in divided doses every 6-8 hours

Adults: Succinate: 100 mg I.V. bolus, then 300 mg/day in divided doses every 8 hours or as a continuous infusion for 48 hours; once patient is stable change to oral, 50 mg every 8 hours for 6 doses, then taper to 30-50 mg/day in divided doses

Chronic adrenal corticoid insufficiency: Adults: Oral: 20-30 mg/day

Anti-inflammatory or immunosuppressive:

Infants and Children:

Oral: 2.5-10 mg/kg/day **or** 75-300 mg/m^2/day every 6-8 hours

I.M., I.V.: Succinate: 1-5 mg/kg/day **or** 30-150 mg/m^2/day divided every 12-24 hours

Adolescents and Adults: Oral, I.M., I.V.: Succinate: 15-240 mg every 12 hours

Congenital adrenal hyperplasia: Oral: Initial: 10-20 mg/m^2/day in 3 divided doses; a variety of dosing schedules have been used. **Note:** Inconsistencies have occurred with liquid formulations; tablets may provide more reliable levels. Doses must be individualized by monitoring growth, bone age, and hormonal levels. Mineralocorticoid and sodium supplementation may be required based upon electrolyte regulation and plasma renin activity.

Physiologic replacement: Children:

Oral: 0.5-0.75 mg/kg/day **or** 20-25 mg/m^2/day every 8 hours

I.M.: Succinate: 0.25-0.35 mg/kg/day **or** 12-15 mg/m^2/day once daily

Shock: I.M., I.V.: Succinate:

Children: Initial: 50 mg/kg, then repeated in 4 hours and/or every 24 hours as needed

Adolescents and Adults: 500 mg to 2 g every 2-6 hours

Status asthmaticus: Children and Adults: I.V.: Succinate: 1-2 mg/kg/dose every 6 hours for 24 hours, then maintenance of 0.5-1 mg/kg every 6 hours

Adults:

Rheumatic diseases:

Intralesional, intra-articular, soft tissue injection: Acetate:

Large joints: 25 mg (up to 37.5 mg)

Small joints: 10-25 mg

Tendon sheaths: 5-12.5 mg

(Continued)

Hydrocortisone *(Continued)*

Soft tissue infiltration: 25-50 mg (up to 75 mg)

Bursae: 25-37.5 mg

Ganglia: 12.5-25 mg

Stress dosing (surgery) in patients known to be adrenally-suppressed or on chronic systemic steroids: I.V.:

Minor stress (ie, inguinal herniorrhaphy): 25 mg/day for 1 day

Moderate stress (ie, joint replacement, cholecystectomy): 50-75 mg/day (25 mg every 8-12 hours) for 1-2 days

Major stress (pancreatoduodenectomy, esophagogastrectomy, cardiac surgery): 100-150 mg/day (50 mg every 8-12 hours) for 2-3 days

Dermatosis: Children >2 years and Adults: Topical: Apply to affected area 2-4 times/day (Buteprate: Apply once or twice daily). Therapy should be discontinued when control is achieved; if no improvement is seen, reassessment of diagnosis may be necessary.

Ulcerative colitis: Adults: Rectal: 10-100 mg 1-2 times/day for 2-3 weeks

Combination Regimens

Prostate cancer:

Estramustine + Docetaxel + Hydrocortisone *on page 882*

Mitoxantrone + Hydrocortisone *on page 910*

Administration

Oral: Administer with food or milk to decrease GI upset

Parenteral: Hydrocortisone sodium succinate may be administered by I.M. or I.V. routes

I.V. bolus: Dilute to 50 mg/mL and administer over 30 seconds to several minutes (depending on the dose)

I.V. intermittent infusion: Dilute to 1 mg/mL and administer over 20-30 minutes

Topical: Apply a thin film to clean, dry skin and rub in gently

Dosage Forms [DSC] = Discontinued product

Aerosol, rectal, as acetate (Cortifoam®): 10% (15 g) [90 mg/applicator]

Cream, rectal, as acetate (Nupercainal® Hydrocortisone Cream): 1% (30 g) [strength expressed as base]

Cream, rectal, as base:

Cortizone®-10: 1% (30g) [contains aloe]

Preparation H® Hydrocortisone: 1% (27 g)

Cream, topical, as acetate: 0.5% (9 g, 30 g, 60 g) [available with aloe]; 1% (30 g, 454 g) [available with aloe]

Cream, topical, as base: 0.5% (30 g); 1% (1.5 g, 30 g, 114 g, 454 g); 2.5% (20 g, 30 g, 454 g)

Anusol-HC®: 2.5% (30 g) [contains benzyl alcohol]

Caldecort®: 1% (30 g) [contains aloe vera gel]

Cortaid® Intensive Therapy: 1% (60 g)

Cortaid® Maximum Strength: 1% (15 g, 30 g, 40 g, 60 g) [contains aloe vera gel and benzyl alcohol]

Cortaid® Sensitive Skin: 0.5% (15 g) [contains aloe vera gel]

Cortizone®-10 Maximum Strength: 1% (15 g, 30 g, 60 g) [contains aloe]

Cortizone®-10 Plus Maximum Strength: 1% (30 g, 60 g) [contains vitamins A, D, E and aloe]

Dermarest® Dricort®: 1% (15 g, 30 g)

HydroZone Plus, Proctocort®, Procto-Pak™: 1% (30 g)

Hytone®: 2.5% (30 g, 60 g)

IvySoothe®: 1% (30 g) [contains aloe]

Post Peel Healing Balm: 1% (23 g)

ProctoCream® HC: 2.5% (30 g) [contains benzyl alcohol]

Procto-Kit™: 1% (30 g) [packaged with applicator tips and finger cots]; 2.5% (30g) [packaged with applicator tips and finger cots]

Proctosol-HC®, Proctozone-HC™: 2.5% (30 g)

Summer's Eve® SpecialCare™ Medicated Anti-Itch Cream: 1% (30 g)

Cream, topical, as butyrate (Locoid®, Locoid Lipocream®): 0.1% (15 g, 45 g)

Cream, topical, as probutate (Pandel®): 0.1% (15 g, 45 g, 80 g)

Cream, topical, as valerate (Westcort®): 0.2% (15 g, 45 g, 60 g)

Gel, topical, as base:

Corticool®: 1% (45 g)

CortaGel® Maximum Strength: 1% (15 g, 30 g) [contains aloe vera gel] [DSC]

Injection, powder for reconstitution, as sodium succinate (Solu-Cortef®): 100 mg, 250 mg, 500 mg, 1 g [diluent contains benzyl alcohol; strength expressed as base]

Lotion, topical, as base: 1% (120 mL); 2.5% (60 mL)

Aquanil™ HC: 1% (120 mL)

Beta-HC®, Cetacort®, Sarnol®-HC: 1% (60 mL)

HydroZone Plus: 1% (120 mL)

Hytone®: 2.5% (60 mL)

LactiCare-HC®: 1% (120 mL); 2.5% (60 mL, 120 mL) [DSC]

Nutracort®: 1% (60 mL, 120 mL); 2.5% (60 mL, 120 mL)

Ointment, topical, as acetate: 1% (30 g) [strength expressed as base; available with aloe]

Anusol® HC-1: 1% (21 g) [strength expressed as base]

Cortaid® Maximum Strength: 1% (15 g, 30 g) [strength expressed as base]

Ointment, topical, as base: 0.5% (30 g); 1% (30 g, 454 g); 2.5% (20 g, 30 g, 454 g)

Cortizone®-10 Maximum Strength: 1% (30 g, 60 g)

Hytone®: 2.5% (30 g)

Ointment, topical, as butyrate (Locoid®): 0.1% (15 g, 45 g)

Ointment, topical, as valerate (Westcort®): 0.2% (15 g, 45 g, 60 g)

Solution, otic, as base (EarSol® HC): 1% (30 mL) [contains alcohol 44%, benzyl benzoate, yerba santa]

Solution, topical, as base (Texacort®): 2.5% (30 mL) [contains alcohol]

Solution, topical, as butyrate (Locoid®): 0.1% (20 mL, 60 mL) [contains alcohol 50%]

Solution, topical spray, as base:

Cortaid® Intensive Therapy: 1% (60 mL) [contains alcohol]

Cortizone® 10 Quick Shot: 1% (44 mL) [contains benzyl alcohol]

Dermtex® HC: 1% (52 mL) [contains menthol 1%]

Suppository, rectal, as acetate: 25 mg (12s, 24s, 100s)

Anucort-HC®: 25 mg (12s, 24s, 100s)

Anusol-HC®, Proctosol-HC®: 25 mg (12s, 24s)

Encort™: 30 mg (12s)

Hemril®-30, Proctocort®, Proctosert: 30 mg (12s, 24s)

Suspension, rectal, as base: 100 mg/60 mL (7s)

Colocort®: 100 mg/60 mL (1s, 7s)

Tablet, as base: 20 mg

Cortef®: 5 mg, 10 mg, 20 mg

Hydrocortone®: 10 mg [DSC]

(Continued)

Hydrocortisone *(Continued)*

Monitoring Parameters Blood pressure, weight, serum glucose, and electrolytes

Dietary Considerations Systemic use of corticosteroids may require a diet with increased potassium, vitamins A, B_6, C, D, folate, calcium, zinc, phosphorus, and decreased sodium. Sodium content of 1 g (sodium succinate injection): 47.5 mg (2.07 mEq)

Patient Information Notify surgeon or dentist before surgical repair; oral formulation may cause GI upset, take with food; report if any sign of infection occurs; avoid abrupt withdrawal when on long-term therapy. Before applying, gently wash area to reduce risk of infection; apply a thin film to cleansed area and rub in gently and thoroughly until medication vanishes; avoid exposure to sunlight, severe sunburn may occur.

Additional Information Hydrocortisone base topical cream, lotion, and ointments in concentrations of 0.25%, 0.5%, and 1% may be OTC or prescription depending on the product labeling.

Selected Readings

Abraham E and Evans T, "Corticosteroids and Septic Shock [editorial]," *JAMA*, 2002, 288(7):886-7.

Annane D, Sebille V, Charpentier C, et al, "Effect of Treatment With Low Doses of Hydrocortisone and Fludrocortisone on Mortality in Patients With Septic Shock," *JAMA*, 2002, 288(7):862-71.

Cooper MS and Stewart PM, "Corticosteroid Insufficiency in Acutely Ill Patients," *N Engl J Med*, 2003, 348(8):727-34.

Coursin DB and Wood KE, "Corticosteroid Supplementation for Adrenal Insufficiency," *JAMA*, 2002, 287(2):236-40.

de Jonghe B, Sharshar T, Lefaucheur JP, et al, "Paresis Acquired in the Intensive Care Unit. A Prospective Multicenter Study," *JAMA*, 2002, 288(22):2859-67.

Gamsu HR, Mullinger BM, Donnai P, et al, "Antenatal Administration of Betamethasone to Prevent Respiratory Distress Syndrome in Preterm Infants: Report of a UK Multicentre Trial," *Br J Obstet Gynaecol*, 1989, 96(4):401-10.

Hotchkiss RS and Karl IE, "The Pathophysiology and Treatment of Sepsis," *N Engl J Med*, 2003, 348(2):138-50.

Liggins GC and Howie RN, "A Controlled Trial of Antepartum Glucocorticoid Treatment of Respiratory Distress Syndrome in Premature Infants," *Pediatrics*, 1972, 50:515-25.

Salem M, Tainsh RE Jr, Bromberg J, et al, "Perioperative Glucocorticoid Coverage. A Reassessment 42 Years After Emergence of a Problem," *Ann Surg*, 1994, 219(4):416-25.

"Technical Report: Congenital Adrenal Hyperplasia," American Academy of Pediatrics, Section on Endocrinology and Committee on Genetics, *Pediatrics*, 2000, 106(6):1511-8.

♦ **Hydrocortisone Acetate** *see* Hydrocortisone *on page 419*

♦ **Hydrocortisone Butyrate** *see* Hydrocortisone *on page 419*

♦ **Hydrocortisone Probutate** *see* Hydrocortisone *on page 419*

♦ **Hydrocortisone Sodium Succinate** *see* Hydrocortisone *on page 419*

♦ **Hydrocortisone Valerate** *see* Hydrocortisone *on page 419*

♦ **Hydrocortone® [DSC]** *see* Hydrocortisone *on page 419*

♦ **Hydromorph Contin® (Can)** *see* Hydromorphone *on page 426*

Hydromorphone *(hye droe MOR fone)*

Medication Safety Issues

Sound-alike/look-alike issues:

Dilaudid® may be confused with Demerol®, Dilantin®

Hydromorphone may be confused with morphine; significant overdoses have occurred when hydromorphone products have been inadvertently administered instead of morphine sulfate. Commercially available prefilled syringes of both products looks similar and are often stored in close proximity to each other. **Note:** Hydromorphone 1 mg oral is approximately equal to morphine 4 mg oral; hydromorphone 1 mg I.V. is approximately equal to morphine 5 mg I.V..

Dilaudid®, Dilaudid-HP®: Extreme caution should be taken to avoid confusing the highly-concentrated (Dilaudid-HP®) injection with the less-concentrated (Dilaudid®) injectable product.

U.S. Brand Names Dilaudid®; Dilaudid-HP®; Palladone™

Canadian Brand Names Dilaudid®; Dilaudid-HP®; Dilaudid-HP-Plus®; Dilaudid® Sterile Powder; Dilaudid-XP®; Hydromorph Contin®; Hydromorphone HP; PMS-Hydromorphone

Generic Available Yes: Excludes capsule, liquid, powder for injection

Synonyms Dihydromorphinone; Hydromorphone Hydrochloride

Pharmacologic Category Analgesic, Narcotic

Pregnancy Risk Factor C/D (prolonged use or high doses at term)

Lactation Excretion in breast milk unknown/not recommended

Use Management of moderate-to-severe pain

Unlabeled/Investigational Use Antitussive

Mechanism of Action Binds to opiate receptors in the CNS, causing inhibition of ascending pain pathways, altering the perception of and response to pain; causes cough supression by direct central action in the medulla; produces generalized CNS depression

Restrictions C-II; An FDA-approved medication guide is available at www.fda.gov/cder/Offices/ODS/labeling.htm; distribute to each patient to whom this medication is dispensed.

Labeled Contraindications Hypersensitivity to hydromorphone, any component of the formulation, or other phenanthrene derivative; increased intracranial pressure; acute or severe asthma, severe respiratory depression (in absence of resuscitative equipment or ventilatory support); severe CNS depression; pregnancy (prolonged use or high doses at term)

Palladone™ is also contraindicated with known or suspected paralytic ileus.

Warnings/Precautions Controlled release capsules should only be used when continuous analgesia is required over an extended period of time. Palladone™ should only be used in opioid tolerant patients requiring doses of hydromorphone >12 mg/day (or equianalgesic dose of another opioid) and who have been at that dose for >7 days. Controlled release products are not to be used on an as needed basis. Hydromorphone shares toxic potential of opiate agonists, and precaution of opiate agonist therapy should be observed; use with caution in patients with hypersensitivity to other phenanthrene opiates, respiratory disease, biliary tract disease, acute pancreatitis, or severe liver or renal failure; tolerance or drug dependence may result from extended use. Those at risk for opioid abuse include patients with a history of substance abuse or mental illness.

An opioid-containing analgesic regimen should be tailored to each patient's needs and based upon the type of pain being treated (acute versus chronic), the route of administration, degree of tolerance for (Continued)

Hydromorphone *(Continued)*

opioids (naive versus chronic user), age, weight, and medical condition. The optimal analgesic dose varies widely among patients. Doses should be titrated to pain relief/prevention. I.M. use may result in variable absorption and a lag time to peak effect.

Some dosage forms contain trace amounts of sodium bisulfite which may cause allergic reactions in susceptible individuals.

Adverse Reactions Frequency not defined.

Cardiovascular: Palpitations, hypotension, peripheral vasodilation, tachycardia, bradycardia, facial flushing

Central nervous system: CNS depression, increased intracranial pressure, fatigue, headache, nervousness, restlessness, dizziness, lightheadedness, drowsiness, hallucinations, mental depression, seizure

Dermatologic: Pruritus, rash, urticaria

Endocrine & metabolic: Antidiuretic hormone release

Gastrointestinal: Nausea, vomiting, constipation, stomach cramps, xerostomia, anorexia, biliary tract spasm, paralytic ileus

Genitourinary: Decreased urination, ureteral spasm, urinary tract spasm

Hepatic: LFTs increased, AST increased, ALT increased

Local: Pain at injection site (I.M.)

Neuromuscular & skeletal: Trembling, weakness, myoclonus

Ocular: Miosis

Respiratory: Respiratory depression, dyspnea

Miscellaneous: Histamine release, physical and psychological dependence

Vesicant No

Overdosage/Toxicology Symptoms of overdose include CNS depression, respiratory depression, miosis, apnea, pulmonary edema, and convulsions. Along with supportive measures, naloxone, 2 mg I.V. with repeat administration as necessary up to a total of 10 mg, can also be used to reverse toxic effects of the opiate.

Drug Interactions

Increased Effect/Toxicity: Effects may be additive with CNS depressants; hypotensive effects may be increased with phenothiazines; serotonergic effects may be additive with SSRIs

Decreased Effect: Hydromorphone may diminish the effects of pegvisomant.

Ethanol/Nutrition/Herb Interactions

Ethanol: Avoid ethanol (may increase CNS depression).

Herb/Nutraceutical: Avoid valerian, St John's wort, kava kava, gotu kola (may increase CNS depression).

Storage/Stability Store injection and oral dosage forms at 25°C (77°F). Protect tablets from light. A slightly yellowish discoloration has not been associated with a loss of potency.

Compatibility Stable in D_5LR, D_5W, $D_5^1/_2NS$, D_5NS, LR, $^1/_2NS$, NS

Y-site administration: Compatible: Acyclovir, allopurinol, amifostine, amikacin, amsacrine, aztreonam, cefamandole, cefepime, cefoperazone, cefotaxime, cefoxitin, ceftazidime, ceftizoxime, cefuroxime, chloramphenicol, cisatracurium, cisplatin, cladribine, clindamycin, cyclophosphamide, cytarabine, diltiazem, dobutamine, docetaxel, dopamine, doxorubicin, doxorubicin liposome, doxycycline, epinephrine, erythromycin lactobionate, etoposide, famotidine, fentanyl, filgrastim, fludarabine, foscarnet, furosemide, gatifloxacin, gemcitabine, gentamicin, granisetron, heparin, kanamycin, labetalol, linezolid, lorazepam, magnesium sulfate, melphalan, methotrexate, metronidazole, midazolam, milrinone, morphine, nafcillin, nicardipine, nitroglycerin, norepinephrine, ondansetron, oxacillin, paclitaxel, penicillin G potassium, piperacillin, piperacillin/tazobactam, propofol, ranitidine, remifentanil, tacrolimus, teniposide, thiotepa, ticarcillin, tobramycin, trimethoprim/sulfamethoxazole, vancomycin, vecuronium, vinorelbine. **Incompatible:** Amphotericin B cholesteryl sulfate complex, diazepam, minocycline, phenobarbital, phenytoin, sargramostim, tetracycline, thiopental. **Variable (consult detailed reference):** Ampicillin, cefazolin

Compatibility in syringe: Compatible: Albuterol, atropine, bupivacaine, ceftazidime, chlorpromazine, cimetidine, dimenhydrinate, diphenhydramine, fentanyl, glycopyrrolate, haloperidol, hydroxyzine, lorazepam, midazolam, pentazocine, pentobarbital, prochlorperazine mesylate, promethazine, ranitidine, scopolamine, thiethylperazine, trimethobenzamide. **Incompatible:** Ampicillin, diazepam, hyaluronidase, phenobarbital, phenytoin. **Variable (consult detailed reference):** Cefazolin, dexamethasone sodium phosphate, ketorolac, prochlorperazine edisylate

Compatibility when admixed: Compatible: Bupivacaine, fluorouracil, midazolam, ondansetron, promethazine, verapamil. **Incompatible:** Sodium bicarbonate, thiopental. **Variable (consult detailed reference):** Tetracaine

Pharmacodynamics/Kinetics

Onset of action: Analgesic: Immediate release formulations:
Oral: 15-30 minutes
Peak effect: Oral: 30-60 minutes
Duration: Immediate release formulations: 4-5 hours
Absorption: I.M.: Variable and delayed; Palladone™: Biphasic
Distribution: V_d: 4 L/kg
Protein binding: ~20%
Metabolism: Hepatic; to inactive metabolites
Bioavailability: 62%
Half-life elimination:
Immediate release formulations: 1-3 hours
Palladone™: 18.6 hours
Excretion: Urine (primarily as glucuronide conjugates)

Dosage

Acute pain (moderate to severe): **Note:** These are guidelines and do not represent the maximum doses that may be required in all patients. Doses should be titrated to pain relief/prevention.

Young Children ≥6 months and <50 kg:
Oral: 0.03-0.08 mg/kg/dose every 3-4 hours as needed
I.V.: 0.015 mg/kg/dose every 3-6 hours as needed
Older Children >50 kg and Adults:
Oral: Initial: Opiate-naive: 2-4 mg every 3-4 hours as needed; patients with prior opiate exposure may require higher initial doses; usual dosage range: 2-8 mg every 3-4 hours as needed
I.V.: Initial: Opiate-naive: 0.2-0.6 mg every 2-3 hours as needed; patients with prior opiate exposure may tolerate higher initial doses
Note: More frequent dosing may be needed.

(Continued)

Hydromorphone *(Continued)*

Mechanically-ventilated patients (based on 70 kg patient): 0.7-2 mg every 1-2 hours as needed; infusion (based on 70 kg patient): 0.5-1 mg/hour

Patient-controlled analgesia (PCA): (Opiate-naive: Consider lower end of dosing range)

Usual concentration: 0.2 mg/mL

Demand dose: Usual: 0.1-0.2 mg; range: 0.05-0.5 mg

Lockout interval: 5-15 minutes

4-hour limit: 4-6 mg

Epidural:

Bolus dose: 1-1.5 mg

Infusion concentration: 0.05-0.075 mg/mL

Infusion rate: 0.04-0.4 mg/hour

Demand dose: 0.15 mg

Lockout interval: 30 minutes

I.M., SubQ: **Note:** I.M. use may result in variable absorption and a lag time to peak effect.

Initial: Opiate-naive: 0.8-1 mg every 4-6 hours as needed; patients with prior opiate exposure may require higher initial doses; usual dosage range: 1-2 mg every 3-6 hours as needed

Rectal: 3 mg every 4-8 hours as needed

Chronic pain: Adults: Oral: **Note:** Patients taking opioids chronically may become tolerant and require doses higher than the usual dosage range to maintain the desired effect. Tolerance can be managed by appropriate dose titration. There is no optimal or maximal dose for hydromorphone in chronic pain. The appropriate dose is one that relieves pain throughout its dosing interval without causing unmanageable side effects.

Controlled release formulation (Hydromorph Contin®, not available in U.S.): 3-30 mg every 12 hours. **Note:** A patient's hydromorphone requirement should be established using prompt release formulations; conversion to long acting products may be considered when chronic, continuous treatment is required. Higher dosages should be reserved for use only in opioid-tolerant patients.

Extended release formulation (Palladone™): For use only in opioid-tolerant patients requiring extended treatment of pain. Initial Palladone™ dose should be calculated using standard conversion estimates based on previous total daily opioid dose, rounding off to the most appropriate strength available. Doses should be administered once every 24 hours. Discontinue all previous around-the-clock opioids when treatment is initiated. Dose may be adjusted every 2 days as needed.

Conversion from transdermal fentanyl to oral Palladone™ (limited clinical experience): Initiate Palladone™ 18 hours after removal of patch; substitute Palladone™ 12 mg/day for each fentanyl 50 mcg/hour patch; monitor closely

Conversion from opioid combination drugs: Initial dose: Palladone™ 12 mg/day in patients receiving around-the-clock fixed combination-opioid analgesics with a total dose greater than or equal to oxycodone 45 mg/day, hydrocodone 45 mg/day, or codeine 300 mg/day

Antitussive (unlabeled use): Oral:

Children 6-12 years: 0.5 mg every 3-4 hours as needed

Children >12 years and Adults: 1 mg every 3-4 hours as needed

Dosing adjustment in hepatic impairment: Should be considered

Administration

Parenteral: May be given SubQ or I.M.; for IVP, must be given slowly over 2-3 minutes (rapid IVP has been associated with an increase in side effects, especially respiratory depression and hypotension). Vial stopper contains latex.

Oral: Capsule should be swallowed whole; do not crush or chew; contents may be sprinkled on soft food and swallowed

Dosage Forms [CAN] = Canadian brand name

Capsule, controlled release (Hydromorph Contin®) [CAN]: 3 mg, 6 mg, 12 mg, 18 mg, 24 mg, 30 mg [not available in U.S.]

Capsule, extended release, as hydrochloride (Palladone™): 12 mg, 16 mg, 24 mg, 32 mg

Injection, powder for reconstitution, as hydrochloride (Dilaudid-HP®): 250 mg

Injection, solution, as hydrochloride: 1 mg/mL (1 mL); 2 mg/mL (1 mL, 20 mL); 4 mg/mL (1 mL); 10 mg/mL (1 mL, 5 mL, 10 mL)

Dilaudid®: 1 mg/mL (1 mL); 2 mg/mL (1 mL, 20 mL) [20 mL size contains edetate sodium; vial stopper contains latex]; 4 mg/mL (1 mL)

Dilaudid-HP®: 10 mg/mL (1 mL, 5 mL, 50 mL)

Liquid, oral, as hydrochloride (Dilaudid®): 1 mg/mL (480 mL) [may contain trace amounts of sodium bisulfite]

Suppository, rectal, as hydrochloride (Dilaudid®): 3 mg (6s)

Tablet, as hydrochloride (Dilaudid®): 2 mg, 4 mg, 8 mg (8 mg tablets may contain trace amounts of sodium bisulfite)

Monitoring Parameters Pain relief, respiratory and mental status, blood pressure

Patient Information May cause drowsiness; avoid alcohol; take with food or milk to minimize GI distress

Additional Information Equianalgesic doses: Morphine 10 mg I.M. = hydromorphone 1.5 mg I.M.

Special Geriatric Considerations Elderly may be particularly susceptible to the CNS depressant and constipating effects of narcotics.

Selected Readings

Agency for Health Care Policy and Research, "Acute Pain Management in Infants, Children and Adolescents: Operative and Medical Procedures," *Am Fam Physician*, 1992, 46(2):469-79.

"Clinical Practice Guidelines for the Sustained Use of Sedatives and Analgesics in the Critically Ill Adult. Task Force of the American College of Critical Care Medicine (ACCM) of the Society of Critical Care Medicine (SCCM), American Society of Health-System Pharmacists (ASHP), American College of Chest Physicians," *Am J Health Syst Pharm*, 2002, 59(2):150-78.

"Drugs for Pain," *Med Lett Drugs Ther*, 2000, 42(1085):73-8.

Ferrell BA, "Pain Management in Elderly People," *J Am Geriatr Soc*, 1991, 39(1):64-73.

Honigberg IL, and Stewart JT, "Radioimmunoassay of Hydromorphone and Hydrocodone in Human Plasma," *J Pharm Sci*, 1980, 69(10):1171-3.

Inturrisi CE, "Narcotic Drugs," *Med Clin North Am*, 1982, 66(5):1061-71.

Jacobi J, Fraser GL, Coursin DB, et al, "Clinical Practice Guidelines for the Sustained Use of Sedatives and Analgesics in the Critically Ill Adult," *Crit Care Med*, 2002, 30(1):119-41. Available at: http://www.sccm.org/pdf/sedatives.pdf. Accessed August 2, 2003.

Kaiko RF, Wallenstein SL, Rogers AG, et al, "Narcotics in the Elderly," *Med Clin North Am*, 1982, 66(5):1079-89.

(Continued)

Hydromorphone *(Continued)*

Levy MH, "Pharmacologic Treatment of Cancer Pain," *N Engl J Med*, 1996, 335(15):1124-32.

Mokhlesi B, Leikin JB, Murray P, et al, "Adult Toxicology in Critical Care: Part II: Specific Poisonings," *Chest*, 2003, 123(3):897-922.

Nasraway SA, "Use of Sedative Medications in the Intensive Care Unit," *Sem Resp Crit Care Med*, 2001, 22(2):165-74.

"Principles of Analgesic Use in the Treatment of Acute Pain and Cancer Pain," 4th ed, Glenview, IL: American Pain Society, 1999.

+ **Hydromorphone HP (Can)** *see* Hydromorphone *on page 426*
+ **Hydromorphone Hydrochloride** *see* Hydromorphone *on page 426*
+ **HydroVal® (Can)** *see* Hydrocortisone *on page 419*
+ **Hydroxycarbamide** *see* Hydroxyurea *on page 432*
+ **Hydroxydaunomycin Hydrochloride** *see* DOXOrubicin *on page 280*
+ **Hydroxyldaunorubicin Hydrochloride** *see* DOXOrubicin *on page 280*

Hydroxyurea (hye droks ee yoor EE a)

Medication Safety Issues

Sound-alike/look-alike issues:

Hydroxyurea may be confused with hydrOXYzine

Related Information

Safe Handling of Hazardous Drugs *on page 1034*

U.S. Brand Names Droxia™; Hydrea®; Mylocel™

Canadian Brand Names Gen-Hydroxyurea; Hydrea®

Generic Available Yes: Capsule

Synonyms Hydroxycarbamide

Pharmacologic Category Antineoplastic Agent, Antimetabolite

Pregnancy Risk Factor D

Lactation Enters breast milk/contraindicated

Use CML in chronic phase; radiosensitizing agent in the treatment of primary brain tumors, head and neck tumors, uterine cervix and nonsmall cell lung cancer, and psoriasis; treatment of hematologic conditions such as essential thrombocythemia, polycythemia vera, hypereosinophilia, and hyperleukocytosis due to acute leukemia. Has shown activity against renal cell cancer, melanoma, ovarian cancer, head and neck cancer (excluding lip cancer), and prostate cancer.

Orphan drug: Droxia™: Sickle cell anemia: Specifically for patients >18 years of age who have had at least three "painful crises" in the previous year - to reduce frequency of these crises and the need for blood transfusions

Unlabeled/Investigational Use Treatment of HIV; treatment of psoriasis

Mechanism of Action Thought to interfere (unsubstantiated hypothesis) with synthesis of DNA, during the S phase of cell division, without interfering with RNA synthesis; inhibits ribonucleoside diphosphate reductase, preventing conversion of ribonucleotides to deoxyribonucleotides; cell-cycle specific for the S phase and may hold other cells in the G_1 phase of the cell cycle.

Labeled Contraindications Hypersensitivity to hydroxyurea or any component of the formulation; severe anemia; severe bone marrow suppression; WBC <2500/mm^3 or platelet count <100,000/mm^3; pregnancy

Warnings/Precautions Use with caution in patients with renal impairment, in patients who have received prior irradiation therapy with exacerbation of postirradiation erythema, bone marrow suppression, erythrocytic abnormalities, mucositis, and in the elderly. The U.S. Food and Drug Administration (FDA) currently recommends that procedures for proper handling and disposal of antineoplastic agents be considered. May cause pancreatitis, neuropathy, or hepatotoxicity; risk is increased in HIV-infected patients receiving didanosine and/or stavudine. Secondary leukemias have been reported with long-term use.

Adverse Reactions Frequency not defined.

Cardiovascular: Edema

Central nervous system: Drowsiness (with high doses), hallucinations, headache, dizziness, disorientation, seizure, fever, chills

Dermatologic: Erythema of the hands and face, maculopapular rash, pruritus, dry skin, dermatomyositis-like skin changes, hyperpigmentation, atrophy of skin and nails, scaling and violet papules (long-term use), nail banding, skin cancer

Endocrine & metabolic: Hyperuricemia

Gastrointestinal: Nausea, vomiting, stomatitis, anorexia, diarrhea, constipation, mucositis (potentiated in patients receiving radiation), pancreatitis, ulceration of buccal mucosa and GI epithelium (severe intoxication)

Emetic potential: Low (10% to 30%)

Genitourinary: Dysuria

Hematologic: Myelosuppression (primarily leukopenia); Dose-limiting toxicity, causes a rapid drop in leukocyte count (seen in 4-5 days in nonhematologic malignancy and more rapidly in leukemia); thrombocytopenia and anemia occur less often

Onset: 24-48 hours

Nadir: 10 days

Recovery: 7 days after stopping drug (reversal of WBC count occurs rapidly but the platelet count may take 7-10 days to recover)

Other hematologic effects include megaloblastic erythropoiesis, macrocytosis, hemolysis, decreased serum iron, persistent cytopenias, secondary leukemias (long-term use)

Hepatic: Elevation of hepatic enzymes, hepatotoxicity, hyperbilirubinemia (polycythemia vera)

Neuromuscular & skeletal: Weakness, peripheral neuropathy

Renal: Increased creatinine and BUN due to impairment of renal tubular function

Respiratory: Acute diffuse pulmonary infiltrates (rare), dyspnea, pulmonary fibrosis

Emetic Potential Low (10% to 30%)

Overdosage/Toxicology Symptoms of overdose include myelosuppression, facial swelling, hallucinations, and disorientation. Treatment is supportive.

Drug Interactions

Increased Effect/Toxicity: Zidovudine, zalcitabine, didanosine may increase synergy. The potential for neurotoxicity may increase with concomitant administration with fluorouracil. Hydroxyurea modulates the metabolism and cytotoxicity of cytarabine; dose reduction is recommended. Hydroxyurea may precipitate didanosine- or

(Continued)

Hydroxyurea *(Continued)*

stavudine-induced pancreatitis, hepatotoxicity, or neuropathy; concomitant use is not recommended.

Storage/Stability Store capsules at room temperature. Capsules may be opened and emptied into water (will not dissolve completely).

Pharmacodynamics/Kinetics

Absorption: Readily ($\geq$80%)

Distribution: Readily crosses blood-brain barrier; well into intestine, brain, lung, kidney tissues, effusions and ascites; enters breast milk

Metabolism: Hepatic and via GI tract; 50% degradation by enzymes of intestinal bacteria

Half-life elimination: 3-4 hours

Time to peak: ~2 hours

Excretion: Urine (80%, 50% as unchanged drug, 30% as urea); exhaled gases (as CO_2)

Dosage Oral (refer to individual protocols): All dosage should be based on ideal or actual body weight, whichever is less:

Children:

No FDA-approved dosage regimens have been established; dosages of 1500-3000 mg/m^2 as a single dose in combination with other agents every 4-6 weeks have been used in the treatment of pediatric astrocytoma, medulloblastoma, and primitive neuroectodermal tumors

CML: Initial: 10-20 mg/kg/day once daily; adjust dose according to hematologic response

Adults: Dose should always be titrated to patient response and WBC counts; usual oral doses range from 10-30 mg/kg/day or 500-3000 mg/day; if WBC count falls to <2500 cells/mm^3, or the platelet count to <100,000/mm^3, therapy should be stopped for at least 3 days and resumed when values rise toward normal

Solid tumors:

Intermittent therapy: 80 mg/kg as a single dose every third day

Continuous therapy: 20-30 mg/kg/day given as a single dose/day

Concomitant therapy with irradiation: 80 mg/kg as a single dose every third day starting at least 7 days before initiation of irradiation

Resistant chronic myelocytic leukemia: Continuous therapy: 20-30 mg/kg as a single daily dose

HIV (unlabeled use; in combination with antiretroviral agents): 1000-1500 mg daily in a single dose or divided doses

Psoriasis (unlabeled use): 1000-1500 mg/day in a single dose or divided doses

Sickle cell anemia (moderate/severe disease): Initial: 15 mg/kg/day, increased by 5 mg/kg every 12 weeks if blood counts are in an acceptable range until the maximum tolerated dose of 35 mg/kg/day is achieved or the dose that does not produce toxic effects

Acceptable range:

Neutrophils $\geq$2500 cells/mm^3

Platelets $\geq$95,000/mm^3

Hemoglobin >5.3 g/dL, and

Reticulocytes $\geq$95,000/mm^3 if the hemoglobin concentration is <9 g/dL

Toxic range:

Neutrophils <2000 cells/mm^3

Platelets <80,000/mm³
Hemoglobin <4.5 g/dL
Reticulocytes <80,000/mm³ if the hemoglobin concentration is <9 g/dL
Monitor for toxicity every 2 weeks; if toxicity occurs, stop treatment until the bone marrow recovers; restart at 2.5 mg/kg/day less than the dose at which toxicity occurs; if no toxicity occurs over the next 12 weeks, then the subsequent dose should be increased by 2.5 mg/kg/day; reduced dosage of hydroxyurea alternating with erythropoietin may decrease myelotoxicity and increase levels of fetal hemoglobin in patients who have not been helped by hydroxyurea alone

Dosing adjustment in renal impairment:
Sickle cell anemia: Cl_{cr} <60 mL/minute or ESRD: Reduce initial dose to 7.5 mg/kg; titrate to response/avoidance of toxicity (refer to usual dosing)
Other indications:
Cl_{cr} 10-50 mL/minute: Administer 50% of normal dose
Cl_{cr} <10 mL/minute: Administer 20% of normal dose
Hemodialysis: Supplemental dose is not necessary. Hydroxyurea is a low molecular weight compound with high aqueous solubility that may be freely dialyzable, however, clinical studies confirming this hypothesis have not been performed; peak serum concentrations are reached within 2 hours after oral administration and by 24 hours, the concentration in the serum is zero
CAPD effects: Unknown
CAVH effects: Dose for GFR 10-50 mL/minute

Combination Regimens
Brain tumors: 8 in 1 (Brain Tumors) *on page 841*
Gestational trophoblastic tumor: CHAMOCA *on page 858*
Head and neck cancer: FU HURT *on page 893*
Neuroblastoma: N4SE Protocol *on page 922*
Retinoblastoma: 8 in 1 (Retinoblastoma) *on page 842*

Administration Capsules may be opened and emptied into water (will not dissolve completely).

Dosage Forms
Capsule: 500 mg
Droxia™: 200 mg, 300 mg, 400 mg
Hydrea®: 500 mg
Tablet (Mylocel™): 1000 mg

Monitoring Parameters CBC with differential, platelets, hemoglobin, renal function and liver function tests, serum uric acid

Patient Information Take capsules exactly on schedule directed by prescriber (dosage and timing will be specific to purpose of therapy). Contents of capsule may be emptied into a glass of water and taken immediately. You will require frequent monitoring and blood tests while taking this medication to assess effectiveness and monitor adverse reactions. You will be susceptible to infection; avoid crowds, infected persons, and persons with contagious diseases. You may experience nausea, vomiting, or loss of appetite (small frequent meals, frequent mouth care, sucking lozenges, or chewing gum may help); constipation (increased exercise, fluid, or dietary fiber may help); diarrhea (buttermilk, boiled milk, or yogurt may help); mouth sores (frequent mouth care will help). Report
(Continued)

435

Hydroxyurea *(Continued)*

persistent vomiting, diarrhea, constipation, stomach pain, or mouth sores; skin rash, redness, irritation, or sores; painful or difficult urination; increased confusion, depression, hallucinations, lethargy, or seizures; persistent fever or chills, unusual fatigue, white plaques in mouth, vaginal discharge, or unhealed sores; unusual lassitude, weakness, or muscle tremors; easy bruising/bleeding; or blood in vomitus, stool, or urine. People not taking hydroxyurea should not be exposed to it; if powder from capsule is spilled, wipe up with damp, disposable towel immediately, and discard the towel in a closed container, such as a plastic bag; wash hands thoroughly. Contraceptive measures are recommended during therapy.

Additional Information Although I.V. use is reported, no parenteral product is commercially available in the U.S.

If WBC decreases to <2500/mm^3 or platelet count to <100,000/mm^3, interrupt therapy until values rise significantly toward normal. Treat anemia with whole blood replacement; do not interrupt therapy. Adequate trial period to determine effectiveness is 6 weeks. Almost all patients receiving hydroxyurea in clinical trials needed to have their medication stopped for a time to allow their low blood count to return to acceptable levels.

Special Geriatric Considerations Elderly may be more sensitive to the effects of this drug. Advance dose slowly and adjust dose for renal function with careful monitoring.

Selected Readings

Donehower RC, "An Overview of the Clinical Experience With Hydroxyurea," *Semin Oncol*, 1992, 19(3 Suppl 9):11-9.

Gwilt PR and Tracewell WG, "Pharmacokinetics and Pharmacodynamics of Hydroxyurea," *Clin Pharmacokinet*, 1998, 34(5):347-58.

Navarra P and Preziosi P, "Hydroxyurea: New Insights on an Old Drug," *Crit Rev Oncol Hematol*, 1999, 29(3):249-55.

Stevens MR, "Hydroxyurea: An Overview," *J Biol Regul Homeost Agents*, 1999, 13(3):172-5.

Timson J, "Hydroxyurea," *Mutat Res*, 1975, 32(2):115-32.

Yarboro JW, "Mechanism of Action of Hydroxyurea," *Semin Oncol*, 1992, 19(3 Suppl 9):1-10.

HydrOXYzine *(hye DROKS i zeen)*

Medication Safety Issues

Sound-alike/look-alike issues:

HydrOXYzine may be confused with hydrALAZINE, hydroxyurea

Atarax® may be confused with amoxicillin, Ativan®

Vistaril® may be confused with Restoril®, Versed, Zestril®

Related Information

Management of Nausea and Vomiting *on page 982*

U.S. Brand Names Atarax®; Vistaril®

Canadian Brand Names Apo-Hydroxyzine®; Atarax®; Novo-Hydroxyzin; PMS-Hydroxyzine; Vistaril®

Generic Available Yes

Synonyms Hydroxyzine Hydrochloride; Hydroxyzine Pamoate

Pharmacologic Category Antiemetic; Antihistamine

Pregnancy Risk Factor C

Lactation Enters breast milk/contraindicated

Use Treatment of anxiety; preoperative sedative; antipruritic

Unlabeled/Investigational Use Antiemetic; ethanol withdrawal symptoms

Mechanism of Action Competes with histamine for H_1-receptor sites on effector cells in the gastrointestinal tract, blood vessels, and respiratory tract. Possesses skeletal muscle relaxing, bronchodilator, antihistamine, antiemetic, and analgesic properties.

Labeled Contraindications Hypersensitivity to hydroxyzine or any component of the formulation; early pregnancy

Warnings/Precautions Causes sedation, caution must be used in performing tasks which require alertness (eg, operating machinery or driving). Sedative effects of CNS depressants or ethanol are potentiated. SubQ and intra-arterial are not recommended since thrombosis and digital gangrene can occur; should be used with caution in patients with narrow-angle glaucoma, prostatic hyperplasia, and bladder neck obstruction; should also be used with caution in patients with asthma or COPD. Not recommended for use as a sedative or anxiolytic in the elderly.

Adverse Reactions Frequency not defined.

Central nervous system: Drowsiness, headache, fatigue, nervousness, dizziness, hallucination

Dermatologic: Pruritus, rash, urticaria

Gastrointestinal: Xerostomia

Neuromuscular & skeletal: Tremor, paresthesia, seizure, involuntary movements

Ocular: Blurred vision

Respiratory: Thickening of bronchial secretions

Miscellaneous: Allergic reaction

Vesicant No; may be an irritant

Emetic Potential Very low (<10%)

Overdosage/Toxicology Symptoms of overdose include seizures, sedation, and hypotension. There is no specific treatment for antihistamine overdose. Clinical toxicity is due to blockade of cholinergic receptors. For anticholinergic overdose with severe life-threatening symptoms, physostigmine 1-2 mg I.V. slowly, may be given to reverse these effects.

Drug Interactions

Cytochrome P450 Effect: Inhibits CYP2D6 (weak)

Increased Effect/Toxicity: CNS depressants, anticholinergics, used in combination with hydroxyzine may result in additive effects.

Ethanol/Nutrition/Herb Interactions

Ethanol: Avoid ethanol (may increase CNS depression).

Herb/Nutraceutical: Avoid valerian, St John's wort, kava kava, gotu kola (may increase CNS depression).

Storage/Stability Protect from light. Store at 15°C to 30°C and protected from freezing.

Reconstitution I.V.: Dilute in 50-250 mL NS or D_5W

Compatibility

Y-site administration: Compatible: Aztreonam, ciprofloxacin, cisatracurium, cladribine, docetaxel, etoposide phosphate, famotidine, filgrastim, foscarnet, gatifloxacin, gemcitabine, granisetron, linezolid, melphalan, ondansetron, propofol, remifentanil, sufentanil, teniposide, thiotepa, vinorelbine. **Incompatible:** Allopurinol, amifostine, amphotericin B cholesteryl sulfate complex, cefepime, doxorubicin liposome, fluconazole, fludarabine, paclitaxel, piperacillin/tazobactam, sargramostim

(Continued)

HydrOXYzine *(Continued)*

Compatibility in syringe: Compatible: Atropine, atropine with meperidine, butorphanol, chlorpromazine, cimetidine, codeine, diphenhydramine, doxapram, droperidol, fentanyl, fluphenazine, glycopyrrolate, hydromorphone, lidocaine, meperidine, methotrimeprazine, metoclopramide, midazolam, morphine, nalbuphine, oxymorphone, pentazocine, perphenazine, procaine, prochlorperazine edisylate, promazine, promethazine, scopolamine, sufentanil. **Incompatible:** Dimenhydrinate, haloperidol, ketorolac, pentobarbital, ranitidine

Compatibility when admixed: Compatible: Cisplatin, cyclophosphamide, cytarabine, dimenhydrinate, etoposide, lidocaine, mesna, methotrexate, nafcillin. **Incompatible:** Aminophylline, amobarbital, chloramphenicol, penicillin G potassium, penicillin G sodium, pentobarbital, phenobarbital

Pharmacodynamics/Kinetics

Onset of action: 15-30 minutes
Duration: 4-6 hours
Absorption: Oral: Rapid
Metabolism: Exact fate unknown
Half-life elimination: 3-7 hours
Time to peak: ~2 hours

Dosage

Children:
Preoperative sedation:
Oral: 0.6 mg/kg/dose every 6 hours
I.M.: 0.5-1.1 mg/kg/dose every 4-6 hours as needed
Manufacturer labeling: Pruritus, anxiety:
<6 years: 50 mg daily in divided doses
≥6 years: 50-100 mg daily in divided doses
Adults:
Antiemetic: I.M.: 25-100 mg/dose every 4-6 hours as needed
Anxiety: Oral: 25-100 mg 4 times/day; maximum dose: 600 mg/day
Preoperative sedation:
Oral: 50-100 mg
I.M.: 25-100 mg
Management of pruritus: Oral: 25 mg 3-4 times/day

Dosing interval in hepatic impairment: Change dosing interval to every 24 hours in patients with primary biliary cirrhosis

Administration
Do not give SubQ or intra-arterial.
I.M., I.V.: Not generally recommended. May be given as a short (30-60 minutes) infusion.

Dosage Forms [DSC] = Discontinued product

Capsule, as pamoate (Vistaril®): 25 mg, 50 mg, 100 mg
Injection, solution, as hydrochloride: 25 mg/mL (1 mL); 50 mg/mL (1 mL, 2 mL, 10 mL)
Suspension, oral, as pamoate (Vistaril®): 25 mg/5 mL (120 mL, 480 mL) [lemon flavor]
Syrup, as hydrochloride: 10 mg/5 mL (120 mL, 480 mL)
Atarax®: 10 mg/5 mL (480 mL) [contains alcohol, sodium benzoate; mint flavor] [DSC]
Tablet, as hydrochloride: 10 mg, 25 mg, 50 mg
Atarax®: 10 mg, 25 mg, 50 mg, 100 mg [DSC]

Monitoring Parameters Relief of symptoms, mental status, blood pressure

Patient Information Will cause drowsiness, avoid alcohol and other CNS depressants, avoid driving and other hazardous tasks until the CNS effects are known

Additional Information

Hydroxyzine hydrochloride: Atarax®, Vistaril® injection

Hydroxyzine pamoate: Vistaril® capsule and suspension

Special Geriatric Considerations Anticholinergic effects are not well tolerated in the elderly. Hydroxyzine may be useful as a short-term antipruritic, but it is not recommended for use as a sedative or anxiolytic in the elderly.

Selected Readings

Simons FE, Simons KJ, and Frith EM, "The Pharmacokinetics and Antihistaminic of the H₁ Receptor Antagonist Hydroxyzine," *J Allergy Clin Immunol*, 1984, 73(1 Pt 1):69-75.

Simons KJ, Watson WT, Chen XY, et al, "Pharmacokinetic and Pharmacodynamic Studies of the H₁-Receptor Antagonist Hydroxyzine in the Elderly," *Clin Pharmacol Ther*, 1989, 45(1):9-14.

◆ **Hydroxyzine Hydrochloride** *see* HydrOXYzine *on page 436*

◆ **Hydroxyzine Pamoate** *see* HydrOXYzine *on page 436*

◆ **HydroZone Plus [OTC]** *see* Hydrocortisone *on page 419*

◆ **Hytone®** *see* Hydrocortisone *on page 419*

◆ **131 I Anti-B1 Antibody** *see* Tositumomab and Iodine I 131 Tositumomab *on page 781*

◆ **131 I-Anti-B1 Monoclonal Antibody** *see* Tositumomab and Iodine I 131 Tositumomab *on page 781*

Ibritumomab (ib ri TYOO mo mab)

U.S. Brand Names Zevalin™

Generic Available No

Synonyms Ibritumomab Tiuxetan; In-111 Zevalin; Y-90 Zevalin

Pharmacologic Category Antineoplastic Agent, Monoclonal Antibody; Radiopharmaceutical

Pregnancy Risk Factor D

Lactation Excretion in breast milk unknown/contraindicated

Use Treatment of relapsed or refractory low-grade, follicular, or transformed B-cell non-Hodgkin's lymphoma

Mechanism of Action Ibritumomab is a monoclonal antibody directed against the CD20 antigen found on B lymphocytes (normal and malignant). Ibritumomab binding induces apoptosis in B lymphocytes *in vitro*. It is combined with the chelator tiuxetan, which acts as a specific chelation site for either Indium-111 (In-111) or Yttrium-90 (Y-90). The monoclonal antibody acts as a delivery system to direct the radioactive isotope to the targeted cells, however, binding has been observed in lymphoid cells throughout the body and in lymphoid nodules in organs such as the large and small intestines. Indium-111 is a gamma-emitter used to assess biodistribution of ibritumomab, while Y-90 emits beta particles. Beta-emission induces cellular damage through the formation of free radicals (in both target cells and surrounding cells).

Labeled Contraindications Known type I hypersensitivity or anaphylactic reactions to murine proteins, rituximab, yttrium chloride, indium chloride, or any component of the formulation; ≥25% lymphoma marrow involvement; prior myeloablative therapies; platelet count <100,000 cells/mm³; (Continued)

Ibritumomab *(Continued)*

neutrophil count <1500 cells/mm3; hypocellular bone marrow (≤15% cellularity of marked reduction in bone marrow precursors); history of failed stem cell collection; pregnancy; breast-feeding. Y-90 ibritumomab should not be administered to patients with altered In-111 ibritumomab biodistribution.

Warnings/Precautions To be used as part of the Zevalin™ therapeutic regimen (in combination with rituximab). The contents of the kit are not radioactive until radiolabeling occurs. During and after radiolabeling, adequate shielding should be used with this product, in accordance with institutional radiation safety practices.

Severe, potentially-fatal infusion reactions (angioedema, bronchospasm, hypotension, hypoxia) have been reported, typically during the first rituximab infusion (during infusion or within 30-120 minutes of infusion). Patients should be screened for human antimouse antibodies (HAMA); may be at increased risk of allergic or serious hypersensitivity reactions.

Safety and efficacy of repeated courses of the therapeutic regimen have not been established. Safety and efficacy have not been established in pediatric patients.

Adverse Reactions Severe, potentially life-threatening allergic reactions have occurred in association with infusions. Also refer to Rituximab monograph.

>10%:

Central nervous system: Chills (24%), fever (17%), pain (13%), headache (12%)

Gastrointestinal: Nausea (31%), abdominal pain (16%), vomiting (12%)

Hematologic: Thrombocytopenia (95%), neutropenia (77%), anemia (61%)

Myelosuppressive:
WBC: Severe
Platelets: Severe
Nadir: 7-9 weeks
Recovery: 22-35 days

Neuromuscular & skeletal: Weakness (43%)

Respiratory: Dyspnea (14%)

Miscellaneous: Infection (29%)

1% to 10%:

Cardiovascular: Peripheral edema (8%), hypotension (6%), flushing (6%), angioedema (5%)

Central nervous system: Dizziness (10%), insomnia (5%), anxiety (4%)

Dermatologic: Pruritus (9%), rash (8%), urticaria (4%), petechia (3%)

Gastrointestinal: Diarrhea (9%), anorexia (8%), abdominal distension (5%), constipation (5%), dyspepsia (4%), melena (2%; life threatening in 1%), gastrointestinal hemorrhage (1%)

Hematologic: Bruising (7%), pancytopenia (2%), secondary malignancies (2%)

Neuromuscular & skeletal: Back pain (8%), arthralgia (7%), myalgia (7%)

Respiratory: Cough (10%), throat irritation (10%), rhinitis (6%), bronchospasm (5%), epistaxis (3%), apnea (1%)

Miscellaneous: Diaphoresis (4%), allergic reaction (2%; life-threatening in 1%)

<1%: Arthritis, encephalopathy, hematemesis, pulmonary edema, pulmonary embolism, stroke (hemorrhagic), subdural hematoma, tachycardia, urticaria, vaginal hemorrhage. Myeloid malignancies and dysplasia have also been reported in patients who had received treatment with ibritumomab.

Overdosage/Toxicology Symptoms may include severe hematological toxicity. Treatment is supportive. In early clinical experience with high dosages, some patients required autologous stem cell transplantation.

Drug Interactions

Increased Effect/Toxicity: Due to the high incidence of thrombocytopenia associated with ibritumomab, the use of agents which decrease platelet function may be associated with a higher risk of bleeding (includes aspirin, NSAIDs, glycoprotein IIb/IIIa antagonists, clopidogrel and ticlopidine). In addition, the risk of bleeding may be increased with anticoagulant agents, including heparin, low molecular weight heparins, thrombolytics, and warfarin. The safety of live viral vaccines has not been established.

Decreased Effect: Response to vaccination may be impaired.

Ethanol/Nutrition/Herb Interactions Herb/Nutraceutical: Avoid cat's claw, dong quai, evening primrose, feverfew, garlic, ginger, ginkgo, red clover, horse chestnut, green tea, ginseng (all have antiplatelet activity).

Storage/Stability Store at 2°C to 8°C (36°F to 46°F). Do not freeze. Kit is not radioactive.

Reconstitution To prepare radiolabeled injection, follow preparation guidelines provided by manufacturer.

Pharmacodynamics/Kinetics

Duration: Beta cell recovery begins in ~12 weeks; generally in normal range within 9 months

Distribution: To lymphoid cells throughout the body and in lymphoid nodules in organs such as the large and small intestines, spleen, testes, and liver

Metabolism: Has not been characterized; the product of yttrium-90 radioactive decay is zirconium-90 (nonradioactive); Indium-111 decays to cadmium-111 (nonradioactive)

Half-life elimination: Y-90 ibritumomab: 30 hours; Indium-111 decays with a physical half-life of 67 hours; Yttrium-90 decays with a physical half-life of 64 hours

Excretion: A median of 7.2% of the radiolabeled activity was excreted in urine over 7 days

Dosage I.V.: Adults: Ibritumomab is administered **only** as part of the Zevalin™ therapeutic regimen (a combined treatment regimen with rituximab). The regimen consists of two steps:

Step 1:

Rituximab infusion: 250 mg/m² at an initial rate of 50 mg/hour. If hypersensitivity or infusion-related events do not occur, increase infusion in increments of 50 mg/hour every 30 minutes, to a maximum of 400 mg/hour. Infusions should be temporarily slowed or interrupted if hypersensitivity or infusion-related events occur. The infusion may be resumed at one-half the previous rate upon improvement of symptoms.

In-111 ibritumomab infusion: Within 4 hours of the completion of rituximab infusion, inject 5 mCi (1.6 mg total antibody dose) over 10 minutes.

(Continued)

Ibritumomab *(Continued)*

Biodistribution of In-111 ibritumomab should be assessed by imaging at 2-24 hours and at 48-72 hours postinjection. An optional third imaging may be performed 90-120 hours following injection. If biodistribution is not acceptable, the patient should not proceed to Step 2.

Step 2 (initiated 7-9 days following Step 1):

Rituximab infusion: 250 mg/m^2 at an initial rate of 100 mg/hour (50 mg/hour if infusion-related events occurred with the first infusion). If hypersensitivity or infusion-related events do not occur, increase infusion in increments of 100 mg/hour every 30 minutes, to a maximum of 400 mg/hour, as tolerated.

Y-90 ibritumomab infusion: Within 4 hours of the completion of rituximab infusion:

Platelet count >150,000 cells/mm^3: Inject 0.4 mCi/kg (14.8 MBq/kg actual body weight) over 10 minutes

Platelet count between 100,000-149,000 cells/mm^3: Inject 0.3 mCi/kg (11.1 MBq/kg actual body weight) over 10 minutes

Platelet count <100,000 cells/mm^3: Do **not** administer

Maximum dose: The prescribed, measured, and administered dose of Y-90 ibritumomab must not exceed 32 mCi (1184 MBq), regardless of the patient's body weight

Administration Ibritumomab: Inject slowly, over 10 minutes.

Dosage Forms Each kit contains 4 vials for preparation of either In-111 or Y-90 conjugate (as indicated on container label)

Injection, solution: 1.6 mg/mL (2 mL) [supplied with sodium acetate solution, formulation buffer vial (includes albumin 750 mg), and an empty reaction vial]

Monitoring Parameters Human antimurine antibody (HAMA) prior to treatment (if positive, may have an allergic or hypersensitivity reaction when treated with this or other murine or chimeric monoclonal antibodies).

Patients must be monitored for infusion-related allergic reactions (typically within 30-120 minutes of administration). Obtain complete blood counts and platelet counts at regular intervals during rituximab therapy (at least weekly and more frequently in patients who develop cytopenia). Platelet count must be obtained prior to step 2. Monitor for up to 3 months after use.

Biodistribution of In-111 ibritumomab should be assessed by imaging at 2-24 hours and at 48-72 hours post injection. An optional third imaging may be performed 90-120 hours following injection. If biodistribution is not acceptable, the patient should not proceed to Step 2.

Additional Information Ibritumomab tiuxetan is produced in Chinese hamster ovary cell cultures. Kit is not radioactive. Radiolabeling of ibritumomab with Yttrium-90 and Indium-111 (not included in kit) must be performed by appropriate personnel in a specialized facility.

Selected Readings

Borghaei H and Schilder RJ, "Safety and Efficacy of Radioimmunotherapy With Yttrium 90 Ibritumomab Tiuxetan (Zevalin)," *Semin Nucl Med*, 2004, 34(1 Suppl 1):4-9.

Krasner C and Joyce RM, "Zevalin: 90yttrium Labeled Anti-CD20 (Ibritumomab Tiuxetan), a New Treatment for Non-Hodgkin's Lymphoma," *Curr Pharm Biotechnol*, 2001, 2(4):341-9.

Smith BE, "Ibritumomab Tiuxetan: The Cancer Smart Bomb," *J Am Pharm Assoc (Wash DC)*, 2003, 43(3):437-8.

Witzig TE, "Yttrium-90-Ibritumomab Tiuxetan Radioimmunotherapy: A New Treatment Approach for B-Cell Non-Hodgkin's Lymphoma," *Drugs Today (Barc)*, 2004, 40(2):111-9.

+ **Ibritumomab Tiuxetan** *see* Ibritumomab *on page 439*
+ **ICI-182,780** *see* Fulvestrant *on page 372*
+ **ICI-46474** *see* Tamoxifen *on page 743*
+ **ICI-118630** *see* Goserelin *on page 403*
+ **ICI-176334** *see* Bicalutamide *on page 131*
+ **ICI-D1033** *see* Anastrozole *on page 85*
+ **ICI-D1694** *see* Raltitrexed *on page 700*
+ **ICRF-187** *see* Dexrazoxane *on page 270*
+ **Idamycin® (Can)** *see* Idarubicin *on page 443*
+ **Idamycin PFS®** *see* Idarubicin *on page 443*

Idarubicin (eye da ROO bi sin)

Medication Safety Issues
Sound-alike/look-alike issues:
Idarubicin may be confused with DOXOrubicin
Idamycin PFS® may be confused with Adriamycin

Related Information
Safe Handling of Hazardous Drugs *on page 1034*

U.S. Brand Names Idamycin PFS®

Canadian Brand Names Idamycin®

Generic Available Yes

Synonyms 4-Demethoxydaunorubicin; 4-DMDR; Idarubicin Hydrochloride; IDR; IMI 30; NSC-256439; SC 33428

Pharmacologic Category Antineoplastic Agent, Anthracycline; Antineoplastic Agent, Antibiotic

Pregnancy Risk Factor D

Lactation Excretion in breast milk unknown

Use Treatment of acute leukemias (AML, ANLL, ALL), accelerated phase or blast crisis of chronic myelogenous leukemia (CML), breast cancer

Unlabeled/Investigational Use Autologous hematopoietic stem cell transplantation

Mechanism of Action Similar to doxorubicin and daunorubicin; inhibition of DNA and RNA synthesis by intercalation between DNA base pairs

Labeled Contraindications Hypersensitivity to idarubicin, other anthracyclines, or any component of the formulation; bilirubin >5 mg/dL; pregnancy

Warnings/Precautions Hazardous agent - use appropriate precautions for handling and disposal. See Safe Handling of Hazardous Drugs *on page 1034* in the Appendix. Can cause myocardial toxicity and is more common in patients who have previously received anthracyclines or have pre-existing cardiac disease; reduce dose in patients with impaired hepatic function.

Adverse Reactions
>10%:
Cardiovascular: Transient ECG abnormalities (supraventricular tachycardia, S-T wave changes, atrial or ventricular extrasystoles); generally asymptomatic and self-limiting. CHF, dose related. The relative cardiotoxicity of idarubicin compared to doxorubicin is unclear. Some
(Continued)

Idarubicin *(Continued)*

investigators report no increase in cardiac toxicity at cumulative oral idarubicin doses up to 540 mg/m^2; other reports suggest a maximum cumulative intravenous dose of 150 mg/m^2.

Central nervous system: Headache

Dermatologic: Alopecia (25% to 30%), radiation recall, skin rash (11%), urticaria

Gastrointestinal: Nausea, vomiting (30% to 60%); diarrhea (9% to 22%); stomatitis (11%); GI hemorrhage (30%)

Genitourinary: Discoloration of urine (darker yellow)

Hematologic: Myelosuppression, primarily leukopenia; thrombocytopenia and anemia. Effects are generally less severe with oral dosing.
Nadir: 10-15 days
Recovery: 21-28 days

Hepatic: Bilirubin and transaminases increased (44%)

1% to 10%:
Central nervous system: Seizures
Neuromuscular & skeletal: Peripheral neuropathy

<1%: Hyperuricemia

Vesicant Yes; see Management of Drug Extravasations *on page 965.*

Emetic Potential Moderate (30% to 60%)

Overdosage/Toxicology Symptoms of overdose include severe myelosuppression and increased GI toxicity. Treatment is supportive. It is unlikely that therapeutic efficacy or toxicity would be altered by conventional peritoneal or hemodialysis.

Drug Interactions

Decreased Effect: Patients may experience impaired immune response to vaccines; possible infection after administration of live vaccines in patients receiving immunosuppressants.

Storage/Stability Store intact vials of solution under refrigeration (2°C to 8°C/36°F to 46°F). Protect from light. Solutions diluted in D$_5$W or NS for infusion are stable for 4 weeks at room temperature, protected from light. Syringe and IVPB solutions are stable for 72 hours at room temperature and 7 days under refrigeration.

Compatibility Stable in D$_5$NS, D$_5$W, LR, NS, sterile water for injection, not stable in bacteriostatic water

Y-site administration: Compatible: Amifostine, amikacin, aztreonam, cimetidine, cladribine, cyclophosphamide, cytarabine, diphenhydramine, droperidol, erythromycin lactobionate, etoposide phosphate, filgrastim, gemcitabine, granisetron, imipenem/cilastatin, magnesium sulfate, mannitol, melphalan, metoclopramide, potassium chloride, ranitidine, sargramostim, thiotepa, vinorelbine. **Incompatible:** Acyclovir, allopurinol, ampicillin/sulbactam, cefazolin, cefepime, ceftazidime, clindamycin, dexamethasone sodium phosphate, etoposide, fluorouracil, furosemide, gentamicin, heparin, hydrocortisone sodium succinate, lorazepam, meperidine, methotrexate, piperacillin/tazobactam, sodium bicarbonate, teniposide, vancomycin, vincristine

Compatibility when admixed: Incompatible: Heparin

Pharmacodynamics/Kinetics

Absorption: Oral: Variable (4% to 77%; mean: ~30%)

Distribution: V$_d$: 64 L/kg (some reports indicate 2250 L); extensive tissue binding; CSF

Protein binding: 94% to 97%

Metabolism: Hepatic to idarubicinol (pharmacologically active)

Half-life elimination: Oral: 14-35 hours; I.V.: 12-27 hours

Time to peak, serum: 1-5 hours

Excretion:

Oral: Urine (~5% of dose; 0.5% to 0.7% as unchanged drug, 4% as idarubicinol); hepatic (8%)

I.V.: Urine (13% as idarubicinol, 3% as unchanged drug); hepatic (17%)

Dosage Refer to individual protocols. I.V.:

Children:

Leukemia: 10-12 mg/m^2/day for 3 days every 3 weeks

Solid tumors: 5 mg/m^2/day for 3 days every 3 weeks

Adults:

Leukemia induction: 12 mg/m^2/day for 3 days

Leukemia consolidation: 10-12 mg/m^2/day for 2 days

Stem cell transplantation (unlabeled use): 20 mg/m^2/24 hours continuous I.V. infusion (with high-dose oral busulfan)

Dosing adjustment in renal impairment: S_{cr}: ≥2 mg/dL: Administer 75% of dose

Hemodialysis: Significant drug removal is unlikely based on physiochemical characteristics

Peritoneal dialysis: Significant drug removal is unlikely based on physiochemical characteristics

Dosing adjustment/comments in hepatic impairment:

Bilirubin 1.5-5.0 mg/dL or AST 60-180 int. units/L: Administer 50% of normal dose

Bilirubin >5.0 mg/dL: Do not administer drug

Combination Regimens

Leukemia, acute myeloid:

7 + 3 (Idarubicin) *on page 840*

Idarubicin, Cytarabine, Etoposide (ICE Protocol) *on page 900*

Idarubicin, Cytarabine, Etoposide (IDA-Based BF12) *on page 901*

Leukemia, acute promyelocytic:

M-3 *on page 906*

Tretinoin/Idarubicin *on page 941*

Administration Do not administer I.M. or SubQ; administer as slow push over 3-5 minutes, preferably into the side of a freely-running saline or dextrose infusion **or** as intermittent infusion over 10-15 minutes into a free-flowing I.V. solution of NS or D$_5$W; also occasionally administered as a bladder lavage.

Dosage Forms Injection, solution, as hydrochloride [preservative free] (Idamycin PFS®): 1 mg/mL (5 mL, 10 mL, 20 mL)

Monitoring Parameters CBC with differential, platelet count, cardiac function, serum electrolytes, creatinine, uric acid, ALT, AST, bilirubin, signs of extravasation

Patient Information This drug can only be administered I.V. Maintain adequate nutrition and hydration (2-3 L/day of fluids unless instructed to restrict fluid intake). May cause hair loss (will grow back); nausea or vomiting (consult prescriber for antiemetic medication); you will be susceptible to infection (avoid crowds and exposure to infection); or urine may turn darker (normal). Report immediately any pain, burning, or stinging at infusion site; difficulty breathing; or swelling of extremities. Contraceptive measures are recommended during therapy.

(Continued)

Idarubicin *(Continued)*

Special Geriatric Considerations During induction therapy, patients >60 years of age experience CHF, arrhythmias, MI, and decline in LVEF more frequently than younger populations.

Selected Readings

Berman E, "A Review of Idarubicin in Acute Leukemia," *Oncology (Huntingt)*, 1993, 7(10):91-8, 104.

Borchmann P, Hubel K, Schnell R, et al, "Idarubicin: A Brief Overview on Pharmacology and Clinical Use," *Int J Clin Pharmacol Ther*, 1997, 35(2):80-3.

Buckley MM and Lamb HM, "Oral Idarubicin. A Review of its Pharmacological Properties and Clinical Efficacy in the Treatment of Haematological Malignancies and Advanced Breast Cancer," *Drugs Aging*, 1997, 11(1):61-86.

Goebel M, "Oral Idarubicin - An Anthracycline Derivative With Unique Properties," *Ann Hematol*, 1993, 66(1):33-43.

Hollingshead LM and Faulds D, "Idarubicin. A Review of its Pharmacodynamic and Pharmacokinetic Properties, and Therapeutic Potential in the Chemotherapy of Cancer," *Drugs*, 1991, 42(4):690-719.

Robert J, "Clinical Pharmacokinetics of Idarubicin," *Clin Pharmacokinet*, 1993, 24(4):275-88.

♦ **Idarubicin Hydrochloride** *see* Idarubicin *on page 443*

♦ **IDEC-C2B8** *see* Rituximab *on page 709*

♦ **IDR** *see* Idarubicin *on page 443*

♦ **Ifex®** *see* Ifosfamide *on page 446*

♦ **IFLrA** *see* Interferon Alfa-2a *on page 466*

Ifosfamide *(eye FOSS fa mide)*

Related Information

Safe Handling of Hazardous Drugs *on page 1034*
Transplantation *on page 1019*

U.S. Brand Names Ifex®

Canadian Brand Names Ifex®

Generic Available Yes

Synonyms Isophosphamide; NSC-109724; Z4942

Pharmacologic Category Antineoplastic Agent, Alkylating Agent; Antineoplastic Agent, Alkylating Agent (Nitrogen Mustard)

Pregnancy Risk Factor D

Lactation Enters breast milk/contraindicated

Use Treatment of lung cancer, Hodgkin's and non-Hodgkin's lymphoma, breast cancer, acute and chronic lymphocytic leukemias, ovarian cancer, sarcomas, pancreatic and gastric carcinomas

Orphan drug: Treatment of testicular cancer

Mechanism of Action Causes cross-linking of strands of DNA by binding with nucleic acids and other intracellular structures; inhibits protein synthesis and DNA synthesis

Labeled Contraindications Hypersensitivity to ifosfamide or any component of the formulation; patients with severely depressed bone marrow function; pregnancy

Warnings/Precautions Hazardous agent - use appropriate precautions for handling and disposal. See Safe Handling of Hazardous Drugs *on page 1034* in the Appendix. Used in combination with mesna as a prophylactic agent to protect against hemorrhagic cystitis. Use with caution in patients with impaired renal function or those with compromised bone marrow reserve. Carcinogenic in rats.

Adverse Reactions

>10%:

Central nervous system: Somnolence, confusion, hallucinations (12%)

Dermatologic: Alopecia (75% to 100%)

Endocrine & metabolic: Metabolic acidosis (31%)

Gastrointestinal: Nausea and vomiting (58%), may be more common with higher doses or bolus infusions; constipation

Genitourinary: Hemorrhagic cystitis (40% to 50%), patients should be vigorously hydrated (at least 2 L/day) and receive mesna

Hematologic: Myelosuppression, leukopenia (65% to 100%), thrombocytopenia (10%) - dose related

Onset: 7-14 days

Nadir: 21-28 days

Recovery: 21-28 days

Renal: Hematuria (6% to 92%)

1% to 10%:

Central nervous system: Hallucinations, depressive psychoses, polyneuropathy

Dermatologic: Dermatitis, nail banding/ridging, hyperpigmentation

Endocrine & metabolic: SIADH, sterility

Hematologic: Anemia

Hepatic: Transaminases increased (3%)

Local: Phlebitis

Renal: BUN increased (6%), creatinine increased (6%)

Respiratory: Nasal stuffiness

<1%: Anorexia, cardiotoxicity, diarrhea, stomatitis, acute tubular necrosis, pulmonary fibrosis

Vesicant No

Emetic Potential Moderate (30% to 60%)

Overdosage/Toxicology Symptoms of overdose include myelosuppression, nausea, vomiting, diarrhea, and alopecia; direct extensions of the drug's pharmacologic effect. Treatment is supportive.

Drug Interactions

Cytochrome P450 Effect: Substrate of CYP2A6 (minor), 2B6 (minor), 2C8/9 (minor), 2C19 (minor), 3A4 (major); **Inhibits** CYP3A4 (weak); **Induces** CYP2C8/9 (weak)

Increased Effect/Toxicity: CYP3A4 inducers may increase the levels/effects of acrolein (the active metabolite of ifosfamide); example inducers include aminoglutethimide, carbamazepine, nafcillin, nevirapine, phenobarbital, phenytoin, and rifamycins.

Decreased Effect: CYP3A4 inhibitors may decrease the levels/effects of acrolein (the active metabolite of ifosfamide); example inhibitors include azole antifungals, ciprofloxacin, clarithromycin, diclofenac, doxycycline, erythromycin, imatinib, isoniazid, nefazodone, nicardipine, propofol, protease inhibitors, quinidine, and verapamil.

Ethanol/Nutrition/Herb Interactions Herb/Nutraceutical: St John's wort may decrease ifosfamide levels.

Storage/Stability Store intact vials at room temperature. Reconstituted solutions may be stored under refrigeration for up to 21 days. Solutions diluted for administration are stable for 7 days at room temperature and for 6 weeks under refrigeration.

(Continued)

Ifosfamide *(Continued)*

Reconstitution Dilute powder with SWI or NS to a concentration of 50 mg/mL. Further dilution in 50-1000 mL D_5W or NS is recommended for I.V. infusion.

Compatibility Stable in D_5LR, D_5NS, D_5W, LR, $\frac{1}{2}NS$, NS

Y-site administration: Compatible: Allopurinol, amifostine, amphotericin B cholesteryl sulfate complex, aztreonam, doxorubicin liposome, etoposide phosphate, filgrastim, fludarabine, gatifloxacin, gemcitabine, granisetron, linezolid, melphalan, ondansetron, paclitaxel, piperacillin/ tazobactam, propofol, sargramostim, sodium bicarbonate, teniposide, thiotepa, topotecan, vinorelbine. **Incompatible:** Cefepime, methotrexate

Compatibility in syringe: Compatible: Epirubicin, mesna. **Incompatible:** Mesna with epirubicin

Compatibility when admixed: Compatible: Carboplatin, carboplatin with etoposide, cisplatin, cisplatin with etoposide, epirubicin, etoposide, fluorouracil, mesna. **Incompatible:** Mesna with epirubicin

Pharmacodynamics/Kinetics Pharmacokinetics are dose dependent

Distribution: V_d: 5.7-49 L; does penetrate CNS, but not in therapeutic levels

Protein binding: Negligible

Metabolism: Hepatic to active metabolites phosphoramide mustard, acrolein, and inactive dichloroethylated and carboxy metabolites; acrolein is the agent implicated in development of hemorrhagic cystitis

Bioavailability: Estimated at 100%

Half-life elimination: Beta: High dose: 11-15 hours (3800-5000 mg/m^2); Lower dose: 4-7 hours (1800 mg/m^2)

Time to peak, plasma: Oral: Within 1 hour

Excretion: Urine (15% to 50% as unchanged drug, 41% as metabolites)

Dosage Refer to individual protocols. To prevent bladder toxicity, ifosfamide should be given with the urinary protector mesna and hydration of at least 2 L of oral or I.V. fluid per day. I.V.:

Children:

1200-1800 mg/m^2/day for 3-5 days every 21-28 days **or**

5 g/m^2 once every 21-28 days **or**

3 g/m^2/day for 2 days every 21-28 days

Adults:

50 mg/kg/day or 700-2000 mg/m^2 for 5 days every 3-4 weeks

Alternatives: 2400 mg/m^2/day for 3 days or 5000 mg/m^2 as a single dose every 3-4 weeks

Dosing adjustment in renal impairment: Limited experience in renal impairment; manufacturer does not provide adjustment. Several published recommendations include dose reductions between 20% and 30% in significant renal impairment. Consult individual protocols.

Dosing adjustment in hepatic impairment: Although no specific guidelines are available from the manufacturer, it is possible that adjusted doses are indicated in hepatic disease. One suggestion in the literature: AST >300 or bilirubin >3.0 mg/dL: Decrease ifosfamide dose by 75%

Combination Regimens

Esophageal cancer: TIP *on page 940*

Head and neck cancer: TIP *on page 940*

Hepatoblastoma: IPA *on page 903*

Lymphoma, non-Hodgkin's:
ICE (Lymphoma, non-Hodgkin's) *on page 899*
IMVP-16 *on page 902*
IVAC *on page 904*
MINE *on page 909*
MINE-ESHAP *on page 909*
Lung cancer (small cell): VIP (Small Cell Lung Cancer) *on page 947*
Neuroblastoma:
CI (Neuroblastomas) *on page 860*
HIPE-IVAD *on page 898*
Osteosarcoma: ICE (Sarcoma) *on page 899*
Sarcoma, soft tissue:
ICE (Sarcoma) *on page 899*
ICE-T *on page 900*
IE *on page 901*
MAID *on page 908*
Testicular cancer:
VIP (Etoposide) (Testicular Cancer) *on page 946*
VIP (Vinblastine) (Testicular Cancer) *on page 948*

Administration Administer slow I.V. push, IVPB over 30 minutes to several hours or continuous I.V. over 5 days

Dosage Forms Injection, powder for reconstitution: 1 g, 3 g [packaged with Mesnex® (mesna) 1 g]

High Dose Considerations
High Dose: I.V.: $7.5\text{-}16\ g/m^2$ in divided doses over several days; generally combined with other high-dose chemotherapy

Monitoring Parameters CBC with differential, hemoglobin, and platelet count, urine output, urinalysis, liver function, and renal function tests

Patient Information This drug can only be administered I.V. Report immediately any pain, stinging, or burning at infusion site. It is vital to maintain adequate hydration (2-3 L/day of fluids unless instructed to restrict fluid intake) for 3 days prior to infusion and each day of therapy. May cause hair loss (will grow back); nausea or vomiting (consult prescriber for antiemetic medication); and you will be susceptible to infection (avoid crowds and exposure to infection). Report immediately pain or irritation on urination, severe diarrhea, CNS changes (eg, hallucinations, confusion, somnolence), signs of opportunistic infection (eg, fever, chills, easy bruising or unusual bleeding), difficulty breathing, swelling of extremities, or any other adverse effects. Contraceptive measures are recommended during therapy.

Selected Readings
Furlanut M and Franceschi L, "Pharmacology of Ifosfamide," *Oncology*, 2003, 65 (Suppl 2):2-6.
Kerbusch T, de Kraker J, Keizer HJ, et al, "Clinical Pharmacokinetics and Pharmacodynamics of Ifosfamide and its Metabolites," *Clin Pharmacokinet*, 2001, 40(1):41-62.
Klastersky J, "Side Effects of Ifosfamide," *Oncology*, 2003, 65 (Suppl 2):7-10.

♦ **IL-2** *see* Aldesleukin *on page 32*
♦ **IL-11** *see* Oprelvekin *on page 627*

Imatinib (eye MAT eh nib)
U.S. Brand Names Gleevec®
Canadian Brand Names Gleevec®
Generic Available No
(Continued)

Imatinib *(Continued)*

Synonyms CGP 57148B; Glivec; Imatinib Mesylate; STI571

Pharmacologic Category Antineoplastic Agent, Tyrosine Kinase Inhibitor

Pregnancy Risk Factor D

Lactation Excretion in breast milk unknown/not recommended

Use Treatment of adult patients with Philadelphia chromosome-positive (Ph+) chronic myeloid leukemia (CML); treatment of pediatric patients with Ph+ CML (chronic phase) recurring following stem cell transplant or who are resistant to interferon-alpha therapy; treatment of Kit-positive (CD117) unresectable and/or (metastatic) malignant gastrointestinal stromal tumors (GIST)

Mechanism of Action Inhibits Bcr-Abl tyrosine kinase, the constitutive abnormal gene product of the Philadelphia chromosome in chronic myeloid leukemia (CML). Inhibition of this enzyme blocks proliferation and induces apoptosis in Bcr-Abl positive cell lines as well as in fresh leukemic cells in Philadelphia chromosome positive CML. Also inhibits tyrosine kinase for platelet-derived growth factor (PDGF), stem cell factor (SCF), c-kit, and events mediated by PDGF and SCF.

Labeled Contraindications Hypersensitivity to imatinib or any component of the formulation; pregnancy

Warnings/Precautions Hazardous agent - use appropriate precautions for handling and disposal. See Safe Handling of Hazardous Drugs *on page 1034* in the Appendix. Often associated with fluid retention, weight gain, and edema; occasionally leading to significant complications, including pleural effusion, pericardial effusion, pulmonary edema, and ascites. Use caution in patients where fluid accumulation may be poorly tolerated, such as in cardiovascular disease (CHF or hypertension) and pulmonary disease. Severe dermatologic reactions have been reported; reintroduction has been attempted following resolution. Successful resumption at a lower dose (with corticosteroids and/or antihistamine) has been described; however, some patients may experience recurrent reactions.

Use with caution in renal impairment, hematologic impairment, or hepatic disease. May cause GI irritation, hematologic toxicity (neutropenia, or thrombocytopenia), or hepatotoxicity. Hepatotoxic reactions may be severe. Has been associated with development of opportunistic infections. Use with caution in patients receiving concurrent therapy with drugs which alter cytochrome P450 activity or require metabolism by these isoenzymes. Safety and efficacy in patients <3 years of age have not been established.

Adverse Reactions Adverse reactions listed were established in patients with a wide variation in level of illness or specific diagnosis. In many cases, other medications were used concurrently (relationship to imatinib not specific). Effects reported in children were similar to adults, except that musculoskeletal pain was less frequent and peripheral edema was not reported.

>10%:

Central nervous system: Fatigue (29% to 41%), pyrexia (5% to 41%), headache (25% to 35%), dizziness (11% to 13%), insomnia (10% to 13%)

Dermatologic: Rash (26% to 44%), pruritus (8% to 13%), bruising (2% to 11%)

Endocrine & metabolic: Fluid retention (3% to 22% includes aggravated edema, anasarca, ascites, pericardial effusion, pleural effusion, pulmonary edema, excludes GIST); hypokalemia (5% to 13%)

Gastrointestinal: Nausea (42% to 71%), diarrhea (30% to 60%), vomiting (15% to 56%), abdominal pain (23% to 37%), weight increased (3% to 30%), dyspepsia (11% to 24), flatulence (16% to 23%), anorexia (6% to 17%), constipation (6% to 15%), taste disturbance (1% to 14%)

Hematologic: Hemorrhage (18% to 52%), neutropenia (grade 3 or 4: 2% to 48%), thrombocytopenia (grade 3 or 4: <1% to 31%)

Neuromuscular & skeletal: Muscle cramps (27% to 55%), musculoskeletal pain (11% to 46%), arthralgia (25% to 36%), joint pain (27%), myalgia (8% to 25%), weakness (5% to 12%), back pain (10% to 11%), rigors (8% to 11%)

Ocular: Lacrimation (6% to 11%)

Respiratory: Cough (12% to 26%), dyspnea (9% to 20%), nasopharyngitis (8% to 19%), upper respiratory tract infection (3% to 15%), pharyngolaryngeal pain (14%), epistaxis (5% to 13%), pneumonia (3% to 12%), sore throat (8% to 11%)

Miscellaneous: Superficial edema (53% to 76%), night sweats (10% to 14%)

1% to 10%:

Central nervous system: Paresthesia (1% to 10%)

Hematologic: Anemia (grade 3 or 4: <1% to 4%)

Hepatic: Ascites or pleural effusion (GIST: 4% to 6%), alkaline phosphatase increased (grade 3 or 4: <1% to 5%), ALT increased (grade 3 or 4: <1% to 4%), bilirubin increased (grade 3 or 4: <1% to 4%), AST increased (grade 3 or 4: <1% to 3%)

Renal: Albumin decreased (grade 3 or 4: 3% to 4%), creatine increased (grade 3 or 4: <1% to 3%)

Miscellaneous: Flu-like syndrome (<1% to 10%)

<1%, postmarketing, and/or case reports (limited to important or life-threatening): Acute generalized exanthematous pustulosis, angioedema, aplastic anemia, bullous eruption, cardiac failure, cerebral edema, embolism, erythema multiforme, exfoliative dermatitis, glaucoma, ileus, intestinal obstruction, intracranial pressure increased, interstitial pneumonitis, pancytopenia, papilledema, pancreatitis, paresthesia, pericarditis, photosensitivity, pulmonary fibrosis, seizure, Stevens-Johnson syndrome, thrombosis, vitreous hemorrhage

Emetic Potential Moderate (30% to 60%)

Overdosage/Toxicology Experience with overdose is limited (>800 mg/day). Hematologic adverse effects are more common at dosages >750 mg/day. Treatment is symptomatic and supportive.

Drug Interactions

Cytochrome P450 Effect: Substrate of CYP1A2 (minor), 2D6 (minor), 2C8/9 (minor), 2C19 (minor), 3A4 (major), **Inhibits** CYP2C8/9 (weak), 2D6 (weak), 3A4 (strong)

Increased Effect/Toxicity: Note: Drug interaction data are limited. Few clinical studies have been conducted. Many interactions listed here are derived by extrapolation from *in vitro* inhibition of cytochrome P450 isoenzymes. Chronic use of acetaminophen may increase potential for
(Continued)

Imatinib *(Continued)*

hepatotoxic reaction with imatinib (case report of hepatic failure with concurrent therapy).

Imatinib may increase the levels/effects of amiodarone, selected benzodiazepines, calcium channel blockers, cisapride, cyclosporine, ergot derivatives, fluoxetine, glimepiride, glipizide, HMG-CoA reductase inhibitors, nateglinide, phenytoin, phenytoin, propranolol, sertraline, mirtazapine, nateglinide, nefazodone, pioglitazone, rosiglitazone, sertraline, sildenafil (and other PDE-5 inhibitors), tacrolimus, venlafaxine, warfarin, and other substrates of CYP2C8/9 or 3A4. Selected benzodiazepines (midazolam and triazolam), cisapride, ergot alkaloids, selected HMG-CoA reductase inhibitors (lovastatin and simvastatin), mesoridazine, pimozide, and thioridazine are generally contraindicated with strong CYP3A4 inhibitors. When used with strong CYP3A4 inhibitors, dosage adjustment/limits are recommended for sildenafil and other PDE-5 inhibitors; consult individual monographs.

The levels/effects of imatinib may be increased by azole antifungals, ciprofloxacin, clarithromycin, diclofenac, doxycycline, erythromycin, isoniazid, nefazodone, nicardipine, propofol, protease inhibitors, quinidine, telithromycin, verapamil, and other CYP3A4 inhibitors.

Decreased Effect: The levels/effects of imatinib may be decreased by aminoglutethimide, carbamazepine, nafcillin, nevirapine, phenobarbital, phenytoin, rifamycins, and other CYP3A4 inducers. Dosage of imatinib should be increased by at least 50% (with careful monitoring) when used concurrently with a strong inducer.

Ethanol/Nutrition/Herb Interactions

Ethanol: Avoid ethanol.

Food: Food may reduce gastrointestinal irritation.

Herb/Nutraceutical: Avoid St John's wort (may increase metabolism and decrease imatinib plasma concentration).

Storage/Stability Store at 25°C (77°F); excursions permitted to 15°C to 30°C (59°F to 86°F).

Pharmacodynamics/Kinetics

Protein binding: 95% to albumin and alpha$_1$-acid glycoprotein

Metabolism: Hepatic via CYP3A4 (minor metabolism via CYP1A2, CYP2D6, CYP2C9, CYP2C19); primary metabolite (active): N-demethylated piperazine derivative

Bioavailability: 98%

Half-life elimination: Parent drug: 18 hours; N-demethyl metabolite: 40 hours

Time to peak: 2-4 hours

Excretion: Feces (68% primarily as metabolites, 20% as unchanged drug); urine (13% primarily as metabolites, 5% as unchanged drug)

Clearance: Highly variable; Mean: 8-14 L/hour (for 50 kg and 100 kg male, respectively)

Dosage Oral:

Children ≥3 years: CML (chronic phase): 260 mg/m^2/day; may be increased to 340 mg/m^2/day

Adults:

CML:

Chronic phase: 400 mg once daily; may be increased to 600 mg daily

Accelerated phase or blast crisis: 600 mg once daily; may be increased to 800 mg daily (400 mg twice daily)

Gastrointestinal stromal tumors: 400-600 mg/day

Note: Dosage should be increased by at least 50% when used concurrently with a potent enzyme-inducing agent (ie, rifampin, phenytoin).

Dosage adjustment for hepatotoxicity or other nonhematologic adverse reactions: If elevations of bilirubin >3 times upper limit of normal (ULN) or transaminases (ALT/AST) >5 times ULN occur, withhold until bilirubin <1.5 times ULN or transaminases <2.5 times ULN. Resume treatment at a reduced dose:

Children:

If initial dose 260 mg/m^2/day, reduce dose to 200 mg/m^2/day

If initial dose 340 mg/m^2/day, reduce dose to 260 mg/m^2/day

Adults:

If initial dose 400 mg, reduce dose to 300 mg

If initial dose 600 mg, reduce dose to 400 mg

Dosage adjustment for hematologic adverse reactions:

Chronic phase (initial dose 400 mg/day in adults or 260 mg/m^2/day in children) or GIST (initial dose 400 mg or 600 mg): If ANC <1.0 x 10^9/L and/or platelets <50 x 10^9/L: Discontinue until ANC ≥1.5 x 10^9/L and platelets ≥75 x 10^9/L; resume treatment at original initial dose of 400 or 600 mg/day (260 mg/m^2/day in children). If depression in neutrophils or platelets recurs, withhold until recovery, and reinstitute treatment at a reduced dose:

Children:

If initial dose 260 mg/m^2/day, reduce dose to 200 mg/m^2/day

If initial dose 340 mg/m^2/day, reduce dose to 260 mg/m^2/day

Adults:

If initial dose 400 mg, reduce dose to 300 mg

If initial dose 600 mg, reduce dose to 400 mg

Accelerated phase or blast crisis: Adults: Check to establish whether cytopenia is related to leukemia (bone marrow aspirate). If unrelated to leukemia, reduce dose of imatinib by 25%. If cytopenia persists for an additional 2 weeks, further reduce dose to 50% of original dose. If cytopenia persists for 4 weeks and is still unrelated to leukemia, stop treatment until ANC ≥1.0 x 10^9/L and platelets ≥20 x 10^9/L, resume treatment at 50% of original dose.

Administration Should be administered with food and a large glass of water. Tablets may be dispersed in water or apple juice, stir until dissolved and use immediately.

Dosage Forms Tablet: 100 mg, 400 mg

Monitoring Parameters CBC (weekly for first month, biweekly for second month, then periodically thereafter), liver function tests (at baseline and monthly or as clinically indicated), renal function, weight, and edema/fluid status.

Dietary Considerations Should be taken with food and a large glass of water to decrease gastrointestinal irritation.

Patient Information Take exactly as directed; do not alter or discontinue dose without consulting prescriber. Take with food and a large glass of water. Avoid alcohol, chronic use of acetaminophen or aspirin, OTC or prescription medications, or herbal products unless approved by prescriber. Maintain adequate hydration (2-3 L/day) unless instructed to restrict fluids. You will be required to have regularly scheduled laboratory (Continued)

Imatinib *(Continued)*

tests while on this medication. You will be more susceptible to infection (avoid crowds or contagious persons, and do not receive any vaccination unless approved by prescriber). You may experience headache or fatigue (use caution when driving or engaged in tasks requiring alertness until response to drug in known); loss of appetite, nausea, vomiting, or mouth sores (small frequent meals, frequent mouth care, chewing gum, or sucking lozenges may help); constipation (increased dietary fiber and fluids, exercise may help); or diarrhea (buttermilk, boiled milk, or yogurt may reduce diarrhea). Report chest pain, palpitations, or swelling of extremities; cough, difficulty breathing, or wheezing; weight gain greater than 5 lb; skin rash; muscle or bone pain, tremors, or cramping; persistent fatigue or weakness; easy bruising or unusual bleeding (eg, tarry stools, blood in vomitus, stool, urine, or mouth); persistent gastrointestinal problems or pain; or other adverse effects.

Additional Information Median time to hematologic response was one month; only short-term studies have been completed. Follow-up is insufficient to estimate duration of cytogenic response.

Special Geriatric Considerations Incidence of edema and edema-related adverse effects is increased in elderly patients.

- ◆ **Imatinib Mesylate** *see Imatinib on page 449*
- ◆ **IMC-C225** *see Cetuximab on page 172*
- ◆ **IMI 30** *see Idarubicin on page 443*
- ◆ **Imidazole Carboxamide** *see Dacarbazine on page 239*
- ◆ **Imidazole Carboxamide Dimethyltriazene** *see Dacarbazine on page 239*
- ◆ **Imipemide** *see Imipenem and Cilastatin on page 454*

Imipenem and Cilastatin (i mi PEN em & sye la STAT in)

Medication Safety Issues
Sound-alike/look-alike issues:
Primaxin® may be confused with Premarin®, Primacor®

Related Information
Management of Infections *on page 978*

U.S. Brand Names Primaxin®

Canadian Brand Names Primaxin®

Generic Available No

Synonyms Imipemide

Pharmacologic Category Antibiotic, Carbapenem

Pregnancy Risk Factor C

Lactation Enters breast milk (small amounts)/use caution

Use Treatment of respiratory tract, urinary tract, intra-abdominal, gynecologic, bone and joint, skin structure, and polymicrobic infections as well as bacterial septicemia and endocarditis. Antibacterial activity includes resistant gram-negative bacilli (*Pseudomonas aeruginosa* and *Enterobacter* sp), gram-positive bacteria (methicillin-sensitive *Staphylococcus aureus* and *Streptococcus* sp) and anaerobes.

Mechanism of Action Inhibits bacterial cell wall synthesis by binding to one or more of the penicillin binding proteins (PBPs); which in turn inhibits the final transpeptidation step of peptidoglycan synthesis in bacterial cell walls, thus inhibiting cell wall biosynthesis. Bacteria eventually lyse due to ongoing activity of cell wall autolytic enzymes (autolysins and murein hydrolases) while cell wall assembly is arrested. Cilastatin prevents renal metabolism of imipenem by competitive inhibition of dehydropeptidase along the brush border of the renal tubules.

Labeled Contraindications Hypersensitivity to imipenem/cilastatin or any component of the formulation

Warnings/Precautions Dosage adjustment is required in patients with impaired renal function. Prolonged use may result in superinfection. Has been associated with CNS adverse events. Use with caution in patients with a history of seizures or hypersensitivity to beta-lactams. Elderly patients often require lower doses (adjust carefully to renal function). Doses for I.M. administration are mixed with lidocaine, consult information on lidocaine for associated warnings/precautions.

Adverse Reactions
1% to 10%:
Gastrointestinal: Nausea/diarrhea/vomiting (1% to 2%)
Local: Phlebitis (3%), pain at I.M. injection site (1.2%)
<1%: Abnormal urinalysis, anaphylaxis, anemia, confusion (acute), dizziness, emergence of resistant strains of *P. aeruginosa* eosinophilia, fever, hypersensitivity, hypotension, increased BUN/creatine, increased LFTs, increased PT, neutropenia (including agranulocytosis), pain at injection site, palpitation, positive Coombs' test, pruritus, pseudomembranous colitis, rash, seizure, somnolence, thrombocytopenia, urticaria
Postmarketing reports and/or case reports: Hemorrhagic colitis, hepatitis, jaundice, abdominal pain, staining of teeth, glossitis, pancytopenia, leukopenia, hemolytic anemia, encephalopathy, tremor, confusion, myoclonus, paresthesia, vertigo, headache, psychic disturbances, hallucinations, tinnitus, taste perversion, dyspnea, thoracic spine pain, tachycardia, Stevens-Johnson syndrome, toxic epidermal necrolysis, erythema multiforme, angioneurotic edema, flushing, cyanosis, hyperhidrosis, candidiasis, pruritus vulvae, polyarthralgia, drug fever, asthenia, acute renal failure, polyuria, urine discoloration

Vesicant No

Emetic Potential Very low (<10%)

Overdosage/Toxicology Symptoms of overdose include neuromuscular hypersensitivity and seizures. Hemodialysis may be helpful to aid in removal of the drug from blood; otherwise, treatment is supportive or symptom-directed.

Drug Interactions
Decreased Effect: Imipenem may decrease valproic acid concentrations to subtherapeutic levels; monitor.

Storage/Stability Imipenem/cilastatin powder for injection should be stored at <30°C. Stable for 4 hours at room temperature if reconstituted with 5% or 10% dextrose injection, 5% dextrose and sodium bicarbonate, 5% dextrose and 0.9% sodium chloride, and 24 hours when refrigerated.

Reconstitution
I.M.: Prepare 500 mg vial with 2 mL 1% lidocaine; prepare 750 mg vial with 3 mL 1% lidocaine **(do not use lidocaine with epinephrine)**. Final concentration should not exceed 5 mg/mL.

Standard diluent: 500 mg/100 mL NS; 1 g/250 mL NS

Compatibility Variable stability (consult detailed reference) in D_5W, D_5LR, $D_5^{1}/_4NS$, $D_5^{1}/_2NS$, D_5NS, $D_{10}W$, mannitol 2.5%, mannitol 5%, mannitol 10%, LR, sodium bicarbonate 5%, NS, TPN
(Continued)

Imipenem and Cilastatin *(Continued)*

Y-site administration: Compatible: Acyclovir, amifostine, aztreonam, cefepime, cisatracurium, diltiazem, docetaxel, famotidine, fludarabine, foscarnet, gatifloxacin, granisetron, idarubicin, insulin (regular), linezolid, melphalan, methotrexate, ondansetron, propofol, remifentanil, tacrolimus, teniposide, thiotepa, vinorelbine, zidovudine. **Incompatible:** Allopurinol, amphotericin B cholesteryl sulfate complex, etoposide phosphate, fluconazole, gemcitabine, lorazepam, meperidine, midazolam, sargramostim, sodium bicarbonate. **Variable (consult detailed reference):** Filgrastim, TPN

Pharmacodynamics/Kinetics

Absorption: I.M.: Imipenem: 60% to 75%; cilastatin: 95% to 100%

Distribution: Rapidly and widely to most tissues and fluids including sputum, pleural fluid, peritoneal fluid, interstitial fluid, bile, aqueous humor, reproductive organs, and bone; highest concentrations in pleural fluid, interstitial fluid, peritoneal fluid, and reproductive organs; low concentrations in CSF; crosses placenta; enters breast milk

Metabolism: Renally by dehydropeptidase; activity is blocked by cilastatin; cilastatin is partially metabolized renally

Half-life elimination: Both drugs: 60 minutes; prolonged with renal impairment

Excretion: Both drugs: Urine (~70% as unchanged drug)

Dosage Dosage based on **imipenem** content:

Neonates: Non-CNS infections: I.V.:

<1 week: 25 mg/kg every 12 hours

1-4 weeks: 25 mg/kg every 8 hours

4 weeks to 3 months: 25 mg/kg every 6 hours

Children: >3 months: Non-CNS infections: I.V.: 15-25 mg/kg every 6 hours

Maximum dosage: Susceptible infections: 2 g/day; moderately susceptible organisms: 4 g/day

Children: Cystic fibrosis: I.V.: Doses up to 90 mg/kg/day have been used

Adults:

Moderate infections:

I.M.: 750 mg every 12 hours

I.V.:

Fully-susceptible organisms: 500 mg every 6-8 hours (1.5-2 g/day)

Moderately-susceptible organisms: 500 mg every 6 hours or 1 g every 8 hours (2-3 g/day)

Severe infections: I.V.: **Note:** I.M. administration is not intended for severe or life-threatening infections (eg, septicemia, endocarditis, shock):

Fully-susceptible organisms: 500 mg every 6 hours (2 g/day)

Moderately-susceptible organisms: 1 g every 6-8 hours (3-4 g/day)

Maximum daily dose should not exceed 50 mg/kg or 4 g/day, whichever is lower

Urinary tract infection, uncomplicated: I.V.: 250 mg every 6 hours (1 g/day)

Urinary tract infection, complicated: I.V.: 500 mg every 6 hours (2 g/day)

Mild infections: **Note:** Rarely a suitable option in mild infections; normally reserved for moderate-severe cases:

I.M.: 500 mg every 12 hours; intra-abdominal infections: 750 mg every 12 hours

I.V.:

Fully-susceptible organisms: 250 mg every 6 hours (1g/day)

Moderately-susceptible organisms: 500 mg every 6 hours (2 g/day)

Dosage adjustment in renal impairment: I.V.: **Note:** Adjustments have not been established for I.M. dosing:

Patients with a Cl_{cr} <5 mL/minute/1.73 m^2 should not receive imipenem/cilastatin unless hemodialysis is instituted within 48 hours.

Patients weighing <30 kg with impaired renal function should not receive imipenem/cilastatin.

Hemodialysis: Use the dosing recommendation for patients with a Cl_{cr} 6-20 mL/minute

Peritoneal dialysis: Dose as for Cl_{cr} <10 mL/minute

Continuous arteriovenous or venovenous hemofiltration: Dose as for Cl_{cr} 20-30 mL/minute; monitor for seizure activity; imipenem is well removed by CAVH but cilastatin is not; removes 20 mg of imipenem per liter of filtrate per day

Administration

I.M.: **Note:** I.M. administration is not intended for severe or life-threatening infections (eg, septicemia, endocarditis, shock). Administer by deep injection into a large muscle (gluteal or lateral thigh).

I.V.: Not for direct infusion; infuse each 250-500 mg dose over 20-30 minutes; infuse each 1 g dose over 40-60 minutes

Dosage Forms

Injection, powder for reconstitution [I.M.]: Imipenem 500 mg and cilastatin 500 mg [contains sodium 32 mg (1.4 mEq)]

Injection, powder for reconstitution [I.V.]: Imipenem 250 mg and cilastatin 250 mg [contains sodium 18.8 mg (0.8 mEq)]; imipenem 500 mg and cilastatin 500 mg [contains sodium 37.5 mg (1.6 mEq)]

Monitoring Parameters Periodic renal, hepatic, and hematologic function tests; monitor for signs of anaphylaxis during first dose

Dietary Considerations Sodium content of 1 g injection:

I.M.: 64.4 mg (2.8 mEq)

I.V.: 73.6 mg (3.2 mEq)

Special Geriatric Considerations Many of the seizures attributed to imipenem/cilastatin were in elderly patients. Dose must be carefully adjusted for creatinine clearance.

Selected Readings

Balfour JA, Bryson HM, and Brogden RN, "Imipenem/Cilastatin: An Update of Its Antibacterial Activity, Pharmacokinetics, and Therapeutic Efficacy in the Treatment of Serious Infections," *Drugs*, 1996, 51(1):99-136.

Barza M, "Imipenem: First of a New Class of Beta-Lactam Antibiotics," *Ann Intern Med*, 1985, 103(4):552-60.

Finch RG, Craddock C, Kelly J, et al, "Pharmacokinetic Studies of Imipenem/Cilastatin in Elderly Patients," *J Antimicrob Chemother*, 1986, 18(Suppl E):103-7.

Overturf GD, "Use of Imipenem-Cilastatin in Pediatrics," *Pediatr Infect Dis J*, 1989, 8(11):792-4.

Park SY and Parker RH, "Review of Imipenem," *Infect Control*, 1986, 7(6):333-7.

♦ **ImmuCyst® (Can)** see BCG Vaccine on page 120

Immune Globulin (Intravenous)
(i MYUN GLOB yoo lin, IN tra VEE nus)

Medication Safety Issues
Sound-alike/look-alike issues:
Gamimune® N may be confused with CytoGam®

Related Information
Management of Infections *on page 978*

U.S. Brand Names Carimune™ [DSC]; Carimune™ NF; Flebogamma®; Gamimune® N; Gammagard® S/D; Gammar®-P I.V.; Gamunex®; Iveegam EN; Octagam®; Panglobulin®; Panglobulin® NF; Polygam® S/D; Venoglobulin®-S [DSC]

Canadian Brand Names Gamimune® N; Gammagard® S/D; Gamunex®; Iveegam Immuno®

Generic Available No

Synonyms IVIG

Pharmacologic Category Immune Globulin

Pregnancy Risk Factor C

Lactation Excretion in breast milk unknown

Use
Treatment of primary immunodeficiency syndromes (congenital agammaglobulinemia, severe combined immunodeficiency syndromes [SCIDS], common variable immunodeficiency, X-linked immunodeficiency, Wiskott-Aldrich syndrome); idiopathic thrombocytopenic purpura (ITP); Kawasaki disease (in combination with aspirin)

Prevention of bacterial infection in B-cell chronic lymphocytic leukemia (CLL); pediatric HIV infection; bone marrow transplant (BMT)

Unlabeled/Investigational Use Autoimmune diseases (myasthenia gravis, SLE, bullous pemphigoid, severe rheumatoid arthritis), Guillain-Barré syndrome; used in conjunction with appropriate anti-infective therapy to prevent or modify acute bacterial or viral infections in patients with iatrogenically-induced or disease-associated immunodepression; autoimmune hemolytic anemia or neutropenia, refractory dermatomyositis/polymyositis

Mechanism of Action Replacement therapy for primary and secondary immunodeficiencies; interference with F_c receptors on the cells of the reticuloendothelial system for autoimmune cytopenias and ITP; possible role of contained antiviral-type antibodies

Labeled Contraindications Hypersensitivity to immune globulin or any component of the formulation; selective IgA deficiency

Warnings/Precautions Anaphylactic hypersensitivity reactions can occur, especially in IgA-deficient patients; studies indicate that the currently available products have no discernible risk of transmitting HIV or hepatitis B; aseptic meningitis may occur with high doses (≥2 g/kg). Use with caution in the elderly, patients with renal disease, diabetes mellitus, volume depletion, sepsis, paraproteinemia, and nephrotoxic medications due to risk of renal dysfunction. Patients should be adequately hydrated prior to therapy. Acute renal dysfunction (increased serum creatinine, oliguria, acute renal failure) can rarely occur; usually within 7 days of use (more likely with products stabilized with sucrose). Use caution in patients with a history of thrombotic events or cardiovascular disease; there is clinical evidence of a possible association between thrombotic events and administration of intravenous immune globulin. For intravenous administration only.

Adverse Reactions Frequency not defined.

Cardiovascular: Flushing of the face, tachycardia, hyper-/hypotension, chest tightness, angioedema, lightheadedness, chest pain, MI, CHF, pulmonary embolism

Central nervous system: Anxiety, chills, dizziness, drowsiness, fatigue, fever, headache, irritability, lethargy, malaise, aseptic meningitis syndrome

Dermatologic: Pruritus, rash, urticaria

Gastrointestinal: Abdominal cramps, diarrhea, nausea, sore throat, vomiting

Hematologic: Autoimmune hemolytic anemia, mild hemolysis

Hepatic: Liver function test increased

Local: Pain or irritation at the infusion site

Neuromuscular & skeletal: Arthralgia, back or hip pain, myalgia, nuchal rigidity

Ocular: Photophobia, painful eye movements

Renal: Acute renal failure, acute tubular necrosis, anuria, BUN increased, creatinine increased, nephrotic syndrome, oliguria, proximal tubular nephropathy, osmotic nephrosis

Respiratory: Cough, dyspnea, wheezing, nasal congestion, rhinorrhea, sinusitis

Miscellaneous: Diaphoresis, hypersensitivity reactions, anaphylaxis

Postmarketing and/or case reports: Abdominal pain, apnea, ARDS, bronchospasm, bullous dermatitis, cardiac arrest, Coombs' test positive, cyanosis, epidermolysis, erythema multiforme, hepatic dysfunction, hypoxemia, leukopenia, loss of consciousness, pancytopenia, pulmonary edema, rigors, seizure, Stevens-Johnson syndrome, thromboembolism, transfusion-related acute lung injury (TRALI), tremor, vascular collapse

Vesicant No

Emetic Potential Low

Drug Interactions

Decreased Effect: Decreased effect of live virus vaccines (eg, measles, mumps, rubella); separate administration by at least 3 months

Storage/Stability Stability and dilution is dependent upon the manufacturer and brand; do not freeze

Carimune™ NF, Panglobulin® NF: Prior to reconstitution, store at or below 30°C (86°F). Following reconstitution, store under refrigeration; use within 24 hours. Do not freeze.

Flebogamma®: Store at 2°C to 25°C (36°F to 77°F).

Gamimune® N, Iveegam EN: Store at 2°C to 8°C (36°F to 46°F).

Gammar®-P I.V., Gammagard® S/D, Polygam® S/D, Venoglobulin®-S: Store below 25°C (77°F).

Gamunex®: May be stored for up to 5 months at room temperature up to 25°C (up to 77°F) within 18 months of manufacture date.

Octagam®: Store at 2°C to 8°C (36°F to 46°F) for 24 months or ≤25°C (77°F) for 18 months.

Panglobulin®: Store at room temperature, below 30°C (86°F).

Polygam® S/D: Store at room temperature at or below 25°C (77°F); do not freeze.

(Continued)

Immune Globulin (Intravenous) *(Continued)*

Reconstitution Dilution is dependent upon the manufacturer and brand; do not shake, avoid foaming; discard unused portion:

Carimune™ NF, Panglobulin® NF: Reconstitute with NS, D_5W, or SWFI.

Iveegam EN: Reconstitute with SWFI; use immediately after reconstitution

Gammagard® S/D, Polygam® S/D: Reconstitute with sterile water for injection; store diluted solution under refrigeration for up to 24 hours.

Panglobulin®: Reconstitute with NS, D_5W, or SWFI; may store diluted solution under refrigeration for up to 24 hours.

Gammar®-P I.V.: Reconstitute with SWFI.

Gamunex®: Dilute in D_5W only.

Compatibility Stable in D_5W, $D_{15}W$, $D_5^1/_4NS$; **variable stability (consult detailed reference)** in TPN. Gamunex® should be diluted in D_5W only.

Y-site administration: Compatible: Fluconazole, sargramostim

Pharmacodynamics/Kinetics

Onset of action: I.V.: Provides immediate antibody levels

Duration: Immune effect: 3-4 weeks (variable)

Distribution: V_d: 0.09-0.13 L/kg

Intravascular portion (primarily): Healthy subjects: 41% to 57%; Patients with congenital humoral immunodeficiencies: ~70%

Half-life elimination: IgG (variable among patients): Healthy subjects: 14-24 days; Patients with congenital humoral immunodeficiencies: 26-40 days; hypermetabolism associated with fever and infection have coincided with a shortened half-life

Dosage Approved doses and regimens may vary between brands; check manufacturer guidelines. **Note:** Some clinicians dose IVIG on ideal body weight or an adjusted ideal body weight in morbidly obese patients. The volume of distribution of IVIG preparations in healthy subjects is similar to that observed with endogenous IgG. IVIG remains primarily in the intravascular space. Patients with congenital humoral immunodeficiencies appear to have about 70% of the IVIG available in the intravascular space.

Infants and Children: Prevention of gastroenteritis (unlabeled use): Oral: 50 mg/kg/day divided every 6 hours

Children: I.V.:

Pediatric HIV: 400 mg/kg every 28 days

Severe systemic viral and bacterial infections (unlabeled use): 500-1000 mg/kg/week

Children and Adults: I.V.:

Primary immunodeficiency disorders: 200-400 mg/kg every 4 weeks or as per monitored serum IgG concentrations

Flebogamma®, Gamunex®, Octagam®: 300-600 mg/kg every 3-4 weeks; adjusted based on dosage and interval in conjunction with monitored serum IgG concentrations.

B-cell chronic lymphocytic leukemia (CLL): 400 mg/kg/dose every 3 weeks

Idiopathic thrombocytopenic purpura (ITP):

Acute: 400 mg/kg/day for 5 days or 1000 mg/kg/day for 1-2 days

Chronic: 400 mg/kg as needed to maintain platelet count >30,000/ mm^3; may increase dose to 800 mg/kg (1000 mg/kg if needed)

Kawasaki disease: Initiate therapy within 10 days of disease onset: 2 g/kg as a single dose administered over 10 hours, or 400 mg/kg/day for 4 days. **Note:** Must be used in combination with aspirin: 80-100 mg/kg/day in 4 divided doses for 14 days; when fever subsides, dose aspirin at 3-5 mg/kg once daily for ≥6-8 weeks

Acquired immunodeficiency syndrome (patients must be symptomatic) (unlabeled use): Various regimens have been used, including:

200-250 mg/kg/dose every 2 weeks

or

400-500 mg/kg/dose every month or every 4 weeks

Autoimmune hemolytic anemia and neutropenia (unlabeled use): 1000 mg/kg/dose for 2-3 days

Autoimmune diseases (unlabeled use): 400 mg/kg/day for 4 days

Bone marrow transplant: 500 mg/kg beginning on days 7 and 2 pretransplant, then 500 mg/kg/week for 90 days post-transplant

Adjuvant to severe cytomegalovirus infections (unlabeled use): 500 mg/kg/dose every other day for 7 doses

Guillain-Barré syndrome (unlabeled use): Various regimens have been used, including:

400 mg/kg/day for 4 days

or

1000 mg/kg/day for 2 days

or

2000 mg/kg/day for one day

Refractory dermatomyositis (unlabeled use): 2 g/kg/dose every month x 3-4 doses

Refractory polymyositis (unlabeled use): 1 g/kg/day x 2 days every month x 4 doses

Chronic inflammatory demyelinating polyneuropathy (unlabeled use): Various regimens have been used, including:

400 mg/kg/day for 5 doses once each month

or

800 mg/kg/day for 3 doses once each month

or

1000 mg/kg/day for 2 days once each month

Dosing adjustment/comments in renal impairment: Cl_{cr} <10 mL/minute: Avoid use; in patients at risk of renal dysfunction, consider infusion at a rate less than maximum.

Administration I.V. infusion over 2-24 hours; for initial treatment, a lower concentration and/or a slower rate of infusion should be used. Administer in separate infusion line from other medications; if using primary line, flush with saline prior administration (**Note:** Venoglobulin®-S: Flush with D_5W). Decrease dose, rate and/or concentration of infusion in patients who may be at risk of renal failure. Decreasing the rate or stopping the infusion may help relieve some adverse effects (flushing, changes in pulse rate, changes in blood pressure). Epinephrine should be available during administration.

Dosage Forms [DSC] = Discontinued product

Injection, powder for reconstitution [preservative free]:

Carimune™: 1 g, 3 g, 6 g, 12 g [contains sucrose] [DSC]

Gammar®-P I.V.: 1 g [DSC], 2.5 g [DSC], 5 g, 10 g [stabilized with human albumin and sucrose]

(Continued)

Immune Globulin (Intravenous) *(Continued)*

Iveegam EN: 0.5 g [DSC], 1 g [DSC], 2.5 g [DSC], 5 g [stabilized with glucose]

Panglobulin®: 6 g, 12 g [contains sucrose]

Injection, powder for reconstitution [preservative free, nanofiltered]:

Carimune™ NF: 3 g, 6 g, 12 g [contains sucrose]

Panglobulin® NF: 6 g, 12 g [contains sucrose]

Injection, powder for reconstitution [preservative free, solvent detergent treated]

Gammagard® S/D: 2.5 g, 5 g, 10 g [stabilized with human albumin, glycine, glucose, and polyethylene glycol]

Polygam® S/D: 5 g, 10 g [stabilized with human albumin, glycine, glucose, and polyethylene glycol]

Injection, solution [preservative free; solvent detergent-treated]:

Gamimune® N: 10% [100 mg/mL] (10 mL, 25 mL, 50 mL, 100 mL, 200 mL)

Octagam®: 5% [50 mg/mL] (20 mL, 50 mL, 100 mL, 200 mL) [sucrose free; contains sodium 30 mmol/L and maltose]

Venoglobulin®-S: 5% [50 mg/mL] (50 mL, 100 mL, 200 mL); 10% [100 mg/mL] (50 mL, 100 mL, 200 mL) [stabilized with human albumin] [DSC]

Injection, solution [preservative free]:

Flebogamma®: 5% (10 mL, 50 mL, 100 mL, 200 mL) [PEG precipitated/ chromatography purified]

Gamunex®: 10% (10 mL, 25 mL, 50 mL, 100 mL, 200 mL) [caprylate/ chromatography purified]

Monitoring Parameters Renal function, urine output, hemoglobin and hematocrit, infusion-related adverse reactions, anaphylaxis

Dietary Considerations Octagam® contains sodium 30 mmol/L

Additional Information

Intravenous Immune Globulin Product Comparison:

Carimune™ NF, Panglobulin® NF:

FDA indication: Primary immunodeficiency, ITP

Contraindication: IgA deficiency

IgA content: 720 mcg/mL

Plasma source: Pooled donors

Half-life: 23 days

IgG subclass (%):

IgG1 (60-70): 60.5

IgG2 (19-31): 30.2

IgG3 (5-8.4): 6.6

IgG4 (0.7-4): 2.8

Storage: Room temperature at or below 30°C (86°F); refrigerate after reconstitution

Recommendations for **initial** infusion rate: 0.5-1 mL/minute

Maximum infusion rate: 2 mg/kg/minute

Flebogamma®:

FDA indication: Primary immunodeficiency

Contraindication: IgA deficiency, intolerance to fructose/sorbitol, history of anaphylaxis with blood products

IgA content: <50 mcg/mL

Plasma source: Pooled donors

Half-life: 30-45 days
IgG subclass (%):
  IgG$_1$ (60-70): 70
  IgG$_2$ (19-31): 25
  IgG$_3$ (5-8.4): 3
  IgG$_4$ (0.7-4): 2
Storage: 2°C to 25°C
Recommendations for **initial** infusion rate: 0.01 mL/kg/minute
Maximum infusion rate: 0.1 mL/kg/minute (0.06 mL/kg/minute in renal impairment)

Gamimune® N:
FDA indication: Primary immunodeficiency, ITP
Contraindication: IgA deficiency
IgA content: 270 mcg/mL
Adverse reactions (%): 5.2
Plasma source: >2000 paid donors
Half-life: 21 days
IgG subclass (%):
  IgG$_1$ (60-70): 60
  IgG$_2$ (19-31): 29.4
  IgG$_3$ (5-8.4): 6.5
  IgG$_4$ (0.7-4): 4.1
Monomers (%): >95
Gamma globulin (%): >98
Storage: Refrigerate
Recommendations for **initial** infusion rate: 0.01-0.02 mL/kg/minute
Maximum infusion rate: 0.08 mL/kg/minute
Maximum concentration for infusion (%): 10

Gammagard® SD:
FDA indication: Primary immunodeficiency, ITP, CLL prophylaxis
Contraindication: None (caution with IgA deficiency)
IgA content: 0.92-1.6 mcg/mL
Adverse reactions (%): 6
Plasma source: 4000-5000 paid donors
Half-life: 24 days
IgG subclass (%):
  IgG$_1$ (60-70): 67 (66.8)*
  IgG$_2$ (19-31): 25 (25.4)
  IgG$_3$ (5-8.4): 5 (7.4)
  IgG$_4$ (0.7-4): 3 (0.3)
Monomers (%): >95
Gamma globulin (%): >90
Storage: Room temperature
Recommendations for **initial** infusion rate: 0.5 mL/kg/hour
Maximum infusion rate: 4 mL/kg/hour
Maximum concentration for infusion (%): 5

Gammar®-P I.V.:
FDA indication: Primary immunodeficiency
Contraindication: IgA deficiency
IgA content: <20 mcg/mL
Adverse reactions (%): 15
Plasma source: >8000 paid donors
Half-life: 21-24 days
(Continued)

Immune Globulin (Intravenous) *(Continued)*

IgG subclass (%):
IgG$_1$ (60-70): 69
IgG$_2$ (19-31): 23
IgG$_3$ (5-8.4): 6
IgG$_4$ (0.7-4): 2
Monomers (%): >98
Gamma globulin (%): >98
Storage: Room temperature
Recommendations for **initial** infusion rate: 0.01-0.02 mL/kg/minute
Maximum infusion rate: 0.06 mL/kg/minute
Maximum concentration for infusion (%): 5

Gamunex®:
FDA indication: Primary immunodeficiency, ITP
Contraindication: Caution in severe, selective IgA deficiency
IgA content: 40 mcg/mL
IgM content: <2 mcg/mL
Plasma source: Pooled donors
Half-life: 36 days
IgG subclass (%):
IgG$_1$ (60-70): 65
IgG$_2$ (19-31): 26
IgG$_3$ (5-8.4): 5.6
IgG$_4$ (0.7-4): 2.6
Monomer + dimer (%): 100
Gamma globulin (%): >98
Storage: 2°C to 8°C; may be stored at room temperature for 5 months
(only during first 18 months after manufacture)
Recommendations for **initial** infusion rate: 0.01 mL/kg/minute
Maximum infusion rate: 0.08 mL/kg/minute
Maximum concentration for infusion (%): 10

Octagam®:
FDA indication: Primary immunodeficiency
Contraindications: IgA deficiency
IgA content: 100 mcg/mL
Half-life: Immunodeficiency: 40 days
IgG subclass (%):
IgG$_1$ (60-70): 65
IgG$_2$ (19-31): 30
IgG$_3$ (5-8.4): 3
IgG$_4$ (0.7-4): 2
Monomers (%): ≥90
Gamma globulin (%): 96
Storage: Refrigerated or room temperature
Recommendations for initial infusion rate: 0.6 mL/kg/hour
Maximum infusion rate: 4 mL/kg/hour
Maximum concentration for infusion: 5%

Polygam®:
FDA indication: Primary immunodeficiency, ITP, CLL
Contraindication: None (caution with IgA deficiency)
IgA content: 0.74 ± 0.33 mcg/mL
Adverse reactions (%): 6

Plasma source: 50,000 voluntary donors
Half-life: 21-25 days
IgG subclass (%):
    IgG_1 (60-70): 67
    IgG_2 (19-31): 25
    IgG_3 (5-8.4): 5
    IgG_4 (0.7-4): 3
Monomers (%): >95
Gamma globulin (%): >90
Storage: Room temperature
Recommendations for **initial** infusion rate: 0.5 mL/kg/hour
Maximum infusion rate: 4 mL/kg/hour
Maximum concentration for infusion (%): 10

Venoglobulin®-S:
FDA indication: Primary immunodeficiency, ITP
Contraindication: IgA deficiency
IgA content: 20-24 mcg/mL
Adverse reactions (%): 6
Plasma source: 6000-9000 paid donors
Half-life: 29 days
IgG subclass (%):
    IgG_1 (60-70): 62.3**
    IgG_2 (19-31): 32.8
    IgG_3 (5-8.4): 2.9
    IgG_4 (0.7-4): 2
Monomers (%): >98
Gamma globulin (%): >98
Storage: Room temperature
Recommendations for **initial** infusion rate: 0.01-0.02 mL/kg/minute
Maximum infusion rate: 0.04 mL/kg/minute
Maximum concentration for infusion (%):10

*Skvaril F and Gardi A, "Differences Among Available Immunoglobulin Preparations for Intravenous Use," *Pediatr Infect Dis J*, 1988, 7:543-48.
**Roomer J, Morgenthaler JJ, Scherz R, et al, "Characterization of Various Immunoglobulin Preparations for Intravenous Application," *Vox Sang*, 1982, 42:62-73.

Selected Readings
ASHP Commission on Therapeutics, "ASHP Therapeutic Guidelines for Intravenous Immune Globulin," *Am J Hosp Pharm*, 1992, 49(3):652-4.

Blanchette VS, Luke B, Andrew M, et al, "A Prospective Randomized Trial of High-Dose Intravenous Immune Globulin G Therapy, Oral Prednisone Therapy, and No Therapy in Childhood Acute Immune Thrombocytopenic Purpura," *J Pediatr*, 1993, 123(6):989-95.

Grillo JA, Gorson, KC, Ropper AH, et al, "Rapid Infusion of Intravenous Immune Globulin in Patients With Neuromuscular Disorders," *Neurology*, 2001; 57:1699-1701.

Morrell A, "Pharmacokinetics of Intravenous Immunoglobulin Preparations," *Intravenous Immunoglobulins in Clinical Practice*, Lee ML and Strand V eds, New York, NY: Marcel Dekker, Inc, 1997, 1-18.

NIH Consensus Conference, "Intravenous Immunoglobulin, Prevention and Treatment of Disease," *JAMA*, 1990, 264(24):3189-93.

"University Hospital Consortium Expert Panel for Off-Label Use of Polyvalent Intravenously Administered Immunoglobulin Preparations Consensus Statement," *JAMA*, 1995, 273(23):1865-70.

♦ **Immunine® VH (Can)** *see* Factor IX *on page 327*

♦ **In-111 Zevalin** *see* Ibritumomab *on page 439*

♦ **Inapsine®** *see* Droperidol *on page 294*

- **INF-alpha 2** *see* Interferon Alfa-2b *on page 471*
- **INFeD®** *see* Iron Dextran Complex *on page 484*
- **Inflamase® Forte (Can)** *see* PrednisoLONE *on page 679*
- **Inflamase® Mild (Can)** *see* PrednisoLONE *on page 679*
- **Infufer® (Can)** *see* Iron Dextran Complex *on page 484*
- **Infumorph®** *see* Morphine Sulfate *on page 588*
- **α-2-Interferon** *see* Interferon Alfa-2b *on page 471*

Interferon Alfa-2a (in ter FEER on AL fa too aye)

Medication Safety Issues
Sound-alike/look-alike issues:
   Interferon alfa-2a may be confused with interferon alfa-2b
   Roferon-A® may be confused with Rocephin®

Related Information
Safe Handling of Hazardous Drugs *on page 1034*

U.S. Brand Names Roferon-A®

Canadian Brand Names Roferon-A®

Generic Available No

Synonyms IFLrA; rIFN-A

Pharmacologic Category Interferon

Pregnancy Risk Factor C

Lactation Enters breast milk/contraindicated (AAP rates "compatible")

Use

Patients >18 years of age: Hairy cell leukemia, AIDS-related Kaposi's sarcoma, chronic hepatitis C

Children and Adults: Chronic myelogenous leukemia (CML), Philadelphia chromosome positive, within 1 year of diagnosis (limited experience in children)

Unlabeled/Investigational Use Adjuvant therapy for malignant melanoma, AIDS-related thrombocytopenia, cutaneous ulcerations of Behçet's disease, brain tumors, metastatic ileal carcinoid tumors, cervical and colorectal cancers, genital warts, idiopathic mixed cryoglobulinemia, hemangioma, hepatitis D, hepatocellular carcinoma, idiopathic hypereosinophilic syndrome, mycosis fungoides, Sézary syndrome, low-grade non-Hodgkin's lymphoma, macular degeneration, multiple myeloma, renal cell carcinoma, basal and squamous cell skin cancer, essential thrombocythemia, cutaneous T-cell lymphoma

Mechanism of Action Following activation, multiple effects can be detected including induction of gene transcription. Inhibits cellular growth, alters the state of cellular differentiation, interferes with oncogene expression, alters cell surface antigen expression, increases phagocytic activity of macrophages, and augments cytotoxicity of lymphocytes for target cells

Restrictions An FDA-approved medication guide is available at www.fda.gov/cder/Offices/ODS/labeling.htm; distribute to each patient to whom this medication is dispensed.

Labeled Contraindications Hypersensitivity to alfa interferon, benzyl alcohol, or any component of the formulation; autoimmune hepatitis; visceral AIDS-related Kaposi's sarcoma associated with rapidly-progressing or life-threatening disease; hepatic decompensation (Child-Pugh Class B or C)

Warnings/Precautions Use caution in patients with a history of depression. May cause severe psychiatric adverse events (psychosis, mania, depression, suicidal behavior/ideation) in patients with and without previous psychiatric symptoms; careful neuropsychiatric monitoring is required during therapy. Use with caution in patients with seizure disorders, brain metastases, or compromised CNS function. Higher doses in the elderly or in malignancies other than hairy cell leukemia may result in severe obtundation.

Use caution in patients with autoimmune diseases, pre-existing cardiac disease (ischemic or thromboembolic), arrhythmias, renal impairment (Cl_{cr} <50 mL/minute), mild hepatic impairment, or myelosuppression. Also use caution in patients receiving therapeutic immunosuppression. Use caution in patients with diabetes or pre-existing thyroid disease. Discontinue if persistent unexplained pulmonary infiltrates are noted. Gastrointestinal ischemia, ulcerative colitis and hemorrhage have been associated rarely with alpha interferons; some cases are severe and life-threatening. Ophthalmologic disorders have occurred in patients receiving alpha interferons; close monitoring is warranted.

Treatment should be discontinued in patients with worsening or persistently severe signs/symptoms of autoimmune, infectious, ischemic, or neuropsychiatric disorders (including depression and/or suicidal thoughts/behavior). Discontinue treatment if neutrophils <0.5 x 10^9/L or platelets <25 x 10^9/L. **Due to differences in dosage, patients should not change brands of interferons.** Injection solution contains benzyl alcohol; do not use in neonates or infants. Safety and efficacy in children <18 years of age have not been established.

Adverse Reactions Note: A flu-like syndrome (fever, chills, tachycardia, malaise, myalgia, arthralgia, headache) occurs within 1-2 hours of administration; may last up to 24 hours and may be dose-limiting (symptoms in up to 92% of patients). For the listing below, the percentage of incidence noted generally corresponds to highest reported ranges. Incidence depends upon dosage and indication.

>10%:

Cardiovascular: Chest pain (4% to 11%), edema (11%), hypertension (11%)

Central nervous system: Psychiatric disturbances (including depression and suicidal behavior/ideation; reported incidence highly variable, generally >15%), fatigue (90%), headache (52%), dizziness (21%), irritability (15%), insomnia (14%), somnolence, lethargy, confusion, mental impairment, and motor weakness (most frequently seen at high doses [>100 million units], usually reverses within a few days); vertigo (19%); mental status changes (12%)

Dermatologic: Rash (usually maculopapular) on the trunk and extremities (7% to 18%), alopecia (19% to 22%), pruritus (13%), dry skin

Endocrine & metabolic: Hypocalcemia (10% to 51%), hyperglycemia (33% to 39%), transaminases increased (25% to 30%), alkaline phosphatase increased (48%)

Gastrointestinal: Loss of taste, anorexia (30% to 70%), nausea (28% to 53%), vomiting (10% to 30%, usually mild), diarrhea (22% to 34%, may be severe), taste change (13%), dry throat, xerostomia, abdominal cramps, abdominal pain

Hematologic (often due to underlying disease): Myelosuppression; neutropenia (32% to 70%); thrombocytopenia (22% to 70%); anemia

(Continued)

Interferon Alfa-2a *(Continued)*

(24% to 65%, may be dose-limiting, usually seen only during the first 6 months of therapy)

Onset: 7-10 days

Nadir: 14 days, may be delayed 20-40 days in hairy cell leukemia

Recovery: 21 days

Hepatic: Elevation of AST (SGOT) (77% to 80%), LDH (47%), bilirubin (31%)

Local: Injection site reaction (29%)

Neuromuscular & skeletal: Weakness (may be severe at doses >20,000,000 units/day); arthralgia and myalgia (5% to 73%, usually during the first 72 hours of treatment); rigors

Renal: Proteinuria (15% to 25%)

Respiratory: Cough (27%), irritation of oropharynx (14%)

Miscellaneous: Flu-like syndrome (up to 92% of patients), diaphoresis (15%)

1% to 10%:

Cardiovascular: Hypotension (6%), supraventricular tachyarrhythmia, palpitation (<3%), acute MI (<1% to 1%)

Central nervous system: Confusion (10%), delirium

Dermatologic: Erythema (diffuse), urticaria

Endocrine & metabolic: Hyperphosphatemia (2%)

Gastrointestinal: Stomatitis, pancreatitis (<5%), flatulence, liver pain

Genitourinary: Impotence (6%), menstrual irregularities

Neuromuscular & skeletal: Leg cramps; peripheral neuropathy, paresthesia (7%), and numbness (4%) are more common in patients previously treated with vinca alkaloids or receiving concurrent vinblastine

Ocular: Conjunctivitis (4%)

Respiratory: Dyspnea (7.5%), epistaxis (4%), rhinitis (3%)

Miscellaneous: Antibody production to interferon (10%)

<1%: Abdominal fullness, angioedema, aplastic anemia, arthritis, ascites, autoimmune reaction with worsening of liver disease, bronchospasm, bronchiolitis obliterans, BUN/creatinine increased, cardiomyopathy, coagulopathy, coma, CHF, cutaneous eruptions, distal cyanosis, diffuse encephalopathy, dysphasia, eczema, EEG abnormalities, hallucinations, hemolytic anemia, hyper-/hypothyroidism, hypermotility, hypertriglyceridemia, hyponatremia (SIADH), mania, gait disturbance, gastrointestinal hemorrhage, hepatic failure, idiopathic thrombocytopenia purpura, interstitial nephritis, interstitial pneumonitis, ischemic colitis, leukopenia, libido decreased, lupus erythematosus syndrome, myositis, nasal congestion, nephrotic syndrome, optic neuritis, pneumonia, pneumonitis, presenile dementia, proteinuria, psoriasis, psychotic episodes, Raynaud's phenomenon, renal failure (acute), rhabdomyolysis, sarcoidosis, seborrhea, seizure, stroke, syncope, tachypnea, ulcerative colitis, urticaria, vasculitis, visual acuity decreased

Vesicant No

Emetic Potential Moderate (30% to 60%); usually mild to moderate, aggressive therapy with serotonin antagonists is usually not necessary

Overdosage/Toxicology Symptoms of overdose include CNS depression, obtundation, flu-like symptoms, and myelosuppression. Treatment is supportive.

Drug Interactions

Cytochrome P450 Effect: Inhibits CYP1A2 (weak)

Increased Effect/Toxicity: Note: May exacerbate the toxicity of other agents with respect to CNS, myelotoxicity, or cardiotoxicity. Theophylline clearance has been reported to be decreased in hepatitis patients receiving interferon. Interferons may increase the adverse/toxic effects of ACE inhibitors, specifically the development of granulocytopenia. Agranulocytosis has been reported with concurrent use of clozapine (case report). Interferons may increase the anticoagulant effects of warfarin, and interferons may increase serum levels of zidovudine.

Decreased Effect: Prednisone may decrease the therapeutic effects of interferon alpha. A decreased response to erythropoietin has been reported (case reports) in patients receiving interferons. Interferon alpha may decrease the serum concentrations of melphalan (may or may not decrease toxicity of melphalan).

Storage/Stability Refrigerate (2°C to 8°C/36°F to 46°F); do not freeze; do not shake. After reconstitution, the solution is stable for 24 hours at room temperature and for 1 month when refrigerated.

Reconstitution Reconstitute vial with the diluent provided, or SWFI, NS, or D_5W; concentrations $\geq 3 \times 10^6$ units/mL are hypertonic.

Compatibility Stable in LR, NS; not stable in D_5W

Pharmacodynamics/Kinetics

Absorption: Filtered and absorbed at the renal tubule

Distribution: V_d: 0.223-0.748 L/kg

Metabolism: Primarily renal; filtered through glomeruli and undergoes rapid proteolytic degradation during tubular reabsorption

Bioavailability: I.M.: 83%; SubQ: 90%

Half-life elimination: I.V.: 3.7-8.5 hours (mean ~5 hours)

Time to peak, serum: I.M., SubQ: ~6-8 hours

Dosage Refer to individual protocols

Children (limited data):

Chronic myelogenous leukemia (CML): I.M.: 2.5-5 million units/m²/day; **Note:** In juveniles, higher dosages (30 million units/m²/day) have been associated with severe adverse events, including death

Adults:

Hairy cell leukemia: SubQ, I.M.: 3 million units/day for 16-24 weeks, then 3 million units 3 times/week for up to 6-24 months

Chronic myelogenous leukemia (CML): SubQ, I.M.: 9 million units/day, continue treatment until disease progression

AIDS-related Kaposi's sarcoma: SubQ, I.M.: 36 million units/day for 10-12 weeks, then 36 million units 3 times/week; to minimize adverse reactions, can use escalating dose (3-, 9-, then 18 million units each day for 3 days, then 36 million units daily thereafter).

Hepatitis C: SubQ, I.M.: 3 million units 3 times/week for 12 months

Dosage adjustment in renal impairment: Not removed by hemodialysis

Combination Regimens

Melanoma: Dacarbazine-Carboplatin-Aldesleukin-Interferon *on page 871*

Renal cell cancer:

Interleukin 2-Interferon Alfa 2 *on page 902*

Interleukin 2-Interferon Alfa 2-Fluorouracil *on page 903*

(Continued)

Interferon Alfa-2a *(Continued)*

Administration SubQ administration is suggested for those who are at risk for bleeding or are thrombocytopenic; rotate SubQ injection site; patient should be well hydrated

Dosage Forms Injection, solution, [single-dose prefilled syringe; SubQ use only]: 3 million units/0.5 mL (0.5 mL); 6 million units/0.5 mL (0.5 mL); 9 million units/0.5 mL (0.5 mL) [contains benzyl alcohol]

Monitoring Parameters Baseline ophthalmologic exam should be performed in all patients, with periodic reassessment in patients with impairment. Patients with thyroid dysfunction should be monitored by TSH levels at baseline and every 3 months during therapy.

Chronic hepatitis C: Monitor ALT (at baseline, after 2 weeks, and monthly thereafter) and HCV-RNA (particularly in first 3 months of therapy)

CML/hairy cell leukemia: Hematologic monitoring should be performed monthly

Patient Information Use as directed; do not change dosage or schedule of administration without consulting prescriber. Maintain adequate hydration (2-3 L/day of fluids unless instructed to restrict fluid intake). You may experience flu-like syndrome (acetaminophen may help); this syndrome subsides after several weeks of continuous dosing, but usually recurs during each cycle of intermittent therapy. You may also experience nausea, vomiting, dry mouth, or metallic taste (frequent small meals, frequent mouth care, sucking lozenges, or chewing gum may help); drowsiness, dizziness, agitation, abnormal thinking (use caution when driving or engaging in tasks requiring alertness until response to drug is known). Inform prescriber **immediately** if you feel depressed or have any thoughts of suicide. Report unusual bruising or bleeding; persistent abdominal disturbances; unusual fatigue; muscle pain or tremors; chest pain or palpitation; swelling of extremities or unusual weight gain; difficulty breathing; pain, swelling, or redness at injection site; or other unusual symptoms.

Special Geriatric Considerations No specific data is available for the elderly; however, pay close attention to Warnings/Precautions since the elderly often have reduced Cl_{cr} (<50 mL/minute), diabetes, and hyper-/hypothyroidism.

Selected Readings

"American Academy of Pediatrics Committee on Drugs. The Transfer of Drugs and Other Chemicals Into Human Milk," *Pediatrics*, 2001, 108(3):776-89.

Gresser I, "Biologic Effects of Interferons," *J Invest Dermatol*, 1990, 95(6 Suppl):66-71.

Haria M and Benfield P, "Interferon-Alpha-2a. A Review of Its Pharmacological Properties and Therapeutic Use in the Management of Viral Hepatitis," *Drugs*, 1995, 50(5):873-96.

Hirsch MS, Tolkoff-Rubin NE, Kelly AP, et al, "Pharmacokinetics of Human and Recombinant Leukocyte Interferon in Patients With Chronic Renal Failure Who Are Undergoing Hemodialysis," *J Infect Dis*, 1983, 148(2):335.

Legha SS, "The Role of Interferon Alfa in the Treatment of Metastatic Melanoma," *Semin Oncol*, 1997, 24(1 Suppl 4):24-31.

Morris DJ, "Adverse Effects and Drug Interactions of Clinical Importance With Antiviral Drugs," *Drug Saf*, 1994, 10(4):281-91.

Read SJ, Crawford DH, and Pender MP, "Trigeminal Sensory Neuropathy Induced by Interferon-Alpha Therapy," *Aust N Z J Med*, 1995, 25(1):54.

Soto Alvarez J, Sacristan JA, and Alsar MJ, "Interferon Alpha-2a-Induced Impotence," *DICP*, 1991, 25(12):1397.

Tilg H, "New Insights Into the Mechanisms of Interferon Alfa: An Immunoregulatory and Anti-Inflammatory Cytokine," *Gastroenterology*, 1997, 112(3):1017-21.

Vial T and Descotes J, "Clinical Toxicity of the Interferons," *Drug Saf*, 1994, 10(2):115-50.

White CW, Sondheimer HM, Crouch EC, et al, "Treatment of Pulmonary Hemangiomatosis With Recombinant Interferon Alfa-2a," *N Engl J Med*, 1989, 320(18):1197-200.

Williams CD and Linch DC, "Interferon Alfa-2a," *Br J Hosp Med*, 1997, 57(9):436-9.

Wills RJ, "Clinical Pharmacokinetics of Interferons," *Clin Pharmacokinet*, 1990, 19(5):390-9.

Interferon Alfa-2b (in ter FEER on AL fa too bee)

Medication Safety Issues

Sound-alike/look-alike issues:

Interferon alfa-2b may be confused with interferon alfa-2a

Related Information

Safe Handling of Hazardous Drugs *on page 1034*

U.S. Brand Names Intron® A

Canadian Brand Names Intron® A

Generic Available No

Synonyms INF-alpha 2; α-2-Interferon; rLFN-α2

Pharmacologic Category Interferon

Pregnancy Risk Factor C

Lactation Enters breast milk/not recommended (AAP rates "compatible")

Use

Patients ≥1 year of age: Chronic hepatitis B

Patients ≥18 years of age: Condyloma acuminata, chronic hepatitis C, hairy cell leukemia, malignant melanoma, AIDS-related Kaposi's sarcoma, follicular non-Hodgkin's lymphoma

Unlabeled/Investigational Use AIDS-related thrombocytopenia, cutaneous ulcerations of Behçet's disease, carcinoid syndrome, cervical cancer, lymphomatoid granulomatosis, genital herpes, hepatitis D, chronic myelogenous leukemia (CML), non-Hodgkin's lymphomas (other than follicular lymphoma, see approved use), polycythemia vera, medullary thyroid carcinoma, multiple myeloma, renal cell carcinoma, basal and squamous cell skin cancers, essential thrombocytopenia, thrombocytopenic purpura

Investigational: West Nile virus

Mechanism of Action Following activation, multiple effects can be detected including induction of gene transcription. Inhibits cellular growth, alters the state of cellular differentiation, interferes with oncogene expression, alters cell surface antigen expression, increases phagocytic activity of macrophages, and augments cytotoxicity of lymphocytes for target cells

Labeled Contraindications Hypersensitivity to interferon alfa or any component of the formulation; decompensated liver disease; autoimmune hepatitis; history of autoimmune disease; immunosuppressed transplant patients

Warnings/Precautions Suicidal ideation or attempts may occur more frequently in pediatric patients when compared to adults. May cause severe psychiatric adverse events (psychosis, mania, depression, suicidal behavior/ideation) in patients with and without previous psychiatric symptoms, avoid use in severe psychiatric disorders or in patients with a history of depression; careful neuropsychiatric monitoring is required during therapy. Use with caution in patients with a history of seizures, brain metastases, multiple sclerosis, cardiac disease (ischemic or thromboembolic), arrhythmias, myelosuppression, hepatic impairment, or renal dysfunction (use is not recommended if Cl$_{cr}$<50 mL/minute). Use caution in patients with a history of pulmonary disease, coagulopathy, (Continued)

Interferon Alfa-2b *(Continued)*

thyroid disease (monitor thyroid function), hypertension, or diabetes mellitus (particularly if prone to DKA). Caution in patients receiving drugs that may cause lactic acidosis (eg, nucleoside analogues).

Avoid use in patients with autoimmune disorders; worsening of psoriasis and/or development of autoimmune disorders has been associated with alpha interferons. Higher doses in elderly patients, or diseases other than hairy cell leukemia, may result in increased CNS toxicity. Treatment should be discontinued in patients who develop severe pulmonary symptoms with chest x-ray changes, autoimmune disorders, worsening of hepatic function, psychiatric symptoms (including depression and/or suicidal thoughts/behaviors), ischemic and/or infectious disorders. Ophthalmologic disorders (including retinal hemorrhages, cotton wool spots and retinal artery or vein obstruction) have occurred in patients receiving alpha interferons. Hypertriglyceridemia has been reported (discontinue if severe).

Safety and efficacy in children <1 year of age have not been established. Do not treat patients with visceral AIDS-related Kaposi's sarcoma associated with rapidly-progressing or life-threatening disease. A transient increase in SGOT (>2x baseline) is common in patients treated with interferon alfa-2b for chronic hepatitis. Therapy generally may continue, however, functional indicators (albumin, prothrombin time, bilirubin) should be monitored at 2-week intervals. **Due to differences in dosage, patients should not change brands of interferons.**

Intron® A may cause bone marrow suppression, including very rarely, aplastic anemia. Hemolytic anemia (hemoglobin <10 g/dL) was observed in 10% of treated patients in clinical trials; anemia occurred within 1-2 weeks of initiation of therapy.

Adverse Reactions Note: In a majority of patients, a flu-like syndrome (fever, chills, tachycardia, malaise, myalgia, headache), occurs within 1-2 hours of administration; may last up to 24 hours and may be dose-limiting.

>10%:

Cardiovascular: Chest pain (2% to 28%)

Central nervous system: Fatigue (8% to 96%), headache (21% to 62%), fever (34% to 94%), depression (4% to 40%), somnolence (1% to 33%), irritability (1% to 22%), paresthesia (1% to 21%, more common in patients previously treated with vinca alkaloids or receiving concurrent vinblastine), dizziness (7% to 23%), confusion (1% to 12%), malaise (3% to 14%), pain (3% to 15%), insomnia (1% to 12%), impaired concentration (1% to 14%, usually reverses within a few days), amnesia (1% to 14%), chills (45% to 54%)

Dermatologic: Alopecia (8% to 38%), rash (usually maculopapular) on the trunk and extremities (1% to 25%), pruritus (3% to 11%), dry skin (1% to 10%)

Endocrine & metabolic: Alkaline phosphatase increased (48%), hypocalcemia (10% to 51%), hyperglycemia (33% to 39%), amenorrhea (up to 12% in lymphoma)

Gastrointestinal: Anorexia (1% to 69%), nausea (19% to 66%), vomiting (2% to 32%, usually mild), diarrhea (2% to 45%, may be severe), taste change (2% to 24%), xerostomia (1% to 28%), abdominal pain (2% to 23%), gingivitis (2% to 14%), constipation (1% to 14%)

Hematologic: Myelosuppression; neutropenia (30% to 66%); thrombocytopenia (5% to 15%); anemia (15% to 32%, may be dose-limiting, usually seen only during the first 6 months of therapy)

Onset: 7-10 days

Nadir: 14 days, may be delayed 20-40 days in hairy cell leukemia

Recovery: 21 days

Hepatic: Right upper quadrant pain (15% in hepatitis C), transaminases increased (increased SGOT in up to 63%)

Local: Injection site reaction (1% to 20%)

Neuromuscular & skeletal: Weakness (5% to 63%) may be severe at doses >20,000,000 units/day; mild arthralgia and myalgia (5% to 75% - usually during the first 72 hours of treatment), rigors (2% to 42%), back pain (1% to 19%), musculoskeletal pain (1% to 21%), paresthesia (1% to 21%)

Renal: Urinary tract infection (up to 5% in hepatitis C)

Respiratory: Dyspnea (1% to 34%), cough (1% to 31%), pharyngitis (1% to 31%),

Miscellaneous: Loss of smell, flu-like symptoms (5% to 79%), diaphoresis (2% to 21%)

5% to 10%:

Cardiovascular: Hypertension (9% in hepatitis C)

Central nervous system: Anxiety (1% to 9%), nervousness (1% to 3%), vertigo (up to 8% in lymphoma)

Dermatologic: Dermatitis (1% to 8%)

Endocrine & metabolic: Decreased libido (1% to 5%)

Gastrointestinal: Loose stools (1% to 21%), dyspepsia (2% to 8%)

Neuromuscular & skeletal: Hypoesthesia (1% to 10%)

Respiratory: Nasal congestion (1% to 10%)

<5% (Limited to important or life-threatening):

Cardiovascular: Angina, arrhythmia, atrial fibrillation, bradycardia, tachycardia, vasculitis, CHF, cardiomegaly, cardiomyopathy, hypotension, Raynaud's phenomenon, thrombosis, pulmonary embolism, MI

Central nervous system: Abnormal coordination, aggravated depression, aphasia, ataxia, Bell's palsy, coma, seizure, dysphonia, extrapyramidal disorder, flushing, hallucinations, manic reaction, migraine, neuropathy, paranoia, psychosis, stroke, suicidal ideation, suicide attempt, syncope, tremor

Dermatologic: Diffuse erythema, eczema, epidermal necrolysis, hirsutism, psoriasis, urticaria

Endocrine & metabolic: Diabetes mellitus, hyperthyroidism, hypothyroidism, hypertriglyceridemia, hyperglycemia, goiter, pancreatitis

Gastrointestinal: Ascites, colitis, esophagitis, gastritis, gastrointestinal hemorrhage, gingival hyperplasia, mucositis, rectal hemorrhage, stomatitis, taste loss

Genitourinary: Cystitis, incontinence, dysuria

Hematologic: Anemia, granulocytopenia, leukopenia, hemolytic anemia, thrombocytopenic purpura

Hepatic: Hyperbilirubinemia, jaundice, hepatic encephalopathy (rare), hepatic failure (rare), hepatotoxic reaction

Neuromuscular & skeletal: Arthritis, leg cramps, polyarteritis nodosa, tendonitis, rheumatoid arthritis, spondylitis, lupus erythematosus

Ocular: Abnormal vision, nystagmus

(Continued)

Interferon Alfa-2b *(Continued)*

Renal: Proteinuria, hematuria, increased BUN, nephrotic syndrome, renal failure

Respiratory: Asthma, bronchospasm, hemoptysis, hypoventilation, pulmonary fibrosis, pleural effusion, pneumonitis, respiratory insufficiency

Miscellaneous: Acute hypersensitivity reactions, allergic reactions

Vesicant No

Emetic Potential Moderate (10% to 30%); usually mild to moderate, aggressive therapy with serotonin antagonists is usually not necessary

Overdosage/Toxicology Symptoms of overdose include CNS depression, obtundation, flu-like symptoms, and myelosuppression. Treatment is supportive.

Drug Interactions

Cytochrome P450 Effect: Inhibits CYP1A2 (weak)

Increased Effect/Toxicity: Theophylline clearance has been reported to be decreased in hepatitis patients receiving interferon. Interferons may increase the adverse/toxic effects of ACE inhibitors, specifically the development of granulocytopenia. Agranulocytosis has been reported with concurrent use of clozapine (case report). Interferons may increase the anticoagulant effects of warfarin, and interferons may increase serum levels of zidovudine.

Storage/Stability Store powder and solution for injection (vials and pens) under refrigeration (2°C to 8°C).

Powder for injection: Following reconstitution, should be used immediately, but may be stored under refrigeration for up to 24 hours.

Prefilled pens: After first use, discard unused portion after 1 month.

Reconstitution The manufacturer recommends reconstituting vial with the diluent provided (SWFI). To prepare solution for infusion, further dilute appropriate dose in NS 100 mL. Final concentration should not be <10 million units/100 mL.

Compatibility Stable in LR, NS; not stable in D_5W

Pharmacodynamics/Kinetics

Distribution: V_d: 31 L; but has been noted to be much greater (370-720 L) in leukemia patients receiving continuous infusion IFN; IFN does not penetrate the CSF

Metabolism: Primarily renal

Bioavailability: I.M.: 83%; SubQ: 90%

Half-life elimination: I.M., I.V.: 2 hours; SubQ: 3 hours

Time to peak, serum: I.M., SubQ: ~3-12 hours

Dosage Refer to individual protocols

Children 1-17 years: Chronic hepatitis B: SubQ: 3 million units/m² 3 times/week for 1 week; then 6 million units/m² 3 times/week; maximum: 10 million units 3 times/week; total duration of therapy 16-24 weeks

Adults:

Hairy cell leukemia: I.M., SubQ: 2 million units/m² 3 times/week for 2-6 months

Lymphoma (follicular): SubQ: 5 million units 3 times/week for up to 18 months

Malignant melanoma: 20 million units/m² I.V. for 5 consecutive days per week for 4 weeks, then 10 million units/m² SubQ 3 times/week for 48 weeks

AIDS-related Kaposi's sarcoma: I.M., SubQ: 30 million units/m^2 3 times/week

Chronic hepatitis B: I.M., SubQ: 5 million units/day or 10 million units 3 times/week for 16 weeks

Chronic hepatitis C: I.M., SubQ: 3 million units 3 times/week for 16 weeks. In patients with normalization of ALT at 16 weeks, continue treatment for 18-24 months; consider discontinuation if normalization does not occur at 16 weeks. **Note:** May be used in combination therapy with ribavirin in previously untreated patients or in patients who relapse following alpha interferon therapy; refer to Interferon Alfa-2b and Ribavirin Combination Pack monograph.

Condyloma acuminata: Intralesionally: 1 million units/lesion (maximum: 5 lesions/treatment) 3 times/week (on alternate days) for 3 weeks; may administer a second course at 12-16 weeks

Dosage adjustment in renal impairment: Combination therapy with ribavirin (hepatitis C) should not be used in patients with reduced renal function (Cl$_{cr}$ <50 mL/minute).

Not removed by peritoneal or hemodialysis

Dosage adjustment for toxicity: Manufacturer-recommended adjustments, listed according to indication:

Lymphoma (follicular):

Severe toxicity (neutrophils <1000 cells/mm^3 or platelets <50,000 cells/mm^3): Reduce dose by 50% or temporarily discontinue

AST/ALT >5 times ULN: Permanently discontinue

Hairy cell leukemia:

Severe toxicity: Reduce dose by 50% or temporarily discontinue; permanently discontinue if persistent or recurrent severe toxicity is noted

Hepatitis B or C:

WBC <1500 cells/mm^3, granulocytes <750 cells/mm^3, or platelet count <50,000 cells/mm^3: Reduce dose by 50%

WBC <1000 cells/mm^3, granulocytes <500 cells/mm^3, or platelet count <25,000 cells/mm^3: Permanently discontinue

Kaposi sarcoma: Severe toxicity: Reduce dose by 50% or temporarily discontinue

Malignant melanoma:

Severe toxicity (neutrophils <500 cells/mm^3 or AST/ALT >5 times ULN): Reduce dose by 50% or temporarily discontinue

Neutrophils <250 cells/mm^3 or AST/ALT >10 times ULN: Permanently discontinue

Combination Regimens

Head and neck cancer: PFL + IFN *on page 930*

Melanoma: IL-2 + IFN *on page 902*

Renal cell cancer:

Interleukin 2-Interferon Alfa 2 *on page 902*

Interleukin 2-Interferon Alfa 2-Fluorouracil *on page 903*

Administration

Injection: Do not use 3-, 5-, 18-, and 25 million unit strengths intralesionally, solutions are hypertonic; 50 million unit strength is not for use in condylomata, hairy cell leukemia, or chronic hepatitis. Patients with platelet count <50,000/mm^3 should receive doses SubQ, not I.M.

Oral: Capsules should not be crushed, chewed, or opened.

(Continued)

Interferon Alfa-2b *(Continued)*

Dosage Forms

Injection, powder for reconstitution: 10 million units; 18 million units; 50 million units [contains human albumin]

Injection, solution [multidose prefilled pen]:

Delivers 3 million units/0.2 mL (1.5 mL) [delivers 6 doses; 18 million units]

Delivers 5 million units/0.2 mL (1.5 mL) [delivers 6 doses; 30 million units]

Delivers 10 million units/0.2 mL (1.5 mL) [delivers 6 doses; 60 million units]

Injection, solution [multidose vial]: 6 million units/mL (3 mL); 10 million units/mL (2.5 mL)

Injection, solution [single-dose vial]: 10 million units/ mL (1 mL)

See also Interferon Alfa-2b and Ribavirin Combination Pack monograph.

Monitoring Parameters Baseline chest x-ray, ECG, CBC with differential, liver function tests, electrolytes, thyroid function tests, platelets, weight; patients with pre-existing cardiac abnormalities, or in advanced stages of cancer should have ECGs taken before and during treatment.

Patient Information Without the advice of prescriber, do not change brands of interferon as changes in dosage may result; do not operate heavy machinery while on therapy since changes in mental status may occur; report any persistent or severe sore throat, fever, fatigue, unusual bleeding, or bruising. You may experience flu-like syndrome (acetaminophen may help); this syndrome subsides after several weeks of continuous dosing, but usually recurs during each cycle of intermittent therapy.

Selected Readings

"American Academy of Pediatrics Committee on Drugs. The Transfer of Drugs and Other Chemicals Into Human Milk," *Pediatrics*, 2001, 108(3):776-89.

Balkwill FR and Smyth JF, "Interferons in Cancer Therapy: A Reappraisal," *Lancet*, 1987, 2(8554):317-9.

Gresser I, "Biologic Effects of Interferons," *J Invest Dermatol*, 1990, 95(6 Suppl):66-71.

Houglum JE, "Interferon: Mechanisms of Action and Clinical Value," *Clin Pharm*, 1983, 2(1):20-8.

Jeffrey LP, Chairman, National Study Commission on Cytotoxic Exposure. Position Statement. "The Handling of Cytotoxic Agents by Women Who Are Pregnant, Attempting to Conceive, or Breast-Feeding," January 12, 1987.

Kirkwood JM, Bender C, Agarwala S, et al, "Mechanisms and Management of Toxicities Associated With High-Dose Interferon Alfa-2b Therapy," *J Clin Oncol*, 2002, 20(17):3703-18.

Koeller JM, "Biologic Response Modifiers: The Interferon Alfa Experience," *Am J Hosp Pharm*, 1989, 46(11 Suppl 2):11-5.

Legha SS, "The Role of Interferon Alfa in the Treatment of Metastatic Melanoma," *Semin Oncol*, 1997, 24(1 Suppl 4):24-31.

Meaeda T, Onishi S, Miura T, et al, "Exacerbation of Primary Biliary Cirrhosis During Interferon-Alpha-2b Therapy for Chronic Active Hepatitis C," *Dig Dis Sci*, 1995, 40(6):1226-30.

Murakami CS, Zeller K, Bodenheimer HC Jr, et al, "Idiopathic Thrombocytopenic Purpura During Interferon-Alpha 2B Treatment for Chronic Hepatitis," *Am J Gastroenterol*, 1994, 89(12):2244-5.

Parker MG, Atkins MB, Ucci AA, et al, "Rapidly Progressive Glomerulonephritis After Immunotherapy for Cancer," *J Am Soc Nephrol*, 1995, 5(10):1740-4.

Perrillo RP, "Interferon in the Management of Chronic Hepatitis B," *Dig Dis Sci*, 1993, 38(4):577-93.

Sakane N, Yoshida T, Yoshioka K, et al, "Reversible Hypopituitarism After Interferon alfa Therapy," *Lancet*, 1995, 345(8960):1305.

Tilg H, "New Insights Into the Mechanisms of Interferon Alfa: An Immunoregulatory and Anti-Inflammatory Cytokine," *Gastroenterology*, 1997, 112(3):1017-21.

Vial T and Descotes J, "Clinical Toxicity of the Interferons," *Drug Saf*, 1994, 10(2):115-50.

Wills RJ, "Clinical Pharmacokinetics of Interferons," *Clin Pharmacokinet*, 1990, 19(5):390-9.

Zimmerman S, Adkins D, Graham M, et al, "Irreversible, Severe, Congestive Cardiomyopathy Occurring in Association With Interferon Alpha Therapy," *Cancer Biother*, 1994, 9(4):291-9.

Interferon Gamma-1b (in ter FEER on GAM ah won bee)

Related Information

Safe Handling of Hazardous Drugs *on page 1034*

U.S. Brand Names Actimmune®

Canadian Brand Names Actimmune®

Generic Available No

Pharmacologic Category Interferon

Pregnancy Risk Factor C

Lactation Excretion in breast milk unknown/contraindicated

Use Reduce frequency and severity of serious infections associated with chronic granulomatous disease; delay time to disease progression in patients with severe, malignant osteopetrosis

Labeled Contraindications Hypersensitivity to interferon gamma, *E. coli* derived proteins, or any component of the formulation

Warnings/Precautions Patients with pre-existing cardiac disease, seizure disorders, CNS disturbances, or myelosuppression should be carefully monitored; long-term effects on growth and development are unknown; safety and efficacy in children <1 year of age have not been established.

Adverse Reactions Based on 50 mcg/m^2 dose administered 3 times weekly for chronic granulomatous disease

>10%:

Central nervous system: Fever (52%), headache (33%), chills (14%), fatigue (14%)

Dermatologic: Rash (17%)

Gastrointestinal: Diarrhea (14%), vomiting (13%)

Local: Injection site erythema or tenderness (14%)

1% to 10%:

Central nervous system: Depression (3%)

Gastrointestinal: Nausea (10%), abdominal pain (8%)

Neuromuscular & skeletal: Myalgia (6%), arthralgia (2%), back pain (2%)

Vesicant No

Emetic Potential Very low (<10%)

Drug Interactions

Cytochrome P450 Effect: Inhibits CYP1A2 (weak), 2E1 (weak)

Increased Effect/Toxicity: Interferon gamma-1b may increase hepatic enzymes or enhance myelosuppression when taken with other myelosuppressive agents. May decrease cytochrome P450 concentrations leading to increased serum concentrations of drugs metabolized by this pathway.

Ethanol/Nutrition/Herb Interactions Herb/Nutraceutical: Dietary supplements containing aristolochic acid (found most often in Chinese medicines/herbal therapies); cases of nephropathy and ESRD associated with their use.

Storage/Stability Store in refrigerator. Do not freeze. Do not shake. Discard if left unrefrigerated for >12 hours.

(Continued)

Interferon Gamma-1b *(Continued)*

Pharmacodynamics/Kinetics

Absorption: I.M., SubQ: Slowly

Half-life elimination: I.V.: 38 minutes; I.M., SubQ: 3-6 hours

Time to peak, plasma: I.M.: 4 hours (1.5 ng/mL); SubQ: 7 hours (0.6 ng/mL)

Dosage

Chronic granulomatous disease: Children >1 year and Adults: SubQ:

BSA ≤0.5 m^2: 1.5 mcg/kg/dose 3 times/week

BSA >0.5 m^2: 50 mcg/m^2 (1 million int. units/m^2) 3 times/week

Severe, malignant osteopetrosis: Children >1 year: SubQ:

BSA ≤0.5 m^2: 1.5 mcg/kg/dose 3 times/week

BSA >0.5 m^2: 50 mcg/m^2 (1 million int. units/m^2) 3 times/week

Note: Previously expressed as 1.5 million units/m^2; 50 mcg is equivalent to 1 million int. units/m^2.

Dosage adjustment: If severe reactions occur, modify dose (50% reduction) or therapy should be discontinued until adverse reactions abate.

Administration Interferon γ may be administered intravenously, intramuscularly, or subcutaneously.

Dosage Forms Injection, solution [preservative free]: 100 mcg [2 million int. units] (0.5 mL)

Previously, 100 mcg was expressed as 3 million units. This is equivalent to 2 million int. units.

Monitoring Parameters CBC with differential, platelets, LFTs, electrolytes, BUN, creatinine, and urinalysis prior to therapy and at 3-month intervals

Patient Information Use as directed; do not change the dosage or schedule of administration without consulting prescriber. Maintain adequate hydration (2-3 L/day of fluids unless instructed to restrict fluid intake). You may experience flu-like syndrome (acetaminophen may help or can administer dose at bedtime); nausea, vomiting, or loss of appetite (frequent small meals, frequent mouth care, sucking lozenges, or chewing gum may help); drowsiness, dizziness, agitation, or abnormal thinking (use caution when driving or engaging in tasks requiring alertness until response to drug is known). Report unusual bruising or bleeding; persistent abdominal disturbances; unusual fatigue; muscle pain or tremors; chest pain or palpitations; swelling of extremities; visual disturbances; pain, swelling, or redness at injection site; or other unusual symptoms.

- **Interleukin-2** *see* Aldesleukin *on page 32*
- **Interleukin-11** *see* Oprelvekin *on page 627*
- **Intron® A** *see* Interferon Alfa-2b *on page 471*
- **Investigational Drug Service** *see page 1031*
- **Iodine I 131 Tositumomab and Tositumomab** *see* Tositumomab and Iodine I 131 Tositumomab *on page 781*
- **Iquix®** *see* Levofloxacin *on page 504*
- **Iressa™** *see* Gefitinib *on page 386*

Irinotecan *(eye rye no TEE kan)*

Related Information

Management of Nausea and Vomiting *on page 982*

Safe Handling of Hazardous Drugs *on page 1034*

U.S. Brand Names Camptosar®

Canadian Brand Names Camptosar®

Generic Available No

Synonyms Camptothecin-11; CPT-11; NSC-616348

Pharmacologic Category Antineoplastic Agent, Natural Source (Plant) Derivative

Pregnancy Risk Factor D

Lactation Enters breast milk/contraindicated

Use Treatment of metastatic carcinoma of the colon or rectum

Unlabeled/Investigational Use Lung cancer (small cell and nonsmall cell), cervical cancer, gastric cancer, pancreatic cancer, leukemia, lymphoma, breast cancer

Mechanism of Action Irinotecan and its active metabolite (SN-38) bind reversibly to topoisomerase I and stabilize the cleavable complex so that religation of the cleaved DNA strand cannot occur. This results in the accumulation of cleavable complexes and single-strand DNA breaks. This interaction results in single-stranded DNA breaks and cell death consistent with S-phase cell cycle specificity.

Labeled Contraindications Hypersensitivity to irinotecan or any component of the formulation; concurrent use of atazanavir, ketoconazole, St John's wort; pregnancy

Warnings/Precautions Hazardous agent - use appropriate precautions for handling and disposal. See Safe Handling of Hazardous Drugs *on page 1034* in the Appendix. Irinotecan can induce both early and late forms of diarrhea (mediated by different mechanisms). The administration of irinotecan should be delayed until the patient recovers and subsequent doses should be decreased. Premedication with loperamide is not recommended.

Severe diarrhea may be dose-limiting and potentially fatal; deaths due to sepsis following severe myelosuppression have been reported. Therapy should be discontinued if neutropenic fever occurs or if the absolute neutrophil count is <500/mm³. The dose of irinotecan should be reduced if there is a clinically significant decrease in the total WBC (<200/mm³), neutrophil count (<1000/mm³), hemoglobin (<8 g/dL), or platelet count (<100,000/mm³). Routine administration of a colony-stimulating factor is generally not necessary.

Patients with even modest elevations in total serum bilirubin levels (1.0-2.0 mg/dL) have a significantly greater likelihood of experiencing first-course grade 3 or 4 neutropenia than those with bilirubin levels that were <1.0 mg/dL. Patients with abnormal glucuronidation of bilirubin, such as those with Gilbert's syndrome, may also be at greater risk of myelosuppression when receiving therapy with irinotecan. Hold diuretics during dosing due to potential risk of dehydration secondary to vomiting and/or diarrhea induced by irinotecan.

Use caution in patients who previously received pelvic/abdominal radiation, elderly patients with comorbid conditions, or baseline performance status of 2; close monitoring is recommended.

Adverse Reactions

>10%:

Cardiovascular: Vasodilation

Central nervous system: Insomnia, dizziness, fever (45.4%)

(Continued)

Irinotecan *(Continued)*

Dermatologic: Alopecia (60.5%), rash

Gastrointestinal: Diarrhea, overall, 56.9%, abdominal pain and/or cramping during therapy, (dose -limiting toxicity with weekly dosing regimen). Anorexia, constipation, flatulence, stomatitis, and dyspepsia have also been reported.

Early diarrhea (50.7% incidence, grade 3/4 8%) usually occurs during or within 24 hours of administration. Can be successfully managed with atropine.

Late diarrhea (87.8% incidence) usually occurs >24 hours after treatment. The incidence of grade 3 or 4 late diarrhea is significantly higher in patients ≥65 years of age; close monitoring and prompt initiation of high-dose loperamide therapy is prudent.

Nausea and vomiting: 86.2%

Emetic potential: Moderately high (86.2% incidence, however, only 12.5% grade 3 or 4 vomiting)

Hematologic: Myelosuppressive: May be dose-limiting

White blood cell count nadir is 15 days after administration and is more frequent than thrombocytopenia. Recovery is usually within 24-28 days and cumulative toxicity has not been observed.

WBC: Mild to severe

Platelets: Mild

Onset: 10 days

Nadir: 14-16 days

Recovery: 21-28 days

Neuromuscular & skeletal: Weakness (75.7%)

Respiratory: Dyspnea (22%), cough, rhinitis, decreased DLCO (in a few patients)

Miscellaneous: Diaphoresis

1% to 10%: Thrombophlebitis has been reported

<1%, postmarketing and/or case reports: Anaphylactoid reaction, anaphylaxis, bleeding, colitis, ileus, renal failure (acute), renal impairment; pulmonary toxicity (dyspnea, fever, reticulonodular infiltrates on chest x-ray)

Note: In limited pediatric experience, dehydration (often associated with severe hypokalemia and hyponatremia) was among the most significant grade 3/4 adverse events, with a frequency up to 29%. In addition, grade 3/4 infection was reported in 24%.

Vesicant No

Emetic Potential High (60% to 90%, usually mild)

Overdosage/Toxicology Symptoms of overdose include bone marrow suppression, leukopenia, thrombocytopenia, nausea, and vomiting. Treatment is supportive.

Drug Interactions

Cytochrome P450 Effect: Substrate (major) of CYP2B6, 3A4

Increased Effect/Toxicity: CYP2B6 inhibitors may increase the levels/effects of irinotecan; example inhibitors include desipramine, paroxetine, and sertraline. CYP3A4 inhibitors may increase the levels/effects of irinotecan; example inhibitors include azole antifungals, ciprofloxacin, clarithromycin, diclofenac, doxycycline, erythromycin, imatinib, isoniazid, nefazodone, nicardipine, propofol, protease inhibitors, quinidine, and verapamil. Bevacizumab may increase the adverse effects of irinotecan (eg, diarrhea, neutropenia). Ketoconazole increases the levels/effects of irinotecan and active metabolite; discontinue ketoconazole 1 week prior to irinotecan therapy; **concurrent use during irinotecan therapy is contraindicated.**

Decreased Effect: CYP2B6 inducers may decrease the levels/effects of irinotecan; example inducers include carbamazepine, nevirapine, phenobarbital, phenytoin, and rifampin. CYP3A4 inducers may decrease the levels/effects of irinotecan; example inducers include aminoglutethimide, carbamazepine, nafcillin, nevirapine, phenobarbital, phenytoin, and rifamycins. St John's wort decreases therapeutic effect of irinotecan; discontinue ≥2 weeks prior to irinotecan therapy; **concurrent use during irinotecan therapy is contraindicated.**

Ethanol/Nutrition/Herb Interactions Herb/Nutraceutical: St John's wort decreases the efficacy of irinotecan.

Storage/Stability Store intact vials of injection at room temperature; protect from light. Solutions diluted in NS may precipitate if refrigerated. Solutions diluted in D_5W are stable for 24 hours at room temperature or 48 hours under refrigeration.

Reconstitution Dilute in 250-500 mL D_5W or NS to a final concentration of 0.12-2.8 mg/mL. Due to the relatively acidic pH, irinotecan appears to be more stable in D_5W than NS.

Compatibility Stable in D_5W, NS

Y-site administration: Incompatible: Gemcitabine

Compatibility when admixed: Incompatible: Methylprednisolone sodium succinate

Pharmacodynamics/Kinetics

Distribution: V_d: 33-150 L/m^2

Protein binding, plasma: Parent drug: 30% to 68%; SN-38 (active drug): 95%

Metabolism: Via intestinal mucosa, plasma, hepatic, and perhaps in some tumors; converted to SN-38 by carboxylesterase enzymes; undergoes glucuronidation. Enterohepatic recirculation results in a second peak in the concentration of SN-38. The lactones of both irinotecan and SN-38 undergo hydrolysis to inactive hydroxy acid forms.

Half-life elimination: Parent drug: Alpha: 0.2 hours, Beta: 2.5 hours, Gamma: 14.2 hours; SN-38: 3-23.9 hours

Time to peak: SN-38: 30-minute infusion: ~1 hour

Excretion: Urine (~20% of dose) within 24 hours; SN-38 excretion in 24 hours accounted for 0.25% of administered dose

Dosage Refer to individual protocols.

Single-agent therapy:

125 mg/m^2 over 90 minutes on days 1, 8, 15, and 22, followed by a 2-week rest

350 mg/m^2 over 90 minutes, once every 3 weeks

Dosing adjustment in renal impairment: Effects have not been evaluated

Dosing adjustment in hepatic impairment:

The manufacturer recommends that no change in dosage or administration be made for patients with liver metastases and normal hepatic function.

Consideration may be given to starting irinotecan at a lower dose (eg, 100 mg/m^2) if bilirubin is 1-2 mg/dL; for total serum bilirubin elevations >2.0 mg/dL, specific recommendations are not available.

(Continued)

Irinotecan *(Continued)*

Dosage adjustment for toxicities: It is recommended that new courses begin only after the granulocyte count recovers to ≥1500/mm³, the platelet counts recovers to ≥100,000/mm³, and treatment-related diarrhea has fully resolved. Depending on the patient's ability to tolerate therapy, doses should be adjusted in increments of 25-50 mg/m². Irinotecan doses may range 50-150 mg/m². Treatment should be delayed 1-2 weeks to allow for recovery from treatment-related toxicities. If the patient has not recovered after a 2-week delay, consideration should be given to discontinuing irinotecan. See tables.

Combination Schedules: Recommended Dosage Modifications[1]

Toxicity NCI[2] Grade (Value)	During a Cycle of Therapy	At the Start of Subsequent Cycles of Therapy (After Adequate Recovery), Compared to the Starting Dose in the Previous Cycle[1]
No toxicity	Maintain dose level	Maintain dose level
Neutropenia		
1 (1500-1999/mm³)	Maintain dose level	Maintain dose level
2 (1000-1499/mm³)	↓ 1 dose level	Maintain dose level
3 (500-999/mm³)	Omit dose until resolved to ≤ grade 2, then ↓ 1 dose level	↓ 1 dose level
4 (<500/mm³)	Omit dose until resolved to ≤ grade 2, then ↓ 2 dose levels	↓ 2 dose levels
Neutropenic Fever (grade 4 neutropenia and ≥ grade 2 fever)	Omit dose until resolved, then ↓ 2 dose levels	
Other Hematologic Toxicities	Dose modifications for leukopenia or thrombocytopenia during a course of therapy and at the start of subsequent courses of therapy are also based on NCI toxicity criteria and are the same as recommended for neutropenia above.	
Diarrhea		
1 (2-3 stools/day > pretreatment)	Delay dose until resolved to baseline, then give same dose	Maintain dose level
2 (4-6 stools/day > pretreatment)	Omit dose until resolved to baseline, then ↓ 1 dose level	Maintain dose level
3 (7-9 stools/day > pretreatment)	Omit dose until resolved to baseline, then ↓ by 1 dose level	↓ 1 dose level
4 (≥10 stools/day > pretreatment)	Omit dose until resolved to baseline, then ↓ 2 dose levels	↓ 2 dose levels
Other Nonhematologic Toxicities[3]		
1	Maintain dose level	Maintain dose level
2	Omit dose until resolved to ≤ grade 1, then ↓ 1 dose level	Maintain dose level
3	Omit dose until resolved to ≤ grade 2, then ↓ 1 dose level	↓ 1 dose level
4	Omit dose until resolved to ≤ grade 2, then ↓ 2 dose levels	↓ 2 dose levels
Mucositis and/or stomatitis	Decrease only 5-FU, not irinotecan	Decrease only 5-FU, not irinotecan

[1]All dose modifications should be based on the worst preceding toxicity.

[2]National Cancer Institute Common Toxicity Criteria (version 1.0).

[3]Excludes alopecia, anorexia, asthenia.

Single-Agent Schedule: Recommended Dosage Modifications[1]

Toxicity NCI Grade[2] (Value)	During a Cycle of Therapy	At Start of Subsequent Cycles of Therapy (After Adequate Recovery), Compared to Starting Dose in Previous Cycle[1]	
	Weekly	Weekly	Once Every 3 Weeks
No toxicity	Maintain dose level	↑ 25 mg/m² up to a maximum dose of 150 mg/m²	Maintain dose level
Neutropenia			
1 (1500-1999/mm³)	Maintain dose level	Maintain dose level	Maintain dose level
2 (1000-1499/mm³)	↓ 25 mg/m²	Maintain dose level	Maintain dose level
3 (500-999/mm³)	Omit dose until resolved to ≤ grade 2, then ↓ 25 mg/m²	↓ 25 mg/m²	↓ 50 mg/m²
4 (<500/mm³)	Omit dose until resolved to ≤ grade 2, then ↓ 50 mg/m²	↓ 50 mg/m²	↓ 50 mg/m²
Neutropenic Fever (grade 4 neutropenia and ≥ grade 2 fever)	Omit dose until resolved, then ↓ 50 mg/m²	↓ 50 mg/m²	↓ 50 mg/m²
Other Hematologic Toxicities	Dose modifications for leukopenia, thrombocytopenia, and anemia during a course of therapy and at the start of subsequent courses of therapy are also based on NCI toxicity criteria and are the same as recommended for neutropenia above.		
Diarrhea			
1 (2-3 stools/day > pretreatment)	Maintain dose level	Maintain dose level	Maintain dose level
2 (4-6 stools/day > pretreatment)	↓ 25 mg/m²	Maintain dose level	Maintain dose level
3 (7-9 stools/day > pretreatment)	Omit dose until resolved to ≤ grade 2, then ↓ 25 mg/m²	↓ 25 mg/m²	↓ 50 mg/m²
4 (≥10 stools/day > pretreatment)	Omit dose until resolved to ≤ grade 2, then ↓ 50 mg/m²	↓ 50 mg/m²	↓ 50 mg/m²
Other Nonhematologic Toxicities[3]			
1	Maintain dose level	Maintain dose level	Maintain dose level
2	↓ 25 mg/m²	↓ 25 mg/m²	↓ 50 mg/m²
3	Omit dose until resolved to ≤ grade 2, then ↓ 25 mg/m²	↓ 25 mg/m²	↓ 50 mg/m²
4	Omit dose until resolved to ≤ grade 2, then ↓ 50 mg/m²	↓ 50 mg/m²	↓ 50 mg/m²

[1]All dose modifications should be based on the worst preceding toxicity.

[2]National Cancer Institute Common Toxicity Criteria (version 1.0).

[3]Excludes alopecia, anorexia, asthenia.

Combination Regimens

Colorectal cancer:

FOIL *on page 890*

FU/LV/CPT-11 *on page 893*

FU/LV/CPT-11 (Saltz Regimen) *on page 894*

Esophageal cancer: Irinotecan/Cisplatin *on page 903*

Pancreatic cancer: Gemcitabine/Irinotecan *on page 897*

Administration I.V. infusion, usually over 90 minutes.

Dosage Forms Injection, solution, as hydrochloride: 20 mg/mL (2 mL, 5 mL)

Monitoring Parameters CBC with differential, platelet count, and hemoglobin with each dose; monitor infusion site for signs of inflammation and avoid extravasation

(Continued)

Irinotecan *(Continued)*

Patient Information Patients and patients' caregivers should be informed of the expected toxic effects of irinotecan, particularly of its gastrointestinal manifestations, such as nausea, vomiting, and diarrhea. Each patient should be instructed to have loperamide readily available and to begin treatment for late diarrhea (occurring >24 hours after administration of irinotecan) at the first episode of poorly formed or loose stools or the earliest onset of bowel movements more frequent than normally expected for the patient. Refer to Warnings/Precautions. The patient should also be instructed to notify the prescriber if diarrhea occurs. Premedication with loperamide is not recommended. The use of drugs with laxative properties should be avoided because of the potential for exacerbation of diarrhea. Patients should be advised to contact their prescriber to discuss any laxative use. Patients should consult their prescriber if vomiting occurs, fever or evidence of infection develops, or if symptoms of dehydration, such as fainting, lightheadedness, or dizziness, are noted following therapy.

Selected Readings

Marsh S and McLeod HL, "Pharmacogenetics of Irinotecan Toxicity," *Pharmacogenomics*, 2004, 5(7):835-43.

Mathijssen RH, Loos WJ, Verweij J, et al, "Pharmacology of Topoisomerase I Inhibitors Irinotecan (CPT-11) and Topotecan," *Curr Cancer Drug Targets*, 2002, 2(2):103-23.

Mathijssen RH, van Alphen RJ, Verweij J, et al, "Clinical Pharmacokinetics and Metabolism of Irinotecan (CPT-11)," *Clin Cancer Res*, 2001, 7(8):2182-94.

Toffoli G, Cecchin E, Corona G, et al, "Pharmacogenetics of Irinotecan," *Curr Med Chem Anti-Canc Agents*, 2003, 3(3):225-37.

Iron Dextran Complex (EYE ern DEKS tran KOM pleks)

Medication Safety Issues

Sound-alike/look-alike issues:

Dexferrum® may be confused with Desferal®

U.S. Brand Names Dexferrum®; INFeD®

Canadian Brand Names Dexiron™; Infufer®

Generic Available No

Pharmacologic Category Iron Salt

Pregnancy Risk Factor C

Lactation Enters breast milk/contraindicated

Use Treatment of microcytic hypochromic anemia resulting from iron deficiency in patients in whom oral administration is infeasible or ineffective

Mechanism of Action The released iron, from the plasma, eventually replenishes the depleted iron stores in the bone marrow where it is incorporated into hemoglobin

Labeled Contraindications Hypersensitivity to iron dextran or any component of the formulation; all anemias that are not involved with iron deficiency; hemochromatosis; hemolytic anemia

Warnings/Precautions Use with caution in patients with history of asthma, hepatic impairment, or rheumatoid arthritis. Not recommended in children <4 months of age. Deaths associated with parenteral administration following anaphylactic-type reactions have been reported. Use only in patients where the iron deficient state is not amenable to oral iron therapy. A test dose of 0.5 mL I.V. or I.M. should be given to observe for adverse reactions. I.V. administration of iron dextran is often preferred.

Adverse Reactions

>10%:

Cardiovascular: Flushing

Central nervous system: Dizziness, fever, headache, pain

Gastrointestinal: Nausea, vomiting, metallic taste

Local: Staining of skin at the site of I.M. injection

Miscellaneous: Diaphoresis

1% to 10%:

Cardiovascular: Hypotension (1% to 2%)

Dermatologic: Urticaria (1% to 2%), phlebitis (1% to 2%)

Gastrointestinal: Diarrhea

Genitourinary: Discoloration of urine

<1%: Cardiovascular collapse, leukocytosis, chills, arthralgia, respiratory difficulty, lymphadenopathy, anaphylaxis, shock

Note: Diaphoresis, urticaria, arthralgia, fever, chills, dizziness, headache, and nausea may be delayed 24-48 hours after I.V. administration or 3-4 days after I.M. administration.

Anaphylactoid reactions: Respiratory difficulties and cardiovascular collapse have been reported and occur most frequently within the first several minutes of administration.

Overdosage/Toxicology Symptoms of overdose include erosion of GI mucosa, pulmonary edema, hyperthermia, convulsions, tachycardia, hepatic and renal impairment, coma, hematemesis, lethargy, tachycardia, and acidosis. Serum iron level >300 mcg/mL requires treatment of overdose due to severe toxicity. If severe iron overdose (when the serum iron concentration exceeds the total iron-binding capacity) occurs, it may be treated with deferoxamine. Deferoxamine may be administered I.V. (80 mg/kg over 24 hours) or I.M. (40-90 mg/kg every 8 hours).

Drug Interactions

Decreased Effect: Decreased effect with chloramphenicol.

Ethanol/Nutrition/Herb Interactions Food: Iron bioavailability may be decreased if taken with dairy products.

Storage/Stability Store at room temperature. Stability of parenteral admixture at room temperature (25°C) is 3 months.

Reconstitution Solutions for I.V. infusion should be diluted in 250-1000 mL NS

Compatibility Stable in D_5W, NS; **variable stability (consult detailed reference)** in TPN

Compatibility when admixed: Compatible: Cyanocobalamin, netilmicin

Pharmacodynamics/Kinetics

Absorption:

I.M.: 50% to 90% is promptly absorbed, balance is slowly absorbed over month

I.V.: Uptake of iron by the reticuloendothelial system appears to be constant at about 10-20 mg/hour

Excretion: Urine and feces via reticuloendothelial system

Dosage I.M. (Z-track method should be used for I.M. injection), I.V.:

A 0.5 mL test dose (0.25 mL in infants) should be given prior to starting iron dextran therapy; total dose should be divided into a daily schedule for I.M., total dose may be given as a single continuous infusion

Iron-deficiency anemia: Dose (mL) = 0.0476 x LBW (kg) x (normal hemoglobin - observed hemoglobin) + (1 mL/5 kg of LBW to maximum of 14 mL for iron stores)

LBW = Lean Body Weight

(Continued)

Iron Dextran Complex *(Continued)*

Iron replacement therapy for blood loss: Replacement iron (mg) = blood loss (mL) x hematocrit

Maximum daily dosage:

Manufacturer's labeling: **Note:** Replacement of larger estimated iron deficits may be achieved by serial administration of smaller incremental dosages. Daily dosages should be limited to:

Children:

5-15 kg: 50 mg iron (1 mL)

15-50 kg: 100 mg iron (2 mL)

Adults >50 kg: 100 mg iron (2 mL)

Total dose infusion (unlabeled): The entire dose (estimated iron deficit) may be diluted and administered as a one-time I.V. infusion.

Administration A 25 mg (0.5 mL) (pediatrics: 12.5 mg [0.25 mL]) test dose is usually given at the beginning of iron dextron therapy. Use Z-track technique into a large muscle for I.M. administration. I.V. bolus at rate ≤50 mg/minute or infused over 1-6 hours

Dosage Forms Note: Strength expressed as elemental iron

Injection, solution:

Dexferrum®: 50 mg/mL (1 mL, 2 mL)

INFeD®: 50 mg/mL (2 mL)

Monitoring Parameters Hemoglobin, hematocrit, reticulocyte count, serum ferritin, serum iron, TIBC

Special Geriatric Considerations Anemia in the elderly is most often caused by "anemia of chronic disease", a result of aging effect in bone marrow, or associated with inflammation rather than blood loss. Iron stores are usually normal or increased, with a serum ferritin >50 ng/mL and a decreased total iron binding capacity. Hence, the anemia is not secondary to iron deficiency but the inability of the reticuloendothelial system to use available iron stores. I.V. administration of iron dextran is often preferred over I.M. in the elderly secondary to a decreased muscle mass and the need for daily injections.

Selected Readings

Auerbach M, Witt D, and Toler W, "Clinical Use of the Total Dose Intravenous Infusion of Iron Dextran," *J Lab Clin Med*, 1988, 111(5):566-70.

Burns DL, Mascioli EA, and Bistrian BR, "Parenteral Iron Dextran Therapy: A Review," *Nutrition*, 1995, 11(2):163-8.

Kumpf VJ and Holland EG, "Parenteral Iron Dextran Therapy," *DICP*, 1990, 24(2):162-6.

♦ **Isonipecaine Hydrochloride** *see* Meperidine *on page 535*

♦ **Isophosphamide** *see* Ifosfamide *on page 446*

♦ **Isopto® Carpine** *see* Pilocarpine *on page 666*

Itraconazole (i tra KOE na zole)

Medication Safety Issues

Sound-alike/look-alike issues:

Sporanox® may be confused with Suprax®

U.S. Brand Names Sporanox®

Canadian Brand Names Sporanox®

Generic Available No

Pharmacologic Category Antifungal Agent, Oral

Pregnancy Risk Factor C

Lactation Enters breast milk/not recommended

Use Treatment of susceptible fungal infections in immunocompromised and immunocompetent patients including blastomycosis and histoplasmosis; indicated for aspergillosis, and onychomycosis of the toenail; treatment of onychomycosis of the fingernail without concomitant toenail infection via a pulse-type dosing regimen; has activity against *Aspergillus*, *Candida*, *Coccidioides*, *Cryptococcus*, *Sporothrix*, tinea unguium

Oral: Useful in superficial mycoses including dermatophytoses (eg, tinea capitis), pityriasis versicolor, sebopsoriasis, vaginal and chronic mucocutaneous candidiases; systemic mycoses including candidiasis, meningeal and disseminated cryptococcal infections, paracoccidioidomycosis, coccidioidomycoses; miscellaneous mycoses such as sporotrichosis, chromomycosis, leishmaniasis, fungal keratitis, alternariosis, zygomycosis

Oral solution: Treatment of oral and esophageal candidiasis

Intravenous solution: Indicated in the treatment of blastomycosis, histoplasmosis (nonmeningeal), and aspergillosis (in patients intolerant or refractory to amphotericin B therapy); empiric therapy of febrile neutropenic fever

Mechanism of Action Interferes with cytochrome P450 activity, decreasing ergosterol synthesis (principal sterol in fungal cell membrane) and inhibiting cell membrane formation

Labeled Contraindications Hypersensitivity to itraconazole, any component of the formulation, or to other azoles; concurrent administration with cisapride, dofetilide, ergot derivatives, levomethadyl, lovastatin, midazolam, pimozide, quinidine, simvastatin, or triazolam; treatment of onychomycosis in patients with evidence of left ventricular dysfunction, CHF, or a history of CHF

Warnings/Precautions Discontinue if signs or symptoms of CHF or neuropathy occur during treatment. Rare cases of serious cardiovascular adverse events (including death), ventricular tachycardia, and torsade de pointes have been observed due to increased cisapride concentrations induced by itraconazole. Use with caution in patients with left ventricular dysfunction or a history of CHF. Not recommended for use in patients with active liver disease, elevated liver enzymes, or prior hepatotoxic reactions to other drugs. Itraconazole has been associated with rare cases of serious hepatotoxicity (including fatal cases and cases within the first week of treatment); treatment should be discontinued in patients who develop clinical symptoms of liver dysfunction or abnormal liver function tests during itraconazole therapy except in cases where expected benefit exceeds risk. Large differences in itraconazole pharmacokinetic parameters have been observed in cystic fibrosis patients receiving the solution; if a patient with cystic fibrosis does not respond to therapy, alternate therapies should be considered. **Due to differences in bioavailability, oral capsules and oral solution cannot be used interchangeably**. Intravenous formulation should be used with caution in renal impairment; consider conversion to oral therapy if renal dysfunction/toxicity is noted. Initiation of treatment with oral solution is not recommended in patients at immediate risk for systemic candidiasis (eg, patients with severe neutropenia).

Adverse Reactions Listed incidences are for higher doses appropriate for systemic fungal infection.

>10%: Gastrointestinal: Nausea (11%)

(Continued)

Itraconazole *(Continued)*

1% to 10%:

Cardiovascular: Edema (4%), hypertension (3%)

Central nervous system: Headache (4%), fatigue (2% to 3%), malaise (1%), fever (3%), dizziness (2%)

Dermatologic: Rash (9%), pruritus (3%)

Endocrine & metabolic: Decreased libido (1%), hypertriglyceridemia, hypokalemia (2%)

Gastrointestinal: Abdominal pain (2%), anorexia (1%), vomiting (5%), diarrhea (3%)

Hepatic: Abnormal LFTs (3%), hepatitis

Renal: Albuminuria (1%)

<1%: Adrenal suppression, constipation, gastritis, gynecomastia, impotence, somnolence, tinnitus

Postmarketing and/or case reports: Allergic reactions (urticaria, angioedema); alopecia, anaphylactoid reactions, anaphylaxis, arrhythmia, CHF, hepatic failure, menstrual disorders, neutropenia, peripheral neuropathy, photosensitivity, pulmonary edema, Stevens-Johnson syndrome

Overdosage/Toxicology Overdoses are well tolerated. Treatment is supportive. Dialysis is not effective.

Drug Interactions

Cytochrome P450 Effect: Substrate of CYP3A4 (major); **Inhibits** CYP3A4 (strong)

Increased Effect/Toxicity: Itraconazole is a strong inhibitor of CYP3A4, and is contraindicated with cisapride, dofetilide, ergot derivatives, lovastatin, midazolam, pimozide, quinidine, simvastatin, and triazolam. Itraconazole may also increase the levels of alfentanil, benzodiazepines (alprazolam, diazepam, and others), buspirone, busulfan, calcium channel blockers (felodipine, nifedipine, verapamil), carbamazepine, corticosteroids, cyclosporine, digoxin, docetaxel, eletriptan, HMG-CoA reductase inhibitors (except fluvastatin, pravastatin), indinavir, oral hypoglycemics (sulfonylureas), phenytoin, rifabutin, ritonavir, saquinavir, sirolimus, tacrolimus, trimetrexate, vincristine, vinblastine, warfarin, and zolpidem. Other medications metabolized by CYP3A4 should be used with caution. Serum concentrations of itraconazole may be increased by strong CYP3A4 inhibitors. Serum concentrations of PDE-5 inhibitors (sildenafil, tadalafil, and vardenafil) are increased by itraconazole; specific dosage reductions/limitations are recommended.

Decreased Effect: Absorption of itraconazole requires gastric acidity; therefore, antacids, H_2 antagonists (cimetidine, famotidine, nizatidine, and ranitidine), proton pump inhibitors (omeprazole, lansoprazole, rabeprazole), and sucralfate may significantly reduce bioavailability resulting in treatment failures and should not be administered concomitantly. Antacids may decrease serum concentration of itraconazole; administer antacids 1 hour before or 2 hours after itraconazole capsules. Serum levels of itraconazole may be decreased with didanosine, isoniazid, and nevirapine. The levels/effects of itraconazole may be reduced by aminoglutethimide, carbamazepine, nafcillin, phenobarbital, phenytoin, rifamycins, and other CYP3A4 inducers. Oral contraceptive efficacy may be reduced (limited data).

Ethanol/Nutrition/Herb Interactions

Food:

Capsules: Enhanced by food and possibly by gastric acidity. cola drinks have been shown to increase the absorption of the capsules in patients with achlorhydria or those taking H_2-receptor antagonists or other gastric acid suppressors. Avoid grapefruit juice.

Solution: Decreased by food, time to peak concentration prolonged by food.

Herb/Nutraceutical: St John's wort may decrease itraconazole levels.

Storage/Stability

Capsule: Store at room temperature, 15°C to 25°C (59°F to 77°F); protect from light and moisture

Oral solution: Store at ≤25°C (77°F); do not freeze

Solution for injection: Store at ≤25°C (77°F); protect from light; do not freeze. Stable for 48 hours at room temperature or under refrigeration.

Reconstitution Dilute with 0.9% sodium chloride. A precise mixing ratio is required to maintain stability (3.33:1) and avoid precipitate formation. Add 25 mL (1 ampul) to 50 mL 0.9% sodium chloride. Mix and withdraw 15 mL of solution before infusing.

Compatibility Compatible: Stable in NS

Pharmacodynamics/Kinetics

Absorption: Requires gastric acidity; capsule better absorbed with food, solution better absorbed on empty stomach.

Distribution: V_d (average): 796 ± 185 L or 10 L/kg; highly lipophilic and tissue concentrations are higher than plasma concentrations. The highest concentrations: adipose, omentum, endometrium, cervical and vaginal mucus, and skin/nails. Aqueous fluids (eg, CSF and urine) contain negligible amounts.

Protein binding, plasma: 99.9%; metabolite hydroxy-itraconazole: 99.5%

Metabolism: Extensively hepatic via CYP3A4 into >30 metabolites including hydroxy-itraconazole (major metabolite); appears to have *in vitro* antifungal activity. Main metabolic pathway is oxidation; may undergo saturation metabolism with multiple dosing.

Bioavailability: Variable, ~ 55% (oral solution) in 1 small study; **Note:** Oral solution has a higher degree of bioavailability (149% ± 68%) relative to oral capsules; should not be interchanged

Half-life elimination: Oral: After single 200 mg dose: 21 ± 5 hours; 64 hours at steady-state; I.V.: steady-state: 35 hours; steady-state concentrations are achieved in 13 days with multiple administration of itraconazole 100-400 mg/day.

Excretion: Feces (~3% to 18%); urine (~0.03% as parent drug, 40% as metabolites)

Dosage Note: Capsule: Absorption is best if taken with food, therefore, it is best to administer itraconazole after meals; Solution: Should be taken on an empty stomach.

Children: Efficacy and safety have not been established; a small number of patients 3-16 years of age have been treated with 100 mg/day for systemic fungal infections with no serious adverse effects reported. A dose of 5 mg/kg once daily was used in a pharmacokinetic study using the oral solution in patients 6 months to 12 years; duration of study was 2 weeks.

(Continued)

Itraconazole *(Continued)*

Adults:

Oral:

Blastomycosis/histoplasmosis: 200 mg once daily, if no obvious improvement or there is evidence of progressive fungal disease, increase the dose in 100 mg increments to a maximum of 400 mg/day; doses >200 mg/day are given in 2 divided doses; length of therapy varies from 1 day to >6 months depending on the condition and mycological response

Aspergillosis: 200-400 mg/day

Onychomycosis: 200 mg once daily for 12 consecutive weeks

Life-threatening infections: Loading dose: 200 mg 3 times/day (600 mg/day) should be given for the first 3 days of therapy

Oropharyngeal candidiasis: Oral solution: 200 mg once daily for 1-2 weeks; in patients unresponsive or refractory to fluconazole: 100 mg twice daily (clinical response expected in 1-2 weeks)

Esophageal candidiasis: Oral solution: 100-200 mg once daily for a minimum of 3 weeks; continue dosing for 2 weeks after resolution of symptoms

I.V.: 200 mg twice daily for 4 doses, followed by 200 mg daily

Dosing adjustment in renal impairment: Not necessary; itraconazole injection is not recommended in patients with Cl_{cr} <30 mL/minute; hydroxypropyl-β-cyclodextrin (the excipient) is eliminated primarily by the kidneys.

Hemodialysis: Not dialyzable

Dosing adjustment in hepatic impairment: May be necessary, but specific guidelines are not available. Risk-to-benefit evaluation should be undertaken in patients who develop liver function abnormalities during treatment.

Administration

Oral: Doses >200 mg/day are given in 2 divided doses; do not administer with antacids. Capsule absorption is best if taken with food, therefore, it is best to administer itraconazole after meals; solution should be taken on an empty stomach. When treating oropharyngeal and esophageal candidiasis, solution should be swished vigorously in mouth, then swallowed.

I.V.: Infuse 60 mL of the dilute solution (3.33 mg/mL = 200 mg itraconazole, pH ~4.8) over 60 minutes; flush with 15-20 mL of 0.9% sodium chloride over 30 seconds to 15 minutes

Dosage Forms

Capsule: 100 mg

Injection, solution: 10 mg/mL (25 mL) [packaged in a kit containing sodium chloride 0.9% (50 mL); filtered infusion set (1)]

Solution, oral: 100 mg/10 mL (150 mL) [cherry flavor]

Monitoring Parameters Liver function in patients with pre-existing hepatic dysfunction, and in all patients being treated for longer than 1 month

Dietary Considerations

Capsule: Administer with food.

Solution: Take without food, if possible.

Patient Information Take capsule with food; take solution on an empty stomach; stop therapy and report any signs and symptoms that may suggest liver dysfunction immediately so that the appropriate laboratory testing can be done; signs and symptoms may include unusual fatigue, anorexia, nausea and/or vomiting, jaundice, dark urine, or pale stool

Additional Information Due to potential toxicity, the manufacturer recommends confirmation of diagnosis testing of nail specimens prior to treatment of onychomycosis.

Selected Readings
Cleary JD, Taylor JW, and Chapman SW, "Itraconazole in Antifungal Therapy," *Ann Pharmacother*, 1992, 26(4):502-9.

Grant SM and Clissold SP, "Itraconazole. A Review of Its Pharmacodynamic and Pharmacokinetic Properties, and Therapeutic Use in Superficial and Systemic Mycoses," *Drugs*, 1989, 37(3):310-44.

Haria M, Bryson HM, and Goa KL, "Itraconazole: A Reappraisal of Its Pharmacological Properties and Therapeutic Use in the Management of Superficial Fungal Infections," *Drugs*, 1996, 51(4):585-620.

♦ **Iveegam EN** *see* Immune Globulin (Intravenous) *on page 458*

♦ **Iveegam Immuno**® **(Can)** *see* Immune Globulin (Intravenous) *on page 458*

♦ **IVIG** *see* Immune Globulin (Intravenous) *on page 458*

♦ **IvySoothe**® **[OTC]** *see* Hydrocortisone *on page 419*

♦ **Kadian**® *see* Morphine Sulfate *on page 588*

♦ **Kepivance**™ *see* Palifermin *on page 646*

♦ **Ketek**® *see* Telithromycin *on page 747*

Ketoconazole (kee toe KOE na zole)

Medication Safety Issues
Sound-alike/look-alike issues:
Nizoral® may be confused with Nasarel®, Neoral®, Nitrol®

U.S. Brand Names Nizoral®; Nizoral® A-D [OTC]

Canadian Brand Names Apo-Ketoconazole®; Ketoderm®; Nizoral®; Novo-Ketoconazole

Generic Available Yes

Pharmacologic Category Antifungal Agent, Oral; Antifungal Agent, Topical

Pregnancy Risk Factor C

Lactation Enters breast milk/not recommended

Use Treatment of susceptible fungal infections, including candidiasis, oral thrush, blastomycosis, histoplasmosis, paracoccidioidomycosis, coccidioidomycosis, chromomycosis, candiduria, chronic mucocutaneous candidiasis, as well as certain recalcitrant cutaneous dermatophytoses; used topically for treatment of tinea corporis, tinea cruris, tinea versicolor, and cutaneous candidiasis, seborrheic dermatitis

Unlabeled/Investigational Use Treatment of prostate cancer (androgen synthesis inhibitor)

Mechanism of Action Alters the permeability of the cell wall by blocking fungal cytochrome P450; inhibits biosynthesis of triglycerides and phospholipids by fungi; inhibits several fungal enzymes that results in a build-up of toxic concentrations of hydrogen peroxide; also inhibits androgen synthesis

Labeled Contraindications Hypersensitivity to ketoconazole or any component of the formulation; CNS fungal infections (due to poor CNS penetration); coadministration with ergot derivatives or cisapride is contraindicated due to risk of potentially fatal cardiac arrhythmias (Continued)

Ketoconazole *(Continued)*

Warnings/Precautions Use with caution in patients with impaired hepatic function; has been associated with hepatotoxicity, including some fatalities; perform periodic liver function tests; high doses of ketoconazole may depress adrenocortical function.

Adverse Reactions

Oral:

1% to 10%:

Dermatologic: Pruritus (2%)

Gastrointestinal: Nausea/vomiting (3% to 10%), abdominal pain (1%)

<1%: Headache, dizziness, somnolence, fever, chills, bulging fontanelles, depression, gynecomastia, diarrhea, impotence, thrombocytopenia, leukopenia, hemolytic anemia, hepatotoxicity, photophobia

Cream: Severe irritation, pruritus, stinging (~5%)

Shampoo: Increases in normal hair loss, irritation (<1%), abnormal hair texture, scalp pustules, mild dryness of skin, itching, oiliness/dryness of hair

Overdosage/Toxicology Oral: Symptoms of overdose include dizziness, headache, nausea, vomiting, diarrhea. Overdoses are well tolerated. Treatment includes supportive measures and gastric decontamination.

Drug Interactions

Cytochrome P450 Effect: Substrate of CYP3A4 (major); **Inhibits** CYP1A2 (strong), 2A6 (moderate), 2B6 (weak), 2C8/9 (strong), 2C19 (moderate), 2D6 (moderate), 3A4 (strong)

Increased Effect/Toxicity: Due to inhibition of hepatic CYP3A4, ketoconazole use is contraindicated with cisapride, lovastatin, midazolam, simvastatin, and triazolam due to large substantial increases in the toxicity of these agents. Ketoconazole may increase the serum levels/effects of amiodarone, amphetamines, benzodiazepines, beta-blockers, buspirone, busulfan, calcium channel blockers, citalopram, dexmedetomidine, dextromethorphan, diazepam, digoxin, docetaxel, fluoxetine, fluvoxamine, glimepiride, glipizide, ifosfamide, inhalational anesthetics, lidocaine, mesoridazine, methsuximide, mexiletine, mirtazapine, nateglinide, nefazodone, paroxetine, phenytoin, pioglitazone, propranolol, risperidone, ritonavir, ropinirole, rosiglitazone, sertraline, sirolimus, tacrolimus, theophylline, thioridazine, tricyclic antidepressants, trifluoperazine, trimetrexate, venlafaxine, vincristine, vinblastine, warfarin, zolpidem, and other substrates of CYP1A2, 2A6, 2C8/9, 2C19, 2D6, or 3A4. Selected benzodiazepines (midazolam and triazolam), cisapride, ergot alkaloids, selected HMG-CoA reductase inhibitors (lovastatin and simvastatin), and pimozide are generally contraindicated with strong CYP3A4 inhibitors. Mesoridazine and thioridazine are generally contraindicated with strong CYP2D6 inhibitors. When used with strong CYP3A4 inhibitors, dosage adjustment/limits are recommended for sildenafil and other PDE-5 inhibitors; consult individual monographs.

Decreased Effect: Oral: Absorption requires gastric acidity; therefore, antacids, H_2 antagonists (cimetidine, famotidine, nizatidine, and ranitidine), proton pump inhibitors (omeprazole, lansoprazole, rabeprazole), and sucralfate may significantly reduce bioavailability resulting in treatment failures and should not be administered concomitantly. Decreased serum levels with didanosine and isoniazid. The levels/effects of keto-conazole may be decreased by aminoglutethimide, carbamazepine, nafcillin, nevirapine, phenobarbital, phenytoin, rifamycins, or other CYP3A4 inducers. **Should not be administered concomitantly with rifampin.** Oral contraceptive efficacy may be reduced (limited data). Ketoconazole may decrease the levels/effects of CYP2D6 prodrug substrates (eg, codeine, hydrocodone, oxycodone, tramadol).

Ethanol/Nutrition/Herb Interactions

Food: Ketoconazole peak serum levels may be prolonged if taken with food.

Herb/Nutraceutical: St John's wort may decrease ketoconazole levels.

Pharmacodynamics/Kinetics

Absorption: Oral: Rapid (~75%); Shampoo: None

Distribution: Well into inflamed joint fluid, saliva, bile, urine, breast milk, sebum, cerumen, feces, tendons, skin and soft tissues, and testes; crosses blood-brain barrier poorly; only negligible amounts reach CSF

Protein binding: 93% to 96%

Metabolism: Partially hepatic via CYP3A4 to inactive compounds

Bioavailability: Decreases as gastric pH increases

Half-life elimination: Biphasic: Initial: 2 hours; Terminal: 8 hours

Time to peak, serum: 1-2 hours

Excretion: Feces (57%); urine (13%)

Dosage

Fungal infections:

Oral:

Children ≥2 years: 3.3-6.6 mg/kg/day as a single dose for 1-2 weeks for candidiasis, for at least 4 weeks in recalcitrant dermatophyte infections, and for up to 6 months for other systemic mycoses

Adults: 200-400 mg/day as a single daily dose for durations as stated above

Shampoo: Apply twice weekly for 4 weeks with at least 3 days between each shampoo

Topical: Rub gently into the affected area once daily to twice daily

Prostate cancer (unlabeled use): Oral: Adults: 400 mg 3 times/day

Dosing adjustment in hepatic impairment: Dose reductions should be considered in patients with severe liver disease

Hemodialysis: Not dialyzable (0% to 5%)

Combination Regimens

Prostate cancer:

Doxorubicin + Ketoconazole *on page 873*

Doxorubicin + Ketoconazole/Estramustine + Vinblastine *on page 874*

Administration Administer tablets 2 hours prior to antacids to prevent decreased absorption due to the high pH of gastric contents.

Dosage Forms

Cream, topical: 2% (15 g, 30 g, 60 g)

Shampoo, topical (Nizoral® A-D): 1% (6 mL, 120 mL, 210 mL)

Tablet (Nizoral®): 200 mg

Monitoring Parameters Liver function tests

Dietary Considerations May be taken with food or milk to decrease GI adverse effects.

Patient Information Cream is for topical application to the skin only; avoid contact with the eye; avoid taking antacids at the same time as
(Continued)

Ketoconazole *(Continued)*

ketoconazole; may take with food; may cause drowsiness, impair judgment or coordination. Report unusual fatigue, anorexia, vomiting, dark urine, or pale stools.

Extemporaneous Preparations A 20 mg/mL suspension may be made by pulverizing twelve 200 mg ketoconazole tablets to a fine powder; add 40 mL Ora-Plus® in small portions with thorough mixing; incorporate Ora-Sweet® to make a final volume of 120 mL and mix thoroughly; refrigerate (no stability information is available)

Allen LV, "Ketoconazole Oral Suspension," *US Pharm*, 1993, 18(2):98-9, 101.

Selected Readings
Como JA and Dismukes WE, "Oral Azole Drugs as Systemic Antifungal Therapy," *N Engl J Med*, 1994, 330(4):263-72.

Ginsburg AM, McCracken GH Jr, and Olsen K, "Pharmacology of Ketoconazole Suspension in Infants and Children," *Antimicrob Agents Chemother*, 1983, 23(5):787-9.

Lyman CA and Walsh TJ, "Systemically Administered Antifungal Agents. A Review of Their Clinical Pharmacology and Therapeutic Applications," *Drugs*, 1992, 44(1):9-35.

- ◆ **Ketoderm® (Can)** *see* Ketoconazole *on page 491*
- ◆ **Kidrolase® (Can)** *see* Asparaginase *on page 106*
- ◆ **Koāte®-DVI** *see* Antihemophilic Factor (Human) *on page 87*
- ◆ **Kogenate® (Can)** *see* Antihemophilic Factor (Recombinant) *on page 92*
- ◆ **Kogenate® FS** *see* Antihemophilic Factor (Recombinant) *on page 92*
- ◆ **Konakion (Can)** *see* Phytonadione *on page 664*
- ◆ **Kytril®** *see* Granisetron *on page 405*
- ◆ **L 754030** *see* Aprepitant *on page 100*
- ◆ **LA 20304a** *see* Gemifloxacin *on page 392*
- ◆ **LactiCare-HC® [DSC]** *see* Hydrocortisone *on page 419*
- ◆ **Ladakamycin** *see* Azacitidine *on page 110*
- ◆ **L-AmB** *see* Amphotericin B (Liposomal) *on page 76*
- ◆ **Lanvis® (Can)** *see* Thioguanine *on page 762*
- ◆ **Largactil® (Can)** *see* ChlorproMAZINE *on page 178*
- ◆ **Lasix®** *see* Furosemide *on page 374*
- ◆ **Lasix® Special (Can)** *see* Furosemide *on page 374*
- ◆ **L-asparaginase** *see* Asparaginase *on page 106*
- ◆ **LCR** *see* VinCRIStine *on page 819*
- ◆ **LDP-341** *see* Bortezomib *on page 138*

Letrozole *(LET roe zole)*

Medication Safety Issues
Sound-alike/look-alike issues:
Femara® may be confused with femhrt®

Related Information
Safe Handling of Hazardous Drugs *on page 1034*

U.S. Brand Names Femara®

Canadian Brand Names Femara®

Generic Available No

Pharmacologic Category Antineoplastic Agent, Aromatase Inhibitor

Pregnancy Risk Factor D

Lactation Excretion in breast milk unknown/not recommended

Use First-line treatment of hormone receptor positive or hormone receptor unknown, locally advanced, or metastatic breast cancer in postmenopausal women; treatment of advanced breast cancer in postmenopausal women with disease progression following antiestrogen therapy; extended adjuvant treatment of early breast cancer in postmenopausal women who have received 5 years of adjuvant tamoxifen therapy

Mechanism of Action Competitive inhibitor of the aromatase enzyme system which binds to the heme group of aromatase, a cytochrome P450 enzyme which catalyzes conversion of androgens to estrogens (specifically, androstenedione to estrone and testosterone to estradiol). This leads to inhibition of the enzyme and a significant reduction in plasma estrogen levels. Does not affect synthesis of adrenal or thyroid hormones, aldosterone, or androgens.

Labeled Contraindications Hypersensitivity to letrozole or any component of the formulation; pregnancy

Warnings/Precautions Increases in transaminases ≥5 times the upper limit of normal and of bilirubin ≥1.5 times the upper limit of normal were most often, but not always, associated with metastatic liver disease. May cause dizziness and fatigue; patients should be cautioned before performing tasks which require mental alertness (eg, operating machinery or driving). For use in postmenopausal women only.

Adverse Reactions

>10%:

Cardiovascular: Hot flushes (5% to 19%)

Central nervous system: Headache (8% to 12%), fatigue (6% to 13%)

Gastrointestinal: Nausea (13% to 17%)

Neuromuscular & skeletal: Musculoskeletal pain, bone pain (22%), back pain (18%), arthralgia (8% to 16%)

Respiratory: Dyspnea (7% to 18%), cough (5% to 13%)

2% to 10%:

Cardiovascular: Chest pain (3% to 8%), peripheral edema (5%), hypertension (5% to 8%)

Central nervous system: Pain (5%), insomnia (7%), dizziness (3% to 5%), somnolence (2% to 3%), depression (<5%), anxiety (<5%), vertigo (<5%)

Dermatologic: Rash (4% to 5%), alopecia (<5%), pruritus (1% to 2%)

Endocrine & metabolic: Breast pain (7%), hypercholesterolemia (3%), hypercalcemia (<5%)

Gastrointestinal: Vomiting (7%), constipation (6% to 10%), diarrhea (5% to 8%), abdominal pain (5% to 6%), anorexia (3% to 5%), dyspepsia (3% to 4%), weight loss (7%), weight gain (2%)

Neuromuscular & skeletal: Weakness (4% to 6%)

Miscellaneous: Flu (6%)

<2%: Angina, cardiac ischemia, coronary artery disease, hemiparesis, hemorrhagic stroke, bilirubin increased, transaminases increased, lymphopenia, MI, portal vein thrombosis, pulmonary embolism, thrombocytopenia, thrombophlebitis, thrombotic stroke, transient ischemic attack, vaginal bleeding, venous thrombosis

Postmarketing and/or case reports: Blurred vision, hepatic enzymes increased

Emetic Potential Low (10% to 30%)

(Continued)

Letrozole *(Continued)*

Overdosage/Toxicology Firm recommendations for treatment are not possible; emesis could be induced if the patient is alert. In general, supportive care and frequent monitoring of vital signs are appropriate.

Drug Interactions

Cytochrome P450 Effect: Substrate (minor) of CYP2A6, 3A4; **Inhibits** CYP2A6 (strong), 2C19 (weak)

Increased Effect/Toxicity: Letrozole may increase the levels/effects of CYP2A6 substrates; example substrates include dexmedetomidine and ifosfamide.

Storage/Stability Store at 15°C to 30°C (59°F to 86°F)

Pharmacodynamics/Kinetics

Absorption: Well absorbed; not affected by food

Distribution: V_d: ~1.9 L/kg

Protein binding, plasma: Weak

Metabolism: Hepatic via CYP3A4 and CYP2A6 to an inactive carbinol metabolite

Half-life elimination: Terminal: ~2 days

Time to steady state, plasma: 2-6 weeks

Excretion: Urine (6% as unchanged drug, 75% as glucuronide carbinol metabolite)

Dosage Oral (refer to individual protocols): Adults: Breast cancer: 2.5 mg once daily

Elderly: No dosage adjustments required

Dosage adjustment in renal impairment: No dosage adjustment is required in patients with renal impairment if Cl_{cr} ≥10 mL/minute

Dosage adjustment in hepatic impairment:

Mild-to-moderate impairment: No adjustment recommended

Severe impairment: Child-Pugh class C: 2.5 mg every other day

Dosage Forms Tablet: 2.5 mg

Monitoring Parameters Monitor periodically during therapy: complete blood counts, thyroid function tests; serum electrolytes, transaminases, and creatinine; bone density

Dietary Considerations May be taken without regard to meals. Calcium and vitamin D supplementation are recommended.

Patient Information May experience nausea, vomiting, hot flashes, or loss of appetite; musculoskeletal pain or headache; sleepiness, fatigue, or dizziness (use caution when driving, climbing stairs, or engaging in tasks that require alertness until response to drug is known); constipation; diarrhea; or loss of hair. Report chest pain, pressure, palpitations, or swollen extremities; weakness, severe headache, numbness, or loss of strength in any part of the body, difficulty speaking; vaginal bleeding; unusual signs of bleeding or bruising; difficulty breathing; severe nausea, or muscle pain; or skin rash. For use in postmenopausal women only.

Selected Readings

Boeddinghaus IM and Dowsett M, "Comparative Clinical Pharmacology and Pharmacokinetic Interactions of Aromatase Inhibitors," *J Steroid Biochem Mol Biol*, 2001, 79(1-5):85-91.

Buzdar AU, Robertson JF, Eiermann W, et al, "An Overview of the Pharmacology and Pharmacokinetics of the Newer Generation Aromatase Inhibitors Anastrozole, Letrozole, and Exemestane," *Cancer*, 2002, 95(9):2006-16.

Haynes BP, Dowsett M, Miller WR, et al, "The Pharmacology of Letrozole," *J Steroid Biochem Mol Biol*, 2003, 87(1):35-45.

Lamb HM and Adkins JC, "Letrozole. A Review of its Use in Postmenopausal Women With Advanced Breast Cancer," *Drugs*, 1998, 56(6):1125-40.

Mays-Holland T, "Drug Update: Letrozole: A New Aromatase Inhibitor for Metastatic Breast Cancer," *Cancer Pract*, 1998, 6(6):349-52.

Njar VC and Brodie AM, "Comprehensive Pharmacology and Clinical Efficacy of Aromatase Inhibitors," *Drugs*, 1999, 58(2):233-55.

Simpson D, Curran MP, and Perry CM, "Letrozole: A Review of Its Use in Postmenopausal Women With Breast Cancer," *Drugs*, 2004, 64(11):1213-30.

Leucovorin (loo koe VOR in)

Medication Safety Issues

Sound-alike/look-alike issues:

Leucovorin may be confused with Leukeran®, Leukine®

Folinic acid may be confused with folic acid

Generic Available Yes

Synonyms Calcium Leucovorin; Citrovorum Factor; Folinic Acid; 5-Formyl Tetrahydrofolate; Leucovorin Calcium

Pharmacologic Category Antidote; Vitamin, Water Soluble

Pregnancy Risk Factor C

Lactation Enters breast milk/compatible

Use Antidote for folic acid antagonists (methotrexate, trimethoprim, pyrimethamine); treatment of megaloblastic anemias when folate is deficient as in infancy, sprue, pregnancy, and nutritional deficiency when oral folate therapy is not possible; in combination with fluorouracil in the treatment of colon cancer

Mechanism of Action A reduced form of folic acid, leucovorin supplies the necessary cofactor blocked by methotrexate, enters the cells via the same active transport system as methotrexate. Stabilizes the binding of 5-dUMP and thymidylate synthetase, enhancing the activity of fluorouracil.

Labeled Contraindications Hypersensitivity to leucovorin or any component of the formulation; pernicious anemia or vitamin B_{12} deficient megaloblastic anemias

Adverse Reactions Frequency not defined.

Dermatologic: Rash, pruritus, erythema, urticaria

Hematologic: Thrombocytosis

Respiratory: Wheezing

Miscellaneous: Anaphylactoid reactions

Vesicant No

Emetic Potential Low

Drug Interactions

Decreased Effect: May decrease efficacy of co-trimoxazole against *Pneumocystis carinii* pneumonitis

Storage/Stability Store at room temperature; protect from light. Reconstituted solution is chemically stable for 7 days; reconstitutions with bacteriostatic water for injection, U.S.P., must be used within 7 days. Parenteral admixture is stable for 24 hours stored at room temperature (25°C) and for 4 days when stored under refrigeration (4°C).

Reconstitution Reconstitute with SWFI, bacteriostatic NS, BWFI, NS, or D_5W; dilute in 100-1000 mL NS, D_5W for infusion

Compatibility Stable in $D_{10}NS$, D_5W, $D_{10}W$, LR, sterile water for injection, bacteriostatic water, bacteriostatic NS; **variable stability (consult detailed reference)** in NS

(Continued)

Leucovorin *(Continued)*

Y-site administration: Compatible: Amifostine, aztreonam, bleomycin, cefepime, cisplatin, cladribine, cyclophosphamide, docetaxel, doxorubicin, doxorubicin liposome, etoposide phosphate, filgrastim, fluconazole, fluorouracil, furosemide, gatifloxacin, gemcitabine, granisetron, heparin, linezolid, methotrexate, metoclopramide, mitomycin, piperacillin/tazobactam, tacrolimus, teniposide, thiotepa, vinblastine, vincristine. **Incompatible:** Amphotericin B cholesteryl sulfate complex, droperidol, foscarnet, sodium bicarbonate

Compatibility in syringe: Compatible: Bleomycin, cisplatin, cyclophosphamide, doxorubicin, fluorouracil, furosemide, heparin, methotrexate, metoclopramide, mitomycin, vinblastine, vincristine. **Incompatible:** Droperidol

Compatibility when admixed: Compatible: Cisplatin, cisplatin with floxuridine, floxuridine. **Incompatible:** Concentrations >2 mg/mL of leucovorin and >25 mg/mL of fluorouracil

Pharmacodynamics/Kinetics

Onset of action: Oral: ~30 minutes; I.V.: ~5 minutes

Absorption: Oral, I.M.: Rapid and well absorbed

Metabolism: Intestinal mucosa and hepatically to 5-methyl-tetrahydrofolate (5MTHF; active)

Bioavailability: 31% following 200 mg dose; 98% following doses ≤25 mg

Half-life elimination: Leucovorin: 15 minutes; 5MTHF: 33-35 minutes

Excretion: Urine (80% to 90%); feces (5% to 8%)

Dosage Children and Adults:

Treatment of folic acid antagonist overdosage: Oral: 2-15 mg/day for 3 days or until blood counts are normal, **or** 5 mg every 3 days; doses of 6 mg/day are needed for patients with platelet counts <100,000/mm^3

Folate-deficient megaloblastic anemia: I.M.: 1 mg/day

Megaloblastic anemia secondary to congenital deficiency of dihydrofolate reductase: I.M.: 3-6 mg/day

Rescue dose: Initial: I.V.: 10 mg/m^2, then:

Oral, I.M., I.V., SubQ: 10-15 10 mg/m^2 every 6 hours until methotrexate level <0.05 µmol/mL; if methotrexate level remains >5 µmol/mL at 48-72 hours after the end of the methotrexate infusion, increase to 20-100 mg/m^2 every 6 hours until methotrexate level <0.05 µmol/mL

Investigational: Post I.T. methotrexate: Oral, I.V.: 12 mg/m^2 as a single dose

Combination Regimens

Breast cancer:

M-VAC (Breast Cancer) *on page 921*

NFL *on page 923*

Colorectal cancer:

F-CL *on page 886*

FOIL *on page 890*

FOLFOX 1 *on page 891*

FOLFOX 2 *on page 891*

FOLFOX 3 *on page 891*

FOLFOX 4 *on page 892*

FOLFOX 6 *on page 892*

FOLFOX 7 *on page 892*

FU/LV/CPT-11 *on page 893*

FU/LV/CPT-11 (Saltz Regimen) *on page 894*

Administration Refer to individual protocols. Leucovorin calcium should be administered I.M. or I.V. Leucovorin should not be administered concurrently with methotrexate. It is commonly initiated 24 hours after the start of methotrexate. Toxicity to normal tissues may be irreversible if leucovorin is not initiated by ~40 hours after the start of methotrexate. **Note:** The manufacturer states that leucovorin should not be given intrathecally/intraventricularly; however, it has been given by these routes.

As a rescue after folate antagonists: Leucovorin may be administered by I.V. bolus injection, I.M. injection, or orally. Doses >25 mg should be administered parenterally.

In combination with fluorouracil: When leucovorin is used to modulate fluorouracil activity, the fluorouracil is usually given after, or at the midpoint, of the leucovorin infusion. Leucovorin is usually administered by I.V. bolus injection or short (10-15 minutes) I.V. infusion. Other administration schedules have been used; refer to individual protocols.

Dosage Forms
Injection, powder for reconstitution, as calcium: 50 mg, 100 mg, 200 mg, 350 mg, 500 mg
Injection, solution, as calcium: 10 mg/mL (50 mL)
Tablet, as calcium: 5 mg, 10 mg, 15 mg, 25 mg

Monitoring Parameters Plasma methotrexate concentration as a therapeutic guide to high-dose methotrexate therapy with leucovorin factor rescue. Leucovorin is continued until the plasma methotrexate level <0.05 µmol/mL.
(Continued)

Leucovorin *(Continued)*

With 4- to 6-hour high-dose methotrexate infusions, plasma drug values in excess of 50 and 1 µmol at 24 and 48 hours after starting the infusion, respectively, are often predictive of delayed methotrexate clearance

Patient Information Contact prescriber immediately if you have an allergic reaction after taking leucovorin calcium (trouble breathing, wheezing, fainting, skin rash, or hives). Inform prescriber if you are pregnant or are trying to get pregnant before taking leucovorin calcium. Leucovorin calcium can be taken with or without food. Take as directed, at evenly spaced intervals around-the-clock. Maintain hydration (2-3 L of water/day while taking for rescue therapy). For folic acid deficiency, eat foods high in folic acid (eg, meat proteins, bran, dried beans, asparagus, green leafy vegetables).

Selected Readings

Bleyer WA, "New Vistas for Leucovorin in Cancer Chemotherapy," *Cancer,* 1989, 63(6 Suppl):995-1007.

Grogan L, Sotos GA, and Allegra CJ, "Leucovorin Modulation of Fluorouracil," *Oncology (Huntingt),* 1993, 7(8):63-72.

Jolivet J, "Role of Leucovorin Dosing and Administration Schedule," *Eur J Cancer,* 1995, 31A(7-8):1311-5.

Rustum YM, "Modulation of Fluoropyrimidines by Leucovorin: Rationale and Status," *J Surg Oncol Suppl,* 1991, 2:116-23.

Stover P and Schirch V, "The Metabolic Role of Leucovorin," *Trends Biochem Sci,* 1993, 18(3):102-6.

- ♦ **Leucovorin Calcium** *see* Leucovorin *on page 497*
- ♦ **Leukeran®** *see* Chlorambucil *on page 175*
- ♦ **Leukine®** *see* Sargramostim *on page 713*

Leuprolide *(loo PROE lide)*

Medication Safety Issues

Sound-alike/look-alike issues:

Lupron® may be confused with Nuprin®

Related Information

Safe Handling of Hazardous Drugs *on page 1034*

U.S. Brand Names Eligard®; Lupron®; Lupron Depot®; Lupron Depot-Ped®; Viadur®

Canadian Brand Names Lupron®; Lupron® Depot®; Viadur®

Generic Available Yes: Injection (solution)

Synonyms Abbott-43818; Leuprolide Acetate; Leuprorelin Acetate; NSC-377526; TAP-144

Pharmacologic Category Gonadotropin Releasing Hormone Agonist

Pregnancy Risk Factor X

Lactation Excretion in breast milk unknown/contraindicated

Use Palliative treatment of advanced prostate carcinoma; management of endometriosis; treatment of anemia caused by uterine leiomyomata (fibroids); central precocious puberty

Unlabeled/Investigational Use Treatment of breast, ovarian, and endometrial cancer; infertility; prostatic hyperplasia

Mechanism of Action Potent inhibitor of gonadotropin secretion; continuous daily administration results in suppression of ovarian and testicular steroidogenesis due to decreased levels of LH and FSH with subsequent decrease in testosterone (male) and estrogen (female) levels. Leuprolide may also have a direct inhibitory effect on the testes, and act by a different mechanism not directly related to reduction in serum testosterone.

Labeled Contraindications Hypersensitivity to leuprolide, GnRH, GnRH-agonist analogs, or any component of the formulation; spinal cord compression (orchiectomy suggested); undiagnosed abnormal vaginal bleeding; pregnancy; breast-feeding

Warnings/Precautions Transient increases in testosterone serum levels occur at the start of treatment. Tumor flare, bone pain, neuropathy, urinary tract obstruction, and spinal cord compression have been reported when used for prostate cancer; closely observe patients for weakness, paresthesias, hematuria, and urinary tract obstruction in first few weeks of therapy. Observe patients with metastatic vertebral lesions or urinary obstruction closely. Exacerbation of endometriosis or uterine leiomyomata may occur initially. Decreased bone density has been reported when used for ≥6 months. Use caution in patients with a history of psychiatric illness; alteration in mood, memory impairment, and depression have been associated with use.

Adverse Reactions

Children:

1% to 10%

Central nervous system: Pain (2%)

Dermatologic: Acne (2%), rash (2%), seborrhea (2%)

Genitourinary: Vaginitis (2%), vaginal bleeding (2%), vaginal discharge (2%)

Local: Injection site reaction (5%)

<1%: Alopecia, cervix disorder, dysphagia, emotional lability, epistaxis, fever, gingivitis, gynecomastia, headache, nausea, nervousness, peripheral edema, personality disorder, sexual maturity accelerated, skin striae, somnolence, syncope, urinary incontinence, vasodilation, vomiting, weight gain

Adults (frequency dependent upon formulation and indication):

Cardiovascular: Angina, atrial fibrillation, CHF, deep vein thrombosis, edema, hot flashes, hypertension, MI, tachycardia

Central nervous system: Abnormal thinking, agitation, amnesia, confusion, convulsion, dementia, depression, dizziness, fatigue, fever, headache, insomnia, pain, vertigo

Dermatologic: Alopecia, bruising, cellulitis

Endocrine & metabolic: Bone density decreased, breast enlargement, breast tenderness, dehydration, hyperglycemia, hyperlipidemia, hyperphosphatemia, libido decreased, menstrual disorders, potassium decreased

Gastrointestinal: Anorexia, appetite increased, diarrhea, dysphagia, eructation, GI hemorrhage, gingivitis, gum hemorrhage, intestinal obstruction, nausea, peptic ulcer

Genitourinary: Balanitis, impotence, nocturia, penile shrinkage, testicular atrophy, urinary disorder, vaginitis

Hematologic: Platelets decreased, PT prolonged, WBC increased

Hepatic: Hepatomegaly, liver function tests abnormal

Local: Abscess, injection site reaction

Neuromuscular & skeletal: Leg cramps, myalgia, paresthesia, weakness

Renal: BUN increased

(Continued)

Leuprolide *(Continued)*

Respiratory: Allergic reaction, emphysema, hemoptysis, hypoxia, lung edema, pulmonary embolism

Miscellaneous: Body odor, flu-like syndrome, neoplasm, night sweats, voice alteration

Children and Adults: Postmarketing/case reports: Anaphylactic reactions, asthmatic reactions, bone density decreased; fibromyalgia-like symptoms (arthralgia/myalgia, headaches, GI distress); hypotension, induration at the injection site, peripheral neuropathy, photosensitivity, prostate pain, rash, spinal fracture/paralysis, tenosynovitis-like symptoms, urticaria, WBC decreased

Vesicant No

Emetic Potential Very low (<10%)

Overdosage/Toxicology Treatment is supportive.

Storage/Stability

Lupron®: Store unopened vials of injection in refrigerator, vial in use can be kept at room temperature of ≤30°C (86°F) for several months with minimal loss of potency. Protect from light and store vial in carton until use. Do not freeze.

Eligard®: Store at 2°C to 8°C (36°F to 46°F). Allow to reach room temperature prior to using; once mixed, must be administered within 30 minutes.

Lupron Depot® may be stored at room temperature of 25°C, excursions permitted to 15°C to 30°C (59°F to 86°F). Upon reconstitution, the suspension does not contain a preservative and should be used immediately.

Viadur® may be stored at room temperature of 15°C to 30°C (59°F and 86°F).

Reconstitution

Eligard®: Packaged in two syringes; one contains the Atrigel® polymer system and the second contains leuprolide acetate powder; follow instructions for mixing

Lupron Depot®: Reconstitute only with diluent provided

Pharmacodynamics/Kinetics

Onset of action: Following transient increase, testosterone suppression occurs in ~2-4 weeks of continued therapy

Distribution: Males: V_d: 27 L

Protein binding: 43% to 49%

Metabolism: Major metabolite, pentapeptide (M-1)

Bioavailability: Oral: None; SubQ: 94%

Half-life elimination: 3 hours

Excretion: Urine (<5% as parent and major metabolite)

Dosage

Children: Precocious puberty (consider discontinuing by age 11 for females and by age 12 for males):

SubQ (Lupron®): 20-45 mcg/kg/day; titrate dose upward by 10 mcg/kg/day if down-regulation is not achieved

I.M. (Lupron Depot-Ped®): 0.3 mg/kg/dose given every 28 days (minimum dose: 7.5 mg)

≤25 kg: 7.5 mg

>25-37.5 kg: 11.25 mg

>37.5 kg: 15 mg

Titrate dose upward in 3.75 mg every 4 weeks if down-regulation is not achieved.

Adults:

Advanced prostatic carcinoma:

SubQ:

Eligard®: 7.5 mg monthly **or** 22.5 mg every 3 months **or** 30 mg every 4 months **or** 45 mg every 6 months

Lupron®: 1 mg/day

Viadur®: 65 mg implanted subcutaneously every 12 months

I.M.:

Lupron Depot®: 7.5 mg/dose given monthly (every 28-33 days) **or**

Lupron Depot-3®: 22.5 mg every 3 months **or**

Lupron Depot-4®: 30 mg every 4 months

Endometriosis: I.M.: Initial therapy may be with leuprolide alone or in combination with norethindrone; if retreatment for an additional 6 months is necessary, norethindrone should be used. Retreatment is not recommended for longer than one additional 6-month course.

Lupron Depot®: 3.75 mg/month for up to 6 months **or**

Lupron Depot-3®: 11.25 mg every 3 months for up to 2 doses (6 months total duration of treatment)

Uterine leiomyomata (fibroids): I.M. (in combination with iron):

Lupron Depot®: 3.75 mg/month for up to 3 months **or**

Lupron Depot-3®: 11.25 mg as a single injection

Combination Regimens

Prostate cancer:

Bicalutamide + LHRH-A *on page 848*

FL *on page 889*

Administration

I.M.: Lupron Depot®: Vary injection site periodically

SubQ:

Eligard®: Vary injection site; choose site with adequate subcutaneous tissue (eg, abdomen, upper buttocks)

Lupron®: Vary injection site; if an alternate syringe from the syringe provided is required, insulin syringes should be used; use disposable syringe once only

Other Viadur® implant: Requires surgical implantation (subcutaneous) and removal at 12-month intervals

Dosage Forms

Implant (Viadur®): 65 mg [released over 12 months; packaged with administration kit]

Injection, solution, as acetate (Lupron®): 5 mg/mL (2.8 mL) [contains benzyl alcohol; packaged with syringes and alcohol swabs]

Injection, powder for reconstitution, as acetate [depot formulation; prefilled syringe]:

Eligard®:

7.5 mg [released over 1 month]

22.5 mg [released over 3 months]

30 mg [released over 4 months]

45 mg [released over 6 months]

Lupron Depot®: 3.75 mg, 7.5 mg [released over 1 month; contains polysorbate 80]

Lupron Depot®-3 Month: 11.25 mg, 22.5 mg [released over 3 months; contains polysorbate 80]

(Continued)

Leuprolide *(Continued)*

Lupron Depot®-4 Month: 30 mg [released over 4 months; contains polysorbate 80]

Lupron Depot-Ped®: 7.5 mg, 11.25 mg, 15 mg [released over 1 month; contains polysorbate 80]

Monitoring Parameters Bone mineral density

Precocious puberty: GnRH testing (blood LH and FSH levels), measurement of bone age every 6-12 months, testosterone in males and estradiol in females; Tanner staging

Prostatic cancer: LH and FSH levels, serum testosterone (2-4 weeks after initiation of therapy), PSA; weakness, paresthesias, and urinary tract obstruction in first few weeks of therapy

Patient Information Do not discontinue medication without prescriber's advice. May cause depression; report changes in mood or memory immediately. For self administration, patient must be taught aseptic technique and SubQ injection technique; rotate SubQ injection sites frequently. Disease flare can briefly occur with initiation of therapy.

Additional Information

Eligard® Atrigel®: A nongelatin-based, biodegradable, polymer matrix

Viadur®: Leuprolide acetate implant containing 72 mg of leuprolide acetate, equivalent to 65 mg leuprolide free base. One Viadur® implant delivers 120 mcg of leuprolide/day over 12 months.

Special Geriatric Considerations Leuprolide has the advantage of not increasing risk of atherosclerotic vascular disease, causing swelling of breasts, fluid retention, and thromboembolism as compared to estrogen therapy.

Selected Readings

Adjei AL and Hsu L, "Leuprolide and Other LH-RH Analogues," *Pharm Biotechnol*, 1993, 5:159-99.

Chrisp P and Sorkin EM, "Leuprorelin. A Review of Its Pharmacology and Therapeutic Use in Prostatic Disorders," *Drugs Aging*, 1991, 1(6):487-509.

Drago JR, Rohner T, Santen R, et al, "Leuprolide: A Review of its Effects in Animals and Man," *Br J Clin Pract*, 1985, 24:4-7, 16-9.

Plosker GL and Brogden RN, "Leuprorelin. A Review of its Pharmacology and Therapeutic Use in Prostate Cancer, Endometriosis and Other Sex Hormone-Related Disorders," *Drugs*, 1994, 48(6):930-67.

- ♦ **Leuprolide Acetate** *see* Leuprolide *on page 500*
- ♦ **Leuprorelin Acetate** *see* Leuprolide *on page 500*
- ♦ **Leurocristine Sulfate** *see* VinCRIStine *on page 819*
- ♦ **Leustatin**® *see* Cladribine *on page 196*
- ♦ **Levaquin**® *see* Levofloxacin *on page 504*
- ♦ **Levo-Dromoran**® *see* Levorphanol *on page 509*

Levofloxacin *(lee voe FLOKS a sin)*

U.S. Brand Names Iquix®; Levaquin®; Quixin™

Canadian Brand Names Levaquin®

Generic Available No

Pharmacologic Category Antibiotic, Quinolone

Pregnancy Risk Factor C

Lactation Excretion in breast milk unknown/not recommended

Use

Systemic: Treatment of mild, moderate, or severe infections caused by susceptible organisms. Includes the treatment of community-acquired pneumonia, including multidrug resistant strains of *S. pneumoniae* (MDRSP); nosocomial pneumonia; chronic bronchitis (acute bacterial exacerbation); acute maxillary sinusitis; urinary tract infection (uncomplicated or complicated), including acute pyelonephritis caused by *E. coli*; prostatitis (chronic bacterial); skin or skin structure infections (uncomplicated or complicated); prevention of inhalational anthrax (postexposure)

Ophthalmic: Treatment of bacterial conjunctivitis caused by susceptible organisms (Quixin™ 0.5% ophthalmic solution); treatment of corneal ulcer caused by susceptible organisms (Iquix® 1.5% ophthalmic solution)

Mechanism of Action As the S (-) enantiomer of the fluoroquinolone, ofloxacin, levofloxacin, inhibits DNA-gyrase in susceptible organisms thereby inhibits relaxation of supercoiled DNA and promotes breakage of DNA strands. DNA gyrase (topoisomerase II), is an essential bacterial enzyme that maintains the superhelical structure of DNA and is required for DNA replication and transcription, DNA repair, recombination, and transposition.

Labeled Contraindications Hypersensitivity to levofloxacin, any component of the formulation, or other quinolones

Warnings/Precautions Systemic: Not recommended in children <18 years of age; CNS stimulation may occur (tremor, restlessness, confusion, and very rarely hallucinations or seizures); use with caution in patients with known or suspected CNS disorders or renal dysfunction; use caution to avoid possible photosensitivity reactions during and for several days following fluoroquinolone therapy

Rare cases of torsade de pointes have been reported in patients receiving levofloxacin. Risk may be minimized by avoiding use in patients with known prolongation of QT interval, bradycardia, hypokalemia, hypomagnesemia, cardiomyopathy, or in those receiving concurrent therapy with Class Ia or Class III antiarrhythmics.

Severe hypersensitivity reactions, including anaphylaxis, have occurred with quinolone therapy. If an allergic reaction occurs (itching, urticaria, dyspnea or facial edema, loss of consciousness, tingling, cardiovascular collapse), discontinue drug immediately. Prolonged use may result in superinfection; pseudomembranous colitis may occur and should be considered in all patients who present with diarrhea. Tendon inflammation and/or rupture has been reported; risk may be increased with concurrent corticosteroids, particularly in the elderly. Discontinue at first sign of tendon inflammation or pain. Peripheral neuropathies have been linked to levofloxacin use; discontinue if numbness, tingling, or weakness develops. Quinolones may exacerbate myasthenia gravis.

Ophthalmic solution: For topical use only. Do not inject subconjunctivally or introduce into anterior chamber of the eye. Contact lenses should not be worn during treatment for bacterial conjunctivitis. Safety and efficacy in children <1 year of age (Quixin™) or <6 years of age (Iquix®) have not been established. **Note:** Indications for ophthalmic solutions are product concentration-specific and should not be used interchangeably.

Adverse Reactions

1% to 10%:

Central nervous system: Dizziness, fever, headache, insomnia

(Continued)

Levofloxacin *(Continued)*

Gastrointestinal: Abdominal pain, constipation, diarrhea, dyspepsia, nausea, vomiting

Ocular (with ophthalmic solution use): Decreased vision (transient), foreign body sensation, transient ocular burning, ocular pain or discomfort, photophobia

Respiratory: Dyspnea, pharyngitis

<1% (Limited to important or life-threatening):

Systemic: Acute renal failure; allergic reaction (including pneumonitis rash, pneumonitis, and anaphylaxis); agranulocytosis, anaphylactoid reaction, arrhythmia (including ventricular tachycardia and torsade de pointes), arthralgia, bradycardia, cardiac failure, dysphonia, eosinophilia, erythema multiforme, granulocytopenia, hemolytic anemia, hepatic failure, hypertension, INR/prothrombin time increased, intracranial hypertension, involuntary muscle contractions, jaundice, leukocytosis, leukopenia, leukorrhea, peripheral neuropathy, photosensitivity (<0.1%), pseudomembraneous colitis, pulmonary embolism, QT_c prolongation, rhabdomyolysis, seizure, Stevens-Johnson syndrome, tachycardia, taste perversion, tendon rupture, transaminases increased, thrombocytopenia, tremor

Ophthalmic solution: Allergic reaction, lid edema, ocular dryness, ocular itching

Postmarketing and/or case reports: Systemic: EEG abnormalities, encephalopathy

Overdosage/Toxicology

Symptoms of overdose include acute renal failure, seizures

Treatment should include GI decontamination and supportive care; not removed by peritoneal or hemodialysis

Drug Interactions

Increased Effect/Toxicity: Levofloxacin may increase the effects/toxicity of glyburide and warfarin. Concomitant use with corticosteroids may increase the risk of tendon rupture. Concomitant use with other QT_c-prolonging agents (eg, Class Ia and Class III antiarrhythmics, erythromycin, cisapride, antipsychotics, and cyclic antidepressants) may result in arrhythmias, such as torsade de pointes. Probenecid may increase levofloxacin levels.

Decreased Effect: Concurrent administration of metal cations, including most antacids, oral electrolyte supplements, quinapril, sucralfate, and some didanosine formulations (chewable/buffered tablets and pediatric powder for oral suspension), may decrease quinolone levels; separate doses.

Storage/Stability

Solution for injection:

Vial: Store at room temperature; protect from light. Diluted solution is stable for 72 hours when stored at room temperature; stable for 14 days when stored under refrigeration. When frozen, stable for 6 months; do not refreeze. Do not thaw in microwave or by bath immersion.

Premixed: Store at ≤25°C (77°F); protect from freezing and light.

Tablet, oral solution: Store at 25°C (77°F); excursions permitted to 15°C to 25°C (59°F to 77°F).

Ophthalmic solution: Store at 15°C to 25°C (59°F to 77°F).

Reconstitution Solution for injection: Single-use vials must be further diluted in compatible solution to a final concentration of 5 mg/mL prior to infusion.

Compatibility Stable in D_5LR, D_5NS, D_5W, NS; **incompatible** with mannitol 20%, sodium bicarbonate 5%

Y-site administration: Compatible: Amikacin, aminophylline, ampicillin, caffeine citrate, cefotaxime, cimetidine, clindamycin, dexamethasone sodium phosphate, dobutamine, dopamine, epinephrine, fentanyl, gentamicin, isoproterenol, lidocaine, linezolid, lorazepam, metoclopramide, morphine, oxacillin, pancuronium, penicillin G sodium, phenobarbital, phenylephrine, sodium bicarbonate, vancomycin. **Incompatible:** Acyclovir, alprostadil, furosemide, heparin, indomethacin, nitroglycerin, sodium nitroprusside. **Variable (consult detailed reference):** Insulin (regular)

Pharmacodynamics/Kinetics

Absorption: Rapid and complete

Distribution: V_d: 1.25 L/kg; CSF concentrations ~15% of serum levels; high concentrations are achieved in prostate, lung, and gynecological tissues, sinus, saliva

Protein binding: 50%

Metabolism: Minimally hepatic

Bioavailability: 99%

Half-life elimination: 6-8 hours

Time to peak, serum: 1-2 hours

Excretion: Primarily urine (as unchanged drug)

Dosage

Oral, I.V.: Adults:

Note: Sequential therapy (intravenous to oral) may be instituted based on prescriber's discretion.

Chronic bronchitis (acute bacterial exacerbation): 500 mg every 24 hours for at least 7 days

Inhalational anthrax: 500 mg every 24 hours for 60 days, beginning as soon as possible after exposure

Maxillary sinusitis (acute): 500 mg every 24 hours for 10-14 days

Pneumonia:

Community-acquired: 500 mg every 24 hours for 7-14 days or 750 mg every 24 hours for 5 days (efficacy of 5-day regimen for MDRSP not established)

Nosocomial: 750 mg every 24 hours for 7-14 days

Prostatitis (chronic bacterial): 500 mg every 24 hours for 28 days

Skin infections:

Uncomplicated: 500 mg every 24 hours for 7-10 days

Complicated: 750 mg every 24 hours for 7-14 days

Urinary tract infections:

Uncomplicated: 250 mg once daily for 3 days

Complicated, including acute pyelonephritis: 250 mg every 24 hours for 10 days

Ophthalmic:

Conjunctivitis (0.5% ophthalmic solution): Children ≥1 year and Adults:

Treatment day 1 and day 2: Instill 1-2 drops into affected eye(s) every 2 hours while awake, up to 8 times/day

Treatment day 3 through day 7: Instill 1-2 drops into affected eye(s) every 4 hours while awake, up to 4 times/day

(Continued)

Levofloxacin *(Continued)*

Corneal ulceration (1.5% ophthalmic solution): Children ≥6 years and Adults:

Treatment day 1 through day 3: Instill 1-2 drops into affected eye(s) every 30 minutes to 2 hours while awake and ~4-6 hours after retiring.

Treatment day 4 to treatment completion: Instill 1-2 drops into affected eye(s) every 1-4 hours while awake.

Dosing adjustment in renal impairment: Administer first dose as indicated in patients with normal renal function, then adjust dose as follows:

Chronic bronchitis, acute maxillary sinusitis, uncomplicated skin infection, community-acquired pneumonia, chronic bacterial prostatitis, or inhalational anthrax:

Cl_{cr} 20-49 mL/minute: 250 mg every 24 hours

Cl_{cr} 10-19 mL/minute: 250 mg every 48 hours

Hemodialysis/CAPD: 250 mg every 48 hours

Uncomplicated UTI: No dosage adjustment required

Complicated UTI, acute pyelonephritis: Cl_{cr} 10-19 mL/minute: 250 mg every 48 hours

Complicated skin infection, community-acquired pneumonia, or nosocomial pneumonia:

Cl_{cr} 20-49 mL/minute: Administer 750 mg every 48 hours

Cl_{cr} 10-19 mL/minute: Administer 500 mg every 48 hours

Hemodialysis/CAPD: 250 mg every 48 hours

Administration

Oral: May be administered without regard to meals.

I.V.: Infuse I.V. solution over 60 minutes. Too rapid of infusion can lead to hypotension. Avoid administration through an intravenous line with a solution containing multivalent cations (ie, magnesium, calcium).

Dosage Forms

Infusion [premixed in D_5W] (Levaquin®): 250 mg (50 mL); 500 mg (100 mL); 750 mg (150 mL)

Injection, solution [preservative free] (Levaquin®): 25 mg/mL (20 mL, 30 mL)

Solution, ophthalmic:

Iquix®: 1.5% (5 mL)

Quixin™: 0.5% (5 mL) [contains benzalkonium chloride]

Solution, oral (Levaquin®): 25 mg/mL (480 mL) [contains benzyl alcohol]

Tablet (Levaquin®): 250 mg, 500 mg, 750 mg

Levaquin® Leva-Pak: 750 mg (5s)

Monitoring Parameters Evaluation of organ system functions (renal, hepatic, ophthalmologic, and hematopoietic) is recommended periodically during therapy; the possibility of crystalluria should be assessed; WBC and signs of infection

Dietary Considerations Tablets may be taken without regard to meals. Oral solution should be administered on an empty stomach (1 hour before or 2 hours after a meal).

Patient Information

Oral: Take per recommended schedule, preferably on an empty stomach (1 hour before or 2 hours after meals). Maintain adequate hydration (2-3 L/day of fluids unless instructed to restrict fluid intake). Take complete prescription; do not skip doses. Do not take with antacids; separate by 2 hours. You may experience dizziness, lightheadedness, or confusion; use caution when driving or engaging in tasks that require alertness until response to drug is known. Small frequent meals and frequent mouth care may reduce nausea or vomiting. You may experience photosensitivity; use sunscreen, wear protective clothing and eyewear, and avoid direct sunlight. Report palpitations or chest pain, persistent diarrhea, GI disturbances or abdominal pain, muscle tremor or pain, yellowing of eyes or skin, easy bruising or bleeding, unusual fatigue, fever, chills, signs of infection, or worsening of condition. Report immediately any rash, itching, unusual CNS changes, or any facial swelling. Report immediately any pain, inflammation, or rupture of tendon.

Ophthalmic: Wash hands before instilling solution. Sit or lie down to instill. Open eye, look at ceiling, and instill prescribed amount of solution. Close eye and roll eye in all directions, and apply gentle pressure to inner corner of eye. Do not let tip of applicator touch eye or contaminate tip of applicator. Temporary stinging or blurred vision may occur. Report persistent pain, burning, vision disturbances, swelling, itching, or worsening of condition. Discontinue medication and contact prescriber immediately if you develop a rash or allergic reaction. Do not wear contact lenses.

Special Geriatric Considerations The risk of torsade de pointes and tendon inflammation and/or rupture associated with the concomitant use of corticosteroids and quinolones is increased in the elderly population. Adjust dose for renal function.

Selected Readings

Ernst ME, Ernst EJ, and Klepser ME, "Levofloxacin and Trovafloxacin: The Next Generation of Fluoroquinolones?" *Am J Health Syst Pharm*, 1997, 54(22):2569-84.

Martin SJ, Meyer JM, Chuck SK, et al, "Levofloxacin and Sparfloxacin: New Quinolone Antibiotics," *Ann Pharmacother*, 1998, 32(3):320-36.

North DS, Fish DN, and Redington JJ, "Levofloxacin, A Second-Generation Fluoroquinolone," *Pharmacotherapy*, 1998, 18(5):915-35.

Levorphanol (lee VOR fa nole)

U.S. Brand Names Levo-Dromoran®

Generic Available Yes: Tablet

Synonyms Levorphanol Tartrate; Levorphan Tartrate

Pharmacologic Category Analgesic, Narcotic

Pregnancy Risk Factor B/D (prolonged use or high doses at term)

Lactation Excretion in breast milk unknown/not recommended

Use Relief of moderate to severe pain; also used parenterally for preoperative sedation and an adjunct to nitrous oxide/oxygen anesthesia

Mechanism of Action Levorphanol tartrate is a synthetic opioid agonist that is classified as a morphinan derivative. Opioids interact with stereospecific opioid receptors in various parts of the central nervous system and other tissues. Analgesic potency parallels the affinity for these binding sites. These drugs do not alter the threshold or responsiveness to pain, but the perception of pain.

Restrictions C-II

Labeled Contraindications Hypersensitivity to levorphanol or any component of the formulation; pregnancy (prolonged use or high doses at term)

Warnings/Precautions An opioid-containing analgesic regimen should be tailored to each patient's needs and based upon the type of pain being treated (acute versus chronic), the route of administration, degree of tolerance for opioids (naive versus chronic user), age, weight, and (Continued)

Levorphanol *(Continued)*

medical condition. The optimal analgesic dose varies widely among patients. Doses should be titrated to pain relief/prevention.

Use with caution in patients with hypersensitivity reactions to other phenanthrene derivative opioid agonists (morphine, hydrocodone, hydromorphone, levorphanol, oxycodone, oxymorphone); respiratory diseases including asthma, emphysema, COPD, or severe liver or renal insufficiency. Some preparations contain sulfites which may cause allergic reactions. May be habit-forming. Dextromethorphan has equivalent antitussive activity but has much lower toxicity in accidental overdose. Elderly may be particularly susceptible to the CNS depressant and constipating effects of narcotics.

Adverse Reactions Frequency not defined.

Cardiovascular: Palpitations, hypotension, bradycardia, peripheral vasodilation, cardiac arrest, shock, tachycardia

Central nervous system: CNS depression, fatigue, drowsiness, dizziness, nervousness, headache, restlessness, anorexia, malaise, confusion, coma, convulsion, insomnia, amnesia, mental depression, hallucinations, paradoxical CNS stimulation, intracranial pressure (increased)

Dermatologic: Pruritus, urticaria, rash

Endocrine & metabolic: Antidiuretic hormone release

Gastrointestinal: Nausea, vomiting, dyspepsia, stomach cramps, xerostomia, constipation, abdominal pain, dry mouth, biliary tract spasm, paralytic ileus

Genitourinary: Decreased urination, urinary tract spasm, urinary retention

Local: Pain at injection site

Neuromuscular & skeletal: Weakness

Ocular: Miosis, diplopia

Respiratory: Respiratory depression, apnea, hypoventilation, cyanosis

Miscellaneous: Histamine release, physical and psychological dependence

Vesicant No

Overdosage/Toxicology Symptoms of overdose include CNS depression, respiratory depression, miosis, apnea, pulmonary edema, and convulsions. Naloxone, 2 mg I.V. with repeat administration as necessary up to a total dose of 10 mg, can be used to reverse opiate effects.

Drug Interactions

Increased Effect/Toxicity: CNS depression is enhanced with coadministration of other CNS depressants.

Ethanol/Nutrition/Herb Interactions

Ethanol: Avoid or limit ethanol (may increase CNS depression). Watch for sedation.

Herb/Nutraceutical: Avoid valerian, St John's wort, kava kava, gotu kola (may increase CNS depression).

Storage/Stability Store at room temperature. Protect from freezing.

Compatibility

Y-site administration: Compatible: Propofol

Compatibility in syringe: Compatible: Glycopyrrolate

Compatibility when admixed: Incompatible: Aminophylline, ammonium chloride, amobarbital, chlorothiazide, heparin, pentobarbital, phenobarbital, phenytoin, sodium bicarbonate, thiopental

Pharmacodynamics/Kinetics
Onset of action: Oral: 10-60 minutes
Duration: 4-8 hours
Metabolism: Hepatic
Half-life elimination: 11-16 hours
Excretion: Urine (as inactive metabolite)

Dosage Adults: **Note:** These are guidelines and do not represent the maximum doses that may be required in all patients. Doses should be titrated to pain relief/prevention.

Acute pain (moderate to severe):
Oral: Initial: Opiate-naive: 2 mg every 6-8 hours as needed; patients with prior opiate exposure may require higher initial doses; usual dosage range: 2-4 mg every 6-8 hours as needed
I.M., SubQ: Initial: Opiate-naive: 1 mg every 6-8 hours as needed; patients with prior opiate exposure may require higher initial doses; usual dosage range: 1-2 mg every 6-8 hours as needed
Slow I.V.: Initial: Opiate-naive: Up to 1 mg/dose every 3-6 hours as needed; patients with prior opiate exposure may require higher initial doses

Chronic pain: Patients taking opioids chronically may become tolerant and require doses higher than the usual dosage range to maintain the desired effect. Tolerance can be managed by appropriate dose titration. **There is no optimal or maximal dose for levorphanol in chronic pain. The appropriate dose is one that relieves pain throughout its dosing interval without causing unmanageable side effects.**

Premedication: I.M., SubQ: 1-2 mg/dose 60-90 minutes prior to surgery; older or debilitated patients usually require less drug

Dosing adjustment in hepatic disease: Reduction is necessary in patients with liver disease

Administration Parenteral levorphanol may be given by SubQ, I.V., or I.M. routes; however, intramuscular is generally not recommended in cancer patients.

Dosage Forms
Injection, solution, as tartrate: 2 mg/mL (1 mL, 10 mL)
Tablet, as tartrate: 2 mg

Monitoring Parameters Pain relief, respiratory and mental status, blood pressure

Patient Information Avoid alcohol, may cause drowsiness, impaired judgment or coordination; may cause physical and psychological dependence with prolonged use

Special Geriatric Considerations The elderly may be particularly susceptible to the CNS depressant and constipating effects of narcotics.

♦ **Levorphanol Tartrate** *see* Levorphanol *on page 509*
♦ **Levorphan Tartrate** *see* Levorphanol *on page 509*
♦ **LH-RH Agonist** *see* Histrelin *on page 415*

Lidocaine and Prilocaine (LYE doe kane & PRIL oh kane)
U.S. Brand Names EMLA®
Canadian Brand Names EMLA®
Generic Available Yes: Cream
Synonyms Prilocaine and Lidocaine
Pharmacologic Category Local Anesthetic
(Continued)

Lidocaine and Prilocaine *(Continued)*

Pregnancy Risk Factor B

Lactation Enters breast milk/compatible

Use Topical anesthetic for use on normal intact skin to provide local anal-gesia for minor procedures such as I.V. cannulation or venipuncture; has also been used for painful procedures such as lumbar puncture and skin graft harvesting; for superficial minor surgery of genital mucous membranes and as an adjunct for local infiltration anesthesia in genital mucous membranes.

Mechanism of Action Local anesthetic action occurs by stabilization of neuronal membranes and inhibiting the ionic fluxes required for the initia-tion and conduction of impulses

Labeled Contraindications

Hypersensitivity to amide type anesthetic agents [ie, lidocaine, prilocaine, dibucaine, mepivacaine, bupivacaine, etidocaine]; hypersensitivity to any component of the formulation selected; application on mucous membranes or broken or inflamed skin; infants <1 month of age if gestational age is <37 weeks; infants <12 months of age receiving therapy with methemoglobin-inducing agents; children with congenital or idiopathic methemoglobinemia, or in children who are receiving medications associated with drug-induced methemoglobinemia [ie, acetaminophen (overdosage), benzocaine, chloroquine, dapsone, nitro-furantoin, nitroglycerin, nitroprusside, phenazopyridine, phenelzine, phenobarbital, phenytoin, quinine, sulfonamides]

Warnings/Precautions Use with caution in patients receiving class I antiarrhythmic drugs, since systemic absorption occurs and synergistic toxicity is possible. Although the incidence of systemic adverse reactions with EMLA® is very low, caution should be exercised, particularly when applying over large areas and leaving on for longer than 2 hours.

Adverse Reactions Frequency not defined.

Cardiovascular: Hypotension, angioedema

Central nervous system: Shock

Dermatologic: Hyperpigmentation, erythema, itching, rash, burning, urti-caria

Genitourinary: Blistering of foreskin (rare)

Local: Burning, stinging, edema

Respiratory: Bronchospasm

Miscellaneous: Alteration in temperature sensation, hypersensitivity reac-tions

Emetic Potential Very low (<10%)

Drug Interactions

Cytochrome P450 Effect: Lidocaine: **Substrate** of CYP1A2 (minor), 2A6 (minor), 2B6 (minor), 2C8/9 (minor), 2D6 (major), 3A4 (major); **Inhibits** CYP1A2 (strong), 2D6 (strong), 3A4 (moderate)

Increased Effect/Toxicity: Class I antiarrhythmic drugs (tocainide, mexiletine): Effects are additive and potentially synergistic. Prilocaine may enhance the effect of other drugs known to induce methemoglobi-nemia.

Storage/Stability Store at room temperature.

Pharmacodynamics/Kinetics

EMLA®:

Onset of action: 1 hour

Peak effect: 2-3 hours

Duration: 1-2 hours after removal

Absorption: Related to duration of application and area where applied

3-hour application: 3.6% lidocaine and 6.1% prilocaine

24-hour application: 16.2% lidocaine and 33.5% prilocaine

See individual agents.

Dosage Although the incidence of systemic adverse effects with EMLA® is very low, caution should be exercised, particularly when applying over large areas and leaving on for >2 hours

Children (intact skin): EMLA® should **not** be used in neonates with a gestation age <37 weeks nor in infants <12 months of age who are receiving treatment with methemoglobin-inducing agents

Dosing is based on child's age and weight:

Age 0-3 months or <5 kg: Apply a maximum of 1 g over no more than 10 cm^2 of skin; leave on for no longer than 1 hour

Age 3 months to 12 months and >5 kg: Apply no more than a maximum 2 g total over no more than 20 cm^2 of skin; leave on for no longer than 4 hours

Age 1-6 years and >10 kg: Apply no more than a maximum of 10 g total over no more than 100 cm^2 of skin; leave on for no longer than 4 hours.

Age 7-12 years and >20 kg: Apply no more than a maximum 20 g total over no more than 200 cm^2 of skin; leave on for no longer than 4 hours.

Note: If a patient greater than 3 months old does not meet the minimum weight requirement, the maximum total dose should be restricted to the corresponding maximum based on patient weight.

Adults (intact skin):

EMLA® cream and EMLA® anesthetic disc: A thick layer of EMLA® cream is applied to intact skin and covered with an occlusive dressing, or alternatively, an EMLA® anesthetic disc is applied to intact skin

Minor dermal procedures (eg, I.V. cannulation or venipuncture): Apply 2.5 g of cream (1/2 of the 5 g tube) over 20-25 cm of skin surface area, or 1 anesthetic disc (1 g over 10 cm^2) for at least 1 hour. **Note:** In clinical trials, 2 sites were usually prepared as there was a technical problem with cannulation or venipuncture at the first site.

Major dermal procedures (eg, more painful dermatological procedures involving a larger skin area such as split thickness skin graft harvesting): Apply 2 g of cream per 10 cm^2 of skin and allow to remain in contact with the skin for at least 2 hours.

Adult male genital skin (eg, pretreatment prior to local anesthetic infiltration): Apply a thick layer of cream (1 g/10 cm^2) to the skin surface for 15 minutes. Local anesthetic infiltration should be performed immediately after removal of EMLA® cream.

Note: Dermal analgesia can be expected to increase for up to 3 hours under occlusive dressing and persist for 1-2 hours after removal of the cream

Adult females: Genital mucous membranes: Minor procedures (eg, removal of condylomata acuminata, pretreatment for local anesthetic infiltration): Apply 5-10 g (thick layer) of cream for 5-10 minutes

Dosage Forms

Cream, topical: Lidocaine 2.5% and prilocaine 2.5% (5 g, 30 g)

(Continued)

Lidocaine and Prilocaine *(Continued)*

EMLA®: Lidocaine 2.5% and prilocaine 2.5% (5 g, 30 g) [each packaged with Tegaderm® dressings]

Disc, topical: Lidocaine 2.5% and prilocaine 2.5% per disc (2s, 10s) [each 1 g disc is 10 cm²]

Patient Information Not for ophthalmic use; for external use only. EMLA® may block sensation in the treated skin.

♦ **Lilly CT-3231** *see* Vindesine *on page 825*

♦ **Lin-Megestrol (Can)** see Megestrol *on page 528*

♦ **Locoid®** *see* Hydrocortisone *on page 419*

♦ **Locoid Lipocream®** *see* Hydrocortisone *on page 419*

♦ **L-OHP** *see* Oxaliplatin *on page 629*

Lomustine (loe MUS teen)

Related Information
Safe Handling of Hazardous Drugs *on page 1034*

U.S. Brand Names CeeNU®

Canadian Brand Names CeeNU®

Generic Available No

Synonyms CCNU

Pharmacologic Category Antineoplastic Agent, Alkylating Agent

Pregnancy Risk Factor D

Lactation Enters breast milk/contraindicated

Use Treatment of brain tumors and Hodgkin's disease, non-Hodgkin's lymphoma, melanoma, renal carcinoma, lung cancer, colon cancer

Mechanism of Action Inhibits DNA and RNA synthesis via carbamylation of DNA polymerase, alkylation of DNA, and alteration of RNA, proteins, and enzymes

Labeled Contraindications Hypersensitivity to lomustine, any component of the formulation, or other nitrosoureas; pregnancy

Warnings/Precautions Hazardous agent - use appropriate precautions for handling and disposal. See Safe Handling of Hazardous Drugs *on page 1034* in the Appendix. Use with caution in patients with depressed platelet, leukocyte or erythrocyte counts. Bone marrow depression, notably thrombocytopenia and leukopenia, may lead to bleeding and overwhelming infections in an already compromised patient; will last for at least 6 weeks after a dose, do not give courses more frequently than every 6 weeks because the toxicity is cumulative. Use with caution in patients with liver function abnormalities.

Adverse Reactions

>10%:

Gastrointestinal: Nausea and vomiting, usually within 3-6 hours after oral administration. Administration of the dose at bedtime, with an antiemetic, significantly reduces both the incidence and severity of nausea.

Hematologic: Myelosuppression, common, dose-limiting, may be cumulative and irreversible

Onset: 10-14 days

Nadir: Leukopenia: 6 weeks

Thrombocytopenia: 4 weeks

Recovery: 6-8 weeks

1% to 10%:

Dermatologic: Rash

Gastrointestinal: Anorexia, stomatitis, diarrhea

Genitourinary: Progressive azotemia, renal failure, decrease in kidney size

Hematologic: Anemia

Hepatic: Elevated liver enzymes, transient, reversible

<1%: Disorientation, lethargy, ataxia, dysarthria, alopecia, nephritis (associated with large cumulative doses), interstitial fibrosis and infiltrates (associated with cumulative doses >600-1000 mg, may be irreversible and fatal)

Emetic Potential Very high (>90%)

Overdosage/Toxicology Symptoms of overdose include nausea, vomiting, and leukopenia. There are no known antidotes. Treatment is symptomatic and supportive.

Drug Interactions

Cytochrome P450 Effect: Substrate of CYP2D6 (major); **Inhibits** CYP2D6 (weak), 3A4 (weak)

Increased Effect/Toxicity: CYP2D6 inhibitors may increase the levels/effects of lomustine; example inhibitors include chlorpromazine, delavirdine, fluoxetine, miconazole, paroxetine, pergolide, quinidine, quinine, ritonavir, and ropinirole. Increased toxicity with cimetidine, reported to cause bone marrow depression or to potentiate the myelosuppressive effects of lomustine.

Decreased Effect: Decreased effect with phenobarbital, resulting in reduced efficacy of both drugs.

Ethanol/Nutrition/Herb Interactions Ethanol: Avoid ethanol (due to GI irritation).

Storage/Stability Refrigerate (<40°C/<104°F).

Pharmacodynamics/Kinetics

Duration: Marrow recovery: ≤6 weeks

Absorption: Complete; appears in plasma within 3 minutes after administration

Distribution: Crosses blood-brain barrier to a greater degree than BCNU; CNS concentrations are equal to that of plasma

Protein binding: 50%

Metabolism: Rapidly hepatic via hydroxylation producing at least two active metabolites; enterohepatically recycled

Half-life elimination: Parent drug: 16-72 hours; Active metabolite: Terminal: 1.3-2 days

Time to peak, serum: Active metabolite: ~3 hours

Excretion: Urine; feces (<5%); expired air (<10%)

Dosage Oral (refer to individual protocols):

Children: 75-150 mg/m^2 as a single dose every 6 weeks; subsequent doses are readjusted after initial treatment according to platelet and leukocyte counts

Adults: 100-130 mg/m^2 as a single dose every 6 weeks; readjust after initial treatment according to platelet and leukocyte counts

With compromised marrow function: Initial dose: 100 mg/m^2 as a single dose every 6 weeks

Repeat courses should only be administered after adequate recovery: WBC >4000 and platelet counts >100,000

(Continued)

Lomustine *(Continued)*

Subsequent dosing adjustment based on nadir:
Leukocytes 2000-2900/mm^3, platelets 25,000-74,999/mm^3: Administer 70% of prior dose

Leukocytes <2000/mm^3, platelets <25,000/mm^3: Administer 50% of prior dose

Dosage adjustment in renal impairment:
Cl$_{cr}$ 10-50 mL/minute: Administer 75% of normal dose

Cl$_{cr}$ <10 mL/minute: Administer 50% of normal dose

Hemodialysis: Supplemental dose is not necessary

Peritoneal dialysis: Significant drug removal is unlikely based on physiochemical characteristics

Combination Regimens
Brain tumors:

8 in 1 (Brain Tumors) *on page 841*

PCV *on page 928*

POC *on page 931*

Lymphoma, Hodgkin's: CAD/MOPP/ABV *on page 850*

Melanoma: BOLD *on page 849*

Retinoblastoma: 8 in 1 (Retinoblastoma) *on page 842*

Administration Orally, on an empty stomach. Administration as a single dose at bedtime, about 30 minutes after an antiemetic, significantly reduces the incidence of nausea and vomiting.

Dosage Forms
Capsule: 10 mg, 40 mg, 100 mg

Capsule [dose pack]: 10 mg (2s); 40 mg (2s); 100 mg (2s)

Monitoring Parameters CBC with differential and platelet count, hepatic and renal function tests, pulmonary function tests

Dietary Considerations Should be taken with fluids on an empty stomach; no food or drink for 2 hours after administration to decrease nausea.

Patient Information Take with fluids on an empty stomach; do not eat or drink for 2 hours following administration. Do not use alcohol, aspirin, or aspirin-containing medications and/or OTC medications without consulting prescriber. Maintain adequate fluid balance (2-3 L/day of fluids unless instructed to restrict fluid intake). May cause hair loss (reversible); easy bleeding or bruising (use soft toothbrush or cotton swabs and frequent mouth care, use electric razor, avoid sharp knives or scissors); increased susceptibility to infection (avoid crowds or exposure to infection - do not have any vaccinations unless approved by prescriber). Report unusual bleeding or bruising or persistent fever or sore throat; blood in urine, stool, or vomitus; delayed healing of any wounds; skin rash; yellowing of skin or eyes; changes in color of urine of stool. Contraceptive measures are recommended during therapy.

Selected Readings
Bono VH, "Review of Mechanism of Action Studies of the Nitrosoureas," *Cancer Treat Rep,* 1976, 60(6):699-702.

Lee FY, Workman P, Roberts JT, et al, "Clinical Pharmacokinetics or Oral CCNU (Lomustine)," *Cancer Chemother Pharmacol,* 1985, 14(2):125-31.

Oliverio VT, "Pharmacology of the Nitrosoureas: An Overview," *Cancer Treat Rep,* 1976, 60(6):703-7.

Weiss RB and Issell BF, "The Nitrosoureas: Carmustine (BCNU) and Lomustine (CCNU)," *Cancer Treat Rev,* 1982, 9(4):313-30.

Lorazepam (lor A ze pam)

Medication Safety Issues

Sound-alike/look-alike issues:

Lorazepam may be confused with alprazolam, clonazepam, diazepam, temazepam

Ativan® may be confused with Atarax®, Atgam®, Avitene®

Related Information

Management of Nausea and Vomiting on page 982

U.S. Brand Names Ativan®; Lorazepam Intensol®

Canadian Brand Names Apo-Lorazepam®; Ativan®; Novo-Lorazepam; Nu-Loraz; PMS-Lorazepam; Riva-Lorazepam

Generic Available Yes

Pharmacologic Category Benzodiazepine

Pregnancy Risk Factor D

Lactation Enters breast milk/contraindicated (AAP rates "of concern")

Use

Oral: Management of anxiety disorders or short-term relief of the symptoms of anxiety or anxiety associated with depressive symptoms

I.V.: Status epilepticus, preanesthesia for desired amnesia, antiemetic adjunct

Unlabeled/Investigational Use Ethanol detoxification; insomnia; psychogenic catatonia; partial complex seizures; agitation (I.V.)

Mechanism of Action Binds to stereospecific benzodiazepine receptors on the postsynaptic GABA neuron at several sites within the central nervous system, including the limbic system, reticular formation. Enhancement of the inhibitory effect of GABA on neuronal excitability results by increased neuronal membrane permeability to chloride ions. This shift in chloride ions results in hyperpolarization (a less excitable state) and stabilization.

Restrictions C-IV

Labeled Contraindications Hypersensitivity to lorazepam or any component of the formulation (cross-sensitivity with other benzodiazepines may exist); acute narrow-angle glaucoma; sleep apnea (parenteral); intra-arterial injection of parenteral formulation; severe respiratory insufficiency (except during mechanical ventilation); pregnancy

Warnings/Precautions Causes CNS depression (dose-related) which may impair physical and mental capabilities. Use with caution in patients receiving other CNS depressants or psychoactive agents. Benzodiazepines have been associated with falls and traumatic injury and should be used with extreme caution in patients who are at risk of these events (especially the elderly). Use with caution in patients with a history of drug dependence.

Use with caution in elderly or debilitated patients, patients with hepatic disease (including alcoholics), renal impairment, respiratory disease, impaired gag reflex, or obese patients. Prolonged lorazepam use may have a possible relationship to GI disease, including esophageal dilation. Use is not recommended in patients with depressive disorders or psychoses. Avoid use in patients with sleep apnea.

The parenteral formulation of lorazepam contains polyethylene glycol and propylene glycol. Also contains benzyl alcohol - avoid in neonates. (Continued)

Lorazepam *(Continued)*

Benzodiazepines have been associated with anterograde amnesia. Paradoxical reactions, including hyperactive or aggressive behavior, have been reported with benzodiazepines, particularly in adolescent/pediatric or psychiatric patients. Does not have analgesic, antidepressant, or antipsychotic properties.

Adverse Reactions

>10%:

Central nervous system: Sedation

Respiratory: Respiratory depression

1% to 10%:

Cardiovascular: Hypotension

Central nervous system: Confusion, dizziness, akathisia, unsteadiness, headache, depression, disorientation, amnesia

Dermatologic: Dermatitis, rash

Gastrointestinal: Weight gain/loss, nausea, changes in appetite

Neuromuscular & skeletal: Weakness

Respiratory: Nasal congestion, hyperventilation, apnea

<1%: Blood dyscrasias, increased salivation, menstrual irregularities, physical and psychological dependence with prolonged use, reflex slowing, polyethylene glycol or propylene glycol poisoning (prolonged I.V. infusion)

Vesicant No

Emetic Potential Very low (<10%)

Overdosage/Toxicology Symptoms of overdose include confusion, coma, hypoactive reflexes, dyspnea, labored breathing. **Note:** Prolonged infusions have been associated with toxicity from propylene glycol and/or polyethylene glycol. Treatment for benzodiazepine overdose is supportive. Flumazenil has been shown to selectively block the binding of benzodiazepines to CNS receptors, resulting in a reversal of benzodiazepine-induced CNS depression but not respiratory depression

Drug Interactions

Increased Effect/Toxicity: Ethanol and other CNS depressants may increase the CNS effects of lorazepam. Scopolamine in combination with parenteral lorazepam may increase the incidence of sedation, hallucinations, and irrational behavior. There are rare reports of significant respiratory depression, stupor, and/or hypotension with concomitant use of loxapine and lorazepam. Use caution if concomitant administration of loxapine and CNS drugs is required.

Decreased Effect: Oral contraceptives may increase the clearance of lorazepam. Lorazepam may decrease the antiparkinsonian efficacy of levodopa. Theophylline and other CNS stimulants may antagonize the sedative effects of lorazepam.

Ethanol/Nutrition/Herb Interactions

Ethanol: Avoid or limit ethanol (may increase CNS depression).

Herb/Nutraceutical: Avoid valerian, St John's wort, kava kava, gotu kola (may increase CNS depression).

Storage/Stability Intact vials should be refrigerated and protected from light. Do not use discolored or precipitate-containing solutions. Injectable vials may be stored at room temperature for up to 60 days. Parenteral admixture is stable at room temperature (25°C) for 24 hours. Store tablets at room temperature.

Reconstitution Infusion: Use 2 mg/mL injectable solution to prepare; dilute ≤1 mg/mL and mix in glass bottle; precipitation may develop; can also be administered undiluted via infusion. Dilute I.V. dose with equal volume of compatible diluent (D_5W, NS, SWI)

Compatibility Variable stability (consult detailed reference) in D_5W, LR, NS

Y-site administration: Compatible: Acyclovir, alatrofloxacin, albumin, allopurinol, amifostine, amikacin, amphotericin B cholesteryl sulfate complex, amsacrine, atracurium, bumetanide, cefepime, cefotaxime, ciprofloxacin, cisatracurium, cisplatin, cladribine, clonidine, co-trimoxazole, cyclophosphamide, cytarabine, dexamethasone sodium phosphate, diltiazem, dobutamine, docetaxel, dopamine, doxorubicin, doxorubicin liposome, epinephrine, erythromycin lactobionate, etomidate, etoposide phosphate, famotidine, fentanyl, filgrastim, fluconazole, fludarabine, fosphenytoin, furosemide, gatifloxacin, gemcitabine, gentamicin, granisetron, haloperidol, heparin, hydrocortisone sodium succinate, hydromorphone, ketanserin, labetalol, levofloxacin, linezolid, melphalan, methotrexate, metronidazole, midazolam, milrinone, morphine, nicardipine, nitroglycerin, norepinephrine, paclitaxel, pancuronium, piperacillin, piperacillin/tazobactam, potassium chloride, propofol, ranitidine, remifentanil, tacrolimus, teniposide, thiotepa, vancomycin, vecuronium, vinorelbine, zidovudine. **Incompatible:** Aldesleukin, aztreonam, floxacillin, idarubicin, imipenem/cilastatin, omeprazole, ondansetron, sargramostim, sufentanil. **Variable (consult detailed reference):** Foscarnet, thiopental, TPN

Compatibility in syringe: Compatible: Cimetidine, hydromorphone. **Incompatible:** Sufentanil. **Variable (consult detailed reference):** Ranitidine

Compatibility when admixed: Incompatible: Buprenorphine, dexamethasone sodium phosphate with diphenhydramine and metoclopramide

Pharmacodynamics/Kinetics

Onset of action:
    Hypnosis: I.M.: 20-30 minutes
    Sedation: I.V.: 5-20 minutes
    Anticonvulsant: I.V.: 5 minutes, oral: 30-60 minutes

Duration: 6-8 hours

Absorption: Oral, I.M.: Prompt

Distribution:
    V_d: Neonates: 0.76 L/kg, Adults: 1.3 L/kg; crosses placenta; enters breast milk

Protein binding: 85%; free fraction may be significantly higher in elderly

Metabolism: Hepatic to inactive compounds

Half-life elimination: Neonates: 40.2 hours; Older children: 10.5 hours; Adults: 12.9 hours; Elderly: 15.9 hours; End-stage renal disease: 32-70 hours

Excretion: Urine; feces (minimal)

Dosage

Antiemetic:
    Children 2-15 years: I.V.: 0.05 mg/kg (up to 2 mg/dose) prior to chemotherapy
    Adults: Oral, I.V. (**Note:** May be administered sublingually; not a labeled route): 0.5-2 mg every 4-6 hours as needed

(Continued)

Lorazepam *(Continued)*

Anxiety and sedation:

Infants and Children: Oral, I.M., I.V.: Usual: 0.05 mg/kg/dose (range: 0.02-0.09 mg/kg) every 4-8 hours

I.V.: May use smaller doses (eg, 0.01-0.03 mg/kg) and repeat every 20 minutes, as needed to titrate to effect

Adults: Oral: 1-10 mg/day in 2-3 divided doses; usual dose: 2-6 mg/day in divided doses

Elderly: 0.5-4 mg/day; initial dose not to exceed 2 mg

Insomnia: Adults: Oral: 2-4 mg at bedtime

Preoperative: Adults:

I.M.: 0.05 mg/kg administered 2 hours before surgery (maximum: 4 mg/dose)

I.V.: 0.044 mg/kg 15-20 minutes before surgery (usual maximum: 2 mg/dose)

Operative amnesia: Adults: I.V.: Up to 0.05 mg/kg (maximum: 4 mg/dose)

Sedation (preprocedure): Infants and Children:

Oral, I.M., I.V.: Usual: 0.05 mg/kg (range: 0.02-0.09 mg/kg);

I.V.: May use smaller doses (eg, 0.01-0.03 mg/kg) and repeat every 20 minutes, as needed to titrate to effect

Status epilepticus: I.V.:

Infants and Children: 0.1 mg/kg slow I.V. over 2-5 minutes; do not exceed 4 mg/single dose; may repeat second dose of 0.05 mg/kg slow I.V. in 10-15 minutes if needed

Adolescents: 0.07 mg/kg slow I.V. over 2-5 minutes; maximum: 4 mg/dose; may repeat in 10-15 minutes

Adults: 4 mg/dose slow I.V. over 2-5 minutes; may repeat in 10-15 minutes; usual maximum dose: 8 mg

Rapid tranquilization of agitated patient (administer every 30-60 minutes):

Oral: 1-2 mg

I.M.: 0.5-1 mg

Average total dose for tranquilization: Oral, I.M.: 4-8 mg

Agitation in the ICU patient (unlabeled):

I.V.: 0.02-0.06 mg/kg every 2-6 hours

I.V. infusion: 0.01-0.1 mg/kg/hour

Administration Lorazepam may be administered by I.M., I.V., or orally

I.M.: Should be administered deep into the muscle mass

I.V.: Do not exceed 2 mg/minute or 0.05 mg/kg over 2-5 minutes; dilute I.V. dose with equal volume of compatible diluent (D_5W, NS, SWI)

Dosage Forms

Injection, solution (Ativan®): 2 mg/mL (1 mL, 10 mL); 4 mg/mL (1 mL, 10 mL) [contains benzyl alcohol]

Solution, oral concentrate (Lorazepam Intensol®): 2 mg/mL (30 mL) [alcohol free, dye free]

Tablet (Ativan®): 0.5 mg, 1 mg, 2 mg

Monitoring Parameters Respiratory and cardiovascular status, blood pressure, heart rate, symptoms of anxiety

Patient Information Advise patient of potential for physical and psychological dependence with chronic use; advise patient of possible retrograde amnesia after I.V. or I.M. use; will cause drowsiness, impairment of judgment or coordination

Additional Information Oral doses >0.09 mg/kg produced increased ataxia without increased sedative benefit vs lower doses; preferred anxiolytic when I.M. route needed. Abrupt discontinuation after sustained use (generally >10 days) may cause withdrawal symptoms.

Special Geriatric Considerations Because lorazepam is relatively short-acting with an inactive metabolite, it is a preferred agent to use in elderly patients when a benzodiazepine is indicated. Use with caution since elderly patients have decreased pulmonary reserve and are more prone to hypoxia.

Selected Readings

Ameer B and Greenblatt DJ, "Lorazepam: A Review of Its Clinical Pharmacological Properties and Therapeutic Uses," *Drugs*, 1981, 21(3):162-200.

Greenblatt DJ, Allen MD, Locniskar A, et al, "Lorazepam Kinetics in the Elderly," *Clin Pharmacol Ther*, 1979, 26(1):103-13.

◆ **Lorazepam Intensol**® *see* Lorazepam *on page 517*

◆ **Lotrimin® AF Athlete's Foot Cream [OTC]** *see* Clotrimazole *on page 203*

◆ **Lotrimin® AF Athlete's Foot Solution [OTC]** *see* Clotrimazole *on page 203*

◆ **Lotrimin® AF Jock Itch Cream [OTC]** *see* Clotrimazole *on page 203*

◆ **L-PAM** *see* Melphalan *on page 530*

◆ **L-Sarcolysin** *see* Melphalan *on page 530*

◆ **Lupron**® *see* Leuprolide *on page 500*

◆ **Lupron Depot**® *see* Leuprolide *on page 500*

◆ **Lupron Depot-Ped**® *see* Leuprolide *on page 500*

◆ **LY231514** *see* Pemetrexed *on page 655*

◆ **Lymphocyte Immune Globulin** *see* Antithymocyte Globulin (Equine) *on page 96*

◆ **Lymphocyte Mitogenic Factor** *see* Aldesleukin *on page 32*

◆ **Lysodren**® *see* Mitotane *on page 582*

◆ **m-AMSA** *see* Amsacrine *on page 80*

◆ **Management of Drug Extravasations** *see page 965*

◆ **Management of Infections** *see page 978*

◆ **Management of Nausea and Vomiting** *see page 982*

◆ **Marinol**® *see* Dronabinol *on page 292*

◆ **Matulane**® *see* Procarbazine *on page 688*

◆ **Maxidex**® *see* Dexamethasone *on page 263*

◆ **Maxipime**® *see* Cefepime *on page 162*

◆ **MDL 73,147EF** *see* Dolasetron *on page 277*

Mechlorethamine (me klor ETH a meen)

U.S. Brand Names Mustargen®

Canadian Brand Names Mustargen®

Generic Available No

Synonyms Chlorethazine; Chlorethazine Mustard; HN_2; Mechlorethamine Hydrochloride; Mustine; Nitrogen Mustard; NSC-762

Pharmacologic Category Antineoplastic Agent, Alkylating Agent (Nitrogen Mustard)

Pregnancy Risk Factor D

Lactation Excretion in breast milk unknown/not recommended

(Continued)

Mechlorethamine *(Continued)*

Use Hodgkin's disease; non-Hodgkin's lymphoma; intracavitary injection for treatment of metastatic tumors; pleural and other malignant effusions; topical treatment of mycosis fungoides

Mechanism of Action Bifunctional alkylating agent that inhibits DNA and RNA synthesis via formation of carbonium ions; cross-links strands of DNA, causing miscoding, breakage, and failure of replication; produces interstrand and intrastrand cross-links in DNA resulting in miscoding, breakage, and failure of replication. Although not cell phase-specific *per se,* mechlorethamine effect is most pronounced in the S phase, and cell proliferation is arrested in the G_2 phase.

Labeled Contraindications Hypersensitivity to mechlorethamine or any component of the formulation; pre-existing profound myelosuppression or infection; pregnancy

Warnings/Precautions Hazardous agent - use appropriate precautions for handling and disposal. See Safe Handling of Hazardous Drugs *on page 1034* in the Appendix. Mechlorethamine is a potent vesicant; if extravasation occurs, severe tissue damage (leading to ulceration and necrosis) and pain may occur. Urate precipitation should be anticipated especially with lymphomas.

Adverse Reactions

>10%:

Dermatologic: Alopecia; hyperpigmentation of veins; contact and allergic dermatitis (50% with topical use)

Endocrine & metabolic: Chromosomal abnormalities, delayed menses, oligomenorrhea, amenorrhea, impaired spermatogenesis

Gastrointestinal: Nausea and vomiting (almost 100%), onset may be within minutes of drug administration

Genitourinary: Azoospermia

Hematologic: Myelosuppression, leukopenia, and thrombocytopenia

Onset: 4-7 days

Nadir: 14 days

Recovery: 21 days

1% to 10%:

Central nervous system: Fever

Gastrointestinal: Diarrhea, anorexia, metallic taste

Otic: Tinnitus

<1%: Vertigo, rash, hemolytic anemia, hepatotoxicity, weakness, peripheral neuropathy

Vesicant Yes; see Management of Drug Extravasations *on page 965.*

Emetic Potential Very high (>90%)

Overdosage/Toxicology Suppression of all formed elements of blood, uric acid crystals, nausea, vomiting, and diarrhea. Sodium thiosulfate is the specific antidote for nitrogen mustard extravasations. Treatment of systemic overdose is supportive.

Drug Interactions

Decreased Effect: Patients may experience impaired immune response to vaccines; possible infection after administration of live vaccines in patients receiving immunosuppressants.

Ethanol/Nutrition/Herb Interactions Ethanol: Avoid ethanol (due to GI irritation).

Storage/Stability Store intact vials at room temperature.

Reconstitution Must be prepared immediately before use; solution is stable for only 15-60 minutes after dilution. Dilute powder with 10 mL SWI to a final concentration of 1 mg/mL. May be diluted in up to 100 mL NS for intracavitary administration.

Compatibility Stable in sterile water for injection; not stable in D_5W; **variable stability (consult detailed reference)** in NS

   Y-site administration: Compatible: Amifostine, aztreonam, filgrastim, fludarabine, granisetron, melphalan, ondansetron, sargramostim, teniposide, vinorelbine. **Incompatible:** Allopurinol, cefepime

   Compatibility when admixed: Incompatible: Methohexital

Pharmacodynamics/Kinetics

   Duration: Unchanged drug is undetectable in blood within a few minutes

   Absorption: Intracavitary administration: Incomplete secondary to rapid deactivation by body fluids

   Metabolism: Rapid hydrolysis and demethylation, possibly in plasma

   Half-life elimination: <1 minute

   Excretion: Urine (50% as metabolites, <0.01% as unchanged drug)

Dosage Refer to individual protocols.

   Children and Adults: I.V.: 6 mg/m^2 on days 1 and 8 of a 28-day cycle (MOPP regimen)

   Adults:

   I.V.: 0.4 mg/kg **or** 12-16 mg/m^2 for one dose **or** divided into 0.1 mg/kg/day for 4 days, repeated at 4- to 6-week intervals

   Intracavitary: 0.2-0.4 mg/kg (10-20 mg) as a single dose; may be repeated if fluid continues to accumulate.

   Intrapericardially: 0.2-0.4 mg/kg as a single dose; may be repeated if fluid continues to accumulate.

   Topical: 0.01% to 0.02% solution, lotion, or ointment

   Hemodialysis: Not removed; supplemental dosing is not required.

   Peritoneal dialysis: Not removed; supplemental dosing is not required.

Combination Regimens

   Brain tumors:

   MOP *on page 910*

   MOPP (Medulloblastoma) *on page 912*

   Lymphoma, Hodgkin's:

   CAD/MOPP/ABV *on page 850*

   MOPP (Lymphoma, Hodgkin's Disease) *on page 911*

   MOPP/ABV Hybrid *on page 913*

   MOPP/ABVD *on page 913*

   MVPP *on page 922*

   Stanford V *on page 937*

Administration I.V. as a slow push through the side of a freely-flowing saline or dextrose solution. Due to the limited stability of the drug, and the increased risk of phlebitis and venous irritation and blistering with increased contact time, infusions of the drug are not recommended.

   Intracavitary: Technique and route vary

Dosage Forms Injection, powder for reconstitution, as hydrochloride: 10 mg

High Dose Considerations

   High Dose: I.V.: 0.3-2 mg/kg

Monitoring Parameters CBC with differential, hemoglobin, and platelet count

(Continued)

Mechlorethamine *(Continued)*

Patient Information This medication can only be given by infusion, usually in cycles of therapy. You will need frequent laboratory and medical monitoring during treatment. Do not use alcohol, aspirin or aspirin-containing medications, and/or OTC medications without consulting prescriber. Maintain adequate fluid balance (2-3 L/day of fluids unless instructed to restrict fluid intake) and adequate nutrition (small frequent meals, frequent mouth care, sucking lozenges, or chewing gum may reduce anorexia and nausea). May cause discoloration (brown color) of veins used for infusion, hair loss (reversible); easy bleeding or bruising (use soft toothbrush or cotton swabs and frequent mouth care, use electric razor, avoid sharp knives or scissors); increased susceptibility to infection (avoid crowds or exposure to infection - do not have any vaccinations unless approved by prescriber). This drug may cause menstrual irregularities, permanent sterility, and birth defects. Report changes in auditory or visual acuity; unusual bleeding or bruising or persistent fever or sore throat; blood in urine, stool, or vomitus; delayed healing of any wounds; skin rash; yellowing of skin or eyes; changes in color of urine or stool; acute or unresolved nausea or vomiting; diarrhea; or loss of appetite. The drug may be excreted in breast milk, therefore, an alternative form of feeding your baby should be used. Contraceptive measures are recommended during therapy.

Selected Readings

Bonadonna G, Valagussa P, and Santoro A, "Alternating Non-Cross-Resistant Combination Chemotherapy or MOPP in Stage IV Hodgkin's Disease. A Report of 8-Year Results," *Ann Intern Med*, 1986, 104(6):739-46.

DeVita VT, Serpick A, and Carbone PP, "Combination Chemotherapy in the Treatment of Advanced Hodgkin's Disease," *Ann Intern Med*, 1970, 73:881-95.

Dorr RT, Soble M, and Alberts DS, "Efficacy of Sodium Thiosulfate as a Local Antidote to Mechlorethamine Skin Toxicity in the Mouse," *Cancer Chemother Pharmacol*, 1988, 22(4):299-302.

Loutsidis A, Bellenis I, Argiriou M, et al, "Tetracycline Compared With Mechlorethamine in the Treatment of Malignant Pleural Effusions. A Randomized Trial," *Respir Med*, 1994, 88(7):523-6.

Price NM, Hoppe RT, and Deneau DG, "Ointment Based Mechlorethamine Treatment for Mycosis Fungoides," *Cancer*, 1983, 52:2214-9.

Taylor JR, Halprin KM, Levine V, et al, "Mechlorethamine Hydrochloride Solutions and Ointments," *Arch Dermatol*, 1980, 116:783-5.

Vonderheid EC, "Topical Mechlorethamine Chemotherapy: Considerations on its Use in Mycosis Fungoides ," *Int J Dermatol*, 1984, 23(3):180-6.

♦ **Mechlorethamine Hydrochloride** *see* Mechlorethamine *on page 521*

♦ **Medrol**® *see* MethylPREDNISolone *on page 558*

MedroxyPROGESTERone *(me DROKS ee proe JES te rone)*

Medication Safety Issues

Sound-alike/look-alike issues:

MedroxyPROGESTERone may be confused with hydroxyprogesterone, methylPREDNISolone, methylTESTOSTERone

Provera® may be confused with Covera®, Parlodel®, Premarin®

U.S. Brand Names Depo-Provera®; Depo-Provera® Contraceptive; depo-subQ provera 104™; Provera®

Canadian Brand Names Alti-MPA; Apo-Medroxy®; Depo-Prevera®; Gen-Medroxy; Novo-Medrone; Provera®

Generic Available Yes

Synonyms Acetoxymethylprogesterone; Medroxyprogesterone Acetate; Methylacetoxyprogesterone; MPA

Pharmacologic Category Contraceptive; Progestin

Pregnancy Risk Factor X

Lactation Enters breast milk/compatible

Use Endometrial carcinoma or renal carcinoma; secondary amenorrhea or abnormal uterine bleeding due to hormonal imbalance; reduction of endometrial hyperplasia in nonhysterectomized postmenopausal women receiving conjugated estrogens; prevention of pregnancy; management of endometriosis-associated pain

Mechanism of Action Inhibits secretion of pituitary gonadotropins, which prevents follicular maturation and ovulation; causes endometrial thinning

Labeled Contraindications Hypersensitivity to medroxyprogesterone or any component of the formulation; history of or current thrombophlebitis or venous thromboembolic disorders (including DVT, PE); cerebral vascular disease; severe hepatic dysfunction or disease; carcinoma of the breast or genital organs, undiagnosed vaginal bleeding; missed abortion, diagnostic test for pregnancy, pregnancy

Warnings/Precautions Prolonged use of medroxyprogesterone contraceptive injection may result in a loss of bone mineral density (BMD). Loss is related to the duration of use, and may not be completely reversible on discontinuation of the drug. The impact on peak bone mass in adolescents should be considered in treatment decisions. Long-term use (ie, >2 years) should be limited to situations where other birth control methods are inadequate.

Use caution with cardiovascular disease or dysfunction. MPA used in combination with estrogen may increase the risks of hypertension, myocardial infarction (MI), stroke, pulmonary emboli (PE), and deep vein thrombosis; incidence of these effects was shown to be significantly increased in postmenopausal women using conjugated equine estrogens (CEE) in combination with MPA. MPA in combination with estrogens should not be used to prevent coronary heart disease.

The risk of dementia may be increased in postmenopausal women; increased incidence was observed in women ≥65 years of age taking MPA in combination with CEE. An increased risk of invasive breast cancer was observed in postmenopausal women using MPA in combination with CEE. An increase in abnormal mammograms has also been reported with estrogen and progestin therapy.

Discontinue pending examination in cases of sudden partial or complete vision loss, sudden onset of proptosis, diplopia, or migraine; discontinue permanently if papilledema or retinal vascular lesions are observed on examination. Use with caution in patients with diseases that may be exacerbated by fluid retention (including asthma, epilepsy, migraine, diabetes, or renal dysfunction). Use caution with history of depression. Whenever possible, progestins in combination with estrogens should be discontinued at least 4-6 weeks prior to surgeries associated with an increased risk of thromboembolism or during periods of prolonged immobilization. Progestins used in combination with estrogen should be used for shortest duration possible consistent with treatment goals. Conduct periodic risk:benefit assessments.

Adverse Reactions Adverse effects as reported with any dosage form; percent ranges presented are noted with the MPA contraceptive injection: (Continued)

MedroxyPROGESTERone *(Continued)*

>5%:

Central nervous system: Dizziness, headache, nervousness

Endocrine & metabolic: Libido decreased, menstrual irregularities (includes bleeding, amenorrhea, or both)

Gastrointestinal: Abdominal pain/discomfort, weight changes (average 3-5 pounds after 1 year, 8 pounds after 2 years)

Neuromuscular & skeletal: Weakness

1% to 5%:

Cardiovascular: Edema

Central nervous system: Depression, fatigue, insomnia, irritability, pain

Dermatologic: Acne, alopecia, rash

Endocrine & metabolic: Anorgasmia, breast pain, hot flashes

Gastrointestinal: Bloating, nausea

Genitourinary: Cervical smear abnormal, leukorrhea, menometrorrhagia, menorrhagia, pelvic pain, urinary tract infection, vaginitis, vaginal infection, vaginal hemorrhage

Local: Injection site atrophy, injection site reaction, injection site pain

Neuromuscular & skeletal: Arthralgia, backache, leg cramp

Respiratory: Respiratory tract infections

<1%: Allergic reaction, anemia, angioedema, appetite changes, asthma, axillary swelling, blood dyscrasia, body odor, breast cancer, breast changes, cervical cancer, chest pain, chills, chloasma, convulsions, deep vein thrombosis, diaphoresis, drowsiness, dry skin, dysmenorrhea, dyspareunia, dyspnea, facial palsy, fever, galactorrhea, genitourinary infections, glucose tolerance decreased, hirsutism, hoarseness, jaundice, lack of return to fertility, lactation decreased, libido increased, melasma, nipple bleeding, osteoporosis, paralysis, paresthesia, pruritus, pulmonary embolus, rectal bleeding, scleroderma, sensation of pregnancy, somnolence, syncope, tachycardia, thirst, thrombophlebitis, uterine hyperplasia, vaginal cysts, varicose veins; residual lump, sterile abscess, or skin discoloration at the injection site

Postmarketing and/or case reports: Anaphylaxis, anaphylactoid reactions, bone mineral density decreased, osteoporotic fractures

Vesicant No

Emetic Potential Very low (<10%)

Overdosage/Toxicology Toxicity is unlikely following single exposure of excessive doses. Supportive treatment is adequate in most cases.

Drug Interactions

Cytochrome P450 Effect: Substrate of CYP3A4 (major); **Induces** CYP3A4 (weak)

Decreased Effect: CYP3A4 inducers may decrease the levels/effects of medroxyprogesterone; example inducers include aminoglutethimide, carbamazepine, nafcillin, nevirapine, phenobarbital, phenytoin, and rifamycins.

Ethanol/Nutrition/Herb Interactions

Food: Bioavailability of the oral tablet is increased when taken with food; half-life is unchanged

Pharmacodynamics/Kinetics

Absorption: Oral: Well absorbed; I.M.: Slow

Protein binding: 86% to 90% primarily to albumin; does not bind to sex hormone-binding globulin

Metabolism: Extensively hepatic via hydroxylation and conjugation; forms metabolites

Time to peak: Oral: 2-4 hours

Half-life elimination: Oral: 12-17 hours; I.M. (Depo-Provera® Contraceptive): 50 days; SubQ: ~40 days

Excretion: Urine

Dosage

Adolescents and Adults:

Amenorrhea: Oral: 5-10 mg/day for 5-10 days

Abnormal uterine bleeding: Oral: 5-10 mg for 5-10 days starting on day 16 or 21 of cycle

Contraception:

Depo-Provera® Contraceptive: I.M.: 150 mg every 3 months

depo-subQ provera 104™: SubQ: 104 mg every 3 months (every 12-14 weeks)

Endometriosis: depo-subQ provera 104™: SubQ: 104 mg every 3 months (every 12-14 weeks)

Adults:

Endometrial or renal carcinoma (Depo-Provera®): I.M.: 400-1000 mg/week

Accompanying cyclic estrogen therapy, postmenopausal: Oral: 5-10 mg for 12-14 consecutive days each month, starting on day 1 or day 16 of the cycle; lower doses may be used if given with estrogen continuously throughout the cycle

Dosing adjustment in hepatic impairment: Use is contraindicated with severe impairment. Consider lower dose or less frequent administration with mild-to-moderate impairment. Use of the contraceptive injection has not been studied in patients with hepatic impairment; consideration should be given to not readminister if jaundice develops

Dosage Forms

Injection, suspension, as acetate: 150 mg/mL (1 mL)

Depo-Provera®: 400 mg/mL (2.5 mL)

Depo-Provera® Contraceptive: 150 mg/mL (1 mL) [prefilled syringe or vial]

depo-subQ provera 104™: 104 mg/0.65 mL (0.65 mL) [prefilled syringe]

Tablet, as acetate (Provera®): 2.5 mg, 5 mg, 10 mg

Monitoring Parameters Before starting therapy, a physical exam with reference to the breasts and pelvis are recommended, including a Papanicolaou smear. Exam may be deferred if appropriate prior to administration of MPA contraceptive injection; pregnancy should be ruled out prior to use. Monitor patient closely for loss of vision, sudden onset of proptosis, diplopia, migraine; signs and symptoms of thromboembolic disorders; signs or symptoms of depression; glucose in diabetics; blood pressure

Dietary Considerations Ensure adequate calcium and vitamin D intake when used for the prevention of pregnancy

Patient Information Follow dosage schedule and do not take more than prescribed. You may experience sensitivity to sunlight (use sunblock, wear protective clothing and eyewear, and avoid extensive exposure to direct sunlight); dizziness, anxiety, depression (use caution when driving or engaging in tasks that require alertness until response to drug is known); changes in appetite (maintain adequate hydration and diet - 2-3 L/day of fluids unless instructed to restrict fluid intake); decreased libido (Continued)

MedroxyPROGESTERone *(Continued)*

or increased body hair (reversible when drug is discontinued); hot flashes (cool clothes and environment may help). May cause discoloration of stool (green). Report swelling of face, lips, or mouth; absent or altered menses; abdominal pain; vaginal itching, irritation, or discharge; heat, warmth, redness, or swelling of extremities; or sudden change in vision.

Injection for contraception: This product does not protect against HIV or other sexually-transmitted diseases.

Special Geriatric Considerations No specific recommendations for dosage adjustments. Monitor closely for adverse effects when starting therapy.

♦ **Medroxyprogesterone Acetate** *see MedroxyPROGESTERone on page 524*

♦ **Megace®** *see Megestrol on page 528*

♦ **Megace® OS (Can)** *see Megestrol on page 528*

Megestrol *(me JES trole)*

Medication Safety Issues
   Sound-alike/look-alike issues:
      Megace® may be confused with Reglan®

U.S. Brand Names Megace®

Canadian Brand Names Apo-Megestrol®; Lin-Megestrol; Megace®; Megace® OS; Nu-Megestrol

Generic Available Yes

Synonyms 5071-1DL(6); Megestrol Acetate; NSC-10363

Pharmacologic Category Antineoplastic Agent, Hormone; Appetite Stimulant; Progestin

Pregnancy Risk Factor X

Lactation Enters breast milk/contraindicated

Use Palliative treatment of breast and endometrial carcinoma
   Orphan drug: Treatment of anorexia, cachexia, or significant weight loss ($\geq$10% baseline body weight) and confirmed diagnosis of AIDS

Unlabeled/Investigational Use Uterine bleeding

Mechanism of Action A synthetic progestin with antiestrogenic properties which disrupt the estrogen receptor cycle. Megestrol interferes with the normal estrogen cycle and results in a lower LH titer. May also have a direct effect on the endometrium. Megestrol is an antineoplastic progestin thought to act through an antileutenizing effect mediated via the pituitary.

Labeled Contraindications Hypersensitivity to megestrol or any component of the formulation; pregnancy

Warnings/Precautions Use with caution in patients with a history of thrombophlebitis. Elderly females may have vaginal bleeding or discharge. May suppress hypothalamic-pituitary-adrenal (HPA) axis during chronic administration. Consider the possibility of adrenal suppression in any patient receiving or being withdrawn from chronic therapy when signs/symptoms suggestive of hypoadrenalism are noted (during stress or in unstressed state). Laboratory evaluation and replacement/stress doses of rapid-acting glucocorticoid should be considered.

Adverse Reactions
   Cardiovascular: Edema, hypertension ($\leq$8%), cardiomyopathy, palpitation

Central nervous system: Insomnia, fever (2% to 6%), headache (≤10%), pain (≤6%, similar to placebo), confusion (1% to 3%), convulsions (1% to 3%), depression (1% to 3%)

Dermatologic: Allergic rash (2% to 12%) with or without pruritus, alopecia

Endocrine & metabolic: Breakthrough bleeding and amenorrhea, spotting, changes in menstrual flow, changes in cervical erosion and secretions, increased breast tenderness, changes in vaginal bleeding pattern, edema, fluid retention, hyperglycemia (≤6%), diabetes, HPA axis suppression, adrenal insufficiency, Cushing's syndrome

Gastrointestinal: Weight gain (not attributed to edema or fluid retention), nausea, vomiting (7%), diarrhea (8% to 15%, similar to placebo), flatulence (≤10%), constipation (1% to 3%)

Genitourinary: Impotence (4% to 14%), decreased libido (≤5%)

Hepatic: Cholestatic jaundice, hepatotoxicity, hepatomegaly (1% to 3%)

Local: Thrombophlebitis

Neuromuscular & skeletal: Carpal tunnel syndrome, weakness, paresthesia (1% to 3%)

Respiratory: Hyperpnea, dyspnea (1% to 3%), cough (1% to 3%)

Miscellaneous: Diaphoresis

Emetic Potential Very low (<10%)

Overdosage/Toxicology Toxicity is unlikely following single exposure of excessive doses.

Ethanol/Nutrition/Herb Interactions Herb/Nutraceutical: Avoid black cohosh, dong quai in estrogen-dependent tumors.

Storage/Stability Store at 25°C (77°F); excursions permitted at 15°C to 30°C (59°F to 86°F)

Pharmacodynamics/Kinetics

Absorption: Well absorbed orally

Metabolism: Completely hepatic to free steroids and glucuronide conjugates

Time to peak, serum: 1-3 hours

Half-life elimination: 15-100 hours

Excretion: Urine (57% to 78% as steroid metabolites and inactive compound); feces (8% to 30%)

Dosage Adults: Oral (refer to individual protocols):

Female:

Breast carcinoma: 40 mg 4 times/day

Endometrial carcinoma: 40-320 mg/day in divided doses; use for 2 months to determine efficacy; maximum doses used have been up to 800 mg/day

Uterine bleeding (unlabeled use): 40 mg 2-4 times/day

Male/Female: HIV-related cachexia: Initial dose: 800 mg/day; daily doses of 400 and 800 mg/day were found to be clinically effective

Dosing adjustment in renal impairment: No data available; however, the urinary excretion of megestrol acetate administered in doses of 4-90 mg ranged from 56% to 78% within 10 days

Hemodialysis: Megestrol acetate has not been tested for dialyzability; however, due to its low solubility, it is postulated that dialysis would not be an effective means of treating an overdose

Administration Megestrol acetate (Megace®) oral suspension is compatible with water, orange juice, apple juice, or Sustacal H.C. for immediate consumption.

(Continued)

Megestrol *(Continued)*

Dosage Forms

Suspension, oral, as acetate: 40 mg/mL (240 mL) [contains alcohol 0.06% and sodium benzoate; lemon-lime flavor]

Tablet, as acetate: 20 mg, 40 mg

Monitoring Parameters
Observe for signs of thromboembolic phenomena

Patient Information
Follow dosage schedule and do not take more than prescribed. You may experience sensitivity to sunlight (use sunblock, wear protective clothing, and avoid extended exposure to direct sunlight); dizziness, anxiety, depression (use caution when driving or engaging in tasks that require alertness until response to drug is known); change in appetite (maintain adequate hydration and diet - 2-3 L/day of fluids unless instructed to restrict fluid intake); decreased libido or increased body hair (reversible when drug is discontinued); hot flashes (cool clothes and environment may help). Report swelling of face, lips, or mouth; absence or altered menses; abdominal pain; vaginal itching, irritation, or discharge; heat, warmth, redness, or swelling of extremities; or sudden onset change in vision.

Special Geriatric Considerations
Elderly females may have vaginal bleeding or discharge and need to be forewarned of this side effect and inconvenience. No specific changes in dose are required for elderly. Megestrol has been used in the treatment of the failure to thrive syndrome in cachectic elderly in addition to proper nutrition.

Selected Readings

Canetta R, Florentine S, Hunter H, et al, "Megestrol Acetate," *Cancer Treat Rev*, 1983, 10(3):141-57.

Chang AY, "Megestrol Acetate as a Biomodulator," *Semin Oncol*, 1998, 25(2 Suppl 6):58-61.

Farrar DJ, "Megestrol Acetate: Promises and Pitfalls," *AIDS Patient Care STDS*, 1999, 13(3):149-52.

Schacter L, Rozencweig M, Canetta R, et al, "Megestrol Acetate: Clinical Experience," *Cancer Treat Rev*, 1989, 16(1):49-63.

♦ **Megestrol Acetate** *see* Megestrol *on page 528*

Melphalan (MEL fa lan)

Medication Safety Issues

Sound-alike/look-alike issues:

Melphalan may be confused with Mephyton®, Myleran®

Alkeran® may be confused with Alferon®, Leukeran®

Related Information

Safe Handling of Hazardous Drugs *on page 1034*

Transplantation *on page 1019*

U.S. Brand Names Alkeran®

Canadian Brand Names Alkeran®

Generic Available No

Synonyms L-PAM; L-Sarcolysin; Phenylalanine Mustard

Pharmacologic Category Antineoplastic Agent, Alkylating Agent

Pregnancy Risk Factor D

Lactation Excretion in breast milk unknown/not recommended

Use Palliative treatment of multiple myeloma and nonresectable epithelial ovarian carcinoma; neuroblastoma, rhabdomyosarcoma, breast cancer

Mechanism of Action Alkylating agent which is a derivative of mechlorethamine that inhibits DNA and RNA synthesis via formation of carbonium ions; cross-links strands of DNA

Labeled Contraindications Hypersensitivity to melphalan or any component of the formulation; severe bone marrow suppression; patients whose disease was resistant to prior therapy; pregnancy

Warnings/Precautions Hazardous agent - use appropriate precautions for handling and disposal. See Safe Handling of Hazardous Drugs *on page 1034* in the Appendix. Melphalan is potentially mutagenic, carcinogenic, and teratogenic; produces amenorrhea. Discontinue therapy if leukocyte count is <3000/mm^3 or platelet count is <100,000/mm^3; use with caution in patients with bone marrow suppression, impaired renal function, or who have received prior chemotherapy or irradiation; will cause amenorrhea. Toxicity to immunosuppressives is increased in the elderly. Start with lowest recommended adult doses. Signs of infection, such as fever and WBC rise, may not occur. Lethargy and confusion may be more prominent signs of infection.

Adverse Reactions

>10%: Hematologic: Myelosuppressive: Leukopenia and thrombocytopenia are the most common effects of melphalan; irreversible bone marrow failure has been reported

WBC: Moderate

Platelets: Moderate

Onset: 7 days

Nadir: 8-10 days and 27-32 days

Recovery: 42-50 days

1% to 10%:

Cardiovascular: Vasculitis

Dermatologic: Vesiculation of skin, alopecia, pruritus, rash

Endocrine & metabolic: SIADH, sterility, amenorrhea

Gastrointestinal: Nausea and vomiting are mild; stomatitis and diarrhea are infrequent

Genitourinary: Hemorrhagic cystitis, bladder irritation

Hematologic: Anemia, agranulocytosis, hemolytic anemia

Hepatic: Transaminases increased (hepatitis, jaundice have been reported)

Respiratory: Pulmonary fibrosis, interstitial pneumonitis

Miscellaneous: Hypersensitivity, secondary malignancy

Vesicant No

Emetic Potential

Oral: Very low (<10%)

I.V.: Very high (>90%)

Overdosage/Toxicology Symptoms of overdose include hypocalcemia, pulmonary fibrosis, nausea and vomiting, and bone marrow suppression. Treatment is symptomatic and supportive.

Drug Interactions

Increased Effect/Toxicity: Risk of nephrotoxicity of cyclosporine is increased by melphalan. Concomitant use of I.V. melphalan may cause serious GI toxicity.

Decreased Effect: Cimetidine and other H_2 antagonists: The reduction in gastric pH has been reported to decrease bioavailability of melphalan by 30%.

(Continued)

Melphalan *(Continued)*

Ethanol/Nutrition/Herb Interactions

Ethanol: Avoid ethanol (due to GI irritation).

Food: Food interferes with oral absorption.

Storage/Stability The time between reconstitution/dilution and administration of parenteral melphalan must be kept to a minimum (<60 minutes) because reconstituted and diluted solutions are unstable. Must be prepared fresh; solution is stable for 1 hour after dilution.

Tablet: Store in refrigerator at 2°C to 8°C (36°F to 46°F); protect from light.

Injection: Store at room temperature (15°C to 30°C). Protect from light.

Reconstitution

Injection: Preparation: Dissolve powder initially with 10 mL of diluent to a concentration of 5 mg/mL. Shake vigorously to dissolve. **Immediately dilute dose in NS to a concentration ≤0.45 mg/mL. Do not refrigerate solution; precipitation occurs.**

Standard I.V. dilution: 250-500 mL NS (concentration ≤0.45 mg/mL)

Compatibility Not stable in D_5W, LR; **variable stability (consult detailed reference)** in NS

Y-site administration: Compatible: Acyclovir, amikacin, aminophylline, ampicillin, aztreonam, bleomycin, bumetanide, buprenorphine, butorphanol, calcium gluconate, carboplatin, carmustine, cefazolin, cefepime, cefoperazone, cefotaxime, cefotetan, ceftazidime, ceftizoxime, ceftriaxone, cefuroxime, cimetidine, cisplatin, clindamycin, co-trimoxazole, cyclophosphamide, cytarabine, dacarbazine, dactinomycin, daunorubicin, dexamethasone sodium phosphate, diphenhydramine, doxorubicin, doxycycline, droperidol, enalaprilat, etoposide, famotidine, floxuridine, fluconazole, fludarabine, fluorouracil, furosemide, ganciclovir, gentamicin, granisetron, haloperidol, heparin, hydrocortisone sodium phosphate, hydrocortisone sodium succinate, hydromorphone, hydroxyzine, idarubicin, ifosfamide, imipenem/cilastatin, lorazepam, mannitol, mechlorethamine, meperidine, mesna, methotrexate, methylprednisolone sodium succinate, metoclopramide, metronidazole, minocycline, mitomycin, mitoxantrone, morphine, nalbuphine, netilmicin, ondansetron, pentostatin, piperacillin, plicamycin, potassium chloride, prochlorperazine edisylate, promethazine, ranitidine, sodium bicarbonate, streptozocin, teniposide, thiotepa, ticarcillin, ticarcillin/clavulanate, tobramycin, vancomycin, vinblastine, vincristine, vinorelbine, zidovudine. **Incompatible:** Amphotericin B, chlorpromazine

Pharmacodynamics/Kinetics

Absorption: Oral: Variable and incomplete

Distribution: V_d: 0.5-0.6 L/kg throughout total body water

Bioavailability: Unpredictable, decreasing from 85% to 58% with repeated doses

Half-life elimination: Terminal: 1.5 hours

Time to peak, serum: ~2 hours

Excretion: Oral: Feces (20% to 50%); urine (10% to 30% as unchanged drug)

Dosage Refer to individual protocols.

Oral: Dose should always be adjusted to patient response and weekly blood counts:

Children: 4-20 mg/m²/day for 1-21 days

Adults:

Multiple myeloma: 6 mg/day initially adjusted as indicated **or** 0.15 mg/kg/day for 7 days **or** 0.25 mg/kg/day for 4 days; repeat at 4- to 6-week intervals.

Ovarian carcinoma: 0.2 mg/kg/day for 5 days, repeat every 4-5 weeks.

I.V.:

Children:

Pediatric rhabdomyosarcoma: 10-35 mg/m²/dose every 21-28 days

High-dose melphalan with bone marrow transplantation for neuroblastoma: I.V.: 100-220 mg/m² as a single dose or divided into 2-5 daily doses. Infuse over 20-60 minutes.

Adults: Multiple myeloma: 16 mg/m² administered at 2-week intervals for 4 doses, then repeat monthly as per protocol for multiple myeloma.

Dosing adjustment in renal impairment:

Cl_{cr} 10-50 mL/minute: Administer at 75% of normal dose

Cl_{cr} <10 mL/minute: Administer at 50% of normal dose

or

BUN >30 mg/dL: Reduce dose by 50%

Serum creatinine >1.5 mg/dL: Reduce dose by 50%

Hemodialysis: Unknown

CAPD effects: Unknown

CAVH effects: Dose for GFR 10-50 mL/minute

Combination Regimens

Lymphoma, Hodgkin's:

CAD/MOPP/ABV *on page 850*

mini-BEAM *on page 910*

Multiple myeloma:

M-2 *on page 906*

MP (Multiple Myeloma) *on page 916*

VBMCP *on page 945*

Administration

Oral: Administer on an empty stomach (1 hour prior to or 2 hours after meals)

Parenteral: Due to limited stability, complete administration of I.V. dose should occur within 60 minutes of reconstitution

I.V. infusion: Infusion over 15-20 minutes

I.V. bolus:

Central line: I.V. bolus doses of 17-200 mg/m² (reconstituted and not diluted) have been infused over 2-20 minutes

Peripheral line: I.V. bolus doses of 2-23 mg/m² (reconstituted and not diluted) have been infused over 1-4 minutes

Dosage Forms

Injection, powder for reconstitution: 50 mg [diluent contains ethanol and propylene glycol]]

Tablet: 2 mg

High Dose Considerations

High Dose: I.V.: 100-240 mg/m² administered as a single dose or divided into 2-4 daily doses. Maximum dose as a single agent: 200-400

(Continued)

Melphalan *(Continued)*

mg/m². Maximum dose with total body irradiation (TBI): 110-140 mg/m²; other high-dose chemotherapeutic drugs: 100-180 mg/m². Generally infused over 20-60 minutes.

Unique Toxicities:

Cardiovascular: Atrial fibrillation, left ventricular heart failure

Dermatologic: Alopecia

Gastrointestinal: Mucositis (severity increases with Cl_{cr} ≤40 mL/minute; pretreatment with amifostine or glutamine may decrease mucositis), nausea and vomiting (moderate), diarrhea

Hematologic: Myelosuppression, secondary leukemia

Renal: Increased serum creatinine and azotemia possible without adequate hydration

Rare side effects: Abnormal LFTs, atrial fibrillation, interstitial pneumonitis, secondary leukemia, SIADH, vasculitis

Comments: Saline-based hydration (100-125 mg/m²/hour) preceding (2-4 hours), during, and following (6-12 hours) administration reduces risk of drug precipitation in renal tubules. Hydrolysis causes loss of 1% melphalan injection per 10 minutes. Infusion of admixture must be completed within 100 minutes of preparation to deliver ordered dose. Reconstitute dose to 5 mg/mL in diluent provided by manufacturer. Dose may be infused via central or peripheral venous access without further dilution to minimize volume of infusion.

Monitoring Parameters CBC with differential and platelet count, serum electrolytes, serum uric acid

Dietary Considerations Should be taken on an empty stomach (1 hour prior to or 2 hours after meals).

Patient Information

Do not take alcohol, aspirin or aspirin-containing medications, and/or OTC medications without consulting prescriber. Inform prescriber of all prescription medication you are taking. Maintain adequate fluid balance (2-3 L/day of fluids unless instructed to restrict fluid intake). May cause hair loss (reversible); easy bleeding or bruising (use a soft toothbrush or cotton swabs and frequent mouth care, use electric razor, avoid sharp knives or scissors); increased susceptibility to infection (avoid crowds or exposure to infection - do not have any vaccinations unless approved by prescriber). Report unusual bleeding or bruising or persistent fever or sore throat; blood in urine, stool, or vomitus; delayed healing of any wounds; skin rash; yellowing of skin or eyes; changes in color of urine or black stool; pain or burning on urination; respiratory difficulty; or other severe adverse reactions. Contraceptive measures should be used during therapy. The drug may be excreted in breast milk, therefore, an alternative form of feeding your baby should be used.

I.V.: Report promptly any pain, irritation, or redness at infusion site.

Oral: Preferable to take on an empty stomach, 1 hour prior to or 2 hours after meals.

Special Geriatric Considerations Toxicity to immunosuppressives is increased in the elderly. Start with lowest recommended adult doses. Signs of infection, such as fever and WBC rise, may not occur. Lethargy and confusion may be more prominent signs of infection.

Selected Readings

Jones RB, "Clinical Pharmacology of Melphalan and its Implications for Clinical Resistance to Anticancer Agents," *Cancer Treat Res*, 2002, 112:305-22.

Samuels BL and Bitran JD, "High-Dose Intravenous Melphalan: A Review," *J Clin Oncol*, 1995, 13(7):1786-99.

Sarosy G, Leyland-Jones B, Soochan P, et al, "The Systemic Administration of Intravenous Melphalan," *J Clin Oncol*, 1988, 6(11):1768-82.

Meperidine (me PER i deen)

Medication Safety Issues

Sound-alike/look-alike issues:

Meperidine may be confused with meprobamate

Demerol® may be confused with Demulen®, Desyrel®, dicumarol, Dilaudid®, Dymelor®, Pamelor®

U.S. Brand Names Demerol®; Meperitab®

Canadian Brand Names Demerol®

Generic Available Yes

Synonyms Isonipecaine Hydrochloride; Meperidine Hydrochloride; Pethidine Hydrochloride

Pharmacologic Category Analgesic, Narcotic

Pregnancy Risk Factor C/D (prolonged use or high doses at term)

Lactation Enters breast milk/contraindicated (AAP rates "compatible")

Use Management of moderate to severe pain; adjunct to anesthesia and preoperative sedation

Mechanism of Action Binds to opiate receptors in the CNS, causing inhibition of ascending pain pathways, altering the perception of and response to pain; produces generalized CNS depression

Restrictions C-II

Labeled Contraindications Hypersensitivity to meperidine or any component of the formulation; patients receiving MAO inhibitors presently or in the past 14 days; pregnancy (prolonged use or high doses near term)

Warnings/Precautions An opioid-containing analgesic regimen should be tailored to each patient's needs and based upon the type of pain being treated (acute versus chronic), the route of administration, degree of tolerance for opioids (naive versus chronic user), age, weight, and medical condition. The optimal analgesic dose varies widely among patients. Doses should be titrated to pain relief/prevention. Use for chronic pain management not recommended. Oral meperidine not recommended for acute pain management.

Use with caution in patients with pulmonary, hepatic, renal disorders, or increased intracranial pressure; use with caution in patients with renal failure or seizure disorders or those receiving high-dose meperidine; normeperidine (an active metabolite and CNS stimulant) may accumulate and precipitate twitches, tremors, or seizures; some preparations contain sulfites which may cause allergic reaction; not recommended as a drug of first choice for the treatment of chronic pain in the elderly due to the accumulation of normeperidine; for acute pain, its use should be limited to 1-2 doses; tolerance or drug dependence may result from extended use. Use only with extreme caution **(if at all)** in patients with head injury or increased intracranial pressure (ICP); potential to elevate ICP may be greatly exaggerated in these patients.

Adverse Reactions Frequency not defined.

Cardiovascular: Hypotension

(Continued)

Meperidine *(Continued)*

Central nervous system: Fatigue, drowsiness, dizziness, nervousness, headache, restlessness, malaise, confusion, mental depression, hallucinations, paradoxical CNS stimulation, increased intracranial pressure, seizure (associated with metabolite accumulation)

Dermatologic: Rash, urticaria

Gastrointestinal: Nausea, vomiting, constipation, anorexia, stomach cramps, xerostomia, biliary spasm, paralytic ileus

Genitourinary: Ureteral spasms, decreased urination

Local: Pain at injection site

Neuromuscular & skeletal: Weakness

Respiratory: Dyspnea

Miscellaneous: Histamine release, physical and psychological dependence

Vesicant No

Overdosage/Toxicology Symptoms of overdose include CNS depression, respiratory depression, mydriasis, bradycardia, pulmonary edema, chronic tremor, CNS excitability, and seizures. Treatment is symptomatic. Naloxone, 2 mg I.V. with repeat administration as necessary up to a total dose of 10 mg, can be used to reverse opiate effects. Naloxone should not be used to treat meperidine-induced seizures.

Drug Interactions

Increased Effect/Toxicity: MAO inhibitors greatly potentiate the effects of meperidine; acute opioid overdosage symptoms can be seen, including severe toxic reactions. Concurrent use within 14 days of an MAO inhibitor is contraindicated. CNS depressants may potentiate the sedative effects of meperidine or increase respiratory depression. Phenothiazines may potentiate the sedative effects of meperidine and may increase the incidence of hypotension. Serotonin agonists, serotonin reuptake inhibitors, and tricyclic antidepressants may potentiate the effects of meperidine. In addition, concurrent therapy with these drugs potentially may increase the risk of serotonin syndrome. A number of drugs may increase meperidine metabolite concentrations (including acyclovir, cimetidine, and ritonavir).

Decreased Effect: Barbiturates may decrease the analgesic efficacy and increase the sedative effects of meperidine. Phenytoin may decrease the analgesic effects of meperidine.

Ethanol/Nutrition/Herb Interactions

Ethanol: Avoid or limit ethanol (may increase CNS depression). Watch for sedation.

Food: Glucose may cause hyperglycemia; monitor blood glucose concentrations.

Herb/Nutraceutical: Avoid valerian, St John's wort, kava kava, gotu kola (may increase CNS depression).

Storage/Stability Meperidine injection should be stored at room temperature and protected from light and freezing. Protect oral dosage forms from light.

Compatibility Stable in dextran 6% in NS, D_5LR, $D_5^{1/4}NS$, $D_5^{1/2}NS$, D_5NS, D_5W, $D_{10}W$, LR, $^{1/2}NS$, NS

Y-site administration: Compatible: Amifostine, amikacin, ampicillin, ampicillin/sulbactam, atenolol, aztreonam, bumetanide, cefamandole, cefazolin, cefotaxime, cefotetan, cefoxitin, ceftazidime, ceftizoxime, ceftriaxone, cefuroxime, chloramphenicol, cisatracurium, cladribine, clindamycin, co-trimoxazole, dexamethasone sodium phosphate, diltiazem, diphenhydramine, dobutamine, docetaxel, dopamine, doxycycline, droperidol, erythromycin lactobionate, etoposide phosphate, famotidine, filgrastim, fluconazole, fludarabine, gatifloxacin, gemcitabine, gentamicin, granisetron, heparin, hydrocortisone sodium succinate, insulin (regular), kanamycin, labetalol, lidocaine, linezolid, magnesium sulfate, melphalan, methyldopate, methylprednisolone sodium succinate, metoclopramide, metoprolol, metronidazole, ondansetron, oxacillin, oxytocin, paclitaxel, penicillin G potassium, piperacillin, piperacillin/tazobactam, potassium chloride, propofol, propranolol, ranitidine, remifentanil, sargramostim, teniposide, thiotepa, ticarcillin, ticarcillin/clavulanate, tobramycin, vancomycin, verapamil, vinorelbine. **Incompatible:** Allopurinol, amphotericin B cholesteryl sulfate complex, cefepime, cefoperazone, doxorubicin liposome, idarubicin, imipenem/cilastatin, minocycline. **Variable (consult detailed reference):** Acyclovir, furosemide, nafcillin

Compatibility in syringe: Compatible: Atropine, atropine with hydroxyzine, atropine with promethazine, butorphanol, chlorpromazine, cimetidine, dimenhydrinate, diphenhydramine, droperidol, fentanyl, glycopyrrolate, hydroxyzine, ketamine, metoclopramide, midazolam, ondansetron, pentazocine, pentazocine with perphenazine, perphenazine, prochlorperazine edisylate, promazine, promethazine, ranitidine, scopolamine. **Incompatible:** Heparin, morphine, pentobarbital

Compatibility when admixed: Compatible: Cefazolin, dobutamine, metoclopramide, ondansetron, scopolamine, succinylcholine, triflupromazine, verapamil. **Incompatible:** Aminophylline, amobarbital, floxacillin, furosemide, heparin, morphine, phenobarbital, phenytoin, thiopental. **Variable (consult detailed reference):** Sodium bicarbonate

Pharmacodynamics/Kinetics

Onset of action: Analgesic: Oral, SubQ, I.M.: 10-15 minutes; I.V.: ~5 minutes

Peak effect: Oral, SubQ, I.M.: ~1 hour

Duration: Oral, SubQ, I.M.: 2-4 hours

Distribution: Crosses placenta; enters breast milk

Protein binding: 65% to 75%

Metabolism: Hepatic; active metabolite (normeperidine)

Bioavailability: ~50% to 60%; increased with liver disease

Half-life elimination:

Parent drug: Terminal phase: Neonates: 23 hours (range: 12-39 hours); Adults: 2.5-4 hours, Liver disease: 7-11 hours

Normeperidine (active metabolite): 15-30 hours; can accumulate with high doses or with decreased renal function

Dosage Note: Doses should be titrated to necessary analgesic effect. When changing route of administration, note that oral doses are about half as effective as parenteral dose. Oral route not recommended for chronic pain. These are guidelines and do not represent the maximum doses that may be required in all patients.

Children: Pain: Oral, I.M., I.V., SubQ: 1-1.5 mg/kg/dose every 3-4 hours as needed; 1-2 mg/kg as a single dose preoperative medication may be used; maximum 100 mg/dose

Adults: Pain:

Oral: Initial: Opiate-naive: 50 mg every 3-4 hours as needed; usual dosage range: 50-150 mg every 2-4 hours as needed

(Continued)

Meperidine *(Continued)*

I.M., SubQ: Initial: Opiate-naive: 50-75 mg every 3-4 hours as needed; patients with prior opiate exposure may require higher initial doses; usual dosage range: 50-150 mg every 2-4 hours as needed

Preoperatively: 50-100 mg given 30-90 minutes before the beginning of anesthesia

Slow I.V.: Initial: 5-10 mg every 5 minutes as needed

Patient-controlled analgesia (PCA): Usual concentration: 10 mg/mL
Initial dose: 10 mg
Demand dose: 1-5 mg (manufacturer recommendations); range 5-25 mg
Lockout interval: 5-10 minutes

Elderly:
Oral: 50 mg every 4 hours
I.M.: 25 mg every 4 hours

Dosing adjustment in renal impairment: Avoid repeated administration of meperidine in renal dysfunction:
Cl_{cr} 10-50 mL/minute: Administer at 75% of normal dose
Cl_{cr} <10 mL/minute: Administer at 50% of normal dose

Dosing adjustment/comments in hepatic disease: Increased narcotic effect in cirrhosis; reduction in dose more important for oral than I.V. route

Administration Meperidine may be administered I.M. (preferably), SubQ, or I.V.; I.V. push should be administered slowly, use of a 10 mg/mL concentration has been recommended. For continuous I.V. infusions, a more dilute solution (eg, 1 mg/mL) should be used.

Dosage Forms

Injection, solution, as hydrochloride [ampul]: 25 mg/0.5 mL (0.5 mL); 25 mg/mL (1 mL); 50 mg/mL (1 mL, 1.5 mL, 2 mL); 75 mg/mL (1 mL); 100 mg/mL (1 mL)

Injection, solution, as hydrochloride [prefilled syringe]: 25 mg/mL (1 mL); 50 mg/mL (1 mL); 75 mg/mL (1 mL); 100 mg/mL (1 mL)

Injection, solution, as hydrochloride [for PCA pump]: 10 mg/mL (30 mL, 50 mL, 60 mL)

Injection, solution, as hydrochloride [vial]: 25 mg/mL (1 mL); 50 mg/mL (1 mL, 30 mL); 75 mg/mL (1 mL); 100 mg/mL (1 mL, 20 mL) [may contain sodium metabisulfite]

Syrup, as hydrochloride: 50 mg/5 mL (500 mL) [contains sodium benzoate]
Demerol®: 50 mg/5 mL (480 mL) [contains benzoic acid; banana flavor]

Tablet, as hydrochloride (Demerol®, Meperitab®): 50 mg, 100 mg

Monitoring Parameters Pain relief, respiratory and mental status, blood pressure; observe patient for excessive sedation, CNS depression, seizures, respiratory depression

Patient Information Avoid alcohol; may cause drowsiness

Special Geriatric Considerations Meperidine is not recommended as a drug of first choice for the treatment of chronic pain in the elderly due to the accumulation of its metabolite, normeperidine, which leads to serious CNS side effects (eg, tremor, seizures). For acute pain, its use should be limited to 1-2 doses.

♦ **Meperidine Hydrochloride** *see* Meperidine *on page 535*

♦ **Meperitab®** *see* Meperidine *on page 535*

♦ **Mephyton**® *see* Phytonadione *on page 664*

Mercaptopurine (mer kap toe PYOOR een)
Medication Safety Issues
Sound-alike/look-alike issues:
Purinethol® may be confused with propylthiouracil

To avoid potentially serious dosage errors, the terms "6-mercaptopurine" or "6-MP" should be avoided; use of these terms has been associated with sixfold overdosages.

Related Information
Investigational Drug Service *on page 1031*
Safe Handling of Hazardous Drugs *on page 1034*
U.S. Brand Names Purinethol®
Canadian Brand Names Purinethol®
Generic Available Yes
Synonyms 6-Mercaptopurine; 6-MP; NSC-755
Pharmacologic Category Antineoplastic Agent, Antimetabolite
Pregnancy Risk Factor D
Lactation Enters breast milk/contraindicated
Use Treatment (maintenance and induction) of acute lymphoblastic leukemia (ALL)
Mechanism of Action Purine antagonist which inhibits DNA and RNA synthesis; acts as false metabolite and is incorporated into DNA and RNA, eventually inhibiting their synthesis; specific for the S phase of the cell cycle
Restrictions Note: I.V. formulation is not commercially available in the U.S.
Labeled Contraindications Hypersensitivity to mercaptopurine or any component of the formulation; patients whose disease showed prior resistance to mercaptopurine or thioguanine; severe liver disease, severe bone marrow suppression; pregnancy
Warnings/Precautions Hazardous agent - use appropriate precautions for handling and disposal. See Safe Handling of Hazardous Drugs *on page 1034* in the Appendix. Mercaptopurine is potentially carcinogenic, and may be teratogenic; use with caution in patients with prior bone marrow suppression. Common signs of infection, such as fever and leukocytosis may not occur; lethargy and confusion may be more prominent signs of infection. Use caution with other hepatotoxic drugs or in dosages >2.5 mg/kg/day; hepatotoxicity may occur. Patients with genetic deficiency of thiopurine methyltransferase (TPMT) or concurrent therapy with drugs which may inhibit TPMT (eg, olsalazine) or xanthine oxidase (eg, allopurinol) may be sensitive to myelosuppressive effects.

To avoid potentially serious dosage errors, the terms "6-mercaptopurine" or "6-MP" should be avoided; use of these terms has been associated with sixfold overdosages.

Adverse Reactions
>10%:
Hematologic: Myelosuppression; leukopenia, thrombocytopenia, anemia
Onset: 7-10 days
Nadir: 14-16 days
Recovery: 21-28 days
(Continued)

Mercaptopurine *(Continued)*

Hepatic: Intrahepatic cholestasis and focal centralobular necrosis (40%), characterized by hyperbilirubinemia, increased alkaline phosphatase and AST, jaundice, ascites, encephalopathy; more common at doses >2.5 mg/kg/day. Usually occurs within 2 months of therapy but may occur within 1 week, or be delayed up to 8 years.

1% to 10%:

Central nervous system: Drug fever

Dermatologic: Hyperpigmentation, rash

Endocrine & metabolic: Hyperuricemia

Gastrointestinal: Nausea, vomiting, diarrhea, stomatitis, anorexia, stomach pain, mucositis

Renal: Renal toxicity

<1%: Alopecia, dry and scaling rash, glossitis, oligospermia, tarry stools, eosinophilia

Vesicant No

Emetic Potential Very low (<10%)

Overdosage/Toxicology Symptoms of overdose include nausea and vomiting (immediate); bone marrow suppression, hepatic necrosis, and gastroenteritis (delayed). Treatment is supportive. Efforts to minimize absorption (charcoal, gastric lavage) may be ineffective unless instituted within 60 minutes of ingestion.

Drug Interactions

Increased Effect/Toxicity: Allopurinol can cause increased levels of mercaptopurine by inhibition of xanthine oxidase. Decrease dose of mercaptopurine by 75% when both drugs are used concomitantly. Seen only with oral mercaptopurine usage, not with I.V. May potentiate effect of bone marrow suppression (reduce mercaptopurine to 25% of dose). Synergistic liver toxicity between doxorubicin and mercaptopurine has been reported. Any agent which could potentially alter the metabolic function of the liver could produce higher drug levels and greater toxicities from either mercaptopurine or thioguanine (6-TG). Aminosalicylates (eg, olsalazine, mesalamine, sulfasalazine) may inhibit TPMT, increasing toxicity/myelosuppression of mercaptopurine.

Decreased Effect: Mercaptopurine inhibits the anticoagulation effect of warfarin by an unknown mechanism.

Storage/Stability Store at room temperature.

Reconstitution Further dilute the 10 mg/mL reconstituted solution in normal saline or D_5W to a final concentration for administration of 1-2 mg/mL.

Pharmacodynamics/Kinetics

Absorption: Variable and incomplete (16% to 50%)

Distribution: V_d = total body water; CNS penetration is poor

Protein binding: 19%

Metabolism: Hepatic and in GI mucosa; hepatically via xanthine oxidase and methylation via TPMT to sulfate conjugates, 6-thiouric acid, and other inactive compounds; first-pass effect

Half-life elimination (age dependent): Children: 21 minutes; Adults: 47 minutes

Time to peak, serum: ~2 hours

Excretion: Urine; following high (1 g/m²) I.V. doses, 20% to 40% excreted unchanged; at lower doses renal elimination minor

Dosage Oral (refer to individual protocols):

Children:

Induction: 2.5-5 mg/kg/day **or** 70-100 mg/m^2/day given once daily

Maintenance: 1.5-2.5 mg/kg/day **or** 50-75 mg/m^2/day given once daily

Adults:

Induction: 2.5-5 mg/kg/day (100-200 mg)

Maintenance: 1.5-2.5 mg/kg/day **or** 80-100 mg/m^2/day given once daily

Dosage adjustment with concurrent allopurinol: Reduce mercaptopurine dosage to $\frac{1}{3}$ to $\frac{1}{2}$ the usual dose.

Dosage adjustment in TPMT-deficiency: Not established; substantial reductions are generally required only in homozygous deficiency.

Elderly: Due to renal decline with age, start with lower recommended doses for adults

Note: In ALL, administration in the evening (vs morning administration) may lower the risk of relapse.

Dosing adjustment in renal or hepatic impairment: Dose should be reduced to avoid accumulation, but specific guidelines are not available.

Hemodialysis: Removed; supplemental dosing is usually required

Combination Regimens

Leukemia, acute lymphocytic:

IDMTX/6-MP *on page 901*

MM *on page 910*

MTX/6-MP/VP (Maintenance) *on page 916*

PVA (POG 8602) *on page 932*

PVA (POG 9005) *on page 934*

Leukemia, acute myeloid: POMP *on page 931*

Leukemia, acute promyelocytic:

M-3 *on page 906*

Tretinoin/Idarubicin *on page 941*

Administration I.V.: Administer by slow I.V. continuous infusion.

Dosage Forms Tablet [scored]: 50 mg

Monitoring Parameters CBC with differential and platelet count, liver function tests, uric acid, urinalysis; TPMT genotyping may identify individuals at risk for toxicity

Dietary Considerations Should not be administered with meals.

Patient Information Take daily dose at the same time each day. Preferable to take on an empty stomach (1 hour before or 2 hours after meals). Maintain adequate hydration (2-3 L/day of fluids unless instructed to restrict fluid intake). You may experience nausea and vomiting, diarrhea, or loss of appetite (frequent small meals may help/request medication) or weakness or lethargy (use caution when driving or engaging in tasks that require alertness until response to drug is known). Use good oral care to reduce incidence of mouth sores. You may be more susceptible to infection (avoid crowds or exposure to infection). May cause headache (request medication). Report signs of opportunistic infection (eg, fever, chills, sore throat, burning urination, fatigue); bleeding (eg, tarry stools, easy bruising); unresolved mouth sores, nausea, or vomiting; swelling of extremities, difficulty breathing, or unusual weight gain. The drug may be excreted in breast milk, therefore, an alternative form of feeding your baby should be used. Contraceptive measures are recommended during therapy.

(Continued)

Mercaptopurine *(Continued)*

Special Geriatric Considerations Toxicity to immunosuppressives is increased in the elderly. Start with lowest recommended adult doses. Signs of infection, such as fever and WBC rise, may not occur. Lethargy and confusion may be more prominent signs of infection.

Extemporaneous Preparations A 50 mg/mL oral suspension can be prepared by crushing thirty 50 mg tablets in a mortar, and then mixing in a small amount of vehicle (a 1:1 combination of methylcellulose 1% and syrup) to create a uniform paste. Add a sufficient quantity of vehicle to make 30 mL of suspension. Label "shake well." Room temperature stability is 14 days.

> Dressman JB and Poust RI, "Stability of Allopurinol and of Five Antine-oplastics in Suspension," *Am J Hosp Pharm*, 1983, 40:616-8.

> Nahata MC, Morosco RS, and Hipple TF, 4th ed, *Pediatric Drug Formulations*, Cincinnati, OH: Harvey Whitney Books Co, 2000.

Selected Readings

Bostrom B and Erdmann G, "Cellular Pharmacology of 6-Mercaptopurine in Acute Lympho-blastic Leukemia," *Am J Pediatr Hematol Oncol*, 1993, 15(1):80-6.

Elgemeie GH, "Thioguanine, Mercaptopurine: Their Analogs and Nucleosides as Antime-tabolites," *Curr Pharm Des*, 2003, 9(31):2627-42.

Grindey GB, "Clinical Pharmacology of the 6-Thiopurines," *Cancer Treat Rev*, 1979, 6(Suppl):19-25.

Lennard L, "The Clinical Pharmacology of 6-Mercaptopurine," *Eur J Clin Pharmacol*, 1992, 43(4):329-39.

Mosesso P and Palitti F, "The Genetic Toxicology of 6-Mercaptopurine," *Mutat Res*, 1993, 296(3):279-94.

Pinkel D, "Intravenous Mercaptopurine: Life Begins at 40," *J Clin Oncol*, 1993, 11(9):1826-31.

Van Scoik KG, Johnson CA, and Porter WR, "The Pharmacology and Metabolism of the Thiopurine Drugs 6-Mercaptopurine and Azathioprine," *Drug Metab Rev*, 1985, 16(1-2):157-74.

◆ **6-Mercaptopurine** *see* Mercaptopurine *on page 539*

◆ **M-Eslon® (Can)** *see* Morphine Sulfate *on page 588*

Mesna *(MES na)*

Related Information

Safe Handling of Hazardous Drugs *on page 1034*

U.S. Brand Names Mesnex®

Canadian Brand Names Mesnex®; Uromitexan

Generic Available Yes

Synonyms Sodium 2-Mercaptoethane Sulfonate

Pharmacologic Category Antidote

Pregnancy Risk Factor B

Lactation Excretion in breast milk unknown/not recommended

Use Orphan drug: Prevention of hemorrhagic cystitis induced by ifos-famide

Unlabeled/Investigational Use Prevention of hemorrhagic cystitis induced by cyclophosphamide

Mechanism of Action In blood, mesna is oxidized to dimesna which in turn is reduced in the kidney back to mesna, supplying a free thiol group which binds to and inactivates acrolein, the urotoxic metabolite of ifos-famide and cyclophosphamide

Labeled Contraindications Hypersensitivity to mesna or other thiol compounds, or any component of the formulation

Warnings/Precautions Examine morning urine specimen for hematuria prior to ifosfamide or cyclophosphamide treatment; if hematuria (>50 RBC/HPF) develops, reduce the ifosfamide/cyclophosphamide dose or discontinue the drug; will not prevent or alleviate other toxicities associated with ifosfamide or cyclophosphamide and will not prevent hemorrhagic cystitis in all patients. Allergic reactions have been reported; patients with autoimmune disorders may be at increased risk. Symptoms ranged from mild hypersensitivity to systemic anaphylactic reactions. I.V. formulation contains benzyl alcohol; do not use in neonates or infants.

Adverse Reactions It is difficult to distinguish reactions from those caused by concomitant chemotherapy.

>10%: Gastrointestinal: Bad taste in mouth with oral administration (100%), vomiting (secondary to the bad taste after oral administration, or with high I.V. doses)

<1%: Anaphylaxis, hypersensitivity, hypertonia, injection site reaction, limb pain, myalgia, platelet count decreased, tachycardia, tachypnea

Vesicant No

Emetic Potential Low (10% to 30%); when administered orally, the unpleasant taste may result in vomiting

Drug Interactions

Decreased Effect: Warfarin: Questionable alterations in coagulation control.

Storage/Stability Store intact vials and tablets at controlled room temperature of 20°C to 25°C (68°F to 77°F). Opened multidose vials may be stored and used for use to 8 days after opening. Infusion solutions diluted in D_5W or lactated Ringer's are stable for at least 48 hours at room temperature. Solutions in NS are stable for at least 24 hours at room temperature. Solutions in plastic syringes are stable for 9 days under refrigeration, or at room or body temperature. Solutions of mesna and ifosfamide in lactated Ringer's are stable for 7 days in a PVC ambulatory infusion pump reservoir. Mesna injection is stable for at least 7 days when diluted 1:2 or 1:5 with grape- and orange-flavored syrups or 11:1 to 1:100 in carbonated beverages for oral administration.

Reconstitution Dilute in 50-1000 mL NS, D_5W, or lactated Ringer's.

Compatibility Stable in $D_5^{1/4}NS$, $D_5^{1/3}NS$, $D_5^{1/2}NS$, D_5W, LR, NS

Y-site administration: Compatible: Allopurinol, amifostine, aztreonam, cefepime, cladribine, docetaxel, doxorubicin liposome, etoposide phosphate, filgrastim, fludarabine, gatifloxacin, gemcitabine, granisetron, linezolid, melphalan, methotrexate, ondansetron, paclitaxel, piperacillin/tazobactam, sargramostim, sodium bicarbonate, teniposide, thiotepa, vinorelbine. Incompatible: Amphotericin B cholesteryl sulfate complex

Compatibility in syringe: Compatible: Ifosfamide. Incompatible: Ifosfamide with epirubicin

Compatibility when admixed: Compatible: Cyclophosphamide, hydroxyzine, ifosfamide. Incompatible: Carboplatin, cisplatin, ifosfamide with epirubicin

Pharmacodynamics/Kinetics

Distribution: No tissue penetration

Protein binding: 69% to 75%

Metabolism: Rapidly oxidized intravascularly to mesna disulfide; mesna disulfide is reduced in renal tubules back to mesna following glomerular filtration.

Bioavailability: Oral: 45% to 79%

(Continued)

Mesna *(Continued)*

Half-life elimination: Parent drug: 24 minutes; Mesna disulfide: 72 minutes

Time to peak, plasma: 2-3 hours

Excretion: Urine; as unchanged drug (18% to 26%) and metabolites

Dosage Children and Adults (refer to individual protocols):

I.V.: Recommended dose is 60% of the ifosfamide dose given in 3 divided doses (0, 4, and 8 hours after the start of ifosfamide)

Alternative I.V. regimens include 80% of the ifosfamide dose given in 4 divided doses (0, 3, 6, and 9 hours after the start of ifosfamide) and continuous infusions

I.V./Oral: Recommended dose is 100% of the ifosfamide dose, given as 20% of the ifosfamide dose I.V. at hour 0, followed by 40% of the ifosfamide dose given orally 2 and 6 hours after start of ifosfamide

Combination Regimens

Esophageal cancer: TIP *on page 940*

Head and neck cancer: TIP *on page 940*

Leukemia, acute myeloid: Hyper-CVAD *on page 898*

Lung cancer (small cell): VIP (Small Cell Lung Cancer) *on page 947*

Lymphoma, non-Hodgkin's:

ICE (Lymphoma, non-Hodgkin's) *on page 899*

IMVP-16 *on page 902*

IVAC *on page 904*

MINE *on page 909*

MINE-ESHAP *on page 909*

Neuroblastoma: HIPE-IVAD *on page 898*

Osteosarcoma; soft tissue sarcoma: ICE (Sarcoma) *on page 899*

Sarcoma, soft tissue:

ICE-T *on page 900*

IE *on page 901*

MAID *on page 908*

Testicular cancer: VIP (Etoposide) (Testicular Cancer) *on page 946*

Administration

Oral: Administer orally in tablet formulation or parenteral solution diluted in water, milk, juice, or carbonated beverages; patients who vomit within 2 hours of taking oral mesna should repeat the dose or receive I.V. mesna

I.V.: Administer by short (15-30 minutes) infusion or continuous (24 hour) infusion

Dosage Forms

Injection, solution: 100 mg/mL (10 mL) [contains benzyl alcohol]

Tablet: 400 mg

Monitoring Parameters Urinalysis

Additional Information A parenteral formulation without benzyl alcohol can be requested directly from the manufacturer. Test interactions: May cause a false positive result on dipsticks for urinary ketones.

Selected Readings

Goren MP, "Oral Administration of Mesna With Ifosfamide," *Semin Oncol*, 1996, 23(3 Suppl 6):91-6.

Goren MP, "Oral Mesna: A Review," *Semin Oncol*, 1992, 19(6 Suppl 12):65-71.

Shaw IC and Graham MI, "Mesna - A Short Review," *Cancer Treat Rev*, 1987, 14(2):67-86.

Siu LL and Moore MJ, "Use of Mesna to Prevent Ifosfamide-Induced Urotoxicity," *Support Care Cancer*, 1998, 6(2):144-54.

♦ **Mesnex**® *see Mesna on page 542*

♦ **Metacortandralone** *see PrednisoLONE on page 679*

♦ **Metadol**™ **(Can)** *see Methadone on page 545*

♦ **Metastron**® *see Strontium-89 on page 726*

Methadone (METH a done)

Medication Safety Issues

Sound-alike/look-alike issues:

Methadone may be confused with Mephyton®, methylphenidate

U.S. Brand Names Dolophine®; Methadone Diskets®; Methadone Intensol™; Methadose®

Canadian Brand Names Dolophine®; Metadol™; Methadose®

Generic Available Yes

Synonyms Methadone Hydrochloride

Pharmacologic Category Analgesic, Narcotic

Pregnancy Risk Factor C/D (prolonged use or high doses at term)

Lactation Enters breast milk/not recommended (AAP rates "compatible")

Use Management of severe pain; detoxification and maintenance treatment of narcotic addiction (if used for detoxification and maintenance treatment of narcotic addiction, it must be part of an FDA-approved program)

Mechanism of Action Binds to opiate receptors in the CNS, causing inhibition of ascending pain pathways, altering the perception of and response to pain; produces generalized CNS depression

Restrictions C-II

Treatment of narcotic addiction: May only be dispensed by pharmacies or maintenance programs approved by the FDA and designated state authority. Prior approval must be obtained for doses >120 mg administered at a clinic or >100 mg to be taken at home.

Labeled Contraindications Hypersensitivity to methadone or any component of the formulation; respiratory depression (in the absence of resuscitative equipment or in an unmonitored setting); acute bronchial asthma or hypercarbia; pregnancy (prolonged use or high doses near term)

Warnings/Precautions An opioid-containing analgesic regimen should be tailored to each patient's needs and based upon the type of pain being treated (acute versus chronic), the route of administration, degree of tolerance for opioids (naive versus chronic user), age, weight, and medical condition. The optimal analgesic dose varies widely among patients. Doses should be titrated to pain relief/prevention. Patients maintained on stable doses of methadone may need higher and/or more frequent doses in case of acute pain (eg, postoperative pain, physical trauma).

May prolong the QT interval; use caution in patients at risk for QT prolongation, with medications known to prolong the QT interval, or history of conduction abnormalities. QT interval prolongation and torsade de pointes may be associated with doses >200 mg/day, but have also been observed with lower doses. May cause severe hypotension; use caution with severe volume depletion or other conditions which may compromise maintenance of normal blood pressure. Use caution with cardiovascular disease or patients predisposed to dysrhythmias.
(Continued)

Methadone *(Continued)*

Methadone has a long half-life and risk of accumulation; because methadone's effects on respiration last much longer than its analgesic effects, the dose must be titrated slowly. May cause respiratory depression; use caution in patients with respiratory disease or pre-existing respiratory depression. Potential for drug dependency exists, abrupt cessation may precipitate withdrawal. Use caution in elderly, debilitated, or pediatric patients. Use with caution in patients with depression or suicidal tendencies, or in patients with a history of drug abuse. Tolerance or psychological and physical dependence may occur with prolonged use.

Use with caution in patients with hepatic, pulmonary, or renal function impairment. May cause CNS depression, which may impair physical or mental abilities. Patients must be cautioned about performing tasks which require mental alertness (eg, operating machinery or driving). Effects with other sedative drugs or ethanol may be potentiated. Elderly may be more sensitive to CNS depressant and constipating effects. Use with caution in patients with head injury or increased ICP, biliary tract dysfunction or pancreatitis; history of ileus or bowel obstruction, glaucoma, hyperthyroidism, hypothyroidism, adrenal insufficiency, prostatic hyperplasia or urinary stricture, CNS depression, toxic psychosis, alcoholism, delirium tremens, or kyphoscoliosis. Tablets contain excipients to deter use by injection.

Adverse Reactions Frequency not defined. During prolonged administration, adverse effects may decrease over several weeks; however, constipation and sweating may persist.

Cardiovascular: Bradycardia, peripheral vasodilation, cardiac arrest, syncope, faintness, shock, hypotension, edema, arrhythmia, bigeminal rhythms, extrasystoles, tachycardia, torsade de pointes, ventricular fibrillation, ventricular tachycardia, ECG changes, QT interval prolonged, T-wave inversion, cardiomyopathy, flushing, heart failure, palpitation, phlebitis, orthostatic hypotension

Central nervous system: Euphoria, dysphoria, headache, insomnia, agitation, disorientation, drowsiness, dizziness, lightheadedness, sedation, confusion, seizure

Dermatologic: Pruritus, urticaria, rash, hemorrhagic urticaria

Endocrine & metabolic: Libido decreased, hypokalemia, hypomagnesemia, antidiuretic effect, amenorrhea

Gastrointestinal: Nausea, vomiting, constipation, anorexia, stomach cramps, xerostomia, biliary tract spasm, abdominal pain, glossitis, weight gain

Genitourinary: Urinary retention or hesitancy, impotence

Hematologic: Thrombocytopenia (reversible, reported in patients with chronic hepatitis)

Neuromuscular & skeletal: Weakness

Local: I.M./SubQ injection: Pain, erythema, swelling; I.V. injection: pruritus, urticaria, rash, hemorrhagic urticaria (rare)

Ocular: Miosis, visual disturbances

Respiratory: Respiratory depression, respiratory arrest, pulmonary edema

Miscellaneous: Physical and psychological dependence, death, diaphoresis

Vesicant No

Overdosage/Toxicology Symptoms include respiratory depression, CNS depression, miosis, hypothermia, circulatory collapse, and convulsions. Treatment includes naloxone 2 mg I.V. (0.01 mg/kg for children), with repeat administration as necessary, up to a total of 10 mg, or as a continuous infusion. Nalmefene may also be used to reverse signs of intoxication.

Drug Interactions

Cytochrome P450 Effect: Substrate of CYP2C8/9 (minor), 2C19 (minor), 2D6 (minor), 3A4 (major); **Inhibits** CYP2D6 (moderate), 3A4 (weak)

Increased Effect/Toxicity: CYP3A4 inhibitors may increase the levels/effects of methadone (eg, azole antifungals, ciprofloxacin, clarithromycin, diclofenac, doxycycline, erythromycin, imatinib, isoniazid, nefazodone, nicardipine, propofol, protease inhibitors, quinidine, verapamil). Methadone may increase the levels/effects of CYP2D6 substrates (eg, amphetamines, selected beta-blockers, dextromethorphan, fluoxetine, lidocaine, mirtazapine, nefazodone, paroxetine, risperidone, ritonavir, thioridazine, tricyclic antidepressants, venlafaxine). Methadone may increase bioavailability and toxic effects of zidovudine. CNS depressants (including but not limited to opioid analgesics, general anesthetics, sedatives, hypnotics, ethanol) may cause respiratory depression, hypotension, profound sedation, or coma. Levels of desipramine may be increased by methadone. Effects/toxicity of QT_c interval-prolonging agents may be increased; use with caution (including but may not be limited to amitriptyline, astemizole, bepridil, disopyramide, erythromycin, haloperidol, imipramine, quinidine, pimozide, procainamide, sotalol, thioridazine).

Decreased Effect: Agonist/antagonist analgesics (buprenorphine, butorphanol, nalbuphine, pentazocine) may decrease analgesic effect of methadone and precipitate withdrawal symptoms; use is not recommended. Efavirenz and nevirapine may decrease levels of methadone (opioid withdrawal syndrome has been reported). Methadone may decrease bioavailability of didanosine and stavudine. Ritonavir (and combinations) may decrease levels of methadone; withdrawal symptoms have inconsistently been observed, monitor. CYP3A4 inducers may decrease the levels/effects of methadone (eg, aminoglutethimide, carbamazepine, nafcillin, nevirapine, phenobarbital, phenytoin, rifamycins). Monitor for methadone withdrawal. Larger doses of methadone may be required. Methadone may decrease the levels/effects of CYP2D6 prodrug substrates (eg, codeine, hydrocodone, oxycodone, tramadol).

Ethanol/Nutrition/Herb Interactions

Ethanol: Avoid ethanol (may increase CNS effects). Watch for sedation.

Herb/Nutraceutical: Avoid St John's wort (may decrease methadone levels; may increase CNS depression). Avoid valerian, kava kava, gotu kola (may increase CNS depression). Methadone is metabolized by CYP3A4 in the intestines; avoid concurrent use of grapefruit juice.

Storage/Stability

Injection: Store at controlled room temperature of 15°C to 30°C (59°F to 86°F). Protect from light.

Oral concentrate, oral solution, tablet: Store at controlled room temperature of 15°C to 30°C (59°F to 86°F).

Compatibility Stable in NS

(Continued)

Methadone *(Continued)*

Pharmacodynamics/Kinetics

Onset of action: Oral: Analgesic: 0.5-1 hour; Parenteral: 10-20 minutes

Peak effect: Parenteral: 1-2 hours

Duration: Oral: 6-8 hours, increases to 22-48 hours with repeated doses

Distribution: V_d: 2-6 L/kg; crosses placenta; enters breast milk

Protein binding: 85% to 90%

Metabolism: Hepatic; N-demethylation via CYP3A4 and 2D6 to inactive metabolites

Half-life elimination: 8-59 hours; may be prolonged with alkaline pH, decreased during pregnancy

Excretion: Urine (<10% as unchanged drug); increased with urine pH <6

Dosage Note: These are guidelines and do not represent the maximum doses that may be required in all patients. Methadone accumulates with repeated doses and dosage may need reduction after 3-5 days to prevent CNS depressant effects. Some patients may benefit from every 8-12 hour dosing interval for chronic pain management. Doses should be titrated to appropriate effects.

Children:

Pain (analgesia):

Oral (unlabeled use): Initial: 0.1-0.2 mg/kg 4-8 hours initially for 2-3 doses, then every 6-12 hours as needed. Dosing interval may range from 4-12 hours during initial therapy; decrease in dose or frequency may be required (~ days 2-5) due to accumulation with repeated doses (maximum dose: 5-10 mg)

I.V. (unlabeled use): 0.1 mg/kg every 4-8 hours initially for 2-3 doses, then every 6-12 hours as needed. Dosing interval may range from 4-12 hours during initial therapy; decrease in dose or frequency may be required (~ days 2-5) due to accumulation with repeated doses (maximum dose: 5-8 mg)

Iatrogenic narcotic dependency (unlabeled): Oral: General guidelines: Initial: 0.05-0.1 mg/kg/dose every 6 hours; increase by 0.05 mg/kg/dose until withdrawal symptoms are controlled; after 24-48 hours, the dosing interval can be lengthened to every 12-24 hours; to taper dose, wean by 0.05 mg/kg/day; if withdrawal symptoms recur, taper at a slower rate

Adults:

Pain (analgesia):

Oral: Initial: 5-10 mg; dosing interval may range from 4-12 hours during initial therapy; decrease in dose or frequency may be required (~days 2-5) due to accumulation with repeated doses

Manufacturer's labeling: 2.5-10 mg every 3-4 hours as needed

I.V.: Manufacturers labeling: Initial: 2.5-10 mg every 8-12 hours in opioid-naive patients; titrate slowly to effect; may also be administered by SubQ or I.M. injection

Conversion from oral to parenteral dose: Initial dose: Oral: parenteral: 2:1 ratio

Detoxification: Oral: 15-40 mg/day

Maintenance treatment of opiate dependence: Oral: 20-120 mg/day

Dosage adjustment in renal impairment: Cl_{cr} <10 mL/minute: Administer 50% to 75% of normal dose

Dosage adjustment in hepatic impairment: Avoid in severe liver disease

Administration Oral dose for detoxification and maintenance may be administered in fruit juice or water.

Dosage Forms

Injection, solution, as hydrochloride: 10 mg/mL (20 mL)

Solution, oral, as hydrochloride: 5 mg/5 mL (500 mL); 10 mg/5 mL (500 mL) [contains alcohol 8%; citrus flavor]

Solution, oral concentrate, as hydrochloride: 10 mg/mL (946 mL)

Methadone Intensol™: 10 mg/mL (30 mL)

Methadose®: 10 mg/mL (1000 mL) [cherry flavor or dye free, sugar free, unflavored]

Tablet, as hydrochloride (Dolophine®, Methadose®): 5 mg, 10 mg

Tablet, dispersible, as hydrochloride:

Methadose®: 40 mg

Methadone Diskets®: 40 mg [orange-pineapple flavor]

Monitoring Parameters Pain relief, respiratory and mental status, blood pressure

Patient Information May cause drowsiness, avoid alcohol and other CNS depressants

Special Geriatric Considerations Because of its long half-life and risk of accumulation, methadone is not considered a drug of first choice in the elderly. The elderly may be particularly susceptible to the CNS depressant and constipating effects of narcotics. Adjust dose for renal function.

♦ **Methadone Diskets®** *see* Methadone *on page 545*

♦ **Methadone Hydrochloride** *see* Methadone *on page 545*

♦ **Methadone Intensol™** *see* Methadone *on page 545*

♦ **Methadose®** *see* Methadone *on page 545*

Methotrexate (meth oh TREKS ate)

Medication Safety Issues

Sound-alike/look-alike issues:

Methotrexate may be confused with metolazone, mitoxantrone

High alert medication: The Institute for Safe Medication Practices (ISMP) includes this medication among its list of drugs which have a heightened risk of causing significant patient harm when used in error.

Errors have occurred (resulting in death) when oral methotrexate was administered as "daily" dose instead of the recommended "weekly" dose.

Related Information

Fertility and Cancer Therapy *on page 962*

Safe Handling of Hazardous Drugs *on page 1034*

Transplantation *on page 1019*

U.S. Brand Names Rheumatrex®; Trexall™

Canadian Brand Names Apo-Methotrexate®; ratio-Methotrexate

Generic Available Yes

Synonyms Amethopterin; Methotrexate Sodium; MTX; NSC-740

Pharmacologic Category Antineoplastic Agent, Antimetabolite (Antifolate)

Pregnancy Risk Factor X (psoriasis, rheumatoid arthritis)

Lactation Enters breast milk/contraindicated

(Continued)

Methotrexate *(Continued)*

Use Treatment of trophoblastic neoplasms; leukemias; psoriasis; rheumatoid arthritis (RA), including polyarticular-course juvenile rheumatoid arthritis (JRA); breast, head and neck, and lung carcinomas; osteosarcoma; soft-tissue sarcomas; carcinoma of gastrointestinal tract, esophagus, testes; lymphomas

Mechanism of Action Methotrexate is a folate antimetabolite that inhibits DNA synthesis. Methotrexate irreversibly binds to dihydrofolate reductase, inhibiting the formation of reduced folates, and thymidylate synthetase, resulting in inhibition of purine and thymidylic acid synthesis. Methotrexate is cell cycle specific for the S phase of the cycle.

The MOA in the treatment of rheumatoid arthritis is unknown, but may affect immune function. In psoriasis, methotrexate is thought to target rapidly proliferating epithelial cells in the skin.

Labeled Contraindications Hypersensitivity to methotrexate or any component of the formulation; severe renal or hepatic impairment; pre-existing profound bone marrow suppression in patients with psoriasis or rheumatoid arthritis, alcoholic liver disease, AIDS, pre-existing blood dyscrasias; pregnancy (in patients with psoriasis or rheumatoid arthritis); breast-feeding

Warnings/Precautions Hazardous agent - use appropriate precautions for handling and disposal. See Safe Handling of Hazardous Drugs *on page 1034* in the Appendix.

May cause potentially life-threatening pneumonitis (may occur at any time during therapy and at any dosage); monitor closely for pulmonary symptoms, particularly dry, nonproductive cough. Methotrexate may cause photosensitivity and/or severe dermatologic reactions which are not dose-related. Methotrexate has been associated with acute and chronic hepatotoxicity, fibrosis, and cirrhosis. Risk is related to cumulative dose and prolonged exposure. Ethanol abuse, obesity, advanced age, and diabetes may increase the risk of hepatotoxic reactions.

Methotrexate may cause renal failure, gastrointestinal toxicity, or bone marrow depression. Use with caution in patients with renal impairment, peptic ulcer disease, ulcerative colitis, or pre-existing bone marrow suppression. Diarrhea and ulcerative stomatitis may require interruption of therapy; death from hemorrhagic enteritis or intestinal perforation has been reported. Methotrexate penetrates slowly into 3rd space fluids, such as pleural effusions or ascites, and exits slowly from these compartments (slower than from plasma). Dosage reduction may be necessary in patients with renal or hepatic impairment, ascites, and pleural effusion. Toxicity from methotrexate or any immunosuppressive is increased in the elderly.

Severe bone marrow suppression, aplastic anemia, and GI toxicity have occurred during concomitant administration with NSAIDs. Use caution when used with other hepatotoxic agents (azathioprine, retinoids, sulfasalazine). Methotrexate given concomitantly with radiotherapy may increase the risk of soft tissue necrosis and osteonecrosis. Immune suppression may lead to opportunistic infections.

For rheumatoid arthritis and psoriasis, immunosuppressive therapy should only be used when disease is active and less toxic; traditional therapy is ineffective. Discontinue therapy in RA or psoriasis if a significant decrease in hematologic components is noted. Methotrexate formulations and/or diluents containing preservatives should not be used for intrathecal or high-dose therapy. Methotrexate injection may contain benzyl alcohol and should not be used in neonates.

Adverse Reactions Note: Adverse reactions vary by route and dosage. Hematologic and/or gastrointestinal toxicities may be common at dosages used in chemotherapy; these reactions are much less frequent when used at typical dosages for rheumatic diseases.

>10%:

Central nervous system (with I.T. administration or very high-dose therapy):

Arachnoiditis: Acute reaction manifested as severe headache, nuchal rigidity, vomiting, and fever; may be alleviated by reducing the dose

Subacute toxicity: 10% of patients treated with 12-15 mg/m² of I.T. methotrexate may develop this in the second or third week of therapy; consists of motor paralysis of extremities, cranial nerve palsy, seizure, or coma. This has also been seen in pediatric cases receiving very high-dose I.V. methotrexate.

Demyelinating encephalopathy: Seen months or years after receiving methotrexate; usually in association with cranial irradiation or other systemic chemotherapy

Dermatologic: Reddening of skin

Endocrine & metabolic: Hyperuricemia, defective oogenesis or spermatogenesis

Gastrointestinal: Ulcerative stomatitis, glossitis, gingivitis, nausea, vomiting, diarrhea, anorexia, intestinal perforation, mucositis (dose dependent; appears in 3-7 days after therapy, resolving within 2 weeks)

Hematologic: Leukopenia, thrombocytopenia

Renal: Renal failure, azotemia, nephropathy

Respiratory: Pharyngitis

1% to 10%:

Cardiovascular: Vasculitis

Central nervous system: Dizziness, malaise, encephalopathy, seizure, fever, chills

Dermatologic: Alopecia, rash, photosensitivity, depigmentation or hyperpigmentation of skin

Endocrine & metabolic: Diabetes

Genitourinary: Cystitis

Hematologic: Hemorrhage

Myelosuppressive: This is the primary dose-limiting factor (along with mucositis) of methotrexate; occurs about 5-7 days after methotrexate therapy, and should resolve within 2 weeks

WBC: Mild

Platelets: Moderate

Onset: 7 days

Nadir: 10 days

Recovery: 21 days

Hepatic: Cirrhosis and portal fibrosis have been associated with chronic methotrexate therapy; acute elevation of liver enzymes are common after high-dose methotrexate, and usually resolve within 10 days.

Neuromuscular & skeletal: Arthralgia

Ocular: Blurred vision

(Continued)

Methotrexate *(Continued)*

Renal: Renal dysfunction: Manifested by an abrupt rise in serum creatinine and BUN and a fall in urine output; more common with high-dose methotrexate, and may be due to precipitation of the drug.

Respiratory: Pneumonitis: Associated with fever, cough, and interstitial pulmonary infiltrates; treatment is to withhold methotrexate during the acute reaction; interstitial pneumonitis has been reported to occur with an incidence of 1% in patients with RA (dose 7.5-15 mg/week)

<1% (Limited to important or life-threatening): Acute neurologic syndrome (at high dosages - symptoms include confusion, hemiparesis, transient blindness, and coma); anaphylaxis, alveolitis, cognitive dysfunction (has been reported at low dosage), decreased resistance to infection, erythema multiforme, hepatic failure, leukoencephalopathy (especially following craniospinal irradiation or repeated high-dose therapy), lymphoproliferative disorders, osteonecrosis and soft tissue necrosis (with radiotherapy), pericarditis, plaque erosions (psoriasis), seizure (more frequent in pediatric patients with ALL), Stevens-Johnson syndrome, thromboembolism

Vesicant No

Emetic Potential

Very low (<10%): $\leq$50 mg/m^2

Low (10% to 30%): $\leq$250 mg/m^2

Moderate (30% to 60%): $\leq$1000 mg/m^2

High (60% to 90%): >1000 mg/m^2

Overdosage/Toxicology Symptoms of overdose include nausea, vomiting, alopecia, melena, and renal failure. Administer leucovorin (see Dosage).

Hydration and alkalinization may be used to prevent precipitation of methotrexate or methotrexate metabolites in the renal tubules. Severe bone marrow toxicity can result from overdose. Generally, neither peritoneal nor hemodialysis have been shown to increase elimination. However, effective clearance of methotrexate has been reported with acute, intermittent hemodialysis using a high-flux dialyzer.

Drug Interactions

Increased Effect/Toxicity: Concurrent therapy with NSAIDs has resulted in severe bone marrow suppression, aplastic anemia, and GI toxicity. NSAIDs should not be used during moderate or high-dose methotrexate due to increased and prolonged methotrexate levels (may increase toxicity); NSAID use during treatment of rheumatoid arthritis has not been fully explored, but continuation of prior regimen has been allowed in some circumstances, with cautious monitoring. Salicylates may increase methotrexate levels, however salicylate doses used for prophylaxis of cardiovascular events are not likely to be of concern.

Penicillins, probenecid, sulfonamides, tetracyclines may increase methotrexate concentrations due to a reduction in renal tubular secretion; primarily a concern with high doses of methotrexate. Hepatotoxic agents (acitretin, azathioprine, retinoids, sulfasalazine) may increase the risk of hepatotoxic reactions with methotrexate.

Concomitant administration of cyclosporine with methotrexate may increase levels and toxicity of each. Methotrexate may increase mercaptopurine or theophylline levels. Methotrexate, when administered prior to cytarabine, may enhance the efficacy and toxicity of cytarabine; some combination treatment regimens (eg, hyper-CVAD) have been designed to take advantage of this interaction.

Concurrent use of live virus vaccines may result in infections.

Decreased Effect: Cholestyramine may decrease levels of methotrexate. Corticosteroids may decrease uptake of methotrexate into leukemia cells. Administration of these drugs should be separated by 12 hours. Dexamethasone has been reported to not affect methotrexate influx into cells.

Ethanol/Nutrition/Herb Interactions

Ethanol: Avoid ethanol (may be associated with increased liver injury).

Food: Methotrexate peak serum levels may be decreased if taken with food. Milk-rich foods may decrease methotrexate absorption. Folate may decrease drug response.

Herb/Nutraceutical: Avoid echinacea (has immunostimulant properties).

Storage/Stability Store tablets and intact vials at room temperature (15°C to 25°C); protect from light. Solution diluted in D_5W or NS is stable for 24 hours at room temperature (21°C to 25°C). Reconstituted solutions with a preservative may be stored under refrigeration for up to 3 months, and up to 4 weeks at room temperature. Intrathecal dilutions are stable at room temperature for 7 days, but it is generally recommended that they be used within 4-8 hours.

Reconstitution Dilute powder with D_5W or NS to a concentration of ≤25 mg/mL (20 mg and 50 mg vials) and 50 mg/mL (1 g vial). Intrathecal solutions may be reconstituted to 2.5-5 mg/mL with NS, D_5W, lactated Ringer's, or Elliott's B solution. **Use preservative free preparations for intrathecal or high-dose administration.**

Compatibility Stable in D_5NS, D_5W, NS

Y-site administration: Compatible: Allopurinol, amifostine, amphotericin B cholesteryl sulfate complex, asparaginase, aztreonam, bleomycin, cefepime, ceftriaxone, cimetidine, cisplatin, cyclophosphamide, cytarabine, daunorubicin, dexchlorpheniramine, diphenhydramine, doxorubicin, doxorubicin liposome, etoposide, etoposide phosphate, famotidine, filgrastim, fludarabine, fluorouracil, furosemide, ganciclovir, gatifloxacin, granisetron, heparin, hydromorphone, imipenem/cilastatin, leucovorin, linezolid, lorazepam, melphalan, mesna, methylprednisolone sodium succinate, metoclopramide, mitomycin, morphine, ondansetron, oxacillin, paclitaxel, piperacillin/tazobactam, prochlorperazine edisylate, ranitidine, sargramostim, teniposide, thiotepa, vinblastine, vincristine, vindesine, vinorelbine. **Incompatible:** Chlorpromazine, gemcitabine, idarubicin, ifosfamide, midazolam, nalbuphine, promethazine, propofol. **Variable (consult detailed reference):** Dexamethasone sodium phosphate, droperidol, vancomycin

Compatibility in syringe: Compatible: Bleomycin, cisplatin, cyclophosphamide, doxapram, doxorubicin, fluorouracil, furosemide, heparin, leucovorin, mitomycin, vinblastine, vincristine. **Incompatible:** Droperidol. **Variable (consult detailed reference):** Metoclopramide

Compatibility when admixed: Compatible: Cyclophosphamide, cyclophosphamide with fluorouracil, cytarabine, dacarbazine, fluorouracil, hydrocortisone, hydroxyzine, mercaptopurine, ondansetron, sodium bicarbonate, vincristine. **Incompatible:** Bleomycin

(Continued)

Methotrexate *(Continued)*

Pharmacodynamics/Kinetics

Onset of action: Antirheumatic: 3-6 weeks; additional improvement may continue longer than 12 weeks

Absorption: Oral: Rapid; well absorbed at low doses (<30 mg/m^2), incomplete after large doses; I.M.: Complete

Distribution: Penetrates slowly into 3rd space fluids (eg, pleural effusions, ascites), exits slowly from these compartments (slower than from plasma); crosses placenta; small amounts enter breast milk; sustained concentrations retained in kidney and liver

Protein binding: 50%

Metabolism: <10%; degraded by intestinal flora to DAMPA by carboxypeptidase; hepatic aldehyde oxidase converts methotrexate to 7-OH methotrexate; polyglutamates are produced intracellularly and are just as potent as methotrexate; their production is dose- and duration-dependent and they are slowly eliminated by the cell once formed

Half-life elimination: Low dose: 3-10 hours; High dose: 8-12 hours

Time to peak, serum: Oral: 1-2 hours; I.M.: 30-60 minutes

Excretion: Urine (44% to 100%); feces (small amounts)

Dosage Refer to individual protocols.

Note: Doses between 100-500 mg/m^2 **may require** leucovorin rescue. Doses >500 mg/m^2 **require** leucovorin rescue: I.V., I.M., Oral: Leucovorin 10-15 mg/m^2 every 6 hours for 8 or 10 doses, starting 24 hours after the start of methotrexate infusion. Continue until the methotrexate level is ≤0.1 micromolar (10^{-7} M). Some clinicians continue leucovorin until the methotrexate level is <0.05 micromolar (5×10^{-8} M) or 0.01 micromolar (10^{-8} M).

If the 48-hour methotrexate level is >1 micromolar (10^{-7} M) or the 72-hour methotrexate level is >0.2 micromolar (2×10^{-7} M): Leucovorin 100 mg/m^2 I.V./I.M./Oral every 6 hours until the methotrexate level is ≤0.1 micromolar (10^{-7} M). Some clinicians continue leucovorin until the methotrexate level is <0.05 micromolar (5×10^{-8} M) or 0.01 micromolar (10^{-8} M).

Methotrexate Dosing Schedules

Dose	Route	Frequency
Conventional		
15-20 mg/m^2	P.O.	Twice weekly
30-50 mg/m^2	P.O., I.V.	Weekly
15 mg/day for 5 days	P.O., I.M.	Every 2-3 weeks
Intermediate		
50-150 mg/m^2*	I.V. push	Every 2-3 weeks
240 mg/m^2*	I.V. infusion	Every 4-7 days
0.5-1 g/m^2**	I.V. infusion	Every 2-3 weeks
High		
1-25 g/m^2*	I.V. infusion	Every 1-3 weeks

*Doses between 100-500 mg/m^2 may require leucovorin rescue in some patients.

**Followed with leucovorin rescue - refer to Leucovorin monograph for details.

Children:

Dermatomyositis: Oral: 15-20 mg/m^2/week as a single dose once weekly **or** 0.3-1 mg/kg/dose once weekly

Juvenile rheumatoid arthritis: Oral, I.M.: 10 mg/m^2 once weekly, then 5-15 mg/m^2/week as a single dose **or** as 3 divided doses given 12 hours apart

Antineoplastic dosage range:

Oral, I.M.: 7.5-30 mg/m^2/week **or** every 2 weeks

I.V.: 10-18,000 mg/m^2 bolus dosing **or** continuous infusion over 6-42 hours

For dosing schedules, see table on previous page.

Pediatric solid tumors (high-dose): I.V.:

<12 years: 12-25 g/m^2

≥12 years: 8 g/m^2

Acute lymphocytic leukemia (intermediate-dose): I.V.: Loading: 100 mg/m^2 bolus dose, followed by 900 mg/m^2/day infusion over 23-41 hours.

Meningeal leukemia: I.T.: 10-15 mg/m^2 (maximum dose: 15 mg) **or** an age-based dosing regimen; one possible system is:

≤3 months: 3 mg/dose

4-11 months: 6 mg/dose

1 year: 8 mg/dose

2 years: 10 mg/dose

≥3 years: 12 mg/dose

Adults: I.V.: Range is wide from 30-40 mg/m^2/week to 100-12,000 mg/m^2 with leucovorin rescue

Trophoblastic neoplasms:

Oral, I.M.: 15-30 mg/day for 5 days; repeat in 7 days for 3-5 courses

I.V.: 11 mg/m^2 days 1 through 5 every 3 weeks

Head and neck cancer: Oral, I.M., I.V.: 25-50 mg/m^2 once weekly

Mycosis fungoides (cutaneous T-cell lymphoma): Oral, I.M.: Initial (early stages):

5-50 mg once weekly **or**

15-37.5 mg twice weekly

Bladder cancer: I.V.:

30 mg/m^2 day 1 and 8 every 3 weeks **or**

30 mg/m^2 day 1, 15, and 22 every 4 weeks

Breast cancer: I.V.: 30-60 mg/m^2 days 1 and 8 every 3-4 weeks

Gastric cancer: I.V.:1500 mg/m^2 every 4 weeks

Lymphoma, non-Hodgkin's: I.V.:

30 mg/m^2 days 3 and 10 every 3 weeks **or**

120 mg/m^2 day 8 and 15 every 3-4 weeks **or**

200 mg/m^2 day 8 and 15 every 3 weeks **or**

400 mg/m^2 every 4 weeks for 3 cycles **or**

1 g/m^2 every 3 weeks **or**

1.5 g/m^2 every 4 weeks

Sarcoma: I.V.: 8-12 g/m^2 weekly for 2-4 weeks

Rheumatoid arthritis: Oral: 7.5 mg once weekly **or** 2.5 mg every 12 hours for 3 doses/week, not to exceed 20 mg/week

Psoriasis:

Oral: 2.5-5 mg/dose every 12 hours for 3 doses given weekly **or**

Oral, I.M.: 10-25 mg/dose given once weekly

Ectopic pregnancy: I.M., I.V.: 50 mg/m^2 as a single dose

(Continued)

Methotrexate *(Continued)*

Elderly: Rheumatoid arthritis/psoriasis: Oral: Initial: 5-7.5 mg/week, not to exceed 20 mg/week

Dosing adjustment in renal impairment:

Cl_{cr} 61-80 mL/minute: Reduce dose to 75% of usual dose

Cl_{cr} 51-60 mL/minute: Reduce dose to 70% of usual dose

Cl_{cr} 10-50 mL/minute: Reduce dose to 30% to 50% of usual dose

Cl_{cr} <10 mL/minute: Avoid use

Hemodialysis: Not dialyzable (0% to 5%); supplemental dose is not necessary

Peritoneal dialysis: Supplemental dose is not necessary

Dosage adjustment in hepatic impairment:

Bilirubin 3.1-5 mg/dL **or** AST >180 units: Administer 75% of usual dose

Bilirubin >5 mg/dL: Do not use

Combination Regimens

Bladder cancer:

CMV *on page 863*

M-VAC (Bladder Cancer) *on page 917*

Breast cancer:

CMF *on page 862*

CMF-IV *on page 863*

M-VAC (Breast Cancer) *on page 921*

Cervical cancer: M-VAC (Cervical Cancer) *on page 921*

Endometrial cancer: M-VAC (Endometrial Cancer) *on page 921*

Gastric cancer: FAMTX *on page 886*

Gestational trophoblastic tumor:

CHAMOCA *on page 858*

EMA/CO *on page 877*

EP/EMA *on page 879*

Head and neck cancer:

CABO *on page 849*

M-VAC (Head and Neck Cancer) *on page 922*

Leukemia, acute lymphocytic:

IDMTX/6-MP *on page 901*

Linker Protocol *on page 904*

MM *on page 910*

MTX/6-MP/VP (Maintenance) *on page 916*

PVA (POG 8602) *on page 932*

PVA (POG 9005) *on page 934*

Leukemia, acute myeloid:

Hyper-CVAD *on page 898*

POMP *on page 931*

Leukemia, acute promyelocytic:

M-3 *on page 906*

Tretinoin/Idarubicin *on page 941*

Lymphoma, Hodgkin's: COMP *on page 866*

Lymphoma, non-Hodgkin's:

CODOX-M *on page 865*

COMLA *on page 865*

IMVP-16 *on page 902*

IVAC *on page 904*

MACOP-B *on page 908*

m-BACOD *on page 908*

Pro-MACE-CytaBOM *on page 931*
Osteosarcoma:
HDMTX (Osteosarcoma) *on page 898*
MTX-CDDPAdr *on page 916*

Administration Methotrexate may be administered I.M., I.V., or I.T.; I.V. administration may be as slow push, short bolus infusion, or 24- to 42-hour continuous infusion

Specific dosing schemes vary, but high dose should be followed by leucovorin calcium to prevent toxicity; refer to Leucovorin monograph *on page 497*

Dosage Forms
Injection, powder for reconstitution [preservative free]: 20 mg, 1 g

Injection, solution, as sodium: 25 mg/mL (2 mL, 10 mL) [contains benzyl alcohol]

Injection, solution, as sodium [preservative free]: 25 mg/mL (2 mL, 4 mL, 8 mL, 10 mL)

Tablet, as sodium: 2.5 mg

Rheumatrex®: 2.5 mg

Trexall™: 5 mg, 7.5 mg, 10 mg, 15 mg

Tablet, as sodium [dose pack] (Rheumatrex® Dose Pack): 2.5 mg (4 cards with 2, 3, 4, 5, or 6 tablets each)

Monitoring Parameters For prolonged use (especially rheumatoid arthritis, psoriasis) a baseline liver biopsy, repeated at each 1-1.5 g cumulative dose interval, should be performed; WBC and platelet counts every 4 weeks; CBC and creatinine, LFTs every 3-4 months; chest x-ray

Dietary Considerations
Sodium content of 100 mg injection: 20 mg (0.86 mEq)

Sodium content of 100 mg (low sodium) injection: 15 mg (0.65 mEq)

Patient Information Avoid alcohol to prevent serious side effects. Avoid intake of extra dietary folic acid, maintain adequate hydration (2-3 L/day of fluids unless instructed to restrict fluid intake) and adequate nutrition (frequent small meals may help). You may experience nausea and vomiting (small frequent meals may help or request antiemetic from prescriber); drowsiness, tingling, numbness, or blurred vision (avoid driving or engaging in tasks that require alertness until response to drug is known); mouth sores (frequent oral care is necessary); loss of hair; skin rash; photosensitivity (use sunscreen, wear protective clothing and eyewear, and avoid direct sunlight). Report black or tarry stools, fever, chills, unusual bleeding or bruising, shortness of breath or difficulty breathing, yellowing of skin or eyes, dark or bloody urine, or acute joint pain or other side effects you may experience. The drug may cause permanent sterility and may cause birth defects; contraceptive measures are recommended during therapy. Pregnancy should be avoided for a minimum of 3 months after completion of therapy in male patients, and at least one ovulatory cycle in female patients. The drug is excreted in breast milk, therefore, an alternative form of feeding your baby should be used.

Additional Information Latex-free products: 50 mg/2 mL, 100 mg/4 mL, and 250 mg/10 mL vials with and without preservatives by Immunex

Special Geriatric Considerations Toxicity to methotrexate or any immunosuppressive is increased in the elderly. Must monitor carefully. For rheumatoid arthritis and psoriasis, immunosuppressive therapy should only be used when disease is active and less toxic, traditional
(Continued)

Methotrexate *(Continued)*

therapy is ineffective. Recommended doses should be reduced when initiating therapy in the elderly due to possible decreased metabolism, reduced renal function, and presence of interacting diseases and drugs. Adjust dose as needed for renal function (Cl_{cr}).

Selected Readings

Evans WE, Pratt CB, Taylor RH, et al, "Pharmacokinetic Monitoring of High-Dose Methotrexate: Early Recognition of High-Risk Patients," *Cancer Chemother Pharmacol*, 1979, 3:161-6.

Furst DE, "Methotrexate: New Mechanisms and Old Toxicities," *Agents Actions Suppl*, 1993, 44:131-7.

Grem JL, King SA, Wittes RE, et al, "The Role of Methotrexate in Osteosarcoma," *J Natl Cancer Inst*, 1988, 80(9):626-55.

Jolivet J, Cowan KH, Curt GA, et al, "The Pharmacology and Clinical Use of Methotrexate," *N Engl J Med*, 1983, 309(18):1094-104.

Treon SP and Chabner BA, "Concepts in Use of High-Dose Methotrexate Therapy," *Clin Chem*, 1996, 42(8 Pt 2):1322-9.

♦ **Methotrexate Sodium** *see* Methotrexate *on page 549*

♦ **Methylacetoxyprogesterone** *see* MedroxyPROGESTERone *on page 524*

♦ **Methylmorphine** *see* Codeine *on page 205*

♦ **Methylphytyl Napthoquinone** *see* Phytonadione *on page 664*

MethylPREDNISolone *(meth il pred NIS oh lone)*

Medication Safety Issues

Sound-alike/look-alike issues:

MethylPREDNISolone may be confused with medroxyPROGESTERone, predniSONE

Depo-Medrol® may be confused with Solu-Medrol®

Medrol® may be confused with Mebaral®

Solu-Medrol® may be confused with Depo-Medrol®

Related Information

Transplantation *on page 1019*

U.S. Brand Names Depo-Medrol®; Medrol®; Solu-Medrol®

Canadian Brand Names Depo-Medrol®; Medrol®; Solu-Medrol®

Generic Available Yes: Sodium succinate injection, tablet

Synonyms A-Methapred; 6-α-Methylprednisolone; Methylprednisolone Acetate; Methylprednisolone Sodium Succinate

Pharmacologic Category Corticosteroid, Systemic

Pregnancy Risk Factor C

Lactation Excretion in breast milk unknown

Use Primarily as an anti-inflammatory or immunosuppressant agent in the treatment of a variety of diseases including those of hematologic, allergic, inflammatory, neoplastic, and autoimmune origin. Prevention and treatment of graft-versus-host disease following allogeneic bone marrow transplantation.

Unlabeled/Investigational Use Treatment of fibrosing-alveolitis phase of adult respiratory distress syndrome (ARDS)

Mechanism of Action In a tissue-specific manner, corticosteroids regulate gene expression subsequent to binding specific intracellular receptors and translocation into the nucleus. Corticosteroids exert a wide array of physiologic effects including modulation of carbohydrate, protein, and lipid metabolism and maintenance of fluid and electrolyte homeostasis. Moreover cardiovascular, immunologic, musculoskeletal, endocrine, and neurologic physiology are influenced by corticosteroids. Decreases inflammation by suppression of migration of polymorphonuclear leukocytes and reversal of increased capillary permeability.

Labeled Contraindications Hypersensitivity to methylprednisolone or any component of the formulation; viral, fungal, or tubercular skin lesions; administration of live virus vaccines; serious infections, except septic shock or tuberculous meningitis. Methylprednisolone formulations containing benzyl alcohol preservative are contraindicated in infants.

Warnings/Precautions Use with caution in patients with hyperthyroidism, cirrhosis, nonspecific ulcerative colitis, hypertension, osteoporosis, thromboembolic tendencies, CHF, convulsive disorders, myasthenia gravis, thrombophlebitis, peptic ulcer, diabetes, glaucoma, cataracts, or tuberculosis. Use caution in hepatic impairment. Acute adrenal insufficiency may occur with abrupt withdrawal after long-term therapy or with stress. Because of the risk of adverse effects, systemic corticosteroids should be used cautiously in the elderly, in the smallest possible dose, and for the shortest possible time.

Adverse Reactions Frequency not defined.

Cardiovascular: Edema, hypertension, arrhythmia

Central nervous system: Insomnia, nervousness, vertigo, seizure, psychoses, pseudotumor cerebri, headache, mood swings, delirium, hallucinations, euphoria

Dermatologic: Hirsutism, acne, skin atrophy, bruising, hyperpigmentation

Endocrine & metabolic: Diabetes mellitus, adrenal suppression, hyperlipidemia, Cushing's syndrome, pituitary-adrenal axis suppression, growth suppression, glucose intolerance, hypokalemia, alkalosis, amenorrhea, sodium and water retention, hyperglycemia

Gastrointestinal: Increased appetite, indigestion, peptic ulcer, nausea, vomiting, abdominal distention, ulcerative esophagitis, pancreatitis

Hematologic: Transient leukocytosis

Neuromuscular & skeletal: Arthralgia, muscle weakness, osteoporosis, fractures

Ocular: Cataracts, glaucoma

Miscellaneous: Infections, hypersensitivity reactions, avascular necrosis, secondary malignancy, intractable hiccups

Vesicant No

Emetic Potential Very low (<10%)

Overdosage/Toxicology When consumed in high doses for prolonged periods, systemic hypercorticism and adrenal suppression may occur. In these cases, discontinuation should be done judiciously. Arrhythmias and cardiovascular collapse are possible with rapid intravenous infusion of high-dose methylprednisolone. May mask signs and symptoms of infection.

Drug Interactions

Cytochrome P450 Effect: Substrate of CYP3A4 (minor); **Inhibits** CYP3A4 (weak)

Increased Effect/Toxicity: Methylprednisolone may increase circulating glucose levels; may need adjustments of insulin or oral hypoglycemics. Methylprednisolone increases cyclosporine and tacrolimus blood levels. Itraconazole increases corticosteroid levels.

Decreased Effect: Phenytoin, phenobarbital, rifampin increase clearance of methylprednisolone. Potassium-depleting diuretics enhance

(Continued)

MethylPREDNISolone *(Continued)*

potassium depletion. Skin test antigens, immunizations decrease antibody response and increase potential infections.

Ethanol/Nutrition/Herb Interactions

Ethanol: Avoid ethanol (may increase gastric mucosal irritation).

Food: Methylprednisolone interferes with calcium absorption. Limit caffeine.

Herb/Nutraceutical: St John's wort may decrease methylprednisolone levels. Avoid cat's claw, echinacea (have immunostimulant properties).

Storage/Stability Intact vials of methylprednisolone sodium succinate should be stored at controlled room temperature. Reconstituted solutions of methylprednisolone sodium succinate should be stored at room temperature (15°C to 30°C) and used within 48 hours. Stability of parenteral admixture at room temperature (25°C) and at refrigeration temperature (4°C) is 48 hours.

Reconstitution

Standard diluent (Solu-Medrol®): 40 mg/50 mL D_5W; 125 mg/50 mL D_5W

Minimum volume (Solu-Medrol®): 50 mL D_5W

Compatibility Not stable in $D_5^{1/2}NS$; **variable stability (consult detailed reference)** in D_5NS, D_5W, LR, NS

Y-site administration: Compatible: Acyclovir, amifostine, amphotericin B cholesteryl sulfate complex, aztreonam, cefepime, cisplatin, cladribine, cyclophosphamide, cytarabine, dopamine, doxorubicin, doxorubicin liposome, enalaprilat, famotidine, fludarabine, gatifloxacin, granisetron, heparin, inamrinone, linezolid, melphalan, meperidine, methotrexate, metronidazole, midazolam, morphine, piperacillin/tazobactam, remifentanil, sodium bicarbonate, tacrolimus, teniposide, theophylline, thiotepa, topotecan. **Incompatible:** Allopurinol, amsacrine, ciprofloxacin, docetaxel, etoposide phosphate, filgrastim, gemcitabine, ondansetron, paclitaxel, propofol, sargramostim, vinorelbine. **Variable (consult detailed reference):** Cisatracurium, diltiazem, heparin with hydrocortisone sodium succinate, potassium chloride, vitamin B complex with C

Compatibility in syringe: Compatible: Diatrizoate meglumine 52% and diatrizoate sodium 8%, diatrizoate sodium 60%, granisetron, iohexol, iopamidol, iothalamate meglumine 60%, ioxaglate meglumine 39.3% and ioxaglate sodium 19.6%, metoclopramide. **Incompatible:** Doxapram

Compatibility when admixed: Compatible: Chloramphenicol, cimetidine, clindamycin, dopamine, granisetron, heparin, norepinephrine, penicillin G potassium, ranitidine, theophylline, verapamil. **Incompatible:** Calcium gluconate, glycopyrrolate, insulin (regular), metaraminol, nafcillin, penicillin G sodium. **Variable (consult detailed reference):** Aminophylline, amphotericin B, cytarabine

Pharmacodynamics/Kinetics

Onset of action: Peak effect (route dependent): Oral: 1-2 hours; I.M.: 4-8 days; Intra-articular: 1 week; methylprednisolone sodium succinate is highly soluble and has a rapid effect by I.M. and I.V. routes

Duration (route dependent): Oral: 30-36 hours; I.M.: 1-4 weeks; Intra-articular: 1-5 weeks; methylprednisolone acetate has a low solubility and has a sustained I.M. effect

Distribution: V_d: 0.7-1.5 L/kg

Half-life elimination: 3-3.5 hours; reduced in obese

Excretion: Clearance: Reduced in obese

Dosage Dosing should be based on the lesser of ideal body weight or actual body weight

Only sodium succinate may be given I.V.; methylprednisolone sodium succinate is highly soluble and has a rapid effect by I.M. and I.V. routes. Methylprednisolone acetate has a low solubility and has a sustained I.M. effect.

Children:

Anti-inflammatory or immunosuppressive: Oral, I.M., I.V. (sodium succinate): 0.5-1.7 mg/kg/day **or** 5-25 mg/m^2/day in divided doses every 6-12 hours; "Pulse" therapy: 15-30 mg/kg/dose over ≥30 minutes given once daily for 3 days

Status asthmaticus: I.V. (sodium succinate): Loading dose: 2 mg/kg/ dose, then 0.5-1 mg/kg/dose every 6 hours for up to 5 days

Acute spinal cord injury: I.V. (sodium succinate): 30 mg/kg over 15 minutes, followed in 45 minutes by a continuous infusion of 5.4 mg/ kg/hour for 23 hours

Lupus nephritis: I.V. (sodium succinate): 30 mg/kg over ≥30 minutes every other day for 6 doses

Adults: **Only sodium succinate may be given I.V.;** methylprednisolone sodium succinate is highly soluble and has a rapid effect by I.M. and I.V. routes. Methylprednisolone acetate has a low solubility and has a sustained I.M. effect.

Acute spinal cord injury: I.V. (sodium succinate): 30 mg/kg over 15 minutes, followed in 45 minutes by a continuous infusion of 5.4 mg/kg/ hour for 23 hours

Anti-inflammatory or immunosuppressive:

Oral: 2-60 mg/day in 1-4 divided doses to start, followed by gradual reduction in dosage to the lowest possible level consistent with maintaining an adequate clinical response.

I.M. (sodium succinate): 10-80 mg/day once daily

I.M. (acetate): 10-80 mg every 1-2 weeks

I.V. (sodium succinate): 10-40 mg over a period of several minutes and repeated I.V. or I.M. at intervals depending on clinical response; when high dosages are needed, give 30 mg/kg over a period ≥30 minutes and may be repeated every 4-6 hours for 48 hours.

Status asthmaticus: I.V. (sodium succinate): Loading dose: 2 mg/kg/dose, then 0.5-1 mg/kg/dose every 6 hours for up to 5 days

High-dose therapy for acute spinal cord injury: I.V. bolus: 30 mg/kg over 15 minutes, followed 45 minutes later by an infusion of 5.4 mg/kg/ hour for 23 hours

Lupus nephritis: High-dose "pulse" therapy: I.V. (sodium succinate): 1 g/ day for 3 days

Aplastic anemia: I.V. (sodium succinate): 1 mg/kg/day or 40 mg/day (whichever dose is higher), for 4 days. After 4 days, change to oral and continue until day 10 or until symptoms of serum sickness resolve, then rapidly reduce over approximately 2 weeks.

Pneumocystis pneumonia in AIDs patients: I.V.: 40-60 mg every 6 hours for 7-10 days

Intra-articular (acetate): Administer every 1-5 weeks.

Large joints: 20-80 mg

Small joints: 4-10 mg

Intralesional (acetate): 20-60 mg every 1-5 weeks

(Continued)

MethylPREDNISolone *(Continued)*

Combination Regimens

Brain tumors: 8 in 1 (Brain Tumors) *on page 841*
Leukemia, acute myeloid: Hyper-CVAD *on page 898*
Lymphoma, non-Hodgkin's: ESHAP *on page 880*
Retinoblastoma: 8 in 1 (Retinoblastoma) *on page 842*

Administration

Oral: Administer after meals or with food or milk

Parenteral: Methylprednisolone sodium succinate may be administered I.M. or I.V.; I.V. administration may be IVP over one to several minutes or IVPB or continuous I.V. infusion. **Acetate salt should not be given I.V.**

I.V.: Succinate:
Low dose: ≤1.8 mg/kg or ≤125 mg/dose: I.V. push over 3-15 minutes
Moderate dose: ≥2 mg/kg or 250 mg/dose: I.V. over 15-30 minutes
High dose: 15 mg/kg or ≥500 mg/dose: I.V. over ≥30 minutes
   Doses >15 mg/kg or ≥1 g: Administer over 1 hour
Do **not** administer high-dose I.V. push; hypotension, cardiac arrhythmia, and sudden death have been reported in patients given high-dose methylprednisolone I.V. push over <20 minutes; intermittent infusion over 15-60 minutes; maximum concentration: I.V. push 125 mg/mL

Dosage Forms

Injection, powder for reconstitution, as sodium succinate: 125 mg [strength expressed as base]
   Solu-Medrol®: 40 mg, 125 mg, 500 mg, 1 g, 2 g [packaged with diluent; diluent contains benzyl alcohol; strength expressed as base]
   Solu-Medrol®: 500 mg, 1 g
Injection, suspension, as acetate (Depo-Medrol®): 20 mg/mL (5 mL); 40 mg/mL (5 mL); 80 mg/mL (5 mL) [contains benzyl alcohol; strength expressed as base]
Injection, suspension, as acetate [single-dose vial] (Depo-Medrol®): 40 mg/mL (1 mL, 10 mL); 80 mg/mL (1 mL)
Tablet: 4 mg
   Medrol®: 2 mg, 4 mg, 8 mg, 16 mg, 32 mg
Tablet, dose-pack: 4 mg (21s)
   Medrol® Dosepack™: 4 mg (21s)

Monitoring Parameters Blood pressure, blood glucose, electrolytes

Dietary Considerations Should be taken after meals or with food or milk; need diet rich in pyridoxine, vitamin C, vitamin D, folate, calcium, phosphorus, and protein.
   Sodium content of 1 g sodium succinate injection: 2.01 mEq; 53 mg of sodium succinate salt is equivalent to 40 mg of methylprednisolone base
   Methylprednisolone acetate: Depo-Medrol®
   Methylprednisolone sodium succinate: Solu-Medrol®

Patient Information Do not discontinue or decrease the drug without contacting your prescriber; carry an identification card or bracelet advising that you are on steroids; may take with meals to decrease GI upset

Additional Information Sodium content of 1 g sodium succinate injection: 2.01 mEq; 53 mg of sodium succinate salt is equivalent to 40 mg of methylprednisolone base

Methylprednisolone acetate: Depo-Medrol®

Methylprednisolone sodium succinate: Solu-Medrol®

Special Geriatric Considerations Because of the risk of adverse effects, systemic corticosteroids should be used cautiously in the elderly, in the smallest possible dose, and for the shortest possible time.

♦ **6-α-Methylprednisolone** *see* MethylPREDNISolone *on page 558*

♦ **Methylprednisolone Acetate** *see* MethylPREDNISolone *on page 558*

♦ **Methylprednisolone Sodium Succinate** *see* MethylPREDNISolone *on page 558*

Metoclopramide (met oh kloe PRA mide)

Medication Safety Issues

Sound-alike/look-alike issues:

Metoclopramide may be confused with metolazone

Reglan® may be confused with Megace®, Regonol®, Renagel®

Related Information

Management of Nausea and Vomiting *on page 982*

U.S. Brand Names Reglan®

Canadian Brand Names Apo-Metoclop®; Nu-Metoclopramide

Generic Available Yes

Pharmacologic Category Antiemetic; Gastrointestinal Agent, Prokinetic

Pregnancy Risk Factor B

Lactation Enters breast milk/not recommended (AAP rates "of concern")

Use Symptomatic treatment of diabetic gastric stasis; gastroesophageal reflux

Unlabeled/Investigational Use Postpyloric placement of enteral feeding tubes; prevention and/or treatment of nausea and vomiting associated with chemotherapy, radiation therapy, or postsurgery

Mechanism of Action Blocks dopamine receptors and (when given in higher doses) also blocks serotonin receptors in chemoreceptor trigger zone of the CNS; enhances the response to acetylcholine of tissue in upper GI tract causing enhanced motility and accelerated gastric emptying without stimulating gastric, biliary, or pancreatic secretions; increases lower esophageal sphincter tone

Labeled Contraindications Hypersensitivity to metoclopramide or any component of the formulation; GI obstruction, perforation or hemorrhage; pheochromocytoma; history of seizures

Warnings/Precautions Use with caution in patients with Parkinson's disease and in patients with a history of mental illness; has been associated with extrapyramidal symptoms and depression. The frequency of EPS is higher in pediatric patients and adults <30 years of age; risk is increased at higher dosages. Extrapyramidal reactions typically occur within the initial 24-48 hours of treatment. Use caution with concurrent use of other drugs associated with EPS. Neuroleptic malignant syndrome (NMS) has been reported (rarely) with metoclopramide. Use lowest recommended doses initially; may cause transient increase in serum aldosterone; use caution in patients who are at risk of fluid overload (CHF, cirrhosis). Use caution in patients with hypertension or following (Continued)

Metoclopramide *(Continued)*

surgical anastomosis/closure. Patients with NADH-cytochrome b5 reductase deficiency are at increased risk of methemoglobinemia and/or sulf-hemoglobinemia. Use caution in patients with a history of seizures. Abrupt discontinuation may (rarely) result in withdrawal symptoms (dizziness, headache, nervousness). Use caution and adjust dose in renal impairment.

Adverse Reactions Adverse reactions are more common/severe at dosages used for prophylaxis of chemotherapy-induced emesis.

>10%:

Central nervous system: Restlessness, drowsiness, extrapyramidal symptoms (high-dose, up to 34%; 0.2% at doses of 30-40 mg/day)

Gastrointestinal: Diarrhea (may be dose-limiting)

Neuromuscular & skeletal: Weakness

1% to 10%:

Central nervous system: Insomnia, depression, confusion, headache

Dermatologic: Rash

Endocrine & metabolic: Breast tenderness, prolactin stimulation

Gastrointestinal: Nausea, xerostomia

<1%: Agitation, agranulocytosis, allergic reaction, amenorrhea, angioedema, anxiety, AV block, bradycardia, bronchospasm, CHF, constipation, fatigue, fluid retention, galactorrhea, gynecomastia, hepatotoxicity, hyper-/hypotension, hyperprolactinemia, jaundice, laryngeal edema, methemoglobinemia, neuroleptic malignant syndrome (NMS), neutropenia, porphyria, seizure, suicidal ideation, sulfhemoglobinemia, tachycardia, tardive dyskinesia, urticaria

Vesicant No

Emetic Potential Very low (<10%)

Overdosage/Toxicology Symptoms of overdose include drowsiness, ataxia, extrapyramidal symptoms, seizures, methemoglobinemia (in infants). Disorientation, muscle hypertonia, irritability, and agitation are common. Metoclopramide often causes extrapyramidal symptoms (eg, dystonic reactions) requiring management with diphenhydramine 1-2 mg/kg (adults) up to a maximum of 50-100 mg I.M. or I.V. slow push followed by a maintenance dose (25-50 mg orally every 4-6 hours) for 48-72 hours. When these reactions are unresponsive to diphenhydramine, benztropine mesylate I.V. 1-2 mg (adults) may be effective. These agents are generally effective within 2-5 minutes. Methylene blue is not recommended in patients with G6PD deficiency who experience methemoglobinemia due to metoclopramide.

Drug Interactions

Cytochrome P450 Effect: Substrate (minor) of CYP1A2, 2D6; **Inhibits** CYP2D6 (weak)

Increased Effect/Toxicity: Opiate analgesics may increase CNS depression. Metoclopramide may increase extrapyramidal symptoms (EPS) or risk when used concurrently with antipsychotic agents.

Decreased Effect: Anticholinergic agents antagonize metoclopramide's actions.

Ethanol/Nutrition/Herb Interactions Ethanol: Avoid ethanol (may increase CNS depression).

Storage/Stability

Injection: Store intact vial at controlled room temperature; injection is photosensitive and should be protected from light during storage; parenteral admixtures in D_5W or NS are stable for at least 24 hours, and do not require light protection if used within 24 hours.

Tablet: Store at controlled room temperature; protect from freezing

Reconstitution Stability of parenteral admixture at room temperature (25°C) and at refrigeration temperature (4°C) is 24 hours.

Compatibility Stable in $D_5{}^1/_2NS$, D_5W, mannitol 20%, LR, NS; **variable stability (consult detailed reference)** in TPN

Y-site administration: Compatible: Acyclovir, aldesleukin, amifostine, aztreonam, bleomycin, ciprofloxacin, cisatracurium, cisplatin, cladribine, clarithromycin, cyclophosphamide, cytarabine, diltiazem, docetaxel, doxorubicin, droperidol, etoposide phosphate, famotidine, filgrastim, fluconazole, fludarabine, fluorouracil, foscarnet, gatifloxacin, gemcitabine, granisetron, heparin, idarubicin, leucovorin, levofloxacin, linezolid, melphalan, meperidine, meropenem, methotrexate, mito-mycin, morphine, ondansetron, paclitaxel, piperacillin/tazobactam, remifentanil, sargramostim, sufentanil, tacrolimus, teniposide, thiotepa, topotecan, vinblastine, vincristine, vinorelbine, zidovudine. **Incompatible:** Allopurinol, amphotericin B cholesteryl sulfate complex, amsacrine, cefepime, doxorubicin liposome, furosemide, propofol. **Variable (consult detailed reference):** TPN

Compatibility in syringe: Compatible: Aminophylline, ascorbic acid injection, atropine, benztropine, bleomycin, butorphanol, chlorproma-zine, cisplatin, cyclophosphamide, cytarabine, dexamethasone sodium phosphate, diamorphine, dimenhydrinate, diphenhydramine, doxoru-bicin, droperidol, fentanyl, fluorouracil, heparin, hydrocortisone sodium phosphate, hydrocortisone sodium succinate, hydroxyzine, insulin (regular), leucovorin, lidocaine, magnesium sulfate, meperidine, metho-trimeprazine, methylprednisolone sodium succinate, midazolam, mito-mycin, morphine, ondansetron, pentazocine, perphenazine, prochlorperazine edisylate, promazine, promethazine, ranitidine, scopolamine, sufentanil, vinblastine, vincristine, vitamin B complex with C. **Incompatible:** Ampicillin, calcium gluconate, chloramphenicol, furo-semide, penicillin G potassium, sodium bicarbonate. **Variable (consult detailed reference):** Methotrexate

Compatibility when admixed: Compatible: Cimetidine, clindamycin, diamorphine, meperidine, meropenem, morphine, multivitamins, potas-sium acetate, potassium chloride, potassium phosphate, verapamil. **Incompatible:** Dexamethasone sodium phosphate with lorazepam and diphenhydramine, erythromycin lactobionate, floxacillin, fluorouracil, furosemide

Pharmacodynamics/Kinetics

Onset of action: Oral: 0.5-1 hour; I.V.: 1-3 minutes

Duration: Therapeutic: 1-2 hours, regardless of route

Distribution: V_d: 2-4 L/kg; Crosses placenta; enters breast milk

Protein binding: 30% to 40%, primarily to α_1-acid glycoprotein

Bioavailability: 80%

Half-life elimination: Normal renal function: 4-7 hours (may be dose dependent)

Time to peak, serum: Oral: 1-3 hours; I.M.: 2-3 hours; I.V.: Within 5 minutes; Rectal: 1-8 hours

(Continued)

Metoclopramide *(Continued)*

Excretion: Urine (70% to 85%, ~19% as unchanged drug); feces (2% to 3%)

Dosage

Children:

Gastroesophageal reflux: Oral: 0.1-0.2 mg/kg/dose up to 4 times/day; efficacy of continuing metoclopramide beyond 12 weeks in reflux has not been determined; total daily dose should not exceed 0.5 mg/kg/day

Gastrointestinal hypomotility (gastroparesis): Oral, I.M., I.V.: 0.1 mg/kg/dose up to 4 times/day, not to exceed 0.5 mg/kg/day

Antiemetic (chemotherapy-induced emesis) (unlabeled): I.V.: 1-2 mg/kg 30 minutes before chemotherapy and every 2-4 hours, for a total of 5 doses (5-10 mg/kg) daily

Postpyloric feeding tube placement (unlabeled): I.V.:
<6 years: 0.1 mg/kg
6-14 years: 2.5-5 mg

Adults:

Gastroesophageal reflux: Oral: 10-15 mg/dose up to 4 times/day 30 minutes before meals or food and at bedtime; single doses of 20 mg are occasionally needed for provoking situations

Gastrointestinal hypomotility (gastroparesis):
Oral: 10 mg 30 minutes before each meal and at bedtime for 2-8 weeks

I.V. (for severe symptoms): 10 mg over 1-2 minutes; 10 days of I.V. therapy may be necessary for best response

Antiemetic (chemotherapy-induced emesis) (unlabeled): I.V.: 1-2 mg/kg 30 minutes before chemotherapy and every 2-4 hours, for a total of 5 doses (5-10 mg/kg) daily

Postoperative nausea and vomiting (unlabeled): I.M., I.V.: 10 mg near end of surgery; 20 mg doses may be used

Postpyloric feeding tube placement (unlabeled): I.M., I.V.: 10 mg

Elderly:

Gastroesophageal reflux: Oral: 5 mg 4 times/day (30 minutes before meals and at bedtime); increase dose to 10 mg 4 times/day if no response at lower dose

Gastrointestinal hypomotility:
Oral: Initial: 5 mg 30 minutes before meals and at bedtime for 2-8 weeks; increase if necessary to 10 mg doses

I.V.: Initiate at 5 mg over 1-2 minutes; increase to 10 mg if necessary

Postoperative nausea and vomiting (unlabeled): I.M.: 5 mg near end of surgery; may repeat dose if necessary

Dosing adjustment in renal impairment:

Cl_{cr} 10-40 mL/minute: Administer at 50% of normal dose

Cl_{cr} <10 mL/minute: Administer at 25% of normal dose

Hemodialysis: Not dialyzable (0% to 5%); supplemental dose is not necessary

Administration Injection solution may be given I.M., direct I.V. push, short infusion (15-30 minutes), or continuous infusion; lower doses (≤10 mg) of metoclopramide can be given I.V. push undiluted over 1-2 minutes; higher doses to be given IVPB over at least 15 minutes; continuous SubQ infusion and rectal administration have been reported

Dosage Forms

Injection, solution, as hydrochloride (Reglan®): 5 mg/mL (2 mL, 10 mL, 30 mL)

Syrup, as hydrochloride: 5 mg/5 mL (10 mL, 480 mL) [some products contain sodium benzoate; sugar free]

Tablet, as hydrochloride (Reglan®): 5 mg, 10 mg

Monitoring Parameters Periodic renal function test; monitor for dystonic reactions; monitor for signs of hypoglycemia in patients using insulin and those being treated for gastroparesis; monitor for agitation and irritable confusion

Patient Information May impair mental alertness or physical coordination; avoid alcohol, barbiturates or other CNS depressants; take 30 minutes before meals; report if involuntary movements occur

Special Geriatric Considerations Elderly are more likely to develop tardive dyskinesia syndrome (especially elderly females) reactions than younger adults. Use lowest recommended doses initially. Must consider renal function (estimate creatinine clearance). It is recommended to do involuntary movement assessments on elderly using this medication at high doses and for long-term therapy.

Extemporaneous Preparations

Metoclophen nausea suppository:

Metoclopramide powder (USP) 40 mg
Haloperidol powder (USP) 1 mg
Dexamethasone powder (USP) 10 mg
Diphenhydramine HCl (USP) 25 mg
Benztropine mesylate (USP) 1 mg
Silica gel powder 200 mg
Fatty base (emulsifying type) qs 2.2 g

Metoclophen-modified nausea suppository:

Metoclopramide powder (USP) 40 mg
Haloperidol powder (USP) 1 mg
Lorazepam (USP) 1 mg
Benztropine mesylate (USP) 1 mg
Fatty base (emulsifying type) qs 2.2 g

Grind all powders (and/or tablets) into a fine uniform powder. Melt the fatty base on low temperature, then add the powder. Stir the mixture until uniform. With continuous stirring, draw up part of the mixture and instill into calibrated suppository molds. Refrigerate.

Francom M, "Compounding Nausea Aid," *Am Pharm*, 1991, NS31(7):7.

Selected Readings

Desmond PV and Watson KJ, "Metoclopramide - A Review," *Med J Aust*, 1986, 144(7):366-9.

DiPalma JR, "Metoclopramide: A Dopamine Receptor Antagonist," *Am Fam Physician*, 1990, 41(3):919-24.

Harrington RA, Hamilton CW, Brogden RN, et al, "Metoclopramide. An Updated Review of Its Pharmacological Properties and Clinical Use," *Drugs*, 1983, 25(5):451-94.

McGovern EM, Grevel J, and Bryson SM, "Pharmacokinetics of High-Dose Metoclopramide in Cancer Patients," *Clin Pharmacokinet*, 1986, 11(6):415-24.

Schulze-Delrieu K, "Drug Therapy. Metoclopramide," *N Engl J Med*, 1981, 305(1):28-33.

♦ **MetroCream®** *see* Metronidazole *on page 568*

♦ **MetroGel®** *see* Metronidazole *on page 568*

♦ **MetroGel-Vaginal®** *see* Metronidazole *on page 568*

♦ **MetroLotion®** *see* Metronidazole *on page 568*

Metronidazole (me troe NI da zole)

Medication Safety Issues

Sound-alike/look-alike issues:

Metronidazole may be confused with metformin.

Related Information

Management of Infections *on page 978*

U.S. Brand Names Flagyl®; Flagyl ER®; Flagyl® I.V. RTU™; MetroCream®; MetroGel®; MetroGel-Vaginal®; MetroLotion®; Noritate®; Rozex™ [DSC]

Canadian Brand Names Apo-Metronidazole®; Flagyl®; Florazole® ER; MetroCream®; Metrogel®; Nidagel™; Noritate®; Novo-Nidazol; Trikacide

Generic Available Yes: Cream, infusion, tablet

Synonyms Metronidazole Hydrochloride

Pharmacologic Category Amebicide; Antibiotic, Topical; Antibiotic, Miscellaneous; Antiprotozoal

Pregnancy Risk Factor B (may be contraindicated in 1st trimester)

Lactation Enters breast milk/not recommended (AAP rates "of concern")

Use Treatment of susceptible anaerobic bacterial and protozoal infections in the following conditions: Amebiasis, symptomatic and asymptomatic trichomoniasis; skin and skin structure infections; CNS infections; intra-abdominal infections (as part of combination regimen); systemic anaerobic infections; treatment of antibiotic-associated pseudomembranous colitis (AAPC), bacterial vaginosis; as part of a multidrug regimen for *H. pylori* eradication to reduce the risk of duodenal ulcer recurrence

Topical: Treatment of inflammatory lesions and erythema of rosacea

Unlabeled/Investigational Use Crohn's disease

Mechanism of Action After diffusing into the organism, interacts with DNA to cause a loss of helical DNA structure and strand breakage resulting in inhibition of protein synthesis and cell death in susceptible organisms

Labeled Contraindications Hypersensitivity to metronidazole, nitroimidazole derivatives, or any component of the formulation; pregnancy (1st trimester - found to be carcinogenic in rats)

Warnings/Precautions Use with caution in patients with liver impairment due to potential accumulation, blood dyscrasias; history of seizures, CHF, or other sodium retaining states; reduce dosage in patients with severe liver impairment, CNS disease, and severe renal failure (Cl$_{cr}$ <10 mL/minute); if *H. pylori* is not eradicated in patients being treated with metronidazole in a regimen, it should be assumed that metronidazole-resistance has occurred and it should not again be used; seizures and neuropathies have been reported especially with increased doses and chronic treatment; if this occurs, discontinue therapy

Adverse Reactions

Systemic: Frequency not defined:

Cardiovascular: Flattening of the T-wave, flushing

Central nervous system: Ataxia, confusion, coordination impaired, dizziness, fever, headache, insomnia, irritability, seizure, vertigo

Dermatologic: Erythematous rash, urticaria

Endocrine & metabolic: Disulfiram-like reaction, dysmenorrhea, libido decreased

Gastrointestinal: Nausea (~12%), anorexia, abdominal cramping, constipation, diarrhea, furry tongue, glossitis, proctitis, stomatitis, unusual/metallic taste, vomiting, xerostomia

Genitourinary: Cystitis, darkened urine (rare), dysuria, incontinence, polyuria, vaginitis

Hematologic: Neutropenia (reversible), thrombocytopenia (reversible, rare)

Neuromuscular & skeletal: Peripheral neuropathy, weakness

Respiratory: Nasal congestion, rhinitis, sinusitis, pharyngitis

Miscellaneous: Flu-like syndrome, moniliasis

Topical: Frequency not defined:

Central nervous system: Headache

Dermatologic: Burning, contact dermatitis, dryness, erythema, irritation, pruritus, rash

Gastrointestinal: Unusual/metallic taste, nausea, constipation

Local: Local allergic reaction

Neuromuscular & skeletal: Tingling/numbness of extremities

Ocular: Eye irritation

Vaginal:

>10%: Genitourinary: Vaginal discharge (12%)

1% to 10%:

Central nervous system: Headache (5%), dizziness (2%)

Gastrointestinal: Gastrointestinal discomfort (7%), nausea and/or vomiting (4%), unusual/metallic taste (2%), diarrhea (1%)

Genitourinary: Vaginitis (10%), vulva/vaginal irritation (9%), pelvic discomfort (3%)

Hematologic: WBC increased (2%)

<1%: Abdominal bloating, abdominal gas, darkened urine, depression, fatigue, itching, rash, thirst, xerostomia

Vesicant No

Emetic Potential Low (10% to 30%)

Overdosage/Toxicology Symptoms of overdose include nausea, vomiting, ataxia, seizures, and peripheral neuropathy. Treatment is symptomatic and supportive.

Drug Interactions

Cytochrome P450 Effect: Inhibits CYP2C8/9 (weak), 3A4 (moderate)

Increased Effect/Toxicity: Ethanol may cause a disulfiram-like reaction. Warfarin and metronidazole may increase bleeding times (PT) which may result in bleeding. Cimetidine may increase metronidazole levels. Metronidazole may inhibit metabolism of cisapride, causing potential arrhythmias; avoid concurrent use. Metronidazole may increase lithium levels/toxicity. Metronidazole may increase the levels/effects of selected benzodiazepines, calcium channel blockers, cyclosporine, ergot derivatives, selected HMG-CoA reductase inhibitors, mirtazapine, nateglinide, nefazodone, sildenafil (and other PDE-5 inhibitors), tacrolimus, venlafaxine, and other CYP3A4 substrates.

Decreased Effect: Phenytoin, phenobarbital (potentially other enzyme inducers) may decrease metronidazole half-life and effects.

Ethanol/Nutrition/Herb Interactions

Ethanol: The manufacturer recommends to avoid all ethanol or any ethanol-containing drugs (may cause disulfiram-like reaction characterized by flushing, headache, nausea, vomiting, sweating or tachycardia). (Continued)

Metronidazole *(Continued)*

Food: Peak antibiotic serum concentration lowered and delayed, but total drug absorbed not affected.

Storage/Stability Metronidazole injection should be stored at 15°C to 30°C and protected from light. Product may be refrigerated but crystals may form; crystals redissolve on warming to room temperature. Prolonged exposure to light will cause a darkening of the product. However, short-term exposure to normal room light does not adversely affect metronidazole stability. Direct sunlight should be avoided. Stability of parenteral admixture at room temperature (25°C): Out of overwrap stability: 30 days.

Reconstitution Standard diluent: 500 mg/100 mL NS

Compatibility Stable in D_5W, NS

Y-site administration: Compatible: Acyclovir, allopurinol, amiodarone, amifostine, cefepime, cisatracurium, clarithromycin, cyclophosphamide, diltiazem, docetaxel, dopamine, doxorubicin liposome, enalaprilat, esmolol, etoposide phosphate, fluconazole, foscarnet, gatifloxacin, gemcitabine, granisetron, heparin, hydromorphone, labetalol, linezolid, lorazepam, magnesium sulfate, melphalan, meperidine, methylprednisolone sodium succinate, midazolam, morphine, perphenazine, piperacillin/tazobactam, remifentanil, sargramostim, tacrolimus, teniposide, theophylline, thiotepa, vinorelbine. **Incompatible:** Amphotericin B cholesteryl sulfate complex, aztreonam, filgrastim, meropenem, warfarin

Compatibility when admixed: Compatible: Amikacin, aminophylline, ampicillin, cefazolin, cefotaxime, cefoxitin, ceftazidime, ceftizoxime, ceftriaxone, cefuroxime, chloramphenicol, ciprofloxacin, clindamycin, disopyramide, floxacillin, fluconazole, gentamicin, heparin, hydrocortisone sodium succinate, multivitamins, netilmicin, penicillin G potassium, tobramycin. **Incompatible:** Aztreonam, dopamine, meropenem. **Variable (consult detailed reference):** Cefamandole, cefepime

Pharmacodynamics/Kinetics

Absorption: Oral: Well absorbed; Topical: Concentrations achieved systemically after application of 1 g topically are 10 times less than those obtained after a 250 mg oral dose

Distribution: To saliva, bile, seminal fluid, breast milk, bone, liver, and liver abscesses; lung and vaginal secretions; crosses placenta and blood-brain barrier

CSF:blood level ratio: Normal meninges: 16% to 43%; Inflamed meninges: 100%

Protein binding: <20%

Metabolism: Hepatic (30% to 60%)

Half-life elimination: Neonates: 25-75 hours; Others: 6-8 hours, prolonged with hepatic impairment; End-stage renal disease: 21 hours

Time to peak, serum: Oral: Immediate release: 1-2 hours

Excretion: Urine (20% to 40% as unchanged drug); feces (6% to 15%)

Dosage

Infants and Children:

Amebiasis: Oral: 35-50 mg/kg/day in divided doses every 8 hours for 10 days

Trichomoniasis: Oral: 15-30 mg/kg/day in divided doses every 8 hours for 7 days

Anaerobic infections:
Oral: 15-35 mg/kg/day in divided doses every 8 hours
I.V.: 30 mg/kg/day in divided doses every 6 hours
Clostridium difficile (antibiotic-associated colitis): Oral: 20 mg/kg/day divided every 6 hours
Maximum dose: 2 g/day

Adults:
Amebiasis: Oral: 500-750 mg every 8 hours for 5-10 days
Trichomoniasis: Oral: 250 mg every 8 hours for 7 days **or** 375 mg twice daily for 7 days **or** 2 g as a single dose
Anaerobic infections: Oral, I.V.: 500 mg every 6-8 hours, not to exceed 4 g/day
Antibiotic-associated pseudomembranous colitis: Oral: 250-500 mg 3-4 times/day for 10-14 days
Helicobacter pylori eradication: Oral: 250-500 mg with meals and at bedtime for 14 days; requires combination therapy with at least one other antibiotic and an acid-suppressing agent (proton pump inhibitor or H_2 blocker)
Bacterial vaginosis:
Oral: 750 mg (extended release tablet) once daily for 7 days
Vaginal: 1 applicatorful ($\sim$37.5 mg metronidazole) intravaginally once or twice daily for 5 days; apply once in morning and evening if using twice daily, if daily, use at bedtime
Acne rosacea: Topical:
0.75%: Apply and rub a thin film twice daily, morning and evening, to entire affected areas after washing. Significant therapeutic results should be noticed within 3 weeks. Clinical studies have demonstrated continuing improvement through 9 weeks of therapy.
1%: Apply thin film to affected area once daily
Elderly: Use lower end of dosing recommendations for adults, do not administer as a single dose

Dosing adjustment in renal impairment: Cl_{cr} <10 mL/minute: Administer 50% of dose or every 12 hours
Hemodialysis: Extensively removed by hemodialysis and peritoneal dialysis (50% to 100%); administer dose posthemodialysis
Peritoneal dialysis: Dose as for Cl_{cr} <10 mL/minute
Continuous arteriovenous or venovenous hemofiltration: Administer usual dose
Dosing adjustment/comments in hepatic disease: Unchanged in mild liver disease; reduce dosage in severe liver disease

Administration
Oral: May be taken with food to minimize stomach upset. Extended release tablets should be taken on an empty stomach (1 hour before or 2 hours after meals).
Topical: No disulfiram-like reactions have been reported after **topical** application, although metronidazole can be detected in the blood. Apply to clean, dry skin. Cosmetics may be used after application (wait at least 5 minutes after using lotion).

Dosage Forms [DSC] = Discontinued product
Capsule (Flagyl®): 375 mg
Cream, topical: 0.75% (45 g)
MetroCream®: 0.75% (45 g) [contains benzyl alcohol]
Noritate®: 1% (60 g)
(Continued)

Metronidazole *(Continued)*

Emulsion, topical (Rozex™): 0.75% (60 g) [contains benzyl alcohol] [DSC]

Gel, topical (MetroGel®): 0.75% (45 g)

Gel, vaginal (MetroGel-Vaginal®): 0.75% (70 g)

Infusion (Flagyl® I.V. RTU™) [premixed iso-osmotic sodium chloride solution]: 500 mg (100 mL) [contains sodium 14 mEq]

Lotion, topical (MetroLotion®): 0.75% (60 mL) [contains benzyl alcohol]

Tablet (Flagyl®): 250 mg, 500 mg

Tablet, extended release (Flagyl® ER): 750 mg

Dietary Considerations Take on an empty stomach. Drug may cause GI upset; if GI upset occurs, take with food. Extended release tablets should be taken on an empty stomach (1 hour before or 2 hours after meals). Sodium content of 500 mg (I.V.): 322 mg (14 mEq). The manufacturer recommends that ethanol be avoided during treatment and for 3 days after therapy is complete.

Patient Information Urine may be discolored to a dark or reddish-brown; do not take alcohol for at least 24 hours after the last dose; avoid beverage alcohol or any topical products containing alcohol during therapy; may cause metallic taste; may be taken with food to minimize stomach upset; report numbness or tingling in extremities; avoid contact of the topical product with the eyes; cleanse areas to be treated well before application

Special Geriatric Considerations Adjust dose based on renal function.

Extemporaneous Preparations A 20 mg/mL oral suspension can be prepared by crushing ten 250 mg tablets in a mortar, and then adding 10 mL purified water USP to create a uniform paste. Add a small quantity of syrup, then transfer to a graduate and add a sufficient quantity of syrup to make 125 mL. Label "shake well" and "refrigerate." Refrigerated stability is 10 days.

Irwin DB, Dupuis LL, Prober CG, et al, "The Acceptability, Stability, and Relative Bioavailability of an Extemporaneous Metronidazole Suspension," *Can J Hosp Pharm*, 1987, 40:42-6.

Nahata MC, Morosco RS, and Hipple TF, 4th ed, *Pediatric Drug Formulations*, Cincinnati, OH: Harvey Whitney Books Co, 2000.

Selected Readings

Abramowicz M, "Antimicrobial Prophylaxis in Surgery," *Medical Letter on Drugs and Therapeutics, Handbook of Antimicrobial Therapy*, 16th ed, New York, NY: Medical Letter, 2002.

Brodgen RN, Heel RC, Speight TM, et al, "Metronidazole in Anaerobic Infections: A Review of Its Activity, Pharmacokinetics and Therapeutic Use," *Drugs*, 1978, 16(5):387-417.

Falagas ME and Gorbach SL, "Clindamycin and Metronidazole," *Med Clin North Am*, 1995, 79(4):845-67.

Fekety R and Shah AB, "Diagnosis and Treatment of *Clostridium difficile* Colitis," *JAMA*, 1993, 269(1):71-5.

Freeman CD, Klutman NE, and Lamp KC, "Metronidazole. A Therapeutic Review and Update," *Drugs*, 1997, 54(5):679-708.

Hager WD and Rapp RP, "Metronidazole," *Obstet Gynecol Clin North Am*, 1992, 19(3):497-510.

Oldenburg B and Speck WT, "Metronidazole," *Pediatr Clin North Am*, 1983, 30(1):71-5.

Patterson BD, "Possible Interaction Between Metronidazole and Carbamazepine," *Ann Pharmacother*, 1994, 28(11):1303-4.

Ralph ED, "Clinical Pharmacokinetics of Metronidazole," *Clin Pharmacokinet*, 1983, 8:43-62.

"Treatment of *Clostridium difficile* Diarrhea," *Med Lett Drugs Ther*, 1989, 31(803):94-5.

♦ **Metronidazole Hydrochloride** *see* Metronidazole *on page 568*

♦ **M-FA-142** *see* Amonafide *on page 65*

♦ **Miacalcin**® *see* Calcitonin *on page 145*
♦ **Miacalcin**® **NS (Can)** *see* Calcitonin *on page 145*

Micafungin (mi ka FUN gin)

U.S. Brand Names Mycamine™
Synonyms Echinocandin; Micafungin Sodium
Pharmacologic Category Antifungal Agent, Parenteral; Echinocandin
Pregnancy Risk Factor C
Lactation Excretion in breast milk unknown/use caution
Use Esophageal candidiasis; *Candida* prophylaxis in patients undergoing hematopoietic stem cell transplant
Unlabeled/Investigational Use Treatment of infections due to *Aspergillus* spp; prophylaxis of HIV-related esophageal candidiasis
Mechanism of Action Concentration-dependent inhibition of 1,3-beta-D-glucan synthase resulting in reduced formation of 1,3-beta-D-glucan, an essential polysaccharide comprising 30% to 60% of *Candida* cell walls (absent in mammalian cells); decreased glucan content leads to osmotic instability and cellular lysis
Labeled Contraindications Hypersensitivity to micafungin or any component of the formulation
Warnings/Precautions Anaphylactic reactions, including shock, have been reported. New onset or worsening hepatic failure has been reported; use caution in pre-existing mild-moderate hepatic impairment; safety in severe liver failure has not been evaluated. Hemolytic anemia and hemoglobinuria have been reported. Safety and efficacy in pediatric patients have not been established.

Adverse Reactions
1% to 10%:
  Cardiovascular: Phlebitis (2%), hypertension (1%), flushing (1%)
  Central nervous system: Headache (2%), pyrexia (2%), delirium (1%), dizziness (1%), somnolence (1%)
  Dermatologic: Rash (2%), pruritus (1%), febrile neutropenia (1%)
  Endocrine & metabolic: Hypokalemia (1%), hypocalcemia (1%), hypomagnesemia (1%), hypophosphatemia (1%)
  Gastrointestinal: Nausea (3%), diarrhea (2%), vomiting (2%), abdominal pain (1%), appetite decreased (1%), dysgeusia (1%), dyspepsia (1%)
  Hematologic: Leukopenia (2%), neutropenia (1%), thrombocytopenia (1%), anemia (1%), lymphopenia (1%), eosinophilia (1%)
  Hepatic: Transaminase increased (2% to 3%), serum alkaline phosphatase increased (2%), hyperbilirubinemia (1%)
  Local: Infusion site inflammation (1%)
  Neuromuscular & skeletal: Rigors (1%), lactate dehydrogenase increased (1%)
  Renal: Serum creatinine increased (1%), serum urea increased (1%)
  <1%, postmarketing and/or case reports, or frequency not defined: Acidosis, anorexia, anuria, apnea, arrhythmia, arthralgia, cardiac arrest, coagulopathy, constipation, convulsions, cyanosis, dyspnea, deep vein thrombosis, hypoxia, encephalopathy, erythema multiforme, facial edema, hemoglobinuria, hemolysis, hemolytic anemia, hepatic failure, hepatocellular damage, hepatomegaly, hiccups, hyponatremia, hypotension, infection, injection site necrosis, intracranial hemorrhage, jaundice, MI, mycosal inflammation, oliguria, pancytopenia, pneumonia,
(Continued)

Micafungin *(Continued)*

pulmonary embolism, renal failure, renal tubular necrosis, sepsis, shock, tachycardia, skin necrosis, thrombotic thrombocytopenia purpura, thrombophlebitis, urticaria, vasodilatation

Overdosage/Toxicology Treatment should be symptom-directed and supportive. Not removed by dialysis.

Storage/Stability Store at 25°C (77°F). Reconstituted and diluted solutions are stable for 24 hours at room temperature. Protect from light.

Reconstitution Aseptically add 5 mL of NS (preservative-free) to each 50 mg vial; swirl to dissolve; do not shake. Further dilute 50-150 mg in 100 mL NS; protect from light. Alternatively, D_5W may be used for reconstitution and dilution.

Pharmacodynamics/Kinetics

Distribution: 0.28-0.5 L/kg

Protein binding: >99%

Metabolism: Hepatic; forms M-1 (catechol) and M-2 (methoxy) metabolites (activity unknown)

Half-life elimination: 11-21 hours

Excretion: Primarily feces (71%), urine (<15%, unchanged drug)

Dosage I.V.: Adults:

Esophageal candidiasis: 150 mg daily; median duration of therapy (from clinical trials) was 14 days

Prophylaxis of *Candida* infection in hematopoietic stem cell transplantation: 50 mg daily; median duration of therapy (from clinical trials) was 18 days

Dosage Forms Injection, powder for reconstitution, as sodium [preservative-free]: Micafungin 50 mg [contains lactose]

Monitoring Parameters Liver function tests

Patient Information Inform prescriber of all prescriptions, OTC medications, or herbal products you are taking, and any allergies you have. This medication can only be administered by infusion. Report immediately any pain, burning, or swelling at infusion site, or any signs of allergic reaction (eg, respiratory difficulty or swallowing, back pain, chest tightness, rash, hives, or swelling of lips or mouth). Report nausea, vomiting, abdominal pain, or diarrhea.

Selected Readings

Carver PL, "Micafungin," *Ann Pharmacother*, 2004, 38(10):1707-21.

de Wet N, Llanos-Cuentas A, Suleiman J, et al, "A Randomized, Double-Blind, Parallel-Group, Dose-Response Study of Micafungin Compared with Fluconazole for the Treatment of Esophageal Candidiasis in HIV-Positive Patients," *Clin Infect Dis*, 2004, 39(6):842-9.

Kohno S, Masaoka T, Yamaguchi H, et al, "A Multicenter, Open-Label Clinical Study of Micafungin (FK463) in the Treatment of Deep-Seated Mycosis in Japan," *Scand J Infect Dis*, 36(5):372-9.

Pettengell K, Mynhardt J, Kluyts T, et al, "Successful Treatment of Oesophageal Candidiasis by Micafungin: A Novel Systemic Antifungal Agent," *Aliment Pharmacol Ther*, 2004, 20(4):475-81.

Yokote T, Akioka T, Oka S, et al, "Successful Treatment With Micafungin of Invasive Pulmonary Aspergillosis in Acute Myeloid Leukemia, With Renal Failure Due to Amphotericin B Therapy," *Ann Hematol*, 2004, 83(1):64-6.

◆ **Micafungin Sodium** *see* Micafungin *on page 573*

◆ **MICRhoGAM®** *see* Rh$_o$(D) Immune Globulin *on page 705*

◆ **Mifeprex®** *see* Mifepristone *on page 575*

Mifepristone (mi FE pris tone)

Medication Safety Issues
Sound-alike/look-alike issues:
Mifeprex® may be confused with Mirapex®

Related Information
Investigational Drug Service *on page 1031*

U.S. Brand Names Mifeprex®

Generic Available No

Synonyms RU-486; RU-38486

Pharmacologic Category Abortifacient; Antineoplastic Agent, Hormone Antagonist; Antiprogestin

Pregnancy Risk Factor X

Lactation Excretion in breast milk unknown/contraindicated

Use Medical termination of intrauterine pregnancy, through day 49 of pregnancy. Patients may need treatment with misoprostol and possibly surgery to complete therapy

Unlabeled/Investigational Use Treatment of unresectable meningioma; has been studied in the treatment of breast cancer, ovarian cancer, and adrenal cortical carcinoma

Mechanism of Action Mifepristone, a synthetic steroid, competitively binds to the intracellular progesterone receptor, blocking the effects of progesterone. When used for the termination of pregnancy, this leads to contraction-inducing activity in the myometrium. In the absence of progesterone, mifepristone acts as a partial progesterone agonist. Mifepristone also has weak antiglucocorticoid and antiandrogenic properties; it blocks the feedback effect of cortisol on corticotropin secretion.

Restrictions Investigators wishing to obtain the agent for use in oncology patients must apply for a patient-specific IND from the FDA. Mifepristone will be supplied only to licensed physicians who sign and return a "Prescriber's Agreement." Distribution of mifepristone will be subject to specific requirements imposed by the distributor. Mifepristone will **not** be available to the public through licensed pharmacies. A patient medication guide is available and must be dispensed with the medication; the FDA-approved medication guide is available at www.fda.gov/cder/Offices/ODS/labeling.htm.

Labeled Contraindications Hypersensitivity to mifepristone, misoprostol, other prostaglandins, or any component of the formulation; chronic adrenal failure; porphyrias; hemorrhagic disorder or concurrent anticoagulant therapy; pregnancy termination >49 days; intrauterine device (IUD) in place; ectopic pregnancy or undiagnosed adnexal mass; concurrent long-term corticosteroid therapy; inadequate or lack of access to emergency medical services; inability to understand effects and/or comply with treatment

Warnings/Precautions Patient must be instructed of the treatment procedure and expected effects. A signed agreement form must be kept in the patient's file. Physicians may obtain patient agreement forms, physician enrollment forms, and medical consultation directly from Danco Laboratories at 1-877-432-7596. Adverse effects (including blood transfusions, hospitalization, ongoing pregnancy, and other major complications) must be reported in writing to the medication distributor. To be administered only by physicians who can date pregnancy, diagnose ectopic pregnancies, provide access to surgical abortion (if needed), and can provide
(Continued)

Mifepristone *(Continued)*

access to emergency care. Medication will be distributed directly to these physicians following signed agreement with the distributor. Must be administered under supervision by the qualified physician. Pregnancy is dated from day 1 of last menstrual period (presuming a 28-day cycle, ovulation occurring midcycle). Pregnancy duration can be determined using menstrual history and clinical examination. Ultrasound should be used if an ectopic pregnancy is suspected or if duration of pregnancy is uncertain. Ultrasonography may not identify all ectopic pregnancies, and healthcare providers should be alert for signs and symptoms which may be related to undiagnosed ectopic pregnancy in any patient who receives mifepristone

Bleeding occurs and should be expected (average 9-16 days, may be ≥30 days). In some cases, bleeding may be prolonged and heavy, potentially leading to hypovolemic shock. Patients should be counseled to seek medical attention in cases of excessive bleeding; the manufacturer cites soaking through two thick sanitary pads per hour for two consecutive hours as an example of excessive bleeding. Bleeding may require blood transfusion (rare), curettage, saline infusions, and/or vasoconstrictors. Use caution in patients with severe anemia. Confirmation of pregnancy termination by clinical exam or ultrasound must be made 14 days following treatment. Manufacturer recommends surgical termination of pregnancy when medical termination fails or is not complete. Prescriber should determine in advance whether they will provide such care themselves or through other providers. Preventative measures to prevent rhesus immunization must be taken prior to surgical abortion. Prescriber should also give the patient clear instructions on whom to call and what to do in the event of an emergency following administration of mifepristone.

Bacterial infection has been reported following use of this product. In rare cases, these infections may be serious and/or fatal, with septic shock as a potential complication. A causal relationship has not been established. Sustained fever, abdominal pain, or pelvic tenderness should prompt evaluation; however, healthcare professionals are warned that atypical presentations of serious infection without these symptoms have also been noted.

Safety and efficacy have not been established for use in women with chronic cardiovascular, hypertensive, hepatic, respiratory, or renal disease, insulin-dependent diabetes mellitus, severe anemia, or heavy smokers. Women >35 years of age and smokers (>10 cigarettes/day) were excluded from clinical trials. Safety and efficacy in pediatric patients have not been established.

Adverse Reactions Vaginal bleeding and uterine cramping are expected to occur when this medication is used to terminate a pregnancy; 90% of women using this medication for this purpose also report adverse reactions. Bleeding or spotting occurs in most women for a period of 9-16 days. Up to 8% of women will experience some degree of bleeding or spotting for 30 days or more. In some cases, bleeding may be prolonged and heavy, potentially leading to hypovolemic shock.

>10%:

Central nervous system: Headache (2% to 31%), dizziness (1% to 12%)

Gastrointestinal: Abdominal pain (cramping) (96%), nausea (43% to 61%), vomiting (18% to 26%), diarrhea (12% to 20%)

Genitourinary: Uterine cramping (83%)

1% to 10%:

Cardiovascular: Syncope (1%)

Central nervous system: Fatigue (10%), fever (4%), insomnia (3%), anxiety (2%), fainting (2%)

Gastrointestinal: Dyspepsia (3%)

Genitourinary: Endometriosis/salpingitis/pelvic inflammatory disease (1%), pelvic pain (2%), uterine hemorrhage (5%), vaginitis (3%)

Hematologic: Decreased hemoglobin >2 g/dL (6%), anemia (2%), leukorrhea (2%)

Neuromuscular & skeletal: Back pain (9%), rigors (3%), leg pain (2%), weakness (2%)

Respiratory: Sinusitis (2%)

Miscellaneous: Viral infection (4%)

<1%: Significant SGOT, SGPT, alkaline phosphatase, and GT changes have been reported rarely

Postmarketing and/or case reports: Allergic reaction, dyspnea, hypotension, lightheadedness, loss of consciousness, MI, ruptured ectopic pregnancy, bacterial infection, postabortal infection, sepsis, septic shock, tachycardia

In trials for unresectable meningioma, the most common adverse effects included fatigue, hot flashes, gynecomastia or breast tenderness, hair thinning, and rash. In premenopausal women, vaginal bleeding may be seen shortly after beginning therapy and cessation of menses is common. Thyroiditis and effects related to antiglucocorticoid activity have also been noted.

Vesicant No

Emetic Potential Mild

Overdosage/Toxicology In studies using 3 times the recommended dose for termination of pregnancy, no serious maternal adverse effects were reported. This medication is supplied in single-dose containers to be given under physician supervision, therefore, the risk of overdose should be low. In case of massive ingestion, treat symptomatically and monitor for signs of adrenal failure.

Drug Interactions

Cytochrome P450 Effect: Substrate of CYP3A4 (minor); **Inhibits** CYP2D6 (weak), 3A4 (weak)

Increased Effect/Toxicity: There are no reported interactions. It might be anticipated that the concurrent administration of mifepristone and a progestin would result in an attenuation of the effects of one or both agents.

Ethanol/Nutrition/Herb Interactions

Food: Do not take with grapefruit juice; grapefruit juice may inhibit mifepristone metabolism leading to increased levels.

Herb/Nutraceutical: Avoid St John's wort (may induce mifepristone metabolism, leading to decreased levels).

Storage/Stability Store at room temperature of 25°C (77°F).

Pharmacodynamics/Kinetics

Protein binding: 98% to albumin and α_1-acid glycoprotein

Metabolism: Hepatic via CYP3A4 to three metabolites (may possess some antiprogestin and antiglucocorticoid activity)

(Continued)

Mifepristone *(Continued)*

Half-life elimination: Terminal: 18 hours following a slower phase where 50% eliminated between 12-72 hours

Time to peak: 90 minutes

Excretion: Feces (83%); urine (9%)

Dosage Oral:

Adults:

Termination of pregnancy: Treatment consists of three office visits by the patient; the patient must read medication guide and sign patient agreement prior to treatment:

Day 1: 600 mg (three 200 mg tablets) taken as a single dose under physician supervision

Day 3: Patient must return to the healthcare provider 2 days following administration of mifepristone; if termination of pregnancy cannot be confirmed using ultrasound or clinical examination: 400 mcg (two 200 mcg tablets) of misoprostol; patient may need treatment for cramps or gastrointestinal symptoms at this time

Day 14: Patient must return to the healthcare provider ~14 days after administration of mifepristone; confirm complete termination of pregnancy by ultrasound or clinical exam. Surgical termination is recommended to manage treatment failures.

Meningioma (unlabeled use): Refer to individual protocols. The dose used in meningioma is usually 200 mg/day, continued based on toxicity and response.

Elderly: Safety and efficacy have not been established

Dosage adjustment in renal impairment: Safety and efficacy have not been established

Dosage adjustment in hepatic impairment: Safety and efficacy have not been established; use with caution due to CYP3A4 metabolism

Administration Orally once daily

Dosage Forms Tablet: 200 mg

Monitoring Parameters Clinical exam and/or ultrasound to confirm complete termination of pregnancy; hemoglobin, hematocrit, and red blood cell count in cases of heavy bleeding

Patient Information This medication is used to terminate pregnancy. It is not to be used for pregnancies >49 days (7 weeks). Vaginal bleeding and cramping are expected to occur and may require medical treatment if severe. Most women report that this is heavier bleeding than experienced during a heavy menstrual period. Other side effects that may be expected include abdominal pain, nausea, vomiting, and diarrhea. Follow-up with prescriber at approximately 3 days and 14 days following initial treatment. Surgical termination of pregnancy may be required if medication fails. There is a risk of fetal malformation if treatment fails. Your prescriber will give you a phone number to call for problems, questions, or emergencies; you should not use this medication if you do not have access to emergency care. It is possible to become pregnant again following treatment with this medication but before your next period starts. Contraception should be started once the pregnancy's end has been proven and before resuming sexual intercourse. You will be given a medication guide to help you understand this medication and its effects. It is important to review this carefully. Ask any questions you may have. You will also be required to sign a form saying that you understand the effects of this treatment and are able to return to the prescriber for follow-up appointments. Do not breast feed while using this medication.

Additional Information Medication will be distributed directly to qualified physicians following signed agreement with the distributor, Danco Laboratories. It will not be available through pharmacies.

Selected Readings
Spitz IM and Bardin CW, "Mifepristone (RU486) - A Modulator of Progestin and Glucocorticoid Action," *N Engl J Med*, 1993, 329(6):404-12.

♦ **Milliequivalent and Millimole Calculations and Conversions** *see page 1042*

♦ **Minim's Gentamicin 0.3% (Can)** *see Gentamicin on page 398*

♦ **Minirin® (Can)** *see Desmopressin on page 259*

Mitomycin (mye toe MYE sin)

Medication Safety Issues
Sound-alike/look-alike issues:
Mitomycin may be confused with mithramycin, mitotane, mitoxantrone, Mutamycin®
Mutamycin® may be confused with mitomycin

Related Information
Management of Drug Extravasations *on page 965*
Safe Handling of Hazardous Drugs *on page 1034*

U.S. Brand Names Mutamycin®

Canadian Brand Names Mutamycin®

Generic Available Yes

Synonyms Mitomycin-C; Mitomycin-X; MTC; NSC-26980

Pharmacologic Category Antineoplastic Agent, Antibiotic

Pregnancy Risk Factor D

Lactation Enters breast milk/contraindicated

Use Treatment of adenocarcinoma of stomach or pancreas, bladder cancer, breast cancer, or colorectal cancer

Unlabeled/Investigational Use Prevention of excess scarring in glaucoma filtration procedures in patients at high risk of bleb failure

Mechanism of Action Acts like an alkylating agent and produces DNA cross-linking (primarily with guanine and cytosine pairs); cell-cycle nonspecific; inhibits DNA and RNA synthesis; degrades preformed DNA, causes nuclear lysis and formation of giant cells. While not phase-specific *per se*, mitomycin has its maximum effect against cells in late G and early S phases.

Labeled Contraindications Hypersensitivity to mitomycin or any component of the formulation; thrombocytopenia; coagulation disorders; increased bleeding tendency; pregnancy

Warnings/Precautions Hazardous agent - use appropriate precautions for handling and disposal. See Safe Handling of Hazardous Drugs *on page 1034* in the Appendix. Use with caution in patients who have received radiation therapy or in the presence of hepatobiliary dysfunction; reduce dosage in patients who are receiving radiation therapy simultaneously. Hemolytic-uremic syndrome, potentially fatal, occurs in some patients receiving long-term therapy. It is correlated with total dose (single doses ≥60 mg or cumulative doses ≥50 mg/m^2) and total duration of therapy (>5-11 months). **Mitomycin is a potent vesicant, may cause ulceration, necrosis, cellulitis, and tissue sloughing if infiltrated.**
(Continued)

Mitomycin *(Continued)*

Adverse Reactions

>10%:

Cardiovascular: CHF (3% to 15%) (doses >30 mg/m^2)

Central nervous system: Fever (14%)

Dermatologic: Alopecia, nail banding/discoloration

Gastrointestinal: Nausea, vomiting and anorexia (14%)

Hematologic: Anemia (19% to 24%); myelosuppression, common, dose-limiting, delayed

Onset: 3 weeks

Nadir: 4-6 weeks

Recovery: 6-8 weeks

1% to 10%:

Dermatologic: Rash

Gastrointestinal: Stomatitis

Neuromuscular: Paresthesias

Renal: Creatinine increased (2%)

Respiratory: Interstitial pneumonitis, infiltrates, dyspnea, cough (7%)

<1%: Malaise, pruritus, extravasation reactions, hemolytic uremic syndrome, renal failure, bladder fibrosis/contraction (intravesical administration)

Vesicant Yes; see Management of Drug Extravasations *on page 965.*

Emetic Potential Mild (10% to 30%)

Overdosage/Toxicology Symptoms of overdose include bone marrow suppression, nausea, vomiting, and alopecia. Treatment is symptom-directed and supportive.

Drug Interactions

Increased Effect/Toxicity: *Vinca* alkaloids or doxorubicin may enhance cardiac toxicity when coadministered with mitomycin.

Ethanol/Nutrition/Herb Interactions Herb/Nutraceutical: Avoid black cohosh, dong quai in estrogen-dependent tumors.

Storage/Stability Store intact vials at controlled room temperature. Mitomycin solution is stable for 7 days at room temperature and 14 days when refrigerated if protected from light. Solution of 0.5 mg/mL in a syringe is stable for 7 days at room temperature and 14 days when refrigerated and protected from light.

Further dilution to 20-40 mcg/mL:

In normal saline: Stable for 12 hours at room temperature.

In sodium lactate: Stable for 24 hours at room temperature.

Reconstitution Dilute powder with SWFI or 0.9% sodium chloride to a concentration of 0.5-1 mg/mL.

Compatibility Stable in LR; **variable stability (consult detailed reference)** in D$_5$W, NS

Y-site administration: Compatible: Amifostine, bleomycin, cisplatin, cyclophosphamide, doxorubicin, droperidol, fluorouracil, furosemide, granisetron, heparin, leucovorin, melphalan, methotrexate, metoclopramide, ondansetron, teniposide, thiotepa, vinblastine, vincristine. **Incompatible:** Aztreonam, cefepime, etoposide phosphate, filgrastim, gemcitabine, piperacillin/tazobactam, sargramostim, topotecan, vinorelbine

Compatibility in syringe: Compatible: Bleomycin, cisplatin, cyclophos-phamide, doxorubicin, droperidol, fluorouracil, furosemide, heparin, leucovorin, methotrexate, metoclopramide, vinblastine, vincristine

Compatibility when admixed: Compatible: Dexamethasone sodium phosphate, hydrocortisone sodium succinate. **Incompatible:** Bleo-mycin. **Variable (consult detailed reference):** Heparin

Pharmacodynamics/Kinetics

Distribution: V_d: 22 L/m²; high drug concentrations found in kidney, tongue, muscle, heart, and lung tissue; probably not distributed into the CNS

Metabolism: Hepatic

Half-life elimination: 23-78 minutes; Terminal: 50 minutes

Excretion: Urine (<10% as unchanged drug), with elevated serum concentrations

Dosage Refer to individual protocols. Children and Adults:

Single agent therapy: I.V.: 20 mg/m² every 6-8 weeks

Combination therapy: I.V.: 10 mg/m² every 6-8 weeks

Bladder carcinoma: Intravesicular instillation (unapproved route): 20-40 mg/dose instilled into the bladder for 3 hours repeated up to 3 times/week for up to 20 procedures per course

Glaucoma surgery (unlabeled use): Dosages and techniques vary; 0.2-0.5 mg may be applied to a pledget (using a 0.2-0.5 mg/mL solu-tion), and placed in contact with the surgical wound for 2-5 minutes; other protocols have been reported

Dosage adjustment in renal impairment: Varying approaches to dosing adjustments have been published; one representative recommenda-tion: Cl_{cr} <10 mL/minute: Administer 75% of normal dose

Note: The manufacturers state that products should not be given to patients with serum creatinine >1.7 mg/dL.

Hemodialysis: Unknown

CAPD effects: Unknown

CAVH effects: Unknown

Dosage adjustment in hepatic impairment: Although some mitomycin may be excreted in the bile, no specific guidelines regarding dosage adjustment in hepatic impairment can be made.

Combination Regimens

Gastric cancer: FAM *on page 885*

Pancreatic cancer: FAM *on page 885*

Administration Administer slow I.V. push or by slow (15-30 minute) infusion via a freely-running dextrose or saline infusion. Consider using a central venous catheter.

Dosage Forms Injection, powder for reconstitution (Mutamycin®): 5 mg, 20 mg, 40 mg

Monitoring Parameters Platelet count, CBC with differential, hemo-globin, prothrombin time, renal and pulmonary function tests

Patient Information Make note of scheduled return dates. You may experience, rash, skin lesions, loss of hair, or permanent sterility. Small frequent meals may help if you experience nausea, vomiting, or loss of appetite. Frequent mouth care will help reduce the incidence of mouth sores. Use caution when driving or engaging in tasks that require alert-ness because you may experience dizziness, drowsiness, syncope, or blurred vision. Report difficulty breathing, swelling of extremities, or sudden weight gain; burning, pain, or redness at infusion site; unusual (Continued)

Mitomycin *(Continued)*

bruising or bleeding; pain on urination; or other adverse effects. The drug may be excreted in breast milk, therefore, an alternative form of feeding your baby should be used. Contraceptive measures are recommended during therapy.

Selected Readings

Bradner WT, "Mitomycin C: A Clinical Update," *Cancer Treat Rev*, 2001, 27(1):35-50.

Gibson NW, Phillips M, and Ross D, "Mitomycin C," *Cancer Chemother Biol Response Modif*, 1994, 15:51-7.

Rodriguez JA, Ferrari C, and Hernandez GA, "Intraoperative Application of Topical Mitomycin C 0.05% for Pterygium Surgery," *Bol Asoc Med P R*, 2004, 96(2):100-2.

Verweij J and Pinedo HM, "Mitomycin C: Mechanism of Action, Usefulness and Limitations," *Anticancer Drugs*, 1990, 1(1):5-13.

Wilkins M, Indar A, and Wormald R, "Intra-Operative Mitomycin C for Glaucoma Surgery," *Cochrane Database Syst Rev*, 2001, (1):CD002897.

♦ **Mitomycin-C** *see* Mitomycin *on page 579*

♦ **Mitomycin-X** *see* Mitomycin *on page 579*

Mitotane (MYE toe tane)

Medication Safety Issues

Sound-alike/look-alike issues:

Mitotane may be confused with mitomycin

Related Information

Safe Handling of Hazardous Drugs *on page 1034*

U.S. Brand Names Lysodren®

Canadian Brand Names Lysodren®

Generic Available No

Synonyms NSC-38721; o,p'-DDD

Pharmacologic Category Antineoplastic Agent, Miscellaneous

Pregnancy Risk Factor C

Lactation Enters breast milk/contraindicated

Use Treatment of adrenocortical carcinoma

Unlabeled/Investigational Use Treatment of Cushing's syndrome

Mechanism of Action Causes adrenal cortical atrophy; drug affects mitochondria in adrenal cortical cells and decreases production of cortisol; also alters the peripheral metabolism of steroids

Labeled Contraindications Hypersensitivity to mitotane or any component of the formulation

Warnings/Precautions Hazardous agent - use appropriate precautions for handling and disposal. See Safe Handling of Hazardous Drugs *on page 1034* in the Appendix. Steroid replacement with glucocorticoid, and sometimes mineralocorticoid, is necessary. It has been recommended that replacement therapy be initiated at the start of therapy, rather than waiting for evidence of adrenal insufficiency. Because mitotane can increase the metabolism of hydrocortisone, higher than usual replacement doses of the latter may be required. Acute adrenal insufficiency may occur in the face of shock, trauma, or infection. Mitotane should be discontinued temporarily in this setting and appropriate steroid coverage should be administered.

Adverse Reactions

>10%:

Central nervous system: CNS depression (32%), dizziness (15%)

Dermatologic: Skin rash (12%)

Gastrointestinal: Anorexia (24%), nausea (39%), vomiting (37%), diarrhea (13%)

Neuromuscular & skeletal: Weakness (12%)

1% to 10%:

Central nervous system: Headache (5%), confusion (3%)

Neuromuscular & skeletal: Muscle tremor (3%)

Emetic Potential Moderate (30% to 60%)

Overdosage/Toxicology Symptoms of overdose include diarrhea, vomiting, numbness of limbs, and weakness. Treatment is symptom-directed and supportive.

Drug Interactions

Increased Effect/Toxicity: CNS depressants taken with mitotane may enhance CNS depression.

Decreased Effect: Mitotane may enhance the clearance of barbiturates and warfarin by induction of the hepatic microsomal enzyme system resulting in a decreased effect. Coadministration of spironolactone has resulted in negation of mitotane's effect. Mitotane may increase clearance of phenytoin by microsomal enzyme stimulation.

Ethanol/Nutrition/Herb Interactions Ethanol: Avoid ethanol (may increase CNS depression).

Storage/Stability Protect from light. Store at room temperature.

Pharmacodynamics/Kinetics

Absorption: Oral: ~35% to 40%

Distribution: Stored mainly in fat tissue but is found in all body tissues

Metabolism: Hepatic and other tissues

Half-life elimination: 18-159 days

Time to peak, serum: 3-5 hours

Excretion: Urine and feces (as metabolites)

Dosage Oral:

Children: 0.1-0.5 mg/kg or 1-2 g/day in divided doses increasing gradually to a maximum of 5-7 g/day

Adults: Start at 1-6 g/day in divided doses, then increase incrementally to 8-10 g/day in 3-4 divided doses (maximum daily dose: 18 g)

Dosing adjustment in hepatic impairment: Dose may need to be decreased in patients with liver disease

Dosage Forms Tablet [scored]: 500 mg

Patient Information Desired effects of this drug may not be seen for 2-3 months. Wear identification that alerts medical personnel that you are taking this drug in event of shock or trauma. Maintain adequate hydration (2-3 L/day of fluids unless instructed to restrict fluid intake) and nutrition. May cause dizziness and vertigo (avoid driving or performing tasks requiring alertness until response to drug is known); nausea, vomiting, or loss of appetite (small frequent meals, frequent mouth care, sucking lozenges, or chewing gum may help); orthostatic hypotension (use caution when rising from sitting or lying position or climbing stairs); muscle aches or pain (if severe, request medication from prescriber). Report severe vomiting or acute loss of appetite, muscular twitching, fever or infection, blood in urine or pain on urinating, or darkening of skin. Contraceptive measures are recommended during therapy.

Mitoxantrone (mye toe ZAN trone)

Medication Safety Issues
Sound-alike/look-alike issues:
Mitoxantrone may be confused with methotrexate, mitomycin

Related Information
Safe Handling of Hazardous Drugs *on page 1034*
Transplantation *on page 1019*

U.S. Brand Names Novantrone®

Canadian Brand Names Novantrone®

Generic Available No

Synonyms DAD; DHAD; DHAQ; Dihydroxyanthracenedione Dihydrochloride; Mitoxantrone Hydrochloride CL-232315; Mitozantrone; NSC-301739

Pharmacologic Category Antineoplastic Agent, Anthracenedione

Pregnancy Risk Factor D

Lactation Enters breast milk/contraindicated

Use Treatment of acute leukemias, lymphoma, breast cancer, pediatric sarcoma, progressive or relapsing-remitting multiple sclerosis, prostate cancer

Mechanism of Action Analogue of the anthracyclines, mitoxantrone intercalates DNA; binds to nucleic acids and inhibits DNA and RNA synthesis by template disordering and steric obstruction; replication is decreased by binding to DNA topoisomerase II and seems to inhibit the incorporation of uridine into RNA and thymidine into DNA; active throughout entire cell cycle

Labeled Contraindications Hypersensitivity to mitoxantrone or any component of the formulation; multiple sclerosis with left ventricular ejection fraction (LVEF) <50% or clinically significant decrease in LVEF; pregnancy

Warnings/Precautions Hazardous agent - use appropriate precautions for handling and disposal. See Safe Handling of Hazardous Drugs *on page 1034* in the Appendix.

Dosage should be reduced in patients with impaired hepatobiliary function; not for treatment of multiple sclerosis in patients with concurrent hepatic impairment. Treatment may lead to severe myelosuppression; use with caution in patients with pre-existing myelosuppression. Do not use if baseline neutrophil count <1500 cells/mm^3 (except for treatment of ANLL). May cause myocardial toxicity and potentially-fatal CHF; risk increases with cumulative dosing. Predisposing factors for mitoxantrone-induced cardiotoxicity include prior anthracycline therapy, prior cardiovascular disease, and mediastinal irradiation. Not for treatment of primary progressive multiple sclerosis. Has been associated with the development of secondary acute myelogenous leukemia and myelodysplasia. May cause urine, saliva, tears, and sweat to turn blue-green for 24 hours postinfusion. Whites of eyes may have blue-green tinge.

Adverse Reactions Reported with any indication; incidence varies based on treatment/dose
>10%:
Cardiovascular: Arrhythmia (3% to 18%), edema, nail bed changes
Central nervous system: Fatigue, fever, headache (6% to 13%)
Dermatologic: Alopecia (20% to 61%)
Endocrine & metabolic: Amenorrhea, menstrual disorder

Gastrointestinal: Abdominal pain, anorexia, nausea (29% to 76%), constipation, diarrhea (16% to 47%), GI bleeding, mucositis (10% to 29%), stomatitis, vomiting, weight gain/loss

Genitourinary: Abnormal urine, urinary tract infection

Hematologic: Hemoglobin decreased, leukopenia, lymphopenia, petechiae/bruising; myelosuppressive effects of chemotherapy:

WBC: Mild

Platelets: Mild

Onset: 7-10 days

Nadir: 14 days

Recovery: 21 days

Hepatic: Increased GGT

Neuromuscular & skeletal: Weakness (24%)

Respiratory: Cough, dyspnea, upper respiratory tract infection

Miscellaneous: Fungal infection, infection, sepsis

1% to 10%:

Cardiovascular: CHF (2% to 3%; risk is much lower with anthracyclines, some reports suggest cumulative doses >160 mg/mL cause CHF in ~10% of patients), ECG changes, hypotension, ischemia, LVEF decreased (≤5%)

Central nervous system: Chills, anxiety, depression, seizure

Dermatologic: Skin infection

Endocrine & metabolic: Hypocalcemia, hypokalemia, hyponatremia, hyperglycemia

Gastrointestinal: Dyspepsia, aphthosis

Genitourinary: Impotence, proteinuria, renal failure, sterility

Hematologic: Anemia, granulocytopenia, hemorrhage

Hepatic: Jaundice, increased SGOT, increased SGPT

Neuromuscular & skeletal: Back pain, myalgia, arthralgia

Ocular: Blurred vision, conjunctivitis

Renal: Hematuria

Respiratory: Pneumonia, rhinitis, sinusitis

Miscellaneous: Systemic infection, sweats, development of secondary leukemia (~1% to 2%)

<1% or frequency not defined: Acute leukemia, allergic reaction, anaphylactoid reactions, anaphylaxis, extravasation and phlebitis at the infusion site, interstitial pneumonitis (has occurred during combination chemotherapy), irritant chemotherapy with blue skin discoloration, rash, tachycardia

Vesicant No; may be an irritant

Emetic Potential Moderate (30% to 60%)

Overdosage/Toxicology Symptoms of overdose include leukopenia, tachycardia, and marrow hypoplasia. No known antidote. Treatment is symptom-directed and supportive.

Drug Interactions

Cytochrome P450 Effect: Inhibits CYP3A4 (weak)

Decreased Effect: Patients may experience impaired immune response to vaccines; possible infection after administration of live vaccines in patients receiving immunosuppressants.

Ethanol/Nutrition/Herb Interactions Herb/Nutraceutical: Avoid black cohosh, dong quai in estrogen-dependent tumors.

Storage/Stability Store intact vials at 15°C to 25°C (59°F to 77°F); do not freeze. Opened vials may be stored at room temperature for 7 days or (Continued)

Mitoxantrone *(Continued)*

under refrigeration for up to 14 days. Solutions diluted for administration are stable for 7 days at room temperature or under refrigeration.

Reconstitution Dilute in at least 50 mL of NS or D_5W.

Compatibility Stable in in D_5NS, D_5W, NS

Y-site administration: Compatible: Allopurinol, amifostine, cladribine, etoposide phosphate, filgrastim, fludarabine, gatifloxacin, gemcitabine, granisetron, linezolid, melphalan, ondansetron, sargramostim, teniposide, thiotepa, vinorelbine. **Incompatible:** Amphotericin B cholesteryl sulfate complex, aztreonam, cefepime, doxorubicin liposome, paclitaxel, piperacillin/tazobactam, propofol

Compatibility when admixed: Compatible: Cyclophosphamide, cytarabine, fluorouracil, hydrocortisone sodium succinate, potassium chloride. **Incompatible:** Heparin. **Variable (consult detailed reference):** Hydrocortisone sodium phosphate

Pharmacodynamics/Kinetics

Absorption: Oral: Poor

Distribution: V_d: 14 L/kg; distributes into pleural fluid, kidney, thyroid, liver, heart, and red blood cells

Protein binding: >95%, 76% to albumin

Metabolism: Hepatic; pathway not determined

Half-life elimination: Terminal: 23-215 hours; may be prolonged with hepatic impairment

Excretion: Urine (6% to 11%) and feces as unchanged drug and metabolites

Dosage

Refer to individual protocols. I.V. (dilute in D_5W or NS):

Acute leukemias:

Children ≤2 years: 0.4 mg/kg/day once daily for 3-5 days

Children >2 years and Adults: 8-12 mg/m^2/day once daily for 4-5 days

Solid tumors:

Children: 18-20 mg/m^2 every 3-4 weeks **or** 5-8 mg/m^2 every week

Adults: 12-14 mg/m^2 every 3-4 weeks **or** 2-4 mg/m^2/day for 5 days every 4 weeks

Hormone-refractory prostate cancer: Adults: 12-14 mg/m^2

Multiple sclerosis: Adults: 12 mg/m^2

Dosing adjustment in renal impairment: Safety and efficacy have not been established

Hemodialysis: Supplemental dose is not necessary

Peritoneal dialysis: Supplemental dose is not necessary

Elderly: Clearance is decreased in elderly patients; use with caution

Dosing adjustment in hepatic impairment: Official dosage adjustment recommendations have not been established.

Moderate dysfunction (bilirubin 1.5-3 mg/dL): Some clinicians recommend a 50% dosage reduction

Severe dysfunction (bilirubin >3.0 mg/dL) may require a dosage adjustment to 8 mg/m^2; some clinicians recommend a dosage reduction to 25% of dose

Combination Regimens

Breast cancer:

CNF *on page 863*

NFL *on page 923*

Leukemia, acute lymphocytic: FIS-HAM *on page 889*

Leukemia, acute myeloid:
5 + 2 *on page 840*
7 + 3 (Mitoxantrone) *on page 841*
EMA 86 *on page 877*
FIS-HAM *on page 889*
MV *on page 917*
Leukemia, acute promyelocytic:
M-3 *on page 906*
Tretinoin/Idarubicin *on page 941*
Lymphoma, non-Hodgkin's:
CNOP *on page 864*
MINE *on page 909*
MINE-ESHAP *on page 909*
Prostate cancer:
Mitoxantrone + Hydrocortisone *on page 910*
MP (Prostate Cancer) *on page 916*

Administration Administered as a short (15-30 minutes) I.V. infusion; continuous 24-hour infusions are occasionally used. Although not generally recommended, mitoxantrone has been given as a rapid bolus over 1-3 minutes. High doses for bone marrow transplant are usually given as 1- to 4-hour infusions.

Dosage Forms Injection, solution: 2 mg/mL (10 mL, 12.5 mL, 15 mL)

High Dose Considerations

High Dose: I.V.: 24-48 mg/m^2 as a single dose; duration of infusion is 1-4 hours; total doses of 75-90 mg/m^2 have been used. Generally combined with other high-dose chemotherapeutic drugs.

Unique Toxicities:

Cardiovascular: Bradycardia (infusion-related), heart failure

Dermatologic: Alopecia

Gastrointestinal: Severe mucositis, skin discoloration

Comments: Extensive pretreatment with anthracyclines increases risk of cardiac toxicity.

Monitoring Parameters CBC, serum uric acid (for treatment of leukemia), liver function tests, signs and symptoms of CHF; evaluate LVEF prior to start of therapy and regularly during treatment. In addition, for the treatment of multiple sclerosis, monitor LVEF prior to all doses following cumulative dose of ≥100 mg/m^2.

Patient Information This drug can only be given I.V. Make note of scheduled return dates. Your urine may turn blue-green for 24 hours after infusion and the whites of your eyes may have a blue-green tinge; this is normal. Maintain adequate hydration (2-3 L/day of fluids unless instructed to restrict fluid intake) and nutrition. You may experience rash, skin lesions, or loss of hair. Small frequent meals may help if you experience nausea, vomiting, or loss of appetite. Frequent mouth care will help reduce the incidence of mouth sores. Use caution when driving or engaging in tasks that require alertness because you may experience dizziness, drowsiness, syncope, or blurred vision. Report chest pain or heart palpitations; difficulty breathing or constant cough; swelling of extremities or sudden weight gain; burning, pain, or redness at the I.V. infusion site; persistent fever or chills; unusual bruising or bleeding; twitching or tremors; or pain on urination. Contraceptive measures are recommended during therapy.

(Continued)

Mitoxantrone *(Continued)*

Selected Readings

Ehninger G, Schuler U, Proksch B, et al, "Pharmacokinetics and Metabolism of Mitoxantrone. A Review," *Clin Pharmacokinet*, 1990, 18(5):365-80.

Faulds D, Balfour JA, Chrisp P, et al, "Mitoxantrone. A Review of Its Pharmacodynamic and Pharmacokinetic Properties, and Therapeutic Potential in the Chemotherapy of Cancer," *Drugs*, 1991, 41(3):400-49.

Koeller J and Eble M, "Mitoxantrone: A Novel Anthracycline Derivative," *Clin Pharm*, 1988, 7(8):574-81.

Poirier TI, "Mitoxantrone," *Drug Intell Clin Pharm*, 1986, 20(2):97-105.

Scott LJ and Figgitt DP, "Mitoxantrone: A Review of its Use in Multiple Sclerosis," *CNS Drugs*, 2004, 18(6):379-96.

Shenkenberg TD and Von Hoff DD, "Mitoxantrone: A New Anticancer Drug With Significant Clinical Activity," *Ann Intern Med*, 1986, 105(1):67-81.

Wiseman LR and Spencer CM, "Mitoxantrone. A Review of its Pharmacology and Clinical Efficacy in the Management of Hormone-Resistant Advanced Prostate Cancer," *Drugs Aging*, 1997, 10(6):473-85.

- ◆ **Mitoxantrone Hydrochloride CL-232315** *see* Mitoxantrone *on page 584*
- ◆ **Mitozantrone** *see* Mitoxantrone *on page 584*
- ◆ **MK 869** *see* Aprepitant *on page 100*
- ◆ **MLN341** *see* Bortezomib *on page 138*
- ◆ **MMF** *see* Mycophenolate *on page 598*
- ◆ **Modane Tablets® [OTC]** *see* Bisacodyl *on page 133*
- ◆ **Monarc® M** *see* Antihemophilic Factor (Human) *on page 87*
- ◆ **Monoclate-P®** *see* Antihemophilic Factor (Human) *on page 87*
- ◆ **Monoclonal Antibody** *see* Muromonab-CD3 *on page 595*
- ◆ **Mononine®** *see* Factor IX *on page 327*
- ◆ **Morphine HP® (Can)** *see* Morphine Sulfate *on page 588*
- ◆ **Morphine LP® Epidural (Can)** *see* Morphine Sulfate *on page 588*

Morphine Sulfate *(MOR feen SUL fate)*

Medication Safety Issues

Sound-alike/look-alike issues:

Morphine may be confused with hydromorphone

Morphine sulfate may be confused with magnesium sulfate

Avinza™ may be confused with Evista®, Invanz®

Roxanol™ may be confused with Roxicet™

Avoid the MSO$_4$ abbreviation; errors have occurred with its use.

Use care when prescribing and/or administering morphine solutions. These products are available in different concentrations. Always prescribe dosage in mg; **not** by volume (mL).

U.S. Brand Names Astramorph/PF™; Avinza™; DepoDur™; Duramorph®; Infumorph®; Kadian®; MS Contin®; MSIR®; Oramorph SR®; RMS®; Roxanol™; Roxanol 100™; Roxanol™-T

Canadian Brand Names Kadian®; M-Eslon®; Morphine HP®; Morphine LP® Epidural; M.O.S.-Sulfate®; MS Contin®; MS-IR®; PMS-Morphine Sulfate SR; ratio-Morphine SR; Statex®

Generic Available Yes: Excludes capsule, controlled release tablet, sustained release tablet, extended release liposomal suspension for injection

Pharmacologic Category Analgesic, Narcotic

Pregnancy Risk Factor C/D (prolonged use or high doses at term)

Lactation Enters breast milk/use caution (AAP rates "compatible")

Use Relief of moderate to severe acute and chronic pain; relief of pain of myocardial infarction; relief of dyspnea of acute left ventricular failure and pulmonary edema; preanesthetic medication

DepoDur™: Epidural (lumbar) single-dose management of surgical pain

Orphan drug: Infumorph®: Used in microinfusion devices for intraspinal administration in treatment of intractable chronic pain

Mechanism of Action Binds to opiate receptors in the CNS, causing inhibition of ascending pain pathways, altering the perception of and response to pain; produces generalized CNS depression

Restrictions C-II

Labeled Contraindications Hypersensitivity to morphine sulfate or any component of the formulation; increased intracranial pressure; severe respiratory depression; acute or severe asthma; known or suspected paralytic ileus; sustained release products are not recommended in acute/postoperative pain; pregnancy (prolonged use or high doses at term)

Warnings/Precautions An opioid-containing analgesic regimen should be tailored to each patient's needs and based upon the type of pain being treated (acute versus chronic), the route of administration, degree of tolerance for opioids (naive versus chronic user), age, weight, and medical condition. The optimal analgesic dose varies widely among patients. Doses should be titrated to pain relief/prevention. When used as an epidural injection, monitor for delayed sedation.

May cause respiratory depression; use with caution in patients with impaired respiratory function or severe hepatic dysfunction and in patients with hypersensitivity reactions to other phenanthrene derivative opioid agonists (codeine, hydrocodone, hydromorphone, levorphanol, oxycodone, oxymorphone). Infants <3 months of age are more susceptible to respiratory depression, use with caution and generally in reduced doses in this age group. May cause hypotension in patients with acute myocardial infarction. Tolerance or drug dependence may result from extended use. MS Contin® 200 mg tablets are for use only in opioid-tolerant patients requiring >400 mg/day. Infumorph® solutions are **for use in microinfusion devices only**; not for I.V., I.M., or SubQ administration.

Use caution in CNS depression, toxic psychosis, delirium tremens, or convulsive disorders. Sedation and psychomotor impairment are likely, and are additive with other CNS depressants or ethanol. Extended or sustained release dosage forms should not be crushed or chewed. Controlled-, extended-, or sustained-release products are not intended for "as needed (PRN)" use. Some preparations contain sulfites which may cause allergic reactions.

Use caution in renal impairment; gastrointestinal motility disturbances, thyroid disorders (Addison's disease, myxedema, or hypothyroidism), prostatic hyperplasia, or urethral stricture.

Elderly and/or debilitated may be particularly susceptible to the CNS depressant and constipating effects of narcotics. May mask diagnosis or clinical course in patients with acute abdominal conditions.

Adverse Reactions Note: Individual patient differences are unpredictable, and percentage may differ in acute pain (surgical) treatment. (Continued)

Morphine Sulfate *(Continued)*

Frequency not defined: Flushing, CNS depression, sedation, antidiuretic hormone release, physical and psychological dependence, diaphoresis

>10%:

Cardiovascular: Palpitations, hypotension, bradycardia

Central nervous system: Drowsiness (48%, tolerance usually develops to drowsiness with regular dosing for 1-2 weeks); dizziness (20%); confusion

Dermatologic: Pruritus (may be secondary to histamine release)

Gastrointestinal: Nausea (28%, tolerance usually develops to nausea and vomiting with chronic use); constipation (40%, tolerance develops very slowly if at all); xerostomia (78%)

Genitourinary: Urinary retention (16%)

Local: Pain at injection site

Neuromuscular & skeletal: Weakness

Miscellaneous: Histamine release

1% to 10%:

Central nervous system: Restlessness, headache, false feeling of well being

Gastrointestinal: Anorexia, GI irritation, paralytic ileus, vomiting (9%)

Genitourinary: Decreased urination

Neuromuscular & skeletal: Trembling

Ocular: Vision problems

Respiratory: Respiratory depression, dyspnea

<1%: Anaphylaxis, intestinal obstruction, peripheral vasodilation, insomnia, mental depression, hallucinations, paradoxical CNS stimulation, intracranial pressure increased, biliary tract spasm, urinary tract spasm, muscle rigidity, miosis, liver function tests increased, transaminases increased

Vesicant No

Emetic Potential High (60% to 90%)

Overdosage/Toxicology Symptoms of overdose include respiratory depression, miosis, hypotension, bradycardia, apnea, and pulmonary edema. Treatment is symptomatic. Naloxone, 2 mg I.V. with repeat administration as necessary up to a total dose of 10 mg, can be used to reverse opiate effects.

Drug Interactions

Cytochrome P450 Effect: Substrate of CYP2D6 (minor)

Increased Effect/Toxicity: CNS depressants (phenothiazines, tranquilizers, anxiolytics, sedatives, hypnotics, or alcohol), tricyclic antidepressants may potentiate the effects of morphine and other opiate agonists. Dextroamphetamine may enhance the analgesic effect of morphine and other opiate agonists. Concurrent use of MAO inhibitors and meperidine has been associated with significant adverse effects. Use caution with morphine. Some manufacturers recommend avoiding use within 14 days of MAO inhibitors.

Decreased Effect: Diuretic effects may be decreased (due to antidiuretic hormone release).

Ethanol/Nutrition/Herb Interactions

Ethanol: Avoid ethanol (may increase CNS depression).

Food: Administration of oral morphine solution with food may increase bioavailability (ie, a report of 34% increase in morphine AUC when morphine oral solution followed a high-fat meal). The bioavailability of Oramorph SR® does not appear to be affected by food.

Herb/Nutraceutical: Avoid valerian, St John's wort, kava kava, gotu kola (may increase CNS depression).

Storage/Stability

Suppositories: Store at controlled room temperature 25°C (77°F). Protect from light.

Injection: Store at controlled room temperature. Protect from light. Degradation depends on pH and presence of oxygen; relatively stable in pH ≤4; darkening of solutions indicate degradation.

DepoDur™: Store under refrigeration, 2°C to 8°C (36°F to 46°F). Do not freeze. May store at room temperature for up to 7 days. Once vial is opened, use within 4 hours.

Reconstitution Usual concentration for continuous I.V. infusion: 0.1-1 mg/mL in D_5W. DepoDur™ may be diluted in preservative-free NS to a volume of 5 mL.

Compatibility Stable in dextran 6% in dextrose, dextran 6% in NS, D_5LR, $D_5^1/_4NS$, $D_5^1/_2NS$, D_5NS, D_5W, $D_{10}W$, LR, $^1/_2NS$, NS; **variable stability (consult detailed reference)** in TPN

Y-site administration: Compatible: Allopurinol, amifostine, amikacin, aminophylline, amiodarone, ampicillin, ampicillin/sulbactam, amsacrine, atenolol, atracurium, aztreonam, bumetanide, calcium chloride, cefamandole, cefazolin, cefoperazone, cefotaxime, cefotetan, cefoxitin, ceftazidime, ceftizoxime, ceftriaxone, cefuroxime, chloramphenicol, cisatracurium, cisplatin, cladribine, clindamycin, co-trimoxazole, cyclophosphamide, cytarabine, dexamethasone sodium phosphate, digoxin, diltiazem, dobutamine, docetaxel, dopamine, doxorubicin, doxycycline, enalaprilat, epinephrine, erythromycin lactobionate, esmolol, etomidate, etoposide phosphate, famotidine, fentanyl, filgrastim, fluconazole, fludarabine, foscarnet, gatifloxacin, gemcitabine, gentamicin, granisetron, heparin, hydrocortisone sodium succinate, hydromorphone, IL-2, insulin (regular), kanamycin, labetalol, levofloxacin, lidocaine, linezolid, lorazepam, magnesium sulfate, melphalan, meropenem, methotrexate, methyldopa, methylprednisolone sodium succinate, metoclopramide, metoprolol, metronidazole, midazolam, milrinone, nafcillin, nicardipine, nitroglycerin, norepinephrine, ondansetron, oxacillin, oxytocin, paclitaxel, pancuronium, penicillin G potassium, piperacillin, piperacillin/tazobactam, potassium chloride, propofol, propranolol, ranitidine, remifentanil, sodium bicarbonate, sodium nitroprusside, tacrolimus, teniposide, thiotepa, ticarcillin, ticarcillin/clavulanate, tobramycin, vancomycin, vecuronium, vinorelbine, vitamin B complex with C, warfarin, zidovudine. Incompatible: Alatrofloxacin, amphotericin B cholesteryl sulfate complex, cefepime, doxorubicin liposome, minocycline, sargramostim. Variable (consult detailed reference): Acyclovir, furosemide, thiopental, TPN

Compatibility in syringe: Compatible: Atropine, bupivacaine, bupivacaine with clonidine, butorphanol, cimetidine, dimenhydrinate, diphenhydramine, droperidol, fentanyl, glycopyrrolate, hydroxyzine, hyoscine, ketamine, ketamine with lidocaine, metoclopramide, midazolam, milrinone, ondansetron, pentazocine, perphenazine, promazine, ranitidine, Sthf067200albuterol, scopolamine. Incompatible: Meperidine, thiopental. Variable (consult detailed reference): Chlorpromazine, haloperidol, heparin, pentobarbital, prochlorperazine edisylate, promethazine

(Continued)

Morphine Sulfate *(Continued)*

Compatibility when admixed: Compatible: Alteplase, atracurium, baclofen, bupivacaine, dobutamine, fluconazole, furosemide, ketamine, meropenem, metoclopramide, ondansetron, succinylcholine, verapamil. **Incompatible:** Aminophylline, amobarbital, chlorothiazide, floxacillin, fluorouracil, heparin, meperidine, phenobarbital, phenytoin, sodium bicarbonate, thiopental

DepoDur™: Do not mix with other medications.

Pharmacodynamics/Kinetics

Onset of action: Oral: 1 hour; I.V.: 5-10 minutes

Duration: Pain relief:

Immediate release formulations: 4 hours

Extended release epidural injection (DepoDur™): >48 hours

Absorption: Variable

Distribution: Binds to opioid receptors in the CNS and periphery (eg, GI tract)

Metabolism: Hepatic via conjugation with glucuronic acid to morphine-3-glucuronide (inactive), morphine-6-glucuronide (active), and in lesser amounts, morphine-3-6-diglucuronide; other minor metabolites include normorphine (active) and the 3-ethereal sulfate

Bioavailability: Oral: 17% to 33% (first-pass effect limits oral bioavailability; oral:parenteral effectiveness reportedly varies from 1:6 in opioid naive patients to 1:3 with chronic use)

Half-life elimination: Adults: 2-4 hours (immediate release forms)

Excretion: Urine (primarily as morphine-3-glucuronide, ~2% to 12% excreted unchanged); feces (~7% to 10%). It has been suggested that accumulation of morphine-6-glucuronide might cause toxicity with renal insufficiency. All of the metabolites (ie, morphine-3-glucuronide, morphine-6-glucuronide, and normorphine) have been suggested as possible causes of neurotoxicity (eg, myoclonus).

Dosage Note: These are guidelines and do not represent the doses that may be required in some patients. Doses should be titrated to pain relief/prevention.

Children >6 months and <50 kg: Acute pain (moderate-to-severe):

Oral (prompt release): 0.15-0.3 mg/kg every 3-4 hours as needed

I.M.: 0.1 mg/kg every 3-4 hours as needed

I.V.: 0.05-0.1 mg/kg every 3-4 hours as needed

I.V. infusion: Range: 10-30 mcg/kg/hour

Adolescents >12 years: Sedation/analgesia for procedures: I.V.: 3-4 mg and repeat in 5 minutes if necessary

Adults: Acute pain (moderate-to-severe):

Oral: Prompt release formulations: Opiate-naive: Initial: 10 mg every 3-4 hours as needed; patients with prior opiate exposure may require higher initial doses: usual dosage range: 10-30 mg every 3-4 hours as needed

Oral: Controlled-, extended-, or sustained-release formulations: **Note:** A patient's morphine requirement should be established using prompt-release formulations. Conversion to long-acting products may be considered when chronic, continuous treatment is required. Higher dosages should be reserved for use only in opioid-tolerant patients.

Capsules, extended release (Avinza™): Daily dose administered once daily (for best results, administer at same time each day)

Capsules, sustained release (Kadian®): Daily dose administered once daily or in 2 divided doses daily (every 12 hours)

Tablets, controlled release (MS Contin®), sustained release (Oramorph SR®), or extended release: Daily dose divided and administered every 8 or every 12 hours

I.V.: Initial: Opiate-naive: 2.5-5 mg every 3-4 hours; patients with prior opiate exposure may require higher initial doses. **Note:** Repeated doses (up to every 5 minutes if needed) in small increments (eg, 1-4 mg) may be preferred to larger and less frequent doses.

I.V., SubQ continuous infusion: 0.8-10 mg/hour; usual range: Up to 80 mg/hour

Mechanically-ventilated patients (based on 70 kg patient): 0.7-10 mg every 1-2 hours as needed; infusion: 5-35 mg/hour

Patient-controlled analgesia (PCA): (Opiate-naive: Consider lower end of dosing range):

Usual concentration: 1 mg/mL

Demand dose: Usual: 1 mg; range: 0.5-2.5 mg

Lockout interval: 5-10 minutes

Epidural: **Note:** Administer with extreme caution and in reduced dosage to geriatric or debilitated patients.

Infusion:

Bolus dose: 1-6 mg

Infusion rate: 0.1-1 mg/hour

Maximum dose: 10 mg/24 hours

Single-dose (extended release, Depo-Dur™):

Cesarean section: 10 mg

Lower abdominal/pelvic surgery: 10-15 mg

Note: Some patients may benefit from a 20 mg dose, however, the incidence of adverse effects may be increased.

Intrathecal (I.T.): One-tenth of epidural dose; **Note:** Administer with extreme caution and in reduced dosage to geriatric or debilitated patients.

Opiate-naive: 0.2-1 mg/dose (may provide adequate relief for 24 hours); repeat doses **not** recommended except to establish initial IT dose.

I.M., SubQ: **Note:** Repeated SubQ administration causes local tissue irritation, pain, and induration.

Initial: Opiate-naive: 5-10 mg every 3-4 hours as needed; patients with prior opiate exposure may require higher initial doses; usual dosage range: 5-20 mg every 3-4 hours as needed

Rectal: 10-20 mg every 3-4 hours

Chronic pain: Patients taking opioids chronically may become tolerant and require doses higher than the usual dosage range to maintain the desired effect. Tolerance can be managed by appropriate dose titration. There is no optimal or maximal dose for morphine in chronic pain. The appropriate dose is one that relieves pain throughout its dosing interval without causing unmanageable side effects.

Elderly or debilitated patients: Use with caution; may require dose reduction

Dosing adjustment in renal impairment:

Cl_{cr} 10-50 mL/minute: Administer at 75% of normal dose

Cl_{cr} <10 mL/minute: Administer at 50% of normal dose

(Continued)

Morphine Sulfate *(Continued)*

Dosing adjustment/comments in hepatic disease: Unchanged in mild liver disease; substantial extrahepatic metabolism may occur; excessive sedation may occur in cirrhosis

Administration

Oral: Do not crush controlled release drug product, swallow whole. Kadian® can be opened and sprinkled on applesauce. Avinza™ can also be opened and sprinkled on applesauce; do not crush or chew the beads. Administration of oral morphine solution with food may increase bioavailability (not observed with Oramorph SR®).

I.V.: When giving morphine I.V. push, it is best to first dilute in 4-5 mL of sterile water, and then to administer slowly (eg, 15 mg over 3-5 minutes)

Epidural or intrathecal: Use preservative-free solutions

Dosage Forms

Capsule (MSIR®): 15 mg, 30 mg

Capsule, extended release (Avinza™): 30 mg, 60 mg, 90 mg, 120 mg

Capsule, sustained release (Kadian®): 20 mg, 30 mg, 50 mg, 60 mg, 100 mg

Infusion [premixed in D_5W]: 0.2 mg/mL (250 mL, 500 mL); 1 mg/mL (100 mL, 250 mL, 500 mL)

Injection, extended release liposomal suspension [lumbar epidural injection, preservative free] (DepoDur™): 10 mg/mL (1 mL, 1.5 mL, 2 mL)

Injection, solution: 2 mg/mL (1 mL); 4 mg/mL (1 mL); 5 mg/mL (1 mL); 8 mg/mL (1 mL); 10 mg/mL (1 mL, 2 mL, 10 mL); 15 mg/mL (1 mL, 20 mL); 25 mg/mL (4 mL, 10 mL, 20 mL, 40 mL) [some preparations contain sodium metabisulfite]

Injection, solution [epidural, intrathecal, or I.V. infusion; preservative free]:
Astramorph/PF™: 0.5 mg/mL (2 mL, 10 mL); 1 mg/mL (2 mL, 10 mL)
Duramorph®: 0.5 mg/mL (10 mL); 1 mg/mL (10 mL)

Injection, solution [epidural or intrathecal infusion via microinfusion device; preservative free] (Infumorph®): 10 mg/mL (20 mL); 25 mg/mL (20 mL)

Injection, solution [I.V. infusion via PCA pump]: 1 mg/mL (50 mL); 5 mg/mL (50 mL)

Injection, solution [preservative free]: 0.5 mg/mL (10 mL); 1 mg/mL (10 mL, 30 mL); 10 mg/mL (10 mL); 15 mg/mL (20 mL); 25 mg/mL (4 mL, 10 mL, 20 mL); 50 mg/mL (10 mL, 20 mL, 50 mL)

Solution, oral: 10 mg/5 mL (5 mL, 10 mL, 100 mL, 500 mL); 20 mg/5 mL (100 mL, 500 mL); 20 mg/mL (30 mL, 120 mL, 240 mL)
MSIR®: 10 mg/5 mL (120 mL); 20 mg/5 mL (120 mL); 20 mg/mL (30 mL, 120 mL) [contains sodium benzoate] [DSC]
Roxanol™: 20 mg/mL (30 mL, 120 mL)
Roxanol 100™: 100 mg/5 mL (240 mL) [with calibrated spoon]
Roxanol™-T: 20 mg/mL (30 mL, 120 mL) [tinted, flavored]

Suppository, rectal (RMS®): 5 mg (12s), 10 mg (12s), 20 mg (12s), 30 mg (12s)

Tablet (MSIR®): 15 mg, 30 mg

Tablet, controlled release (MS Contin®): 15 mg, 30 mg, 60 mg, 100 mg, 200 mg

Tablet, extended release: 15 mg, 30 mg, 60 mg, 100 mg, 200 mg

Tablet, sustained release (Oramorph SR®): 15 mg, 30 mg, 60 mg, 100 mg

Monitoring Parameters Pain relief, respiratory and mental status, blood pressure

Infumorph®: Patients should be observed in a fully-equipped and staffed environment for at least 24 hours following initiation, and as appropriate for the first several days after catheter implantation.

Dietary Considerations Morphine may cause GI upset; take with food if GI upset occurs. Be consistent when taking morphine with or without meals.

Patient Information Avoid alcohol, may cause drowsiness, impaired judgment or coordination; may cause physical and psychological dependence with prolonged use

Special Geriatric Considerations The elderly may be particularly susceptible to the CNS depressant and constipating effects of narcotics. For chronic administration of narcotic analgesics, morphine is preferable in the elderly due to its pharmacokinetics and side effect profile as compared to meperidine and methadone.

Selected Readings

Mignault GG, Latreille J, Viguie F, et al, "Control of Cancer-Related Pain With MS Contin: A Comparison Between 12-Hourly and 8-Hourly Administration," *J Pain Symptom Manage*, 1995, 10(6):416-22.

♦ **M.O.S.-Sulfate**® **(Can)** *see* Morphine Sulfate *on page 588*

♦ **6-MP** *see* Mercaptopurine *on page 539*

♦ **MPA** *see* MedroxyPROGESTERone *on page 524*

♦ **MPA** *see* Mycophenolate *on page 598*

♦ **MS Contin**® *see* Morphine Sulfate *on page 588*

♦ **MSIR**® *see* Morphine Sulfate *on page 588*

♦ **MTA** *see* Pemetrexed *on page 655*

♦ **MTC** *see* Mitomycin *on page 579*

♦ **MTX** *see* Methotrexate *on page 549*

♦ **Mucositis/Stomatitis** *see page 995*

♦ **Multitargeted Antifolate** *see* Pemetrexed *on page 655*

Muromonab-CD3 (myoo roe MOE nab see dee three)

Related Information

Safe Handling of Hazardous Drugs *on page 1034*

U.S. Brand Names Orthoclone OKT® 3

Canadian Brand Names Orthoclone OKT® 3

Generic Available No

Synonyms Monoclonal Antibody; OKT3

Pharmacologic Category Immunosuppressant Agent

Pregnancy Risk Factor C

Lactation Excretion in breast milk unknown/contraindicated

Use Treatment of acute allograft rejection in renal transplant patients; treatment of acute hepatic, kidney, and pancreas rejection episodes resistant to conventional treatment. Acute graft-versus-host disease following bone marrow transplantation resistant to conventional treatment.

Mechanism of Action Reverses graft rejection by binding to T cells and interfering with their function by binding T-cell receptor-associated CD3 glycoprotein

(Continued)

Muromonab-CD3 *(Continued)*

Labeled Contraindications Hypersensitivity to OKT3 or any murine product; patients in fluid overload or those with >3% weight gain within 1 week prior to start of OKT3; mouse antibody titers >1:1000

Warnings/Precautions It is imperative, especially prior to the first few doses, that there be no clinical evidence of volume overload, uncontrolled hypertension, or uncompensated heart failure, including a clear chest x-ray and weight restriction of ≤3% above the patient's minimum weight during the week prior to injection.

May result in an increased susceptibility to infection; dosage of concomitant immunosuppressants should be reduced during OKT3 therapy; cyclosporine should be decreased to 50% usual maintenance dose and maintenance therapy resumed about 4 days before stopping OKT3.

Severe pulmonary edema has occurred in patients with fluid overload.

First dose effect (flu-like symptoms, anaphylactic-type reaction): may occur within 30 minutes to 6 hours up to 24 hours after the first dose and may be minimized by using the recommended regimens. See table.

Suggested Prevention/Treatment of Muromonab-CD3 First-Dose Effects

Adverse Reaction	Effective Prevention or Palliation	Supportive Treatment
Severe pulmonary edema	Clear chest x-ray within 24 hours preinjection; weight restriction to ≤3% gain over 7 days preinjection	Prompt intubation and oxygenation; 24 hours close observation
Fever, chills	15 mg/kg methylprednisolone sodium succinate 1 hour preinjection; fever reduction to <37.8°C (100°F) 1 hour preinjection; acetaminophen (1 g orally) and diphenhydramine (50 mg orally) 1 hour preinjection	Cooling blanket Acetaminophen prn
Respiratory effects	100 mg hydrocortisone sodium succinate 30 minutes postinjection	Additional 100 mg hydrocortisone sodium succinate prn for wheezing; if respiratory distress, give epinephrine 1:1000 (0.3 mL SubQ)

Cardiopulmonary resuscitation may be needed. If the patient's temperature is >37.8°C, reduce before administering OKT3

Adverse Reactions

>10%:

Cardiovascular: Tachycardia (including ventricular)

Central nervous system: Chills, dizziness, faintness, headache, pyrexia

Gastrointestinal: Diarrhea, nausea, vomiting

Hematologic: Transient lymphopenia

Neuromuscular & skeletal: Tremor

Respiratory: Dyspnea

1% to 10%:
  Cardiovascular: Tachycardia, hypertension
  Central nervous system: Headache
  Neuromuscular & skeletal: Stiff neck
  Ocular: Photophobia
  Respiratory: Chest pain, pulmonary edema, wheezing
  <1%: Hypertension, hypotension, chest pain, tightness, aseptic menin-
    gitis, seizure, fatigue, confusion, coma, hallucinations, pyrexia, pruritus,
    rash, arthralgia, tremor, increased BUN and creatinine, dyspnea,
    wheezing. Sensitivity reactions: Anaphylactic-type reactions, flu-like
    symptoms (ie, fever, chills), infection, pancytopenia, secondary
    lymphoproliferative disorder or lymphoma, thrombosis of major vessels
    in renal allograft.

Vesicant No

Emetic Potential Moderate (30% to 60%)

Drug Interactions
  Increased Effect/Toxicity: Recommend decreasing dose of predni-
    sone to 0.5 mg/kg, azathioprine to 0.5 mg/kg (approximate 50%
    decrease in dose), and discontinuing cyclosporine while patient is
    receiving OKT3.
  Decreased Effect: Decreased effect with immunosuppressive drugs.

Storage/Stability Refrigerate; do not shake or freeze. Stable in Becton
Dickinson syringe for 16 hours at room temperature or refrigeration.

Pharmacodynamics/Kinetics
  Duration: 7 days after discontinuation
  Time to peak: Steady-state: Trough: 3-14 days

Dosage I.V. (refer to individual protocols):
  Children <30 kg: 2.5 mg/day once daily for 7-14 days
  Children >30 kg: 5 mg/day once daily for 7-14 days
    OR
  Children <12 years: 0.1 mg/kg/day once daily for 10-14 days
  Children ≥12 years and Adults: 5 mg/day once daily for 10-14 days
  Hemodialysis: Molecular size of OKT3 is 150,000 daltons; not dialyzed by
    most standard dialyzers; however, may be dialyzed by high flux dial-
    ysis; OKT3 will be removed by plasmapheresis; administer following
    dialysis treatments
  Peritoneal dialysis: Significant drug removal is unlikely based on physi-
    ochemical characteristics

Administration Filter each dose through a low protein-binding 0.22
micron filter (Millex GV) before administration; administer I.V. push over
<1 minute at a final concentration of 1 mg/mL

Children and Adults:
  Methylprednisolone sodium succinate 15 mg/kg I.V. administered prior
    to first muromonab-CD3 administration and I.V. hydrocortisone
    sodium succinate 50-100 mg given 30 minutes after administration
    are strongly recommended to decrease the incidence of reactions to
    the first dose
  Patient temperature should not exceed 37.8°C (100°F) at time of
    administration

Dosage Forms Injection, solution: 1 mg/mL (5 mL) [contains sodium 43
mg/5 mL]
(Continued)

Muromonab-CD3 *(Continued)*

Monitoring Parameters Chest x-ray, weight gain, CBC with differential, temperature, vital signs (blood pressure, temperature, pulse, respiration); immunologic monitoring of T cells, serum levels of OKT3

Dietary Considerations Injection solution contains sodium 43 mg/5 mL.

Patient Information Inform patient of expected first dose effects which are markedly reduced with subsequent treatments

Selected Readings

Hooks MA, Wade CS, and Millikan WJ Jr, "Muromonab CD-3: A Review of Its Pharmacology, Pharmacokinetics, and Clinical Use in Transplantation," *Pharmacotherapy*, 1991, 11(1):26-37.

Todd PA and Brogden RN, "Muromonab CD3 A Review of Its Pharmacology and Therapeutic Potential," *Drugs*, 1989, 37(6):871-99.

+ **Mustargen**® *see Mechlorethamine on page 521*
+ **Mustine** *see Mechlorethamine on page 521*
+ **Mutamycin**® *see Mitomycin on page 579*
+ **Mycamine**™ *see Micafungin on page 573*
+ **Mycelex**® *see Clotrimazole on page 203*
+ **Mycelex**®-7 [OTC] *see Clotrimazole on page 203*
+ **Mycelex**® Twin Pack [OTC] *see Clotrimazole on page 203*

Mycophenolate *(mye koe FEN oh late)*

Related Information

Safe Handling of Hazardous Drugs *on page 1034*
Transplantation *on page 1019*

U.S. Brand Names CellCept®; Myfortic®

Canadian Brand Names CellCept®

Generic Available No

Synonyms MMF; MPA; Mycophenolate Mofetil; Mycophenolate Sodium; Mycophenolic Acid

Pharmacologic Category Immunosuppressant Agent

Pregnancy Risk Factor C (manufacturer)

Lactation Excretion in breast milk unknown/not recommended

Use Prophylaxis of organ rejection concomitantly with cyclosporine and corticosteroids in patients receiving allogenic renal (CellCept®, Myfortic®), cardiac (CellCept®), or hepatic (CellCept®) transplants

Unlabeled/Investigational Use Treatment of rejection in liver transplant patients unable to tolerate tacrolimus or cyclosporine due to neurotoxicity; mild rejection in heart transplant patients; treatment of moderate-severe psoriasis; treatment of proliferative lupus nephritis

Mechanism of Action MPA exhibits a cytostatic effect on T and B lymphocytes. It is an inhibitor of inosine monophosphate dehydrogenase (IMPDH) which inhibits *de novo* guanosine nucleotide synthesis. T and B lymphocytes are dependent on this pathway for proliferation.

Labeled Contraindications Hypersensitivity to mycophenolate mofetil, mycophenolic acid, mycophenolate sodium, or any component of the formulation; intravenous formulation is contraindicated in patients who are allergic to polysorbate 80

Warnings/Precautions Hazardous agent - use appropriate precautions for handling and disposal. See Safe Handling of Hazardous Drugs *on page 1034* in the Appendix. Risk for infection and development of lymphoproliferative disorders is increased. Use caution with active peptic ulcer disease.

Mycophenolate mofetil is a potential teratogen; tablets should not be crushed, and capsules should not be opened or crushed. Avoid inhalation or direct contact with skin or mucous membranes of the powder contained in the capsules and the powder for oral suspension.

Theoretically, use should be avoided in patients with the rare hereditary deficiency of hypoxanthine-guanine phosphoribosyltransferase (such as Lesch-Nyhan or Kelley-Seegmiller syndrome). Intravenous solutions should be given over at least 2 hours; **never** administer intravenous solution by rapid or bolus injection.

CellCept® and Myfortic® dosage forms should not be used interchangeably due to differences in absorption.

Adverse Reactions As reported in adults following oral dosing of CellCept® alone in renal, cardiac, and hepatic allograft rejection studies. In general, lower doses used in renal rejection patients had less adverse effects than higher doses. Rates of adverse effects were similar for each indication, except for those unique to the specific organ involved. The type of adverse effects observed in pediatric patients was similar to those seen in adults; abdominal pain, anemia, diarrhea, fever, hypertension, infection, pharyngitis, respiratory tract infection, sepsis, and vomiting were seen in higher proportion; lymphoproliferative disorder was the only type of malignancy observed. Percentages of adverse reactions were similar in studies comparing CellCept® to Myfortic® in patients following renal transplant.

>20%:

Cardiovascular: Hypertension (28% to 77%), peripheral edema (27% to 64%), edema (27% to 28%), tachycardia (20% to 22%)

Central nervous system: Pain (31% to 76%), headache (16% to 54%), insomnia (41% to 52%), fever (21% to 52%), anxiety (28%)

Dermatologic: Rash (22%)

Endocrine & metabolic: Hypercholesterolemia (41%), hypokalemia (32% to 37%)

Gastrointestinal: Abdominal pain (25% to 62%), nausea (20% to 54%), diarrhea (31% to 52%), constipation (18% to 41%), vomiting (33% to 34%), anorexia (25%), dyspepsia (22%)

Genitourinary: Urinary tract infection (37%)

Hematologic: Leukopenia (23% to 46%), leukocytosis (22% to 40%), hypochromic anemia (25%)

Hepatic: Liver function tests abnormal (25%), ascites (24%)

Neuromuscular & skeletal: Back pain (35% to 47%), weakness (35% to 43%), tremor (24% to 34%), paresthesia (21%)

Respiratory: Dyspnea (31% to 37%), respiratory tract infection (22% to 37%), cough (31%), lung disorder (22% to 30%)

Miscellaneous: Infection (18% to 27%), *Candida* (11% to 22%), herpes simplex (10% to 21%)

3% to <20%:

Cardiovascular: Angina, arrhythmia, arterial thrombosis, atrial fibrillation, atrial flutter, bradycardia, cardiac arrest, cardiac failure, CHF, extrasystole, facial edema, hypervolemia, hypotension, pallor, palpitation, pericardial effusion, peripheral vascular disorder, postural hypotension, supraventricular extrasystoles, supraventricular tachycardia,

(Continued)

Mycophenolate *(Continued)*

syncope, thrombosis, vasodilation, vasospasm, venous pressure increased, ventricular extrasystole, ventricular tachycardia

Central nervous system: Agitation, chills with fever, confusion, convulsion, delirium, depression, emotional lability, hallucinations, hypoesthesia, malaise, nervousness, psychosis, somnolence, thinking abnormal, vertigo

Dermatologic: Acne, alopecia, bruising, cellulitis, hirsutism, pruritus, skin carcinoma, skin hypertrophy

Endocrine & metabolic: Acidosis, Cushing's syndrome, dehydration, diabetes mellitus, gout, hypercalcemia, hyperlipemia, hyperphosphatemia, hyperuricemia, hypothyroidism, parathyroid disorder

Gastrointestinal: Abdomen enlarged, dry mouth, dysphagia, esophagitis, flatulence, gastritis, gastroenteritis, gastrointestinal hemorrhage, gastrointestinal moniliasis, gingivitis, gum hyperplasia, melena, mouth ulceration, oral moniliasis, stomach disorder, stomatitis

Genitourinary: Impotence, pelvic pain, prostatic disorder, urinary frequency, urinary incontinence, urinary retention, urinary tract disorder

Hematologic: Coagulation disorder, hemorrhage, pancytopenia, polycythemia, prothrombin time increased, thromboplastin increased

Hepatic: Alkaline phosphatase increased, alkalosis, bilirubinemia, cholangitis, cholestatic jaundice, GGT increased, hepatitis, jaundice, liver damage

Local: Abscess, ALT increased, AST increased

Neuromuscular & skeletal: Arthralgia, hypertonia, joint disorder, leg cramps, myalgia, myasthenia, neck pain, neuropathy, osteoporosis

Ocular: Amblyopia, cataract, conjunctivitis, eye hemorrhage, lacrimation disorder, vision abnormal

Otic: Deafness, ear disorder, ear pain, tinnitus

Renal: Albuminuria, creatinine increased, dysuria, hematuria, hydronephrosis, kidney failure, kidney tubular necrosis, oliguria

Respiratory: Apnea, asthma, atelectasis, bronchitis, epistaxis, hemoptysis, hiccup, hyperventilation, hypoxia, respiratory acidosis, lung edema, pharyngitis, pleural effusion, pneumonia, pneumothorax, pulmonary hypertension, respiratory moniliasis, rhinitis, sinusitis, sputum increased, voice alteration

Miscellaneous: CMV viremia/syndrome (12% to 14%), CMV tissue invasive disease (6% to 11%), herpes zoster cutaneous disease (4% to 10%), cyst, diaphoresis, flu-like syndrome, fungal dermatitis, healing abnormal, hernia, ileus infection, lactic dehydrogenase increased, peritonitis, pyelonephritis, scrotal edema, thirst

Postmarketing and/or case reports: Atypical mycobacterial infection, colitis, infectious endocarditis, interstitial lung disorder, intestinal villous atrophy, meningitis, pancreatitis, pulmonary fibrosis (fatal), tuberculosis

Overdosage/Toxicology There are no reported overdoses with mycophenolate. At plasma concentrations >100 mcg/mL, small amounts of the inactive metabolite MPAG are removed by hemodialysis. Excretion of the active metabolite, MPA, may be increased by using bile acid sequestrants (cholestyramine).

Drug Interactions

Increased Effect/Toxicity: Acyclovir and ganciclovir levels may increase due to competition for tubular secretion of these drugs.

Probenecid may increase mycophenolate levels due to inhibition of tubular secretion. High doses of salicylates may increase free fraction of mycophenolic acid. Azathioprine's bone marrow suppression may be potentiated; do not administer together.

Decreased Effect: Antacids decrease serum levels (C_{max} and AUC); **do not administer together**. Cholestyramine resin decreases serum levels; **do not administer together**. Avoid use of live vaccines; vaccinations may be less effective. Influenza vaccine may be of value. During concurrent use of oral contraceptives, progesterone levels are not significantly affected, however, effect on estrogen component varies; an additional form of contraception should be used.

Ethanol/Nutrition/Herb Interactions

Food: Decreases C_{max} of MPA by 40% following CellCept® administration and 33% following Myfortic® use; the extent of absorption is not changed

Herb/Nutraceutical: Avoid cat's claw, echinacea (have immunostimulant properties)

Storage/Stability

Capsules: Store at room temperature of 15°C to 39°C (59°F to 86°F).

Tablets: Store at room temperature of 15°C to 39°C (59°F to 86°F). Protect from light.

Oral suspension: Store powder for oral suspension at room temperature of 15°C to 39°C (59°F to 86°F). Once reconstituted, the oral solution may be stored at room temperature or under refrigeration. Do not freeze. The mixed suspension is stable for 60 days.

Injection: Store intact vials at room temperature 15°C to 30°C (59°F to 86°F). Stability of the infusion solution: 4 hours from reconstitution and dilution of the product. Store solutions at 15°C to 30°C (59°F to 86°F).

Reconstitution

Oral suspension: Should be constituted prior to dispensing to the patient and **not** mixed with any other medication. Add 47 mL of water to the bottle and shake well for ~1 minute. Add another 47 mL of water to the bottle and shake well for an additional minute. Final concentration is 200 mg/mL of mycophenolate mofetil.

I.V.: Reconstitute the contents of each vial with 14 mL of 5% dextrose injection; dilute the contents of a vial with 5% dextrose in water to a final concentration of 6 mg mycophenolate mofetil per mL.

Compatibility Compatible: Stable in D_5W

Pharmacodynamics/Kinetics

Onset of action: Peak effect: Correlation of toxicity or efficacy is still being developed, however, one study indicated that 12-hour AUCs >40 mcg/mL/hour were correlated with efficacy and decreased episodes of rejection

T_{max}: Oral: MPA:
CellCept®: 1-1.5 hours
Myfortic®: 1.5-2.5 hours

Absorption: AUC values for MPA are lower in the early post-transplant period versus later (>3 months) post-transplant period. The extent of absorption in pediatrics is similar to that seen in adults, although there was wide variability reported.

Oral: Myfortic®: 93%

Distribution:
CellCept®: MPA: Oral: 4 L/kg; I.V.: 3.6 L/kg

(Continued)

Mycophenolate *(Continued)*

Myfortic®: MPA: Oral: 54 L (at steady state); 112 L (elimination phase)

Protein binding: MPA: 97%, MPAG 82%

Metabolism: Hepatic and via GI tract; CellCept® is completely hydrolyzed in the liver to mycophenolic acid (MPA; active metabolite); enterohepatic recirculation of MPA may occur; MPA is glucuronidated to MPAG (inactive metabolite)

Bioavailability: Oral: CellCept®: 94%; Myfortic®: 72%

Half-life elimination:

CellCept®: MPA: Oral: 18 hours; I.V.: 17 hours

Myfortic®: MPA: Oral: 8-16 hours; MPAG: 13-17 hours

Excretion:

CellCept®: MPA: Urine (<1%), feces (6%); MPAG: Urine (87%)

Myfortic®: MPA: Urine (3%), feces; MPAG: Urine (>60%)

Dosage

Children: Renal transplant: Oral:

CellCept® suspension: 600 mg/m^2/dose twice daily; maximum dose: 1 g twice daily

Alternatively, may use solid dosage forms according to BSA as follows:

BSA 1.25-1.5 m^2: 750 mg capsule twice daily

BSA >1.5 m^2: 1 g capsule or tablet twice daily

Myfortic®:

BSA <1.19 m^2: Use of this formulation is not recommended

BSA 1.19-1.58 m^2: 400 mg/m^2 twice daily (maximum: 1080 mg/day)

BSA >1.58 m^2: 400 mg/m^2 twice daily (maximum: 1440 mg/day)

Adults:

Renal transplant:

CellCept®:

Oral: 1 g twice daily. Doses >2 g/day are not recommended.

I.V.: 1 g twice daily

Myfortic®: Oral: 720 mg twice daily (1440 mg/day)

Cardiac transplantation:

Oral (CellCept®): 1.5 g twice daily

I.V. (CellCept®): 1.5 g twice daily

Hepatic transplantation:

Oral (CellCept®): 1.5 g twice daily

I.V. (CellCept®): 1 g twice daily

Dosing adjustment in renal impairment:

Renal transplant: GFR <25 mL/minute in patients outside the immediate post-transplant period:

CellCept®: Doses of >1 g administered twice daily should be avoided; patients should also be carefully observed; no dose adjustments are needed in renal transplant patients experiencing delayed graft function postoperatively

Myfortic®: Cl$_{cr}$ <25 mL/minute: Monitor carefully

Cardiac or liver transplant: No data available; mycophenolate may be used in cardiac or hepatic transplant patients with severe chronic renal impairment if the potential benefit outweighs the potential risk

Hemodialysis: Not removed; supplemental dose is not necessary

Peritoneal dialysis: Supplemental dose is not necessary

Dosage adjustment in hepatic impairment: No dosage adjustment is recommended for renal patients with severe hepatic parenchymal

disease; however, it is not currently known whether dosage adjustments are necessary for hepatic disease with other etiologies

Elderly: Dosage is the same as younger patients, however, dosing should be cautious due to possibility of increased hepatic, renal or cardiac dysfunction; elderly patients may be at an increased risk of certain infections, gastrointestinal hemorrhage, and pulmonary edema, as compared to younger patients

Dosing adjustment for toxicity (neutropenia): ANC <1.3 x 10^3/μL: Dosing should be interrupted or the dose reduced, appropriate diagnostic tests performed and patients managed appropriately

Administration

Oral dosage formulations (tablet, capsule, suspension) should be administered on an empty stomach to avoid variability in MPA absorption. The oral solution may be administered via a nasogastric tube (minimum 8 French, 1.7 mm interior diameter) and cannot be mixed with other medications. Delayed release tablets should not be crushed, cut, or chewed.

Intravenous solutions should be administered over at least 2 hours (either peripheral or central vein); do **not** administer intravenous solution by rapid or bolus injection.

Dosage Forms

Capsule, as mofetil (CellCept®): 250 mg

Injection, powder for reconstitution, as mofetil hydrochloride (CellCept®): 500 mg [contains polysorbate 80]

Powder for oral suspension, as mofetil (CellCept®): 200 mg/mL (225 mL) [provides 175 mL suspension following reconstitution; contains phenylalanine 0.56 mg/mL; mixed fruit flavor]

Tablet, as mofetil [film coated] (CellCept®): 500 mg [may contain ethyl alcohol]

Tablet, delayed release, as mycophenolic acid [film coated] (Myfortic®): 180 mg, 360 mg [formulated as a sodium salt]

Monitoring Parameters Complete blood count; signs and symptoms of infection

Dietary Considerations Oral dosage formulations should be taken on an empty stomach to avoid variability in MPA absorption. However, in stable renal transplant patients, may be administered with food if necessary. Oral suspension contains 0.56 mg phenylalanine/mL; use caution if administered to patients with phenylketonuria.

Patient Information Take as directed, preferably 1 hour before or 2 hours after meals. Do not take within 1 hour before or 2 hours after antacids or cholestyramine medications. Do not alter dose and do not discontinue without consulting prescriber. Maintain adequate hydration (2-3 L/day of fluids unless instructed to restrict fluid intake) during entire course of therapy. You will be susceptible to infection (avoid crowds and people with infections or contagious diseases). If you are diabetic, monitor glucose levels closely (may alter glucose levels). You may experience dizziness or trembling (use caution until response to medication is known); nausea or vomiting (frequent small meals, frequent mouth care may help); diarrhea (boiled milk, yogurt, or buttermilk may help); sores or white plaques in mouth (frequent rinsing of mouth and frequent mouth care may help); or muscle or back pain (mild analgesics may be recommended). Report chest pain; acute headache or dizziness; symptoms of (Continued)

Mycophenolate *(Continued)*

respiratory infection, cough, or difficulty breathing; unresolved gastrointestinal effects; fatigue, chills, fever unhealed sores, white plaques in mouth; irritation in genital area or unusual discharge; unusual bruising or bleeding; or other unusual effects related to this medication. May be at increased risk for skin cancer; wear protective clothing and use sunscreen with high protective factor to help limit exposure to sunlight and UV light. Two reliable forms of contraception should be used prior to, during, and for 6 weeks after therapy.

Selected Readings
Gabardi S, Tran JL, and Clarkson MR, "Enteric-Coated Mycophenolate sodium," *Ann Pharmacother*, 2003, 37(11):1685-93.

Lipsky JJ, "Mycophenolate Mofetil," *Lancet*, 1996, 348(9038):1357-9.

Shaw LM, Sollinger HW, Halloran P, et al, "Mycophenolate Mofetil: A Report of the Consensus Panel," *Ther Drug Monit*, 1995, 17(6):690-9.

- ♦ **Mycophenolate Mofetil** *see* Mycophenolate *on page 598*
- ♦ **Mycophenolate Sodium** *see* Mycophenolate *on page 598*
- ♦ **Mycophenolic Acid** *see* Mycophenolate *on page 598*
- ♦ **Mycostatin®** *see* Nystatin *on page 613*
- ♦ **Myfortic®** *see* Mycophenolate *on page 598*
- ♦ **Myleran®** *see* Busulfan *on page 141*
- ♦ **Mylocel™** *see* Hydroxyurea *on page 432*
- ♦ **Mylotarg®** *see* Gemtuzumab Ozogamicin *on page 395*

Nabilone *(NA bi lone)*

Related Information
Management of Nausea and Vomiting *on page 982*

Generic Available No

Pharmacologic Category Antiemetic

Pregnancy Risk Factor C

Lactation Excretion in breast milk unknown

Use Treatment of nausea and vomiting associated with cancer chemotherapy

Mechanism of Action Unknown; animal studies suggest some activity may involve the chemoreceptor trigger zone.

Restrictions C-II

Labeled Contraindications Hypersensitivity to nabilone, cannabinoids, tetrahydrocannabinol, or any component of the formulation

Warnings/Precautions Use with caution in the elderly, those with pre-existing CNS depression, or a history of mental illness.

Adverse Reactions

>10%:
  Cardiovascular: Orthostatic hypotension (5% to 42%)
  Central nervous system: Dizziness (36%), drowsiness (47% to 65%), vertigo (65%), euphoria (27%), clumsiness
  Gastrointestinal: Dry mouth (29%)

1% to 10%:
  Central nervous system: Ataxia, depression
  Ocular: Blurred vision (13%)

<1%: Changes of mood, confusion, dyspnea, hallucinations, headache, loss of appetite

Emetic Potential Very low (<10%)

Overdosage/Toxicology Symptoms of overdose include nausea, vomiting, disorientation, CNS, respiratory depression, dysphoria, and euphoria. Treatment is supportive and symptomatic.

Drug Interactions

Increased Effect/Toxicity: Increased toxicity: CNS depression is potentiated with ethanol and other CNS depressants.

Storage/Stability Store capsules at room temperature.

Pharmacodynamics/Kinetics
Absorption: Rapid
Bioavailability: 95.8%
Distribution: Rapid and extensive to various tissues
Metabolism: To several active metabolites by oxidation and stereospecific reduction
Half-life elimination: Parent compound: 2 hours; Metabolites: 35 hours
Time to peak, serum: Within 2 hours
Excretion: Feces (65%); renal (20%)

Dosage Refer to individual protocols. Oral:
Children >4 years:
    <18 kg: 0.5 mg twice daily
    18-30 kg: 1 mg twice daily
    >30 kg: 1 mg 3 times/day
Adults: 1-2 mg twice daily (maximum: 6 mg divided in 3 doses daily)

Administration Oral; I.V. use is reported, but a parenteral formulation is not available in the U.S.

Dosage Forms Capsule: 1 mg

Patient Information May cause drowsiness, impaired judgment or coordination. Avoid alcohol and other CNS depressants. Can cause disorientation.

Selected Readings
Ward A and Holmes B, "Nabilone: A Preliminary Review of Its Pharmacological Properties and Therapeutic Use," *Drugs*, 1985, 30(2):127-44.

♦ **NAB-Paclitaxel** *see* Paclitaxel (Protein Bound) *on page 644*

Nafcillin (naf SIL in)

Canadian Brand Names Nallpen®; Unipen®

Generic Available Yes

Synonyms Ethoxynaphthamido Penicillin Sodium; Nafcillin Sodium; Nallpen; Sodium Nafcillin

Pharmacologic Category Antibiotic, Penicillin

Pregnancy Risk Factor B

Lactation Enters breast milk/use caution

Use Treatment of infections such as osteomyelitis, septicemia, endocarditis, and CNS infections caused by susceptible strains of staphylococci species

Mechanism of Action Interferes with bacterial cell wall synthesis during active multiplication, causing cell wall death and resultant bactericidal activity against susceptible bacteria

Labeled Contraindications Hypersensitivity to nafcillin, or any component of the formulation, or penicillins

Warnings/Precautions Extravasation of I.V. infusions should be avoided. Modification of dosage is necessary in patients with both severe renal and hepatic impairment. Elimination rate will be slow in neonates.

Adverse Reactions Frequency not defined.
(Continued)

Nafcillin *(Continued)*

Central nervous system: Pain, fever

Dermatologic: Rash

Gastrointestinal: Nausea, diarrhea

Hematologic: Agranulocytosis, bone marrow depression, neutropenia

Local: Pain, swelling, inflammation, phlebitis, skin sloughing, and thrombophlebitis at the injection site; oxacillin (less likely to cause phlebitis) is often preferred in pediatric patients

Renal: Interstitial nephritis (acute)

Miscellaneous: Hypersensitivity reactions

Vesicant Yes; see Management of Drug Extravasations *on page 965.*

Emetic Potential Very low (<10%)

Overdosage/Toxicology Symptoms of penicillin overdose include neuromuscular hypersensitivity (eg, agitation, hallucinations, asterixis, encephalopathy, confusion, and seizures). Electrolyte imbalance may occur if the preparation contains potassium or sodium salts, especially in renal failure. Treatment is supportive or symptom-directed.

Drug Interactions

Cytochrome P450 Effect: Induces CYP3A4 (strong)

Increased Effect/Toxicity: Probenecid may cause an increase in nafcillin levels. Penicillins may increase the exposure to methotrexate during concurrent therapy; monitor.

Decreased Effect: Chloramphenicol may decrease nafcillin efficacy. If taken concomitantly with warfarin, nafcillin may inhibit the anticoagulant response to warfarin. This effect may persist for up to 30 days after nafcillin has been discontinued. Subtherapeutic cyclosporine levels may result when taken concomitantly with nafcillin. Although anecdotal reports suggest oral contraceptive efficacy could be reduced by penicillins, this has been refuted by more rigorous scientific and clinical data. Nafcillin may decrease the levels/effects of benzodiazepines, calcium channel blockers, clarithromycin, cyclosporine, erythromycin, estrogens, mirtazapine, nateglinide, nefazodone, nevirapine, protease inhibitors, tacrolimus, venlafaxine, and other CYP3A4 substrates.

Storage/Stability Reconstituted parenteral solution is stable for 3 days at room temperature, 7 days when refrigerated, or 12 weeks when frozen. For I.V. infusion in NS or D_5W, solution is stable for 24 hours at room temperature and 96 hours when refrigerated.

Compatibility Stable in dextran 40 10% in dextrose, D_5LR, $D_5^1/_4NS$, $D_5^1/_2NS$, D_5NS, D_5W, $D_{10}NS$, $D_{10}W$, LR, NS; **variable stability (consult detailed reference)** in peritoneal dialysis solution, TPN

Y-site administration: Compatible: Acyclovir, atropine, cyclophosphamide, diazepam, enalaprilat, esmolol, famotidine, fentanyl, fluconazole, foscarnet, hydromorphone, magnesium sulfate, morphine, perphenazine, propofol, theophylline, zidovudine. **Incompatible:** Droperidol, fentanyl and droperidol, insulin (regular), labetalol, midazolam, nalbuphine, pentazocine, verapamil. **Variable (consult detailed reference):** Diltiazem, meperidine, TPN, vancomycin

Compatibility in syringe: Compatible: Cimetidine, heparin

Compatibility when admixed: Compatible: Chloramphenicol, chlorothiazide, dexamethasone sodium phosphate, diphenhydramine, ephedrine, heparin, hydroxyzine, lidocaine, potassium chloride, prochlorperazine edisylate, sodium bicarbonate, sodium lactate.

Incompatible: Ascorbic acid injection, aztreonam, bleomycin, cytarabine, gentamicin, hydrocortisone sodium succinate, methylprednisolone sodium succinate, promazine. **Variable (consult detailed reference):** Aminophylline, verapamil, vitamin B complex with C

Pharmacodynamics/Kinetics

Distribution: Widely distributed; CSF penetration is poor but enhanced by meningeal inflammation; crosses placenta

Protein binding: 70% to 90%

Metabolism: Primarily hepatic; undergoes enterohepatic recirculation

Half-life elimination:

Neonates: <3 weeks: 2.2-5.5 hours; 4-9 weeks: 1.2-2.3 hours

Children 3 months to 14 years: 0.75-1.9 hours

Adults: 30 minutes to 1.5 hours with normal renal and hepatic function

Time to peak, serum: I.M.: 30-60 minutes

Excretion: Primarily feces; urine (10% to 30% as unchanged drug)

Dosage

Neonates:

<2000 g, <7 days: 50 mg/kg/day divided every 12 hours

<2000 g, >7 days: 75 mg/kg/day divided every 8 hours

>2000 g, <7 days: 50 mg/kg/day divided every 8 hours

>2000 g, >7 days: 75 mg/kg/day divided every 6 hours

Children:

I.M.: 25 mg/kg twice daily

I.V.:

Mild to moderate infections: 50-100 mg/kg/day in divided doses every 6 hours

Severe infections: 100-200 mg/kg/day in divided doses every 4-6 hours

Maximum dose: 12 g/day

Adults:

I.M.: 500 mg every 4-6 hours

I.V.: 500-2000 mg every 4-6 hours

Dosing adjustment in renal impairment: Not necessary

Dosing adjustment in hepatic impairment: In patients with both hepatic and renal impairment, modification of dosage may be necessary; no data available.

Dialysis: Not dialyzable (0% to 5%) via hemodialysis; supplemental dosage not necessary with hemo- or peritoneal dialysis or continuous arteriovenous or venovenous hemofiltration

Administration

I.M.: Rotate injection sites

I.V.: Vesicant. Administer around-the-clock to promote less variation in peak and trough serum levels; infuse over 30-60 minutes

Dosage Forms

Infusion [premixed iso-osmotic dextrose solution]: 1 g (50 mL); 2 g (100 mL)

Injection, powder for reconstitution, as sodium: 1 g, 2 g, 10 g

Monitoring Parameters Periodic CBC, urinalysis, BUN, serum creatinine, AST and ALT; observe for signs and symptoms of anaphylaxis during first dose

Dietary Considerations Sodium content of 1 g: 76.6 mg (3.33 mEq)

Special Geriatric Considerations Nafcillin has not been studied exclusively in the elderly, however, given its route of elimination, dosage

(Continued)

607

Nafcillin *(Continued)*

adjustments based upon age and renal function are not necessary. Consider sodium content in patients who may be sensitive to volume expansion (ie, CHF).

Selected Readings
Banner W Jr, Gooch WM 3d, Burckart G, et al, "Pharmacokinetics of Nafcillin in Infants With Low Birth Weights," *Antimicrob Agents Chemother*, 1980, 17(4):691-4.

Donowitz GR and Mandell GL, "Beta-Lactam Antibiotics," *N Engl J Med*, 1988, 318(7):419-26 and 318(8):490-500.

Wright AJ, "The Penicillins," *Mayo Clin Proc*, 1999, 74(3):290-307.

- ◆ **Nafcillin Sodium** *see* Nafcillin *on page 605*
- ◆ **Nafidimide** *see* Amonafide *on page 65*
- ◆ **Nallpen** *see* Nafcillin *on page 605*
- ◆ **Naphuride Sodium** *see* Suramin *on page 733*
- ◆ **Natulan® (Can)** *see* Procarbazine *on page 688*
- ◆ **Navelbine®** *see* Vinorelbine *on page 826*
- ◆ **Nebcin® [DSC]** *see* Tobramycin *on page 771*
- ◆ **NebuPent®** *see* Pentamidine *on page 659*
- ◆ **Neoral®** *see* CycloSPORINE *on page 216*
- ◆ **Neumega®** *see* Oprelvekin *on page 627*
- ◆ **Neupogen®** *see* Filgrastim *on page 341*
- ◆ **NeuTrexin®** *see* Trimetrexate Glucuronate *on page 799*
- ◆ **Niastase® (Can)** *see* Factor VIIa (Recombinant) *on page 326*
- ◆ **Nidagel™ (Can)** *see* Metronidazole *on page 568*
- ◆ **Niftolid** *see* Flutamide *on page 366*
- ◆ **Nilandron®** *see* Nilutamide *on page 608*
- ◆ **Nilstat (Can)** *see* Nystatin *on page 613*

Nilutamide *(ni LOO ta mide)*

Related Information
Safe Handling of Hazardous Drugs *on page 1034*

U.S. Brand Names Nilandron®

Canadian Brand Names Anandron®

Generic Available No

Synonyms RU-23908

Pharmacologic Category Antiandrogen; Antineoplastic Agent, Antiandrogen

Pregnancy Risk Factor C

Lactation Not indicated for use in women

Use Treatment of metastatic prostate cancer

Mechanism of Action Nonsteroidal antiandrogen that inhibits androgen uptake or inhibits binding of androgen in target tissues. It specifically blocks the action of androgens by interacting with cytosolic androgen receptor F sites in target tissue

Labeled Contraindications Hypersensitivity to nilutamide or any component of the formulation; severe hepatic impairment; severe respiratory insufficiency

Warnings/Precautions Hazardous agent - use appropriate precautions for handling and disposal. See Safe Handling of Hazardous Drugs *on page 1034* in the Appendix. May cause interstitial pneumonitis; the suggestive signs of pneumonitis most often occurred within the first 3

months of nilutamide treatment. Has been associated with severe hepatitis, which has resulted in fatality. In addition, foreign postmarketing surveillance has revealed isolated cases of aplastic anemia (a causal relationship with nilutamide could not be ascertained).

May alter time for visual adaptation to darkness, ranging from seconds to a few minutes. This effect sometimes does not abate as drug treatment is continued. Caution patients who experience this effect about driving at night or through tunnels. This effect can be alleviated by wearing tinted glasses.

Adverse Reactions
>10%:
Central nervous system: Headache, insomnia

Endocrine & metabolic: Hot flashes (30% to 67%), gynecomastia (10%)

Gastrointestinal: Nausea (mild - 10% to 32%), abdominal pain (10%), constipation, anorexia

Genitourinary: Testicular atrophy (16%), libido decreased

Hepatic: Transaminases increased (8% to 13%; transient)

Ocular: Impaired dark adaptation (13% to 57%), usually reversible with dose reduction, may require discontinuation of the drug in 1% to 2% of patients

Respiratory: Dyspnea (11%)

1% to 10%:
Cardiovascular: Chest pain, edema, heart failure, hypertension, syncope

Central nervous system: Dizziness, drowsiness, malaise, hypoesthesia, depression

Dermatologic: Pruritus, alopecia, dry skin, rash

Endocrine & metabolic: Disulfiram-like reaction (hot flashes, rash) (5%); Flu-like syndrome, fever

Gastrointestinal: Vomiting, diarrhea, dyspepsia, GI hemorrhage, melena, weight loss, xerostomia

Genitourinary: Hematuria, nocturia

Hematologic: Anemia

Hepatic: Hepatitis (1%)

Neuromuscular & skeletal: Arthritis, paresthesia

Ocular: Chromatopsia (9%), abnormal vision (6% to 7%), cataracts, photophobia

Respiratory: Interstitial pneumonitis (2% - typically exertional dyspnea, cough, chest pain, and fever; most often occurring within the first 3 months of treatment); rhinitis

Miscellaneous: Diaphoresis

<1%: Aplastic anemia

Emetic Potential Low (10% to 30)

Overdosage/Toxicology Symptoms of overdose may include nausea, vomiting, malaise, headache, dizziness, and elevated liver enzymes. Management is supportive. Dialysis is of no benefit.

Drug Interactions
Cytochrome P450 Effect: Substrate of CYP2C19 (major); **Inhibits** CYP2C19 (weak)

Increased Effect/Toxicity: CYP2C19 inhibitors may increase the levels/effects of nilutamide; example inhibitors include delavirdine, fluconazole, fluvoxamine, gemfibrozil, isoniazid, omeprazole, and ticlopidine.

(Continued)

Nilutamide *(Continued)*

Decreased Effect: CYP2C19 inducers may decrease the levels/effects of nilutamide; example inducers include aminoglutethimide, carbamazepine, phenytoin, and rifampin.

Ethanol/Nutrition/Herb Interactions

Ethanol: Avoid ethanol. Up to 5% of patients may experience a systemic reaction (flushing, hypotension, malaise) when combined with nilutamide.

Herb/Nutraceutical: St John's wort may decrease nilutamide levels.

Storage/Stability Store at room temperature of 15°C to 30°C (59°F to 86°F). Protect from light.

Pharmacodynamics/Kinetics

Absorption: Rapid and complete

Protein binding: 72% to 85%

Metabolism: Hepatic, forms active metabolites

Half-life elimination: Terminal: 23-87 hours; Metabolites: 35-137 hours

Excretion: Urine (up to 78% at 120 hours; <1% as unchanged drug); feces (1% to 7%)

Dosage Refer to individual protocols.

Adults: Oral: 300 mg daily for 30 days starting the same day or day after surgical castration, then 150 mg/day

Administration Nilutamide is administered orally, usually in 3 divided doses.

Dosage Forms Tablet: 150 mg

Monitoring Parameters Obtain a chest x-ray if a patient reports dyspnea; if there are findings suggestive of interstitial pneumonitis, discontinue treatment with nilutamide. Measure serum hepatic enzyme levels at baseline and at regular intervals (3 months); if transaminases increase over 2-3 times the upper limit of normal, discontinue treatment. Perform appropriate laboratory testing at the first symptom/sign of liver injury (eg, jaundice, dark urine, fatigue, abdominal pain or unexplained GI symptoms).

Dietary Considerations May be taken without regard to food.

Patient Information Take as prescribed; do not change dosing schedule or stop taking without consulting prescriber. May cause a severe reaction with alcohol. Use alcohol cautiously while taking this medication; if the reaction occurs, avoid alcohol. Periodic laboratory tests are necessary while taking this medication. You may experience dizziness, confusion, or blurred vision (avoid driving or engaging in tasks that require alertness until response to drug is known); loss of light accommodation (avoid night driving and use caution in poorly lighted or changing light situations); impotence; or loss of libido (discuss with prescriber). Report yellowing of skin or eyes; change in color of urine or stool; unusual bruising or bleeding; chest pain; difficulty or painful voiding. Report immediately any shortness of breath, difficulty breathing, or increased cough.

Selected Readings

Creaven PJ, Pendyala L, and Tremblay D, "Pharmacokinetics and Metabolism of Nilutamide," *Urology*, 1991, 37(2 Suppl):13-9.

Dole EJ and Holdsworth MT, "Nilutamide: An Antiandrogen for the Treatment of Prostate Cancer," *Ann Pharmacother*, 1997, 31(1):65-75.

Harris MG, Coleman SG, Faulds D, et al, "Nilutamide. A Review of Its Pharmacodynamic and Pharmacokinetic Properties, and Therapeutic Efficacy in Prostate Cancer," *Drugs Aging*, 1993, 3(1):9-25.

- **NSC-85998** *see* Streptozocin *on page 724*
- **NSC-89199** *see* Estramustine *on page 310*
- **NSC-102816** *see* Azacitidine *on page 110*
- **NSC-106977 (*Erwinia*)** *see* Asparaginase *on page 106*
- **NSC-109229 (*E. coli*)** *see* Asparaginase *on page 106*
- **NSC-109724** *see* Ifosfamide *on page 446*
- **NSC-122758** *see* Tretinoin (Oral) *on page 792*
- **NSC-123127** *see* DOXOrubicin *on page 280*
- **NSC-125066** *see* Bleomycin *on page 134*
- **NSC-125973** *see* Paclitaxel *on page 638*
- **NSC-147834** *see* Flutamide *on page 366*
- **NSC-180973** *see* Tamoxifen *on page 743*
- **NSC-218321** *see* Pentostatin *on page 661*
- **NSC-245467** *see* Vindesine *on page 825*
- **NSC-249992** *see* Amsacrine *on page 80*
- **NSC-256439** *see* Idarubicin *on page 443*
- **NSC-266046** *see* Oxaliplatin *on page 629*
- **NSC-296961** *see* Amifostine *on page 53*
- **NSC-301739** *see* Mitoxantrone *on page 584*
- **NSC-308847** *see* Amonafide *on page 65*
- **NSC-352122** *see* Trimetrexate Glucuronate *on page 799*
- **NSC-362856** *see* Temozolomide *on page 750*
- **NSC-373364** *see* Aldesleukin *on page 32*
- **NSC-377526** *see* Leuprolide *on page 500*
- **NSC-409962** *see* Carmustine *on page 154*
- **NSC-603071** *see* Aminocamptothecin *on page 59*
- **NSC-606864** *see* Goserelin *on page 403*
- **NSC-609699** *see* Topotecan *on page 776*
- **NSC-616348** *see* Irinotecan *on page 478*
- **NSC-628503** *see* Docetaxel *on page 272*
- **NSC-639186** *see* Raltitrexed *on page 700*
- **NSC-644954** *see* Pegaspargase *on page 652*
- **NSC-698037** *see* Pemetrexed *on page 655*
- **NSC-706363** *see* Arsenic Trioxide *on page 102*
- **NSC-715055** *see* Gefitinib *on page 386*
- **NSC-718781** *see* Erlotinib *on page 308*
- **N-Trifluoroacetyladriamycin-14-Valerate** *see* Valrubicin *on page 808*
- **Nu-Acyclovir (Can)** *see* Acyclovir *on page 26*
- **Nu-Cotrimox (Can)** *see* Sulfamethoxazole and Trimethoprim *on page 727*
- **Nu-Loraz (Can)** *see* Lorazepam *on page 517*
- **Nu-Megestrol (Can)** *see* Megestrol *on page 528*
- **Nu-Metoclopramide (Can)** *see* Metoclopramide *on page 563*
- **Numorphan®** *see* Oxymorphone *on page 636*
- **Nupercainal® Hydrocortisone Cream [OTC]** *see* Hydrocortisone *on page 419*
- **Nu-Prochlor (Can)** *see* Prochlorperazine *on page 691*

♦ **Nutracort®** *see* Hydrocortisone *on page 419*
♦ **NVB** *see* Vinorelbine *on page 826*
♦ **Nyaderm (Can)** *see* Nystatin *on page 613*

Nystatin (nye STAT in)

Medication Safety Issues
Sound-alike/look-alike issues:
Nystatin may be confused with Nilstat®, Nitrostat®
Nilstat may be confused with Nitrostat®, nystatin

Related Information
Management of Infections *on page 978*
Mucositis/Stomatitis *on page 995*

U.S. Brand Names Bio-Statin®; Mycostatin®; Nystat-Rx®; Nystop®; Pedi-Dri®

Canadian Brand Names Candistatin®; Mycostatin®; Nilstat; Nyaderm; PMS-Nystatin

Generic Available Yes: Cream, ointment, powder, suspension, tablet

Pharmacologic Category Antifungal Agent, Oral Nonabsorbed; Antifungal Agent, Topical; Antifungal Agent, Vaginal

Pregnancy Risk Factor B/C (oral)

Lactation Does not enter breast milk/compatible (not absorbed orally)

Use Treatment of susceptible cutaneous, mucocutaneous, and oral cavity fungal infections normally caused by the *Candida* species

Mechanism of Action Binds to sterols in fungal cell membrane, changing the cell wall permeability allowing for leakage of cellular contents

Labeled Contraindications Hypersensitivity to nystatin or any component of the formulation

Adverse Reactions
Frequency not defined: Dermatologic: Contact dermatitis, Stevens-Johnson syndrome
1% to 10%: Gastrointestinal: Nausea, vomiting, diarrhea, stomach pain
<1%: Hypersensitivity reactions

Emetic Potential Low (10% to 30%)

Overdosage/Toxicology Symptoms of overdose include nausea, vomiting, and diarrhea. Treatment is supportive.

Storage/Stability
Vaginal inserts: Store in refrigerator. Protect from temperature extremes, moisture, and light.
Oral tablets, lozenges, ointment, topical powder, and oral suspension: Store at controlled room temperature 15°C to 25°C (59°F to 77°F)

Pharmacodynamics/Kinetics
Onset of action: Symptomatic relief from candidiasis: 24-72 hours
Absorption: Topical: None through mucous membranes or intact skin; Oral: Poorly absorbed
Excretion: Feces (as unchanged drug)

Dosage
Oral candidiasis:
Suspension (swish and swallow orally):
Premature infants: 100,000 units 4 times/day
Infants: 200,000 units 4 times/day or 100,000 units to each side of mouth 4 times/day
(Continued)

Nystatin (Continued)

Children and Adults: 400,000-600,000 units 4 times/day

Troche: Children and Adults: 200,000-400,000 units 4-5 times/day

Powder for compounding: Children and Adults: $1/8$ teaspoon (500,000 units) to equal approximately $1/2$ cup of water; give 4 times/day

Mucocutaneous infections: Children and Adults: Topical: Apply 2-3 times/day to affected areas; very moist topical lesions are treated best with powder

Intestinal infections: Adults: Oral: 500,000-1,000,000 units every 8 hours

Vaginal infections: Adults: Vaginal tablets: Insert 1 tablet/day at bedtime for 2 weeks

Administration Oral, topical, vaginal

Dosage Forms [DSC] = Discontinued product

Capsule (Bio-Statin®): 500,000 units, 1 million units

Cream: 100,000 units/g (15 g, 30 g)

Mycostatin®: 100,000 units/g (30 g)

Lozenge (Mycostatin®): 200,000 units [DSC]

Ointment, topical: 100,000 units/g (15 g, 30 g)

Powder, for prescription compounding: 50 million units (10 g); 150 million units (30 g); 500 million units (100 g); 2 billion units (400 g)

Nystat-Rx®: 50 million units (10 g); 150 million units (30 g); 500 million units (100 g); 1 billion units (190 g); 2 billion units (350 g)

Powder, topical:

Mycostatin®: 100,000 units/g (15 g)

Nystop®: 100,000 units/g (15 g, 30 g, 60 g)

Pedi-Dri®: 100,000 units/g (56.7 g)

Suspension, oral: 100,000 units/mL (5 mL, 60 mL, 480 mL)

Mycostatin® [DSC]: 100,000 units/mL (60 mL, 480 mL) [contains alcohol ≤1%; cherry-mint flavor]

Tablet: 500,000 units

Tablet, vaginal: 100,000 units (15s) [packaged with applicator]

Patient Information The oral suspension should be swished about the mouth and retained in the mouth for as long as possible (several minutes) before swallowing. For neonates and infants, paint nystatin suspension into recesses of the mouth. Troches must be allowed to dissolve slowly and should not be chewed or swallowed whole. If topical irritation occurs, discontinue; for external use only; do not discontinue therapy even if symptoms are gone

Special Geriatric Considerations For oral infections, patients who wear dentures must have them removed and cleaned in order to eliminate source of reinfection.

Selected Readings

Dismukes WE, Wade JS, Lee JY, et al, "A Randomized, Double-Blind Trial of Nystatin Therapy for the Candidiasis Hypersensitivity Syndrome," *N Engl J Med*, 1990, 323(25):1717-23.

Epstein JB, Vickars L, Spinelli J, et al, "Efficacy of Chlorhexidine and Nystatin Rinses in Prevention of Oral Complications in Leukemia and Bone Marrow Transplantation," *Oral Surg Oral Med Oral Pathol*, 1992, 73(6):682-9.

Meunier-Carpentier F, "Symposium on Infectious Complications of Neoplastic Disease (Part II). Chemoprophylaxis of Fungal Infections," *Am J Med*, 1984, 76(4):652-6.

Poland JM, "Oral Thrush in the Oncologic Patient. Therapy Must Be Tailored," *Am J Hosp Care* 1987, 4(5):30-2.

Wasilewski C Jr, "Allergic Contact Dermatitis From Nystatin," *Arch Dermatol*, 1971, 104(4):437.

♦ **Nystat-Rx**® *see* Nystatin *on page 613*
♦ **Nystop**® *see* Nystatin *on page 613*
♦ **Octagam**® *see* Immune Globulin (Intravenous) *on page 458*
♦ **Octostim**® **(Can)** *see* Desmopressin *on page 259*

Octreotide (ok TREE oh tide)

Medication Safety Issues

Sound-alike/look-alike issues:
Sandostatin® may be confused with Sandimmune®

U.S. Brand Names Sandostatin®; Sandostatin LAR®

Canadian Brand Names Sandostatin®; Sandostatin LAR®

Generic Available No

Synonyms Octreotide Acetate

Pharmacologic Category Antidiarrheal; Somatostatin Analog

Pregnancy Risk Factor B

Lactation Enters breast milk/contraindicated

Use Control of symptoms in patients with metastatic carcinoid and vasoactive intestinal peptide-secreting tumors (VIPomas); pancreatic tumors, gastrinoma, secretory diarrhea, acromegaly

Unlabeled/Investigational Use AIDS-associated secretory diarrhea, control of bleeding of esophageal varices, breast cancer, cryptosporidiosis, Cushing's syndrome, insulinomas, small bowel fistulas, postgastrectomy dumping syndrome, chemotherapy-induced diarrhea, graft-versus-host disease (GVHD) induced diarrhea, Zollinger-Ellison syndrome, congenital hyperinsulinism

Mechanism of Action Mimics natural somatostatin by inhibiting serotonin release, and the secretion of gastrin, VIP, insulin, glucagon, secretin, motilin, and pancreatic polypeptide. Decreases growth hormone and IGF-1 in acromegaly.

Labeled Contraindications Hypersensitivity to octreotide or any component of the formulation

Warnings/Precautions Insulin requirements may be reduced as well as sulfonylurea requirements. Monitor patients for cholelithiasis. Use with caution in patients with renal impairment. Somatostatin analogs may affect glucose regulation; in type I diabetes, severe hypoglycemia may occur; in type II diabetes or nondiabetic patients, hyperglycemia may occur.

Adverse Reactions

>10%:

Cardiovascular: Sinus bradycardia (19% to 25%)

Endocrine & metabolic: Hyperglycemia (15% acromegaly, 27% carcinoid)

Gastrointestinal: Diarrhea (36% to 58% acromegaly), abdominal pain (30% to 44% acromegaly), flatulence (13% to 26% acromegaly), constipation (9% to 19% acromegaly), nausea (10% to 30%)

1% to 10%:

Cardiovascular: Flushing, edema, conduction abnormalities (9% to 10%), arrhythmia (3% to 9%)

Central nervous system: Fatigue, headache, dizziness, vertigo, anorexia, depression

Endocrine & metabolic: Hypoglycemia (2% acromegaly, 4% carcinoid), hyperglycemia (1%), hypothyroidism, galactorrhea

(Continued)

Octreotide *(Continued)*

Gastrointestinal: Nausea, vomiting, diarrhea, constipation, abdominal pain, cramping, discomfort, fat malabsorption, loose stools, flatulence, tenesmus

Hepatic: Jaundice, hepatitis, increase LFTs, cholelithiasis has occurred, presumably by altering fat absorption and decreasing the motility of the gallbladder

Local: Pain at injection site (dose related)

Neuromuscular & skeletal: Weakness

<1%: Chest pain, hypertensive reaction, anxiety, fever, hyperesthesia, alopecia, wheal/erythema, rash, thrombophlebitis, leg cramps, Bell's palsy, muscle cramping, burning eyes, throat discomfort, rhinorrhea, dyspnea, gallstones

Vesicant No

Emetic Potential Very low (<10%)

Overdosage/Toxicology Symptoms of overdose include hypo- or hyperglycemia, blurred vision, dizziness, drowsiness, and loss of motor function. Well tolerated bolus doses up to 1000 mcg have failed to produce adverse effects.

Drug Interactions

Increased Effect/Toxicity: Octreotide may increase the effect of insulin or sulfonylurea agents which may result in hypoglycemia. Octreotide may increase serum levels of bromocriptine.

Decreased Effect: Octreotide may lower cyclosporine serum levels (case report of a transplant rejection due to reduction of serum cyclosporine levels). Codeine effect may be reduced.

Storage/Stability

Solution: Octreotide is a clear solution and should be stored under refrigeration; may be stored at room temperature for up to 14 days when protected from light. Stability of parenteral admixture is stable in NS for 96 hours at room temperature (25°C) and in D_5W for 24 hours.

Suspension: Prior to dilution, store under refrigeration and protect from light; may be at room temperature for 30-60 minutes prior to use; use suspension immediately after preparation.

Compatibility Stable in D_5W, NS; not stable in fat emulsion 10%; **variable stability** in TPN (The manufacturer states that octreotide solution is not compatible in TPN solutions due to the formation of a glycosyl octreotide conjugate which may have decreased activity; other sources give it limited compatibility.)

Y-site administration: Variable (consult detailed reference): TPN

Compatibility when admixed: Compatible: Heparin

Pharmacodynamics/Kinetics

Duration: SubQ: 6-12 hours

Absorption: SubQ: Rapid

Distribution: V_d: 14 L

Protein binding: 65% to lipoproteins

Metabolism: Extensively hepatic

Bioavailability: SubQ: 100%

Half-life elimination: 60-110 minutes

Excretion: Urine (32%)

Dosage

Infants and Children:

Diarrhea: I.V., SubQ: Doses of 1-10 mcg/kg every 12 hours have been used in children beginning at the low end of the range and increasing by 0.3 mcg/kg/dose at 3-day intervals. Suppression of growth hormone (animal data) is of concern when used as long-term therapy.

Congenital hyperinsulinism (unlabeled use): SubQ: Doses of 3-40 mcg/kg/day have been used

Adults: SubQ: Initial: 50 mcg 1-2 times/day and titrate dose based on patient tolerance and response

Carcinoid: 100-600 mcg/day in 2-4 divided doses

VIPomas: 200-300 mcg/day in 2-4 divided doses

Diarrhea: Initial: I.V.: 50-100 mcg every 8 hours; increase by 100 mcg/dose at 48-hour intervals; maximum dose: 500 mcg every 8 hours

Esophageal varices bleeding: I.V. bolus: 25-50 mcg followed by continuous I.V. infusion of 25-50 mcg/hour

Acromegaly: Initial: SubQ: 50 mcg 3 times/day; titrate to achieve growth hormone levels <5 ng/mL or IGF-I (somatomedin C) levels <1.9 U/mL in males and <2.2 U/mL in females; usual effective dose 100 mcg 3 times/day; range 300-1500 mcg/day

Note: Should be withdrawn yearly for a 4-week interval in patients who have received irradiation. Resume if levels increase and signs/symptoms recur.

Acromegaly, carcinoid tumors, and VIPomas (depot injection): Patients must be stabilized on subcutaneous octreotide for at least 2 weeks before switching to the long-acting depot: Upon switch: 20 mg I.M. intragluteally every 4 weeks for 2-3 months, then the dose may be modified based upon response

Dosage adjustment for acromegaly: After 3 months of depot injections the dosage may be continued or modified as follows:

GH ≤2.5 ng/mL, IGF-1 is normal, symptoms controlled: Maintain octreotide LAR® at 20 mg I.M. every 4 weeks

GH >2.5 ng/mL, IGF-1 is elevated, and/or symptoms uncontrolled: Increase octreotide LAR® to 30 mg I.M. every 4 weeks

GH ≤1 ng/mL, IGF-1 is normal, symptoms controlled: Reduce octreotide LAR® to 10 mg I.M. every 4 weeks

Dosages >40 mg are not recommended

Dosage adjustment for carcinoid tumors and VIPomas: After 2 months of depot injections the dosage may be continued or modified as follows:

Increase to 30 mg I.M. every 4 weeks if symptoms are inadequately controlled

Decrease to 10 mg I.M. every 4 weeks, for a trial period, if initially responsive to 20 mg dose

Dosage >30 mg is not recommended

Administration

Regular injection formulation (do not use if solution contains particles or is discolored): Administer SubQ or I.V.; I.V. administration may be IVP, IVPB, or continuous I.V. infusion:

IVP should be administered undiluted over 3 minutes

IVPB should be administered over 15-30 minutes

Continuous I.V. infusion rates have ranged from 25-50 mcg/hour for the treatment of esophageal variceal bleeding

(Continued)

Octreotide *(Continued)*

Depot formulation: Administer I.M. intragluteal; must be administered immediately after mixing

Dosage Forms

Injection, microspheres for suspension, as acetate [depot formulation] (Sandostatin LAR®): 10 mg, 20 mg, 30 mg [with diluent and syringe]

Injection, solution, as acetate (Sandostatin®): 0.05 mg/mL (1 mL); 0.1 mg/mL (1 mL); 0.2 mg/mL (5 mL); 0.5 mg/mL (1 mL); 1 mg/mL (5 mL)

Dietary Considerations
Schedule injections between meals to decrease GI effects.

Selected Readings

Heikenen JB, Pohl JF, Werlin SL, et al, "Octreotide in Pediatric Patients," *J Pediatr Gastroenterol Nutr*, 2002, 35(5):600-9.

Oberg K, "Established Clinical Use of Octreotide and Lanreotide in Oncology," *Chemotherapy*, 2001, 47 Suppl 2:40-53.

Szilagyi A and Shrier I, "Systematic Review: The Use of Somatostatin or Octreotide in Refractory Diarrhoea," *Aliment Pharmacol Ther*, 2001, 15(12):1889-97.

♦ **Octreotide Acetate** *see Octreotide on page 615*

♦ **Ocuflox®** *see Ofloxacin on page 618*

Ofloxacin *(oh FLOKS a sin)*

Medication Safety Issues

Sound-alike/look-alike issues:

Floxin® may be confused with Flexeril®

Ocuflox® may be confused with Ocufen®

U.S. Brand Names Floxin®; Ocuflox®

Canadian Brand Names Apo-Oflox®; Floxin®; Ocuflox®

Generic Available Yes: Tablet, ophthalmic solution

Synonyms Floxin Otic Singles

Pharmacologic Category Antibiotic, Quinolone

Pregnancy Risk Factor C

Lactation Enters breast milk/not recommended (AAP rates "compatible")

Use Quinolone antibiotic for the treatment of acute exacerbations of chronic bronchitis, community-acquired pneumonia, skin and skin structure infections (uncomplicated), urethral and cervical gonorrhea (acute, uncomplicated), urethritis and cervicitis (nongonococcal), mixed infections of the urethra and cervix, pelvic inflammatory disease (acute), cystitis (uncomplicated), urinary tract infections (complicated), prostatitis

Ophthalmic: Treatment of superficial ocular infections involving the conjunctiva or cornea due to strains of susceptible organisms

Otic: Otitis externa, chronic suppurative otitis media, acute otitis media

Unlabeled/Investigational Use Epididymitis (gonorrhea)

Mechanism of Action Ofloxacin is a DNA gyrase inhibitor. DNA gyrase is an essential bacterial enzyme that maintains the superhelical structure of DNA. DNA gyrase is required for DNA replication and transcription, DNA repair, recombination, and transposition; bactericidal

Labeled Contraindications Hypersensitivity to ofloxacin or other members of the quinolone group such as nalidixic acid, oxolinic acid, cinoxacin, norfloxacin, and ciprofloxacin; hypersensitivity to any component of the formulation

Warnings/Precautions Use with caution in patients with epilepsy or other CNS diseases which could predispose seizures. Use with caution in patients with renal or hepatic impairment. Has been associated with rare tendonitis or ruptured tendons (discontinue immediately with signs of inflammation or tendon pain). Risk may be increased with concurrent corticosteroids, particularly in the elderly. Discontinue at first sign of tendon inflammation or pain. Peripheral neuropathies have been linked to ofloxacin use; discontinue if numbness, tingling, or weakness develops.

Rare cases of torsade de pointes have been reported in patients receiving ofloxacin and other quinolones. Risk may be minimized by avoiding use in patients with known prolongation of the QT interval, bradycardia, hypokalemia, hypomagnesemia, cardiomyopathy, or in those receiving concurrent therapy with Class Ia or Class III antiarrhythmics.

Severe hypersensitivity reactions, including anaphylaxis, have occurred with quinolone therapy. Discontinue immediately if an allergic reaction occurs. Prolonged use may result in superinfection; pseudomembranous colitis may occur and should be considered in all patients who present with diarrhea. Quinolones may exacerbate myasthenia gravis.

Adverse Reactions
Systemic:
1% to 10%:

Cardiovascular: Chest pain (1% to 3%)

Central nervous system: Headache (1% to 9%), insomnia (3% to 7%), dizziness (1% to 5%), fatigue (1% to 3%), somnolence (1% to 3%), sleep disorders (1% to 3%), nervousness (1% to 3%), pyrexia (1% to 3%)

Dermatologic: Rash/pruritus (1% to 3%)

Gastrointestinal: Diarrhea (1% to 4%), vomiting (1% to 4%), GI distress (1% to 3%), abdominal cramps (1% to 3%), flatulence (1% to 3%), abnormal taste (1% to 3%), xerostomia (1% to 3%), decreased appetite (1% to 3%), nausea (3% to 10%), constipation (1% to 3%)

Genitourinary: Vaginitis (1% to 5%), external genital pruritus in women (1% to 3%)

Ocular: Visual disturbances (1% to 3%)

Respiratory: Pharyngitis (1% to 3%)

Miscellaneous: Trunk pain

<1%, postmarketing, and/or case reports (limited to important or life-threatening): Anaphylaxis reactions, anxiety, blurred vision, chills, cognitive change, cough, depression, dream abnormality, ecchymosis, edema, erythema nodosum, euphoria, extremity pain, hallucinations, hearing acuity decreased, hepatic dysfunction, hepatitis, hyper/hypoglycemia, hypertension, interstitial nephritis, lightheadedness, malaise, myasthenia gravis exacerbation, palpitation, paresthesia, peripheral neuropathy, photophobia, photosensitivity, psychotic reactions, rhabdomyolysis, seizure, Stevens-Johnson syndrome, syncope, tendonitis and tendon rupture, thirst, tinnitus, torsade de pointes, Tourette's syndrome, toxic epidermal necrolysis, vasculitis, vasodilation, vertigo, weakness, weight loss

Ophthalmic: Frequency not defined:

Central nervous system: Dizziness

Gastrointestinal: Nausea

Ocular: Blurred vision, burning, chemical conjunctivitis/keratitis, discomfort, dryness, edema, eye pain, foreign body sensation, itching, photophobia, redness, stinging, tearing

(Continued)

Ofloxacin *(Continued)*

Otic:
>10%: Local: Application site reaction (<1% to 17%)

1% to 10%:

Central nervous system: Dizziness (≤1%), vertigo (≤1%)

Dermatologic: Pruritus (1% to 4%), rash (1%)

Gastrointestinal: Taste perversion (7%)

Neuromuscular & skeletal: Paresthesia (1%)

<1% (Limited to important or life-threatening): Diarrhea, fever, headache, hearing loss, hypertension, nausea, otorrhagia, tinnitus, tremor, vomiting, xerostomia

Postmarketing and/case reports: Transient neuropsychiatric disturbances

Vesicant No

Emetic Potential Very low (<10%)

Overdosage/Toxicology Symptoms of overdose include acute renal failure, seizures, nausea, and vomiting. Treatment includes GI decontamination, if possible, and supportive care. Not removed by peritoneal or hemodialysis.

Drug Interactions
Cytochrome P450 Effect: Inhibits CYP1A2 (strong)

Increased Effect/Toxicity: Ofloxacin may increase the effects/toxicity of CYP1A2 substrates (eg, aminophylline, fluvoxamine, mexiletine, mirtazapine, ropinirole, and trifluoperazine), glyburide, theophylline and warfarin. Concomitant use with corticosteroids may increase the risk of tendon rupture. Concomitant use with other QT_c-prolonging agents (eg, Class Ia and Class III antiarrhythmics, erythromycin, cisapride, antipsychotics, and cyclic antidepressants) may result in arrhythmias such as torsade de pointes. Probenecid may increase ofloxacin levels.

Decreased Effect: Concurrent administration of metal cations, including most antacids, oral electrolyte supplements, quinapril, sucralfate, and some didanosine formulations (chewable/buffered tablets and pediatric powder for oral suspension), may decrease quinolone levels; separate doses.

Ethanol/Nutrition/Herb Interactions
Food: Ofloxacin average peak serum concentrations may be decreased by 20% if taken with food.

Herb/Nutraceutical: Avoid dong quai, St John's wort (may also cause photosensitization).

Storage/Stability
Opthalmic and otic solution: Store between 15°C-25°C (59°F-77°F)

Otic singles: Store between 15°C-30°C (59°F-86°F) in pouch to protect from light

Tablets: Store below 30°C (86°F)

I.V.: Single use vials should be stored at controlled room temperature and protected from light. Once diluted, may be stored at room temperature or under refrigeration. Premixed bags should be stored at ≤25°C (77°F); protect from freezing and light. Single use vials, once diluted, are stable for 72 hours when stored at or below 24°C (72°F), for 14 days when stored under refrigeration, and for 6 months when frozen (glass or plastic). If frozen, solutions are stable under refrigeration for 14 days.

Reconstitution I.V.:

Single use vials: Desired dose should be diluted with D_5W or NS to a final concentration of 4 mg/mL

Premixed bags: No further dilution is necessary

Pharmacodynamics/Kinetics

Absorption: Well absorbed; food causes only minor alterations

Distribution: V_d: 2.4-3.5 L/kg

Protein binding: 20%

Bioavailability: Oral: 98%

Half-life elimination: Biphasic: 5-7.5 hours and 20-25 hours (accounts for <5%); prolonged with renal impairment

Excretion: Primarily urine (as unchanged drug)

Dosage

Oral: Adults:

Chronic bronchitis (acute exacerbation), community-acquired pneumonia, skin and skin structure infections (uncomplicated): 400 mg every 12 hours for 10 days

Urethral and cervical gonorrhea (acute, uncomplicated): 400 mg as a single dose

Cervicitis/urethritis (nongonococcal) due to *C. trachomatis*, mixed infection of urethra and cervix due to *C. trachomatis* and *N. gonorrhoeae*: 300 mg every 12 hours for 7 days

Pelvic inflammatory disease (acute): 400 mg every 12 hours for 10-14 days

Cystitis (uncomplicated):

Due to *E. coli* or *K. pneumoniae*: 200 mg every 12 hours for 3 days

Due to other organisms: 200 mg every 12 hours for 7 days

UTI (complicated): 200 mg every 12 hours for 10 days

Prostatitis: 200 mg every 12 hours for 6 weeks

Epididymitis (gonorrhea; unlabeled use): 300 mg twice daily for 10 days

Ophthalmic: Children >1 year and Adults:

Conjunctivitis: Instill 1-2 drops in affected eye(s) every 2-4 hours for the first 2 days, then use 4 times/day for an additional 5 days

Corneal ulcer: Instill 1-2 drops every 30 minutes while awake and every 4-6 hours after retiring for the first 2 days; beginning on day 3, instill 1-2 drops every hour while awake for 4-6 additional days; thereafter, 1-2 drops 4 times/day until clinical cure.

Otic:

Acute otitis media with tympanostomy tubes: Children 1-12 years: Instill 5 drops (or the contents of 1 single-dose container) into affected ear(s) twice daily for 10 days

Chronic suppurative otitis media with perforated tympanic membranes: Children >12 years and Adults: Instill 10 drops (or the contents of 2 single-dose containers) into affected ear twice daily for 14 days

Otitis externa:

Children 6 months to 13 years: Instill 5 drops (or the contents of 1 single-dose container) into affected ear(s) once daily for 7 days

Children ≥13 years and Adults: Instill 10 drops (or the contents of 2 single-dose containers) into affected ear(s) once daily for 7 days

Dosing adjustment/interval in renal impairment: Adults: Oral: After a normal initial dose, adjust as follows:

Cl_{cr} 20-50 mL/minute: Administer usual dose every 24 hours

Cl_{cr} <20 mL/minute: Administer half the usual dose every 24 hours

(Continued)

Ofloxacin *(Continued)*

Continuous arteriovenous or venovenous hemodiafiltration effects: Administer 300 mg every 24 hours

Dosing adjustment in hepatic impairment: Severe impairment: Maximum dose: 400 mg/day

Administration

I.V.: Administer over at least 60 minutes. Infuse separately. Do not infuse through lines containing solutions with magnesium or calcium.

Ophthalmic: For ophthalmic use only; avoid touching tip of applicator to eye or other surfaces.

Oral: Do not take within 2 hours of food or any antacids which contain zinc, magnesium, or aluminum.

Otic: Prior to use, warm solution by holding bottle in hands for 1-2 minutes. Patient should lie down with affected ear upward and medication instilled. Pump tragus 4 times to ensure penetration of medication. Patient should remain in this position for 5 minutes.

Dosage Forms

Solution, ophthalmic (Ocuflox®): 0.3% (5 mL, 10 mL) [contains benzalkonium chloride]

Solution, otic:

Floxin®: 0.3% (5 mL, 10 mL) [contains benzalkonium chloride]

Floxin® Otic Singles™: 0.3% (0.25 mL) [contains benzalkonium chloride; packaged as 2 single-dose containers per pouch, 10 pouches per carton, total net volume 5 mL]

Tablet (Floxin®): 200 mg, 300 mg, 400 mg

Patient Information Report any skin rash or other allergic reactions; avoid excessive sunlight; do not take with food; do not take within 2 hours of any products including antacids which contain calcium, magnesium, or aluminum; contact your prescriber immediately with signs of inflammation or tendon pain

Special Geriatric Considerations The risk of torsade de pointes and tendon inflammation and/or rupture associated with the concomitant use of corticosteroids and quinolones is increased in the elderly population. Dosage must be carefully adjusted to renal function. The half-life of ofloxacin may be prolonged, and serum concentrations are elevated in elderly patients even in the absence of overt renal impairment.

Selected Readings

Abramowicz M, "Antimicrobial Prophylaxis in Surgery," *Medical Letter on Drugs and Therapeutics, Handbook of Antimicrobial Therapy*, 16th ed, New York, NY: Medical Letter, 2002.

Monk JP and Campoli-Richards DM, "Ofloxacin. A Review of Its Antibacterial Activity, Pharmacokinetic Properties and Therapeutic Use," *Drugs*, 1987, 33(4):346-91.

- ◆ **OKT3** *see* Muromonab-CD3 *on page 595*
- ◆ **Oncaspar®** *see* Pegaspargase *on page 652*
- ◆ **Oncotice™ (Can)** *see* BCG Vaccine *on page 120*

Ondansetron *(on DAN se tron)*

Medication Safety Issues

Sound-alike/look-alike issues:

Zofran® may be confused with Zantac®, Zosyn®

Related Information

Management of Nausea and Vomiting *on page 982*

U.S. Brand Names Zofran®; Zofran® ODT

Canadian Brand Names Zofran®; Zofran® ODT

Generic Available No

Synonyms GR38032R; Ondansetron Hydrochloride

Pharmacologic Category Antiemetic; Selective 5-HT₃ Receptor Antagonist

Pregnancy Risk Factor B

Lactation Excretion in breast milk unknown/opportunity for use is minimal

Use Prevention of nausea and vomiting associated with moderately- to highly-emetogenic cancer chemotherapy; radiotherapy in patients receiving total body irradiation or fractions to the abdomen; prevention and treatment of postoperative nausea and vomiting

Not recommended for treatment of existing chemotherapy-induced emesis (CIE).

Unlabeled/Investigational Use Treatment of early-onset alcoholism

Mechanism of Action Selective 5-HT₃-receptor antagonist, blocking serotonin, both peripherally on vagal nerve terminals and centrally in the chemoreceptor trigger zone

Labeled Contraindications Hypersensitivity to ondansetron, other selective 5-HT₃ antagonists, or any component of the formulation

Warnings/Precautions Ondansetron should be used on a scheduled basis, not on an "as needed" (PRN) basis, since data support the use of this drug only in the prevention of nausea and vomiting (due to antineoplastic therapy) and not in the rescue of nausea and vomiting. Ondansetron should only be used in the first 24-48 hours of chemotherapy. Data do not support any increased efficacy of ondansetron in delayed nausea and vomiting. Does not stimulate gastric or intestinal peristalsis; may mask progressive ileus and/or gastric distension. Orally-disintegrating tablets contain phenylalanine.

Adverse Reactions

>10%:
  Cardiovascular: Malaise/fatigue (9% to 13%)
  Central nervous system: Headache (9% to 27%)
1% to 10%:
  Central nervous system: Drowsiness (8%), fever (2% to 8%), dizziness (4% to 7%), anxiety (6%), cold sensation (2%)
  Dermatologic: Pruritus (2% to 5%), rash (1%)
  Gastrointestinal: Constipation (6% to 9%), diarrhea (3% to 7%)
  Genitourinary: Gynecological disorder (7%), urinary retention (5%)
  Hepatic: Increased ALT/AST (1% to 2%)
  Local: Injection site reaction (4%)
  Neuromuscular & skeletal: Paresthesia (2%)
  Respiratory: Hypoxia (9%)
<1%: Anaphylaxis, angina, bronchospasm, ECG changes, extrapyramidal symptoms, grand mal seizure, hypokalemia, tachycardia, vascular occlusive events
Postmarketing and/or case reports: Angioedema, cardiopulmonary arrest, dystonic reactions, flushing, hiccups, hypersensitivity reactions, hypotension, laryngeal edema, laryngospasm, oculogyric crisis, shock, dyspnea, stridor, urticaria

Vesicant No

Emetic Potential Very low (<10%)

(Continued)

Ondansetron *(Continued)*

Overdosage/Toxicology Sudden transient blindness, severe constipation, hypotension, and vasovagal episode with transient secondary heart block have been reported in some cases of overdose. I.V. doses of up to 252 mg/day have been inadvertently given without adverse effects. There is no specific antidote. Treatment is symptom-directed and supportive.

Drug Interactions

Cytochrome P450 Effect: Substrate of CYP1A2 (minor), 2C8/9 (minor), 2D6 (minor), 2E1 (minor), 3A4 (major); **Inhibits** CYP1A2 (weak), 2C8/9 (weak), 2D6 (weak)

Decreased Effect: CYP3A4 inducers may decrease the levels/effects of ondansetron; example inducers include aminoglutethimide, carbamazepine, nafcillin, nevirapine, phenobarbital, phenytoin, and rifamycins. The manufacturer does not recommend dosage adjustment in patients receiving CYP3A4 inducers.

Ethanol/Nutrition/Herb Interactions

Food: Food increases the extent of absorption. The C_{max} and T_{max} do not change much.

Herb/Nutraceutical: St John's wort may decrease ondansetron levels.

Storage/Stability

Oral solution: Store between 15°C and 30°C (59°F and 86°F). Protect from light.

Tablet: Store between 2°C and 30°C (36°F and 86°F)

Vial: Store between 2°C and 30°C (36°F and 86°F). Protect from light. Stable when mixed in 5% dextrose or 0.9% sodium chloride for 48 hours at room temperature.

Reconstitution Prior to I.V. infusion, dilute in 50-100 mL D_5W or NS.

Compatibility Stable in $D_5^1/_2NS$, D_5NS, D_5W, mannitol 10%, LR, NS, sodium chloride 3%

Y-site administration: Compatible: Alatrofloxacin, aldesleukin, amifostine, amikacin, aztreonam, bleomycin, carboplatin, carmustine, cefazolin, cefotaxime, cefoxitin, ceftazidime, ceftizoxime, cefuroxime, chlorpromazine, cimetidine, cisatracurium, cisplatin, cladribine, clindamycin, cyclophosphamide, cytarabine, dacarbazine, dactinomycin, daunorubicin, dexamethasone sodium phosphate, diphenhydramine, docetaxel, dopamine, doxorubicin, doxorubicin liposome, doxycycline, droperidol, etoposide, etoposide phosphate, famotidine, filgrastim, floxuridine, fluconazole, fludarabine, gatifloxacin, gemcitabine, gentamicin, haloperidol, heparin, hydrocortisone sodium phosphate, hydrocortisone sodium succinate, hydromorphone, hydroxyzine, ifosfamide, imipenem/cilastatin, linezolid, magnesium sulfate, mannitol, mechlorethamine, melphalan, meperidine, mesna, methotrexate, metoclopramide, mitomycin, mitoxantrone, morphine, paclitaxel, paclitaxel with ranitidine, pentostatin, piperacillin/tazobactam, potassium chloride, prochlorperazine edisylate, promethazine, ranitidine, remifentanil, sodium acetate, streptozocin, teniposide, thiotepa, ticarcillin, ticarcillin/clavulanate, topotecan, vancomycin, vinblastine, vincristine, vinorelbine, zidovudine. **Incompatible:** Acyclovir, allopurinol, aminophylline, amphotericin B, amphotericin B cholesteryl sulfate complex, ampicillin, ampicillin/sulbactam, amsacrine, cefepime, cefoperazone, furosemide, ganciclovir, lorazepam, methylprednisolone sodium succinate, piperacillin, sargramostim, sodium bicarbonate. **Variable (consult detailed reference):** Fluorouracil, meropenem

Pharmacodynamics/Kinetics
Onset of action: ~30 minutes

Distribution: V_d: 2.2-2.5 L/kg

Protein binding, plasma: 70% to 76%

Metabolism: Extensively hepatic via hydroxylation, followed by glucuronide or sulfate conjugation; CYP1A2, CYP2D6, and CYP3A4 substrate; some demethylation occurs

Bioavailability: Oral: 56% to 71%; Rectal: 58% to 74%

Half-life elimination: Children <15 years: 2-3 hours; Adults: 3-6 hours

Time to peak: Oral: ~2 hours

Excretion: Urine (44% to 60% as metabolites, 5% to 10% as unchanged drug); feces (~25%)

Dosage Note: Administration of a single daily dose of 8-12 mg I.V. or 8-24 mg orally is now generally accepted in place of mg/kg dosing. See Management of Nausea and Vomiting *on page 982* in the Appendix.

Children:

I.V.:

Chemotherapy-induced emesis: 4-18 years: 0.15 mg/kg/dose administered 30 minutes prior to chemotherapy, 4 and 8 hours after the first dose **or** 0.45 mg/kg/day as a single dose

Postoperative nausea and vomiting: 2-12 years:

≤40 kg: 0.1 mg/kg

>40 kg: 4 mg

Oral: Chemotherapy-induced emesis:

4-11 years: 4 mg 30 minutes before chemotherapy; repeat 4 and 8 hours after initial dose, then 4 mg every 8 hours for 1-2 days after chemotherapy completed

≥12 years: Refer to adult dosing.

Adults:

I.V.: Chemotherapy-induced emesis:

0.15 mg/kg 3 times/day beginning 30 minutes prior to chemotherapy **or**

0.45 mg/kg once daily **or**

8-10 mg 1-2 times/day **or**

24 mg or 32 mg once daily

I.M., I.V.: Postoperative nausea and vomiting: 4 mg as a single dose approximately 30 minutes before the end of anesthesia, or as treatment if vomiting occurs after surgery

Oral:

Chemotherapy-induced emesis:

Highly-emetogenic agents/single-day therapy: 24 mg given 30 minutes prior to the start of therapy

Moderately-emetogenic agents: 8 mg every 12 hours beginning 30 minutes before chemotherapy, continuously for 1-2 days after chemotherapy completed

Total body irradiation: 8 mg 1-2 hours before daily each fraction of radiotherapy

Single high-dose fraction radiotherapy to abdomen: 8 mg 1-2 hours before irradiation, then 8 mg every 8 hours after first dose for 1-2 days after completion of radiotherapy

Daily fractionated radiotherapy to abdomen: 8 mg 1-2 hours before irradiation, then 8 mg 8 hours after first dose for each day of radiotherapy

(Continued)

Ondansetron *(Continued)*

Postoperative nausea and vomiting: 16 mg given 1 hour prior to induction of anesthesia

Elderly: No dosing adjustment required

Dosage adjustment in renal impairment: No dosing adjustment required

Dosage adjustment in hepatic impairment: Maximum daily dose: 8 mg in patients with severe liver disease (Child-Pugh score ≥10)

Administration

Oral: Oral dosage forms should be administered 30 minutes prior to chemotherapy; 1-2 hours before radiotherapy; 1 hour prior to the induction of anesthesia

Orally-disintegrating tablets: Do not remove from blister until needed. Peel backing off the blister, do not push tablet through. Using dry hands, place tablet on tongue and allow to dissolve. Swallow with saliva.

I.M.: Should be administered undiluted

I.V.: Give first dose 30 minutes prior to beginning chemotherapy; the I.V. preparation has been successful when administered orally

IVPB: Infuse over 15-30 minutes; 24-hour continuous infusions have been reported, but are rarely used

Dosage Forms

Infusion, as hydrochloride [premixed in D_5W] (Zofran®): 32 mg (50 mL)

Injection, solution, as hydrochloride (Zofran®): 2 mg/mL (2 mL, 20 mL)

Solution, as hydrochloride (Zofran®): 4 mg/5 mL (50 mL) [contains sodium benzoate; strawberry flavor]

Tablet, as hydrochloride (Zofran®): 4 mg, 8 mg, 24 mg

Tablet, orally-disintegrating (Zofran® ODT): 4 mg, 8 mg [each strength contains phenylalanine <0.03 mg/tablet; strawberry flavor]

Dietary Considerations Take without regard to meals.

Potassium: Hypokalemia; monitor potassium serum concentration

Orally-disintegrating tablet contains <0.03 mg phenylalanine

Patient Information Orally-disintegrating tablets: Do not remove from blister until needed. Peel backing off the blister, do not push tablet through. Using dry hands, place tablet on tongue and allow to dissolve. Swallow with saliva. Contains <0.03 mg phenylalanine/tablet.

Special Geriatric Considerations Elderly have a slightly decreased hepatic clearance rate. This does not, however, require a dose adjustment.

Extemporaneous Preparations A 0.8 mg/mL syrup may be made by crushing ten 8 mg tablets; flaking of the tablet coating occurs. Mix thoroughly with 50 mL of the suspending vehicle, Ora-Plus® (Paddock), in 5 mL increments. Add sufficient volume of any of the following syrups: Cherry syrup USP, Syrpalta® (Humco), Ora-Sweet® (Paddock), or Ora-Sweet® Sugar-Free (Paddock) to make a final volume of 100 mL. Stability is 42 days refrigerated.

Trissel LA, "Trissel's Stability of Compounded Formulations," American Pharmaceutical Association, 1996.

Rectal suppositories: Calibrate a suppository mold for the base being used. Determine the displacement factor (DF) for ondansetron for the base being used (Fattibase® = 1.1; Polybase® = 0.6). Weigh the ondansetron tablet. Divide the tablet weight by the DF. Subtract the weight of base displaced from the calculated weight of base required for each supposi-tory. Grind the ondansetron tablets to a fine powder in a mortar. Weigh out the appropriate weight of suppository base. Melt the base over a water bath (<55°C). Add the ondansetron powder to the suppository base and mix well. Pour the mixture into the suppository mold and cool. Stable for at least 30 days under refrigeration.

Allen LV, "Ondansetron Suppositories," *US Pharm*, 20(7):84-6.

Selected Readings

Chaffee BJ and Tankanow RM, "Ondansetron - the First of a New Class of Antiemetic Agents," *Clin Pharm*, 1991, 10(6):430-6.

Culy CR, Bhana N, and Plosker GL, "Ondansetron: A Review of its Use as an Antiemetic in Children," *Paediatr Drugs*, 2001, 3(6):441-79.

Markham A and Sorkin EM, "Ondansetron. An Update of Its Therapeutic Use in Chemo-therapy-Induced and Postoperative Nausea and Vomiting," *Drugs*, 1993, 45(6):931-52.

Milne RJ and Heel RC, "Ondansetron: Therapeutic Use as an Antiemetic," *Drugs*, 1991, 41(4):574-95.

Roila F and Del Favero A, "Ondansetron Clinical Pharmacokinetics," *Clin Pharmacokinet*, 1995, 29(2):95-109.

Tramer MR, Moore RA, Reynolds DJ, et al, "A Quantitative Systematic Review of Ondanse-tron in Treatment of Established Postoperative Nausea and Vomiting," *BMJ*, 1997, 314(7087):1088-92.

Wilde MI and Markham A, "Ondansetron. A Review of Its Pharmacology and Preliminary Clinical Findings in Novel Application," *Drugs*, 1996, 52(5):773-94.

Oprelvekin (oh PREL ve kin)

Medication Safety Issues

Sound-alike/look-alike issues:

Oprelvekin may be confused with aldesleukin, Proleukin®

Neumega® may be confused with Neupogen®

U.S. Brand Names Neumega®

Generic Available No

Synonyms IL-11; Interleukin-11; Recombinant Human Interleukin-11; Recombinant Interleukin-11; rhIL-11; rIL-11

Pharmacologic Category Biological Response Modulator; Human Growth Factor

Pregnancy Risk Factor C

Lactation Excretion in breast milk unknown

Use Prevention of severe thrombocytopenia and the reduction of the need for platelet transfusions following myelosuppressive chemotherapy

Mechanism of Action Oprelvekin stimulates multiple stages of mega-karyocytopoiesis and thrombopoiesis, resulting in proliferation of mega-karyocyte progenitors and megakaryocyte maturation

Labeled Contraindications Hypersensitivity to oprelvekin or any component of the formulation

Warnings/Precautions Oprelvekin may cause serious fluid retention and should be used cautiously in patients with conditions where expansion of plasma volume should be avoided (eg, left ventricular dysfunction, CHF, hypertension). Use caution in patients with cardiac arrhythmias or conduction defects, respiratory disease; history of thromboembolic prob-lems; hepatic or renal dysfunction. Not indicated following myeloablative (Continued)

Oprelvekin *(Continued)*

chemotherapy. Severe hypokalemia and/or sudden death have been reported in patients receiving chronic diuretic therapy. Permanently discontinue oprelvekin in any patient developing an allergic reaction. Although used in pediatric patients in clinical trials, safety and efficacy have not been established in pediatric patients. Papilledema, more frequently associated with use in children and dose limiting, has occurred; use caution in patients with pre-existing papilledema or with tumors involving the central nervous system.

Adverse Reactions

>10%:

Cardiovascular: Tachycardia (19% to 30%), palpitation (14% to 24%), atrial arrhythmia (12%), peripheral edema (60% to 75%), syncope (6% to 13%)

Central nervous system: Headache (41%), dizziness (38%), insomnia (33%), fatigue (30%), fever (36%)

Dermatologic: Rash (25%)

Endocrine & metabolic: Fluid retention

Gastrointestinal: Nausea (50% to 77%), vomiting, anorexia

Hematologic: Anemia (100%), probably a dilutional phenomena; appears within 3 days of initiation of therapy, resolves in about 1 week after cessation of oprelvekin

Neuromuscular & skeletal: Arthralgia, myalgia

Ocular: Papilledema (16% in pediatric patients, 1% in adults)

Respiratory: Dyspnea (48%), pleural effusion (10%)

1% to 10%: Gastrointestinal: Weight gain (5%)

Postmarketing and/or case reports: Allergic reaction, anaphylaxis/anaphylactoid reactions, capillary leak syndrome, injection site reactions, renal failure

Vesicant No

Emetic Potential Moderate (30% to 60%)

Overdosage/Toxicology Doses of oprelvekin >50 mcg/kg may be associated with an increased incidence of cardiovascular events. If an overdose is administered, discontinue oprelvekin and closely observe patient for signs of toxicity. Base reinstitution of therapy on individual patient factors (evidence of toxicity and continued need for therapy).

Drug Interactions

Increased Effect/Toxicity: Oprelvekin may increase the risk of hypokalemia in patients receiving chronic diuretic therapy.

Storage/Stability Store vials under refrigeration between 2°C to 8°C (36°F to 46°F); do not freeze. Use reconstituted oprelvekin within 3 hours of reconstitution and store in the vial at either 2°C to 8°C (36°F to 46°F) or room temperature (≤25°C/70°F). Do not freeze or shake reconstituted solution.

Reconstitution Reconstitute to a final concentration of 5 mg/mL with SWFI.

Pharmacodynamics/Kinetics

Metabolism: Uncertain

Half-life elimination: Terminal: 5-8 hours

Time to peak, serum: 1-6 hours

Excretion: Urine (primarily as metabolites)

Dosage SubQ: First dose should not be administered until 24-36 hours after the end of chemotherapy. Discontinue the drug at least 48 hours before beginning the next cycle of chemotherapy.

Children: 75-100 mcg/kg once daily for 10-21 days (until postnadir platelet count ≥50,000 cells/µL)

> **Note:** The manufacturer states that, until efficacy/toxicity parameters are established, the use of oprelvekin in pediatric patients (particularly those <12 years of age) should be restricted to use in controlled clinical trials.

Adults: 50 mcg/kg once daily for 10-21 days (until postnadir platelet count ≥50,000 cells/µL)

Administration Subcutaneously in either the abdomen, thigh, or hip (or upper arm if not self-injected).

Dosage Forms Injection, powder for reconstitution: 5 mg [packaged with diluent]

Monitoring Parameters Monitor electrolytes and fluid balance during therapy; obtain a CBC at regular intervals during therapy; monitor platelet counts until adequate recovery has occurred

Patient Information Report any swelling in the arms or legs (peripheral edema), shortness of breath (congestive failure, anemia), irregular heartbeat, headaches

Selected Readings

Du X and Williams DA, "Interleukin-11: Review of Molecular, Cell Biology, and Clinical Use," *Blood*, 1997, 89(11):3897-908.

Gordon MS, "Thrombopoietic Activity of Recombinant Human Interleukin 11 in Cancer Patients Receiving Chemotherapy," *Cancer Chemother Pharmacol*, 1996, 38 (Suppl):96-8.

Sitaraman SV and Gewirtz AT, "Oprelvekin. Genetics Institute," *Curr Opin Investig Drugs*, 2001, 2(10):1395-400.

Tepler I, Elias L, Smith JW 2d, et al, "A Randomized Placebo-Controlled Trial of Recombinant Human Interleukin-11 in Cancer Patients With Severe Thrombocytopenia Due to Chemotherapy," *Blood*, 1996, 87(9):3607-14.

Teramura M, Kobayashi S, Yoshinaga K, et al, "Effect of Interleukin 11 on Normal and Pathological Thrombopoiesis," *Cancer Chemother Pharmacol*, 1996, 38 (Suppl):99-102.

♦ **Oramorph SR**® *see* Morphine Sulfate *on page 588*

♦ **Orapred**® *see* PrednisoLONE *on page 679*

♦ **Orthoclone OKT**® **3** *see* Muromonab-CD3 *on page 595*

♦ **Orzel**® *see* UFT *on page 804*

♦ **OSI-774** *see* Erlotinib *on page 308*

♦ **Ostac**® **(Can)** *see* Clodronate *on page 199*

Oxaliplatin (ox AL i pla tin)

Medication Safety Issues

Sound-alike/look-alike issues:

Oxaliplatin may be confused with Aloxi™

Related Information

Investigational Drug Service *on page 1031*

Safe Handling of Hazardous Drugs *on page 1034*

U.S. Brand Names Eloxatin™

Generic Available No

Synonyms Diaminocyclohexane Oxalatoplatinum; L-OHP; NSC-266046

Pharmacologic Category Antineoplastic Agent, Alkylating Agent

Pregnancy Risk Factor D

Lactation Excretion in breast milk unknown/not recommended

(Continued)

Oxaliplatin *(Continued)*

Use Treatment of advanced colon cancer and advanced rectal carcinoma

Unlabeled/Investigational Use Head and neck cancer, nonsmall cell lung cancer, non-Hodgkin's lymphoma, ovarian cancer

Mechanism of Action Oxaliplatin is an alkylating agent. Following intracellular hydrolysis, the platinum compound binds to DNA, RNA, or proteins. Cytotoxicity is cell-cycle nonspecific.

Labeled Contraindications Hypersensitivity to oxaliplatin, other platinum-containing compounds, or any component of the formulation; pregnancy

Warnings/Precautions Hazardous agent - use appropriate precautions for handling and disposal. See Safe Handling of Hazardous Drugs *on page 1034* in the Appendix. Anaphylactic-like reaction may occur within minutes of oxaliplatin administration. Two different types of neuropathy may occur: First, acute (within first 2 days), reversible (resolves within 14 days), primarily peripheral symptoms that are often exacerbated by cold (may include pharyngolaryngeal dysesthesia); and secondly, a more persistent (>14 days) presentation that often interferes with daily activities (eg, writing, buttoning, swallowing), these symptoms may improve upon discontinuing treatment. May cause pulmonary fibrosis or hepatotoxicity. The presence of hepatic vascular disorders (including veno-occlusive disease) should be considered, especially in individuals developing portal hypertension or who present with increased liver function tests. Caution in renal dysfunction. Safety and efficacy in pediatric patients have not been established.

Adverse Reactions Based on clinical trial data using oxaliplatin alone. Some adverse effects (eg, thrombocytopenia, hemorrhagic events, neutropenia) may be increased when therapy is combined with fluorouracil/leucovorin.

>10%:

  Central nervous system: Fatigue (61%), fever (25%), pain (14%), headache (13%), insomnia (11%)

  Gastrointestinal: Nausea (64%), diarrhea (46%), vomiting (37%), abdominal pain (31%), constipation (31%), anorexia (20%), stomatitis (14%)

  Hematologic: Anemia (64%), thrombocytopenia (30%), leukopenia (13%)

  Hepatic: SGOT increased (54%), SGPT increased (36%); total bilirubin increased (13%)

  Neuromuscular & skeletal: Neuropathy (may be dose-limiting), peripheral (acute 56%, persistent 48%), back pain (11%)

  Respiratory: Dyspnea (13%), cough (11%)

1% to 10%:

  Cardiovascular: Edema (10%), chest pain (5%), flushing (3%), thrombosis (2% to 6%), thromboembolism (6% to 9%)

  Central nervous system: Rigors (9%), dizziness (7%), hand-foot syndrome (1%)

  Dermatologic: Rash (5%), alopecia (3%)

  Endocrine & metabolic: Dehydration (5%), hypokalemia (3%)

  Gastrointestinal: Dyspepsia (7%), taste perversion (5%), flatulence (3%), mucositis (2%), gastroesophageal reflux (1%), dysphagia (acute 1% to 2%)

  Genitourinary: Dysuria (1%)

Hematologic: Neutropenia (7%)
Local: Injection site reaction (9%)
Neuromuscular & skeletal: Arthralgia (7%)
Ocular: Abnormal lacrimation (1%)
Renal: Serum creatinine increased (10%)
Respiratory: URI (7%), rhinitis (6%), epistaxis (2%), pharyngitis (2%), pharyngolaryngeal dysesthesia (1% to 2%)
Miscellaneous: Allergic reactions (3%), hiccup (2%)

Postmarketing and/or case reports: Anaphylactic shock, angioedema, colitis, cranial nerve palsies, deep tendon reflex loss, deafness, dysarthria, fasciculations, hemolytic anemia (immuno-allergic), hemolytic uremia syndrome, ileus, interstitial lung diseases, intestinal obstruction, Lhermittes' sign, metabolic acidosis, optic neuritis, pancreatitis, pulmonary fibrosis, thrombocytopenia (immuno-allergic), veno-occlusive disease of the liver, visual acuity decreased, visual field disturbance

Vesicant No

Emetic Potential High (60% to 90%)

Overdosage/Toxicology Overdose symptoms are extensions of known side effects (eg, thrombocytopenia, myelosuppression, nausea, vomiting, neurotoxicity, respiratory symptoms). Treatment should be supportive.

Drug Interactions

Increased Effect/Toxicity: Taxane derivatives may increase oxaliplatin toxicity if administered before the platin as a sequential infusion. Nephrotoxic agents may increase oxaliplatin toxicity. Prolonged prothrombin time and increased INR associated with hemorrhage have been reported in patients receiving oxaliplatin/fluorouracil/leucovorin concomitantly with oral anticoagulants.

Storage/Stability Store in original outer carton at room temperature of 15°C to 30°C (59°F to 86°F); do not freeze. Protect from light. Diluted solution is stable up to 6 hours at room temperature of 20°C to 25°C (68°F to 77°F) or up to 24 hours under refrigeration at 2°C to 8°C (36°F to 46°F).

Reconstitution Do not reconstitute using a chloride-containing solution (eg, NaCl). Further dilution with D_5W (250 or 500 mL) is required prior to administration. Reconstituted solution does not require protection from light.

Compatibility Incompatible with alkaline solutions (eg, fluorouracil) and chloride-containing solutions. Flush infusion line with D_5W prior to, and following, administration of concomitant medications via same I.V. line.

Y-site administration: Compatible: Allopurinol, aminophylline, bumetanide, buprenorphine, butorphanol, calcium gluconate, carboplatin, chlorpromazine, cimetidine, cyclophosphamide, dexamethasone, diphenhydramine, dobutamine, docetaxel, dolasetron, dopamine, doxorubicin, droperidol, enalaprilat, epirubicin, etoposide phosphate, famotidine, fentanyl, furosemide, gemcitabine, granisetron, haloperidol, heparin, hydrocortisone sodium succinate, hydromorphone, hydroxyzine, ifosfamide, irinotecan, leucovorin, lorazepam, magnesium sulfate, mannitol, meperidine, mesna, methotrexate, methylprednisolone sodium succinate, metoclopramide, mitoxantrone, morphine, nalbuphine, ondansetron, paclitaxel, potassium chloride, prochlorperazine, promethazine, ranitidine, sodium bicarbonate, theophylline, topotecan, verapamil, vincristine, vinorelbine. **Incompatible:** Diazepam
(Continued)

Oxaliplatin *(Continued)*

Pharmacodynamics/Kinetics

Distribution: V_d: 440 L

Protein binding: >90% primarily albumin and gamma globulin (irreversible binding to platinum)

Metabolism: Nonenzymatic (rapid and extensive), forms active and inactive derivatives

Half-life elimination: 391 hours; Distribution: Alpha phase: 0.4 hours, Beta phase: 16.8 hours

Excretion: Primarily urine

Dosage I.V.: Colorectal cancer (labeled dosing): Refer to individual protocols.

Adults:

85 mg/m² every 2 weeks **or**

20-25 mg/m² days 1-5 every 3 weeks **or**

100-130 mg/m² every 2-3 weeks

Elderly: No dosing adjustment recommended

Dosage adjustments for toxicity: Longer infusion times may mitigate acute toxicities. In patients experiencing persistent neurosensory events (grade 2) which do not resolve, a dose reduction may be considered. Grade 3 neurosensory events may prompt consideration to discontinue oxaliplatin (while fluorouracil/leucovorin are continued or decreased). After recovery from grade 3/4 gastrointestinal toxicity, grade 4 neutropenia, or grade 3/4 thrombocytopenia, a dosage reduction is recommended.

Dosage adjustment in renal impairment: Use with caution; specific guidelines not established

Combination Regimens

Colorectal cancer:

FOIL *on page 890*

FOLFOX 1 *on page 891*

FOLFOX 2 *on page 891*

FOLFOX 3 *on page 891*

FOLFOX 4 *on page 892*

FOLFOX 6 *on page 892*

FOLFOX 7 *on page 892*

XelOx *on page 949*

Lymphoma, non-Hodgkin's: DHAP *on page 872*

Administration Administer as I.V. infusion over 2-6 hours. Flush infusion line with D_5W prior to administration of any concomitant medication.

Dosage Forms

Injection, powder for reconstitution: 50 mg, 100 mg [contains lactose]

Injection, solution [preservative free]: 5 mg/mL (10 mL, 20 mL)

Monitoring Parameters CBC, serum creatinine, liver function tests; signs of neuropathy, hypersensitivity, and/or respiratory effects; delay dosage until recover of neutrophils ≥1.5 x 10⁹/L and platelets ≥75 x 10⁹/L

Patient Information Maintain adequate nutrition (frequent small meals may help) and adequate hydration (2-3 L/day of fluids unless instructed to restrict fluid intake). Nausea and vomiting may be severe; request antiemetic. You will be susceptible to infection; avoid crowds or exposure to infection. Report sore throat, fever, chills, unusual fatigue or unusual bruising/bleeding, difficulty breathing, muscle cramps or twitching, tingling/numbness in arms, fingers, legs, or toes (may be increased by cold temperature). Inform prescriber if you are pregnant. Do not get pregnant during or for 1 month following therapy. Male: Do not cause a female to become pregnant. Male/female: Consult prescriber for instruction on appropriate barrier contraceptive measures. This drug may cause severe fetal defects. Do not breast-feed.

Selected Readings

Cassidy J and Misset JL, "Oxaliplatin-Related Side Effects: Characteristics and Management," *Semin Oncol*, 2002, 29(5 Suppl 15):11-20

Culy CR, Clemett D, and Wiseman LR, "Oxaliplatin. A Review of its Pharmacological Properties and Clinical Efficacy in Metastatic Colorectal Cancer and its Potential in Other Malignancies," *Drugs*, 2000, 60(4):895-924.

Graham MA, Lockwood GF, Greenslade D, et al, "Clinical Pharmacokinetics of Oxaliplatin: A Critical Review," *Clin Cancer Res*, 2000, 6(4):1205-18.

Mani S, Graham MA, Bregman DB, et al, "Oxaliplatin: A Review of Evolving Concepts," *Cancer Invest*, 2002, 20(2):246-63.

Misset JL, Bleiberg H, Sutherland W, et al, "Oxaliplatin Clinical Activity: A Review," *Crit Rev Oncol Hematol*, 2000, 35(2):75-93.

Raymond E, Faivre S, Chaney S, et al, "Cellular and Molecular Pharmacology of Oxaliplatin," *Mol Cancer Ther*, 2002, 1(3):227-35.

Oxycodone (oks i KOE done)

Medication Safety Issues

Sound-alike/look-alike issues:

Oxycodone may be confused with OxyContin®

OxyContin® may be confused with oxybutynin, oxycodone

U.S. Brand Names OxyContin®; Oxydose™; OxyFast®; OxyIR®; Roxicodone™; Roxicodone™ Intensol™

Canadian Brand Names OxyContin®; Oxy.IR®; Supeudol®

Generic Available Yes

Synonyms Dihydrohydroxycodeinone; Oxycodone Hydrochloride

Pharmacologic Category Analgesic, Narcotic

Pregnancy Risk Factor B/D (prolonged use or high doses at term)

Lactation Enters breast milk/use caution

Use Management of moderate to severe pain, normally used in combination with non-narcotic analgesics

OxyContin® is indicated for around-the-clock management of moderate to severe pain when an analgesic is needed for an extended period of time. **Note:** OxyContin® is not intended for use as an "as needed" analgesic or for immediately-postoperative pain management (should be used postoperatively only if the patient has received it prior to surgery or if severe, persistent pain is anticipated).

Mechanism of Action Binds to opiate receptors in the CNS, causing inhibition of ascending pain pathways, altering the perception of and response to pain; produces generalized CNS depression

Restrictions C-II

Labeled Contraindications Hypersensitivity to oxycodone or any component of the formulation; significant respiratory depression; hypercarbia; acute or severe bronchial asthma; OxyContin® is also contraindicated in paralytic ileus (known or suspected); pregnancy (prolonged use or high doses at term)

Warnings/Precautions Use with caution in patients with hypersensitivity reactions to other phenanthrene derivative opioid agonists (morphine, hydrocodone, hydromorphone, levorphanol, oxycodone, oxymorphone), respiratory diseases including asthma, emphysema, or COPD. Use with (Continued)

Oxycodone *(Continued)*

caution in pancreatitis or biliary tract disease, acute alcoholism (including delirium tremens), adrenocortical insufficiency, CNS depression/coma, kyphoscoliosis (or other skeletal disorder which may alter respiratory function), hypothyroidism (including myxedema), prostatic hyperplasia, urethral stricture, and toxic psychosis.

Use with caution in the elderly, debilitated, severe hepatic or renal function. Hemodynamic effects (hypotension, orthostasis) may be exaggerated in patients with hypovolemia, concurrent vasodilating drugs, or in patients with head injury. Respiratory depressant effects and capacity to elevate CSF pressure may be exaggerated in presence of head injury, other intracranial lesion, or pre-existing intracranial pressure. Tolerance or drug dependence may result from extended use. Healthcare provider should be alert to problems of abuse, misuse, and diversion. Do **not** crush controlled-release tablets. Some preparations contain sulfites which may cause allergic reactions. OxyContin® 80 mg and 160 mg strengths are for use only in opioid-tolerant patients requiring high daily dosages >160 mg (80 mg formulation) or >320 mg (160 mg formulation).

Adverse Reactions

>10%:

Central nervous system: Fatigue, drowsiness, dizziness, somnolence

Dermatologic: Pruritus

Gastrointestinal: Nausea, vomiting, constipation

Neuromuscular & skeletal: Weakness

1% to 10%:

Cardiovascular: Postural hypotension

Central nervous system: Nervousness, headache, restlessness, malaise, confusion, anxiety, abnormal dreams, euphoria, thought abnormalities

Dermatologic: Rash

Gastrointestinal: Anorexia, stomach cramps, xerostomia, biliary spasm, abdominal pain, dyspepsia, gastritis

Genitourinary: Ureteral spasms, decreased urination

Local: Pain at injection site

Respiratory: Dyspnea, hiccups

Miscellaneous: Diaphoresis

<1% (Limited to important or life-threatening): Anaphylaxis, anaphylactoid reaction, dysphagia, exfoliative dermatitis, hallucinations, histamine release, hyponatremia, ileus, intracranial pressure increased, mental depression, paradoxical CNS stimulation, paralytic ileus, physical and psychological dependence, SIADH, syncope, urinary retention, urticaria, vasodilation, withdrawal syndrome (may include seizure)

Note: Deaths due to overdose have been reported due to misuse/abuse after crushing the sustained release tablets.

Overdosage/Toxicology Symptoms of toxicity include CNS depression, respiratory depression, and miosis. Naloxone, 2 mg I.V. with repeat administration as necessary up to a total of 10 mg, can also be used to reverse toxic effects of the opiate.

Drug Interactions

Cytochrome P450 Effect: Substrate of CYP2D6 (major)

Increased Effect/Toxicity: MAO inhibitors may increase adverse symptoms. Cimetidine may increase narcotic analgesic serum levels resulting in toxicity. CNS depressants (barbiturates, ethanol) and TCAs may potentiate the sedative and respiratory depressive effects of morphine and other opiate agonists. Dextroamphetamine may enhance the analgesic effect of morphine and other opiate agonists.

Ethanol/Nutrition/Herb Interactions
Ethanol: Avoid ethanol (may increase CNS depression).

Food: When taken with a high-fat meal, peak concentration is 25% greater following a single OxyContin® 160 mg tablet as compared to two 80 mg tablets.

Herb/Nutraceutical: Avoid valerian, St John's wort, kava kava, gotu kola (may increase CNS depression).

Storage/Stability Tablets should be stored at room temperature.

Pharmacodynamics/Kinetics
Onset of action: Pain relief: 10-15 minutes

Peak effect: 0.5-1 hour

Duration: 3-6 hours; Controlled release: ≤12 hours

Metabolism: Hepatic

Half-life elimination: 2-3 hours

Excretion: Urine

Dosage Oral:
Immediate release:

Children:

6-12 years: 1.25 mg every 6 hours as needed

>12 years: 2.5 mg every 6 hours as needed

Adults: 5 mg every 6 hours as needed

Controlled release: Adults:

Opioid naive (not currently on opioid): 10 mg every 12 hours

Currently on opioid/ASA or acetaminophen or NSAID combination:

1-5 tablets: 10-20 mg every 12 hours

6-9 tablets: 20-30 mg every 12 hours

10-12 tablets: 30-40 mg every 12 hours

May continue the nonopioid as a separate drug.

Currently on opioids: Use standard conversion chart to convert daily dose to oxycodone equivalent. Divide daily dose in 2 (for every 12-hour dosing) and round down to nearest dosage form.

Note: 80 mg or 160 mg tablets are for use **only** in opioid-tolerant patients. Special safety considerations must be addressed when converting to OxyContin® doses ≥160 mg every 12 hours. Dietary caution must be taken when patients are initially titrated to 160 mg tablets.

Dosing adjustment in hepatic impairment: Reduce dosage in patients with severe liver disease

Administration Do not crush controlled-release tablets; 80 mg and 160 mg tablets are for use **only** in opioid-tolerant patients. Do not administer OxyContin® 160 mg tablet with a high-fat meal.

Dosage Forms
Capsule, immediate release, as hydrochloride (OxyIR®): 5 mg

Solution, oral, as hydrochloride: 5 mg/5 mL (500 mL)

Roxicodone™: 5 mg/5 mL (5 mL, 500 mL) [contains alcohol]

Solution, oral concentrate, as hydrochloride: 20 mg/mL (30 mL)

Oxydose™: 20 mg/mL (30 mL) [contains sodium benzoate; berry flavor]

OxyFast®, Roxicodone™ Intensol™: 20 mg/mL (30 mL) [contains sodium benzoate]

(Continued)

Oxycodone *(Continued)*

Tablet, as hydrochloride: 5 mg
 Roxicodone™: 5 mg, 15 mg, 30 mg
Tablet, controlled release, as hydrochloride (OxyContin®): 10 mg, 20 mg, 40 mg, 80 mg, 160 mg
Tablet, extended release, as hydrochloride: 80 mg

Monitoring Parameters Pain relief, respiratory and mental status, blood pressure

Dietary Considerations Instruct patient to avoid high-fat meals when taking OxyContin® 160 mg tablets.

Patient Information Avoid alcohol; may cause drowsiness, impaired judgment or coordination; may be addicting if used for prolonged periods; do not crush or chew the controlled-release product

Additional Information Prophylactic use of a laxative should be considered. OxyContin® 80 mg and 160 mg tablets are for use in opioid-tolerant patients only.

Special Geriatric Considerations The elderly may be particularly susceptible to the CNS depressant and constipating effects of narcotics. Serum levels at a given dose may also be increased relative to concentrations in younger patients.

♦ **Oxycodone Hydrochloride** *see* Oxycodone *on page 633*

♦ **OxyContin®** *see* Oxycodone *on page 633*

♦ **Oxydose™** *see* Oxycodone *on page 633*

♦ **OxyFast®** *see* Oxycodone *on page 633*

♦ **OxyIR®** *see* Oxycodone *on page 633*

Oxymorphone *(oks i MOR fone)*

Medication Safety Issues
Sound-alike/look-alike issues:
 Oxymorphone may be confused with oxymetholone

U.S. Brand Names Numorphan®

Canadian Brand Names Numorphan®

Generic Available No

Synonyms Oxymorphone Hydrochloride

Pharmacologic Category Analgesic, Narcotic

Pregnancy Risk Factor B/D (prolonged use or high doses at term)

Lactation Excretion in breast milk unknown/use caution

Use Management of moderate to severe pain and preoperatively as a sedative and a supplement to anesthesia

Mechanism of Action Oxymorphone hydrochloride (Numorphan®) is a potent narcotic analgesic with uses similar to those of morphine. The drug is a semisynthetic derivative of morphine (phenanthrene derivative) and is closely related to hydromorphone chemically (Dilaudid®).

Restrictions C-II

Labeled Contraindications Hypersensitivity to oxymorphone or any component of the formulation; increased intracranial pressure; severe respiratory depression; pregnancy (prolonged use or high doses at term)

Warnings/Precautions Some preparations contain sulfites which may cause allergic reactions; infants <3 months of age are more susceptible to respiratory depression, use with caution and generally in reduced doses in this age group; use with caution in patients with impaired respiratory function or severe hepatic dysfunction and in patients with hypersensitivity reactions to other phenanthrene derivative opioid agonists (codeine, hydrocodone, hydromorphone, levorphanol, oxycodone, oxymorphone); tolerance or drug dependence may result from extended use

Adverse Reactions

>10%:

Cardiovascular: Hypotension

Central nervous system: Fatigue, drowsiness, dizziness

Gastrointestinal: Nausea, vomiting, constipation

Neuromuscular & skeletal: Weakness

Miscellaneous: Histamine release

1% to 10%:

Central nervous system: Nervousness, headache, restlessness, malaise, confusion

Gastrointestinal: Anorexia, stomach cramps, xerostomia, biliary spasm

Genitourinary: Decreased urination, ureteral spasms

Local: Pain at injection site

Respiratory: Dyspnea

<1%: Mental depression, hallucinations, paradoxical CNS stimulation, increased intracranial pressure, rash, urticaria, paralytic ileus, histamine release, physical and psychological dependence

Vesicant No

Overdosage/Toxicology Symptoms of overdose include respiratory depression, miosis, hypotension, bradycardia, apnea, and pulmonary edema. Treatment of overdose includes maintaining patent airway and establishing an I.V. line. Naloxone, 2 mg I.V., with repeat administration as necessary up to a total of 10 mg, can also be used to reverse toxic effects of the opiate.

Drug Interactions

Increased Effect/Toxicity: Increased effect/toxicity with CNS depressants (phenothiazines, tranquilizers, anxiolytics, sedatives, hypnotics, alcohol), tricyclic antidepressants, and dextroamphetamine.

Decreased Effect: Decreased effect with phenothiazines.

Ethanol/Nutrition/Herb Interactions

Ethanol: Avoid ethanol (may increase CNS depression).

Herb/Nutraceutical: Avoid valerian, St John's wort, kava kava, gotu kola (may increase CNS depression).

Storage/Stability Refrigerate suppository.

Compatibility Compatibility in syringe: Compatible: Glycopyrrolate, hydroxyzine, ranitidine

Pharmacodynamics/Kinetics

Onset of action: Analgesic: I.V., I.M., SubQ: 5-10 minutes; Rectal: 15-30 minutes

Duration: Analgesic: Parenteral, rectal: 3-4 hours

Metabolism: Hepatic via glucuronidation

Excretion: Urine

Dosage Adults: **Note:** More frequent dosing may be required.

I.M., SubQ: 0.5 mg initially, 1-1.5 mg every 4-6 hours as needed

I.V.: 0.5 mg initially

Rectal: 5 mg every 4-6 hours

Dosage Forms

Injection, solution, as hydrochloride: 1 mg (1 mL); 1.5 mg/mL (10 mL)

Suppository, rectal, as hydrochloride: 5 mg

(Continued)

Oxymorphone *(Continued)*

Monitoring Parameters Respiratory rate, heart rate, blood pressure, CNS activity

Patient Information Avoid alcohol, may cause drowsiness, impaired judgment or coordination; may cause physical and psychological dependence with prolonged use

Special Geriatric Considerations The elderly may be particularly susceptible to the CNS depressant and constipating effects of narcotics.

♦ **Oxymorphone Hydrochloride** *see Oxymorphone on page 636*
♦ **Pacis™ (Can)** *see BCG Vaccine on page 120*

Paclitaxel *(PAK li taks el)*

Medication Safety Issues
Sound-alike/look-alike issues:
Paclitaxel may be confused with paroxetine, Paxil®
Paclitaxel (conventional) may be confused with paclitaxel (protein-bound)
Taxol® may be confused with Abraxane™, Paxil®, Taxotere®

Related Information
Safe Handling of Hazardous Drugs *on page 1034*
Transplantation *on page 1019*

U.S. Brand Names Onxol™; Taxol®

Canadian Brand Names Taxol®

Generic Available Yes

Synonyms NSC-125973

Pharmacologic Category Antineoplastic Agent, Antimicrotubular; Antineoplastic Agent, Natural Source (Plant) Derivative

Pregnancy Risk Factor D

Lactation Excretion in breast milk unknown/contraindicated

Use Treatment of breast, lung (small cell and nonsmall cell), and ovarian cancers

Mechanism of Action Paclitaxel promotes microtubule assembly by enhancing the action of tubulin dimers, stabilizing existing microtubules, and inhibiting their disassembly, interfering with the late G_2 mitotic phase, and inhibiting cell replication. In addition, the drug can distort mitotic spindles, resulting in the breakage of chromosomes. Paclitaxel may also suppress cell proliferation and modulate immune response.

Labeled Contraindications Hypersensitivity to paclitaxel, Cremophor® EL (polyoxyethylated castor oil), or any component of the formulation; pregnancy

Warnings/Precautions Hazardous agent - use appropriate precautions for handling and disposal. See Safe Handling of Hazardous Drugs *on page 1034* in the Appendix. All patients should be premedicated prior to paclitaxel administration to prevent severe hypersensitivity reactions. Prolongation of the infusion (to ≥6 hours) plus premedication may minimize this effect.

When administered as sequential infusions, taxane derivatives (docetaxel, paclitaxel) should be administered before platinum derivatives (carboplatin, cisplatin) to limit myelosuppression. Elderly patients have an increased risk of toxicity (neutropenia, neuropathy).

Adverse Reactions

>10%:

Allergic: Appear to be primarily nonimmunologically mediated release of histamine and other vasoactive substances; almost always seen within the first hour of an infusion (~75% occur within 10 minutes of starting the infusion); incidence is significantly reduced by premedication

Cardiovascular: Bradycardia (transient, 25%)

Dermatologic: Alopecia (87%), venous erythema, tenderness, discomfort

Hematologic: Myelosuppression, leukopenia, neutropenia (6% to 21%), thrombocytopenia

Hepatic: Mild increases in liver enzymes

Onset: 8-11 days

Nadir: 15-21 days

Recovery: 21 days

Neurotoxicity: Sensory and/or autonomic neuropathy (numbness, tingling, burning pain), myopathy or myopathic effects (25% to 55%), and central nervous system toxicity. May be cumulative and dose-limiting. **Note:** Motor neuropathy is uncommon at doses <250 mg/m^2; sensory neuropathy is almost universal at doses >250 mg/m^2; myopathic effects are common with doses >250 mg/m^2, generally occurring within 2-3 days of treatment, resolving over 5-6 days; pre-existing neuropathy may increase the risk of neuropathy.

Gastrointestinal: Severe, potentially dose-limiting mucositis, stomatitis (15%), most common at doses >390 mg/m^2

Neuromuscular & skeletal: Arthralgia, myalgia

1% to 10%:

Cardiovascular: Myocardial infarction

Dermatologic: Phlebitis (2%)

Gastrointestinal: Mild nausea and vomiting (5% to 6%), diarrhea (5% to 6%)

Hematologic: Anemia

<1%: Ataxia, atrial fibrillation, enterocolitis, hepatic encephalopathy, intestinal obstruction, interstitial pneumonia, necrotic changes and ulceration following extravasation, neuroencephalopathy, ototoxicity (tinnitus and hearing loss), pancreatitis, paralytic ileus, pruritus, pulmonary fibrosis, radiation recall, radiation pneumonitis, rash, seizure, Stevens-Johnson syndrome, toxic epidermal necrolysis, visual disturbances (scintillating scotomata)

Vesicant No; the drug is an irritant. See Management of Drug Extravasations *on page 965.*

Emetic Potential Very low (<10%)

Drug Interactions

Cytochrome P450 Effect: Substrate (major) of CYP2C8/9, 3A4; **Induces** CYP3A4 (weak)

Increased Effect/Toxicity: CYP2C8/9 inhibitors may increase the levels/effects of paclitaxel; example inhibitors include delavirdine, fluconazole, gemfibrozil, ketoconazole, nicardipine, NSAIDs, pioglitazone, and sulfonamides. CYP3A4 inhibitors may increase the levels/effects of paclitaxel; example inhibitors include azole antifungals, ciprofloxacin, clarithromycin, diclofenac, doxycycline, erythromycin, imatinib, (Continued)

Paclitaxel *(Continued)*

isoniazid, nefazodone, nicardipine, propofol, protease inhibitors, quinidine, and verapamil. In Phase I trials, myelosuppression was more profound when given after cisplatin than with alternative sequence. administered as sequential infusions, studies indicate a potential for increased toxicity when platinum derivatives (carboplatin, cisplatin) are administered before taxane derivatives (docetaxel, paclitaxel). Paclitaxel may increase doxorubicin levels/toxicity.

Decreased Effect: CYP2C8/9 inducers may decrease the levels/effects of paclitaxel; example inducers include carbamazepine, phenobarbital, phenytoin, rifampin, rifapentine, and secobarbital. CYP3A4 inducers may decrease the levels/effects of paclitaxel; example inducers include aminoglutethimide, carbamazepine, nafcillin, nevirapine, phenobarbital, phenytoin, and rifamycins.

Ethanol/Nutrition/Herb Interactions Herb/Nutraceutical: Avoid black cohosh, dong quai in estrogen-dependent tumors. Avoid valerian, St John's wort, kava kava, gotu kola (may increase CNS depression).

Storage/Stability Store intact vials at room temperature of 20°C to 25°C (68°F to 77°F). Protect from light. Per the manufacturer, reconstituted solution is stable for up to 27 hours at room temperature (25°C) and ambient light conditions. Other sources report that solutions in D_5W and NS are stable for up to 3 days at room temperature (25°C).

Paclitaxel should be dispensed in either glass or Excel™/PAB™ containers. Should also use **nonpolyvinyl** (non-PVC) tubing (eg, polyethylene) to minimize leaching. Formulated in a vehicle known as Cremophor® EL (polyoxyethylated castor oil). Cremophor® EL has been found to leach the plasticizer DEHP from polyvinyl chloride infusion bags or administration sets. Contact of the undiluted concentrate with plasticized polyvinyl chloride (PVC) equipment or devices is not recommended.

Reconstitution Dilute in 250-1000 mL D_5W, D_5LR, D_5NS, or NS to a concentration of of 0.3-1.2 mg/mL.

Compatibility Stable in D_5W, D_5LR, D_5NS, NS;

Y-site administration: Compatible: Acyclovir, amikacin, aminophylline, ampicillin/sulbactam, bleomycin, butorphanol, calcium chloride, carboplatin, cefepime, cefotetan, ceftazidime, ceftriaxone, cimetidine, cisplatin, cladribine, cyclophosphamide, cytarabine, dacarbazine, dexamethasone sodium phosphate, diphenhydramine, doxorubicin, droperidol, etoposide, etoposide phosphate, famotidine, floxuridine, fluconazole, fluorouracil, furosemide, ganciclovir, gatifloxacin, gemcitabine, gentamicin, granisetron, haloperidol, heparin, hydrocortisone sodium phosphate, hydrocortisone sodium succinate, hydromorphone, ifosfamide, linezolid, lorazepam, magnesium sulfate, mannitol, meperidine, mesna, methotrexate, metoclopramide, morphine, nalbuphine, ondansetron, ondansetron with ranitidine, pentostatin, potassium chloride, prochlorperazine edisylate, propofol, ranitidine, sodium bicarbonate, thiotepa, topotecan, vancomycin, vinblastine, vincristine, zidovudine. **Incompatible:** Amphotericin B, amphotericin B cholesteryl sulfate complex, chlorpromazine, doxorubicin liposome, hydroxyzine, methylprednisolone sodium succinate, mitoxantrone

Compatibility when admixed: Compatible: Carboplatin, doxorubicin. **Variable (consult detailed reference):** Cisplatin

Pharmacodynamics/Kinetics

Distribution:

V_d: Widely distributed into body fluids and tissues; affected by dose and duration of infusion

V_{dss}:

1- to 6-hour infusion: 67.1 L/m^2

24-hour infusion: 227-688 L/m^2

Protein binding: 89% to 98%

Metabolism: Hepatic via CYP2C8/9 and 3A4; forms metabolites

Half-life elimination:

1- to 6-hour infusion: Mean (beta): 6.4 hours

3-hour infusion: Mean (terminal): 13.1-20.2 hours

24-hour infusion: Mean (terminal): 15.7-52.7 hours

Excretion: Feces (~70%, 5% as unchanged drug); urine (14%)

Clearance: Mean: Total body: After 1- and 6-hour infusions: 5.8-16.3 L/hour/m^2; After 24-hour infusions: 14.2-17.2 L/hour/m^2

Dosage Premedication with dexamethasone (20 mg orally or I.V. at 12 and 6 hours **or** 14 and 7 hours before the dose), diphenhydramine (50 mg I.V. 30-60 minutes prior to the dose), and cimetidine, famotidine or ranitidine (I.V. 30-60 minutes prior to the dose) is recommended

Adults: I.V.: Refer to individual protocols

Ovarian carcinoma: 135-175 mg/m^2 over 3 hours every 3 weeks **or**

50-80 mg/m^2 over 1-3 hours weekly **or**

1.4-4 mg/m^2/day continuous infusion for 14 days every 4 weeks

Metastatic breast cancer: 175-250 mg/m^2 over 3 hours every 3 weeks **or**

50-80 mg/m^2 weekly **or**

1.4-4 mg/m^2/day continuous infusion for 14 days every 4 weeks

Nonsmall cell lung carcinoma: 135 mg/m^2 over 24 hours every 3 weeks

AIDS-related Kaposi's sarcoma: 135 mg/m^2 over 3 hours every 3 weeks **or**

100 mg/m^2 over 3 hours every 2 weeks

Dosage modification for toxicity (solid tumors, including ovary, breast, and lung carcinoma): Courses of paclitaxel should not be repeated until the neutrophil count is ≥1500 cells/mm^3 and the platelet count is ≥100,000 cells/mm^3; reduce dosage by 20% for patients experiencing severe peripheral neuropathy or severe neutropenia (neutrophil <500 cells/mm^3 for a week or longer)

Dosage modification for immunosuppression in advanced HIV disease: Paclitaxel should not be given to patients with HIV if the baseline or subsequent neutrophil count is <1000 cells/mm^3. Additional modifications include: Reduce dosage of dexamethasone in premedication to 10 mg orally; reduce dosage by 20% in patients experiencing severe peripheral neuropathy or severe neutropenia (neutrophil <500 cells/mm^3 for a week or longer); initiate concurrent hematopoietic growth factor (G-CSF) as clinically indicated

Dosage adjustment in hepatic impairment: Note: These recommendations are based upon the patient's first course of therapy where the usual dose would be 135 mg/m^2 dose over 24 hours or the 175 mg/m^2 dose over 3 hours in patients with normal hepatic function. Dosage in subsequent courses should be based upon individual tolerance. Adjustments for other regimens are not available.

(Continued)

Paclitaxel *(Continued)*

24-hour infusion:

If transaminase levels <2 times upper limit of normal (ULN) and bilirubin level ≤1.5 mg/dL: 135 mg/m^2

If transaminase levels 2-<10 times ULN and bilirubin level ≤1.5 mg/dL: 100 mg/m^2

If transaminase levels <10 times ULN and bilirubin level 1.6-7.5 mg/dL: 50 mg/m^2

If transaminase levels ≥10 times ULN and bilirubin level >7.5 mg/dL: Avoid use

3-hour infusion:

If transaminase levels <10 times ULN and bilirubin level ≤1.25 times ULN: 175 mg/m^2

If transaminase levels <10 times ULN and bilirubin level 1.26-2 times ULN: 135 mg/m^2

If transaminase levels <10 times ULN and bilirubin level 2.01-5 times ULN: 90 mg/m^2

If transaminase levels ≥10 times ULN and bilirubin level >5 times ULN: Avoid use

Combination Regimens

Adenocarcinoma, unknown primary:
Carbo-Tax (Adenocarcinoma) *on page 851*
Paclitaxel, Carboplatin, Etoposide *on page 926*
Bladder cancer: PC (Bladder Cancer) *on page 927*
Breast cancer:
AC *on page 843*
Paclitaxel-Vinorelbine *on page 927*
PV *on page 932*
Trastuzumab-Paclitaxel *on page 940*
Esophageal cancer:
TCF *on page 939*
TIP *on page 940*
Head and neck cancer:
FU HURT *on page 893*
TIP *on page 940*
Lung cancer (nonsmall cell):
Carbo-Tax (Nonsmall Cell Lung Cancer) *on page 851*
CaT (Nonsmall Cell Lung Cancer) *on page 852*
PC (Nonsmall Cell Lung Cancer) *on page 927*
Ovarian cancer:
Carbo-Tax (Ovarian Cancer) *on page 852*
CaT (Ovarian Cancer) *on page 853*
CT *on page 868*
Gemcitabine-Paclitaxel *on page 897*
Prostate cancer:
Paclitaxel + Estramustine + Carboplatin *on page 926*
Paclitaxel + Estramustine + Etoposide *on page 926*
PE *on page 928*
Sarcoma, soft tissue: ICE-T *on page 900*

Administration

Corticosteroids (dexamethasone), H$_1$-antagonists (diphenhydramine), and H$_2$-antagonists should be administered prior to paclitaxel administration to minimize potential for anaphylaxis. The following regimen is suggested: Dexamethasone I.V. 10-20 mg, diphenhydramine I.V. 50 mg, and cimetidine I.V. 300 mg **or** ranitidine I.V. 50 mg, all given 30 minutes prior to paclitaxel administration.

Administer I.V. infusion over 1-24 hours; use of a 0.22 micron in-line filter and nonsorbing administration set is recommended during the infusion

Nonpolyvinyl (non-PVC) tubing (eg, polyethylene) should be used to minimize leaching. Formulated in a vehicle known as Cremophor® EL (polyoxyethylated castor oil). Cremophor® EL has been found to leach the plasticizer DEHP from polyvinyl chloride infusion bags or administration sets. Contact of the undiluted concentrate with plasticized polyvinyl chloride (PVC) equipment or devices is not recommended. Administer through I.V. tubing containing an in-line (NOT >0.22 µ) filter; administration through IVEX-2® filters (which incorporate short inlet and outlet polyvinyl chloride-coated tubing) has not resulted in significant leaching of DEHP.

Dosage Forms Injection, solution: 6 mg/mL (5 mL, 16.7 mL, 50 mL) [contains alcohol and purified Cremophor® EL (polyoxyethylated castor oil)]

Onxol™: 6 mg/mL (5 mL, 25 mL, 50 mL) [contains alcohol] [contains alcohol and purified Cremophor® EL (polyoxyethylated castor oil)]

Taxol®: 6 mg/mL (5 mL, 16.7 mL, 50 mL) [contains alcohol and purified Cremophor® EL (polyoxyethylated castor oil)]

High Dose Considerations

High Dose: I.V.: 250-775 mg/m^2; generally combined with other high-dose chemotherapy; maximum dose as single agent: 825 mg/m^2

Comments: Glutamine may decrease mucositis

Monitoring Parameters Monitor for hypersensitivity reactions

Patient Information This medication can only be administered by I.V. infusion, usually on a cyclic basis. Maintain adequate hydration (2-3 L/day of fluids unless instructed to restrict fluid intake) and nutrition (small frequent meals will help). You will most likely lose your hair (will grow back after therapy); experience some nausea or vomiting (request antiemetic); feel weak or lethargic (use caution when driving or engaging in tasks that require alertness until response to drug is known). Use good oral care to reduce incidence of mouth sores. You will be more susceptible to infection; avoid crowds or exposure to infection. Report numbness or tingling in fingers or toes (use care to prevent injury); signs of infection (fever, chills, sore throat, burning urination, fatigue); unusual bleeding (tarry stools, easy bruising, or blood in stool, urine, or mouth); unresolved mouth sores; nausea or vomiting; or skin rash or itching. Contraceptive measures are recommended during therapy.

Additional Information Sensory neuropathy is almost universal at doses >250 mg/m^2; motor neuropathy is uncommon at doses <250 mg/m^2. Myopathic effects are common with doses >200 mg/m^2, generally occur within 2-3 days of treatment, and resolve over 5-6 days. Patients with pre-existing neuropathies from chemotherapy or coexisting conditions (eg, diabetes mellitus) may be at a higher risk.

Special Geriatric Considerations Elderly patients may have a higher incidence of severe neuropathy, severe myelosuppression, or cardiovascular events as compared to younger patients.

Selected Readings

Mekhail TM and Markman M, "Paclitaxel in Cancer Therapy," *Expert Opin Pharmacother*, 2002, 3(6):755-66.

(Continued)

Paclitaxel *(Continued)*

Spencer CM and Faulds D, "Paclitaxel. A Review of Its Pharmacodynamic and Pharmaco-kinetic Properties and Therapeutic Potential in the Treatment of Cancer," *Drugs*, 1994, 48(5):794-847.

Paclitaxel (Protein Bound) (PAK li taks el PROE teen bownd)

Medication Safety Issues

Sound-alike/look-alike issues:

Paclitaxel (protein bound) may be confused with paclitaxel (conventional)

Abraxane™ may be confused with Paxil®, Taxol®, Taxotere®

U.S. Brand Names Abraxane™

Generic Available No

Synonyms BI-007; NAB-Paclitaxel; Protein-Bound Paclitaxel

Pharmacologic Category Antineoplastic Agent, Antimicrotubular; Antineoplastic Agent, Natural Source (Plant) Derivative

Pregnancy Risk Factor D

Lactation Excretion in breast milk unknown/not recommended

Use Treatment of breast cancer (second-line)

Mechanism of Action Paclitaxel promotes microtubule assembly by enhancing the action of tubulin dimers, stabilizing existing microtubules, and inhibiting their disassembly, interfering with the late G_2 mitotic phase, and inhibiting cell replication. In addition, the drug can distort mitotic spindles, resulting in the breakage of chromosomes. Paclitaxel may also suppress cell proliferation and modulate immune response.

Labeled Contraindications Hypersensitivity to paclitaxel or any component of the formulation

Warnings/Precautions Hazardous agent - use appropriate precautions for handling and disposal. See Safe Handling of Hazardous Drugs *on page 1034* in the Appendix.

Paclitaxel (protein-bound) is not interchangeable with Cremophor®-based paclitaxel. Severe sensory neuropathy may occur. Use caution in hepatic and renal dysfunction. When administered as sequential infusions, taxane derivatives (docetaxel, paclitaxel) should be administered before platinum derivatives (carboplatin, cisplatin) to limit myelosuppression.

Adverse Reactions

>10%:

Cardiovascular: EKG abnormal (60%)

Dermatologic: Alopecia (90%)

Gastrointestinal: Nausea (30%; severe 3%), diarrhea (26%; severe <1%), vomiting (18%; severe 4%)

Hematologic: Neutropenia (80%; grade 4 - 9%), anemia (33%; severe 1%)

Hepatic: AST increased (39%), alkaline phosphatase increased (36%)

Neuromuscular & skeletal: Sensory neuropathy (71%; severe 10%), asthenia (47%; severe 8%), myalgia/arthralgia (44%; severe 8%)

Ocular: Vision disturbance (13%; severe 1%)

Respiratory: Dyspnea (12%)

Miscellaneous: Infections (24%; primarily included oral candidiasis, respiratory tract infections, and pneumonia)

1% to 10%:
  Cardiovascular: Edema (10%; severe 0%), hypotension (5%), Grade 3 cardiovascular events (3%; included chest pain, cardiac arrest, supraventricular tachycardia, edema, thrombosis, pulmonary thromboembolism, pulmonary emboli, and hypertension)
  Central nervous system: Febrile neutropenia (2%)
  Gastrointestinal: Mucositis (7%; severe < 1%)
  Hematologic: Thrombocytopenia (2%), bleeding (2%)
  Hepatic: Bilirubin increased (7%)
  Local: Injection site reaction (1%)
  Renal: Creatinine increased (11%; severe 1%)
  Respiratory: Cough (6%)
  Miscellaneous: Hypersensitivity reaction (4%)
  <1%: Bradycardia, cerebral vascular attacks, conjunctivitis, hepatic necrosis, hepatic encephalopathy, interstitial pneumonia, intestinal obstruction, intestinal perforation, ischemic colitis, lacrimation increased, lung fibrosis, maculopapular rash, neutropenic enterocolitis, pancreatitis, pneumothorax, radiation pneumonitis with concurrent radiation therapy, Stevens-Johnson syndrome, toxic epidermal necrolysis, transient ischemic attacks

Vesicant No

Emetic Potential Very low (<10%)

Overdosage/Toxicology Overdose would likely result in severe bone marrow suppression, sensory neuropathy, and mucositis. Treatment should be supportive.

Drug Interactions
  Cytochrome P450 Effect: Substrate (major) of CYP2C8/9, 3A4; **Induces** CYP3A4 (weak)
  Increased Effect/Toxicity: CYP2C8/9 inhibitors may increase the levels/effects of paclitaxel; example inhibitors include delavirdine, fluconazole, gemfibrozil, ketoconazole, nicardipine, NSAIDs, pioglitazone, and sulfonamides. CYP3A4 inhibitors may increase the levels/effects of paclitaxel; example inhibitors include azole antifungals, ciprofloxacin, clarithromycin, diclofenac, doxycycline, erythromycin, imatinib, isoniazid, nefazodone, nicardipine, propofol, protease inhibitors, quinidine, and verapamil. In Phase I trials, myelosuppression was more profound when given after cisplatin than with alternative sequence. administered as sequential infusions, studies indicate a potential for increased toxicity when platinum derivatives (carboplatin, cisplatin) are administered before taxane derivatives (docetaxel, paclitaxel). Paclitaxel may increase doxorubicin levels/toxicity.
  Decreased Effect: CYP2C8/9 inducers may decrease the levels/effects of paclitaxel; example inducers include carbamazepine, phenobarbital, phenytoin, rifampin, rifapentine, and secobarbital. CYP3A4 inducers may decrease the levels/effects of paclitaxel; example inducers include aminoglutethimide, carbamazepine, nafcillin, nevirapine, phenobarbital, phenytoin, and rifamycins.

Ethanol/Nutrition/Herb Interactions
  Herb/Nutraceutical: Avoid black cohosh, dong quai in estrogen-dependent tumors. Avoid valerian, St John's wort, kava kava, gotu kola (may increase CNS depression).

Storage/Stability Store intact vial at room temperature of 20°C to 25°C (68°F to 77°F) and protect from bright light. Reconstituted solution may
(Continued)

Paclitaxel (Protein Bound) *(Continued)*

be stored under refrigeration 2°C to 8°C (36°F to 46°F) for up to 8 hours. The solution for administration is stable for up to 8 hours at room temperature and ambient light.

Reconstitution Reconstitute vial with 20 mL NS to achieve 5 mg/mL solution. Inject dose for infusion into empty, sterile container. **Note:** Use of DEHP-free containers or administration sets is not necessary. **Do not use an in-line filter.**

Pharmacodynamics/Kinetics

Distribution: V_d: 632 L/m^2

Protein binding: 89% to 98%

Metabolism: Hepatic via CYP3A4 and 2C8

Half-life elimination: Terminal: 27 hours

Excretion: Urine (4% as unchanged drug, 1% as metabolites); feces (20%)

Clearance 15 L/hour/m^2

Dosage I.V.: Adults: Breast cancer: 260 mg/m^2 every 3 weeks

Dosage adjustment for toxicity:

Severe neutropenia (<500 cells/mm^3) ≥1 week: Reduce dose to 220 mg/m^2 for subsequent courses

Recurrent severe neutropenia: Reduce dose to 180 mg/m^2

Severe sensory neuropathy: Reduce dose to 180 mg/m^2

Sensory neuropathy grade 3 or 4: Hold treatment until resolved to grade 1 or 2, then resume with reduced dose

Dosage adjustment in renal impairment: Safety not established for serum creatinine >2 mg/dL; use with caution

Dosage adjustment in hepatic impairment: Effects of hepatic dysfunction (serum bilirubin >1.5 mg/dL) unknown; dosage adjustment recommendations are not available

Administration I.V.: Administer over 30 minutes. Do not use an in-line filter

Dosage Forms Injection, powder for reconstitution: 100 mg [contains human albumin 900 mg]

High Dose Considerations

Comments: Glutamine may decrease mucositis.

Monitoring Parameters CBC, BP (during infusion), baseline ECG, infusion site

Palifermin *(pal ee FER min)*

Related Information

Mucositis/Stomatitis *on page 995*

U.S. Brand Names Kepivance™

Generic Available No

Synonyms AMJ 9701; rHu-KGF

Pharmacologic Category Keratinocyte Growth Factor

Pregnancy Risk Factor C

Lactation Excretion in breast milk unknown/use caution

Use Decrease the incidence and severity of severe oral mucositis associated with hematologic malignancies in patients receiving myelotoxic therapy requiring hematopoietic stem cell support

Mechanism of Action Palifermin is a recombinant keratinocyte growth factor (KGF) produced in *E. coli*. Endogenous KGF is produced by mesenchymal cells in response to epithelial tissue injury. KGF binds to the KGF receptor resulting in proliferation, differentiation and migration of epithelial cells in multiple tissues, including (but not limited to) the tongue, buccal mucosa, esophagus, and salivary gland.

Labeled Contraindications Hypersensitivity to palifermin, *E. coli*-derived proteins, or any component of the formulation

Warnings/Precautions Safety and efficacy have not been established with nonhematologic malignancies; effect on the growth of nonhematopoietic human tumors is not known. Palifermin should be administered prior to and following, but not with, chemotherapy. If administered within 24 hours of chemotherapy, palifermin may increase the severity and duration of mucositis due to the increased sensitivity of rapidly-dividing epithelial cells. Safety and efficacy have not been established in children.

Adverse Reactions

>10%:

Cardiovascular: Edema (28%), hypertension (7% to 14%)

Central nervous system: Fever (39%), pain (16%), dysesthesia (12%)

Dermatologic: Rash (62%), pruritus (35%), erythema (32%)

Gastrointestinal: Mouth/tongue discoloration or thickness (17%), taste alteration (16%)

Miscellaneous: Serum amylase increased (grade 3/4, 38%); serum lipase increased (grade 3/4, 11%)

1% to 10%: Neuromuscular & skeletal: Arthralgia (10%)

Overdosage/Toxicology Specific information is not available. Doses higher than those recommended were associated with the reported adverse events, but in general were more severe.

Drug Interactions

Increased Effect/Toxicity: Drug interaction studies have not been conducted.

Storage/Stability Store powder for reconstitution under refrigeration at 2°C to 8°C (36°F to 46°F) and protect from light. Following reconstitution, may store under refrigeration for up to 24 hours; protect from light, do not freeze. Reconstituted solution should not be used if left at room temperature >1 hour.

Reconstitution To reconstitute, slowly add SWFI 1.2 mL to vial; final concentration will be 5 mg/mL. Do not shake or vigorously agitate.

Compatibility Incompatible: Heparin

Pharmacodynamics/Kinetics Half-life elimination: 4.5 hours (range: 3.3-5.7 hours)

Dosage I.V.: Adults: 60 mcg/kg/day for 3 consecutive days before and after myelotoxic therapy; total of 6 doses

Note: Administer first 3 doses prior to myelotoxic therapy, with the 3rd dose given 24-48 hours before therapy begins. The last 3 doses should be administered after myelotoxic therapy, with the first of these doses after but on the same day of hematopoietic stem cell infusion and at least 4 days after the most recent dose of palifermin.

Administration Administer by I.V. bolus. If heparin is used to maintain the patency of the I.V. line, flush line with saline prior to and after palifermin administration. Do not administer palifermin with or within 24 hours of chemotherapy. Allow solution to reach room temperature prior to administration; do not use if at room temperature >1 hour.

Dosage Forms Injection, powder for reconstitution [preservative free]: 6.25 mg [contains mannitol 50 mg, sucrose 25 mg]

(Continued)

Palifermin *(Continued)*

Selected Readings

Finch PW and Rubin JS, "Keratinocyte Growth Factor/Fibroblast Growth Factor 7, a Homeostatic Factor With Therapeutic Potential for Epithelial Protection and Repair," *Adv Cancer Res*, 2004, 91:69-136.

Meropol NJ, Somer RA, Gutheil J, et al, "Randomized Phase I Trial of Recombinant Human Keratinocyte Growth Factor Plus Chemotherapy: Potential Role as Mucosal Protectant," *J Clin Oncol*, 2003, 21(8):1452-8.

"Palifermin: AMJ 9701, KGF-Amgen, Recombinant Human Keratinocyte Growth Factor, rHu-KGF," *Drugs R D*, 2004, 5(6):351-4.

Spielberger R, Stiff P, Bensinger W, et al, "Palifermin for Oral Mucositis After Intensive Therapy for Hematologic Cancers," *N Engl J Med*, 2004, 351(25):2590-8.

◆ Palladone™ *see Hydromorphone on page 426*

Palonosetron *(pal oh NOE se tron)*

Medication Safety Issues

Sound-alike/look-alike issues:

Aloxi™ may be confused with oxaliplatin

U.S. Brand Names Aloxi™

Generic Available No

Synonyms Palonosetron Hydrochloride; RS-25259; RS-25259-197

Pharmacologic Category Antiemetic; Selective 5-HT$_3$ Receptor Antagonist

Pregnancy Risk Factor B

Lactation Excretion in breast milk unknown/not recommended

Use Prevention of acute (within 24 hours) and delayed (2-5 days) chemotherapy-induced nausea and vomiting

Unlabeled/Investigational Use Prevention of postoperative vomiting

Mechanism of Action Selective 5-HT$_3$ receptor antagonist, blocking serotonin, both peripherally on vagal nerve terminals and centrally in the chemoreceptor trigger zone

Labeled Contraindications Hypersensitivity to palonosetron or any component of the formulation

Warnings/Precautions Use caution in patients allergic to other 5-HT$_3$ receptor antagonists; cross-reactivity is possible. Caution in patients with congenital QT syndrome or other risk factors for QT prolongation (eg, drugs, electrolyte abnormalities). Not intended for treatment of nausea and vomiting or for chronic continuous therapy. Safety and efficacy in pediatric patients (<18 years of age) have not been established.

Adverse Reactions

>10%: Dermatologic: Pruritus (8% to 22%)

1% to 10%:

Cardiovascular: Bradycardia (1%), hypotension (1%), tachycardia (nonsustained) (1%)

Central nervous system: Headache (6% to 9%), anxiety (1% to 5%), dizziness (1%)

Endocrine & metabolic: Hyperkalemia (1%)

Gastrointestinal: Constipation (5% to 10%), diarrhea (1%)

Neuromuscular & skeletal: Weakness (1%)

<1%: Abdominal pain, allergic dermatitis, anorexia, appetite decreased, arthralgia, ALT increased, amblyopia, AST increased, bilirubin increased, dyspepsia, electrolyte fluctuations, euphoric mood, eye irritation, extrasystoles, fatigue, fever, flatulence, flu-like syndrome,

glycosuria, hiccups, hot flash, hyperglycemia, hypersomnia, hypertension, insomnia, metabolic acidosis, motion sickness, myocardial ischemia, QT prolongation, paresthesia, rash, sinus arrhythmia, sinus tachycardia, somnolence, supraventricular extrasystoles, tinnitus, urinary retention, vein discoloration, vein distention, xerostomia

Overdosage/Toxicology Dose-ranging studies in humans using doses up to 25 times the recommended dose of 0.25 mg revealed no increase in the incidence of adverse effects compared to lower dose groups. Treatment is supportive.

Drug Interactions

Cytochrome P450 Effect: Substrate (minor) of CYP1A2, 2D6, 3A4

Increased Effect/Toxicity: No drug interactions of concern have been identified.

Storage/Stability Store intact vials at controlled room temperature of 20°C to 25°C (68°F to 77°F); protect from freezing and light. Solutions of 5 mcg/mL and 30 mcg/mL in NS, D_5W, $D_51/2NS$, and D_5LR injection are stable for 48 hours at room temperature and 14 days under refrigeration.

Pharmacodynamics/Kinetics

Distribution: V_d: 8.3 ± 2.5 L/kg

Protein binding: 62%

Metabolism: ~50% metabolized via CYP enzymes (and likely other pathways) to relatively inactive metabolites; CYP1A2, 2D6, and 3A4 contribute to its metabolism

Half-life elimination: Terminal: 40 hours

Excretion: Urine (80%, 40% as unchanged drug)

Dosage I.V.: Adults:

Chemotherapy-induced nausea and vomiting: 0.25 mg 30 minutes prior to chemotherapy administration, day 1 of each cycle (doses should not be given more than once weekly)

Postoperative vomiting (unlabeled use): 30 mcg/kg (used in hysterectomy, lower doses ineffective; no significant reduction in nausea at any dose)

Elderly: No dosage adjustment necessary

Dosage adjustment in renal/hepatic impairment: No dosage adjustment necessary

Administration I.V.: Infuse over 30 seconds; flush I.V. line with NS prior to and following administration.

Dosage Forms Injection, solution: 0.05 mg/mL (5 mL)

Patient Information Inform prescriber of all prescriptions, OTC medications, or herbal products you are taking, and any allergies you have. Do not take anything new during treatment unless approved by prescriber. May cause drowsiness or dizziness (use caution when driving or engaging in tasks that require alertness until response to drug is known): or fatigue, diarrhea, constipation, or headache (request appropriate treatment from prescriber). Do not change position rapidly (rise slowly). Report persistent headache, excessive drowsiness, fever, numbness or tingling, or changes in elimination patterns (constipation or diarrhea); or chest pain or palpitations.

Selected Readings
Grunberg SM and Koeller JM, "Palonosetron: A Unique 5-HT$_3$-Receptor Antagonist for the Prevention of Chemotherapy-Induced Emesis," *Expert Opin Pharmacother*, 2003, 4(12):2297-303.

Siddiqui MA and Scott LJ, "Palonosetron," *Drugs*, 2004, 64(10):1125-32

Stacher G, "Palonosetron (Helsinn)," *Curr Opin Investig Drugs*, 2002, 3(10):1502-7.

◆ **Palonosetron Hydrochloride** *see* Palonosetron *on page 648*

Pamidronate (pa mi DROE nate)

Medication Safety Issues
Sound-alike/look-alike issues:
Aredia® may be confused with Adriamycin

U.S. Brand Names Aredia®

Canadian Brand Names Aredia®

Generic Available Yes

Synonyms Pamidronate Disodium

Pharmacologic Category Antidote; Bisphosphonate Derivative

Pregnancy Risk Factor D

Lactation Excretion in breast milk unknown/use caution

Use Treatment of hypercalcemia associated with malignancy; treatment of osteolytic bone lesions associated with multiple myeloma or metastatic breast cancer; moderate to severe Paget's disease of bone

Mechanism of Action A bisphosphonate which inhibits bone resorption via actions on osteoclasts or on osteoclast precursors. Does not appear to produce any significant effects on renal tubular calcium handling and is poorly absorbed following oral administration (high oral doses have been reported effective); therefore, I.V. therapy is preferred.

Labeled Contraindications Hypersensitivity to pamidronate, other bisphosphonates, or any component of the formulation; pregnancy

Warnings/Precautions Osteonecrosis of the jaw has been reported in patients with cancer who were receiving chemotherapy, corticosteroids, and chronic bisphosphonate therapy; symptoms included nonhealing extraction socket or an exposed jawbone. Dental exams and preventative dentistry should be performed prior to placing patients with risk factors (eg, chemotherapy, corticosteroids, poor oral hygiene) on chronic bisphosphonate therapy. Invasive dental procedures should be avoided during treatment.

May cause deterioration in renal function. Use caution in patients with renal impairment and avoid in severe renal impairment. Assess serum creatinine prior to each dose; withhold dose in patients with bone metastases who experience deterioration in renal function. Leukopenia has been observed with oral pamidronate and monitoring of white blood cell counts is suggested. Vein irritation and thrombophlebitis may occur with infusions. Monitor serum electrolytes, especially in the elderly.

Adverse Reactions As reported with hypercalcemia of malignancy; percentage of adverse effect varies upon dose and duration of infusion.
>10%:
Central nervous system: Fever (18% to 26%), fatigue (12%)
Endocrine & metabolic: Hypophosphatemia (9% to 18%), hypokalemia (4% to 18%), hypomagnesemia (4% to 12%), hypocalcemia (1% to 12%)
Gastrointestinal: Nausea (up to 18%), anorexia (1% to 12%)
Local: Infusion site reaction (up to 18%)
1% to 10%:
Cardiovascular: Atrial fibrillation (up to 6%), hypertension (up to 6%), syncope (up to 6%), tachycardia (up to 6%), atrial flutter (up to 1%), cardiac failure (up to 1%)
Central nervous system: Somnolence (1% to 6%), psychosis (up to 4%), insomnia (up to 1%)

Endocrine & metabolic: Hypothyroidism (6%)

Gastrointestinal: Constipation (4% to 6%), stomatitis (up to 1%)

Hematologic: Leukopenia (up to 4%), neutropenia (up to 1%), thrombocytopenia (up to 1%)

Neuromuscular & skeletal: Myalgia (up to 1%)

Renal: Uremia (up to 4%)

Respiratory: Rales (up to 6%), rhinitis (up to 6%), upper respiratory tract infection (up to 3%)

<1%: Iritis, episcleritis, scleritis, uveitis

Postmarketing and/or case reports: Allergic reaction, anaphylactic shock, angioedema, dyspnea, hypotension, osteonecrosis (primarily jaws)

Vesicant No

Emetic Potential Low

Overdosage/Toxicology Symptoms of overdose include hypocalcemia, ECG changes, seizures, bleeding, paresthesia, carpopedal spasm, and fever. Treat with I.V. calcium gluconate, and general supportive care; fever and hypotension can be treated with corticosteroids.

Drug Interactions

Increased Effect/Toxicity: Aminoglycosides may lower serum calcium levels with prolonged administration; concomitant use may have additive effect. Increased risk of hypocalcemia with concomitant loop diuretic use.

Storage/Stability Do not store powder for reconstitution at temperatures above 30°C (86°F). The reconstituted solution is stable under refrigeration at 2°C to 8°C (36°F to 46°F) for 24 hours. Pamidronate solution for infusion is stable at room temperature for up to 24 hours.

Reconstitution Powder for injection: Reconstitute by adding 10 mL of sterile water for injection to each vial of lyophilized pamidronate disodium powder, the resulting solution will be 30 mg/10 mL or 90 mg/10 mL.

Pamidronate may be further diluted in 250-1000 mL of 0.45% or 0.9% sodium chloride or 5% dextrose.

Compatibility Incompatible with calcium-containing infusion solutions such as Ringer's injection

Pharmacodynamics/Kinetics

Onset of action: 24-48 hours

Peak effect: Maximum: 5-7 days

Absorption: Poor; pharmacokinetic studies lacking

Metabolism: Not metabolized

Half-life elimination: 21-35 hours

Excretion: Biphasic; urine (~50% as unchanged drug) within 120 hours

Dosage Drug must be diluted properly before administration and infused intravenously slowly. Due to risk of nephrotoxicity, doses should not exceed 90 mg. I.V.: Adults:

Hypercalcemia of malignancy:

Moderate cancer-related hypercalcemia (corrected serum calcium: 12-13.5 mg/dL): 60-90 mg, as a single dose

Severe cancer-related hypercalcemia (corrected serum calcium: >13.5 mg/dL): 90 mg, as a single dose

A period of 7 days should elapse before the use of second course; repeat infusions every 2-3 weeks have been suggested, however, could be administered every 2-3 months according to the degree and of severity of hypercalcemia and/or the type of malignancy.

Osteolytic bone lesions with multiple myeloma: 90 mg monthly

(Continued)

Pamidronate *(Continued)*

Osteolytic bone lesions with metastatic breast cancer: 90 mg repeated every 3-4 weeks

Paget's disease: 30 mg for 3 consecutive days

Dosing adjustment in renal impairment: Not recommended in severe renal impairment (patients with bone metastases)

Dosing adjustment in renal toxicity: In patients with bone metastases, treatment should be withheld in patients who experience deterioration in renal function (increase of serum creatinine ≥0.5 mg/dL in patients with normal baseline or ≥1.0 mg/dL in patients with abnormal baseline). Resumption of therapy may be considered when serum creatinine returns to within 10% of baseline.

Administration I.V. infusion over 2-24 hours.

Dosage Forms

Injection, powder for reconstitution, as disodium (Aredia®): 30 mg, 90 mg

Injection, solution: 3 mg/mL (10 mL); 6 mg/mL (10 mL); 9 mg/mL (10 mL)

Monitoring Parameters Serum electrolytes, monitor for hypocalcemia for at least 2 weeks after therapy; serum calcium, phosphate, magnesium, potassium, CBC with differential; monitor serum creatinine prior to each dose; dental exam and preventative dentistry for patients at risk for osteonecrosis

Patient Information This medication can only be administered I.V. Avoid foods high in calcium, or vitamins with minerals, during infusion or for 2-3 hours after completion. You may experience nausea or vomiting (small frequent meals and good mouth care may help); or recurrent bone pain (consult prescriber for analgesic). Report unusual muscle twitching or spasms, severe diarrhea/constipation, or acute bone pain.

Special Geriatric Considerations Has not been studied exclusively in the elderly. Monitor serum electrolytes periodically since elderly are often receiving diuretics which can result in decreases in serum calcium, potassium, and magnesium.

Selected Readings

Fitton A and McTavish D, "Pamidronate: A Review of Its Pharmacological Properties and Therapeutic Efficacy in Resorptive Bone Disease," *Drugs*, 1991, 41(2):289-318.

Kellihan MJ and Mangino PD, "Pamidronate," *Ann Pharmacother*, 1992, 26(10):1262-9.

♦ **Pamidronate Disodium** *see* Pamidronate *on page 650*

♦ **Pan-B Antibody** *see* Rituximab *on page 709*

♦ **Pandel®** *see* Hydrocortisone *on page 419*

♦ **Panglobulin®** *see* Immune Globulin (Intravenous) *on page 458*

♦ **Panglobulin® NF** *see* Immune Globulin (Intravenous) *on page 458*

♦ **Panretin®** *see* Alitretinoin *on page 41*

♦ **Paraplatin®** *see* Carboplatin *on page 151*

♦ **Paraplatin-AQ (Can)** *see* Carboplatin *on page 151*

♦ **Pediapred®** *see* PrednisoLONE *on page 679*

♦ **Pedi-Dri®** *see* Nystatin *on page 613*

Pegaspargase *(peg AS par jase)*

Medication Safety Issues

Sound-alike/look-alike issues:

Pegaspargase may be confused with asparaginase

Related Information

Safe Handling of Hazardous Drugs *on page 1034*

U.S. Brand Names Oncaspar®
Generic Available No
Synonyms NSC-644954; PEG-L-Asparaginase
Pharmacologic Category Antineoplastic Agent, Miscellaneous
Pregnancy Risk Factor C
Lactation Enters breast milk/contraindicated
Use Treatment of acute lymphocytic leukemia, blast crisis of chronic lymphocytic leukemia (CLL), salvage therapy of non-Hodgkin's lymphoma; may be used in some patients who have had hypersensitivity reactions to *E. coli* asparaginase
Mechanism of Action Pegaspargase is a modified version of asparaginase. Leukemic cells, especially lymphoblasts, require exogenous asparagine; normal cells can synthesize asparagine. Asparaginase contains L-asparaginase amidohydrolase type EC-2 which inhibits protein synthesis by deaminating asparagine to aspartic acid and ammonia in the plasma and extracellular fluid and therefore deprives tumor cells of the amino acid for protein synthesis. Asparaginase is cycle-specific for the G_1 phase of the cell cycle.
Labeled Contraindications Hypersensitivity to pegaspargase or any component of the formulation; pancreatitis or a history of pancreatitis; previous serious allergic reactions or other unacceptable adverse reactions to pegaspargase
Warnings/Precautions Hazardous agent - use appropriate precautions for handling and disposal. See Safe Handling of Hazardous Drugs *on page 1034* in the Appendix.

Monitor for severe allergic reactions. Use cautiously in patients with an underlying coagulopathy or previous hematologic complications from asparaginase, hepatic dysfunction, hyperglycemia or diabetes, or pancreatitis. May be used cautiously in patients who have had hypersensitivity reactions to *E. coli* asparaginase; however, up to 33% of patients who have an allergic reaction to *E. coli* asparaginase will also react to pegaspargase.
Adverse Reactions In general, pegaspargase toxicities tend to be less frequent and appear somewhat later than comparable toxicities of asparaginase. Intramuscular rather than intravenous injection may decrease the incidence of coagulopathy; GI, hepatic, and renal toxicity.
>10%:
  Cardiovascular: Edema
  Central nervous system: Fatigue, disorientation (10%)
  Gastrointestinal: Nausea, vomiting (50% to 60%), generally mild to moderate, but may be severe and protracted in some patients; anorexia (33%); abdominal pain (38%); diarrhea (28%); increased serum lipase and amylase
  Hematologic: Hypofibrinogenemia and depression of clotting factors V and VII, variable decreases in factors VII and IX, severe protein C deficiency and decrease in antithrombin III - overt bleeding is uncommon, but may be dose-limiting, or fatal in some patients
  Neuromuscular & skeletal: Weakness (33%)
  Miscellaneous: Acute allergic reactions, including fever, rash, urticaria, arthralgia, hypotension, angioedema, bronchospasm, anaphylaxis (10% to 30%) - dose-limiting in some patients
1% to 10%:
  Cardiovascular: Hypotension, tachycardia, thrombosis
(Continued)

Pegaspargase *(Continued)*

Dermatologic: Urticaria, erythema, lip edema
Endocrine & metabolic: Hyperglycemia (3%)
Gastrointestinal: Acute pancreatitis (1%)
<1%: Agitation, bronchospasm, coma, convulsions, depression, dyspnea, hallucinations, paresthesia, parkinsonian symptoms (tremor, increased muscle tone), seizure, somnolence; transaminases, bilirubin, and alkaline phosphatase increased (transient)
Mild to moderate myelosuppression, leukopenia, anemia, thrombocytopenia; onset: 7 days; nadir: 14 days; recovery: 21 days

Vesicant No

Emetic Potential Very low (<10%)

Overdosage/Toxicology Symptoms of overdose include nausea and diarrhea.

Drug Interactions

Increased Effect/Toxicity:

Aspirin, dipyridamole, heparin, warfarin, NSAIDs: Imbalances in coagulation factors have been noted with the use of pegaspargase - use with caution.

Vincristine and prednisone: An increased toxicity has been noticed when asparaginase is administered with VCR and prednisone.

Cyclophosphamide (decreased metabolism)

Mercaptopurine (increased hepatotoxicity)

Vincristine (increased neuropathy)

Prednisone (hyperglycemia)

Decreased Effect: Asparaginase terminates methotrexate action by inhibition of protein synthesis and prevention of cell entry into the S Phase.

Storage/Stability Refrigerate at 2°C to 8°C (36°F to 46°F). Do not use of cloudy or if precipitate is present. Do not use if stored at room temperature for >48 hours. Do **not** freeze. Do not use product if it is known to have been frozen.

Reconstitution Avoid excessive agitation; do **not** shake.

Standard I.M. dilution: Do not exceed 2 mL volume per injection site

Standard I.V. dilution: Dose/100 mL NS or D_5W; stable for 48 hours at room temperature.

Compatibility Compatible: Stable in NS, D_5W

Pharmacodynamics/Kinetics

Duration: Asparaginase was measurable for at least 15 days following initial treatment with pegaspargase

Distribution: V_d: 4-5 L/kg; 70% to 80% of plasma volume; does not penetrate the CSF

Metabolism: Systemically degraded

Half-life elimination: 5.73 days; unaffected by age, renal or hepatic function

Excretion: Urine (trace amounts)

Dosage Refer to individual protocols.

I.M. administration is **preferred** over I.V. administration

Children: I.M., I.V.:

Body surface area <0.6 m^2: 82.5 int. units/kg every 14 days

Body surface area ≥0.6 m^2: 2500 int. units/m^2 every 14 days

Adults: I.M., I.V.: 2500 int. units/m^2 every 14 days

Hemodialysis: Significant drug removal is unlikely based on physiochemical characteristics

Peritoneal dialysis: Significant drug removal is unlikely based on physiochemical characteristics

Administration I.M.: Must only be administered as a deep intramuscular injection into a large muscle

Dosage Forms Injection, solution [preservative free]: 750 units/mL (5 mL)

Monitoring Parameters Vital signs during administration, coagulation factors, amylase, liver enzymes, prothrombin time, renal function tests, urine dipstick for glucose, blood glucose; monitor for onset of abdominal pain and mental status changes

Patient Information This drug can only be given I.M. or I.V. Inform prescriber if you are using any other medications that may increase risk of bleeding. Possibility of hypersensitivity reactions includes anaphylaxis. Maintain adequate hydration (2-3 L/day of fluids unless instructed to restrict fluid intake) and nutrition (small frequent meals may help if you experience nausea, vomiting, or loss of appetite). You may experience dizziness, drowsiness, syncope, or blurred vision (use caution when driving or engaging in tasks that require alertness until response to drug is known). You may experience increased sweating, decreased sexual drive, or cough. Report immediately chest pain or heart palpitations; difficulty breathing or constant cough; rash, hives, or swelling of lips or mouth; or abdominal pain. Report swelling of extremities or sudden weight gain; burning, pain, or redness at infusion site; persistent fever or chills; unusual bruising or bleeding; twitching or tremors; pain on urination; or persistent nausea or diarrhea.

Selected Readings

Asselin BL, Whitin JC, Cappola DJ, et al, "Comparative Pharmacokinetic Studies of Three Asparaginase Preparations," *J Clin Oncol*, 1993, 11(9):1780-6.

Graham ML, "Pegaspargase: A Review of Clinical Studies," *Adv Drug Deliv Rev*, 2003, 55(10):1293-302.

Keating MJ, Holmes R, Lerner S, et al, "L-Asparaginase and PEG Asparaginase - Past, Present, and Future," *Leuk Lymphoma*, 1993, 10(Suppl):153-7.

Patel SS and Benfield P, "Pegaspargase (Polyethylene Glycol-L-Asparaginase)," *Clin Immunother*, 1996, 5:490-6.

♦ **PEG-L-Asparaginase** *see* Pegaspargase *on page 652*

Pemetrexed (pem e TREKS ed)

U.S. Brand Names Alimta®

Synonyms LY231514; MTA; Multitargeted Antifolate; NSC-698037; Pemetrexed Disodium

Pharmacologic Category Antineoplastic Agent, Antimetabolite; Antineoplastic Agent, Antimetabolite (Antifolate)

Pregnancy Risk Factor D

Lactation Excretion in breast milk unknown/not recommended

Use Treatment of malignant pleural mesothelioma in combination with cisplatin; treatment of nonsmall cell lung cancer

Unlabeled/Investigational Use Bladder, breast, cervical, colorectal, esophageal, gastric, head and neck, ovarian, pancreatic, and renal cell cancers

Mechanism of Action Inhibits thymidylate synthase (TS), dihydrofolate reductase (DHFR), glycinamide ribonucleotide formyltransferase (Continued)

Pemetrexed (Continued)

(GARFT), and aminoimidazole carboxamide ribonucleotide formyltransferase (AICARFT), the enzymes involved in folate metabolism and DNA synthesis, resulting in inhibition of purine and thymidine nucleotide and protein synthesis.

Labeled Contraindications Hypersensitivity to pemetrexed or any component of the formulation

Warnings/Precautions Hazardous agent - use appropriate precautions for handling and disposal. See Safe Handling of Hazardous Drugs *on page 1034* in the Appendix. Prophylactic folic acid and vitamin B_{12} supplements are necessary to reduce hematologic and gastrointestinal toxicity. Folic acid and vitamin B_{12} should be started 1 week before the first dose of pemetrexed. Pretreatment with corticosteroids reduces the incidence and severity of cutaneous reactions. Use caution with hepatic dysfunction not due to metastases and in patients receiving concurrent nephrotoxins. Safety and efficacy have not been established in pediatric patients.

Adverse Reactions Note: Reported frequencies of adverse effects vary by indication/population and concurrent therapy.

>10%:

Cardiovascular: Chest pain (38% to 40%), edema (19%)

Central nervous system: Fatigue (80% to 87%), fever (17% to 26%), depression (11% to 14%)

Dermatologic: Rash (17% to 22%), alopecia (11%)

Gastrointestinal: Nausea (39% to 84%; grade 3/4 in 12%), vomiting (25% to 58%; grade 3/4 in 11%), constipation (30% to 44%), anorexia (35% to 62%), stomatitis/pharyngitis (20% to 28%), diarrhea (21% to 26%)

Hematologic: Neutropenia (11% to 58%), leukopenia (13% to 55%), anemia (33%), thrombocytopenia (9% to 27%)

Nadir: 8-10 days

Recovery: 12-17 days

Neuromuscular & skeletal: Neuropathy (17% to 29%), myalgia (13%)

Renal: Creatinine increased (3% to 16%)

Respiratory: Dyspnea (66%)

Miscellaneous: Infection (17% to 23%)

1% to 10%:

Cardiovascular: Thrombosis/embolism (4% to 7%), cardiac ischemia (3%)

Endocrine & metabolic: Dehydration (3% to 7%)

Gastrointestinal: Dysphagia/esophagitis/odynophagia (5% to 6%)

Renal: Renal failure (<1% to 2%)

Miscellaneous: Allergic reaction (2% to 8%)

Neuromuscular & skeletal: Arthralgia (8%)

Vesicant No

Emetic Potential Moderate (30% to 60%; grade 3 or 4: 10% to 12%)

Overdosage/Toxicology Toxicities include neutropenia, anemia, thrombocytopenia, mucositis, rash, infection, and diarrhea. Treatment is supportive and symptom-directed. Continuing leucovorin may help minimize additional hematologic toxicity. The intravenous leucovorin doses used in clinical trials were 100 mg/m² once, followed by 50 mg/m² every 6 hours for 8 days. It is unknown if pemetrexed is removed by hemodialysis.

Drug Interactions

Increased Effect/Toxicity: NSAIDs may increase the toxicity of pemetrexed.

Ethanol/Nutrition/Herb Interactions Lower ANC nadirs occur in patients with elevated baseline cystathionine or homocysteine concentrations. Levels of these substances can be reduced by folic acid and vitamin B_{12} supplementation.

Storage/Stability Store unopened vials at 25°C (77°F). Reconstituted and infusion solutions are stable for 24 hours when refrigerated or stored at room temperature.

Reconstitution Add 20 mL of 0.9% preservative free sodium chloride injection to make a 25 mg/mL solution. Gently swirl. Solution may be colorless to green-yellow. Further dilute in 50-200 mL of 0.9% sodium chloride for administration.

Compatibility Stable in NS

Y-site administration: Compatible: Acyclovir, amifostine, amikacin sulfate, aminophylline, ampicillin sodium, ampicillin sodium-sulbactam sodium, aztreonam, bumetanide, buprenorphine hydrochloride, butorphanol tartrate, carboplatin, ceftizoxime sodium, ceftriaxone sodium, cefuroxime sodium, cimetidine hydrochloride, cisplatin, clindamycin phosphate, co-trimoxazole, cyclophosphamide, cytarabine, dexamethasone sodium phosphate, dexrazoxane, diphenhydramine hydrochloride, docetaxel, dopamine hydrochloride, enalaprilat, famotidine, fluconazole, fluorouracil, ganciclovir sodium, granisetron hydrochloride, haloperidol lactate, heparin sodium, hydromorphone hydrochloride, hydroxyzine hydrochloride, ifosfamide, leucovorin calcium, lorazepam, mannitol, meperidine hydrochloride, mesna, methylprednisolone sodium succinate, metoclopramide hydrochloride, morphine sulfate, paclitaxel, potassium chloride, promethazine hydrochloride, ranitidine hydrochloride, sodium bicarbonate, ticarcillin disodium, ticarcillin disodium-clavulanate potassium, vancomycin hydrochloride, vinblastine sulfate, vincristine sulfate, zidovudine. **Incompatible:** Amphotericin B, calcium gluconate, cefazolin sodium, cefotaxime sodium, cefotetan disodium, cefoxitin sodium, ceftazidime, chlorpromazine hydrochloride, ciprofloxacin, dobutamine hydrochloride, doxorubicin hydrochloride, doxycycline hyclate, droperidol, gemcitabine hydrochloride, gentamicin sulfate, irinotecan hydrochloride, metronidazole, minocycline hydrochloride, mitoxantrone hydrochloride, nalbuphine hydrochloride, ondansetron hydrochloride, prochlorperazine edisylate, tobramycin sulfate, topotecan hydrochloride

Pharmacodynamics/Kinetics

Duration: V_{dss}: 16.1 L

Protein binding: ~81%

Metabolism: Minimal

Half-life elimination: Normal renal function: 3.5 hours

Excretion: Urine (70% to 90% as unchanged drug)

Dosage I.V.: Adults:

Nonsmall cell lung cancer: 500 mg/m^2 on day 1 of each 21-day cycle

Malignant pleural mesothelioma: 500-600 mg/m^2 on day 1 of each 21-day cycle

Note: Start vitamin supplements 1 week before initial dose of pemetrexed. Folic acid 350-1000 mcg/day orally (continuing for 21 days after last dose of pemetrexed) and vitamin B_{12} 1000 mcg I.M. every 9 weeks. (Continued)

Pemetrexed *(Continued)*

Dexamethasone 4 mg twice daily can be started the day before therapy, and continued the day of and the day after to minimize cutaneous reactions.

Dosage adjustments for toxicities:

Toxicity: Discontinue if patient has any grade 3 or 4 toxicity after two dose reductions (except grade 3 transaminase elevations) or immediately if grade 3 or 4 neurotoxicity develops

Hematologic toxicity: Upon recovery, reinitiate therapy

Nadir ANC <500/mm^3 and nadir platelets ≥50,000/mm^3: Reduce dose to 75% of previous dose of pemetrexed and cisplatin

Nadir platelets <50,000/mm^3: Reduce dose to 50% of previous dose of pemetrexed and cisplatin

Nonhematologic toxicity (excluding neurotoxicity or ≥ grade 3 transaminase elevations): Upon recovery, reinitiate therapy

Grade 3 or 4 toxicity (excluding mucositis or transaminase elevations): Reduce dose to 75% of previous dose of pemetrexed and cisplatin

Diarrhea requiring hospitalization: Reduce dose to 75% of previous dose of pemetrexed and cisplatin

Grade 3 or 4 mucositis: Reduce dose to 50% of previous dose of pemetrexed; continue cisplatin at 100% of previous dose

Neurotoxicity:

Common Toxicity Criteria (CTC) Grade 0-1: Continue at previous dose of pemetrexed and cisplatin.

CTC Grade 2: Continue at previous dose of pemetrexed; Reduce dose to 50% of previous dose of cisplatin.

Dosage adjustment in renal impairment:

Cl$_{cr}$ <45 mL/minute: No dosage adjustment guidelines are available; manufacturer recommends not using the drug.

Cl$_{cr}$ ≥45 mL/minute: No dosage adjustment required.

Dosage adjustment in hepatic impairment: No dosage adjustment required.

Combination Regimens

Malignant pleural mesothelioma: Cisplatin + Pemetrexed *on page 862*

Administration I.V.: Infuse over 10 minutes.

Dosage Forms Injection, powder for reconstitution: 500 mg

Monitoring Parameters CBC (before each dose); serum creatinine, total bilirubin, ALT, AST (day 1 of each, or every other, cycle)

Dietary Considerations Initiate folic acid supplementation 1 week before first dose of pemetrexed, continue for full course of therapy, and for 21 days after last dose. Institute vitamin B$_{12}$ 1 week before the first dose; administer every 9 weeks thereafter.

Selected Readings

Adjei AA, "Pemetrexed (Alimta): A Novel Multitargeted Antifolate Agent," *Expert Rev Anticancer Ther*, 2003, 3(2):145-56.

Goldman ID and Zhao R, "Molecular, Biochemical, and Cellular Pharmacology of Pemetrexed," *Semin Oncol*, 2002, 29(6 Suppl 18):3-17.

Niyikiza C, Hanauske AR, Rusthoven JJ, et al, "Pemetrexed Safety and Dosing Strategy," *Semin Oncol*, 2002, 29(6 Suppl 18):24-9.

Ouellet D, Periclou AP, Johnson RD, et al, "Population Pharmacokinetics of Pemetrexed Disodium (ALIMTA) in Patients With Cancer," *Cancer Chemother Pharmacol*, 2000, 46(3):227-34.

Paz-Ares L, Bezares S, Tabernero JM, et al, "Review of a Promising New Agent - Pemetrexed Disodium," *Cancer*, 2003, 97(8 Suppl):2056-63.

Pentamidine (pen TAM i deen)

Related Information
Safe Handling of Hazardous Drugs *on page 1034*

U.S. Brand Names NebuPent®️; Pentam-300®️

Canadian Brand Names Pentacarinat®️

Generic Available No

Synonyms Pentamidine Isethionate

Pharmacologic Category Antibiotic, Miscellaneous

Pregnancy Risk Factor C

Lactation Excretion in breast milk unknown/contraindicated

Use Treatment and prevention of pneumonia caused by *Pneumocystis carinii* (PCP)

Unlabeled/Investigational Use Treatment of trypanosomiasis and visceral leishmaniasis

Mechanism of Action Interferes with RNA/DNA, phospholipids and protein synthesis, through inhibition of oxidative phosphorylation and/or interference with incorporation of nucleotides and nucleic acids into RNA and DNA, in protozoa

Labeled Contraindications Hypersensitivity to pentamidine isethionate or any component of the formulation (inhalation and injection)

Warnings/Precautions Use with caution in patients with diabetes mellitus, renal or hepatic dysfunction, hyper-/hypotension, leukopenia, thrombocytopenia, asthma, or hypo-/hyperglycemia.

Adverse Reactions Injection (I); Aerosol (A)

>10%:
  Cardiovascular: Chest pain (A - 10% to 23%)
  Central nervous system: Fatigue (A - 50% to 70%); dizziness (A - 31% to 47%)
  Dermatologic: Rash (31% to 47%)
  Endocrine & metabolic: Hyperkalemia
  Gastrointestinal: Anorexia (A - 50% to 70%), nausea (A - 10% to 23%)
  Local: Local reactions at injection site
  Renal: Increased creatinine (I - 23%)
  Respiratory: Wheezing (A - 10% to 23%), dyspnea (A - 50% to 70%), cough (A - 31% to 47%), pharyngitis (10% to 23%)

1% to 10%:
  Cardiovascular: Hypotension (I - 4%)
  Central nervous system: Confusion/hallucinations (1% to 2%), headache (A - 1% to 5%)
  Dermatologic: Rash (I - 3.3%)
  Endocrine & metabolic: Hypoglycemia <25 mg/dL (I - 2.4%)
  Gastrointestinal: Nausea/anorexia (I - 6%), diarrhea (A - 1% to 5%), vomiting
  Hematologic: Severe leukopenia (I - 2.8%), thrombocytopenia <20,000/mm^3 (I - 1.7%), anemia (A - 1% to 5%)
  Hepatic: Increased LFTs (I - 8.7%)

(Continued)

Pentamidine *(Continued)*

<1%: Hypotension <60 mm Hg systolic (I - 0.9%), tachycardia, arrhythmia, dizziness (I), fever, fatigue (I), hyperglycemia or hypoglycemia, hypocalcemia, pancreatitis, megaloblastic anemia, granulocytopenia, leukopenia, renal insufficiency, extrapulmonary pneumocystosis, irritation of the airway, pneumothorax, Jarisch-Herxheimer-like reaction, mild renal or hepatic injury

Vesicant No

Overdosage/Toxicology Symptoms of overdose include hypotension, hypoglycemia, and cardiac arrhythmias. Treatment is supportive.

Drug Interactions

Cytochrome P450 Effect: Substrate of CYP2C19 (major); **Inhibits** CYP2C8/9 (weak), 2C19 (weak), 2D6 (weak), 3A4 (weak)

Increased Effect/Toxicity: CYP2C19 inhibitors may increase the levels/effects of pentamidine; example inhibitors include delavirdine, fluconazole, fluvoxamine, gemfibrozil, isoniazid, omeprazole, and ticlopidine. Pentamidine may potentiate the effect of other drugs which prolong QT interval (cisapride, sparfloxacin, gatifloxacin, moxifloxacin, pimozide, and type Ia and type III antiarrhythmics).

Decreased Effect: CYP2C19 inducers may decrease the levels/effects of pentamidine; example inducers include aminoglutethimide, carbamazepine, phenytoin, and rifampin.

Ethanol/Nutrition/Herb Interactions Ethanol: Avoid ethanol (may increase CNS depression or aggravate hypoglycemia).

Storage/Stability Store intact vials at controlled room temperature and protect from light. Reconstituted vials with SWFI (60-100 mg/mL) are stable for 48 hours at room temperature and do not require light protection. Diluted solutions in 50-250 mL D_5W for infusion (1-2.5 mg/mL) are stable for at least 24 hours at room temperature.

Reconstitution Powder for inhalation should be reconstituted with sterile water for injection (6 mL per 300 mg vial). Powder for injection may be reconstituted with sterile water for injection or D_5W (SWFI should be used for I.M. injections). **Do not use NS as a diluent.**

Compatibility Solutions for injection (1-2.5 mg/mL) in D_5W are stable for at least 24 hours at room temperature. The manufacturer's labeling recommends D_5W, however stability in NS has also been documented.

Y-site administration: Compatible: Diltiazem, gatifloxacin, zidovudine. **Incompatible:** Aldesleukin, cefazolin, cefoperazone, cefotaxime, cefoxitin, ceftazidime, ceftriaxone, fluconazole, foscarnet, linezolid Vials reconstituted with SWFI (60-100 mg/mL) are stable for 48 hours at room temperature protected from light. Solutions for injection (1-2.5 mg/mL) in D_5W are stable for at least 24 hours at room temperature.

Y-site administration: Compatible: Diltiazem, gatifloxacin, zidovudine. **Incompatible:** Aldesleukin, cefazolin, cefoperazone, cefotaxime, cefoxitin, ceftazidime, ceftriaxone, fluconazole, foscarnet, linezolid

Pharmacodynamics/Kinetics

Absorption: I.M.: Well absorbed; Inhalation: Limited systemic absorption

Half-life elimination: Terminal: 6.4-9.4 hours; may be prolonged with severe renal impairment

Excretion: Urine (33% to 66% as unchanged drug)

Dosage

Children:

Treatment of PCP pneumonia: I.M., I.V. (I.V. preferred): 4 mg/kg/day once daily for 10-14 days

Prevention of PCP pneumonia:

I.M., I.V.: 4 mg/kg monthly or every 2 weeks

Inhalation (aerosolized pentamidine in children ≥5 years): 300 mg/ dose given every 3-4 weeks via Respirgard® II inhaler (8 mg/kg dose has also been used in children <5 years)

Treatment of trypanosomiasis (unlabeled use): I.V.: 4 mg/kg/day once daily for 10 days

Adults:

Treatment: I.M., I.V. (I.V. preferred): 4 mg/kg/day once daily for 14-21 days

Prevention: Inhalation: 300 mg every 4 weeks via Respirgard® II nebulizer

Dialysis: Not removed by hemo or peritoneal dialysis or continuous arteriovenous or venovenous hemofiltration; supplemental dosage is not necessary

Dosing adjustment in renal impairment: Adults: I.V.:

Cl_{cr} 10-50 mL/minute: Administer 4 mg/kg every 24-36 hours

Cl_{cr} <10 mL/minute: Administer 4 mg/kg every 48 hours

Administration

Inhalation: Deliver until nebulizer is gone (30-45 minutes)

Infuse I.V. slowly over a period of at least 60 minutes or administer deep I.M.

Dosage Forms

Injection, powder for reconstitution, as isethionate (Pentam-300®): 300 mg

Powder for nebulization, as isethionate (NebuPent®): 300 mg

Monitoring Parameters Liver function tests, renal function tests, blood glucose, serum potassium and calcium, ECG, blood pressure

Patient Information PCP pneumonia may still occur despite pentamidine use; report fever, shortness of breath, or coughing up blood; maintain adequate fluid intake

Additional Information Virtually undetectable amounts are transferred to healthcare personnel during aerosol administration.

Special Geriatric Considerations Ten percent of acquired immunodeficiency syndrome (AIDS) cases are in the elderly and this figure is expected to increase. Pentamidine has not as yet been studied exclusively in this population. Adjust dose for renal function.

Selected Readings

Goa KL and Campoli-Richards DM, "Pentamidine Isethionate. A Review of Its Antiprotozoal Activity, Pharmacokinetic Properties and Therapeutic Use in *Pneumocystis carinii* Pneumonia," *Drugs*, 1987, 33(3):242-58.

Monk JP and Benfield P, "Inhaled Pentamidine. An Overview of Its Pharmacological Properties and a Review of Its Therapeutic Use in *Pneumocystis carinii* Pneumonia," *Drugs*, 1990, 39(5):741-56.

♦ **Pentamidine Isethionate** *see* Pentamidine *on page 659*

Pentostatin (PEN toe stat in)

Medication Safety Issues

Sound-alike/look-alike issues:

Pentostatin may be confused with pentosan

(Continued)

Pentostatin (Continued)

Related Information
Safe Handling of Hazardous Drugs *on page 1034*
U.S. Brand Names Nipent®
Canadian Brand Names Nipent®
Generic Available No
Synonyms CL-825; Co-Vidarabine; dCF; Deoxycoformycin; 2'-Deoxyco-formycin; NSC-218321
Pharmacologic Category Antineoplastic Agent, Antibiotic; Antineoplastic Agent, Antimetabolite (Purine Antagonist)
Pregnancy Risk Factor D
Lactation Excretion in breast milk unknown/contraindicated
Use Treatment of hairy cell leukemia; non-Hodgkin's lymphoma, cutaneous T-cell lymphoma
Mechanism of Action Pentostatin is a purine antimetabolite that inhibits adenosine deaminase, preventing the deamination of adenosine to inosine. Accumulation of deoxyadenosine (dAdo) and deoxyadenosine 5'-triphosphate (dATP) results in a reduction of purine metabolism and DNA synthesis and cell death.
Labeled Contraindications Hypersensitivity to pentostatin or any component; pregnancy
Warnings/Precautions Hazardous agent - use appropriate precautions for handling and disposal. See Safe Handling of Hazardous Drugs *on page 1034* in the Appendix. Use extreme caution in the presence of renal insufficiency. Use with caution in patients with signs or symptoms of impaired hepatic function.
Adverse Reactions
>10%:
  Central nervous system: Fever, chills, headache
  Dermatologic: Skin rash (25% to 30%), alopecia (10%)
  Gastrointestinal: Mild to moderate nausea, vomiting (60%), stomatitis, diarrhea (13%), anorexia
  Genitourinary: Acute renal failure (35%)
  Hematologic: Thrombocytopenia (50%), dose-limiting in 25% of patients; anemia (40% to 45%), neutropenia, mild to moderate, not dose-limiting (11%)
    Nadir: 7 days
    Recovery: 10-14 days
  Hepatic: Transaminases increased, mild-moderate, usually transient (30%); hepatitis (19%), usually reversible
  Respiratory: Pulmonary edema (15%), may be exacerbated by fludarabine
  Miscellaneous: Infection (57%; 35% severe, life-threatening)
1% to 10%:
  Cardiovascular: Chest pain, arrhythmia, peripheral edema
  Central nervous system: Opportunistic infection (8%); anxiety, confusion, depression, dizziness, insomnia, nervousness, somnolence, myalgia, malaise
  Dermatologic: Dry skin, eczema, pruritus
  Gastrointestinal: Constipation, flatulence, weight loss
  Neuromuscular & skeletal: Paresthesia, weakness

Ocular: Moderate to severe keratoconjunctivitis, abnormal vision, eye pain

Otic: Ear pain

Respiratory: Dyspnea, pneumonia, bronchitis, pharyngitis, rhinitis, epistaxis, sinusitis (3% to 7%)

<1%: Dysuria, hematuria, hypersensitivity reactions, BUN increased, thrombophlebitis; lethargy, seizure, coma (uncommon at doses <4 mg/m²)

Vesicant No

Emetic Potential Moderate (30% to 60%)

Overdosage/Toxicology Symptoms of overdose include severe renal, hepatic, pulmonary, and CNS toxicity. Treatment is supportive.

Drug Interactions

Increased Effect/Toxicity: Increased toxicity with vidarabine and allopurinol; combined use with fludarabine may lead to severe, even fatal, pulmonary toxicity

Storage/Stability Vials are stable under refrigeration at 2°C to 8°C; reconstituted vials or further dilutions are stable for 24 hours in D_5W or 48 hours in NS or lactated Ringer's

Reconstitution Reconstitute with SWFI to a concentration of 2 mg/mL. The injection may be further diluted with 25-50 mL NS or D_5W for infusion.

Compatibility Stable in LR, NS; **variable stability (consult detailed reference)** in D_5W

Y-site administration: Compatible: Fludarabine, melphalan, ondansetron, paclitaxel, sargramostim

Pharmacodynamics/Kinetics

Distribution: I.V.: V_d: 36.1 L (20.1 L/m²); rapidly to body tissues

Half-life elimination: Distribution half-life: 30-85 minutes; Terminal: 5-15 hours

Excretion: Urine (~50% to 96%) within 24 hours (30% to 90% as unchanged drug)

Dosage Refractory hairy cell leukemia: Adults (refer to individual protocols):

4 mg/m² every other week **or**

4 mg/m² weekly for 3 weeks, then every 2 weeks **or**

5 mg/m² daily for 3 days every 3 weeks

Dosing interval in renal impairment:

Cl_{cr} <60 mL/minute: Use extreme caution

Cl_{cr} 50-60 mL/minute: 2 mg/m²/dose

Administration Administer I.V. as a 15- to 30-minute infusion; continuous infusion regimens have been reported, but are not commonly used

I.V. bolus over ≥3-5 minutes

Dosage Forms Injection, powder for reconstitution: 10 mg

Selected Readings

Brogden RN and Sorkin EM, "Pentostatin. A Review of Its Pharmacodynamic and Pharmacokinetic Properties, and Therapeutic Potential in Lymphoproliferative Disorders," *Drugs*, 1993, 46(4):652-77.

Catovsky D, "Clinical Experience With 2'-Deoxycoformycin," *Hematol Cell Ther*, 1996, 38(Suppl 2):103-7.

Dillman RO, "A New Chemotherapeutic Agent: Deoxycoformycin (Pentostatin)," *Semin Hematol*, 1994, 31(1):16-27.

Kane BJ, Kuhn JG, and Roush MK, "Pentostatin: An Adenosine Deaminase Inhibitor For the Treatment of Hairy Cell Leukemia," *Ann Pharmacother*, 1992, 26(7-8):939-47.

Margolis J and Grever MR, "Pentostatin (Nipent): A Review of Potential Toxicity and its Management," *Semin Oncol*, 2000, 27(2 Suppl 5):9-14.

Phytonadione (fye toe na DYE one)

Medication Safety Issues
Sound-alike/look-alike issues:
Mephyton® may be confused with melphalan, methadone

U.S. Brand Names Mephyton®

Canadian Brand Names AquaMEPHYTON®; Konakion; Mephyton®

Generic Available Yes: Injection

Synonyms Methylphytyl Napthoquinone; Phylloquinone; Phytomenadione; Vitamin K_1

Pharmacologic Category Vitamin, Fat Soluble

Pregnancy Risk Factor C

Lactation Enters breast milk/compatible

Use Prevention and treatment of hypoprothrombinemia caused by drug-induced or anticoagulant-induced vitamin K deficiency, hemorrhagic disease of the newborn; phytonadione is more effective and is preferred to other vitamin K preparations in the presence of impending hemorrhage; oral absorption depends on the presence of bile salts

Mechanism of Action Promotes liver synthesis of clotting factors (II, VII, IX, X); however, the exact mechanism as to this stimulation is unknown. Menadiol is a water soluble form of vitamin K; phytonadione has a more rapid and prolonged effect than menadione; menadiol sodium diphosphate (K_4) is half as potent as menadione (K_3).

Labeled Contraindications Hypersensitivity to phytonadione or any component of the formulation

Warnings/Precautions Severe reactions resembling anaphylaxis or hypersensitivity have occurred rarely during or immediately after I.V. administration (even with proper dilution and rate of administration), as well as I.M. administration. Restrict I.V. administration for emergency use only. Allergic reactions have also occurred with I.M. and SubQ injection. Ineffective in hereditary hypoprothrombinemia, hypoprothrombinemia caused by severe liver disease. Severe hemolytic anemia has been reported rarely in neonates following large doses (10-20 mg) of phytonadione.

Adverse Reactions <1%: Abnormal taste, anaphylaxis, cyanosis, diaphoresis, dizziness (rarely), dyspnea, GI upset (oral), hemolysis in neonates and in patients with G6PD deficiency, hypersensitivity reactions, hypotension (rarely), pain, tenderness at injection site, transient flushing reaction

Vesicant No

Emetic Potential Very low (<10%)

Drug Interactions
  Decreased Effect: The anticoagulant effects of warfarin, dicumarol, anisindione are reversed by phytonadione.

Storage/Stability Protect injection from light at all times; may be autoclaved.

Reconstitution Dilute in normal saline, D_5W or D_5NS.

Pharmacodynamics/Kinetics
  Onset of action: Increased coagulation factors: Oral: 6-12 hours; Parenteral: 1-2 hours; prothrombin may become normal after 12-14 hours
  Absorption: Oral: From intestines in presence of bile
  Metabolism: Rapidly hepatic
  Excretion: Urine and feces

Dosage SubQ is the preferred (per manufacturer) parenteral route; I.V. route should be restricted for emergency use only
  Minimum daily requirement: Not well established
    Infants: 1-5 mcg/kg/day
    Adults: 0.03 mcg/kg/day
  Hemorrhagic disease of the newborn:
    Prophylaxis: I.M.: 0.5-1 mg within 1 hour of birth
    Treatment: I.M., SubQ: 1-2 mg/dose/day
  Oral anticoagulant overdose:
    Infants and Children:
      No bleeding, rapid reversal needed, patient **will require** further oral anticoagulant therapy: SubQ, I.V.: 0.5-2 mg
      No bleeding, rapid reversal needed, patient **will not require** further oral anticoagulant therapy: SubQ, I.V.: 2-5 mg
      Significant bleeding, not life-threatening: SubQ, I.V.: 0.5-2 mg
      Significant bleeding, life-threatening: I.V.: 5 mg over 10-20 minutes
    Adults: Oral, I.V., SubQ: 1-10 mg/dose depending on degree of INR elevation
      Serious bleeding or major overdose: 10 mg I.V. (slow infusion); may repeat every 12 hours (have required doses up to 25 mg)
  Vitamin K deficiency: Due to drugs, malabsorption, or decreased synthesis of vitamin K
    Infants and Children:
      Oral: 2.5-5 mg/24 hours
      I.M., I.V., SubQ: 1-2 mg/dose as a single dose
    Adults:
      Oral: 5-25 mg/24 hours
      I.M., I.V., SubQ: 10 mg

Administration
  I.V.: Rate of infusion should not exceed 1 mg/minute. **This route should be used only if administration by another route is not feasible.**
  Oral: The parenteral preparation has been administered orally to neonates.
  (Continued)

Phytonadione *(Continued)*

Dosage Forms

Injection, aqueous colloidal: 2 mg/mL (0.5 mL); 10 mg/mL (1 mL) [contains benzyl alcohol]

Tablet (Mephyton®): 5 mg

Monitoring Parameters PT

Extemporaneous Preparations A 1 mg/mL oral suspension was stable for only 3 days when refrigerated when compounded as follows:

Triturate six 5 mg tablets in a mortar, reduce to a fine powder, then add 5 mL each of water and methylcellulose 1% while mixing; then transfer to a graduate and qs to 30 mL with sorbitol

Shake well before using and keep in refrigerator

Nahata MC and Hipple TF, *Pediatric Drug Formulations*, 3rd ed, Cincinnati, OH: Harvey Whitney Books Co, 1997.

♦ **Pidorubicin** *see* Epirubicin *on page 298*

♦ **Pidorubicin Hydrochloride** *see* Epirubicin *on page 298*

♦ **Pilocar®** *see* Pilocarpine *on page 666*

Pilocarpine *(pye loe KAR peen)*

Medication Safety Issues

Sound-alike/look-alike issues:

Isopto® Carpine may be confused with Isopto® Carbachol

Salagen® may be confused with Salacid®

Related Information

Mucositis/Stomatitis *on page 995*

U.S. Brand Names Isopto® Carpine; Pilocar®; Pilopine HS®; Salagen®

Canadian Brand Names Diocarpine; Isopto® Carpine; Pilopine HS®; Salagen®

Generic Available Yes: Hydrochloride solution

Synonyms Pilocarpine Hydrochloride

Pharmacologic Category Cholinergic Agonist; Ophthalmic Agent, Antiglaucoma; Ophthalmic Agent, Miotic

Pregnancy Risk Factor C

Lactation Excretion in breast milk unknown/not recommended

Use

Ophthalmic: Management of chronic simple glaucoma, chronic and acute angle-closure glaucoma

Oral: Symptomatic treatment of xerostomia caused by salivary gland hypofunction resulting from radiotherapy for cancer of the head and neck or Sjögren's syndrome

Unlabeled/Investigational Use Counter effects of cycloplegics

Mechanism of Action Directly stimulates cholinergic receptors in the eye causing miosis (by contraction of the iris sphincter), loss of accommodation (by constriction of ciliary muscle), and lowering of intraocular pressure (with decreased resistance to aqueous humor outflow)

Labeled Contraindications Hypersensitivity to pilocarpine or any component of the formulation; acute inflammatory disease of the anterior chamber of the eye; in addition, tablets are also contraindicated in patients with uncontrolled asthma, angle-closure glaucoma, severe hepatic impairment

Warnings/Precautions Use caution with cardiovascular disease; patients may have difficulty compensating for transient changes in hemodynamics or rhythm induced by pilocarpine.

Ophthalmic products: May cause decreased visual acuity, especially at night or with reduced lighting.

Oral tablets: Use caution with controlled asthma, chronic bronchitis or COPD; may increase airway resistance, bronchial smooth muscle tone, and bronchial secretions. Use caution with cholelithiasis, biliary tract disease, nephrolithiasis; adjust dose with moderate hepatic impairment.

Adverse Reactions
Ophthalmic: Frequency not defined:
Cardiovascular: Hypertension, tachycardia
Gastrointestinal: Diarrhea, nausea, salivation, vomiting
Ocular: Burning, ciliary spasm, conjunctival vascular congestion, corneal granularity (gel 10%), lacrimation, lens opacity, myopia, retinal detachment, supraorbital or temporal headache, visual acuity decreased
Respiratory: Bronchial spasm, pulmonary edema
Miscellaneous: Diaphoresis

Oral (frequency varies by indication and dose):
>10%:
Cardiovascular: Flushing (8% to 13%)
Central nervous system: Chills (3% to 15%), dizziness (5% to 12%), headache (11%)
Gastrointestinal: Nausea (6% to 15%)
Genitourinary: Urinary frequency (9% to 12%)
Neuromuscular & skeletal: Weakness (2% to 12%)
Respiratory: Rhinitis (5% to 14%)
Miscellaneous: Diaphoresis (29% to 68%)
1% to 10%:
Cardiovascular: Edema (<1% to 5%), facial edema, hypertension (3%), palpitation, tachycardia
Central nervous system: Pain (4%), fever, somnolence
Dermatologic: Pruritus, rash
Gastrointestinal: Diarrhea (4% to 7%), dyspepsia (7%), vomiting (3% to 4%), constipation, flatulence, glossitis, salivation increased, stomatitis, taste perversion
Genitourinary: Vaginitis, urinary incontinence
Neuromuscular & skeletal: Myalgias, tremor
Ocular: Lacrimation (6%), amblyopia (4%), abnormal vision, blurred vision, conjunctivitis
Otic: Tinnitus
Respiratory: Cough increased, dysphagia, epistaxis, sinusitis
Miscellaneous: Allergic reaction, voice alteration
<1%: Abnormal dreams, abnormal thinking, alopecia, angina pectoris, anorexia, anxiety, aphasia, appetite increased, arrhythmia, arthralgia, arthritis, bilirubinemia, body odor, bone disorder, bradycardia, breast pain, bronchitis, cataract, cholelithiasis, colitis, confusion, contact dermatitis, cyst, deafness, depression, dry eyes, dry mouth, dry skin, dyspnea, dysuria, ear pain, ECG abnormality, eczema, emotional lability, eructation, erythema nodosum, esophagitis, exfoliative dermatitis, eye hemorrhage, eye pain, gastritis, gastroenteritis, gastrointestinal disorder, gingivitis, glaucoma, hematuria, hepatitis,
(Continued)

Pilocarpine *(Continued)*

herpes simplex, hiccup, hyperkinesias, hypoesthesia, hypoglycemia, hypotension, hypothermia, insomnia, intracranial hemorrhage, laryngismus, laryngitis, leg cramps, leukopenia, liver function test abnormal, lymphadenopathy, mastitis, melena, menorrhagia, metrorrhagia, migraine, moniliasis, myasthenia, MI, neck pain, photosensitivity reaction, nervousness, ovarian disorder, pancreatitis, paresthesia, parotid gland enlargement, peripheral edema, platelet abnormality, pneumonia, pyuria, salivary gland enlargement, salpingitis, seborrhea, skin ulcer, speech disorder, sputum increased, stridor, syncope, taste loss, tendon disorder, tenosynovitis, thrombocythemia, thrombocytopenia, thrombosis, tongue disorder, twitching, urethral pain, urinary impairment, urinary urgency, vaginal hemorrhage, vaginal moniliasis, vesiculobullous rash, WBC abnormality, yawning

Emetic Potential Very low (<10%)

Overdosage/Toxicology Symptoms of overdose include bronchospasm, bradycardia, involuntary urination, vomiting, hypotension, and tremor. Atropine is the treatment of choice for intoxications manifesting with significant muscarinic symptoms. Atropine I.V. 2-4 mg every 3-60 minutes should be repeated to control symptoms and then continued as needed for 1-2 days following acute ingestion. Epinephrine 0.1-1 mg SubQ may be useful for reversing severe cardiovascular or pulmonary sequelae.

Drug Interactions

Cytochrome P450 Effect: Inhibits CYP2A6 (weak), 2E1 (weak), 3A4 (weak)

Increased Effect/Toxicity: Concurrent use with beta-blockers may cause conduction disturbances.

Decreased Effect: May decrease effects of anticholinergic drugs (atropine, ipratropium).

Ethanol/Nutrition/Herb Interactions Food: Avoid administering oral formulation with high-fat meal; fat decreases the rate of absorption, maximum concentration and increases the time it takes to reach maximum concentration.

Storage/Stability

Gel: Store at room temperature of 2°C to 27°C (36°F to 80°F). Do not freeze; avoid excessive heat.

Tablets: Store at controlled room temperature of 15°C to 30°C (59°F to 86°F).

Pharmacodynamics/Kinetics

Onset of action:

Ophthalmic: Miosis: 10-30 minutes; Intraocular pressure reduction: 1 hour

Oral: 20 minutes

Duration:

Ophthalmic: Miosis: 4-8 hours; Intraocular pressure reduction: 4-12 hours

Oral: 3-5 hours

Half-life elimination: Oral: 0.76-1.35 hours; increased with hepatic impairment

Excretion: Urine

Dosage Adults:

Ophthalmic:

Glaucoma:

Solution: Instill 1-2 drops up to 6 times/day; adjust the concentration and frequency as required to control elevated intraocular pressure

Gel: Instill 0.5" ribbon into lower conjunctival sac once daily at bedtime

To counteract the mydriatic effects of sympathomimetic agents (unlabeled use): Solution: Instill 1 drop of a 1% solution in the affected eye

Oral: Xerostomia:

Following head and neck cancer: 5 mg 3 times/day, titration up to 10 mg 3 times/day may be considered for patients who have not responded adequately; do not exceed 2 tablets/dose

Sjögren's syndrome: 5 mg 4 times/day

Dosage adjustment in hepatic impairment: Oral: Patients with moderate impairment: 5 mg 2 times/day regardless of indication; adjust dose based on response and tolerability. Do not use with severe impairment (Child-Pugh score 10-15).

Administration

Oral: Avoid administering with high-fat meal. Fat decreases the rate of absorption, maximum concentration, and increases the time it takes to reach maximum concentration.

Ophthalmic: If both solution and gel are used, the solution should be applied first, then the gel at least 5 minutes later. Following administration of the solution, finger pressure should be applied on the lacrimal sac for 1-2 minutes.

Dosage Forms

Gel, ophthalmic, as hydrochloride (Pilopine HS®): 4% (3.5 g) [contains benzalkonium chloride]

Solution, ophthalmic, as hydrochloride: 1% (15 mL); 2% (15 mL); 4% (15 mL); 6% (15 mL) [may contain benzalkonium chloride]

Isopto® Carpine: 1% (15 mL); 2% (15 mL, 30 mL); 4% (15 mL, 30 mL); 6% (15 mL); 8% (15 mL) [contains benzalkonium chloride]

Pilocar®: 0.5% (15 mL); 1% (1 mL, 15 mL); 2% (1 mL, 15 mL); 3% (15 mL); 4% (1 mL, 15 mL); 6% (15 mL) [contains benzalkonium chloride]

Tablet, as hydrochloride (Salagen®): 5 mg, 7.5 mg

Monitoring Parameters Intraocular pressure, funduscopic exam, visual field testing

Patient Information Ophthalmic: May sting on instillation; report sweating, urinary retention; usually causes difficulty in dark adaptation; advise patients to use caution while night driving or performing hazardous tasks in poor illumination; after topical instillation, finger pressure should be applied to lacrimal sac to decrease drainage into the nose and throat and minimize possible systemic absorption

Special Geriatric Considerations Assure the patient or a caregiver can adequately administer ophthalmic medication dosage form.

Selected Readings

Hawthorne M and Sullivan K, "Pilocarpine for Radiation-Induced Xerostomia in Head and Neck Cancer," *Int J Palliat Nurs*, 2000, 6(5):228-32.

Taylor SE, "Efficacy and Economic Evaluation of Pilocarpine in Treating Radiation-Induced Xerostomia," *Expert Opin Pharmacother*, 2003, 4(9):1489-97.

♦ **Pilocarpine Hydrochloride** *see* Pilocarpine *on page 666*

♦ **Pilopine HS**® *see* Pilocarpine *on page 666*

Piperacillin (pi PER a sil in)

Related Information
Management of Infections *on page 978*

Generic Available Yes

Synonyms Piperacillin Sodium

Pharmacologic Category Antibiotic, Penicillin

Pregnancy Risk Factor B

Lactation Enters breast milk (small amounts - other penicillins are compatible with breast-feeding)

Use Treatment of susceptible infections such as septicemia, acute and chronic respiratory tract infections, skin and soft tissue infections, and urinary tract infections due to susceptible strains of *Pseudomonas*, *Proteus*, and *Escherichia coli* and *Enterobacter*; active against some streptococci and some anaerobic bacteria; febrile neutropenia (as part of combination regimen)

Mechanism of Action Inhibits bacterial cell wall synthesis by binding to one or more of the penicillin binding proteins (PBPs); which in turn inhibits the final transpeptidation step of peptidoglycan synthesis in bacterial cell walls, thus inhibiting cell wall biosynthesis. Bacteria eventually lyse due to ongoing activity of cell wall autolytic enzymes (autolysins and murein hydrolases) while cell wall assembly is arrested.

Labeled Contraindications Hypersensitivity to piperacillin, other penicillins, or any component of the formulation

Warnings/Precautions Dosage modification required in patients with impaired renal function; history of seizure activity; use with caution in patients with a history of beta-lactam allergy

Adverse Reactions Frequency not defined.
Central nervous system: Confusion, convulsions, drowsiness, fever, Jarisch-Herxheimer reaction
Dermatologic: Rash
Endocrine & metabolic: Electrolyte imbalance
Hematologic: Abnormal platelet aggregation and prolonged PT (high doses), hemolytic anemia, Coombs' reaction (positive)
Local: Thrombophlebitis
Neuromuscular & skeletal: Myoclonus
Renal: Acute interstitial nephritis
Miscellaneous: Anaphylaxis, hypersensitivity reactions

Vesicant No

Emetic Potential Very low (<10%)

Overdosage/Toxicology Symptoms of penicillin overdose include neuromuscular hypersensitivity (eg, agitation, hallucinations, asterixis, encephalopathy, confusion, and seizures). Electrolyte imbalance may occur if the preparation contains potassium or sodium salts, especially in renal failure. Hemodialysis may be helpful to aid in removal of the drug from blood; otherwise, treatment is supportive or symptom-directed.

Drug Interactions
Increased Effect/Toxicity: Probenecid may increase penicillin levels. Neuromuscular blockers may increase duration of blockade. Penicillins may increase the exposure to methotrexate during concurrent therapy; monitor.
Decreased Effect: Tetracyclines may decrease penicillin effectiveness. High concentrations of piperacillin may cause physical inactivation of

aminoglycosides and lead to potential toxicity in patients with mild-moderate renal dysfunction. Although anecdotal reports suggest oral contraceptive efficacy could be reduced by penicillins, this has been refuted by more rigorous scientific and clinical data.

Storage/Stability Reconstituted solution is stable (I.V. infusion) in NS or D_5W for 24 hours at room temperature, 7 days when refrigerated, or 4 weeks when frozen. After freezing, thawed solution is stable for 24 hours at room temperature or 48 hours when refrigerated. 40 g bulk vial should **not** be frozen after reconstitution.

Compatibility Stable in dextran 6% in NS, D_5NS, D_5W, LR, NS, sterile water for injection, bacteriostatic water; **variable stability (consult detailed reference)** in peritoneal dialysis solutions

Y-site administration: Compatible: Acyclovir, allopurinol, amifostine, aztreonam, ciprofloxacin, cyclophosphamide, diltiazem, docetaxel, doxorubicin liposome, enalaprilat, esmolol, etoposide phosphate, famotidine, fludarabine, foscarnet, granisetron, heparin, hydromorphone, IL-2, labetalol, linezolid, lorazepam, magnesium sulfate, melphalan, meperidine, midazolam, morphine, perphenazine, propofol, ranitidine, remifentanil, tacrolimus, teniposide, theophylline, thiotepa, verapamil, zidovudine. **Incompatible:** Amphotericin B cholesteryl sulfate complex, filgrastim, fluconazole, gatifloxacin, gemcitabine, ondansetron, sargramostim, vinorelbine. **Variable (consult detailed reference):** Cisatracurium, vancomycin

Compatibility in syringe: Compatible: Heparin

Compatibility when admixed: Compatible: Ciprofloxacin, clindamycin, flucloxacillin, fluconazole, hydrocortisone sodium succinate, linezolid, ofloxacin, potassium chloride, verapamil

Pharmacodynamics/Kinetics

Absorption: I.M.: 70% to 80%

Distribution: Crosses placenta; low concentrations enter breast milk

Protein binding: 22%

Half-life elimination (dose dependent; prolonged with moderately severe renal or hepatic impairment):

Neonates: 1-5 days old: 3.6 hours; >6 days old: 2.1-2.7 hours

Children: 1-6 months: 0.79 hour; 6 months to 12 years: 0.39-0.5 hour

Adults: 36-80 minutes

Time to peak, serum: I.M.: 30-50 minutes

Excretion: Primarily urine; partially feces

Dosage

Neonates: 100 mg/kg every 12 hours

Infants and Children: I.M., I.V.: 200-300 mg/kg/day in divided doses every 4-6 hours

Higher doses have been used in cystic fibrosis: 350-500 mg/kg/day in divided doses every 4-6 hours

Adults: I.M., I.V.:

Moderate infections (urinary tract infections): 2-3 g/dose every 6-12 hours; maximum: 2 g I.M./site

Serious infections: 3-4 g/dose every 4-6 hours; maximum: 24 g/24 hours

Uncomplicated gonorrhea: 2 g I.M. in a single dose accompanied by 1 g probenecid 30 minutes prior to injection

Dosing adjustment in renal impairment: Adults: I.V.:

Cl_{cr} 20-40 mL/minute: Administer 3-4 g every 8 hours

(Continued)

Piperacillin *(Continued)*

Cl$_{cr}$ <20 mL/minute: Administer 3-4 g every 12 hours

Moderately dialyzable (20% to 50%)

Continuous arteriovenous or venovenous hemodiafiltration effects: Dose as for Cl$_{cr}$ 10-50 mL/minute

Administration Administer at least 1 hour apart from aminoglycosides

Dosage Forms Injection, powder for reconstitution: 2 g, 3 g, 4 g, 40 g

Monitoring Parameters Observe for signs and symptoms of anaphylaxis during first dose

Dietary Considerations Sodium content of 1 g: 1.85 mEq

Additional Information As of September 2002, piperacillin is not available from the manufacturer. This product is anticipated to return to the market in 2003.

Special Geriatric Considerations Antipseudomonal penicillins should not be used alone and are often combined with an aminoglycoside as empiric therapy for lower respiratory infection and sepsis in which gram-negative (including *Pseudomonas*) and/or anaerobes are of a high probability. Because of piperacillin's lower sodium content, it is preferred over ticarcillin in patients with a history of heart failure and/or renal or hepatic disease. Adjust dose for renal function.

Selected Readings

Capelli G, Cornette C, Boillot A, et al, "Removal of Piperacillin in Critically Ill Patients Undergoing Continuous Veno-Venous Hemofiltration," *Crit Care Med*, 1998, 26(1):88-91.

Donowitz GR and Mandell GL, "Beta-Lactam Antibiotics," *N Engl J Med*, 1988, 318(7):419-26 and 318(8):490-500.

Keller E, Bohler J, Busse-Grawitz A, et al, "Single Dose Kinetics of Piperacillin During Continuous Arteriovenous Hemodialysis in Intensive Care Patients," *Clin Nephrol*, 1995, 43(Suppl 1):20-3.

Placzek M, Whitelaw A, Want S, et al, "Piperacillin in Early Neonatal Infection," *Arch Dis Child*, 1983, 58(12):1006-9.

Prince AS and Neu HC, "Use of Piperacillin, A Semisynthetic Penicillin, in the Therapy of Acute Exacerbations of Pulmonary Disease in Patients With Cystic Fibrosis," *J Pediatr*, 1980, 97(1):148-51.

Tan JS and File TM Jr, "Antipseudomonal Penicillins," *Med Clin North Am*, 1995, 79(4):679-93.

Thirumoorthi MC, Asmar BI, Buckley JA, et al, "Pharmacokinetics of Intravenously Administered Piperacillin in Preadolescent Children," *J Pediatr*, 1983, 102(6):941-6.

Wright AJ, "The Penicillins," *Mayo Clin Proc*, 1999, 74(3):290-307.

Yoshikawa TT, "Antimicrobial Therapy for the Elderly Patient," *J Am Geriatr Soc*, 1990, 38(12):1353-72.

Piperacillin and Tazobactam Sodium

(pi PER a sil in & ta zoe BAK tam SOW dee um)

Medication Safety Issues

Sound-alike/look-alike issues:

Zosyn® may be confused with Zofran®, Zyvox™

Related Information

Management of Infections *on page 978*

U.S. Brand Names Zosyn®

Canadian Brand Names Tazocin®

Generic Available No

Synonyms Piperacillin Sodium and Tazobactam Sodium

Pharmacologic Category Antibiotic, Penicillin

Pregnancy Risk Factor B

Lactation Enters breast milk/use caution

Use Treatment of infections caused by susceptible organisms, including infections of the lower respiratory tract (community-acquired pneumonia, nosocomial pneumonia); urinary tract; skin and skin structures; gynecologic (endometritis, pelvic inflammatory disease); bone and joint infections; intra-abdominal infections (appendicitis with rupture/abscess, peritonitis); and septicemia. Tazobactam expands activity of piperacillin to include beta-lactamase producing strains of *S. aureus*, *H. influenzae*, *Bacteroides*, and other gram-negative bacteria.

Mechanism of Action Inhibits bacterial cell wall synthesis by binding to one or more of the penicillin binding proteins (PBPs); which in turn inhibits the final transpeptidation step of peptidoglycan synthesis in bacterial cell walls, thus inhibiting cell wall biosynthesis. Bacteria eventually lyse due to ongoing activity of cell wall autolytic enzymes (autolysins and murein hydrolases) while cell wall assembly is arrested. Tazobactam inhibits many beta-lactamases, including staphylococcal penicillinase and Richmond and Sykes types II, III, IV, and V, including extended spectrum enzymes; it has only limited activity against class I beta-lactamases other than class Ic types.

Labeled Contraindications Hypersensitivity to penicillins, beta-lactamase inhibitors, or any component of the formulation

Warnings/Precautions Due to sodium load and to the adverse effects of high serum concentrations of penicillins, dosage modification is required in patients with impaired or underdeveloped renal function; use with caution in patients with seizures or in patients with history of beta-lactam allergy; safety and efficacy have not been established in children <12 years of age

Adverse Reactions

>10%: Gastrointestinal: Diarrhea (11%)

1% to 10%:

Cardiovascular: Hypertension (2%)

Central nervous system: Insomnia (7%), headache (7% to 8%), agitation (2%), fever (2%), dizziness (1%)

Dermatologic: Rash (4%), pruritus (3%)

Gastrointestinal: Constipation (7% to 8%), nausea (7%), vomiting/dyspepsia (3%)

Hepatic: Transaminases increased

Respiratory: Rhinitis/dyspnea (~1%)

Miscellaneous: Serum sickness-like reaction

<1%: Bronchospasm, *Clostridium difficile* colitis, confusion, edema, hepatitis, hepatotoxicity, hypotension, leukopenia, pseudomembranous colitis, seizure, thrombocytopenia

Postmarketing and/or case reports: Agranulocytosis, anaphylaxis, anaphylactoid reactions, cholestatic jaundice, erythema multiforme, hemolytic anemia, hypersensitivity, interstitial nephritis, pancytopenia, Stevens-Johnson syndrome, toxic epidermal necrolysis

Several laboratory abnormalities have rarely been associated with piperacillin/tazobactam including reversible eosinophilia, and neutropenia (associated most often with prolonged therapy), positive direct Coombs' test, prolonged PT and aPTT, transient elevations of LFT, increases in creatinine

Vesicant No

Emetic Potential Very low (<10%)

(Continued)

Piperacillin and Tazobactam Sodium *(Continued)*

Overdosage/Toxicology Symptoms of penicillin overdose include neuromuscular hypersensitivity (eg, agitation, hallucinations, asterixis, encephalopathy, confusion, and seizures). Electrolyte imbalance may occur if the preparation contains potassium or sodium salts, especially in renal dysfunction. Hemodialysis may be helpful to aid in removal of the drug from blood; otherwise, treatment is supportive or symptom-directed.

Drug Interactions

Increased Effect/Toxicity: Probenecid may increase penicillin levels. Neuromuscular blockers may increase duration of blockade. Penicillins may increase methotrexate exposure; clinical significance has not been established.

Decreased Effect: Tetracyclines may decrease penicillin effectiveness. Aminoglycosides may cause physical inactivation of aminoglycosides in the presence of high concentrations of piperacillin and potential toxicity in patients with mild-moderate renal dysfunction. Although anecdotal reports suggest oral contraceptive efficacy could be reduced by penicillins, this has been refuted by more rigorous scientific and clinical data.

Storage/Stability Store at controlled room temperature. After reconstitution, vials and solution are stable in NS or D_5W for 24 hours at room temperature and 48 hours (vials) or 7 days (solution) when refrigerated.

Reconstitution Reconstitute with 5 mL of diluent per 1 g of piperacillin and then further dilute.

Compatibility Stable in dextran 6% in NS, D_5W, NS, sterile water for injection, bacteriostatic water; not stable in LR; **variable stability (consult detailed reference)** in peritoneal dialysis solution

Y-site administration: Compatible: Aminophylline, aztreonam, bleomycin, bumetanide, buprenorphine, butorphanol, calcium gluconate, carboplatin, carmustine, cefepime, cimetidine, clindamycin, co-trimoxazole, cyclophosphamide, cytarabine, dexamethasone sodium phosphate, diphenhydramine, docetaxel, dopamine, enalaprilat, etoposide, etoposide phosphate, floxuridine, fluconazole, fludarabine, fluorouracil, furosemide, granisetron, heparin, hydrocortisone sodium phosphate, hydrocortisone sodium succinate, hydromorphone, ifosfamide, leucovorin, linezolid, lorazepam, magnesium sulfate, mannitol, meperidine, mesna, methotrexate, methylprednisolone sodium succinate, metoclopramide, metronidazole, morphine, ondansetron, plicamycin, potassium chloride, ranitidine, remifentanil, sargramostim, sodium bicarbonate, thiotepa, vinblastine, vincristine, zidovudine. **Incompatible:** Acyclovir, alatrofloxacin, amphotericin B, amphotericin B cholesteryl sulfate complex, chlorpromazine, cisplatin, dacarbazine, daunorubicin, dobutamine, doxorubicin, doxorubicin liposome, doxycycline, droperidol, famotidine, ganciclovir, gatifloxacin, gemcitabine, haloperidol, hydroxyzine, idarubicin, minocycline, mitomycin, mitoxantrone, nalbuphine, prochlorperazine edisylate, promethazine, streptozocin. **Variable (consult detailed reference):** Cisatracurium, vancomycin

Compatibility when admixed: Compatible: Potassium chloride

Pharmacodynamics/Kinetics Both AUC and peak concentrations are dose proportional; hepatic impairment does not affect kinetics

Distribution: Well into lungs, intestinal mucosa, skin, muscle, uterus, ovary, prostate, gallbladder, and bile; penetration into CSF is low in subject with noninflamed meninges

Protein binding: Piperacillin: ~26% to 33%; Tazobactam: 31% to 32%

Metabolism: Piperacillin: 6% to 9%; Tazobactam: ~26%

Half-life elimination: Piperacillin: 1 hour; Metabolite: 1-1.5 hours; Tazobactam: 0.7-0.9 hour

Excretion: Both piperacillin and tazobactam are directly proportional to renal function

Piperacillin: Urine (50% to 70%); feces (10% to 20%)

Tazobactam: Urine (26% as inactive metabolite) within 24 hours

Dosage

Infants and Children ≥6 months: **Note:** Not FDA-approved for use in children <12 years of age:

I.V.: 240 mg of piperacillin component/kg/day in divided doses every 8 hours; higher doses have been used for serious pseudomonal infections: 300-400 mg of piperacillin component/kg/day in divided doses every 6 hours.

Children >12 years and Adults:

Nosocomial pneumonia: I.V.: Piperacillin/tazobactam 4/0.5 g every 6 hours for 7-14 days (when used empirically, combination with an aminoglycoside is recommended; consider discontinuation of aminoglycoside if *P. aeruginosa* is not isolated)

Severe infections: I.V.: Piperacillin/tazobactam 4/0.5 g every 8 hours or 3/0.375 g every 6 hours for 7-10 days

Moderate infections: I.M.: Piperacillin/tazobactam 2/0.25 g every 6-8 hours; treatment should be continued for ≥7-10 days depending on severity of disease (**Note:** I.M. route not FDA-approved)

Dosing interval in renal impairment:

Cl_{cr} 20-40 mL/minute: Administer 2/0.25 g every 6 hours (3/0.375 g every 6 hours for nosocomial pneumonia)

Cl_{cr} <20 mL/minute: Administer 2/0.25 g every 8 hours (2/0.25 g every 6 hours for nosocomial pneumonia)

Hemodialysis: Administer 2/0.25 g every 12 hours (every 8 hours for nosocomial pneumonia) with an additional dose of 0.75 g after each dialysis

Continuous arteriovenous or venovenous hemodiafiltration effects: Dose as for Cl_{cr} 10-50 mL/minute

Administration Administer by I.V. infusion over 30 minutes.

Dosage Forms Note: 8:1 ratio of piperacillin sodium/tazobactam sodium:

Infusion [premixed iso-osmotic solution, frozen]:

2.25 g: Piperacillin 2 g and tazobactam 0.25 g (50 mL) [contains sodium 5.7 mEq (131 mg)]

3.375 g: Piperacillin 3 g and tazobactam 0.375 g (50 mL) [contains sodium 8.6 mEq (197 mg)]

4.5 g: Piperacillin 4 g and tazobactam 0.5 g (50 mL) [contains sodium 11.4 mEq (263 mg)]

Injection, powder for reconstitution:

2.25 g: Piperacillin 2 g and tazobactam 0.25 g [contains sodium 4.69 mEq (108 mg)]

3.375 g: Piperacillin 3 g and tazobactam 0.375 g [contains sodium 7.04 mEq (162 mg)]

4.5 g: Piperacillin 4 g and tazobactam 0.5 g [contains sodium 9.39 mEq (216 mg)]

(Continued)

Piperacillin and Tazobactam Sodium *(Continued)*

40.5 g: Piperacillin 36 g and tazobactam 4.5 g [contains sodium 84.5 mEq (1944 mg); bulk pharmacy vial]

Monitoring Parameters LFTs, creatinine, BUN, CBC with differential, serum electrolytes, urinalysis, PT, PTT; monitor for signs of anaphylaxis during first dose

Dietary Considerations

Infusion, premixed: 2.25 g contains sodium 5.7 mEq (131 mg); 3.375 g contains sodium 8.6 mEq (197 mg); 4.5 g contains sodium 11.4 mEq (263 mg)

Injection, powder for reconstitution: 2.25 g contains sodium 4.69 mEq (108 mg); 3.375 g contains sodium 7.04 mEq (162 mg); 4.5 g contains sodium 9.39 mEq (216 mg); 40.5 g contains sodium 84.5 mEq (1944 mg, bulk pharmacy vial)

Special Geriatric Considerations Has not been studied exclusively in the elderly.

Selected Readings

Bryson HM and Brogden RN, "Piperacillin/Tazobactam. A Review of its Antibacterial Activity, Pharmacokinetic Properties, and Therapeutic Potential," *Drugs*, 1994, 47(3):506-35.

Sanders WE Jr and Sanders CC, "Piperacillin/Tazobactam: A Critical Review of the Evolving Clinical Literature," *Clin Infect Dis*, 1996, 22(1):107-23.

Schoonover LL, Occhipinti DJ, Rodvold KA, et al, "Piperacillin/Tazobactam: A New Beta-Lactam/Beta-Lactamase Inhibitor Combination," *Ann Pharmacother*, 1995, 29(5):501-14.

Sorgel F and Kinzig M, "The Chemistry, Pharmacokinetics and Tissue Distribution of Piperacillin/Tazobactam," *J Antimicrob Chemother*, 1993, 31(Suppl A):39-60.

- **Piperacillin Sodium** *see Piperacillin on page 670*
- **Piperacillin Sodium and Tazobactam Sodium** *see Piperacillin and Tazobactam Sodium on page 672*
- **Platinol®-AQ** *see Cisplatin on page 190*
- **Plenaxis™** *see Abarelix on page 24*
- **PMS-Benzydamine (Can)** *see Benzydamine on page 123*
- **PMS-Deferoxamine (Can)** *see Deferoxamine on page 254*
- **PMS-Dexamethasone (Can)** *see Dexamethasone on page 263*
- **PMS-Flutamide (Can)** *see Flutamide on page 366*
- **PMS-Haloperidol LA (Can)** *see Haloperidol on page 409*
- **PMS-Hydromorphone (Can)** *see Hydromorphone on page 426*
- **PMS-Hydroxyzine (Can)** *see HydrOXYzine on page 436*
- **PMS-Lorazepam (Can)** *see Lorazepam on page 517*
- **PMS-Morphine Sulfate SR (Can)** *see Morphine Sulfate on page 588*
- **PMS-Nystatin (Can)** *see Nystatin on page 613*
- **PMS-Tamoxifen (Can)** *see Tamoxifen on page 743*
- **PMS-Tobramycin (Can)** *see Tobramycin on page 771*
- **Polygam® S/D** *see Immune Globulin (Intravenous) on page 458*

Porfimer *(POR fi mer)*

Related Information

Safe Handling of Hazardous Drugs *on page 1034*

U.S. Brand Names Photofrin®

Canadian Brand Names Photofrin®

Generic Available No

Synonyms CL-184116; Dihematoporphyrin Ether; Porfimer Sodium

Pharmacologic Category Antineoplastic Agent, Miscellaneous

Pregnancy Risk Factor C

Lactation Excretion in breast milk unknown/contraindicated

Use Adjunct to laser light therapy for obstructing esophageal cancer, obstructing endobronchial nonsmall cell lung cancer (NSCLC), ablation of high-grade dysplasia in Barrett's esophagus

Unlabeled/Investigational Use Transitional cell carcinoma *in situ* of the urinary bladder; gastric and rectal cancers

Mechanism of Action Porfimer's cytotoxic activity is dependent on light and oxygen. Following administration, the drug is selectively retained in neoplastic tissues. Exposure of the drug to laser light at wavelengths >630 nm results in the production of oxygen free-radicals. Release of thromboxane A_2, leading to vascular occlusion and ischemic necrosis, may also occur.

Labeled Contraindications Hypersensitivity to porfimer, porphyrins, or any component of the formulation; porphyria; tracheoesophageal or bronchoesophageal fistula; tumors eroding into a major blood vessel

Warnings/Precautions Hazardous agent - use appropriate precautions for handling and disposal. See Safe Handling of Hazardous Drugs *on page 1034* in the Appendix. Photosensitivity reactions are common is patients are exposed to direct sunlight or bright indoor light (eg fluorescent lights, unshaded light bulbs, examination/operating lights). Photosensitivity may last 30-90 days. Ocular discomfort has been reported; for at least 30 days, when outdoors, patients should wear dark sunglasses which have an average white light transmittance of <4%. When treating endobronchial tumors, use caution if treatment-induced inflammation may obstruct airway.

Adverse Reactions

>10%:

Cardiovascular: Atrial fibrillation (10%), chest pain (5% to 22%)

Central nervous system: Insomnia (14%), hyperthermia (31%)

Dermatologic: Photosensitivity reaction (10% to 80%, minor reactions may occur in up to 100%)

Gastrointestinal: Abdominal pain (20%), constipation (23%), dysphagia, nausea (24%), vomiting (17%)

Genitourinary: Urinary tract irritation including frequency, urgency, nocturia, painful urination, or bladder spasm (~100% of bladder cancer patients)

Hematologic: Anemia (26% of esophageal cancer patients)

Neuromuscular & skeletal: Back pain

Respiratory: Dyspnea (20%), pharyngitis (11%), pleural effusion (32% of esophageal cancer patients), pneumonia (18%), respiratory insufficiency

Miscellaneous: Mild-moderate allergic-type reactions (34% of lung cancer patients)

1% to 10%:

Cardiovascular: Hyper-/hypotension (6% to 7%), edema, cardiac failure (6% to 7%), tachycardia (6%), chest pain (substernal)

Central nervous system: Anxiety (7%), confusion (8%)

Dermatologic: Increased hair growth, skin discoloration, skin wrinkles, skin nodules, increased skin fragility

Endocrine & metabolic: Dehydration

(Continued)

677

Porfimer *(Continued)*

Gastrointestinal: Diarrhea (5%), dyspepsia (6%), eructation (5%), esophageal edema (8%), esophageal tumor bleeding, esophageal stricture, esophagitis, hematemesis, melena, weight loss, anorexia

Genitourinary: Urinary tract infection

Neuromuscular & skeletal: Weakness

Respiratory: Coughing, tracheoesophageal fistula

Miscellaneous: Moniliasis, surgical complication

Vesicant No

Emetic Potential Low (10% to 30%)

Overdosage/Toxicology Laser treatment should not be given if an overdose of porfimer is administered. In the event of overdose, patients should protect their eyes and skin from direct sunlight or bright indoor lights for 30 days. Patients should be tested for residual photosensitivity. Porfimer is not dialyzable.

Drug Interactions

Increased Effect/Toxicity: Concomitant administration of other photosensitizing agents (eg, tetracyclines, sulfonamides, phenothiazines, sulfonylureas, thiazide diuretics, griseofulvin) could increase the photosensitivity reaction.

Decreased Effect: Compounds that quench active oxygen species or scavenge radicals (eg, dimethyl sulfoxide, beta-carotene, ethanol, mannitol) would be expected to decrease photodynamic therapy (PDT) activity. Allopurinol, calcium channel blockers, and some prostaglandin synthesis inhibitors could interfere with porfimer. Drugs that decrease clotting, vasoconstriction, or platelet aggregation could decrease the efficacy of PDT. Glucocorticoid hormones may decrease the efficacy of the treatment.

Storage/Stability Store intact vials at controlled room temperature of 20°C to 25°C (68°F to 77°F). Reconstituted solutions are stable for 24 hours under refrigeration and protected from light.

Reconstitution Reconstitute each vial of porfimer with 31.8 mL of either D_5W or NS injection resulting in a final concentration of 2.5 mg/mL. Shake well until dissolved. Protect the reconstituted product from bright light and use immediately.

Compatibility Do not mix porfimer with other drugs in the same solution.

Pharmacodynamics/Kinetics

Distribution: V_{dss}: 0.49 L/kg

Protein binding, plasma: 90%

Half-life elimination: Mean: 21.5 days (range: 11-28 days)

Time to peak, serum: ~2 hours

Excretion: Feces; Clearance: Plasma: Total: 0.051 mL/minute/kg

Dosage I.V. (refer to individual protocols):

Children: Safety and efficacy have not been established

Adults: 2 mg/kg, followed by exposure to the appropriate laser light

Administration Administer slow I.V. injection over 3-5 minutes; eye protection is recommended

Dosage Forms Injection, powder for reconstitution, as sodium: 75 mg

Patient Information This medication can only be administered I.V. and will be followed by laser light therapy. Avoid any exposure to sunlight or bright indoor light for 30 days following therapy (cover skin with protective clothing and wear dark sunglasses with light transmittance <4% when outdoors - severe blistering, burning, and skin/eye damage can result). After 30 days, test a small area of skin (not face) for remaining sensitivity. Retest sensitivity if traveling to a different geographic area with greater sunshine. Exposure to indoor normal light is beneficial since it will help dissipate photosensitivity gradually. Maintain adequate hydration (2-3 L/day of fluids unless instructed to restrict fluid intake); maintain good oral hygiene (use a soft toothbrush or cotton applicators several times a day and rinse mouth frequently). Small frequent meals, frequent mouth care, sucking lozenges, or chewing gum may reduce nausea or vomiting. Report rapid heart rate, chest pain or palpitations, difficulty breathing or air hunger, persistent fever or chills, foul-smelling urine or burning on urination, swelling of extremities, increased anxiety, confusion, or hallucination.

Selected Readings

Evensen JF, "The Use of Porphyrins and Nonionizing Radiation for Treatment of Cancer," *Acta Oncol*, 1995, 34(8):1103-10.

Levy JG, "Photosensitizers in Photodynamic Therapy," *Semin Oncol*, 1994, 21(6 Suppl 15):4-10.

Rosenthal DI and Glatstein E, "Clinical Applications of Photodynamic Therapy," *Ann Med*, 1994, 26(6):405-9.

Van Hillegersberg R, Kort WJ, and Wilson JH, "Current Status of Photodynamic Therapy in Oncology," *Drugs*, 1994, 48(4):510-27.

♦ **Porfimer Sodium** *see* Porfimer *on page 676*

♦ **Post Peel Healing Balm [OTC]** *see* Hydrocortisone *on page 419*

♦ **PPI-149** *see* Abarelix *on page 24*

♦ **Pred Forte®** *see* PrednisoLONE *on page 679*

♦ **Pred Mild®** *see* PrednisoLONE *on page 679*

PrednisoLONE (pred NISS oh lone)

Medication Safety Issues

Sound-alike/look-alike issues:

PrednisoLONE may be confused with predniSONE

Pediapred® may be confused with Pediazole®

U.S. Brand Names AK-Pred®; Bubbli-Pred™; Econopred® Plus; Orapred®; Pediapred®; Pred Forte®; Pred Mild®; Prelone®

Canadian Brand Names Diopred®; Hydeltra T.B.A.®; Inflamase® Forte; Inflamase® Mild; Novo-Prednisolone; Ophtho-Tate®; Pediapred®; Pred Forte®; Pred Mild®; Sab-Prenase

Generic Available Yes

Synonyms Deltahydrocortisone; Metacortandralone; Prednisolone Acetate; Prednisolone Acetate, Ophthalmic; Prednisolone Sodium Phosphate; Prednisolone Sodium Phosphate, Ophthalmic

Pharmacologic Category Corticosteroid, Ophthalmic; Corticosteroid, Systemic

Pregnancy Risk Factor C

Lactation Enters breast milk/use caution (AAP rates "compatible")

Use Treatment of palpebral and bulbar conjunctivitis; corneal injury from chemical, radiation, thermal burns, or foreign body penetration; endocrine disorders, rheumatic disorders, collagen diseases, dermatologic diseases, allergic states, ophthalmic diseases, respiratory diseases, hematologic disorders, neoplastic diseases, edematous states, and gastrointestinal diseases; resolution of acute exacerbations of multiple sclerosis

(Continued)

PrednisoLONE *(Continued)*

Mechanism of Action Decreases inflammation by suppression of migration of polymorphonuclear leukocytes and reversal of increased capillary permeability; suppresses the immune system by reducing activity and volume of the lymphatic system

Labeled Contraindications Hypersensitivity to prednisolone or any component of the formulation; acute superficial herpes simplex keratitis; live or attenuated virus vaccines; systemic fungal infections; varicella

Warnings/Precautions Use with caution in patients with hyperthyroidism, cirrhosis, nonspecific ulcerative colitis, hypertension, osteoporosis, thromboembolic tendencies, CHF, convulsive disorders, myasthenia gravis, thrombophlebitis, peptic ulcer, diabetes, or tuberculosis; acute adrenal insufficiency may occur with abrupt withdrawal after long-term therapy or with stress; young pediatric patients may be more susceptible to adrenal axis suppression from topical therapy.

Prolonged use of corticosteroids may result in glaucoma; damage to the optic nerve (not for treatment of optic neuritis), defects in visual acuity and fields of vision, and posterior subcapsular cataract formation may occur. Prolonged use may increase the incidence of secondary infection, mask acute infection (including fungal) or prolong or exacerbate viral infections. Avoid exposure to chickenpox. Corticosteroids should not treat ocular herpes simplex. Use following cataract surgery may delay healing or increase the incidence of bleb formation.

Corticosteroids should not be used for cerebral malaria. Use cautiously in the elderly.

Adverse Reactions Frequency not defined.

Ophthalmic formulation:

Endocrine & metabolic: Hypercorticoidism (rare)

Ocular: Conjunctival hyperemia, conjunctivitis, corneal ulcers, delayed wound healing, glaucoma, intraocular pressure increased, keratitis, loss of accommodation, optic nerve damage, mydriasis, posterior subcapsular cataract formation, ptosis, secondary ocular infection

Oral formulation:

Cardiovascular: CHF, edema, hypertension

Central nervous system: Convulsions, headache, insomnia, malaise, nervousness, psychic disorders, vertigo

Dermatologic: Bruising, diaphoresis increased, facial erythema, hirsutism, petechiae, skin test reaction suppression, thin fragile skin, urticaria

Endocrine & metabolic: Carbohydrate tolerance decreased, Cushing's syndrome, diabetes mellitus, growth suppression, hyperglycemia, hypokalemic alkalosis, menstrual irregularities, negative nitrogen balance, pituitary adrenal axis suppression, potassium loss

Gastrointestinal: Abdominal distention, increased appetite, indigestion, nausea, peptic ulcer, ulcerative esophagitis, weight gain

Hepatic: LFTs increased (usually reversible)

Neuromuscular & skeletal: Arthralgia, fractures, intracranial pressure with papilledema (usually after discontinuation), muscle mass decreased, muscle weakness, osteoporosis, steroid myopathy, tendon rupture, weakness

Ocular: Cataracts, exophthalmus, glaucoma, intraocular pressure increased

Respiratory: Epistaxis
Miscellaneous: Impaired wound healing

Overdosage/Toxicology When consumed in high doses for prolonged periods, systemic hypercorticism and adrenal suppression may occur, in those cases discontinuation of the corticosteroid should be done judiciously.

Drug Interactions

Cytochrome P450 Effect: Substrate of CYP3A4 (minor); **Inhibits** CYP3A4 (weak)

Increased Effect/Toxicity: Effects of prednisolone may be increased by azole antifungals, calcium channel blockers, cyclosporine, estrogens, ketoconazole, salicylates.

Decreased Effect: Effects of prednisolone may be decreased by aminoglutethimide, antacids, barbiturates, CYP34 inducers, carbamazepine, nafcillin, nevirapine, phenobarbital, phenytoin, rifampin. Prednisolone may decrease the effects of isoniazid, skin tests, toxoids, warfarin, vaccines.

Ethanol/Nutrition/Herb Interactions

Ethanol: Avoid ethanol (may increase gastric mucosal irritation).

Food: Prednisolone interferes with calcium absorption. Limit caffeine.

Herb/Nutraceutical: St John's wort may decrease prednisolone levels. Avoid cat's claw, echinacea (have immunostimulant properties).

Pharmacodynamics/Kinetics

Duration: 18-36 hours

Protein binding (concentration dependent): 65% to 91%; decreased in elderly

Metabolism: Primarily hepatic, but also metabolized in most tissues, to inactive compounds

Half-life elimination: 3.6 hours; End-stage renal disease: 3-5 hours

Excretion: Primarily urine (as glucuronides, sulfates, and unconjugated metabolites)

Dosage Dose depends upon condition being treated and response of patient; dosage for infants and children should be based on severity of the disease and response of the patient rather than on strict adherence to dosage indicated by age, weight, or body surface area. Consider alternate day therapy for long-term therapy. Discontinuation of long-term therapy requires gradual withdrawal by tapering the dose. Patients undergoing unusual stress while receiving corticosteroids, should receive increased doses prior to, during, and after the stressful situation.

Children: Oral:

Acute asthma: 1-2 mg/kg/day in divided doses 1-2 times/day for 3-5 days

Anti-inflammatory or immunosuppressive dose: 0.1-2 mg/kg/day in divided doses 1-4 times/day

Nephrotic syndrome:

Initial (first 3 episodes): 2 mg/kg/day **or** 60 mg/m^2/day (maximum: 80 mg/day) in divided doses 3-4 times/day until urine is protein free for 3 consecutive days (maximum: 28 days); followed by 1-1.5 mg/kg/dose **or** 40 mg/m^2/dose given every other day for 4 weeks

Maintenance (long-term maintenance dose for frequent relapses): 0.5-1 mg/kg/dose given every other day for 3-6 months

Adults: Oral:

Usual range: 5-60 mg/day

(Continued)

PrednisoLONE *(Continued)*

Multiple sclerosis: 200 mg/day for 1 week followed by 80 mg every other day for 1 month

Rheumatoid arthritis: Initial: 5-7.5 mg/day; adjust dose as necessary

Ophthalmic suspension/solution: Conjunctivitis, corneal injury: Children and Adults: Instill 1-2 drops into conjunctival sac every hour during day, every 2 hours at night until favorable response is obtained, then use 1 drop every 4 hours.

Elderly: Use lowest effective dose

Dosing adjustment in hyperthyroidism: Prednisolone dose may need to be increased to achieve adequate therapeutic effects

Hemodialysis: Slightly dialyzable (5% to 20%); administer dose posthemodialysis

Peritoneal dialysis: Supplemental dose is not necessary

Combination Regimens

Lymphoma, Hodgkin's:

LOPP *on page 905*

MOPP (Lymphoma, Hodgkin's Disease) *on page 911*

Lymphoma, non-Hodgkin's: R-CVP *on page 936*

Administration Administer oral formulation with food or milk to decrease GI effects

Dosage Forms

Solution, ophthalmic, as sodium phosphate: 1% (5 mL, 10 mL, 15 mL) [contains benzalkonium chloride]

AK-Pred®: 1% (5 mL, 15 mL) [contains benzalkonium chloride]

Solution, oral, as sodium phosphate: Prednisolone base 5 mg/5 mL (120 mL)

Bubbli-Pred™: Prednisolone base 5 mg/5 mL (120 mL) [bubble gum flavor]

Orapred®: 20 mg/5 mL (240 mL) [equivalent to prednisolone base 15 mg/5 mL; dye free; contains alcohol 2%, sodium benzoate; grape flavor]

Pediapred®: 6.7 mg/5 mL (120 mL) [equivalent to prednisolone base 5 mg/5 mL; dye free; raspberry flavor]

Suspension, ophthalmic, as acetate: 1% (5 mL, 10 mL, 15 mL) [contains benzalkonium chloride]

Econopred® Plus: 1% (5 mL, 10 mL) [contains benzalkonium chloride]

Pred Forte®: 1% (1 mL, 5 mL, 10 mL, 15 mL) [contains benzalkonium chloride and sodium bisulfite]

Pred Mild®: 0.12% (5 mL, 10 mL) [contains benzalkonium chloride and sodium bisulfite]

Syrup, as base: 5 mg/5 mL (120 mL); 15 mg/5 mL (240 mL, 480 mL)

Prelone®: 15 mg/5 mL (240 mL, 480 mL) [contains alcohol 5%, benzoic acid; cherry flavor]

Tablet, as base: 5 mg

Monitoring Parameters Blood pressure; blood glucose, electrolytes; intraocular pressure (use >6 weeks); bone mineral density

Dietary Considerations Should be taken after meals or with food or milk to decrease GI effects; increase dietary intake of pyridoxine, vitamin C, vitamin D, folate, calcium, and phosphorus.

Patient Information Notify surgeon or dentist before surgical repair; may cause GI upset, take orally with food; notify prescriber if any sign of infection occurs; avoid abrupt withdrawal when on long-term therapy

Special Geriatric Considerations Useful in patients with inability to activate prednisone (liver disease). Because of the risk of adverse effects, systemic corticosteroids should be used cautiously in the elderly, in the smallest possible dose, and for the shortest possible time.

Selected Readings

Frey BM and Frey FJ, "Clinical Pharmacokinetics of Prednisone and Prednisolone," *Clin Pharmacokinet*, 1990, 19(2):126-46.

Frey FJ, "Kinetics and Dynamics of Prednisolone," *Endocr Rev*, 1987, 8(4):453-73.

Gambertoglio JG, Amend WJ Jr and Benet LZ, "Pharmacokinetics and Bioavailability of Prednisone and Prednisolone in Healthy Volunteers and Patients: A Review," *J Pharmacokinet Biopharm*, 1980, 8(1):1-52.

♦ **Prednisolone Acetate** *see* PrednisoLONE *on page 679*

♦ **Prednisolone Acetate, Ophthalmic** *see* PrednisoLONE *on page 679*

♦ **Prednisolone Sodium Phosphate** *see* PrednisoLONE *on page 679*

♦ **Prednisolone Sodium Phosphate, Ophthalmic** *see* PrednisoLONE *on page 679*

PredniSONE (PRED ni sone)

Medication Safety Issues

Sound-alike/look-alike issues:

PredniSONE may be confused with methylPREDNISolone, Pramosone®, prazosin, prednisoLONE, Prilosec®, primidone, promethazine

U.S. Brand Names Prednisone Intensol™; Sterapred®; Sterapred® DS

Canadian Brand Names Apo-Prednisone®; Winpred™

Generic Available Yes

Synonyms Deltacortisone; Deltadehydrocortisone

Pharmacologic Category Corticosteroid, Systemic

Pregnancy Risk Factor B

Lactation Enters breast milk/compatible

Use Treatment of a variety of diseases including adrenocortical insufficiency, hypercalcemia, rheumatic, and collagen disorders; dermatologic, ocular, respiratory, gastrointestinal, and neoplastic diseases; organ transplantation and a variety of diseases including those of hematologic, allergic, inflammatory, and autoimmune in origin; not available in injectable form, prednisolone must be used

Unlabeled/Investigational Use Investigational: Prevention of postherpetic neuralgia and relief of acute pain in the early stages

Mechanism of Action Decreases inflammation by suppression of migration of polymorphonuclear leukocytes and reversal of increased capillary permeability; suppresses the immune system by reducing activity and volume of the lymphatic system; suppresses adrenal function at high doses. Antitumor effects may be related to inhibition of glucose transport, phosphorylation, or induction of cell death in immature lymphocytes. Antiemetic effects are thought to occur due to blockade of cerebral innervation of the emetic center via inhibition of prostaglandin synthesis.

Labeled Contraindications Hypersensitivity to prednisone or any component of the formulation; serious infections, except tuberculous meningitis; systemic fungal infections; varicella

(Continued)

PredniSONE *(Continued)*

Warnings/Precautions Use with caution in patients with hypothyroidism, cirrhosis, CHF, ulcerative colitis, thromboembolic disorders, and patients with an increased risk for peptic ulcer disease. Corticosteroids should be used with caution in patients with diabetes, hypertension, osteoporosis, glaucoma, cataracts, or tuberculosis. Use caution in hepatic impairment. May retard bone growth. Gradually taper dose to withdraw therapy. Because of the risk of adverse effects, systemic corticosteroids should be used cautiously in the elderly, in the smallest possible dose, and for the shortest possible time.

Adverse Reactions

>10%:

Central nervous system: Insomnia, nervousness

Gastrointestinal: Increased appetite, indigestion

1% to 10%:

Dermatologic: Hirsutism

Endocrine & metabolic: Diabetes mellitus, glucose intolerance, hyperglycemia

Neuromuscular & skeletal: Arthralgia

Ocular: Cataracts, glaucoma

Respiratory: Epistaxis

<1%: Edema, hypertension, vertigo, seizure, psychoses, pseudotumor cerebri, headache, mood swings, delirium, hallucinations, euphoria, acne, skin atrophy, bruising, hyperpigmentation, Cushing's syndrome, pituitary-adrenal axis suppression, growth suppression, glucose intolerance, hypokalemia, alkalosis, amenorrhea, sodium and water retention, hyperglycemia, peptic ulcer, nausea, vomiting, abdominal distention, ulcerative esophagitis, pancreatitis, muscle weakness, osteoporosis, fractures, muscle wasting, hypersensitivity reactions

Vesicant No

Emetic Potential Very low (<10%)

Overdosage/Toxicology When consumed in high doses for prolonged periods, systemic hypercorticism and adrenal suppression may occur. In those cases, discontinuation of the corticosteroid should be done judiciously.

Drug Interactions

Cytochrome P450 Effect: Substrate of CYP3A4 (minor); **Induces** CYP2C19 (weak), 3A4 (weak)

Increased Effect/Toxicity: Concurrent use with NSAIDs may increase the risk of GI ulceration.

Decreased Effect: Decreased effect with barbiturates, phenytoin, rifampin; decreased effect of salicylates, vaccines, and toxoids.

Ethanol/Nutrition/Herb Interactions

Ethanol: Avoid ethanol (may increase gastric mucosal irritation)

Food: Prednisone interferes with calcium absorption, Limit caffeine.

Herb/Nutraceutical: St John's wort may decrease prednisone levels. Avoid cat's claw, echinacea (have immunostimulant properties).

Pharmacodynamics/Kinetics

Protein binding (concentration dependent): 65% to 91%

Metabolism: Hepatically converted from prednisone (inactive) to prednisolone (active); may be impaired with hepatic dysfunction

Half-life elimination: Normal renal function: 2.5-3.5 hours

See Prednisolone monograph for complete information.

Dosage Oral: Dose depends upon condition being treated and response of patient; dosage for infants and children should be based on severity of the disease and response of the patient rather than on strict adherence to dosage indicated by age, weight, or body surface area. Consider alternate day therapy for long-term therapy. Discontinuation of long-term therapy requires gradual withdrawal by tapering the dose.

Children:

Anti-inflammatory or immunosuppressive dose: 0.05-2 mg/kg/day divided 1-4 times/day

Acute asthma: 1-2 mg/kg/day in divided doses 1-2 times/day for 3-5 days

Alternatively (for 3- to 5-day "burst"):

<1 year: 10 mg every 12 hours

1-4 years: 20 mg every 12 hours

5-13 years: 30 mg every 12 hours

>13 years: 40 mg every 12 hours

Asthma long-term therapy (alternative dosing by age):

<1 year: 10 mg every other day

1-4 years: 20 mg every other day

5-13 years: 30 mg every other day

>13 years: 40 mg every other day

Nephrotic syndrome:

Initial (first 3 episodes): 2 mg/kg/day **or** 60 mg/m^2/day (maximum: 80 mg/day) in divided doses 3-4 times/day until urine is protein free for 3 consecutive days (maximum: 28 days); followed by 1-1.5 mg/kg/dose **or** 40 mg/m^2/dose given every other day for 4 weeks

Maintenance dose (long-term maintenance dose for frequent relapses): 0.5-1 mg/kg/dose given every other day for 3-6 months

Children and Adults: Physiologic replacement: 4-5 mg/m^2/day

Children ≥5 years and Adults: Asthma:

Moderate persistent: Inhaled corticosteroid (medium dose) or inhaled corticosteroid (low-medium dose) with a long-acting bronchodilator

Severe persistent: Inhaled corticosteroid (high dose) and corticosteroid tablets or syrup long term: 2 mg/kg/day, generally not to exceed 60 mg/day

Adults:

Immunosuppression/chemotherapy adjunct: Range: 5-60 mg/day in divided doses 1-4 times/day

Allergic reaction (contact dermatitis):

Day 1: 30 mg divided as 10 mg before breakfast, 5 mg at lunch, 5 mg at dinner, 10 mg at bedtime

Day 2: 5 mg at breakfast, 5 mg at lunch, 5 mg at dinner, 10 mg at bedtime

Day 3: 5 mg 4 times/day (with meals and at bedtime)

Day 4: 5 mg 3 times/day (breakfast, lunch, bedtime)

Day 5: 5 mg 2 times/day (breakfast, bedtime)

Day 6: 5 mg before breakfast

Pneumocystis carinii pneumonia (PCP):

40 mg twice daily for 5 days **followed by**

40 mg once daily for 5 days **followed by**

20 mg once daily for 11 days or until antimicrobial regimen is completed

(Continued)

PredniSONE *(Continued)*

Thyrotoxicosis: Oral: 60 mg/day

Chemotherapy (refer to individual protocols): Oral: Range: 20 mg/day to 100 mg/m^2/day

Rheumatoid arthritis: Oral: Use lowest possible daily dose (often ≤7.5 mg/day)

Idiopathic thrombocytopenia purpura (ITP): Oral: 60 mg daily for 4-6 weeks, gradually tapered over several weeks

Systemic lupus erythematosus (SLE): Oral:

Acute: 1-2 mg/kg/day in 2-3 divided doses

Maintenance: Reduce to lowest possible dose, usually <1 mg/kg/day as single dose (morning)

Elderly: Use the lowest effective dose

Dosing adjustment in hepatic impairment: Prednisone is inactive and must be metabolized by the liver to prednisolone. This conversion may be impaired in patients with liver disease, however, prednisolone levels are observed to be higher in patients with severe liver failure than in normal patients. Therefore, compensation for the inadequate conversion of prednisone to prednisolone occurs.

Dosing adjustment in hyperthyroidism: Prednisone dose may need to be increased to achieve adequate therapeutic effects

Hemodialysis: Supplemental dose is not necessary

Peritoneal dialysis: Supplemental dose is not necessary

Combination Regimens Note: In the U.S. prednisone is the preferred corticosteroid. However, in the British literature prednisolone is often used. The oral doses of these two agents are equivalent (ie, 1 mg prednisone = 1 mg prednisolone). Also, early clinical trials gave prednisone only with the first and fourth cycles. Some clinicians give prednisone with every cycle.

Brain tumors:

MOPP (Medulloblastoma) *on page 912*

POC *on page 931*

Leukemia, acute lymphocytic:

DVP *on page 875*

Larson Regimen *on page 904*

Linker Protocol *on page 904*

MTX/6-MP/VP (Maintenance) *on page 916*

PVA (POG 8602) *on page 932*

PVA (POG 9005) *on page 934*

PVDA *on page 936*

Leukemia, acute myeloid: POMP *on page 931*

Leukemia, chronic lymphocytic:

CHL + PRED *on page 859*

CP (Leukemia) *on page 867*

CVP (Leukemia) *on page 869*

Lymphoma, Hodgkin's:

BEACOPP *on page 846*

CAD/MOPP/ABV *on page 850*

ChIVPP *on page 859*

COMP *on page 866*

LOPP *on page 905*

MOPP (Lymphoma, Hodgkin's Disease) *on page 911*

MOPP/ABV Hybrid *on page 913*

MOPP/ABVD *on page 913*
MVPP *on page 922*
OPA *on page 924*
OPPA *on page 925*
Stanford V *on page 937*
Lymphoma, non-Hodgkin's:
CEPP(B) *on page 857*
CHOP *on page 859*
CNOP *on page 864*
COP-BLAM *on page 866*
COPP *on page 867*
CVP (Lymphoma, non-Hodgkin's) *on page 869*
EPOCH *on page 880*
MACOP-B *on page 908*
Pro-MACE-CytaBOM *on page 931*
R-CHOP *on page 936*
Multiple myeloma:
M-2 *on page 906*
MP (Multiple Myeloma) *on page 916*
VBAP *on page 944*
VBMCP *on page 945*
VCAP *on page 946*
Prostate cancer: MP (Prostate Cancer) *on page 916*

Administration Administer with meals to decrease gastrointestinal upset

Dosage Forms

Solution, oral: 1 mg/mL (5 mL, 120 mL, 500 mL) [contains alcohol 5%, sodium benzoate; vanilla flavor]

Solution, oral concentrate (Prednisone Intensol™): 5 mg/mL (30 mL) [contains alcohol 30%]

Tablet: 1 mg, 2.5 mg, 5 mg, 10 mg, 20 mg, 50 mg

Sterapred®: 5 mg [supplied as 21 tablet 6-day unit-dose package or 48 tablet 12-day unit-dose package]

Sterapred® DS: 10 mg [supplied as 21 tablet 6-day unit-dose package or 48 tablet 12-day unit-dose package]

Monitoring Parameters Blood pressure, blood glucose, electrolytes

Dietary Considerations Should be taken after meals or with food or milk; increase dietary intake of pyridoxine, vitamin C, vitamin D, folate, calcium, and phosphorus.

Patient Information Notify surgeon or dentist before surgical repair; may cause GI upset, take with food; notify prescriber if any sign of infection occurs; avoid abrupt withdrawal when on long-term therapy; do not discontinue or decrease drug without contacting physician, carry an identification card or bracelet advising that you are on steroids

Additional Information Tapering of corticosteroids after a short course of therapy (<7-10 days) is generally not required unless the disease/inflammatory process is slow to respond. Tapering after prolonged exposure is dependent upon the individual patient, duration of corticosteroid treatments, and size of steroid dose. Recovery of the HPA axis may require several months. Subtle but important HPA axis suppression may be present for as long as several months after a course of as few as 10-14 days duration. Testing of HPA axis (cosyntropin) may be required, and signs/symptoms of adrenal insufficiency should be monitored in patients with a history of use.

(Continued)

PredniSONE *(Continued)*

Special Geriatric Considerations Because of the risk of adverse effects, systemic corticosteroids should be used cautiously in the elderly, in the smallest possible dose, and for the shortest possible time.

Selected Readings

Frey BM and Frey FJ, "Clinical Pharmacokinetics of Prednisone and Prednisolone," *Clin Pharmacokinet*, 1990, 19(2):126-46.

Gambertoglio JG, Amend WJ Jr, and Benet LZ, "Pharmacokinetics and Bioavailability of Prednisone and Prednisolone in Healthy Volunteers and Patients: A Review," *J Pharmacokinet Biopharm*, 1980, 8(1):1-52.

Jusko WJ and Rose JQ, "Monitoring Prednisone and Prednisolone," *Ther Drug Monit*, 1980, 2(2):169-76.

♦ **Prednisone Intensol™** *see* PredniSONE *on page 683*

♦ **Prelone®** *see* PrednisoLONE *on page 679*

♦ **Preparation H® Hydrocortisone [OTC]** *see* Hydrocortisone *on page 419*

♦ **Prevex® HC (Can)** *see* Hydrocortisone *on page 419*

♦ **Prialt®** *see* Ziconotide *on page 831*

♦ **Prilocaine and Lidocaine** *see* Lidocaine and Prilocaine *on page 511*

♦ **Primaxin®** *see* Imipenem and Cilastatin *on page 454*

♦ **Primsol®** *see* Trimethoprim *on page 797*

Procarbazine *(proe KAR ba zeen)*

Medication Safety Issues

Sound-alike/look-alike issues:

Procarbazine may be confused with dacarbazine

Matulane® may be confused with Modane®

Related Information

Fertility and Cancer Therapy *on page 962*

Management of Nausea and Vomiting *on page 982*

Safe Handling of Hazardous Drugs *on page 1034*

U.S. Brand Names Matulane®

Canadian Brand Names Matulane®; Natulan®

Generic Available No

Synonyms Benzmethyzin; N-Methylhydrazine; NSC-77213; Procarbazine Hydrochloride

Pharmacologic Category Antineoplastic Agent, Alkylating Agent

Pregnancy Risk Factor D

Lactation Excretion in breast milk unknown/not recommended

Use Treatment of Hodgkin's disease

Unlabeled/Investigational Use Treatment of non-Hodgkin's lymphoma, brain tumors, melanoma, lung cancer, multiple myeloma

Mechanism of Action Mechanism of action is not clear, methylating of nucleic acids; inhibits DNA, RNA, and protein synthesis; may damage DNA directly and suppresses mitosis; metabolic activation required by host

Labeled Contraindications Hypersensitivity to procarbazine or any component of the formulation; pre-existing bone marrow aplasia; ethanol ingestion; pregnancy

Warnings/Precautions Hazardous agent - use appropriate precautions for handling and disposal. See Safe Handling of Hazardous Drugs *on page 1034* in the Appendix. Use with caution in patients with pre-existing renal or hepatic impairment. Procarbazine possesses MAO inhibitor activity. Procarbazine is a carcinogen which may cause acute leukemia. Procarbazine may cause infertility.

Adverse Reactions Frequency not defined.

Central nervous system: Reports of neurotoxicity with procarbazine generally originate from early usage with single agent oral (continuous) or I.V. dosing; CNS depression is commonly reported to be additive with other CNS depressants

Hematologic: Myelosuppression, hemolysis in patients with G6PD deficiency

Gastrointestinal: Nausea and vomiting (60% to 90%); increasing the dose in a stepwise fashion over several days may minimize this

Genitourinary: Reproductive dysfunction >10% (in animals, hormone treatment has prevented azoospermia)

Respiratory: Pulmonary toxicity (<1%); the most commonly reported pulmonary toxicity is a hypersensitivity pneumonitis which responds to steroids and discontinuation of the drug. At least one report of persistent pulmonary fibrosis has been reported, however, a higher incidence (18%) of pulmonary toxicity (fibrosis) was reported when procarbazine was given prior to BCNU (BCNU alone does cause pulmonary fibrosis).

Miscellaneous: Second malignancies (cumulative incidence 2% to 15% reported with MOPP combination therapy)

Emetic Potential Moderately high (60% to 90%)

Overdosage/Toxicology Symptoms of overdose include arthralgia, alopecia, paresthesia, bone marrow suppression, hallucinations, nausea, vomiting, diarrhea, seizures, and coma. Treatment is supportive. Adverse effects such as marrow toxicity may begin as late as 2 weeks after exposure.

Drug Interactions

Increased Effect/Toxicity: Procarbazine exhibits weak MAO inhibitor activity. Foods containing high amounts of tyramine should, therefore, be avoided. When an MAO inhibitor is given with food high in tyramine, hypertensive crisis, intracranial bleeding, and headache have been reported.

Sympathomimetic amines (epinephrine and amphetamines) and antidepressants (tricyclics) should be used cautiously with procarbazine. Barbiturates, narcotics, phenothiazines, and other CNS depressants can cause somnolence, ataxia, and other symptoms of CNS depression. Ethanol has caused a disulfiram-like reaction with procarbazine. May result in headache, respiratory difficulties, nausea, vomiting, sweating, thirst, hypotension, and flushing.

Ethanol/Nutrition/Herb Interactions

Ethanol: Use ethanol and ethanol-containing products cautiously.

Food: Clinically severe and possibly life-threatening elevations in blood pressure may occur if procarbazine is taken with tyramine-containing foods.

Storage/Stability Protect from light

Pharmacodynamics/Kinetics

Absorption: Rapid and complete

Distribution: Crosses blood-brain barrier; distributes into CSF

Metabolism: Hepatic and renal

Half-life elimination: 1 hour

(Continued)

Procarbazine *(Continued)*

Excretion: Urine and respiratory tract (<5% as unchanged drug, 70% as metabolites)

Dosage Refer to individual protocols. Manufacturer states that the dose is based on patient's ideal weight if the patient is obese or has abnormal fluid retention. Other studies suggest that ideal body weight may not be necessary. Oral (may be given as a single daily dose or in 2-3 divided doses):

Children:

BMT aplastic anemia conditioning regimen: 12.5 mg/kg/day every other day for 4 doses

Hodgkin's disease: MOPP/IC-MOPP regimens: 100 mg/m^2/day for 14 days and repeated every 4 weeks

Neuroblastoma and medulloblastoma: Doses as high as 100-200 mg/m^2/day once daily have been used

Adults: Initial: 2-4 mg/kg/day in single or divided doses for 7 days then increase dose to 4-6 mg/kg/day until response is obtained or leukocyte count decreased <4000/mm^3 or the platelet count decreased <100,000/mm^3; maintenance: 1-2 mg/kg/day

Dosing in renal/hepatic impairment: Use with caution, may result in increased toxicity; decrease dose if serum creatinine >2 mg/dL or total bilirubin >3 mg/dL

Combination Regimens

Brain tumors:

8 in 1 (Brain Tumors) *on page 841*

MOP *on page 910*

MOPP (Medulloblastoma) *on page 912*

PCV *on page 928*

Lymphoma, Hodgkin's:

BEACOPP *on page 846*

CAD/MOPP/ABV *on page 850*

ChIVPP *on page 859*

LOPP *on page 905*

MOPP (Lymphoma, Hodgkin's Disease) *on page 911*

MOPP/ABV Hybrid *on page 913*

MOPP/ABVD *on page 913*

MVPP *on page 922*

OPPA *on page 925*

Lymphoma, non-Hodgkin's:

CEPP(B) *on page 857*

COP-BLAM *on page 866*

COPP *on page 867*

Retinoblastoma: 8 in 1 (Retinoblastoma) *on page 842*

Dosage Forms Capsule, as hydrochloride: 50 mg

Monitoring Parameters CBC with differential, platelet and reticulocyte count, urinalysis, liver function test, renal function test.

Patient Information Take as directed. Maintain adequate hydration (2-3 L/day of fluids unless instructed to restrict fluid intake). Avoid aspirin and aspirin-containing substances; use alcohol cautiously, may cause acute disulfiram-like reaction - flushing, headache, acute vomiting, chest and/or abdominal pain; avoid tyramine-containing foods (aged cheese, chocolate, pickles, aged meat, wine, etc). You may experience mental depression, nervousness, insomnia, nightmares, dizziness, confusion, or lethargy (use caution when driving or engaging in tasks that require alertness until response to drug is known); photosensitivity (use sunscreen, wear protective clothing and eyewear, and avoid direct sunlight). You may experience rash or hair loss (reversible), loss of libido, increased sensitivity to infection (avoid crowds and infected persons). Report persistent fever, chills, sore throat; unusual bleeding; blood in urine, stool (black stool), or vomitus; unresolved depression; mania; hallucinations; nightmares; disorientation; seizures; chest pain or palpitations; or difficulty breathing.

Selected Readings

Longo DL, Young RC, Wesley M, et al, "Twenty Years of MOPP Therapy for Hodgkin's Disease," *J Clin Oncol*, 1986, 4(9):1295-306.

Rodriguez LA, Prados M, Silver P, et al, "Re-evaluation of Procarbazine for the Treatment of Recurrent Malignant Central Nervous System Tumors," *Cancer*, 1989, 64(12):2420-3.

Spivack SD, "Procarbazine," *Ann Intern Med*, 1974, 81:795-800.

Toth B, "A Review of the Antineoplastic Action of Certain Hydrazines and Hydrazine-Containing Natural Products," *In Vivo*, 1996, 10(1):65-96.

♦ **Procarbazine Hydrochloride** *see* Procarbazine *on page 688*

Prochlorperazine (proe klor PER a zeen)

Medication Safety Issues

Sound-alike/look-alike issues:

Prochlorperazine may be confused with chlorproMAZINE

Compazine® may be confused with Copaxone®, Coumadin®

U.S. Brand Names Compazine® [DSC]; Compro™

Canadian Brand Names Apo-Prochlorperazine®; Compazine®; Nu-Prochlor; Stemetil®

Generic Available Yes: Injection, tablet, suppository

Synonyms Chlormeprazine; Prochlorperazine Edisylate; Prochlorperazine Maleate

Pharmacologic Category Antiemetic; Antipsychotic Agent, Phenothiazine, Piperazine

Pregnancy Risk Factor C

Lactation Enters breast milk/not recommended

Use Management of nausea and vomiting; psychosis; anxiety

Unlabeled/Investigational Use Behavioral syndromes in dementia

Mechanism of Action Prochlorperazine is a piperazine phenothiazine antipsychotic which blocks postsynaptic mesolimbic dopaminergic D_1 and D_2 receptors in the brain, including the medullary chemoreceptor trigger zone; exhibits a strong alpha-adrenergic and anticholinergic blocking effect and depresses the release of hypothalamic and hypophyseal hormones; believed to depress the reticular activating system, thus affecting basal metabolism, body temperature, wakefulness, vasomotor tone and emesis

Labeled Contraindications Hypersensitivity to prochlorperazine or any component of the formulation (cross-reactivity between phenothiazines may occur); severe CNS depression; coma; should not be used in children <2 years of age or <10 kg

Warnings/Precautions May be sedating; use with caution in disorders where CNS depression is a feature. May impair physical or mental abilities; patients must be cautioned about performing tasks which require
(Continued)

Prochlorperazine *(Continued)*

mental alertness (eg, operating machinery or driving). Effects with other sedative drugs or ethanol may be potentiated. Avoid use in Reye's syndrome. Use with caution in Parkinson's disease; hemodynamic instability; bone marrow suppression; predisposition to seizures; subcortical brain damage; and in severe cardiac, hepatic, renal or respiratory disease. May alter temperature regulation or mask toxicity of other drugs due to antiemetic effects. May alter cardiac conduction - life threatening arrhythmias have occurred with therapeutic doses of phenothiazines. May cause orthostatic hypotension; use with caution in patients at risk of hypotension or where transient hypotensive episodes would be poorly tolerated (cardiovascular disease or cerebrovascular disease). Hypotension may occur following administration, particularly when parenteral form is used or in high dosages.

Due to anticholinergic effects, use with caution in patients with decreased gastrointestinal motility, urinary retention, BPH, xerostomia, visual problems, narrow-angle glaucoma (screening is recommended) and myasthenia gravis. May cause extrapyramidal symptoms, including pseudoparkinsonism, acute dystonic reactions, akathisia and tardive dyskinesia. May be associated with neuroleptic malignant syndrome (NMS).

Adverse Reactions Frequency not defined.

Cardiovascular: Hyper-/hypotension, orthostatic hypotension, tachycardia, bradycardia, dizziness, cardiac arrest

Central nervous system: Extrapyramidal symptoms (pseudoparkinsonism, akathisia, dystonias, tardive dyskinesia), dizziness, cerebral edema, seizure, headache, drowsiness, paradoxical excitement, restlessness, hyperactivity, insomnia, neuroleptic malignant syndrome (NMS), impairment of temperature regulation

Dermatologic: Rash, discoloration of skin (blue-gray), photosensitivity

Endocrine & metabolic: Hypoglycemia, hyperglycemia, galactorrhea, lactation, breast enlargement, gynecomastia, menstrual irregularity, amenorrhea, SIADH, libido (changes in)

Gastrointestinal: Constipation, weight gain, vomiting, stomach pain, nausea, xerostomia, salivation, diarrhea, anorexia, ileus

Genitourinary: Difficulty in urination, ejaculatory disturbances, incontinence, polyuria, ejaculating dysfunction, priapism

Hematologic: Agranulocytosis, leukopenia, eosinophilia, hemolytic anemia, thrombocytopenic purpura, pancytopenia

Hepatic: Cholestatic jaundice, hepatotoxicity

Neuromuscular & skeletal: Tremor

Ocular: Pigmentary retinopathy, blurred vision, cornea and lens changes

Respiratory: Nasal congestion

Miscellaneous: Diaphoresis

Vesicant No

Emetic Potential Very low (<10%)

Overdosage/Toxicology Symptoms of overdose include deep sleep, coma, extrapyramidal symptoms, abnormal involuntary muscle movements, and hypotension. Treatment is symptom-directed and supportive.

Drug Interactions

Increased Effect/Toxicity: Chloroquine, propranolol, and sulfadoxine-pyrimethamine may increase prochlorperazine concentrations.

Concurrent use with TCA may produce increased toxicity or altered therapeutic response. Prochlorperazine plus lithium may rarely produce neurotoxicity. Prochlorperazine may produce additive CNS depressant effects with CNS depressants (ethanol, narcotics). Metoclopramide may increase risk of extrapyramidal symptoms (EPS).

Decreased Effect: Barbiturates and carbamazepine may increase the metabolism of prochlorperazine, lowering its serum levels. Benztropine (and other anticholinergics) may inhibit the therapeutic response to prochlorperazine. Antipsychotics such as prochlorperazine inhibit the ability of bromocriptine to lower serum prolactin concentrations. The antihypertensive effects of guanethidine and guanadrel may be inhibited by prochlorperazine. Prochlorperazine may inhibit the antiparkinsonian effect of levodopa. Prochlorperazine (and possibly other low potency antipsychotics) may reverse the pressor effects of epinephrine.

Ethanol/Nutrition/Herb Interactions

Ethanol: Avoid ethanol (may increase CNS depression).

Food: Limit caffeine.

Herb/Nutraceutical: Avoid dong quai, St John's wort (may also cause photosensitization). Avoid kava kava, gotu kola, valerian, St John's wort (may increase CNS depression).

Storage/Stability

Injection: Intact vials/ampuls for injection are stable at room temperature. Protect from light. Clear or slightly yellow solutions may be used.

I.V. infusion: Injection may be diluted in 50-100 mL NS or D_5W.

Suppository: May require refrigeration.

Tablet: Stable at room temperature.

Compatibility Stable in dextran 6% in dextrose, dextran 6% in NS, D_5W, $D_{10}W$, D_5LR, $D_5^1/_4NS$, $D_5^1/_2NS$, D_5NS, LR, $^1/_2NS$, NS.

Y-site administration: Compatible: Amsacrine, calcium gluconate, cisatracurium, cisplatin, cladribine, clarithromycin, cyclophosphamide, cytarabine, docetaxel, doxorubicin, doxorubicin liposome, fluconazole, gatifloxacin, granisetron, heparin, hydrocortisone sodium succinate, linezolid, melphalan, methotrexate, ondansetron, paclitaxel, potassium chloride, propofol, remifentanil, sargramostim, sufentanil, teniposide, thiotepa, topotecan, vinorelbine, vitamin B complex with C. **Incompatible:** Aldesleukin, allopurinol, amifostine, amphotericin B cholesteryl sulfate complex, aztreonam, cefepime, etoposide phosphate, fludarabine, foscarnet, filgrastim, gemcitabine, piperacillin/tazobactam

Compatibility in syringe: Compatible: Atropine, butorphanol, chlorpromazine, cimetidine, diamorphine, diphenhydramine, droperidol, fentanyl, glycopyrrolate, hydroxyzine, meperidine, metoclopramide, nalbuphine, pentazocine, perphenazine, promazine, promethazine, ranitidine, scopolamine, sufentanil. **Incompatible:** Dimenhydrinate, ketorolac, midazolam, morphine tartrate, pentobarbital, thiopental. **Variable (consult detailed reference):** Hydromorphone, morphine sulfate

Compatibility when admixed: Compatible: Amikacin, ascorbic acid injection, cephalothin, dexamethasone sodium phosphate, dimenhydrinate, erythromycin lactobionate, ethacrynate, lidocaine, nafcillin, sodium bicarbonate, vitamin B complex with C. **Incompatible:** Aminophylline, amphotericin B, ampicillin, chloramphenicol, chlorothiazide, (Continued)

Prochlorperazine *(Continued)*

floxacillin, furosemide, heparin, hydrocortisone sodium succinate, methohexital, penicillin G sodium, phenobarbital, phenytoin, thiopental. **Variable (consult detailed reference):** Calcium gluconate, penicillin G potassium

Pharmacodynamics/Kinetics

Onset of action: Oral: 30-40 minutes; I.M.: 10-20 minutes; Rectal: ~60 minutes

Duration: I.M., oral extended-release: 12 hours; Rectal, immediate release: 3-4 hours

Distribution: V_d: 1400-1548 L; crosses placenta; enters breast milk

Metabolism: Primarily hepatic; N-desmethyl prochlorperazine (major active metabolite)

Bioavailability: Oral: 12.5%

Half-life elimination: Oral: 3-5 hours; I.V.: ~7 hours

Dosage

Antiemetic: Children (not recommended in children <10 kg or <2 years):

Oral, rectal: >10 kg: 0.4 mg/kg/24 hours in 3-4 divided doses; **or**
9-14 kg: 2.5 mg every 12-24 hours as needed; maximum: 7.5 mg/day
14-18 kg: 2.5 mg every 8-12 hours as needed; maximum: 10 mg/day
18-39 kg: 2.5 mg every 8 hours or 5 mg every 12 hours as needed; maximum: 15 mg/day

I.M.: 0.1-0.15 mg/kg/dose; usual: 0.13 mg/kg/dose; change to oral as soon as possible

Antiemetic: Adults:

Oral: 5-10 mg 3-4 times/day; usual maximum: 40 mg/day

I.M.: 5-10 mg every 3-4 hours; usual maximum: 40 mg/day

I.V.: 2.5-10 mg; maximum 10 mg/dose or 40 mg/day; may repeat dose every 3-4 hours as needed

Rectal: 25 mg twice daily

Surgical nausea/vomiting: Adults:

I.M.: 5-10 mg 1-2 hours before induction; may repeat once if necessary

I.V.: 5-10 mg 15-30 minutes before induction; may repeat once if necessary

Antipsychotic:

Children 2-12 years (not recommended in children <10 kg or <2 years):

Oral, rectal: 2.5 mg 2-3 times/day; increase dosage as needed to maximum daily dose of 20 mg for 2-5 years and 25 mg for 6-12 years

I.M.: 0.13 mg/kg/dose; change to oral as soon as possible

Adults:

Oral: 5-10 mg 3-4 times/day; doses up to 150 mg/day may be required in some patients for treatment of severe disturbances

I.M.: 10-20 mg every 4-6 hours may be required in some patients for treatment of severe disturbances; change to oral as soon as possible

Nonpsychotic anxiety: Oral: Adults: Usual dose: 15-20 mg/day in divided doses; do not give doses >20 mg/day or for longer than 12 weeks

Elderly: Behavioral symptoms associated with dementia (unlabeled use): Initial: 2.5-5 mg 1-2 times/day; increase dose at 4- to 7-day intervals by 2.5-5 mg/day; increase dosing intervals (twice daily, 3 times/day, etc) as necessary to control response or side effects; maximum daily dose should probably not exceed 75 mg in elderly; gradual increases (titration) may prevent some side effects or decrease their severity

Hemodialysis: Not dialyzable (0% to 5%)

Administration May be administered orally, I.M., or I.V.: I.V. doses should be given as a short (~30 minute) infusion to avoid orthostatic hypotension.

Dosage Forms [DSC] = Discontinued product

Injection, solution, as edisylate: 5 mg/mL (2 mL, 10 mL) [contains benzyl alcohol]

Suppository, rectal: 2.5 mg (12s), 5 mg (12s), 25 mg (12s) [may contain coconut and palm oil]

Compazine®: 2.5 mg (12s), 5 mg (12s), 25 mg (12s) [contains coconut and palm oils] [DSC]

Compro™: 25 mg (12s) [contains coconut and palm oils]

Tablet, as maleate: 5 mg, 10 mg

Monitoring Parameters Vital signs; lipid profile, fasting blood glucose/Hgb A_{1c}; BMI; mental status, abnormal involuntary movement scale (AIMS); periodic ophthalmic exams (if chronically used); extrapyramidal symptoms (EPS)

Dietary Considerations Increase dietary intake of riboflavin; should be administered with food or water. Rectal suppositories may contain coconut and palm oil.

Patient Information May cause drowsiness, impair judgment and coordination; may cause photosensitivity; avoid excessive sunlight; report involuntary movements or feelings of restlessness

Additional Information Not recommended as an antipsychotic due to inferior efficacy compared to other phenothiazines.

Special Geriatric Considerations Due to side effect profile (dystonias, EPS) this is not a preferred drug in the elderly for antiemetic therapy.

Selected Readings

Goldstein D, Levi JA, Woods RL, et al, "Double-Blind Randomized Cross-Over Trial of Dexamethasone and Prochlorperazine as Antiemetics for Cancer Chemotherapy," *Oncology*, 1989, 46(2):105-8.

Hesketh PJ, Gandara DR, Hesketh AM, et al, "Improved Control of High-Dose-Cisplatin-Induced Acute Emesis With the Addition of Prochlorperazine to Granisetron/Dexamethasone," *Cancer J Sci Am*, 1997, 3(3):180-3.

Lapierre J, Amin M, and Hattangadi S, "Prochlorperazine - A Review of the Literature Since 1956," *Can Psychiatr Assoc J*, 1969, 14(3):267-74.

Olver IN, Webster LK, Bishop JF, et al, "A Dose Finding Study of Prochlorperazine as an Antiemetic for Cancer Chemotherapy," *Eur J Cancer Clin Oncol*, 1989, 25(10):1457-61.

Owens NH, Schauer AR, Nightingale CH, et al, "Antiemetic Efficacy of Prochlorperazine, Haloperidol, Droperidol in Cisplatin-Induced Emesis," *Clin Pharm*, 1984, 3(2):167-70.

Peabody CA, Warner MD, Whiteford HA, et al, "Neuroleptics and the Elderly," *J Am Geriatr Soc*, 1987, 35(3):233-8.

* **Procytox® (Can)** *see* Cyclophosphamide *on page 209*
* **Profilnine® SD** *see* Factor IX Complex (Human) *on page 330*
* **Prograf®** *see* Tacrolimus *on page 734*
* **Proleukin®** *see* Aldesleukin *on page 32*
* **Proloprim®** *see* Trimethoprim *on page 797*

Promethazine (proe METH a zeen)

Medication Safety Issues

Sound-alike/look-alike issues:

Promethazine may be confused with chlorproMAZINE, predniSONE, promazine

Phenergan® may be confused with Phenaphen®, Phrenilin®, Theragran®

Related Information

Management of Nausea and Vomiting *on page 982*

U.S. Brand Names Phenadoz™; Phenergan®; Promethegan™

Canadian Brand Names Phenergan®

Generic Available Yes

Synonyms Promethazine Hydrochloride

Pharmacologic Category Antiemetic; Antihistamine; Phenothiazine Derivative; Sedative

Pregnancy Risk Factor C

Lactation Excretion in breast milk unknown/not recommended

Use Symptomatic treatment of various allergic conditions; antiemetic; motion sickness; sedative; postoperative pain (adjunctive therapy); anesthetic (adjunctive therapy); anaphylactic reactions (adjunctive therapy)

Mechanism of Action Blocks postsynaptic mesolimbic dopaminergic receptors in the brain; exhibits a strong alpha-adrenergic blocking effect and depresses the release of hypothalamic and hypophyseal hormones; competes with histamine for the H_1-receptor; reduces stimuli to the brainstem reticular system

Labeled Contraindications Hypersensitivity to promethazine or any component of the formulation (cross-reactivity between phenothiazines may occur); coma; treatment of lower respiratory tract symptoms, including asthma; children <2 years of age

Warnings/Precautions Do not give SubQ or intra-arterially, necrotic lesions may occur. Injection may contain sulfites which may cause allergic reactions in some patients. Rapid I.V. administration may produce a transient fall in blood pressure; rate of administration should not exceed 25 mg/minute. Slow I.V. administration may produce a slightly elevated blood pressure. Not considered an antihistamine of choice in the elderly.

May be sedating and may impair physical or mental abilities. Use with caution in Parkinson's disease, hemodynamic instability, bone marrow suppression, subcortical brain damage, and in severe cardiac, hepatic, renal, or respiratory disease. Avoid use in Reye's syndrome. Respiratory fatalities have been reported in children <2 years of age. In children ≥2 years, use the lowest possible dose; other drugs with respiratory depressant effects should be avoided. May lower seizure threshold; use caution in persons with seizure disorders or in persons using narcotics or local anesthetics which may also affect seizure threshold. May alter temperature regulation or mask toxicity of other drugs due to antiemetic effects. May alter cardiac conduction (life-threatening arrhythmias have occurred with therapeutic doses of phenothiazines). May cause orthostatic hypotension. Use caution in cardiovascular or cerebrovascular disease.

Due to anticholinergic effects, use caution in patients with decreased gastrointestinal motility, urinary retention, BPH, xerostomia, visual problems, narrow-angle glaucoma, and myasthenia gravis. May cause extrapyramidal symptoms, including pseudoparkinsonism, acute dystonic reactions, akathisia, and tardive dyskinesia. May be associated with neuroleptic malignant syndrome (NMS). Ampuls contain sodium metabisulfite.

Adverse Reactions Frequency not defined.

Cardiovascular: Bradycardia, hypertension, postural hypotension, tachycardia, nonspecific QT changes

Central nervous system: Akathisia, catatonic states, confusion, delirium, disorientation, dizziness, drowsiness, dystonias, euphoria, excitation, extrapyramidal symptoms, fatigue, hallucinations, hysteria, insomnia, lassitude, pseudoparkinsonism, tardive dyskinesia, nervousness, neuroleptic malignant syndrome, nightmares, sedation, seizure, somnolence

Dermatologic: Angioneurotic edema, photosensitivity, dermatitis, skin pigmentation (slate gray), urticaria

Endocrine & metabolic: Lactation, breast engorgement, amenorrhea, gynecomastia, hyper-/hypoglycemia

Gastrointestinal: Xerostomia, constipation, nausea, vomiting

Genitourinary: Urinary retention, ejaculatory disorder, impotence

Hematologic: Agranulocytosis, eosinophilia, leukopenia, hemolytic anemia, aplastic anemia, thrombocytopenia, thrombocytopenic purpura

Hepatic: Jaundice

Neuromuscular & skeletal: Incoordination, tremor

Ocular: Blurred vision, corneal and lenticular changes, diplopia, epithelial keratopathy, pigmentary retinopathy

Otic: Tinnitus

Respiratory: Apnea, asthma, nasal congestion, respiratory depression

Vesicant No

Emetic Potential Very low (<10%)

Overdosage/Toxicology Symptoms of overdose include CNS depression, respiratory depression, possible CNS stimulation, dry mouth, fixed and dilated pupils, and hypotension. Treatment is symptom-directed and supportive. Epinephrine should not be used. Hemodialysis: Not dialyzable (0% to 5%)

Drug Interactions

Cytochrome P450 Effect: Substrate (major) of CYP2B6, 2D6; **Inhibits** CYP2D6 (weak)

Increased Effect/Toxicity: CYP2B6 inhibitors may increase the levels/effects of promethazine; example inhibitors include desipramine, paroxetine, and sertraline. CYP2D6 inhibitors may increase the levels/effects of promethazine; example inhibitors include chlorpromazine, delavirdine, fluoxetine, miconazole, paroxetine, pergolide, quinidine, quinine, ritonavir, and ropinirole. Chloroquine, propranolol, and sulfadoxine-pyrimethamine also may increase promethazine concentrations. Concurrent use with TCA may produce increased toxicity or altered therapeutic response. Promethazine plus lithium may rarely produce neurotoxicity. Concurrent use of promethazine and CNS depressants (ethanol, narcotics) may produce additive depressant effects.

(Continued)

Promethazine (Continued)

Decreased Effect: CYP2B6 inducers may decrease the levels/effects of promethazine; example inducers include carbamazepine, nevirapine, phenobarbital, phenytoin, and rifampin. Benztropine (and other anticholinergics) may inhibit the therapeutic response to promethazine. Promethazine may inhibit the ability of bromocriptine to lower serum prolactin concentrations. The antihypertensive effects of guanethidine and guanadrel may be inhibited by promethazine. Promethazine may inhibit the antiparkinsonian effect of levodopa. Promethazine (and possibly other low potency antipsychotics) may reverse the pressor effects of epinephrine.

Ethanol/Nutrition/Herb Interactions

Ethanol: Avoid ethanol (may increase CNS depression).

Herb/Nutraceutical: Avoid valerian, St John's wort, kava kava, gotu kola (may increase CNS depression).

Storage/Stability

Injection: Prior to dilution, store at room temperature; protect from light. Solutions in NS or D_5W are stable for 24 hours at room temperature.

Suppositories: Store refrigerated at 2°C to 8°C (36°F to 46°F).

Tablets: Store at room temperature. Protect from light.

Compatibility Stable in dextran 6% in dextrose, dextran 6% in NS, D_5W, $D_{10}W$, D_5LR, $D_5^1/_4NS$, $D_5^1/_2NS$, D_5NS, LR, $^1/_2NS$, NS

Y-site administration: Compatible: Amifostine, amsacrine, aztreonam, ciprofloxacin, cisatracurium, cisplatin, cladribine, cyclophosphamide, cytarabine, docetaxel, doxorubicin, etoposide phosphate, filgrastim, fluconazole, fludarabine, gatifloxacin, gemcitabine, granisetron, linezolid, melphalan, ondansetron, remifentanil, sargramostim, teniposide, thiotepa, vinorelbine. **Incompatible:** Aldesleukin, allopurinol, amphotericin B cholesteryl sulfate complex, cefazolin, cefepime, cefoperazone, cefotetan, doxorubicin liposome, foscarnet, methotrexate, piperacillin/tazobactam. **Variable (consult detailed reference):** Cefazolin, ceftizoxime, heparin, hydrocortisone sodium succinate, potassium chloride, vitamin B complex with C

Compatibility in syringe: Compatible: Atropine, atropine with meperidine, butorphanol, chlorpromazine, cimetidine, dihydroergotamine, diphenhydramine, droperidol, fentanyl, glycopyrrolate, hydromorphone, hydroxyzine, meperidine, metoclopramide, midazolam, pentazocine, perphenazine, prochlorperazine edisylate, promazine, ranitidine, scopolamine. **Incompatible:** Cefotetan, chloroquine, diatrizoate sodium 75%, diatrizoate meglumine 52% with diatrizoate sodium 8%, diatrizoate meglumine 34.3% with diatrizoate sodium 35%, dimenhydrinate, heparin, iodipamide meglumine 52%, iothalamate meglumine 60%, iothalamate sodium 80%, ketorolac, pentobarbital, thiopental. **Variable (consult detailed reference):** Morphine, nalbuphine

Compatibility when admixed: Compatible: Amikacin, ascorbic acid injection, buprenorphine, butorphanol, chloroquine, hydromorphone, netilmicin, vitamin B complex with C. **Incompatible:** Aminophylline, chloramphenicol, chlorothiazide, dimenhydrinate, floxacillin, furosemide, heparin, hydrocortisone sodium succinate, methohexital, penicillin G sodium, pentobarbital, phenobarbital, phenytoin, thiopental. **Variable (consult detailed reference):** Penicillin G potassium

Pharmacodynamics/Kinetics

Onset of action: I.M.: ~20 minutes; I.V.: 3-5 minutes

Peak effect: C_{max}: 9.04 ng/mL (suppository); 19.3 ng/mL (syrup)

Duration: 2-6 hours

Absorption:

I.M.: Bioavailability may be greater than with oral or rectal administration

Oral: Rapid and complete; large first pass effect limits systemic bioavailability

Distribution: V_d: 171 L

Protein binding: 93%

Metabolism: Hepatic; primarily oxidation; forms metabolites

Half-life elimination: 9-16 hours

Time to maximum serum concentration: 4.4 hours (syrup); 6.7-8.6 hours (suppositories)

Excretion: Primarily urine and feces (as inactive metabolites)

Dosage

Children ≥2 years:

Allergic conditions: Oral, rectal: 0.1 mg/kg/dose (maximum: 12.5 mg) every 6 hours during the day and 0.5 mg/kg/dose (maximum: 25 mg) at bedtime as needed

Antiemetic: Oral, I.M., I.V., rectal: 0.25-1 mg/kg 4-6 times/day as needed (maximum: 25 mg/dose)

Motion sickness: Oral, rectal: 0.5 mg/kg/dose 30 minutes to 1 hour before departure, then every 12 hours as needed (maximum dose: 25 mg twice daily)

Sedation: Oral, I.M., I.V., rectal: 0.5-1 mg/kg/dose every 6 hours as needed (maximum: 50 mg/dose)

Adults:

Allergic conditions (including allergic reactions to blood or plasma):

Oral, rectal: 25 mg at bedtime **or** 12.5 mg before meals and at bedtime (range: 6.25-12.5 mg 3 times/day)

I.M., I.V.: 25 mg, may repeat in 2 hours when necessary; switch to oral route as soon as feasible

Antiemetic: Oral, I.M., I.V., rectal: 12.5-25 mg every 4-6 hours as needed

Motion sickness: Oral, rectal: 25 mg 30-60 minutes before departure, then every 12 hours as needed

Sedation: Oral, I.M., I.V., rectal: 12.5-50 mg/dose

Administration For oral, rectal, I.M./I.V.; not for SubQ or intra-arterial administration. Administer I.M. into deep muscle (preferred route of administration). I.V. administration is **not** the preferred route. Solution for injection may be diluted in 25-100 mL NS or D_5W (maximum concentration of 25 mg/mL) and infused over 15-30 minutes.

Dosage Forms [DSC] = Discontinued product

Injection, solution, as hydrochloride: 25 mg/mL (1 mL); 50 mg/mL (1 mL)

Phenergan®: 25 mg/mL (1 mL); 50 mg/mL (1 mL) [contains sodium metabisulfite]

Suppository, rectal, as hydrochloride: 12.5 mg, 25 mg, 50 mg

Phenadoz™: 12.5 mg, 25 mg

Phenergan®, Promethegan™: 12.5 mg, 25 mg, 50 mg

Syrup, as hydrochloride: 6.25 mg/5 mL (120 mL, 480 mL) [contains alcohol]

Tablet, as hydrochloride: 12.5 mg, 25 mg, 50 mg

Phenergan®: 12.5 mg [DSC], 25 mg, 50 mg [DSC]

(Continued)

Promethazine *(Continued)*

Monitoring Parameters Relief of symptoms, mental status

Dietary Considerations Increase dietary intake of riboflavin.

Patient Information May cause drowsiness, impair judgment and coordination; may cause photosensitivity; avoid excessive sunlight; report involuntary movements or feelings of restlessness

Special Geriatric Considerations Because promethazine is a phenothiazine (and can, therefore, cause side effects such as extrapyramidal symptoms), it is not considered an antihistamine of choice in the elderly.

Selected Readings

Blanc VF, Ruest P, Milot J, et al, "Antiemetic Prophylaxis With Promethazine or Droperidol in Paediatric Outpatient Strabismus Surgery," *Can J Anaesth*, 1991, 38(1):54-60.

Grunberg SM and Hesketh PJ, "Control of Chemotherapy-Induced Emesis," *N Engl J Med*, 1993, 329(24):1790-6.

McGee JL and Alexander MR, "Phenothiazine Analgesia - Fact or Fantasy?" *Am J Hosp Pharm*, 1979, 36(5):633-40.

Strenkoski-Nix LC, Ermer J, DeCleene S, et al, "Pharmacokinetics of Promethazine Hydrochloride After Administration of Rectal Suppositories and Oral Syrup to Healthy Subjects," *Am J Health Syst Pharm*, 2000, 57(16):1499-505.

Tavorath R and Hesketh PJ, "Drug Treatment of Chemotherapy-Induced Delayed Emesis," *Drugs*, 1996, 52(5):639-48.

Tortorice PV and O'Connell MB, "Management of Chemotherapy-Induced Nausea and Vomiting," *Pharmacotherapy*, 1990, 10(2):129-45.

- **Promethazine Hydrochloride** *see* Promethazine *on page 696*
- **Promethegan**™ *see* Promethazine *on page 696*
- **Propecia**® *see* Finasteride *on page 345*
- **Proplex**® **T** *see* Factor IX Complex (Human) *on page 330*
- **Proscar**® *see* Finasteride *on page 345*
- **Protein-Bound Paclitaxel** *see* Paclitaxel (Protein Bound) *on page 644*
- **Prothrombin Complex Concentrate** *see* Factor IX Complex (Human) *on page 330*
- **Protopic**® *see* Tacrolimus *on page 734*
- **Provera**® *see* MedroxyPROGESTERone *on page 524*
- **PS-341** *see* Bortezomib *on page 138*
- **Purinethol**® *see* Mercaptopurine *on page 539*
- **Quixin**™ *see* Levofloxacin *on page 504*
- **R 14-15** *see* Erlotinib *on page 308*
- **R-3827** *see* Abarelix *on page 24*
- **rAHF** *see* Antihemophilic Factor (Recombinant) *on page 92*

Raltitrexed (ral ti TREX ed)

Related Information

Investigational Drug Service *on page 1031*
Safe Handling of Hazardous Drugs *on page 1034*

Canadian Brand Names Tomudex®

Generic Available No

Synonyms ICI-D1694; NSC-639186; Raltitrexed Disodium; ZD1694

Pharmacologic Category Antineoplastic Agent, Antimetabolite

Pregnancy Risk Factor X

Lactation Excretion in breast milk unknown/contraindicated

Use Treatment of advanced colorectal neoplasms

Unlabeled/Investigational Use Undergoing clinical trials for a variety of neoplasms, including breast, colorectal nonsmall cell lung, ovarian and pancreatic cancers

Mechanism of Action Raltitrexed is a folate analogue that inhibits thymidylate synthase, blocking purine synthesis. This results in an overall inhibition of DNA synthesis.

Restrictions Not available in U.S./Investigational

Labeled Contraindications Hypersensitivity to raltitrexed or any component of the formulation; uncontrolled diarrhea; severe renal or hepatic impairment; pregnancy or breast-feeding

Warnings/Precautions Hazardous agent - use appropriate precautions for handling and disposal. See Safe Handling of Hazardous Drugs *on page 1034* in the Appendix. Use caution in patients heavily pretreated with chemotherapy or radiation, especially if myelosuppression, stomatitis, hepatic or renal toxicities persist. Use caution in elderly and in patients taking folic acid or folate-containing medications (eg, multivitamins), mild to moderate hepatic or renal dysfunction, or a history of gastrointestinal problems (particularly diarrhea). May cause malaise/weakness (caution patients concerning operation of machinery/driving). Safety and efficacy in pediatric patients have not been established.

Adverse Reactions

>10%:

Central nervous system: Fever (2% to 23%), may be delayed until several days after administration

Dermatologic: Rashes (14%), usually pruritic papular lesions on head and thorax

Gastrointestinal: Nausea (58%; grade 3 or 4 in 12%), mucositis/stomatitis (12% to 48%; grade 3 or 4 in 2%), diarrhea (38%; grade 3 or 4 in 11%), vomiting (37%), anorexia (27%), abdominal pain (18%), constipation (13% to 15%; grade 3 or 4 in 2%)

Hematologic: Myelosuppression; leukopenia occurs in about 21% of patients (grade 3 or 4 in 12%), nadirs occur in ~8 days, but may be delayed to day 21, with recovery in ~10 days; thrombocytopenia (5% to 6%; grade 3 or 4 in 4%), anemia (15% to 18%; grade 3 or 4 in 7%)

Hepatic: Transaminases increased (14% to 18%; grade 3 or 4 in 10%)

Neuromuscular & skeletal: Weakness (46% to 48%; grade 3 or 4 in 9%)

1% to 10%:

Cardiovascular: Arrhythmias (3%), edema (9% to 10%), CHF (2%)

Central nervous system: Malaise, headache, pain, chills, insomnia, depression, paresthesia

Dermatologic: Alopecia, cellulitis, exfoliative eruptions

Endocrine & metabolic: Dehydration, hypokalemia

Gastrointestinal: Dyspepsia, flatulence, xerostomia, weight loss, taste perversion

Genitourinary: Urinary tract infection

Hepatic: Alkaline phosphatase increased, bilirubin increased

Neuromuscular & skeletal: Arthralgia, myalgia, hypotonia

Ocular: Conjunctivitis

Renal: Serum creatinine increased

Respiratory: Cough (increased), dyspnea, pharyngitis

Miscellaneous: Flu-like syndrome (6% to 8%), diaphoresis, infection, sepsis

(Continued)

Raltitrexed *(Continued)*

<1%: Hypersensitivity/allergic reaction (including stridor and wheezing following the first dose), desquamation

Vesicant No

Emetic Potential Mild to moderate (30% to 60%)

Overdosage/Toxicology Symptoms may include severe hematologic and gastrointestinal toxicity. Treatment is symptom-directed and supportive. Anecdotal reports suggest potential benefit of folinic acid (25 mg/m^2 every 6 hours) if administered early.

Drug Interactions

Decreased Effect: Folic acid, folinic acid, and multivitamins with folic acid may decrease the effectiveness of raltitrexed.

Ethanol/Nutrition/Herb Interactions Herb/Nutraceutical: Avoid folic acid and multivitamins with folic acid close to and during administration.

Storage/Stability Intact vials should be refrigerated at 2°C to 25°C. Protect from light. Solutions reconstituted with saline or dextrose to a concentrate of 0.5 mg/mL are stable for up to 24 hours under refrigeration at 2°C to 8°C.

Reconstitution Reconstitute 2 mg vial with 4 mL SWFI; add to 50-250 mL NS or D_5W.

Compatibility Compatible: Stable in D_5W, NS

Pharmacodynamics/Kinetics

Distribution: V_{ss}: 548 L

Protein binding: 93%

Metabolism: Undergoes extensive intracellular metabolism to active polyglutamate forms; appears to be little or no systemic metabolism of the drug

Half-life elimination: Triphasic; Beta: 2 hours; Terminal: Up to 198 hours

Excretion: Urine (50% as unchanged drug); feces (15%)

Dosage Refer to individual protocols.

I.V.: 3 mg/m^2 every 3 weeks

Dosage adjustment in renal impairment:

Cl_{cr} 55-65 mL/minute: Administer 75% of dose every 4 weeks

Cl_{cr} 25-54 mL/minute: Administer % of dose equivalent to Cl_{cr} every 4 weeks (ie, 25% of dose for Cl_{cr} of 25 mL/minute)

Cl_{cr} <25 mL/minute: Do not administer

Dosage adjustment for hepatic impairment: No adjustment required for mild-moderate hepatic insufficiency. Patients who develop hepatic toxicity should have treatment until WHO grade 2.

Dosage adjustment for toxicity:

WHO grade 4 gastrointestinal toxicity or grade 3 gastrointestinal toxicity in combination with grade 4 hematologic toxicity: Discontinue therapy

Grade 3 hematologic toxicity or grade 2 gastrointestinal toxicity: Reduce dose by 25%

Grade 4 hematologic toxicity or grade 3 gastrointestinal toxicity: Reduce dose by 50%

Administration Infuse over 15 minutes.

Dosage Forms Injection, powder for reconstitution, as disodium: 2 mg

Monitoring Parameters CBC with differential, hepatic function tests, serum lipids, serum creatinine

Dietary Considerations Avoid folic acid, folinic acid, and multivitamins with folic acid close to and during administration.

Patient Information This medication can only be given intravenously. Avoid folic acid and multivitamins with folate. Inform prescriber if you are pregnant. Do not get pregnant during or for 6 months following therapy. Male: Do not cause a female to become pregnant. Male/female: Consult prescriber for instruction on appropriate contraceptive measures. This drug may cause severe fetal defects. Do not breast-feed.

Selected Readings

Clarke SJ, Beale PJ, and Rivory LP, "Clinical and Preclinical Pharmacokinetics of Raltitrexed," *Clin Pharmacokinet*, 2000, 39(6):429-43.

Taylor SC, "Raltitrexed for Advanced Colorectal Cancer. The Story So Far," *Cancer Pract*, 2000, 8(1):51-4.

Van Cutsem E, Cunningham D, Maroun J, et al, "Raltitrexed: Current Clinical Status and Future Directions," *Ann Oncol*, 2002, 13(4):513-22.

♦ **Raltitrexed Disodium** *see* Raltitrexed *on page 700*

♦ **Rapamune**® *see* Sirolimus *on page 718*

Rasburicase (ras BYOOR i kayse)

U.S. Brand Names Elitek™

Generic Available No

Pharmacologic Category Enzyme; Enzyme, Urate-Oxidase (Recombinant)

Pregnancy Risk Factor C

Lactation Excretion in breast milk unknown/not recommended

Use Initial management of uric acid levels in pediatric patients with leukemia, lymphoma, and solid tumor malignancies receiving anticancer therapy expected to result in tumor lysis and elevation of plasma uric acid

Mechanism of Action Rasburicase is a recombinant urate-oxidase enzyme, which converts uric acid to allantoin (an inactive and soluble metabolite of uric acid); it does not inhibit the formation of uric acid.

Labeled Contraindications Hypersensitivity, hemolytic or methemoglobinemia reactions to rasburicase or any component of the formulation; glucose-6-phosphatase dehydrogenase (G6PD) deficiency

Warnings/Precautions Hypersensitivity reactions (including anaphylaxis), methemoglobinemia, and severe hemolysis have been reported; reactions may occur at any time during treatment (including the initial dose); discontinue **immediately and permanently** in patients developing any of these reactions. Hemolysis may be associated with G6PD deficiency; patients at higher risk for G6PD deficiency should be screened prior to therapy. Enzymatic degradation of uric acid in blood samples will occur if left at room temperature; specific guidelines for the collection of plasma uric acid samples must be followed. Rasburicase is immunogenic and can elicit an antibody response. Administration of more than one course is not recommended. Efficacy in adults has not been established.

Adverse Reactions As reported in patients receiving rasburicase with antitumor therapy versus active-control:

>10%:

Central nervous system: Fever (5% to 46%), headache (26%)

Dermatologic: Rash (13%)

Gastrointestinal: Vomiting (50%), nausea (27%), abdominal pain (20%), constipation (20%), mucositis (2% to 15%), diarrhea (≤1% to 20%)

1% to 10%:

Hematologic: Neutropenia with fever (4%), neutropenia (2%)

Respiratory: Respiratory distress (3%)

(Continued)

Rasburicase *(Continued)*

Miscellaneous: Sepsis (3%)

<1%: Acute renal failure, anaphylaxis, arrhythmia, cardiac arrest, cardiac failure, cellulitis, cerebrovascular disorder, chest pain, convulsions, cyanosis, dehydration, hemolysis, hemorrhage, hot flashes, ileus, infection, intestinal obstruction, methemoglobinemia, MI, pancytopenia, paresthesia, pneumonia, pulmonary edema, pulmonary hypertension, retinal hemorrhage, rigors, thrombosis, thrombophlebitis

Overdosage/Toxicology No cases of overdose have been reported; low or undetectable serum levels of uric acid would be expected. Treatment should be symptom-directed and supportive.

Storage/Stability Both the reconstituted and final solution may be stored up to 24 hours at 2°C to 8°C (36°F to 46°F). Do not freeze; protect from light.

Reconstitution Reconstitute each vial with 1 mL of the provided diluent. Mix by gently swirling; do **not** shake or vortex. Discard if discolored or containing particulate matter. Total dose should be further diluted in NS to a final volume of 50 mL.

Pharmacodynamics/Kinetics

Distribution: Pediatric patients: 110-127 mL/kg

Half-life elimination: Pediatric patients: 18 hours

Dosage I.V.:

Children: Management of uric acid levels: 0.15 mg/kg or 0.2 mg/kg once daily for 5 days (manufacturer-recommended duration); begin chemotherapy 4-24 hours after the first dose

Limited data suggest that a single prechemotherapy dose (versus multiple-day administration) may be sufficiently efficacious. Monitoring electrolytes, hydration status, and uric acid concentrations are necessary to identify the need for additional doses. Other clinical manifestations of tumor lysis syndrome (eg, hyperphosphatemia, hypocalcemia, and hyperkalemia) may occur.

Adults and Elderly: Refer to pediatric dosing; insufficient data collected in adult/geriatric patients to determine response to treatment

Administration I.V. infusion over 30 minutes; do **not** administer as a bolus infusion. Do **not** filter during infusion. If not possible to administer through a separate line, I.V. line should be flushed with at least 15 mL saline prior to and following rasburicase infusion.

Dosage Forms Injection, powder for reconstitution: 1.5 mg [packaged with three 1 mL ampuls of diluent]

Monitoring Parameters Plasma uric acid levels, CBC

Patient Information This medication can only be given by injection. Notify prescriber immediately for chest pain, difficulty breathing, or itching. May cause headache, nausea, vomiting, constipation, or fever.

Selected Readings

Lee AC, Li CH, So KT, et al, "Treatment of Impending Tumor Lysis With Single-Dose Rasburicase," *Ann Pharmacother*, 2003, 37(11):1614-7.

Pui CH, "Rasburicase: A Potent Uricolytic Agent," *Expert Opin Pharmacother*, 2002, 3(4):433-42.

Rh$_o$(D) Immune Globulin

(ar aych oh (dee) i MYUN GLOB yoo lin)

U.S. Brand Names BayRho-D® Full-Dose; BayRho-D® Mini-Dose; MICRhoGAM®; RhoGAM®; Rhophylac®; WinRho SDF®

Canadian Brand Names BayRho-D® Full-Dose

Generic Available No

Synonyms RhIG; Rho(D) Immune Globulin (Human); RhoIGIV; RhoIVIM

Pharmacologic Category Immune Globulin

Pregnancy Risk Factor C

Lactation Does not enter breast milk

Use

Suppression of Rh isoimmunization: Use in the following situations when an Rh$_o$(D)-negative individual is exposed to Rh$_o$(D)-positive blood: During delivery of an Rh$_o$(D)-positive infant; abortion; amniocentesis; chorionic villus sampling; ruptured tubal pregnancy; abdominal trauma; transplacental hemorrhage. Used when the mother is Rh$_o$(D) negative, the father of the child is either Rh$_o$(D) positive or Rh$_o$(D) unknown, the baby is either Rh$_o$(D) positive or Rh$_o$(D) unknown.

Transfusion: Suppression of Rh isoimmunization in Rh$_o$(D)-negative female children and female adults in their childbearing years transfused with Rh$_o$(D) antigen-positive RBCs or blood components containing Rh$_o$(D) antigen-positive RBCs

Treatment of idiopathic thrombocytopenic purpura (ITP): Used in the following nonsplenectomized Rh$_o$(D) positive individuals: Children with acute or chronic ITP, adults with chronic ITP, children and adults with ITP secondary to HIV infection

Mechanism of Action

Rh suppression: Suppresses the immune response and antibody formation of Rh$_o$(D) negative individuals to Rh$_o$(D) positive red blood cells.

ITP: Coats the patients Rh$_o$(D) positive red blood cells with antibody, so that as they are cleared by the spleen, the spleens ability to clear antibody-coated cells is saturated, sparing the platelets.

Labeled Contraindications Hypersensitivity to immune globulins or any component of the formulation; prior sensitization to Rh$_o$(D)

(Continued)

Rhₒ(D) Immune Globulin *(Continued)*

Warnings/Precautions As a product of human plasma, may potentially transmit disease; screening of donors, as well as testing and/or inactivation of certain viruses reduces this risk. Not for replacement therapy in immune globulin deficiency syndromes. Use caution with IgA deficiency, may contain trace amounts of IgA; patients who are IgA deficient may have the potential for developing IgA antibodies, anaphylactic reactions may occur. Administer I.M. injections with caution in patients with thrombocytopenia or coagulation disorders.

ITP: Do not administer I.M. or SubQ; administer dose I.V. only. Safety and efficacy not established in Rhₒ(D) negative or splenectomized patients. Decrease dose with hemoglobin <10 g/dL; use with extreme caution if hemoglobin <8 g/dL

Rhₒ(D) suppression: For use in the mother; do not administer to the neonate.

Adverse Reactions Frequency not defined.

Cardiovascular: Hypotension, pallor, tachycardia, vasodilation

Central nervous system: Chills, dizziness, fever, headache, malaise, somnolence

Dermatologic: Pruritus, rash

Gastrointestinal: Abdominal pain, diarrhea, nausea, vomiting

Hematologic: Hemoglobin decreased (patients with ITP), intravascular hemolysis (patients with ITP)

Hepatic: LDH increased

Local: Injection site reaction: Discomfort, induration, mild pain, redness, swelling

Neuromuscular & skeletal: Back pain, hyperkinesia, myalgia, weakness

Miscellaneous: Anaphylaxis, diaphoresis

Overdosage/Toxicology No symptoms are likely, however, high doses have been associated with a mild, transient hemolytic anemia. Treatment is supportive.

Drug Interactions

Decreased Effect: Rhₒ(D) immune globulin may interfere with the response to live vaccines; vaccines should not be administered within 3 months after Rhₒ(D)

Storage/Stability Store at 2°C to 8°C (35°F to 46°F). Do not freeze. Following reconstitution, may store at room temperature for up to 12 hours.

Rhophylac®: Stored at this temperature, Rhophylac® has a shelf life of 36 months. Protect from light.

Reconstitution WinRho SDF®: Dilute with provided NS only. Inject diluent slowly into vial and gently swirl until dissolved; do not shake.

Pharmacodynamics/Kinetics

Onset of platelet increase: ITP: 1-3 days

Duration: Suppression of Rh isoimmunization: ~12 weeks; Treatment of ITP: 3-4 weeks

Distribution: V_d: I.M.: 8.59 L

Half-life elimination: 21-30 days

Time to peak, plasma: I.M.: 5-10 days

Dosage

ITP: Children and Adults: WinRho SDF®: I.V.:

Initial: 50 mcg/kg as a single injection, or can be given as a divided dose on separate days. If hemoglobin is <10 g/dL: Dose should be reduced to 25-40 mcg/kg.

Subsequent dosing: 25-60 mcg/kg can be used if required to elevate platelet count

Maintenance dosing if patient **did respond** to initial dosing: 25-60 mcg/kg based on platelet and hemoglobin levels:

Maintenance dosing if patient **did not respond** to initial dosing:

Hemoglobin 8-10 g/dL: Redose between 25-40 mcg/kg

Hemoglobin >10 g/dL: Redose between 50-60 mcg/kg

Hemoglobin <8 g/dL: Use with caution

Rh$_o$(D) suppression: Adults: **Note:** One "full dose" (300 mcg) provides enough antibody to prevent Rh sensitization if the volume of RBC entering the circulation is ≤15 mL. When >15 mL is suspected, a fetal red cell count should be performed to determine the appropriate dose.

Pregnancy:

Antepartum prophylaxis: In general, dose is given at 28 weeks. If given early in pregnancy, administer every 12 weeks to ensure adequate levels of passively acquired anti-Rh

BayRho-D® Full Dose, RhoGAM®: I.M.: 300 mcg

Rhophylac®, WinRho SDF®: I.M., I.V.: 300 mcg

Postpartum prophylaxis: In general, dose is administered as soon as possible after delivery, preferably within 72 hours. Can be given up to 28 days following delivery

BayRho-D® Full Dose, RhoGAM®: I.M.: 300 mcg

Rhophylac®: I.M., I.V.: 300 mcg

WinRho SDF®: I.M., I.V.: 120 mcg

Threatened abortion, any time during pregnancy (with continuation of pregnancy):

BayRho-D® Full Dose, RhoGAM®: I.M.: 300 mcg; administer as soon as possible

Rhophylac®, WinRho SDF®: I.M., I.V.: 300 mcg; administer as soon as possible

Abortion, miscarriage, termination of ectopic pregnancy:

BayRho-D®, RhoGAM®: I.M.: ≥13 weeks gestation: 300 mcg.

BayRho-D® Mini Dose, MICRhoGAM®: <13 weeks gestation: I.M.: 50 mcg

Rhophylac®: I.M., I.V.: 300 mcg

WinRho SDF®: I.M., I.V.: After 34 weeks gestation: 120 mcg; administer immediately or within 72 hours

Amniocentesis, chorionic villus sampling:

BayRho-D®, RhoGAM®: I.M.: At 15-18 weeks gestation or during the 3rd trimester: 300 mcg. If dose is given between 13-18 weeks, repeat at 26-28 weeks and within 72 hours of delivery.

Rhophylac®: I.M., I.V.: 300 mcg

WinRho SDF®: I.M., I.V.: Before 34 weeks gestation: 300 mcg; administer immediately, repeat dose every 12 weeks during pregnancy; After 34 weeks gestation: 120 mcg, administered immediately or within 72 hours

(Continued)

Rh₀(D) Immune Globulin *(Continued)*

Abdominal trauma, manipulation:

BayRho-D®, RhoGAM®: I.M.: 2nd or 3rd trimester: 300 mcg. If dose is given between 13-18 weeks, repeat at 26-28 weeks and within 72 hours of delivery

WinRho SDF®: I.M./I.V.: After 34 weeks gestation: 120 mcg; administer immediately or within 72 hours

Transfusion:

Children and Adults: WinRho SDF®: Administer within 72 hours after exposure of incompatible blood transfusions or massive fetal hemorrhage.

I.V.: Calculate dose as follows; administer 600 mcg every 8 hours until the total dose is administered:

Exposure to Rh₀(D) positive whole blood: 9 mcg/mL blood

Exposure to Rh₀(D) positive red blood cells: 18 mcg/mL cells

I.M.: Calculate dose as follows; administer 1200 mcg every 12 hours until the total dose is administered:

Exposure to Rh₀(D) positive whole blood: 12 mcg/mL blood

Exposure to Rh₀(D) positive red blood cells: 24 mcg/mL cells

Adults:

BayRho-D®, RhoGAM®: I.M.: Multiply the volume of Rh positive whole blood administered by the hematocrit of the donor unit to equal the volume of RBCs transfused. The volume of RBCs is then divided by 15 mL, providing the number of 300 mcg doses (vials/syringes) to administer. If the dose calculated results in a fraction, round up to the next higher whole 300 mcg dose (vial/syringe).

Rhophylac®: I.M., I.V.: 20 mcg/2 mL transfused blood or 20 mcg/mL erythrocyte concentrate

Administration The total volume can be administered in divided doses at different sites at one time or may be divided and given at intervals, provided the total dosage is given within 72 hours of the fetomaternal hemorrhage or transfusion.

I.M.: Administer into the deltoid muscle of the upper arm or anterolateral aspect of the upper thigh; avoid gluteal region due to risk of sciatic nerve injury. If large doses (>5 mL) are needed, administration in divided doses at different sites is recommended.

I.V.: WinRho SDF®: Infuse over 3-5 minutes; do not administer with other medications

Dosage Forms

Injection, solution [preservative free]:

BayRho-D® Full-Dose, RhoGAM®: 300 mcg [for I.M. use only]

BayRho-D® Mini-Dose, MICRhoGAM®: 50 mcg [for I.M. use only]

Rhophylac®: 300 mcg/2 mL (2 mL) [1500 int. units; for I.M. or I.V. use]

Injection, powder for reconstitution [preservative free] (WinRho SDF®): 120 mcg [600 int. units], 300 mcg [1500 int. units], 1000 mcg [5000 int. units] [for I.M. or I.V. use]

Monitoring Parameters Signs and symptoms of intravascular hemolysis (IVH), anemia, and renal insufficiency; observe patient for side effects for at least 20 minutes following administration

Patient Information This medication is only given by injection. It may be given as a one-time dose, or may need repeated. You may experience pain at the injection site. Notify prescriber if you experience chills, headache, dizziness, fever or rash.

Additional Information A "full dose" of $Rh_o(D)$ immune globulin has previously been referred to as a 300 mcg dose. It is not the actual anti-D content. Although dosing has traditionally been expressed in mcg, potency is listed in int. units.

Selected Readings

Hartwell EA, "Use of Rh Immune Globulin: ASCP Practice Parameter. American Society of Clinical Pathologists," *Am J Clin Pathol*, 1998, 110(3):281-92.

"$Rh_o(D)$ Immune Globulin I.V. for Prevention of Rh Isoimmunization and for Treatment of ITP," *Med Lett Drugs Ther*, 1996, 38(966):6-8.

Simpson KN, Coughlin CM, Eron J, et al, "Idiopathic Thrombocytopenia Purpura: Treatment Patterns and an Analysis of Cost Associated With Intravenous Immunoglobulin and Anti-D Therapy," *Semin Hematol*, 1998, 35(1 Suppl 1):58-64.

Scaradavou A, Bussel J. "Clinical Experience With Anti-D in the Treatment of Idiopathic Thrombocytopenic Purpura." *Semin Hematol*, 1998, 35(1 Suppl 1):52-7.

Ware RE and Zimmerman SA, "Anti-D: Mechanisms of Action," *Semin Hematol*, 1998, 35(1 Suppl 1):14-22.

+ **Rho(D) Immune Globulin (Human)** *see $Rh_o(D)$ Immune Globulin on page 705*

+ **RhoGAM®** *see $Rh_o(D)$ Immune Globulin on page 705*

+ **RhoIGIV** *see $Rh_o(D)$ Immune Globulin on page 705*

+ **RhoIVIM** *see $Rh_o(D)$ Immune Globulin on page 705*

+ **Rhophylac®** *see $Rh_o(D)$ Immune Globulin on page 705*

+ **Rhoxal-cyclosporine (Can)** *see CycloSPORINE on page 216*

+ **rHuEPO-α** *see Epoetin Alfa on page 302*

+ **rHu-KGF** *see Palifermin on page 646*

+ **rhuMAb-VEGF** *see Bevacizumab on page 124*

+ **rIFN-A** *see Interferon Alfa-2a on page 466*

+ **rIL-11** *see Oprelvekin on page 627*

+ **Rituxan®** *see Rituximab on page 709*

Rituximab (ri TUK si mab)

Medication Safety Issues

Sound-alike/look-alike issues:

Rituxan® may be confused with Remicade®

Related Information

Safe Handling of Hazardous Drugs *on page 1034*

U.S. Brand Names Rituxan®

Canadian Brand Names Rituxan®

Generic Available No

Synonyms Anti-CD20 Monoclonal Antibody; C2B8; C2B8 Monoclonal Antibody; IDEC-C2B8; Pan-B Antibody

Pharmacologic Category Antineoplastic Agent, Monoclonal Antibody

Pregnancy Risk Factor C

Lactation Excretion in breast milk unknown/contraindicated

Use Treatment of relapsed or refractory CD20 positive, B-cell non-Hodgkin's lymphoma

Mechanism of Action Rituximab is a monoclonal antibody directed against the CD20 antigen on B-lymphocytes. CD20 regulates cell cycle initiation; and, possibly, functions as a calcium channel. Rituximab binds
(Continued)

Rituximab *(Continued)*

to the antigen on the cell surface, activating complement-dependent cyto-toxicity; and to human Fc receptors, mediating cell killing through an antibody-dependent cellular toxicity.

Labeled Contraindications Type I hypersensitivity or anaphylactic reactions to murine proteins or any component of the formulation

Warnings/Precautions Hazardous agent - use appropriate precautions for handling and disposal. See Safe Handling of Hazardous Drugs *on page 1034* in the Appendix. Severe infusion related reactions have been reported (77% following the first dose). Hypotension, bronchospasm, and angioedema have occurred as part of an infusion-related symptom complex; hypoxia, pulmonary infiltrates, acute respiratory distress syndrome, myocardial infarction, ventricular fibrillation, or cardiogenic shock may occur in the most severe cases. Risk factors associated with fatal outcomes include chronic lymphocytic leukemia, female gender, mantle cell lymphoma, or pulmonary infiltrates. Treatment of these reactions is symptomatic. Medications for the treatment of hypersensitivity reactions (eg, epinephrine, antihistamines, corticosteroids) should be available for immediate use. Discontinue infusions in the event of serious or life-threatening cardiac arrhythmias. Reactivation of Hepatitis B has been reported in association with rituximab (rare); consider screening in high-risk patients.

Tumor lysis syndrome leading to acute renal failure requiring dialysis may occur 12-24 hours following the first dose. Consider prophylaxis in patients at high risk. Severe and sometimes fatal mucocutaneous reactions have been reported, occurring from 1-13 weeks following exposure. Use caution with cardiac or pulmonary disease, prior cardiopulmonary events and with high numbers of circulating malignant cells ($\geq 25000/mm^3$). Safety and efficacy in pediatric patients have not been established.

Adverse Reactions Note: Abdominal pain, anemia, dyspnea, hypotension, and neutropenia are more common in patients with bulky disease.
>10%:
Central nervous system: Fever (53%), chills (33%), headache (19%), pain (12%)
Dermatologic: Rash (15%), pruritus (14%), angioedema (11%)
Gastrointestinal: Nausea (23%), abdominal pain (14%)
Hematologic: Lymphopenia (48%; Grade 3/ 4: 40%; mean duration 14 days), leukopenia (14%; Grade 3/4: 4%), neutropenia (14%; Grade 3/ 4: 6%; mean duration 13 days), thrombocytopenia (12%; Grade 3/4: 2%)
Neuromuscular & skeletal: Weakness (26%)
Respiratory: Cough (13%), rhinitis (12%)
Miscellaneous: Infection (31%), night sweats (15%)
Infusion-related reactions: Chills, fever, rigors, dizziness, hypertension, myalgia, nausea, pruritus, rash and vomiting (first dose 77%; fourth dose 30%; eighth dose 14%)
1% to 10%:
Cardiovascular: Dizziness (10%), hypotension (10%), peripheral edema (8%), hypertension (6%), anxiety (5%), flushing (5%)
Central nervous system: Agitation (<5%), depression (<5%), edema (<5%), insomnia (<5%), malaise (<5%), nervousness (<5%), somnolence (<5%), vertigo (<5%)

Dermatologic: Urticaria (8%)

Endocrine & metabolic: Hyperglycemia (9%), hypoglycemia (<5%)

Gastrointestinal: Diarrhea (10%), vomiting (10%), anorexia (<5%), weight loss (<5%)

Hematologic: Anemia (8%; Grade 3/4: 3%)

Local: Pain at the injection site (<5%)

Neuromuscular & skeletal: Arthralgia (10%), back pain (10%), myalgia (10%), arthritis (<5%), hyperkinesia (<5%), hypertonia (<5%), hypoesthesia (<5%), neuritis (<5%), neuropathy (<5%), paresthesia (<5%)

Ocular: Conjunctivitis (<5%), lacrimation disorder (<5%)

Respiratory: Throat irritation (9%), bronchospasm (8%), dyspnea (7%), sinusitis (6%), dyspepsia (<5%)

Miscellaneous: LDH increased (7%)

Postmarketing and/or case reports: ARDS, arrhythmia, bronchiolitis obliterans, cardiogenic shock, fatal infusion related reactions, hemolytic anemia, hepatic failure, hepatitis, lichenoid dermatitis, marrow hypoplasia, MI, neutropenia (late onset - occurring >40 days after last dose), optic neuritis, pancytopenia, paraneoplastic pemphigus (uncommon), pleuritis, pneumonitis, pure red cell aplasia, reactivation of hepatitis, serum sickness, Stevens-Johnson syndrome, toxic epidermal necrolysis, uveitis, vasculitis with rash, ventricular fibrillation, ventricular tachycardia, vesiculobullous dermatitis

Vesicant No

Emetic Potential Low (10% to 30%)

Overdosage/Toxicology There has been no experience with overdosage in human clinical trials; single doses higher than 500 mg/m^2 have not been tested

Storage/Stability Store under refrigeration; protect vials from direct sunlight. Solutions for infusion are stable at 2°C to 8°C/36°F to 46°F for 24 hours and at room temperature for an additional 12 hours.

Reconstitution Withdraw necessary amount of rituximab and dilute to a final concentration of 1-4 mg/mL with 0.9% sodium chloride or 5% dextrose in water.

Pharmacodynamics/Kinetics

Duration: Detectable in serum 3-6 months after completion of treatment; B-cell recovery begins ~6 months following completion of treatment; median B-cell levels return to normal by 12 months following completion of treatment

Absorption: I.V.: Immediate and results in a rapid and sustained depletion of circulating and tissue-based B cells

Half-life elimination:

>100 mg/m^2: 4.4 days (range 1.6-10.5 days)

375 mg/m^2: 50 hours (following first dose) to 174 hours (following fourth dose)

Excretion: Uncertain; may undergo phagocytosis and catabolism in the reticuloendothelial system (RES)

Dosage Adults: I.V. infusion (refer to individual protocols):

Manufacturer's labeling: 375 mg/m^2 once weekly for 4-8 weeks

or

100 mg/m^2 I.V. day 1, then 375 mg/m^2 3 times/week for 11 doses has also been reported (cycles may be repeated in patients with refractory or relapsed disease)

(Continued)

Rituximab *(Continued)*

Retreatment following disease progression: 375 mg/m^2 once weekly for 4 doses

Combination therapy with ibritumomab: 250 mg/m^2 I.V. day 1; repeat in 7-9 days with ibritumomab (also see Ibritumomab monograph *on page 439*):

Combination Regimens

Leukemia, chronic lymphocytic: Fludarabine-Rituximab *on page 890*

Lymphoma, non-Hodgkins:

R-CHOP *on page 936*

R-CVP *on page 936*

Administration Do **not** administer as an I.V. push.

Initial infusion: Start rate of 50 mg/hour; if there is no reaction, increase the rate 50 mg/hour every 30 minutes, to a maximum of 400 mg/hour.

Subsequent infusions: Start at 100 mg/hour; if there is no reaction, increase the rate 100 mg/hour every 30 minutes, to a maximum of 400 mg/hour.

Note: If a reaction occurs, slow or stop the infusion. If the reaction abates, restart infusion at 50% of the previous dose.

In most cases, patients who have experienced nonlife-threatening reactions have been able to complete the full course of therapy. Rituximab is associated with hypersensitivity reactions which may respond to adjustments in the infusion rate.

Dosage Forms Injection, solution [preservative free]: 10 mg/mL (10 mL, 50 mL)

Monitoring Parameters CBC with differential, peripheral CD20$^+$ cells; HAMA/HACA titers (high levels may increase the risk of allergic reactions); renal function, fluid balance; cardiac monitoring during and after infusion in patients with pre-existing cardiac disease or if arrhythmias develop during or after subsequent infusions

Screening for Hepatitis B in high-risk persons may be considered prior to initiation of rituximab therapy. In addition, carriers and patients with evidence of recovery from prior hepatitis B infection should be monitored closely for clinical and laboratory signs of HBV infection during therapy and for up to a year following completion of treatment.

Selected Readings

Boye J, Elter T, and Engert A, "An Overview of the Current Clinical Use of the Anti-CD20 Monoclonal Antibody Rituximab," *Ann Oncol*, 2003, 14(4):520-35.

Grillo-Lopez AJ, "Rituximab (Rituxan/MabThera): The First Decade (1993-2003)," *Expert Rev Anticancer Ther*, 2003, 3(6):767-79.

Maloney DG, Smith B, and Rose A, "Rituximab: Mechanism of Action and Resistance," *Semin Oncol*, 2002, 29(1 Suppl 2):2-9.

Multani P and White CA, "Rituximab," *Cancer Chemother Biol Response Modif*, 2003, 21:235-58.

Smith MR, "Rituximab (Monoclonal Anti-CD20 Antibody): Mechanisms of Action and Resistance," *Oncogene*, 2003, 22(47):7359-68.

- ♦ **Riva-Lorazepam (Can)** *see* Lorazepam *on page 517*
- ♦ **rLFN-α2** *see* Interferon Alfa-2b *on page 471*
- ♦ **RMS®** *see* Morphine Sulfate *on page 588*
- ♦ **Ro 5488** *see* Tretinoin (Oral) *on page 792*
- ♦ **Rocephin®** *see* Ceftriaxone *on page 168*
- ♦ **Roferon-A®** *see* Interferon Alfa-2a *on page 466*
- ♦ **Roxanol™** *see* Morphine Sulfate *on page 588*

Sargramostim (sar GRAM oh stim)

Medication Safety Issues
Sound-alike/look-alike issues:
Leukine® may be confused with Leukeran®

Related Information
Management of Infections *on page 978*
Transplantation *on page 1019*

U.S. Brand Names Leukine®

Canadian Brand Names Leukine™

Generic Available No

Synonyms GM-CSF; Granulocyte-Macrophage Colony Stimulating Factor; rGM-CSF

Pharmacologic Category Colony Stimulating Factor

Pregnancy Risk Factor C

Lactation Excretion in breast milk unknown

Use

Myeloid reconstitution after autologous bone marrow transplantation: Non-Hodgkin's lymphoma (NHL), acute lymphoblastic leukemia (ALL), Hodgkin's lymphoma, metastatic breast cancer

Myeloid reconstitution after allogeneic bone marrow transplantation

Peripheral stem cell transplantation: Metastatic breast cancer, non-Hodgkin's lymphoma, Hodgkin's lymphoma, multiple myeloma

Orphan drug:

Acute myelogenous leukemia (AML) following induction chemotherapy in older adults to shorten time to neutrophil recovery and to reduce the incidence of severe and life-threatening infections and infections resulting in death

(Continued)

Sargramostim *(Continued)*

Bone marrow transplant (allogeneic or autologous) failure or engraftment delay

Safety and efficacy of GM-CSF given simultaneously with cytotoxic chemotherapy have not been established. Concurrent treatment may increase myelosuppression.

Mechanism of Action Stimulates proliferation, differentiation and functional activity of neutrophils, eosinophils, monocytes, and macrophages, as indicated: See table.

Comparative Effects — G-CSF vs GM-CSF

Proliferation/Differentiation	G-CSF (Filgrastim)	GM-CSF (Sargramostim)
Neutrophils	Yes	Yes
Eosinophils	No	Yes
Macrophages	No	Yes
Neutrophil migration	Enhanced	Inhibited

Labeled Contraindications Hypersensitivity to sargramostim, yeast-derived products, or any component of the formulation; concurrent myelosuppressive chemotherapy or radiation therapy. The solution for injection contains benzyl alcohol and should not be used in neonates.

Warnings/Precautions Simultaneous administration, or administration 24 hours preceding/following cytotoxic chemotherapy or radiotherapy is not recommended. Use with caution in patients with pre-existing cardiac problems, hypoxia, fluid retention, pulmonary infiltrates or CHF, renal or hepatic impairment, rapid increase in peripheral blood counts. If ANC is >20,000/mm^3, or platelets >500,000/mm^3 decrease dose by 50% or discontinue drug (counts will fall to normal within 3-7 days after discontinuing drug). The manufacturer recommends that precaution should be exercised in the usage of sargramostim in any malignancy with myeloid characteristics. Sargramostim can potentially act as a growth factor for any tumor type, particularly myeloid malignancies. Tumors of nonhematopoietic origin may have surface receptors for sargramostim.

Adverse Reactions

>10%:

Cardiovascular: Hypotension, tachycardia, flushing, and syncope may occur with the first dose of a cycle ("first-dose effect"); peripheral edema (11%)

Central nervous system: Headache (26%)

Dermatologic: Rash, alopecia

Endocrine & metabolic: Polydipsia

Gastrointestinal: Diarrhea (52% to 89%), stomatitis, mucositis

Local: Local reactions at the injection site (~50%)

Neuromuscular & skeletal: Myalgia (18%), arthralgia (21%), bone pain

Renal: Increased serum creatinine (14%)

Respiratory: Dyspnea (28%)

1% to 10%:

Cardiovascular: Transient supraventricular arrhythmia; chest pain; capillary leak syndrome; pericardial effusion (4%)

Central nervous system: Headache

Gastrointestinal: Nausea, vomiting

Hematologic: Leukocytosis, thrombocytopenia

Neuromuscular & skeletal: Weakness

Respiratory: Cough; pleural effusion (1%)

<1%: Anaphylaxis, anorexia, constipation, fever, lethargy, malaise, pericarditis, rigors, sore throat, thrombophlebitis

Postmarketing and/or case reports: Arrhythmia, eosinophilia, thrombosis

Vesicant No

Emetic Potential Very low (<10%)

Overdosage/Toxicology Symptoms of overdose include dyspnea, malaise, nausea, fever, headache, and chills. Discontinue drug and wait for levels to fall. Treatment is supportive. Monitor CBC, respiratory symptoms, and fluid status. Discontinue drug and wait for levels to fall, monitor for pulmonary edema. Toxicity of GM-CSF is dose dependent. Severe reactions such as capillary leak syndrome are seen at higher doses (>15 mcg/kg/day).

Drug Interactions

Increased Effect/Toxicity: Lithium, corticosteroids may potentiate myeloproliferative effects.

Storage/Stability Sargramostim should be stored at 2°C to 8°C (36°F to 46°F). Vials should not be frozen or shaken. Preparations made with SWFI should be administered as soon as possible, and discarded within 6 hours of reconstitution. Preparations made with bacteriostatic water may be stored for up to 20 days at 2°C to 8°C (36°F to 46°F). Preparations diluted with NS are stable for 48 hours at room temperature and refrigeration.

Reconstitution

Solution for injection: May be stored for up to 20 days at 2°C to 8°C (36°F to 46°F) once the vial has been entered. Discard remaining solution after 20 days.

Powder for injection: May be reconstituted with preservative free SWFI or bacteriostatic water for injection (with benzyl alcohol 0.9%). Gently swirl to reconstitute; do not shake.

Sargramostim may also be further diluted in 0.9% sodium chloride to a concentration of ≥10 mcg/mL for I.V. infusion administration.

If the final concentration of sargramostim is <10 mcg/mL, 1 mg of human albumin/1 mL of 0.9% sodium chloride (eg, 1 mL of 5% human albumin/50 mL of 0.9% sodium chloride) should be added.

Standard diluent: 25-100 mL NS

Compatibility Stable in NS, sterile water for injection, bacteriostatic water; **incompatible** with dextrose-containing solutions

Y-site administration: Compatible: Amikacin, aminophylline, aztreonam, bleomycin, butorphanol, calcium gluconate, carboplatin, carmustine, cefazolin, cefepime, cefotaxime, cefotetan, ceftizoxime, ceftriaxone, cefuroxime, cimetidine, cisplatin, clindamycin, co-trimoxazole, cyclophosphamide, cyclosporine, cytarabine, dacarbazine, dactinomycin, dexamethasone sodium phosphate, diphenhydramine, dopamine, doxorubicin, doxycycline, droperidol, etoposide, famotidine, fentanyl, floxuridine, fluconazole, fluorouracil, furosemide, gentamicin, granisetron, heparin, idarubicin, ifosfamide, immune globulin, magnesium sulfate, mannitol, mechlorethamine, meperidine, mesna, methotrexate, metoclopramide, metronidazole, minocycline, mitoxantrone, netilmicin, pentostatin, piperacillin/tazobactam, potassium chloride, prochlorperazine edisylate, promethazine, ranitidine, (Continued)

Sargramostim *(Continued)*

teniposide, ticarcillin, ticarcillin/clavulanate, vinblastine, vincristine, zidovudine. **Incompatible:** Acyclovir, ampicillin, ampicillin/sulbactam, cefoperazone, chlorpromazine, ganciclovir, haloperidol, hydrocortisone sodium phosphate, hydrocortisone sodium succinate, hydromorphone, hydroxyzine, imipenem/cilastatin, lorazepam, methylprednisolone sodium succinate, mitomycin, morphine, nalbuphine, ondansetron, piperacillin, sodium bicarbonate, tobramycin. **Variable (consult detailed reference):** Amphotericin B, amsacrine, ceftazidime, vancomycin

Pharmacodynamics/Kinetics

Onset of action: Increase in WBC: 7-14 days
Duration: WBCs return to baseline within 1 week of discontinuing drug
Half-life elimination: 2 hours
Time to peak, serum: SubQ: 1-2 hours

Dosage

Children and Adults: I.V. infusion over ≥2 hours or SubQ

Rounding the dose to the nearest vial size enhances patient convenience and reduce costs without clinical detriment

Myeloid reconstitution after peripheral stem cell, allogeneic or autologous bone marrow transplant: I.V.: 250 mcg/m^2/day for 21 days to begin 2-4 hours after the marrow infusion or ≥24 hours after chemotherapy or 12 hours after last dose of radiotherapy

If a severe adverse reaction occurs, reduce or temporarily discontinue the dose until the reaction abates

If blast cells appear or progression of the underlying disease occurs, disrupt treatment

Interrupt or reduce the dose by half if ANC is >20,000 cells/mm^3

Patients should not receive sargramostim until the postmarrow infusion ANC is <500 cells/mm^3

Neutrophil recovery following chemotherapy in AML: I.V.: 250 mcg/m^2/day over a 4-hour period starting approximately day 11 or 4 days following the completion of induction chemotherapy, if day 10 bone marrow is hypoblastic with <5% blasts

If a second cycle of chemotherapy is necessary, administer ~4 days after the completion of chemotherapy if the bone marrow is hypoblastic with <5% blasts

Continue sargramostim until ANC is >1500 cells/mm^3 for consecutive days or a maximum of 42 days

Discontinue sargramostim immediately if leukemic regrowth occurs

If a severe adverse reaction occurs, reduce the dose by 50% or temporarily discontinue the dose until the reaction abates

Mobilization of peripheral blood progenitor cells: I.V.: 250 mcg/m^2/day over 24 hours or SubQ once daily

Continue the same dose through the period of PBPC collection

The optimal schedule for PBPC collection has not been established (usually begun by day 5 and performed daily until protocol specified targets are achieved)

If WBC >50,000 cells/mm^3, reduce the dose by 50%

If adequate numbers of progenitor cells are not collected, consider other mobilization therapy

Postperipheral blood progenitor cell transplantation: I.V.: 250 mcg/m^2/day or SubQ once daily beginning immediately following infusion of progenitor cells and continuing until ANC is >1500 for 3 consecutive days is attained

BMT failure or engraftment delay: I.V.: 250 mcg/m^2/day for 14 days

The dose can be repeated after 7 days off therapy if engraftment has not occurred

If engraftment still has not occurred, a third course of 500 mcg/m^2/day for 14 days may be tried after another 7 days off therapy; if there is still no improvement, it is unlikely that further dose escalation will be beneficial

If a severe adverse reaction occurs, reduce or temporarily discontinue the dose until the reaction abates

If blast cells appear or disease progression occurs, discontinue treatment

Combination Regimens

Lymphoma, non-Hodgkin's: CODOX-M *on page 865*

Administration Sargramostim is administered as a subcutaneous injection or intravenous infusion; intravenous infusion should be over at least 2 hours; continuous infusions may be more effective than short infusion or bolus injection. An in-line membrane filter should not be used for intravenous injection.

Dosage Forms

Injection, powder for reconstitution: 250 mcg

Injection, solution: 500 mcg/mL (1 mL) [contains benzyl alcohol]

Monitoring Parameters Vital signs, weight, CBC with differential, platelets, renal/liver function tests, especially with previous dysfunction, WBC with differential, pulmonary function

Patient Information You may experience bone pain (request analgesic), nausea and vomiting (small frequent meals may help), hair loss (reversible). Report fever, chills, unhealed sores, severe bone pain, difficulty breathing, swelling or pain at infusion site. Avoid crowds or exposure to infected persons; you will be susceptible to infection.

Additional Information Reimbursement Hotline (Leukine®): 1-800-321-4669

Selected Readings

Lieschke GJ and Burgess AW, "Granulocyte Colony-Stimulating Factor and Granulocyte-Macrophage Colony-Stimulating Factor," (1) *N Engl J Med*, 1992, 327(1):28-35.

Lieschke GJ and Burgess AW, "Granulocyte Colony-Stimulating Factor and Granulocyte-Macrophage Colony-Stimulating Factor," (2) *N Engl J Med*, 1992, 327(2):99-106.

Stute N, Furman WL, Schell M, et al, "Pharmacokinetics of Recombinant Human Granulocyte - Macrophage Colony - Stimulating Factor in Children After Intravenous and Subcutaneous Administration," *J Pharm Sci*, 1995, 84(7):824-8.

- ◆ **Sarna® HC (Can)** *see* Hydrocortisone *on page 419*
- ◆ **Sarnol®-HC [OTC]** *see* Hydrocortisone *on page 419*
- ◆ **SB-265805** *see* Gemifloxacin *on page 392*
- ◆ **SC 33428** *see* Idarubicin *on page 443*
- ◆ **SCH 13521** *see* Flutamide *on page 366*
- ◆ **Septra®** *see* Sulfamethoxazole and Trimethoprim *on page 727*
- ◆ **Septra® DS** *see* Sulfamethoxazole and Trimethoprim *on page 727*
- ◆ **Septra® Injection (Can)** *see* Sulfamethoxazole and Trimethoprim *on page 727*
- ◆ **Simulect®** *see* Basiliximab *on page 118*

Sirolimus (sir OH li mus)

U.S. Brand Names Rapamune®

Canadian Brand Names Rapamune®

Generic Available No

Pharmacologic Category Immunosuppressant Agent

Pregnancy Risk Factor C

Lactation Excretion in breast milk unknown/not recommended

Use Prophylaxis of organ rejection in patients receiving renal transplants, in combination with corticosteroids and cyclosporine (cyclosporine may be withdrawn in low-to-moderate immunological risk patients after 2-4 months, in conjunction with an increase in sirolimus dosage)

Unlabeled/Investigational Use Investigational: Immunosuppression in other forms of solid organ transplantation

Mechanism of Action Sirolimus inhibits T-lymphocyte activation and proliferation in response to antigenic and cytokine stimulation. Its mechanism differs from other immunosuppressants. It inhibits acute rejection of allografts and prolongs graft survival.

Labeled Contraindications Hypersensitivity to sirolimus or any component of the formulation

Warnings/Precautions Immunosuppressive agents, including sirolimus, increase the risk of infection and may be associated with the development of lymphoma. May increase serum lipids (cholesterol and triglycerides). Use with caution in patients with hyperlipidemia. May decrease GFR and increase serum creatinine. Use caution in patients with renal impairment, or when used concurrently with medications which may alter renal function. Monitor renal function closely when combined with cyclosporine; consider dosage adjustment or discontinue in patients with increasing serum creatinine. Has been associated with an increased risk of lymphocele. Cases of interstitial lung disease (eg, pneumonitis, bronchiolitis obliterans organizing pneumonia, pulmonary fibrosis) have been observed; risk may be increased with higher trough levels. Avoid concurrent use of strong CYP3A4 inhibitors or strong inducers of either CYP3A4 or P-glycoprotein. Anaphylactic reactions have been reported. May increase sensitivity to UV light; use appropriate sun protection.

Sirolimus is not recommended for use in liver transplant patients; studies indicate an association with an increase risk of hepatic artery thrombosis and graft failure in these patients. Cases of bronchial anastomotic dehiscence have been reported in lung transplant patients when sirolimus was used as part of an immunosuppressive regimen; most of these reactions were fatal. Use in patients with lung transplants is not recommended. Safety and efficacy of cyclosporine withdrawal in high-risk patients is not currently recommended. Safety and efficacy in children <13 years of age, or in adolescent patients <18 years of age considered at high immunological risk, have not been established.

Adverse Reactions Incidence of many adverse effects is dose related
>20%:

Cardiovascular: Hypertension (39% to 49%), peripheral edema (54% to 64%), edema (16% to 24%), chest pain (16% to 24%)

Central nervous system: Fever (23% to 34%), headache (23% to 34%), pain (24% to 33%), insomnia (13% to 22%)

Dermatologic: Acne (20% to 31%)

Endocrine & metabolic: Hypercholesterolemia (38% to 46%), hypophosphatemia (15% to 23%), hyperlipidemia (38% to 57%), hypokalemia (11% to 21%)

Gastrointestinal: Abdominal pain (28% to 36%), nausea (25% to 36%), vomiting (19% to 25%), diarrhea (25% to 42%), constipation (28% to 38%), dyspepsia (17% to 25%), weight gain (8% to 21%)

Genitourinary: Urinary tract infection (20% to 33%)

Hematologic: Anemia (23% to 37%), thrombocytopenia (13% to 40%)

Neuromuscular & skeletal: Arthralgia (25% to 31%), weakness (22% to 40%), back pain (16% to 26%), tremor (21% to 31%)

Renal: Serum creatinine increased (35% to 40%)

Respiratory: Dyspnea (22% to 30%), upper respiratory infection (20% to 26%), pharyngitis (16% to 21%)

3% to 20%:

Cardiovascular: Atrial fibrillation, CHF, hypervolemia, hypotension, palpitation, peripheral vascular disorder, postural hypotension, syncope, tachycardia, thrombosis, vasodilation, venous thromboembolism

Central nervous system: Chills, malaise, anxiety, confusion, depression, dizziness, emotional lability, hypoesthesia, hypotonia, insomnia, neuropathy, somnolence

Dermatologic: Dermatitis (fungal), hirsutism, pruritus, skin hypertrophy, dermal ulcer, ecchymosis, cellulitis, rash (10% to 20%)

Endocrine & metabolic: Cushing's syndrome, diabetes mellitus, glycosuria, acidosis, dehydration, hypercalcemia, hyperglycemia, hyperphosphatemia, hypocalcemia, hypoglycemia, hypomagnesemia, hyponatremia, hyperkalemia (12% to 17%)

Gastrointestinal: Enlarged abdomen, anorexia, dysphagia, eructation, esophagitis, flatulence, gastritis, gastroenteritis, gingivitis, gingival hyperplasia, ileus, mouth ulceration, oral moniliasis, stomatitis, weight loss

Genitourinary: Pelvic pain, scrotal edema, testis disorder, impotence

Hematologic: Leukocytosis, polycythemia, TTP, hemolytic-uremic syndrome, hemorrhage, leukopenia (9% to 15%)

Hepatic: Abnormal liver function tests, alkaline phosphatase increased, ascites, LDH increased, transaminases increased

Local: Thrombophlebitis

Neuromuscular & skeletal: Arthrosis, bone necrosis, CPK increased, leg cramps, myalgia, osteoporosis, tetany, hypertonia, paresthesia

Ocular: Abnormal vision, cataract, conjunctivitis

Otic: Ear pain, deafness, otitis media, tinnitus

Renal: Albuminuria, bladder pain, BUN increased, dysuria, hematuria, hydronephrosis, kidney pain, tubular necrosis, nocturia, oliguria, pyuria, nephropathy (toxic), urinary frequency, urinary incontinence, urinary retention

Respiratory: Asthma, atelectasis, bronchitis, cough, epistaxis, hypoxia, lung edema, pleural effusion, pneumonia, rhinitis, sinusitis

Miscellaneous: Abscess, diaphoresis, facial edema, flu-like syndrome, hernia, infection, lymphadenopathy, lymphocele, peritonitis, sepsis

Postmarketing and/or case reports: Anaphylaxis; anaphylactoid reaction; interstitial lung disease (pneumonitis, pulmonary fibrosis, and bronchiolitis obliterans organizing pneumonia) with no identified infectious etiology; fascial dehiscence; hepatic necrosis; neutropenia; pancytopenia; anastomotic disruption. In liver transplant patients (not an

(Continued)

Sirolimus *(Continued)*

approved use), an increase in hepatic artery thrombosis and graft failure were noted in clinical trials. In lung transplant patients (not an approved use), bronchial anastomotic dehiscence has been reported.

Overdosage/Toxicology Experience with overdosage has been limited. Dose-limiting toxicities include immune suppression. Reported symptoms of overdose include atrial fibrillation. Treatment is supportive, dialysis is not likely to facilitate removal.

Drug Interactions

Cytochrome P450 Effect: Substrate of CYP3A4 (major); **Inhibits** CYP3A4 (weak)

Increased Effect/Toxicity: Cyclosporine increases sirolimus concentrations during concurrent therapy, and cyclosporine levels may be increased; sirolimus should be taken 4 hours after cyclosporine oral solution (modified) and/or cyclosporine capsules (modified). CYP3A4 inhibitors may increase the levels/effects of sirolimus; example inhibitors include azole antifungals, ciprofloxacin, clarithromycin, diclofenac, diltiazem, doxycycline, erythromycin, imatinib, isoniazid, nefazodone, nicardipine, propofol, protease inhibitors, quinidine, and verapamil; avoid concurrent use. Vaccination may be less effective and use of live vaccines should be avoided during sirolimus therapy.

Decreased Effect: CYP3A4 inducers may decrease the levels/effects of sirolimus; example inducers include aminoglutethimide, carbamazepine, nafcillin, nevirapine, phenobarbital, phenytoin, and rifamycins.

Ethanol/Nutrition/Herb Interactions

Food: Do not administer with grapefruit juice; may decrease clearance of sirolimus. Ingestion with high-fat meals decreases peak concentrations but increases AUC by 35%. Sirolimus should be taken consistently either with or without food to minimize variability.

Herb/Nutraceutical: St John's wort may decrease sirolimus levels; avoid concurrent use. Avoid cat's claw, echinacea (have immunostimulant properties).

Storage/Stability

Oral solution: Protect from light and store under refrigeration, 2°C to 8°C (36°F to 46°F). A slight haze may develop in refrigerated solutions, but the quality of the product is not affected. After opening, solution should be used in 1 month. If necessary, may be stored at temperatures up to 25°C (77°F) for several days after opening (up to 24 hours for pouches and not >15 days for bottles). Product may be stored in amber syringe for a maximum of 24 hours (at room temperature or refrigerated). Solution should be used immediately following dilution.

Tablet: Store at room temperature of 20°C to 25°C (68°F to 77°F). Protect from light.

Pharmacodynamics/Kinetics

Absorption: Rapid

Distribution: 12 L/kg (range: 4-20 L/kg)

Protein binding: 92%, primarily to albumin

Metabolism: Extensively hepatic via CYP3A; P-glycoprotein-mediated efflux into gut lumen

Bioavailability: Oral solution: 14%; Oral tablet: 18%

Half-life elimination: Mean: 62 hours

Time to peak: 1-2 hours

Excretion: Feces (91%); urine (2%)

Dosage Oral:

Combination therapy with cyclosporine: For *de novo* transplant recipients, a loading dose of 3 times the daily maintenance dose should be administered on day 1 of dosing. Doses should be taken 4 hours after cyclosporine and should be taken consistently either with or without food.

Children ≥13 years and Adults: Dosing by body weight:

<40 kg: Loading dose: 3 mg/m^2 on day 1, followed by maintenance dosing of 1 mg/m^2/day

≥40 kg: Loading dose: 6 mg on day 1; maintenance: 2 mg/day

Maintenance therapy after withdrawal of cyclosporine:

Following 2-4 months of combined therapy, withdrawal of cyclosporine may be considered in low-to-moderate risk patients. Cyclosporine withdrawal in not recommended in high immunological risk patients. Cyclosporine should be discontinued over 4-8 weeks, and a necessary increase in the dosage of sirolimus (up to fourfold) should be anticipated due to removal of metabolic inhibition by cyclosporine and to maintain adequate immunosuppressive effects.

Sirolimus dosages should be adjusted to maintain trough concentrations of 12-24 ng/mL. Dosage should be adjusted at intervals of 7-14 days to account for the long half-life of sirolimus. Considerable increases in dosage may require an additional loading dose, calculated as the difference between the target concentration and the current concentration, multiplied by a factor of 3. Loading doses >40 mg may be administered over two days. Serum concentrations should not be used as the sole basis for dosage adjustment (monitor clinical signs/symptoms, tissue biopsy, and laboratory parameters).

Dosage adjustment in renal impairment: No dosage adjustment is necessary in renal impairment

Dosage adjustment in hepatic impairment: Reduce maintenance dose by approximately 33% in hepatic impairment. Loading dose is unchanged.

Administration The solution should be mixed with at least 2 ounces of water or orange juice. No other liquids should be used for dilution. Patient should drink diluted solution immediately. The cup should then be refilled with an additional 4 ounces of water or orange juice, stirred vigorously, and the patient should drink the contents at once. Sirolimus should be taken 4 hours after cyclosporine oral solution (modified) or cyclosporine capsules (modified)

Dosage Forms

Solution, oral [bottle]: 1 mg/mL (60 mL, 150 mL) [contains ethanol 1.5% to 2.5%; packaged with 1 mL, 2 mL, or 5 mL oral syringes]

Solution, oral [unit-dose pouch]: 1 mg/mL (1 mL, 2 mL, 5 mL) [contains ethanol 1.5% to 2.5%; packaged in cartons of 30]

Tablet: 1 mg, 2 mg, 5 mg

Monitoring Parameters Monitor sirolimus levels in pediatric patients, patients ≥13 years of age weighing <40 kg, patients with hepatic impairment, or on concurrent potent inhibitors or inducers of CYP3A4, and/or if cyclosporine dosing is markedly reduced or discontinued. Also monitor serum cholesterol and triglycerides, blood pressure, and serum creatinine. Serum drug concentrations should be determined 3-4 days after loading doses; however, these concentrations should not be used as the
(Continued)

Sirolimus *(Continued)*

sole basis for dosage adjustment, especially during withdrawal of cyclosporine (monitor clinical signs/symptoms, tissue biopsy, and laboratory parameters).

Dietary Considerations Take consistently, with or without food, to minimize variability of absorption.

Patient Information Do not get pregnant while taking this medication. Use reliable contraception while on this medication and for 3 months after discontinuation. May be taken with or without food but take medication consistently with respect to meals (always take with food or always take on an empty stomach). Wear protective clothing and use sunscreen to limit exposure to sunlight and UV light; decreases risk of skin cancer.

Additional Information Sirolimus tablets and oral solution are not bioequivalent, due to differences in absorption. Clinical equivalence was seen using 2 mg tablet and 2 mg solution. It is not known if higher doses are also clinically equivalent.

Selected Readings

Kahan BD, Keown P, Levy GA, et al, "Therapeutic Drug Monitoring of Immunosuppressant Drugs in Clinical Practice," *Clin Ther*, 2002, 24(3):330-50.

Oberbauer R, Kreis H, Johnson RW, et al, "Long-term Improvement in Renal Function With Sirolimus After Early Cyclosporine Withdrawal in Renal Transplant Recipients: 2-Year Results of the Rapamune Maintenance Regimen Study," *Transplantation*, 2003, 76(2):364-70.

♦ **SK and F 104864** *see* Topotecan *on page 776*

♦ **SKF 104864** *see* Topotecan *on page 776*

♦ **SKF 104864-A** *see* Topotecan *on page 776*

♦ **SMZ-TMP** *see* Sulfamethoxazole and Trimethoprim *on page 727*

♦ **Sodium 2-Mercaptoethane Sulfonate** *see* Mesna *on page 542*

♦ **Sodium Etidronate** *see* Etidronate Disodium *on page 313*

♦ **Sodium Fusidate** *see* Fusidic Acid *on page 378*

♦ **Sodium Hyposulfate** *see* Sodium Thiosulfate *on page 722*

♦ **Sodium Nafcillin** *see* Nafcillin *on page 605*

Sodium Thiosulfate *(SOW dee um thye oh SUL fate)*

Related Information

Management of Drug Extravasations *on page 965*

U.S. Brand Names Versiclear™

Generic Available Yes: Injection

Synonyms Disodium Thiosulfate Pentahydrate; Pentahydrate; Sodium Hyposulfate; Sodium Thiosulphate; Thiosulfuric Acid Disodium Salt

Pharmacologic Category Antidote

Pregnancy Risk Factor C

Use

Parenteral: Used alone or with sodium nitrite or amyl nitrite in cyanide poisoning or arsenic poisoning; reduce the risk of nephrotoxicity associated with cisplatin therapy

Topical: Treatment of tinea versicolor

Unlabeled/Investigational Use Management of I.V. extravasation

Mechanism of Action

Cyanide toxicity: Increases the rate of detoxification of cyanide by the enzyme rhodanese by providing an extra sulfur

Cisplatin toxicity: Complexes with cisplatin to form a compound that is nontoxic to either normal or cancerous cells

Labeled Contraindications Hypersensitivity to sodium thiosulfate or any component of the formulation

Warnings/Precautions Discontinue topical use if irritation or sensitivity occurs. Rapid I.V. infusion has caused transient hypotension and ECG changes in dogs. May increase risk of thiocyanate intoxication.

Adverse Reactions

1% to 10%:

Cardiovascular: Hypotension

Central nervous system: Coma, CNS depression secondary to thiocyanate intoxication, psychosis, confusion

Dermatologic: Contact dermatitis, local irritation

Neuromuscular & skeletal: Weakness

Otic: Tinnitus

<1%: Gastrointestinal: Diarrhea (following large oral doses)

Vesicant No

Emetic Potential Very low (<10%)

Pharmacodynamics/Kinetics

Absorption: Oral: Poor

Distribution: Extracellular fluid

Half-life elimination: 0.65 hour

Excretion: Urine (28.5% as unchanged drug)

Dosage

Cyanide and nitroprusside antidote: I.V.:

Children <25 kg: 50 mg/kg after receiving 4.5-10 mg/kg sodium nitrite; a half dose of each may be repeated if necessary

Children >25 kg and Adults: 12.5 g after 300 mg of sodium nitrite; a half dose of each may be repeated if necessary

Cyanide poisoning: I.V.: Dose should be based on determination as with nitrite, at rate of 2.5-5 mL/minute to maximum of 50 mL.

Variation of sodium nitrite and sodium thiosulfate dose, based on hemoglobin concentration: See table.

Variation of Sodium Nitrite and Sodium Thiosulfate Dose With Hemoglobin Concentration[1]

Hemoglobin (g/dL)	Initial Dose Sodium Nitrite (mg/kg)	Initial Dose Sodium Nitrite 3% (mL/kg)	Initial Dose Sodium Thiosulfate 25% (mL/kg)
7	5.8	0.19	0.95
8	6.6	0.22	1.10
9	7.5	0.25	1.25
10	8.3	0.27	1.35
11	9.1	0.30	1.50
12	10.0	0.33	1.65
13	10.8	0.36	1.80
14	11.6	0.39	1.95

[1]Adapted from Berlin DM Jr, "The Treatment of Cyanide Poisoning in Children," *Pediatrics*, 1970, 46:793.

(Continued)

Sodium Thiosulfate *(Continued)*

Cisplatin rescue should be given before or during cisplatin administration: I.V. infusion (in sterile water): 12 g/m^2 over 6 hours or 9 g/m^2 I.V. push followed by 1.2 g/m^2 continuous infusion for 6 hours

Arsenic poisoning: I.V.: 1 mL first day, 2 mL second day, 3 mL third day, 4 mL fourth day, 5 mL on alternate days thereafter

Children and Adults:

Topical: 20% to 25% solution: Apply a thin layer to affected areas twice daily

SubQ: Drug extravasation (unlabeled use):

2% solution: Infiltrate SubQ into the affected area

1/6 M (~4%) solution: 5-10 mL infused through I.V. line and SubQ into the affected area

Administration

I.V.: Inject slowly, over at least 10 minutes; rapid administration may cause hypotension.

Topical: Do not apply to or near eyes.

Dosage Forms

Injection, solution [preservative free]: 100 mg/mL (10 mL); 250 mg/mL (50 mL)

Lotion (Versiclear™): Sodium thiosulfate 25% and salicylic acid 1% (120 mL) [contains isopropyl alcohol 10%]

Monitoring Parameters Monitor for signs of thiocyanate toxicity

Patient Information Avoid topical application near the eyes, mouth, or other mucous membranes; notify prescriber if condition worsens or burning or irritation occurs; shake well before using

- **Sodium Thiosulphate** *see* Sodium Thiosulfate *on page 722*
- **Solu-Cortef**® *see* Hydrocortisone *on page 419*
- **Solu-Medrol**® *see* MethylPREDNISolone *on page 558*
- **Sporanox**® *see* Itraconazole *on page 486*
- **Statex**® **(Can)** *see* Morphine Sulfate *on page 588*
- **Stemetil**® **(Can)** *see* Prochlorperazine *on page 691*
- **Sterapred**® *see* PredniSONE *on page 683*
- **Sterapred**® **DS** *see* PredniSONE *on page 683*
- **STI571** *see* Imatinib *on page 449*
- **Stimate**™ *see* Desmopressin *on page 259*

Streptozocin (strep toe ZOE sin)

Medication Safety Issues

Sound-alike/look-alike issues:

Streptozocin may be confused with streptomycin

Related Information

Management of Drug Extravasations *on page 965*

Management of Nausea and Vomiting *on page 982*

Safe Handling of Hazardous Drugs *on page 1034*

U.S. Brand Names Zanosar®

Canadian Brand Names Zanosar®

Generic Available No

Synonyms NSC-85998

Pharmacologic Category Antineoplastic Agent, Alkylating Agent

Pregnancy Risk Factor D

Lactation Enters breast milk/contraindicated

Use Treatment of metastatic islet cell carcinoma of the pancreas, carcinoid tumor and syndrome, Hodgkin's disease, palliative treatment of colorectal cancer

Mechanism of Action Interferes with the normal function of DNA by alkylation and cross-linking the strands of DNA, and by possible protein modification

Labeled Contraindications Pregnancy

Warnings/Precautions Hazardous agent - use appropriate precautions for handling and disposal. See Safe Handling of Hazardous Drugs *on page 1034* in the Appendix. Renal toxicity is dose-related and cumulative and may be severe or fatal.

Adverse Reactions
>10%:
Gastrointestinal: Nausea and vomiting (100%)
Hepatic: Increased LFTs
Miscellaneous: Hypoalbuminemia
Renal: BUN increased, Cl_{cr} decreased, hypophosphatemia, nephrotoxicity (25% to 75%), proteinuria, renal dysfunction (65%), renal tubular acidosis
1% to 10%:
Endocrine & metabolic: Hypoglycemia (6%)
Gastrointestinal: Diarrhea (10%)
Local: Pain at injection site
<1%: Confusion, lethargy, depression, leukopenia, thrombocytopenia, liver dysfunction, secondary malignancy
Myelosuppressive:
WBC: Mild
Platelets: Mild
Onset: 7 days
Nadir: 14 days
Recovery: 21 days

Vesicant Yes; see Management of Drug Extravasations *on page 965.*

Emetic Potential Very high (>90%)

Overdosage/Toxicology Symptoms of overdose include bone marrow suppression, nausea, and vomiting. Treatment of bone marrow suppression is supportive.

Drug Interactions
Increased Effect/Toxicity: Doxorubicin toxicity may be increased with concurrent use of streptozocin. Manufacturer recommends doxorubicin dosage adjustment be considered.
Decreased Effect: Phenytoin results in negation of streptozocin cytotoxicity.

Storage/Stability Store intact vials under refrigeration; vials are stable for one year at room temperature. Solution reconstituted with 9.5 mL SWFI or NS to a concentration of 100 mg/mL is stable for 48 hours at room temperature and 96 hours under refrigeration. Further dilution in D_5W or NS is stable for 48 hours at room temperature and 96 hours under refrigeration when protected from light.

Reconstitution Dilute powder with 9.5 mL SWFI or NS to a concentration of 100 mg/mL.

Compatibility Stable in D_5W, NS

(Continued)

Streptozocin *(Continued)*

Y-site administration: Compatible: Amifostine, etoposide phosphate, filgrastim, gemcitabine, granisetron, melphalan, ondansetron, teniposide, thiotepa, vinorelbine. **Incompatible:** Allopurinol, aztreonam, cefepime, piperacillin/tazobactam

Pharmacodynamics/Kinetics

Duration: Disappears from serum in 4 hours

Distribution: Concentrates in liver, intestine, pancreas, and kidney

Metabolism: Rapidly hepatic

Half-life elimination: 35-40 minutes

Excretion: Urine (60% to 70% as metabolites); exhaled gases (5%); feces (1%)

Dosage I.V. (refer to individual protocols):

Children and Adults:

Single agent therapy: 1-1.5 g/m^2 weekly for 6 weeks followed by a 4-week rest period

Combination therapy: 0.5-1 g/m^2 for 5 consecutive days followed by a 4- to 6-week rest period

Dosing adjustment in renal impairment:

Cl_{cr} 10-50 mL/minute: Administer 75% of dose

Cl_{cr} <10 mL/minute: Administer 50% of dose

Hemodialysis: Unknown

CAPD effects: Unknown

CAVH effects: Unknown

Dosing adjustment in hepatic impairment: Dose should be decreased in patients with severe liver disease

Administration Administer as short (30-60 minutes) or 6-hour infusion; may be given by rapid I.V. push

Dosage Forms Injection, powder for reconstitution: 1 g

Monitoring Parameters Monitor renal function closely

Strontium-89 *(STRON shee um atey nine)*

U.S. Brand Names Metastron®

Canadian Brand Names Metastron®

Generic Available No

Synonyms Strontium-89 Chloride

Pharmacologic Category Radiopharmaceutical

Pregnancy Risk Factor D

Use Relief of bone pain in patients with skeletal metastases

Labeled Contraindications Hypersensitivity to any strontium-containing compounds or any other component of the formulation; pregnancy; breast-feeding

Warnings/Precautions Use caution in patients with bone marrow compromise; incontinent patients may require urinary catheterization. Body fluids may remain radioactive up to one week after injection. Not indicated for use in patients with cancer not involving bone and should be used with caution in patients whose platelet counts fall <60,000 or whose white blood cell counts fall <2400. A small number of patients have experienced a transient increase in bone pain at 36-72 hours postdose; this reaction is generally mild and self-limiting. It should be handled cautiously, in a similar manner to other radioactive drugs. Appropriate safety measures to minimize radiation to personnel should be instituted.

Adverse Reactions Most severe reactions of marrow toxicity can be managed by conventional means

Frequency not defined:

Cardiovascular: Flushing (most common after rapid injection)

Central nervous system: Fever and chills (rare)

Hematologic: Thrombocytopenia, leukopenia

Neuromuscular & skeletal: Increase in bone pain may occur (10% to 20% of patients)

Vesicant No

Emetic Potential Low (<10%)

Storage/Stability Store vial and its contents inside its transportation container at room temperature.

Dosage Adults: I.V.: 148 megabecquerel (4 millicurie) administered by slow I.V. injection over 1-2 minutes or 1.5-2.2 megabecquerel (40-60 microcurie)/kg; repeated doses are generally not recommended at intervals <90 days; measure the patient dose by a suitable radioactivity calibration system immediately prior to administration

Administration I.V. bolus injection over 1-2 minutes

Dosage Forms Injection, solution, as chloride [preservative free]: 10.9-22.6 mg/mL [148 megabecquerel, 4 millicurie] (10 mL)

Monitoring Parameters Routine blood tests

Patient Information Eat and drink normally, there is no need to avoid alcohol or caffeine unless already advised to do so; may be advised to take analgesics until Metastron® begins to become effective; the effect lasts for several months, if pain returns before that, notify medical personnel

Additional Information During the first week after injection, strontium-89 will be present in the blood and urine, therefore, the following common sense precautions should be instituted:

1. Where a normal toilet is available, use in preference to a urinal, flush the toilet twice
2. Wipe away any spilled urine with a tissue and flush it away
3. Have patient wash hands after using the toilet
4. Immediately wash any linen or clothes that become stained with blood or urine
5. Wash away any spilled blood if a cut occurs

Selected Readings

Brandi ML, "New Treatment Strategies: Ipriflavone Strontium, Vitamin D Metabolites and Analogs," *Am J Med*, 1993, 95(Suppl 5A):5A-69S-5A-74S.

Lincoln TA, "Importance of Initial Management of Persons Internally Contaminated with Radionuclides," *Am Ind Hyg Assoc J*, 1976, 37(1):16-21.

Robinson RG, Preston DF, Schiefelbein M, et al, "Strontium 89 Therapy for the Palliation of Pain Due to Osseous Metastases," *JAMA*, 1995, 274(5):420-4.

♦ **Strontium-89 Chloride** *see* Strontium-89 *on page 726*

♦ **Sublimaze**® *see* Fentanyl *on page 335*

Sulfamethoxazole and Trimethoprim

(sul fa meth OKS a zole & trye METH oh prim)

Medication Safety Issues

Sound-alike/look-alike issues:

Bactrim™ may be confused with bacitracin, Bactine®

Co-trimoxazole may be confused with clotrimazole

Septra® may be confused with Ceptaz®, Sectral®, Septa®

(Continued)

Sulfamethoxazole and Trimethoprim *(Continued)*

Related Information
Management of Infections *on page 978*

U.S. Brand Names Bactrim™; Bactrim™ DS; Septra®; Septra® DS

Canadian Brand Names Apo-Sulfatrim®; Novo-Trimel; Novo-Trimel D.S.; Nu-Cotrimox; Septra®; Septra® DS; Septra® Injection

Generic Available Yes

Synonyms Co-Trimoxazole; SMZ-TMP; Sulfatrim; TMP-SMZ; Trimethoprim and Sulfamethoxazole

Pharmacologic Category Antibiotic, Sulfonamide Derivative; Antibiotic, Miscellaneous

Pregnancy Risk Factor C/D (at term - expert analysis)

Lactation Enters breast milk/contraindicated (AAP rates "compatible with restrictions")

Use
Oral treatment of urinary tract infections due to *E. coli*, *Klebsiella* and *Enterobacter* sp, *M. morganii*, *P. mirabilis* and *P. vulgaris*; acute otitis media in children and acute exacerbations of chronic bronchitis in adults due to susceptible strains of *H. influenzae* or *S. pneumoniae*; treatment and prophylaxis of *Pneumocystis carinii* pneumonitis (PCP), traveler's diarrhea due to enterotoxigenic *E. coli*; treatment of enteritis caused by *Shigella flexneri* or *Shigella sonnei*

I.V. treatment or severe or complicated infections when oral therapy is not feasible, for documented PCP, empiric treatment of PCP in immune compromised patients; treatment of documented or suspected shigellosis, typhoid fever, *Nocardia asteroides* infection, or other infections caused by susceptible bacteria

Unlabeled/Investigational Use Cholera and *Salmonella*-type infections and nocardiosis; chronic prostatitis; as prophylaxis in neutropenic patients with *P. carinii* infections, in leukemics, and in patients following renal transplantation, to decrease incidence of PCP; treatment of *Cyclospora* infection, typhoid fever, *Nocardia asteroides* infection

Mechanism of Action Sulfamethoxazole interferes with bacterial folic acid synthesis and growth via inhibition of dihydrofolic acid formation from para-aminobenzoic acid; trimethoprim inhibits dihydrofolic acid reduction to tetrahydrofolate resulting in sequential inhibition of enzymes of the folic acid pathway

Labeled Contraindications Hypersensitivity to any sulfa drug, trimethoprim, or any component of the formulation; porphyria; megaloblastic anemia due to folate deficiency; infants <2 months of age; marked hepatic damage; severe renal disease; pregnancy (at term)

Warnings/Precautions Use with caution in patients with G6PD deficiency, impaired renal or hepatic function. Adjust dosage in patients with renal impairment. Injection vehicle contains benzyl alcohol and sodium metabisulfite. Fatalities associated with severe reactions including Stevens-Johnson syndrome, toxic epidermal necrolysis, hepatic necrosis, agranulocytosis, aplastic anemia, and other blood dyscrasias. Discontinue use at first sign of rash. Elderly patients and patients with HIV appear at greater risk for more severe adverse reactions. May cause hypoglycemia (particularly in malnourished, renal, or hepatic impairment). Use caution in patients with porphyria or thyroid dysfunction. May cause hyperkalemia. Slow acetylators may be more prone to adverse reactions.

Chemical similarities are present among sulfonamides, sulfonylureas, carbonic anhydrase inhibitors, thiazides, and loop diuretics (except ethacrynic acid). Use in patients with sulfonamide allergy is specifically contraindicated in product labeling, however, a risk of cross-reaction exists in patients with allergy to any of these compounds; avoid use when previous reaction has been severe.

Adverse Reactions The most common adverse reactions include gastrointestinal upset (nausea, vomiting, anorexia) and dermatologic reactions (rash or urticaria). Rare, life-threatening reactions have been associated with co-trimoxazole, including severe dermatologic reactions and hepatotoxic reactions. Most other reactions listed are rare, however, frequency cannot be accurately estimated.

Cardiovascular: Allergic myocarditis

Central nervous system: Confusion, depression, hallucinations, seizure, aseptic meningitis, peripheral neuritis, fever, ataxia, kernicterus in neonates

Dermatologic: Rashes, pruritus, urticaria, photosensitivity; rare reactions include erythema multiforme, Stevens-Johnson syndrome, toxic epidermal necrolysis, exfoliative dermatitis, and Henoch-Schönlein purpura

Endocrine & metabolic: Hyperkalemia (generally at high dosages), hypoglycemia

Gastrointestinal: Nausea, vomiting, anorexia, stomatitis, diarrhea, pseudomembranous colitis, pancreatitis

Hematologic: Thrombocytopenia, megaloblastic anemia, granulocytopenia, eosinophilia, pancytopenia, aplastic anemia, methemoglobinemia, hemolysis (with G6PD deficiency), agranulocytosis

Hepatic: Hepatotoxicity (including hepatitis, cholestasis, and hepatic necrosis), hyperbilirubinemia, transaminases increased

Neuromuscular & skeletal: Arthralgia, myalgia, rhabdomyolysis

Renal: Interstitial nephritis, crystalluria, renal failure, nephrotoxicity (in association with cyclosporine), diuresis

Respiratory: Cough, dyspnea, pulmonary infiltrates

Miscellaneous: Serum sickness, angioedema, periarteritis nodosa (rare), systemic lupus erythematosus (rare)

Vesicant No

Overdosage/Toxicology Symptoms of overdose include nausea, vomiting, GI distress, hematuria, and crystalluria. Bone marrow suppression may occur. Treatment is supportive. Adequate fluid intake is essential. Peritoneal dialysis is not effective and hemodialysis is only moderately effective in removing co-trimoxazole. Leucovorin 5-15 mg/day may accelerate hematologic recovery.

Drug Interactions

Cytochrome P450 Effect:

Sulfamethoxazole: **Substrate** of CYP2C8/9 (major), 3A4 (minor); **Inhibits** CYP2C8/9 (moderate)

Trimethoprim: **Substrate** (major) of CYP2C8/9, 3A4; **Inhibits** CYP2C8/9 (moderate)

Increased Effect/Toxicity: Sulfamethoxazole/trimethoprim may increase toxicity of methotrexate. Sulfamethoxazole/trimethoprim may increase the serum levels of procainamide. Concurrent therapy with pyrimethamine (in doses >25 mg/week) may increase the risk of megaloblastic anemia. Sulfamethoxazole/trimethoprim may increase the
(Continued)

Sulfamethoxazole and Trimethoprim *(Continued)*

levels/effects of amiodarone, fluoxetine, glimepiride, glipizide, nateglinide, phenytoin, pioglitazone, rosiglitazone, sertraline, warfarin, and other CYP2C8/9 substrates.

ACE Inhibitors, angiotensin receptor antagonists, or potassium-sparing diuretics may increase the risk of hyperkalemia. Concurrent use with cyclosporine may result in an increased risk of nephrotoxicity when used with sulfamethoxazole/trimethoprim. Trimethoprim may increase the serum concentration of dapsone.

Decreased Effect: The levels/effects of sulfamethoxazole may be decreased by carbamazepine, phenobarbital, phenytoin, rifampin, rifapentine, secobarbital, and other CYP2C8/9 inducers. Although occasionally recommended to limit or reverse hematologic toxicity of high-dose sulfamethoxazole/trimethoprim, concurrent use has been associated with a decreased effectiveness in treating *Pneumocystis carinii*.

Ethanol/Nutrition/Herb Interactions Herb/Nutraceutical: Avoid dong quai, St John's wort (may also cause photosensitization).

Storage/Stability

Injection: Store at room temperature; do not refrigerate. Less soluble in more alkaline pH. Protect from light. Following dilution, store at room temperature; do not refrigerate.

Suspension, tablet: Store at room temperature. Protect from light.

Stability of parenteral admixture at room temperature (25°C):

5 mL/125 mL D_5W; stable for 6 hours

5 mL/100 mL D_5W; stable for 4 hours

5 mL/75 mL D_5W; stable for 2 hours

Studies have also confirmed limited stability in NS; detailed references should be consulted.

Reconstitution Injection: Less soluble in more alkaline pH. Solution must be diluted prior to administration.

Compatibility Stable in $D_5\frac{1}{2}NS$, LR, $\frac{1}{2}NS$; **variable stability (consult detailed reference)** in D_5W, NS

Y-site administration: Compatible: Acyclovir, aldesleukin, allopurinol, amifostine, amphotericin B cholesteryl sulfate complex, atracurium, aztreonam, cefepime, cyclophosphamide, diltiazem, docetaxel, doxorubicin liposome, enalaprilat, esmolol, etoposide phosphate, filgrastim, fludarabine, gatifloxacin, gemcitabine, granisetron, hydromorphone, labetalol, linezolid, lorazepam, magnesium sulfate, melphalan, meperidine, morphine, pancuronium, perphenazine, piperacillin/tazobactam, remifentanil, sargramostim, tacrolimus, teniposide, thiotepa, vecuronium, zidovudine. **Incompatible:** Fluconazole, midazolam, vinorelbine. **Variable (consult detailed reference):** Cisatracurium, foscarnet

Compatibility in syringe: Compatible: Heparin

Compatibility when admixed: Incompatible: Fluconazole, verapamil

Pharmacodynamics/Kinetics

Absorption: Oral: Almost completely, 90% to 100%

Protein binding: SMX: 68%, TMP: 45%

Metabolism: SMX: N-acetylated and glucuronidated; TMP: Metabolized to oxide and hydroxylated metabolites

Half-life elimination: SMX: 9 hours, TMP: 6-17 hours; both are prolonged in renal failure

Time to peak, serum: Within 1-4 hours

Excretion: Both are excreted in urine as metabolites and unchanged drug

Effects of aging on the pharmacokinetics of both agents has been variable; increase in half-life and decreases in clearance have been associated with reduced creatinine clearance

Dosage Dosage recommendations are based on the trimethoprim component. Double-strength tablets are equivalent to sulfamethoxazole 800 mg and trimethoprim 160 mg.

Children >2 months:

General dosing guidelines:

Mild-to-moderate infections: Oral: 8-12 mg TMP/kg/day in divided doses every 12 hours

Serious infection:

Oral: 20 mg TMP/kg/day in divided doses every 6 hours

I.V.: 8-12 mg TMP/kg/day in divided doses every 6 hours

Acute otitis media: Oral: 8 mg TMP/kg/day in divided doses every 12 hours for 10 days

Urinary tract infection:

Treatment:

Oral: 6-12 mg TMP/kg/day in divided doses every 12 hours

I.V.: 8-10 mg TMP/kg/day in divided doses every 6, 8, or 12 hours for up to 4 days with serious infections

Prophylaxis: Oral: 2 mg TMP/kg/dose daily or 5 mg TMP/kg/dose twice weekly

Pneumocystis:

Treatment: Oral, I.V.: 15-20 mg TMP/kg/day in divided doses every 6-8 hours

Prophylaxis: Oral, 150 mg TMP/m^2/day in divided doses every 12 hours for 3 days/week; dose should not exceed trimethoprim 320 mg and sulfamethoxazole 1600 mg daily

Alternative prophylaxis dosing schedules include:

150 mg TMP/m^2/day as a single daily dose 3 times/week on consecutive days

or

150 mg TMP/m^2/day in divided doses every 12 hours administered 7 days/week

or

150 mg TMP/m^2/day in divided doses every 12 hours administered 3 times/week on alternate days

Shigellosis:

Oral: 8 mg TMP/kg/day in divided doses every 12 hours for 5 days

I.V.: 8-10 mg TMP/kg/day in divided doses every 6, 8, or 12 hours for up to 5 days

Cyclospora (unlabeled use): Oral, I.V.: 5 mg TMP/kg twice daily for 7-10 days

Adults:

Urinary tract infection:

Oral: One double-strength tablet every 12 hours for 10-14 days

I.V.: 8-10 mg TMP/kg/day in divided doses every 6, 8, or 12 hours for up to 14 days with severe infections

Chronic bronchitis: Oral: One double-strength tablet every 12 hours for 10-14 days

Shigellosis:

Oral: One double strength tablet every 12 hours for 5 days

(Continued)

Sulfamethoxazole and Trimethoprim *(Continued)*

I.V.: 8-10 mg TMP/kg/day in divided doses every 6, 8, or 12 hours for up to 5 days

Travelers' diarrhea: Oral: One double strength tablet every 12 hours for 5 days

Sepsis: I.V.: 20 TMP/kg/day divided every 6 hours

Pneumocystis carinii:

Prophylaxis: Oral: 1 double strength tablet daily or 3 times/week

Treatment: Oral, I.V.: 15-20 mg TMP/kg/day in 3-4 divided doses

Cyclospora (unlabeled use): Oral, I.V.: 160 mg TMP twice daily for 7-10 days

Nocardia (unlabeled use): Oral, I.V.: 640 mg TMP/day in divided doses for several months (duration is controversial; an average of 7 months has been reported)

Dosing adjustment in renal impairment: Oral, I.V.:

Cl_{cr} 15-30 mL/minute: Administer 50% of recommended dose

Cl_{cr} <15 mL/minute: Use is not recommended

Administration

I.V.: Infuse over 60-90 minutes, must dilute well before giving; may be given less diluted in a central line; not for I.M. injection

Oral: May be taken with food and water.

Dosage Forms Note: The 5:1 ratio (SMX:TMP) remains constant in all dosage forms.

Injection, solution: Sulfamethoxazole 80 mg and trimethoprim 16 mg per mL (5 mL, 10 mL, 30 mL, 50 mL) [contains propylene glycol ~400 mg/mL, alcohol, benzyl alcohol, and sodium metabisulfite]

Suspension, oral: Sulfamethoxazole 200 mg and trimethoprim 40 mg per 5 mL (20 mL, 480 mL) [contains alcohol]

Septra®: Sulfamethoxazole 200 mg and trimethoprim 40 mg per 5 mL (100 mL, 480 mL) [contains alcohol 0.26% and sodium benzoate; cherry and grape flavors]

Tablet: Sulfamethoxazole 400 mg and trimethoprim 80 mg

Bactrim™: Sulfamethoxazole 400 mg and trimethoprim 80 mg [contains sodium benzoate]

Septra®: Sulfamethoxazole 400 mg and trimethoprim 80 mg

Tablet, double strength: Sulfamethoxazole 800 mg and trimethoprim 160 mg

Bactrim™ DS: Sulfamethoxazole 800 mg and trimethoprim 160 mg [contains sodium benzoate]

Septra® DS: Sulfamethoxazole 800 mg and trimethoprim 160 mg

Dietary Considerations Should be taken with 8 oz of water on empty stomach.

Patient Information Take oral medication with 8 oz of water on an empty stomach (1 hour before or 2 hours after meals) for best absorption; report any skin rashes immediately; finish all medication, do not skip doses

Special Geriatric Considerations Elderly patients appear at greater risk for more severe adverse reactions. Adjust dose based on renal function.

Selected Readings

Cockerill FR and Edson RS, "Trimethoprim-Sulfamethoxazole," *Mayo Clin Proc*, 1991, 66(12):1260-9.

Naber K, Vergin H, and Weigand W, "Pharmacokinetics of Co-trimoxazole and Co-tetroxazine in Geriatric Patients," *Infection*, 1981, 9(5):239-43.

- **Sulfatrim** *see* Sulfamethoxazole and Trimethoprim *on page 727*
- **Summer's Eve® SpecialCare™ Medicated Anti-Itch Cream [OTC]** *see* Hydrocortisone *on page 419*
- **Sun-Benz® (Can)** *see* Benzydamine *on page 123*
- **Supeudol® (Can)** *see* Oxycodone *on page 633*

Suramin (SUR a min)

Related Information
Investigational Drug Service *on page 1031*
Safe Handling of Hazardous Drugs *on page 1034*

Generic Available No

Synonyms Antrypol; Bayer 205; 309F; Forneau-309; Naphuride Sodium; NSC-34936; Suramin Sodium

Pharmacologic Category Antineoplastic Agent

Unlabeled/Investigational Use Investigational: Treatment of prostate cancer; chemosensitizing agent in treatment of various solid tumors

Mechanism of Action Suramin inhibits a number of growth factors and enzymes essential to cell proliferation including platelet-derived growth factor (PDGF), fibroblast growth factor, DNA polymerase, glycerol phosphate oxidase, reverse transcriptase, and various lysosomal enzymes. Suramin may also have some angiogenic inhibitory activity.

Labeled Contraindications Hypersensitivity to suramin or any component of the formulation

Warnings/Precautions Hazardous agent - use appropriate precautions for handling and disposal. See Safe Handling of Hazardous Drugs *on page 1034* in the Appendix. Use cautiously in patients with significant hepatic dysfunction, malnourishment, or with decreased serum albumin levels.

Adverse Reactions
>10%:
  Central nervous system: Fever (78%), headache; palmar and plantar hyperesthesia occur at levels >350 mcg/mL
  Dermatologic: Rash (48%)
  Endocrine & metabolic: Adrenal insufficiency (23%), patients usually require adrenocorticoid therapy; transaminases increased (transient 14%)
  Gastrointestinal: Nausea (20%), vomiting (35%), metallic taste
  Hematologic: Leukopenia, agranulocytosis, thrombocytopenia (12% to 26%), usually not dose-limiting
  Hepatic: Transient increases in bilirubin levels (14%)
  Neuromuscular & skeletal: Paresthesias, peripheral neuropathies (33%), may be dose-limiting; areflexia and paralysis may occur at levels >375 mcg/mL
  Ocular: Keratopathy (11%), possibly related to dose and/or rate of infusion
  Renal: Mild, nondose-limiting, proteinuria (33%); decrease in creatinine clearance
1% to 10%:
  Gastrointestinal: Stomatitis (5%)
  Neuromuscular & skeletal: Myalgia (3%)
<1%: Abdominal pain, atrial fibrillation, diarrhea; coagulopathy (dose-limiting, inhibits factors V, VIII, IX, X, XI, and XII)
(Continued)

Suramin *(Continued)*

Immediate hypersensitivity reactions, including nausea, vomiting, shock, and loss of consciousness (0.1% to 0.3%); a 100-200 mg (10-20 mg in children) test dose prior to the first treatment cycle is occasionally given

Vesicant No; may be an irritant

Emetic Potential Moderate (30% to 60%)

Storage/Stability Solutions of 10 mg/mL in saline or dextrose solutions are stable for up to 2 weeks at room temperature of 15°C to 30°C (59°F to 86°F).

Pharmacodynamics/Kinetics

Absorption: Not absorbed orally

Distribution: V_d: 31-46 L; does not penetrate the CNS

Protein binding: >99%

Half-life elimination: Triphasic, terminal half-life: 50 days

Excretion: Urine (as unchanged drug); bile (small amounts)

Dosage Refer to individual protocols. I.V.: Adults:

Prostate cancer: 350 mg/m²/day continuous I.V. infusion for 7 days, then titrated to a plasma level of 250-300 mcg/mL for 7 days, repeated after an 8-week interval.

Titrate to a plasma level of 300 mcg/mL for 14 days, repeat after an 8-week interval.

Chemosensitizing agent: Doses are not yet established; anticipated to be significantly lower than cancer treatment doses.

Dosage adjustment in renal impairment: Dosage reductions have been suggested for "severe" renal dysfunction; however, specific guidelines have not been published.

Dosage adjustment in hepatic impairment: Dosage reductions of 50% to 75% have been suggested for "severe" hepatic dysfunction; however, specific guidelines have not been published.

Administration I.V.: Usually administered as a carefully titrated continuous infusion

Dosage Forms Injection, powder for reconstitution: 600 mg

Selected Readings

Eisenberger MA and Reyno LM, "Suramin," *Cancer Treat Rev*, 1994, 20(3):259-73.

Larsen AK, "Suramin: An Anticancer Drug With Unique Biological Effects," *Cancer Chemother Pharmacol*, 1993, 32(2):96-8.

Stein CA, "Suramin: A Novel Antineoplastic Agent With Multiple Potential Mechanisms of Action," *Cancer Res*, 1993, 53(10 Suppl):2239-48.

Voogd TE, Vansterkenburg EL, Wilting J, et al, "Recent Research on the Biological Activity of Suramin," *Pharmacol Rev*, 1993, 45(2):177-203.

♦ **Suramin Sodium** *see* Suramin *on page 733*

♦ **Tabloid**® *see* Thioguanine *on page 762*

Tacrolimus *(ta KROE li mus)*

Medication Safety Issues

Sound-alike/look-alike issues:

Prograf® may be confused with Gengraf®

Related Information

Transplantation *on page 1019*

U.S. Brand Names Prograf®; Protopic®

Canadian Brand Names Prograf®; Protopic®

Generic Available No

Synonyms FK506

Pharmacologic Category Immunosuppressant Agent; Topical Skin Product

Pregnancy Risk Factor C

Lactation Enters breast milk/contraindicated

Use

Oral/injection: Potent immunosuppressive drug used in liver or kidney transplant recipients

Topical: Moderate to severe atopic dermatitis in patients not responsive to conventional therapy or when conventional therapy is not appropriate

Unlabeled/Investigational Use Potent immunosuppressive drug used in heart, lung, small bowel transplant recipients; immunosuppressive drug for peripheral stem cell/bone marrow transplantation

Mechanism of Action Suppresses cellular immunity (inhibits T-lymphocyte activation), possibly by binding to an intracellular protein, FKBP-12

Labeled Contraindications Hypersensitivity to tacrolimus or any component of the formulation

Warnings/Precautions

Oral/injection: Insulin-dependent post-transplant diabetes mellitus (PTDM) has been reported (1% to 20%); risk increases in African-American and Hispanic kidney transplant patients. Increased susceptibility to infection and the possible development of lymphoma may occur after administration of tacrolimus. Nephrotoxicity and neurotoxicity have been reported, especially with higher doses; to avoid excess nephrotoxicity do not administer simultaneously with cyclosporine; monitoring of serum concentrations (trough for oral therapy) is essential to prevent organ rejection and reduce drug-related toxicity; tonic clonic seizures may have been triggered by tacrolimus. A period of 24 hours should elapse between discontinuation of cyclosporine and the initiation of tacrolimus. Use caution in renal or hepatic dysfunction, dosing adjustments may be required. Delay initiation if postoperative oliguria occurs. Use may be associated with the development of hypertension (common). Myocardial hypertrophy has been reported (rare). Each mL of injection contains polyoxyl 60 hydrogenated castor oil (HCO-60) (200 mg) and dehydrated alcohol USP 80% v/v. Anaphylaxis has been reported with the injection, use should be reserved for those patients not able to take oral medications.

Topical: Topical calcineurin agents are considered second-line therapies in the treatment of atopic dermatitis/eczema, and should be limited to use in patients who have failed treatment with other therapies. They should be used for short-term and intermittent treatment using the minimum amount necessary for the control of symptoms should be used.

Infections at the treatment site should be cleared prior to therapy. Patients with atopic dermatitis are predisposed to skin infections, including eczema herpeticum, varicella zoster, and herpes simplex. Discontinue use in patients with unknown cause of lymphadenopathy or acute infectious mononucleosis. Not recommended for use in patients with Netherton's syndrome. Safety not established in patients with generalized erythroderma. The use of Protopic® in children <2 years of age is not recommended, particularly since the effect on immune system development is unknown.
(Continued)

Tacrolimus *(Continued)*

Adverse Reactions

Oral, I.V.:

≥15%

Cardiovascular: Chest pain, hypertension

Central nervous system: Dizziness, headache, insomnia, tremor (headache and tremor are associated with high whole blood concentrations and may respond to decreased dosage)

Dermatologic: Pruritus, rash

Endocrine & metabolic: Diabetes mellitus, hyperglycemia, hyperkalemia, hyperlipemia, hypomagnesemia, hypophosphatemia

Gastrointestinal: Abdominal pain, constipation, diarrhea, dyspepsia, nausea, vomiting

Genitourinary: Urinary tract infection

Hematologic: Anemia, leukocytosis, thrombocytopenia

Hepatic: Ascites

Neuromuscular & skeletal: Arthralgia, back pain, weakness, paresthesia

Renal: Abnormal kidney function, increased creatinine, oliguria, urinary tract infection, increased BUN

Respiratory: Atelectasis, dyspnea, increased cough

3% to 15%:

Cardiovascular: Abnormal ECG, angina pectoris, deep thrombophlebitis, hemorrhage, hypotension, hypervolemia, generalized edema, peripheral vascular disorder, phlebitis, postural hypotension, tachycardia, thrombosis, vasodilation

Central nervous system: Abnormal dreams, abnormal thinking, agitation, amnesia, anxiety, chills, confusion, depression, emotional lability, encephalopathy, hallucinations, nervousness, psychosis, somnolence

Dermatologic: Acne, alopecia, cellulitis, exfoliative dermatitis, fungal dermatitis, hirsutism, increased diaphoresis, photosensitivity reaction, skin discoloration, skin disorder, skin ulcer

Endocrine & metabolic: Acidosis, alkalosis, Cushing's syndrome, decreased bicarbonate, decreased serum iron, diabetes mellitus, hypercalcemia, hypercholesterolemia, hyperphosphatemia, hypoproteinemia, increased alkaline phosphatase

Gastrointestinal: Anorexia, cramps, dysphagia, enlarged abdomen, esophagitis, flatulence, gastritis, GI perforation/hemorrhage, ileus, increased appetite, oral moniliasis, rectal disorder, stomatitis, weight gain

Genitourinary: Urinary frequency, urinary incontinence, vaginitis, cystitis, dysuria

Hematologic: Bruising, coagulation disorder, decreased prothrombin, hypochromic anemia, leukopenia, polycythemia

Hepatic: Abnormal liver function tests, bilirubinemia, cholangitis, cholestatic jaundice, hepatitis, increased ALT, increased AST, increased GGT, jaundice, liver damage, increase LDH

Neuromuscular & skeletal: Hypertonia, incoordination, joint disorder, leg cramps, myalgia, myasthenia, myoclonus, neuropathy, osteoporosis

Ocular: Abnormal vision, amblyopia

Otic: Ear pain, otitis media, tinnitus

Renal: Albuminuria

Respiratory: Asthma, bronchitis, lung disorder, pharyngitis, pneumonia, pneumothorax, pulmonary edema, respiratory disorder, rhinitis, sinusitis, voice alteration

Miscellaneous: Abscess, abnormal healing, allergic reaction, flu-like syndrome, generalized spasm, hernia, herpes simplex, peritonitis, sepsis

Postmarketing and/or case reports: Acute renal failure, anaphylaxis, coma, deafness, delirium, hearing loss, hemolytic-uremic syndrome, leukoencephalopathy, lymphoproliferative disorder (related to EBV), myocardial hypertrophy (associated with ventricular dysfunction; reversible upon discontinuation), pancreatitis, QT_c prolongation, seizure, Stevens-Johnson syndrome, thrombocytopenic purpura, torsade de pointes

Topical (as reported in children and adults, unless otherwise noted):

>10%:

Central nervous system: Headache (5% to 20%), fever (1% to 21%)

Dermatologic: Skin burning (43% to 58%), pruritus (41% to 46%), erythema (12% to 28%)

Respiratory: Increased cough (18% children)

Miscellaneous: Flu-like syndrome (23% to 28%), allergic reaction (4% to 12%)

1% to 10%:

Cardiovascular: Peripheral edema (3% to 4% adults)

Central nervous system: Hyperesthesia (3% to 7% adults), pain (1% to 2%)

Dermatologic: Skin tingling (2% to 8%), acne (4% to 7% adults), localized flushing (following ethanol consumption 3% to 7% adults), folliculitis (2% to 6%), urticaria (1% to 6%), rash (2% to 5%), pustular rash (2% to 4%), vesiculobullous rash (4% children), contact dermatitis (3% to 4%), cyst (1% to 3% adults), eczema herpeticum (1% to 2%), fungal dermatitis (1% to 2% adults), sunburn (1% to 2% adults), dry skin (1% children)

Endocrine & metabolic: Dysmenorrhea (4% women)

Gastrointestinal: Diarrhea (3% to 5%), dyspepsia (1% to 4% adults), abdominal pain (3% children), vomiting (1% adults), gastroenteritis (adults 2%), nausea (1% children)

Neuromuscular & skeletal: Myalgia (2% to 3% adults), weakness (2% to 3% adults), back pain (2% adults)

Ocular: Conjunctivitis (2% adults)

Otic: Otitis media (12% children)

Respiratory: Rhinitis (6% to 10%), sinusitis (2% to 4% adults), bronchitis (2% adults), pneumonia (1% adults)

Miscellaneous: Varicella/herpes zoster (1% to 5%), lymphadenopathy (3% children)

≥1%: Alopecia, increased ALT, increased AST, anaphylactoid reaction, angina pectoris, angioedema, anorexia, anxiety, arrhythmia, arthralgia, arthritis, bilirubinemia, breast pain, cellulitis, cerebrovascular accident, cheilitis, chills, constipation, increased creatinine, dehydration, depression, dizziness, dyspnea, ear pain, ecchymosis, edema, epistaxis, exacerbation of untreated area, eye pain, furunculosis, gastritis, hernia, hyperglycemia, hypertension, hypoglycemia, hypoxia, laryngitis, leukocytosis, leukopenia, abnormal liver function tests, lymphadenopathy

(Continued)

Tacrolimus *(Continued)*

(0.8%), malaise, migraine, neck pain, neuritis, palpitation, paresthesia, peripheral vascular disorder, photosensitivity reaction, skin discoloration, diaphoresis, taste perversion, unintended pregnancy, vaginal moniliasis, vasodilation, vertigo

Vesicant No

Overdosage/Toxicology Symptoms are extensions of immunosuppressive activity and adverse effects. Symptomatic and supportive treatment is required. Hemodialysis is not effective.

Drug Interactions

Cytochrome P450 Effect: Substrate of CYP3A4 (major); **Inhibits** CYP3A4 (weak)

Increased Effect/Toxicity: Amphotericin B and other nephrotoxic antibiotics have the potential to increase tacrolimus-associated nephrotoxicity. Cisapride and metoclopramide may increase tacrolimus levels. Synergistic immunosuppression results from concurrent use of cyclosporine. Voriconazole may increase tacrolimus serum concentrations; decrease tacrolimus dosage by 66% when initiating voriconazole. CYP3A4 inhibitors may increase the levels/effects of tacrolimus; example inhibitors include azole antifungals, ciprofloxacin, clarithromycin, diclofenac, doxycycline, erythromycin, imatinib, isoniazid, nefazodone, nicardipine, propofol, protease inhibitors, quinidine, and verapamil. Calcium channel blockers (dihydropyridine) may increase tacrolimus serum concentrations (monitor).

Decreased Effect: Antacids impair tacrolimus absorption (separate administration by at least 2 hours). St John's wort may reduce tacrolimus serum concentrations (avoid concurrent use). CYP3A4 inducers may decrease the levels/effects of tacrolimus; example inducers include aminoglutethimide, carbamazepine, nafcillin, nevirapine, phenobarbital, phenytoin, and rifamycins. Caspofungin and sirolimus may decrease the serum concentrations of tacrolimus.

Ethanol/Nutrition/Herb Interactions

Ethanol: Localized flushing (redness, warm sensation) may occur at application site of topical tacrolimus following ethanol consumption.

Food: Decreases rate and extent of absorption. High-fat meals have most pronounced effect (35% decrease in AUC, 77% decrease in C_{max}). Grapefruit juice, CYP3A4 inhibitor, may increase serum level and/or toxicity of tacrolimus; avoid concurrent use.

Herb/Nutraceutical: St John's wort: May reduce tacrolimus serum concentrations (avoid concurrent use).

Storage/Stability

Injection: Prior to dilution, store at 5°C to 25°C (41°F to 77°F). Stable for 24 hours in D_5W or NS in glass or polyolefin containers.

Capsules and ointment: Store at room temperature 25°C (77°F).

Reconstitution Dilute with 5% dextrose injection or 0.9% sodium chloride injection to a final concentration between 0.004 mg/mL and 0.02 mg/mL.

Compatibility Variable stability (consult detailed reference) in D_5W, NS

Y-site administration: Compatible: Acyclovir, aminophylline, amphotericin B, ampicillin, ampicillin/sulbactam, benztropine, calcium gluconate, cefazolin, cefotetan, ceftazidime, ceftriaxone, cefuroxime, chloramphenicol, cimetidine, ciprofloxacin, clindamycin, co-trimoxazole, dexamethasone sodium phosphate, digoxin, diphenhydramine, dobutamine, dopamine, doxycycline, erythromycin lactobionate, esmolol, fluconazole, furosemide, ganciclovir, gentamicin, haloperidol, heparin, hydrocortisone sodium succinate, hydromorphone, imipenem/cilastatin, insulin (regular), isoproterenol, leucovorin, lorazepam, methylprednisolone sodium succinate, metoclopramide, metronidazole, morphine, multivitamins, nitroglycerin, oxacillin, penicillin G potassium, perphenazine, phenytoin, piperacillin, potassium chloride, propranolol, ranitidine, sodium bicarbonate, sodium nitroprusside, sodium tetradecyl sulfate, tobramycin, vancomycin

Compatibility when admixed: Compatible: Cimetidine

Pharmacodynamics/Kinetics

Absorption: Better in resected patients with a closed stoma; unlike cyclosporine, clamping of the T-tube in liver transplant patients does not alter trough concentrations or AUC

Oral: Incomplete and variable; food within 15 minutes of administration decreases absorption (27%)

Topical: Serum concentrations range from undetectable to 20 ng/mL (<5 ng/mL in majority of adult patients studied)

Protein binding: 99%

Metabolism: Extensively hepatic via CYP3A4 to eight possible metabolites (major metabolite, 31-demethyl tacrolimus, shows same activity as tacrolimus *in vitro*)

Bioavailability: Oral: Adults: 7% to 28%, Children: 10% to 52%; Topical: <0.5%; Absolute: Unknown

Half-life elimination: Variable, 21-61 hours in healthy volunteers

Time to peak: 0.5-4 hours

Excretion: Feces (~92%); feces/urine (<1% as unchanged drug)

Dosage

Children:

Liver transplant: Patients without pre-existing renal or hepatic dysfunction have required and tolerated higher doses than adults to achieve similar blood concentrations. It is recommended that therapy be initiated at high end of the recommended adult I.V. and oral dosing ranges; dosage adjustments may be required.

Oral: Initial dose: 0.15-0.20 mg/kg/day in 2 divided doses, given every 12 hours; begin oral dose no sooner than 6 hours post-transplant; adjunctive therapy with corticosteroids is recommended; if switching from I.V. to oral, the oral dose should be started 8-12 hours after stopping the infusion

Typical whole blood trough concentrations: Months 1-12: 5-20 ng/mL

I.V.: **Note:** I.V. route should only be used in patients not able to take oral medications, anaphylaxis has been reported. Initial dose: 0.03-0.05 mg/kg/day as a continuous infusion; begin no sooner than 6 hours post-transplant; adjunctive therapy with corticosteroids is recommended; continue only until oral medication can be tolerated

Children ≥2 years: Moderate to severe atopic dermatitis: Topical: Apply 0.03% ointment to affected area twice daily; rub in gently and completely; continue applications for 1 week after symptoms have cleared

(Continued)

Tacrolimus *(Continued)*

Adults:

Kidney transplant:

Oral: Initial dose: 0.2 mg/kg/day in 2 divided doses, given every 12 hours; initial dose may be given within 24 hours of transplant, but should be delayed until renal function has recovered; African-American patients may require larger doses to maintain trough concentration

Typical whole blood trough concentrations: Months 1-3: 7- 20 ng/mL; months 4-12: 5-15 ng/mL

I.V.: **Note:** I.V. route should only be used in patients not able to take oral medications, anaphylaxis has been reported. Initial dose: 0.03-0.05 mg/kg/day as a continuous infusion; begin no sooner than 6 hours post-transplant, starting at lower end of the dosage range; adjunctive therapy with corticosteroids is recommended; continue only until oral medication can be tolerated

Liver transplant:

Oral: Initial dose: 0.1-0.15 mg/kg/day in 2 divided doses, given every 12 hours; begin oral dose no sooner than 6 hours post-transplant; adjunctive therapy with corticosteroids is recommended; if switching from I.V. to oral, the oral dose should be started 8-12 hours after stopping the infusion

Typical whole blood trough concentrations: Months 1-12: 5-20 ng/mL

I.V.: **Note:** I.V. route should only be used in patients not able to take oral medications, anaphylaxis has been reported. Initial dose: 0.03-0.05 mg/kg/day as a continuous infusion; begin no sooner than 6 hours post-transplant starting at lower end of the dosage range; adjunctive therapy with corticosteroids is recommended; continue only until oral medication can be tolerated

Prevention of graft-vs-host disease: I.V.: 0.03 mg/kg/day as continuous infusion

Moderate to severe atopic dermatitis: Topical: Apply 0.03% or 0.1% ointment to affected area twice daily; rub in gently and completely; continue applications for 1 week after symptoms have cleared

Dosing adjustment in renal impairment: Evidence suggests that lower doses should be used; patients should receive doses at the lowest value of the recommended I.V. and oral dosing ranges; further reductions in dose below these ranges may be required

Tacrolimus therapy should usually be delayed up to 48 hours or longer in patients with postoperative oliguria

Hemodialysis: Not removed by hemodialysis; supplemental dose is not necessary

Peritoneal dialysis: Significant drug removal is unlikely based on physiochemical characteristics

Dosing adjustment in hepatic impairment: Use of tacrolimus in liver transplant recipients experiencing post-transplant hepatic impairment may be associated with increased risk of developing renal insufficiency related to high whole blood levels of tacrolimus. The presence of moderate-to-severe hepatic dysfunction (serum bilirubin >2 mg/dL) appears to affect the metabolism of FK506. The half-life of the drug was prolonged and the clearance reduced after I.V. administration. The bioavailability of FK506 was also increased after oral administration.

The higher plasma concentrations as determined by ELISA, in patients with severe hepatic dysfunction are probably due to the accumulation of FK506 metabolites of lower activity. These patients should be monitored closely and dosage adjustments should be considered. Some evidence indicates that lower doses could be used in these patients.

Administration I.V.: Administer by I.V. continuous infusion only. Do not use PVC tubing when administering dilute solutions.

Dosage Forms

Capsule (Prograf®): 0.5 mg, 1 mg, 5 mg

Injection, solution (Prograf®): 5 mg/mL (1 mL) [contains dehydrated alcohol 80% and polyoxyl 60 hydrogenated castor oil]

Ointment, topical (Protopic®): 0.03% (30 g, 60 g, 100 g); 0.1% (30 g, 60 g, 100 g)

Monitoring Parameters Renal function, hepatic function, serum electrolytes, glucose and blood pressure, measure 3 times/week for first few weeks, then gradually decrease frequency as patient stabilizes. Whole blood concentrations should be used for monitoring (trough for oral therapy). Signs/symptoms of anaphylactic reactions during infusion should also be monitored. Patients should be monitored during the first 30 minutes of the infusion, and frequently thereafter.

Dietary Considerations Capsule: Take on an empty stomach; be consistent with timing and composition of meals if GI intolerance occurs (per manufacturer).

Patient Information You will be susceptible to infection (avoid crowds and people with infections or contagious diseases). May lead to diabetes mellitus, notify prescriber if you develop increased urination, increased thirst, or increased hunger. If you are diabetic, monitor glucose levels closely (may alter glucose levels). You may experience nausea, vomiting, loss of appetite (frequent small meals, frequent mouth care may help); diarrhea (boiled milk, yogurt, or buttermilk may help); constipation (increased exercise or dietary fruit, fluid, or fiber may help, if not consult prescriber); muscle or back pain (mild analgesics may be recommended). Report chest pain; acute headache or dizziness; symptoms of respiratory infection, cough, or difficulty breathing; unresolved gastrointestinal effects; fatigue, chills, fever, unhealed sores, white plaques in mouth, irritation in genital area; unusual bruising or bleeding; pain or irritation on urination or change in urinary patterns; rash or skin irritation; or other unusual effects related to this medication.

Oral: Take as directed, preferably 30 minutes before or 30 minutes after meals. Do not take within 2 hours before or after antacids. Do not alter dose and do not discontinue without consulting prescriber. Maintain adequate hydration (2-3 L/day of fluids unless instructed to restrict fluid intake) during entire course of therapy.

Topical: For external use only. Avoid exposure to sunlight or tanning beds. Apply to clean, dry skin. Do not cover with occlusive dressings. Burning and itching are most common in the first few days of use and improve as atopic dermatitis improves. Wash hands after use, unless hands are an area of treatment. Caution with alcohol consumption; may cause localized flushing at application site.

Additional Information Additional dosing considerations:

Switch from I.V. to oral therapy: Threefold increase in dose

Pediatric patients: About 2 times higher dose compared to adults

Liver dysfunction: Decrease I.V. dose; decrease oral dose

(Continued)

Tacrolimus (Continued)

Renal dysfunction: Does not affect kinetics; decrease dose to decrease levels if renal dysfunction is related to the drug

Extemporaneous Preparations Tacrolimus oral suspension can be compounded at a concentration of 0.5 mg/mL; an extemporaneous suspension can be prepared by mixing the contents of six 5-mg tacrolimus capsules with equal amounts of Ora-Plus® and Simple Syrup, N.F., to make a final volume of 60 mL. The Suspension is stable for 56 days at room temperature in glass or plastic amber prescription bottles.

> Esquivel C, So S, McDiarmid S, Andrews W, and Colombani PM, "Suggested Guidelines for the Use of Tacrolimus in Pediatric Liver Transplant Patients," *Transplantation*, 1996, 61(5):847-8.

> Foster JA, Jacobson PA, Johnson CE, et al, "Stability of Tacrolimus in an Extemporaneously Compounded Oral Liquid (Abstract of Meeting Presentation)," *American Society of Health-System Pharmacists Annual Meeting*, 1996, 53:P-52(E).

Selected Readings

Asante-Korang A, Boyle GJ, Webber SA, et al, "Experience of FK506 Immune Suppression in Pediatric Heart Transplantation: A Study of Long-Term Adverse Effects," *J Heart Lung Transplant*, 1996, 15(4):415-22.

Atkison P, Joubert G, Barron A, et al, "Hypertrophic Cardiomyopathy Associated With Tacrolimus in Paediatric Transplant Patients," *Lancet*, 1995, 345(8954):894-6.

Bronster DJ, Yonover P, Stein J, et al, "Demyelinating Sensorimotor Polyneuropathy After Administration of FK506," *Transplantation*, 1995, 59(7):1066-8.

Cerra FB and Gruber SA, "Critical Care of the Transplant Patient," *Crit Care Clin*, 6:813-1034.

Ehst BD and Warshaw EM, "Alcohol-Induced Application Site Erythema After Topical Immunomodulator Use and Its Inhibition by Aspirin," *Arch Dermatol*, 2004, 140(8):1014-5.

Furlan V, Perello L, Jacquemin E, et al, "Interactions Between FK506 and Rifampicin or Erythromycin in Pediatric Liver Recipients," *Transplantation*, 1995, 59(8):1217-8.

Hodak SP, Moubarak JB, Rodriguez I, et al, "QT Prolongation and Near Fatal Cardiac Arrhythmia After Intravenous Tacrolimus Administration: A Case Report," *Transplantation*, 1998, 66(4):535-7.

Johnson MC, So S, March JW, et al, "QT Prolongation and Torsades de Pointes After Administration of FK506," *Transplantation*, 1992, 53(4):929-30.

Jusko WJ, Piekoszewski W, Klintmalm GB, et al, "Pharmacokinetics of Tacrolimus in Liver Transplant Patients," *Clin Pharmacol Ther*, 1995, 57(3):281-96.

Kaufman DB, Kaplan B, Kanwar YS, et al, "The Successful Use of Tacrolimus (FK506) in a Pancreas/Kidney Transplant Recipient With Recurrent Cyclosporine-Associated Hemolytic Uremic Syndrome," *Transplantation*, 1995, 59(12):1737-9.

Kelly PA, Burckart GJ, and Venkataramanan R, "Tacrolimus: A New Immunosuppressive Agent," *Am J Health Syst Pharm*, 1995, 52(14):1521-35.

Lubbe J and Milingou M, "Images in Clinical Medicine. Tacrolimus Ointment, Alcohol, and Facial Flushing," *N Engl J Med*, 2004, 351(26):2740.

MacDonald AS and Sketris IS, "Tacrolimus in Transplantation," *Am J Health Syst Pharm*, 1995, 52(14):1569-71.

McDiarmid SV, Colonna JO, Shaked A, et al, "Differences in Oral FK506 Dose Requirements Between Adults and Pediatric Liver Transplant Patients," *Transplantation*, 1993, 55(6):1328-32.

Menegaux F, Keeffe EB, Andrews BT, et al, "Neurological Complications of Liver Transplantation in Adult Versus Pediatric Patients," *Transplantation*, 1994, 58(4):447-50.

Minematsu T, Ohtani H, Sato H, et al, "Sustained QT Prolongation Induced by Tacrolimus in Guinea Pigs," *Life Sci*, 1999, 65(14):PL197-202.

Mrvos R, Hodgman M, Dean B, et al, "FK506 Overdose: A Report of Four Cases," *Clin Toxicol*, 1995, 33(5):487-8.

Natazuka T, Ogawa R, Kizaki T, et al, "Immunosuppressive Drugs and Hypertrophic Cardiomyopathy," *Lancet*, 1995, 345(8965):1644.

Przepiorka D, Suzuki J, Ippoliti C, et al, "Blood Tacrolimus Concentration Unchanged by Plasmapheresis," *Am J Hosp Pharm*, 1994, 51(13):1708.

Starzl TE, Fung J, Jordan M, et al, "Kidney Transplantation Under FK506," *JAMA*, 1990, 264(1):63-7.

Winkel E, DiSesa VJ, and Costanzo MR, "Advances in Heart Transplantation," *Dis Mon*, 1999, 45(3):62-87.

Winkler M and Christians U, "A Risk-Benefit Assessment of Tacrolimus in Transplantation," *Drug Saf*, 1995, 12(5):348-57.

♦ **TAM** *see* Tamoxifen *on page 743*

♦ **Tamofen® (Can)** *see* Tamoxifen *on page 743*

Tamoxifen (ta MOKS i fen)

Medication Safety Issues
Sound-alike/look-alike issues:
Tamoxifen may be confused with pentoxifylline, Tambocor™

Related Information
Safe Handling of Hazardous Drugs *on page 1034*

U.S. Brand Names Nolvadex®

Canadian Brand Names Apo-Tamox®; Gen-Tamoxifen; Nolvadex®; Nolvadex®-D; Novo-Tamoxifen; PMS-Tamoxifen; Tamofen®

Generic Available Yes

Synonyms ICI-46474; NSC-180973; TAM; Tamoxifen Citrate

Pharmacologic Category Antineoplastic Agent, Estrogen Receptor Antagonist

Pregnancy Risk Factor D

Lactation Excretion in breast milk unknown/contraindicated

Use Palliative or adjunctive treatment of advanced breast cancer; reduce the incidence of breast cancer in women at high risk; reduce risk of invasive breast cancer in women with ductal carcinoma *in situ* (DCIS); metastatic female and male breast cancer; treatment of melanoma, desmoid tumors

Unlabeled/Investigational Use Treatment of mastalgia, gynecomastia, pancreatic carcinoma; induction of ovulation; treatment of precocious puberty in females, secondary to McCune-Albright syndrome

Mechanism of Action Competitively binds to estrogen receptors on tumors and other tissue targets, producing a nuclear complex that decreases DNA synthesis and inhibits estrogen effects; nonsteroidal agent with potent antiestrogenic properties which compete with estrogen for binding sites in breast and other tissues; cells accumulate in the G_0 and G_1 phases; therefore, tamoxifen is cytostatic rather than cytocidal.

Restrictions An FDA-approved medication guide is available at www.AstraZeneca-us.com/pi/Nolvadex.pdf. Distribute to each female patient who is using tamoxifen to decrease risk of developing breast cancer or who has ductal carcinoma *in situ*.

Labeled Contraindications Hypersensitivity to tamoxifen or any component of the formulation; concurrent warfarin therapy (when used for cancer risk reduction); pregnancy

Warnings/Precautions Hazardous agent - use appropriate precautions for handling and disposal. See Safe Handling of Hazardous Drugs *on page 1034* in the Appendix. Serious and life-threatening events (including stroke, pulmonary emboli, and uterine malignancy) have occurred at an incidence greater than placebo during use for cancer risk reduction; these events are rare, but require consideration in risk:benefit evaluation. An increased incidence of thromboembolic events has been associated with use for breast cancer; risk may increase with chemotherapy addition; use
(Continued)

Tamoxifen *(Continued)*

caution in individuals with a history of thromboembolic events. Use with caution in patients with leukopenia, thrombocytopenia, or hyperlipidemias. Decreased visual acuity, retinopathy, corneal changes, and increased incidence of cataracts have been reported. Hypercalcemia has occurred in patients with bone metastasis. Significant bone loss of the lumbar spine and hip was associated with use in premenopausal women. Liver abnormalities such as cholestasis, hepatitis, and hepatic necrosis have occurred; hepatocellular carcinomas have been reported in some studies, relationship to treatment is unclear. Endometrial hyperplasia and polyps have occurred. Increased risk of uterine or endometrial cancer; monitor.

Adverse Reactions Note: Differences in the frequency of some adverse events may be related to use for a specific indication.

>10%:
  Cardiovascular: Flushing (33%)
  Central nervous system: Mood changes (up to 12%)
  Dermatologic: Skin changes (19%)
  Endocrine & metabolic: Hot flashes (3% to 80%), fluid retention (32%), altered menses (13% to 25%), amenorrhea (16%)
  Gastrointestinal: Nausea (5% to 26%), weight loss (23%)
  Genitourinary: Vaginal bleeding (up to 23%), vaginal discharge (30% to 55%)

1% to 10%:
  Cardiovascular: Edema (4%)
  Central nervous system: Fatigue (4%), depression (2%)
  Dermatologic: Alopecia (<1% to 5%)
  Endocrine & metabolic: Oligomenorrhea (9%), menstrual disorder (6%)
  Gastrointestinal: Constipation (up to 4%), abdominal cramps (1%), anorexia (1%)
  Genitourinary: Ovarian cyst (3%)
  Hematologic: Thrombocytopenia (<1% to 10%)
  Hepatic: SGOT increased (5%), serum bilirubin increased (2%)
  Neuromuscular & skeletal: Bone pain (6%), musculoskeletal pain (3%), pain (3%)
  Renal: Serum creatinine increased (up to 2%)
  Respiratory: Cough (4%)
  Miscellaneous: Infection/sepsis (up to 6%), allergic reaction (up to 3%)

<1%, infrequent, or frequency not defined: Cataract, cholestasis, corneal changes, deep vein thrombosis, dizziness, endometriosis, endometrial cancer, endometrial hyperplasia, endometrial polyps, , fatty liver, hepatic necrosis, hepatitis, hypercalcemia, hyperlipidemias, lightheadedness, pancreatitis, peripheral edema, phlebitis, pruritus vulvae, pulmonary embolism, retinal vein thrombosis, retinopathy, second primary tumors, stroke, taste disturbances, tumor pain and local disease flare (including increase in lesion size and erythema) during treatment of metastatic breast cancer (generally resolves with continuation), uterine fibroids, vaginal dryness

Postmarketing and/or case reports: Angioedema, bullous pemphigoid, erythema multiforme, hypersensitivity reactions, headache, hypertriglyceridemia, interstitial pneumonitis, impotence (males), loss of libido (males), rash, Stevens-Johnson syndrome

Emetic Potential Low (10% to 30%)

Overdosage/Toxicology Symptoms of overdose include hypercalcemia and edema. Provide general supportive care.

Drug Interactions

Cytochrome P450 Effect: Substrate of CYP2A6 (minor), 2B6 (minor), 2C8/9 (major), 2D6 (major), 2E1 (minor), 3A4 (major); **Inhibits** CYP2B6 (weak), 2C8/9 (weak), 3A4 (weak)

Increased Effect/Toxicity: Allopurinol and tamoxifen results in exacerbation of allopurinol-induced hepatotoxicity. Cyclosporine serum levels may be increased when taken with tamoxifen. Concomitant use of warfarin is contraindicated when used for risk reduction; results in significant enhancement of the anticoagulant effects of warfarin. CYP2C8/9 inhibitors may increase the levels/effects of tamoxifen; example inhibitors include delavirdine, fluconazole, gemfibrozil, ketoconazole, nicardipine, NSAIDs, pioglitazone, and sulfonamides. CYP2D6 inhibitors may increase the levels/effects of tamoxifen; example inhibitors include chlorpromazine, delavirdine, fluoxetine, miconazole, paroxetine, pergolide, quinidine, quinine, ritonavir, and ropinirole. CYP3A4 inhibitors may increase the levels/effects of tamoxifen; example inhibitors include azole antifungals, ciprofloxacin, clarithromycin, diclofenac, doxycycline, erythromycin, imatinib, isoniazid, nefazodone, nicardipine, propofol, protease inhibitors, quinidine, and verapamil.

Decreased Effect: CYP2C8/9 inducers may decrease the levels/effects of tamoxifen; example inducers include carbamazepine, phenobarbital, phenytoin, rifampin, rifapentine, and secobarbital. CYP3A4 inducers may decrease the levels/effects of tamoxifen; example inducers include aminoglutethimide, carbamazepine, nafcillin, nevirapine, phenobarbital, phenytoin, and rifamycins. Letrozole serum levels may be reduced by tamoxifen.

Ethanol/Nutrition/Herb Interactions Herb/Nutraceutical: Avoid black cohosh, dong quai in estrogen-dependent tumors.

Storage/Stability Store at room temperature of 20°C to 25°C (68°F to 77°F).

Pharmacodynamics/Kinetics

Absorption: Well absorbed

Distribution: High concentrations found in uterus, endometrial and breast tissue

Protein binding: 99%

Metabolism: Hepatic (via CYP3A4) to major metabolites, N-desmethyl tamoxifen (major) and 4-hydroxytamoxifen (minor), and a tamoxifen derivative (minor); undergoes enterohepatic recirculation

Half-life elimination: Distribution: 7-14 hours; Elimination: 5-7 days; Metabolites: 14 days

Time to peak, serum: 5 hours

Excretion: Feces (26% to 51%); urine (9% to 13%)

Dosage Oral (refer to individual protocols):

Children: Female: Precocious puberty and McCune-Albright syndrome (unlabeled use): A dose of 20 mg/day has been reported in patients 2-10 years of age; safety and efficacy have not been established for treatment of longer than 1 year duration

(Continued)

Tamoxifen *(Continued)*

Adults:

Breast cancer:

Metastatic (males and females) or adjuvant therapy (females): 20-40 mg/day; daily doses >20 mg should be given in 2 divided doses (morning and evening)

Prevention (high-risk females): 20 mg/day for 5 years

DCIS (females): 20 mg once daily for 5 years

Note: Higher dosages (up to 700 mg/day) have been investigated for use in modulation of multidrug resistance (MDR), but are not routinely used in clinical practice

Induction of ovulation (unlabeled use): 5-40 mg twice daily for 4 days

Combination Regimens

Breast cancer: Tamoxifen-Epirubicin *on page 939*

Melanoma:

CCDT (Melanoma) *on page 855*

Dacarbazine/Tamoxifen *on page 871*

Administration Oral: Twice daily dosing has been traditional, but once daily dosing is equally effective in most patients. Doses >20 mg/day should be given in divided doses.

Dosage Forms Tablet, as citrate: 10 mg, 20 mg

Monitoring Parameters Monitor WBC and platelet counts, serum calcium, LFTs; abnormal vaginal bleeding; annual gynecologic exams, mammogram

Patient Information Take as directed, morning and night, and maintain adequate hydration (2-3 L/day of fluids unless instructed to restrict fluid intake). You may experience menstrual irregularities, vaginal bleeding, hot flashes, hair loss, loss of libido (these will subside when treatment is completed). Bone pain may indicate a good therapeutic response (consult prescriber for mild analgesics). For nausea/vomiting, small frequent meals, chewing gum, or sucking lozenges may help. You may experience photosensitivity (use sunscreen, wear protective clothing and eyewear, and avoid direct sunlight). Report unusual bleeding or bruising, severe weakness, sedation, mental changes, swelling or pain in calves, difficulty breathing, or any changes in vision.

Additional Information Oral clonidine is being studied for the treatment of tamoxifen-induced "hot flashes." The tumor flare reaction may indicate a good therapeutic response, and is often considered a good prognostic factor.

Special Geriatric Considerations Studies have shown tamoxifen to be effective in the treatment of primary breast cancer in elderly women. Comparative studies with other antineoplastic agents in elderly women with breast cancer had more favorable survival rates with tamoxifen. Initiation of hormone therapy rather than chemotherapy is justified for elderly patients with metastatic breast cancer who are responsive.

Selected Readings

Benson JR and Pitsinis V, "Update on Clinical Role of Tamoxifen," *Curr Opin Obstet Gynecol*, 2003, 15(1):13-23.

Clemons M, Danson S, and Howell A, "Tamoxifen ("Nolvadex"): A Review," *Cancer Treat Rev*, 2002, 28(4):165-80.

Gradishar WJ, "Tamoxifen - What Next?" *Oncologist*, 2004, 9(4):378-84.

Jordan VC, "Tamoxifen: A Most Unlikely Pioneering Medicine," *Nat Rev Drug Discov*, 2003, 2(3):205-13.

Wickerham L, "Tamoxifen - An Update on Current Data and Where it Can Now Be Used," *Breast Cancer Res Treat*, 2002, 75 Suppl 1:S7-12.

- **Tamoxifen Citrate** *see* Tamoxifen *on page 743*
- **Tantum®** **(Can)** *see* Benzydamine *on page 123*
- **TAP-144** *see* Leuprolide *on page 500*
- **Tarceva™** *see* Erlotinib *on page 308*
- **Targretin®** *see* Bexarotene *on page 127*
- **Taxol®** *see* Paclitaxel *on page 638*
- **Taxotere®** *see* Docetaxel *on page 272*
- **Tazicef®** *see* Ceftazidime *on page 165*
- **Tazocin®** **(Can)** *see* Piperacillin and Tazobactam Sodium *on page 672*
- **T-Cell Growth Factor** *see* Aldesleukin *on page 32*
- **TCGF** *see* Aldesleukin *on page 32*

Telithromycin (tel ith roe MYE sin)

U.S. Brand Names Ketek®
Canadian Brand Names Ketek®
Generic Available No
Synonyms HMR 3647
Pharmacologic Category Antibiotic, Ketolide
Pregnancy Risk Factor C
Lactation Excretion in breast milk unknown/use caution
Use Treatment of community-acquired pneumonia (mild-to-moderate) caused by susceptible strains of *Streptococcus pneumoniae* (including multidrug-resistant isolates), *Haemophilus influenzae*, *Chlamydia pneumoniae*, *Moraxella catarrhalis*, and *Mycoplasma pneumoniae*; treatment of bacterial exacerbation of chronic bronchitis caused by susceptible strains of *S. pneumoniae*, *H. influenzae* and *Moraxella catarrhalis*; treatment of acute bacterial sinusitis caused by *Streptococcus pneumoniae*, *Haemophilus influenzae*, *Moraxella catarrhalis*, and *Staphylococcus aureus*
Unlabeled/Investigational Use Approved in Canada for use in the treatment of tonsillitis/pharyngitis due to *S. pyogenes* (as an alternative to beta-lactam antibiotics when necessary/appropriate)
Mechanism of Action Inhibits bacterial protein synthesis by binding to two sites on the 50S ribosomal subunit. Telithromycin has also been demonstrated to alter secretion of IL-1alpha and TNF-alpha; the clinical significance of this immunomodulatory effect has not been evaluated.
Labeled Contraindications Hypersensitivity to telithromycin, macrolide antibiotics, or any component of the formulation; concurrent use of cisapride or pimozide
Warnings/Precautions May prolong QT_c interval, leading to a risk of ventricular arrhythmias; closely-related antibiotics have been associated with malignant ventricular arrhythmias and torsade de pointes. Avoid in patients with prolongation of QT_c interval due to congenital causes, history of long QT syndrome, uncorrected electrolyte disturbances (hypokalemia or hypermagnesemia), significant bradycardia (<50 bpm), or concurrent therapy with QT_c-prolonging drugs (eg, class Ia and class III antiarrhythmics). Avoid use in patients with a prior history of confirmed cardiogenic syncope or ventricular arrhythmias while receiving macrolide antibiotics or other QT_c-prolonging drugs. Use caution in renal impairment. Use caution in patients with myasthenia gravis (use only if suitable
(Continued)

Telithromycin *(Continued)*

alternatives are not available). Inform patients of potential for blurred vision, which may interfere with ability to operate machinery or drive; use caution until effects are known. Safety and efficacy not established in pediatric patients <13 years of age.

Adverse Reactions

2% to 10%:

Central nervous system: Headache (2% to 6%), dizziness (3% to 4%)

Gastrointestinal: Diarrhea (10%), nausea (7% to 8%), vomiting (2% to 3%), loose stools (2%), dysgeusia (2%)

≥0.2% to <2%:

Central nervous system: Vertigo, fatigue, somnolence, insomnia

Dermatologic: Rash

Gastrointestinal: Abdominal distension, abdominal pain, anorexia, constipation, dyspepsia, flatulence, gastritis, gastroenteritis, GI upset, glossitis, stomatitis, watery stools, xerostomia

Genitourinary: Vaginal candidiasis

Hematologic: Platelets increased

Hepatic: Transaminases increased, hepatitis

Ocular: Blurred vision, accommodation delayed, diplopia

Miscellaneous: Candidiasis, diaphoresis increased, exacerbation of myasthenia gravis (rare)

<0.2%: Alkaline phosphatase increased, anxiety, bilirubin increased, bradycardia, eczema, eosinophilia, erythema multiforme, flushing, hypotension, paresthesia, pruritus, urticaria

Postmarketing and/or case reports: Anaphylaxis, angioedema, arrhythmia, edema (facial), hepatocellular injury, muscle cramps

Additional effects also reported with telithromycin:

Cardiovascular: Bundle branch block, palpitation, QT_c prolongation, vasculitis

Central nervous system: Abnormal dreams, nervousness, tremor

Endocrine & metabolic: Appetite decreased, hypokalemia, hyperkalemia

Gastrointestinal: Esophagitis, pharyngolaryngeal pain, pseudomembranous colitis, reflux esophagitis, tooth discoloration

Genitourinary: Vaginal irritation, urine discoloration, polyuria

Hematologic: Anemia, coagulation disorder, leukopenia, neutropenia, thrombocytopenia, lymphopenia

Hepatic: Cholestasis

Neuromuscular & skeletal: Weakness

Renal: Serum creatinine increased

Miscellaneous: Hypersensitivity

Overdosage/Toxicology Treatment should be symptomatic and supportive. ECG and electrolytes should be monitored.

Drug Interactions

Cytochrome P450 Effect: **Substrate** of CYP1A2 (minor), 3A4 (major); **Inhibits** CYP2D6 (weak), 3A4 (strong)

Increased Effect/Toxicity: Concurrent use of cisapride or pimozide is contraindicated. Concurrent use with antiarrhythmics (eg, class Ia and class III) or other drugs which prolong QT_c (eg, gatifloxacin, mesoridazine, moxifloxacin, pimozide, sparfloxacin, thioridazine) may be additive; serious arrhythmias may occur. Neuromuscular-blocking agents may be potentiated by telithromycin.

Telithromycin may increase the levels/effects of selected benzodiazepines, calcium channel blockers, cyclosporine, ergot alkaloids, selected HMG-CoA reductase inhibitors, mirtazapine, nateglinide, nefazodone, pimozide, quinidine, sildenafil (and other PDE-5 inhibitors), tacrolimus, venlafaxine, and other CYP3A4 substrates. Selected benzodiazepines (midazolam, triazolam), and selected HMG-CoA reductase inhibitors (atorvastatin, lovastatin and simvastatin) are generally contraindicated with strong CYP3A4 inhibitors. When used with strong CYP3A4 inhibitors, dosage adjustment/limits are recommended for sildenafil and other PDE-5 inhibitors; refer to individual monographs.

The levels/effects of telithromycin may be increased by azole antifungals, ciprofloxacin, clarithromycin, diclofenac, doxycycline, erythromycin, imatinib, isoniazid, nefazodone, nicardipine, propofol, protease inhibitors, quinidine, verapamil, and other CYP3A4 inhibitors.

Decreased Effect: The levels/effects of telithromycin may be decreased by aminoglutethimide, carbamazepine, nafcillin, nevirapine, phenobarbital, phenytoin, rifamycins, and other CYP3A4 inducers; avoid concurrent use.

Storage/Stability Store at room temperature between 15°C and 30°C.

Pharmacodynamics/Kinetics
Absorption: Rapid
Distribution: 2.9 L/kg
Protein binding: 60% to 70%
Metabolism: Hepatic, via CYP3A4 (50%) and non-CYP-mediated pathways
Bioavailability: 57% (significant first-pass metabolism)
Half-life elimination: 10 hours
Time to peak, plasma: 1 hour
Excretion: Urine (13% unchanged drug, remainder as metabolites); feces (7%)

Dosage Oral:
Children ≥13 years and Adults: Tonsillitis/pharyngitis (unlabeled U.S. indication): 800 mg once daily for 5 days
Adults:
Acute exacerbation of chronic bronchitis, acute bacterial sinusitis: 800 mg once daily for 5 days
Community-acquired pneumonia: 800 mg once daily for 7-10 days

Dosage adjustment in renal impairment:
U.S. product labeling: Cl_{cr} <30 mL/minute: 600 mg once daily; when renal impairment is accompanied by hepatic impairment, reduce dosage to 400 mg once daily
Canadian product labeling: Cl_{cr} <30 mL/minute: Reduce dose to 400 mg once daily
Hemodialysis: Administer following dialysis

Dosage adjustment in hepatic impairment: No adjustment recommended, unless concurrent severe renal impairment is present

Administration May be administered with or without food.

Dosage Forms
Tablet [film coated]: 300 mg [not available in Canada], 400 mg
(Continued)

Telithromycin *(Continued)*

Ketek Pak™ [blister pack]: 400 mg (10s) [packaged as 10 tablets/card; 2 tablets/blister]

Dietary Considerations May be taken with or without food.

Special Geriatric Considerations Bioavailability (57%) equivalent in persons ≥65 years compared to younger adults; although a 1.4- to 2-fold increase in AUC found in older adults. No dosage adjustment required. See dosing information.

Selected Readings

Araujo FG, Slifer TL, and Remington JS, "Inhibition of Secretion of Interleukin-1alpha and Tumor Necrosis Factor Alpha by the Ketolide Antibiotic Telithromycin," *Antimicrob Agents Chemother*, 2002, 46(10):3327-30.

Bhargava V, Lenfant B, Perret C, et al, "Lack of Effect of Food on the Bioavailability of a New Ketolide Antibacterial, Telithromycin," *Scand J Infect Dis*, 2002, 34(11):823-6.

Cantalloube C, Bhargava V, Sultan E, et al, "Pharmacokinetics of the Ketolide Telithromycin After Single and Repeated Doses in Patients With Hepatic Impairment," *Int J Antimicrob Agents*, 2003, 22(2):112-21.

Canton R, Morosini M, Enright MC, et al, "Worldwide Incidence, Molecular Epidemiology and Mutations Implicated in Fluoroquinolone-resistant *Streptococcus pneumoniae*: Data From the Global PROTEKT Surveillance Programme," *J Antimicrob Chemother*, 2003, 52(6):944-52.

Carbon C, "A Pooled Analysis of Telithromycin in the Treatment of Community-Acquired Respiratory Tract Infections in Adults," *Infection*, 2003, 31(5):308-17.

Demolis JL, Vacheron F, Cardus S, et al, "Effect of Single and Repeated Oral Doses of Telithromycin on Cardiac QT Interval in Healthy Subjects," *Clin Pharmacol Ther*, 2003, 73(3):242-52.

Perret C, Lenfant B, Weinling E, et al, "Pharmacokinetics and Absolute Oral Bioavailability of an 800-mg Oral Dose of Telithromycin in Healthy Young and Elderly Volunteers," *Chemotherapy*, 2002, 48(5):217-23.

Nieman RB, Sharma K, Edelberg H, et al, "Telithromycin and Myasthenia Gravis," *Clin Infect Dis*, 2003, 37(11):1579.

Quinn J, Ruoff GE, and Ziter PS, "Efficacy and tolerability of 5-day, once-daily telithromycin compared with 10-day, twice-daily clarithromycin for the treatment of group A beta-hemolytic streptococcal tonsillitis/pharyngitis: a multicenter, randomized, double-blind, parallel-group study," *Clin Ther*, 2003, 25(2):422-43.

Ubukata K, Iwata S, and Sunakawa K, "*In vitro* Activities of New Ketolide, Telithromycin, and Eight Other Macrolide Antibiotics Against *Streptococcus pneumoniae* Having mefA and ermB Genes That Mediate Macrolide Resistance," *J Infect Chemother*, 2003, 9(3):221-6.

Zervos MJ, Heyder AM, and Leroy B, "Oral Telithromycin 800 mg Once Daily for 5 Days Versus Cefuroxime Axetil 500 mg Twice Daily for 10 Days in Adults With Acute Exacerbations of Chronic Bronchitis," *J Int Med Res*, 2003, 31(3):157-69.

♦ **Temodal™ (Can)** *see* Temozolomide *on page 750*

♦ **Temodar®** *see* Temozolomide *on page 750*

Temozolomide *(te moe ZOE loe mide)*

Related Information

Safe Handling of Hazardous Drugs *on page 1034*

U.S. Brand Names Temodar®

Canadian Brand Names Temodal™; Temodar®

Generic Available No

Synonyms NSC-362856; TMZ

Pharmacologic Category Antineoplastic Agent, Alkylating Agent

Pregnancy Risk Factor D

Lactation Excretion in breast milk unknown/not recommended

Use Treatment of adult patients with refractory (first relapse) anaplastic astrocytoma who have experienced disease progression on nitrosourea and procarbazine; newly-diagnosed glioblastoma multiforme

Unlabeled/Investigational Use Glioma, melanoma

Mechanism of Action Like dacarbazine, temozolomide is converted to the active alkylating metabolite MTIC [(methyl-triazene-1-yl)-imidazole - 4 - carboxamide]. Unlike dacarbazine, however, this conversion is spontaneous, nonenzymatic, and occurs under physiologic conditions in all tissues to which the drug distributes.

Labeled Contraindications Hypersensitivity to temozolomide or any component of the formulation; hypersensitivity to dacarbazine (since both drugs are metabolized to MTIC); pregnancy

Warnings/Precautions Hazardous agent - use appropriate precautions for handling and disposal. See Safe Handling of Hazardous Drugs *on page 1034* in the Appendix. *Pneumocystis carinii* pneumonia (PCP) may occur; risk is increased in those receiving steroids or longer dosing regimens; PCP prophylaxis is required with radiotherapy for the 42-day regimen. Myelosuppression may occur; an increased incidence has been reported in geriatric and female patients; prior to dosing, absolute neutrophil count (ANC) should be $\geq$1.5 X 10^9/L and platelet count $\geq$100 X 10^9/L. Use caution in patients with severe hepatic or renal impairment. Safety and efficacy in pediatric patients have not been established.

Adverse Reactions Adverse reactions are listed as the combined incidence in studies for treatment of newly-diagnosed glioblastoma multiforme during the maintenance phase (after radiotherapy) and refractory anaplastic astrocytoma in adults.

>10%:

Cardiovascular: Peripheral edema (up to 11%)

Central nervous system: Fatigue (34% to 61%), headache (23% to 41%), fatigue (34% to 61%), convulsions (11% to 23%), hemiparesis (18%), dizziness (5% to 12%), fever (up to 13%), coordination abnormality (up to 11%). In the case of CNS malignancies, it is difficult to distinguish the relative contributions of temozolomide and progressive disease to CNS symptoms.

Dermatologic: Alopecia (55% - maintenance phase after radiotherapy), rash (8% to 13%)

Gastrointestinal: Nausea (49% to 53%), vomiting (29% to 42%), constipation (22% to 33%), anorexia (9% to 27%), diarrhea (10% to 16%)

Hematologic: Lymphopenia (grade 3/4 in 55%), thrombocytopenia (grade 3/4 in 4% to 19%), neutropenia (grade 3/4 in 8% to 14%), leukopenia (grade 3/4 in 11%)

Neuromuscular & skeletal: Weakness (7% to 13%)

Miscellaneous: Viral infection (up to 11%)

1% to 10%:

Central nervous system: Ataxia (8%), memory impairment (up to 7%), confusion (5%), anxiety (7%), depression (up to 6%), amnesia (up to 10%), paresis (up to 8%), somnolence (up to 9%), insomnia (4% to 10%)

Dermatologic: Rash (8% to 13%), pruritus (5% to 8%), dry skin (up to 5%), radiation injury (2% - maintenance phase after radiotherapy), erythema (1%)

Endocrine & metabolic: Hypercorticism (8%), breast pain (up to 6%)

Gastrointestinal: Dysphagia (up to 7%), abdominal pain (5% to 9%), stomatitis (up to 9%), weight gain (up to 5%)

Genitourinary: Micturition frequency increased (up to 6%), incontinence (up to 8%), urinary tract infection (up to 8%)

(Continued)

751

Temozolomide *(Continued)*

Hematologic: Anemia (8%; grade 3/4 in up to 4%)

Neuromuscular & skeletal: Paresthesia (up to 9%), back pain (up to 8%), arthralgia (up to 6%), abnormal gait (up to 6%), myalgia (up to 5%),

Ocular: Diplopia (5%); vision abnormality (blurred vision, visual deficit, vision changes) (5% to 8%)

Respiratory: Pharyngitis (up to 8%), sinusitis (up to 6%), cough (5% to 8%), upper respiratory tract infection (up to 8%), dyspnea (5%)

Miscellaneous: Taste perversion (up to 5%), allergic reaction (up to 3%)

Postmarketing and/or case reports: Anaphylaxis, erythema multiforme, opportunistic infection (eg, PCP)

Emetic Potential Moderate (30% to 60%)

Overdosage/Toxicology Dose-limiting toxicity is hematological. In the event of an overdose, hematological evaluation is necessary. Treatment is supportive.

Ethanol/Nutrition/Herb Interactions Food: Food reduces rate and extent of absorption.

Storage/Stability Store at controlled room temperature (15°C to 10°C/ 59°F to 86°F).

Pharmacodynamics/Kinetics

Distribution: V_d: Parent drug: 0.4 L/kg

Protein binding: 15%

Metabolism: Prodrug, hydrolyzed to the active form, MTIC; MTIC is eventually eliminated as CO_2 and 5-aminoimidazole-4-carboxamide (AIC), a natural constituent in urine

Bioavailability: 100%

Half-life elimination: Mean: Parent drug: 1.8 hours

Time to peak: Empty stomach: 1 hour

Excretion: Urine (~38%; parent drug 6%); feces 0.8%

Dosage Oral (refer to individual protocols): Adults:

Anaplastic astrocytoma (refractory): Initial dose: 150 mg/m²/day for 5 days; repeat every 28 days. Subsequent doses of 100-200 mg/m²/day; based upon hematologic tolerance. This monthly-cycle regimen may be preceded by a 6- to 7-week regimen of 75 mg/m²/day.

ANC <1000/mm³ or platelets <50,000/mm³ on day 22 or day 29 (day 1 of next cycle): Postpone therapy until ANC >1500/mm³ and platelets >100,000/mm³; reduce dose by 50 mg/m²/day for subsequent cycle

ANC 1000-1500/mm³ or platelets 50,000-100,000/mm³ on day 22 or day 29 (day 1 of next cycle): Postpone therapy until ANC >1500/mm³ and platelets >100,000/mm³; maintain initial dose

ANC >1500/mm³ and platelets >100,000/mm³ on day 22 or day 29 (day 1 of next cycle): Increase dose to or maintain dose at 200 mg/m²/day for 5 days for subsequent cycle

Glioblastoma multiforme (high-grade glioma):

Concomitant phase: 75 mg/m²/day for 42 days with radiotherapy (60Gy administered in 30 fractions). **Note:** PCP prophylaxis is required during concomitant phase and should continue in patients who develop lymphocytopenia until recovery (common toxicity criteria [CTC] ≤1). Obtain weekly CBC.

ANC ≥1500/mm³, platelet count ≥100,000/mm³, and nonhematologic CTC ≤grade 1 (excludes alopecia, nausea/vomiting): Temodar® 75 mg/m²/day may be continued throughout the 42-day concomitant period up to 49 days

Dosage modification:

ANC ≥500/mm³ but <1500/mm³ **or** platelet count ≥10,000/mm³ but <100,000/mm³ **or** nonhematologic CTC grade 2 (excludes alopecia, nausea/vomiting): Interrupt therapy

ANC <500/mm³ **or** platelet count <10,000/mm³ **or** nonhematologic CTC grade 3/4 (excludes alopecia, nausea/vomiting): Discontinue therapy

Maintenance phase (consists of 6 treatment cycles): Begin 4 weeks after concomitant phase completion. **Note:** Each subsequent cycle is 28 days (consisting of 5 days of drug treatment followed by 23 days without treatment). Draw CBC within 48 hours of day 22; hold next cycle and do weekly CBC until ANC >1500/mm³ and platelet count >100,000/mm³; dosing modification should be based on lowest blood counts and worst nonhematologic toxicity during the previous cycle.

Cycle 1: 150 mg/m²/day for 5 days

Dosage modification for next cycle:

ANC <1000/mm³, platelet count <50,000/mm³, or nonhematologic CTC grade 3 (excludes for alopecia, nausea/vomiting) during previous cycle: Decrease dose by 50 mg/m²/day for 5 days, unless dose has already been lowered to 100 mg/m²/day, then discontinue therapy.

If dose reduction <100 mg/m²/day is required or nonhematologic CTC grade 4 (excludes for alopecia, nausea/vomiting), or if the same grade 3 nonhematologic toxicity occurs after dose reduction: Discontinue therapy

Cycle 2: 200 mg/m²/day for 5 days unless prior toxicity, then refer to Dosage Modifications under "Cycle 1" and give adjusted dose for 5 days

Cycles 3-6: Continue with previous cycle's dose for 5 days unless toxicity has occurred then, refer to Dosage Modifications under "Cycle 1" and give adjusted dose for 5 days

Elderly: Patients ≥70 years of age had a higher incidence of grade 4 neutropenia and thrombocytopenia in the first cycle of therapy than patients <70 years of age.

Dosage adjustment in renal impairment: No guidelines exist. Caution should be used when administered to patients with severe renal impairment (Cl_cr <39 mL/minute).

Dosage adjustment in hepatic impairment: Caution should be used when administering to patients with severe hepatic impairment.

Administration Capsules should not be opened or chewed but swallowed whole with a glass of water. May be administered on an empty stomach to reduce nausea and vomiting. Bedtime administration may be advised.

Dosage Forms Capsule: 5 mg, 20 mg, 100 mg, 250 mg

Monitoring Parameters CBC; platelet count >100,000/mm³ and WBC >1500/mm³ before initiating therapy

Dietary Considerations The incidence of nausea/vomiting is decreased when the drug is taken on an empty stomach.

Patient Information Swallow capsules whole with a glass of water. Take on an empty stomach at similar time each day. If you have nausea and vomiting, contact prescriber for medicine to decrease this. Male and (Continued)

753

Temozolomide *(Continued)*

female patients who take temozolomide should protect against pregnancy (use effective contraception). Do not breast-feed while on medicine.

Selected Readings

Agarwala SS and Kirkwood JM, "Temozolomide, A Novel Alkylating Agent With Activity in the Central Nervous System, May Improve the Treatment of Advanced Metastatic Melanoma," *Oncologist*, 2000, 5(2):144-51.

Gaya A, Rees J, Greenstein A, et al, "The Use of Temozolomide in Recurrent Malignant Gliomas," *Cancer Treat Rev*, 2002; 28(2):115-20.

Newlands ES, Stevens MF, Wedge SR, et al, "Temozolomide: A Review of Its Discovery, Chemical Properties, Pre-Clinical Development and Clinical Trials," *Cancer Treat Rev*, 1997, 23(1):35-61.

Schwenka J and Ignoffo RJ, "Temozolomide. A New Option for High-Grade Astrocytomas," *Cancer Pract*, 2000, 8(6):311-3.

Stupp R, Dietrich PY, Ostermann Kraljevic S, et al, "Promising Survival for Patients With Newly Diagnosed Glioblastoma Multiforme Treated With Concomitant Radiation Plus Temozolomide Followed by Adjuvant Temozolomide," *J Clin Oncol*, 2002, 20(5):1375-82.

Stupp R, Gander M, Leyvraz S, et al, "Current and Future Developments in the Use of Temozolomide for the Treatment of Brain Tumours," *Lancet Oncol*, 2001, 2(9):552-60.

Teniposide *(ten i POE side)*

Related Information

Safe Handling of Hazardous Drugs *on page 1034*

U.S. Brand Names Vumon

Canadian Brand Names Vumon®

Generic Available No

Synonyms EPT; VM-26

Pharmacologic Category Antineoplastic Agent, Miscellaneous

Pregnancy Risk Factor D

Lactation Not recommended

Use Treatment of acute lymphocytic leukemia, small cell lung cancer

Mechanism of Action Teniposide does not inhibit microtubular assembly; it has been shown to delay transit of cells through the S phase and arrest cells in late S or early G_2 phase. Teniposide is a topoisomerase II inhibitor, and appears to cause DNA strand breaks by inhibition of strand-passing and DNA ligase action.

Labeled Contraindications Hypersensitivity to teniposide, Cremophor® EL (polyoxyethylated castor oil), or any component of the formulation; pregnancy

Warnings/Precautions Hazardous agent - use appropriate precautions for handling and disposal. See Safe Handling of Hazardous Drugs *on page 1034* in the Appendix. Teniposide injection contains benzyl alcohol and should be avoided in neonates. The injection contains about 43% alcohol; the possible CNS depressant effect, especially with higher doses of teniposide, should be considered.

Adverse Reactions

>10%:

Gastrointestinal: Mucositis (75%); diarrhea, nausea, vomiting (20% to 30%); anorexia

Hematologic: Myelosuppression, leukopenia, neutropenia (95%), thrombocytopenia (65% to 80%), anemia

Onset: 5-7 days

Nadir: 7-10 days

Recovery: 21-28 days

1% to 10%:

Cardiovascular: Hypotension (2%), associated with rapid (<30 minutes) infusions

Dermatologic: Alopecia (9%), rash (3%)

Miscellaneous: Anaphylactoid reactions (5%) (fever, rash, hyper-/hypotension, dyspnea, bronchospasm), usually seen with rapid (<30 minutes) infusions

<1%: Lethargy, peripheral neuropathies, somnolence

Vesicant No; may be an irritant

Emetic Potential Moderate (30% to 60%)

Overdosage/Toxicology Symptoms of overdose include bone marrow suppression, leukopenia, thrombocytopenia, nausea, and vomiting. Treatment is supportive.

Drug Interactions

Cytochrome P450 Effect: Substrate of CYP3A4 (major); **Inhibits** CYP2C8/9 (weak), 3A4 (weak)

Increased Effect/Toxicity: May increase toxicity of methotrexate. Sodium salicylate, sulfamethizole, and tolbutamide displace teniposide from protein-binding sites which could cause substantial increases in free drug levels, resulting in potentiation of toxicity. Concurrent use of vincristine may increase the incidence of peripheral neuropathy. CYP3A4 inhibitors may increase the levels/effects of teniposide; example inhibitors include azole antifungals, ciprofloxacin, clarithromycin, diclofenac, doxycycline, erythromycin, imatinib, isoniazid, nefazodone, nicardipine, propofol, protease inhibitors, quinidine, and verapamil.

Decreased Effect: CYP3A4 inducers may decrease the levels/effects of teniposide; example inducers include aminoglutethimide, carbamazepine, nafcillin, nevirapine, phenobarbital, phenytoin, and rifamycins.

Ethanol/Nutrition/Herb Interactions Herb/Nutraceutical: St John's wort may decrease teniposide levels.

Storage/Stability Store ampuls in refrigerator at 2°C to 8°C (36°F to 46°F). Reconstituted solutions are stable at room temperature for up to 24 hours after preparation. Precipitation may occur at any concentration.

Reconstitution Teniposide must be diluted with either D_5W or 0.9% sodium chloride solutions to a final concentration of 0.1, 0.2, 0.4, or 1 mg/mL. **Solutions should be prepared in non-DEHP-containing containers such as glass or polyolefin containers**.

Compatibility Stable in D_5W, LR, NS

Y-site administration: Compatible: Acyclovir, allopurinol, amifostine, amikacin, aminophylline, amphotericin B, ampicillin, ampicillin/sulbactam, aztreonam, bleomycin, bumetanide, buprenorphine, butorphanol, calcium gluconate, carboplatin, carmustine, cefazolin, cefoperazone, cefotaxime, cefotetan, cefoxitin, ceftazidime, ceftizoxime, ceftriaxone, cefuroxime, chlorpromazine, cimetidine, ciprofloxacin, cisplatin, cladribine, clindamycin, co-trimoxazole, cyclophosphamide, cytarabine, dacarbazine, dactinomycin, daunorubicin, dexamethasone sodium phosphate, diphenhydramine, doxorubicin, doxycycline, droperidol, enalaprilat, etoposide, etoposide phosphate, famotidine, floxuridine, fluconazole, fludarabine, fluorouracil, furosemide, ganciclovir, gemcitabine, gentamicin, granisetron, haloperidol, hydrocortisone sodium phosphate, hydrocortisone sodium succinate, hydromorphone, hydroxyzine, ifosfamide, imipenem/cilastatin, leucovorin, lorazepam, (Continued)

Teniposide *(Continued)*

mannitol, mechlorethamine, melphalan, meperidine, mesna, methotrexate, methylprednisolone sodium succinate, metoclopramide, metronidazole, minocycline, mitomycin, mitoxantrone, morphine, nalbuphine, netilmicin, ondansetron, piperacillin, plicamycin, potassium chloride, prochlorperazine edisylate, promethazine, ranitidine, sargramostim, sodium bicarbonate, streptozocin, thiotepa, ticarcillin, ticarcillin/clavulanate, tobramycin, vancomycin, vinblastine, vincristine, vinorelbine, zidovudine. **Incompatible:** Idarubicin, heparin

Pharmacodynamics/Kinetics

Distribution: V_d: 0.28 L/kg; Adults: 8-44 L; Children: 3-11 L; mainly into liver, kidneys, small intestine, and adrenals; crosses blood-brain barrier to a limited extent

Protein binding: 99.4%

Metabolism: Extensively hepatic

Half-life elimination: 5 hours

Excretion: Urine (44%, 21% as unchanged drug); feces (≤10%)

Dosage I.V.:

Children: 130 mg/m²/week, increasing to 150 mg/m² after 3 weeks and up to 180 mg/m² after 6 weeks

Acute lymphoblastic leukemia (ALL): 165 mg/m² twice weekly for 8-9 doses **or** 250 mg/m² weekly for 4-8 weeks

Adults: 50-180 mg/m² once or twice weekly for 4-6 weeks or 20-60 mg/m²/day for 5 days

Small cell lung cancer: 80-90 mg/m²/day for 5 days every 4-6 weeks

Dosage adjustment in renal/hepatic impairment: Data is insufficient, but dose adjustments may be necessary in patient with significant renal or hepatic impairment

Dosage adjustment in Down syndrome patients: Reduce initial dosing; administer the first course at half the usual dose. Patients with both Down syndrome and leukemia may be especially sensitive to myelosuppressive chemotherapy.

Combination Regimens

Leukemia, acute lymphocytic: Linker Protocol *on page 904*

Neuroblastoma:

CCDDT (Neuroblastomas) *on page 855*

CCT (Neuroblastomas) *on page 855*

OPEC *on page 924*

OPEC-D *on page 924*

PE-CAdO *on page 929*

Administration

Must be administered slowly (over at least 30-60 minutes).

Dosage Forms

Injection, solution: 10 mg/mL (5 mL) [contains benzyl alcohol, dehydrated alcohol, and polyoxyethylated castor oil]

High Dose Considerations

High Dose: I.V.: 750-1000 mg/m²

Selected Readings

Clark PI and Slevin ML, "The Clinical Pharmacology of Etoposide and Teniposide," *Clin Pharmacokinet*, 1987, 12(4):223-52.

Muggia FM, "Teniposide: Overview of Its Therapeutic Potential in Adult Cancers," *Cancer Chemother Pharmacol*, 1994, 34(Suppl):127-33.

O'Dwyer PJ, Alonso MT, Leyland-Jones B, et al, "Teniposide: A Review of 12 Years of Experience," *Cancer Treat Rep*, 1984, 68(12):1455-66.

Rivera GK and Evans WE, "Clinical Trials of Teniposide (VM-26) in Childhood Acute Lymphocytic Leukemia," *Semin Oncol*, 1992, 19(2 Suppl 6):51-8.

Sonneveld P, "Teniposide in Lymphomas and Leukemias," *Semin Oncol*, 1992, 19(2 Suppl 6):59-64.

♦ **Teslac**® *see* Testolactone *on page 757*

♦ **TESPA** *see* Thiotepa *on page 764*

Testolactone (tes toe LAK tone)
Medication Safety Issues
Sound-alike/look-alike issues:
Testolactone may be confused with testosterone
U.S. Brand Names Teslac®
Canadian Brand Names Teslac®
Generic Available No
Pharmacologic Category Androgen
Pregnancy Risk Factor C
Lactation Excretion in breast milk unknown/not recommended
Use Palliative treatment of advanced or disseminated breast carcinoma
Mechanism of Action Testolactone is a synthetic testosterone derivative without significant androgen activity. The drug inhibits steroid aromatase activity, thereby blocking the production of estradiol and estrone from androgen precursors such as testosterone and androstenedione. Unfortunately, the enzymatic block provided by testolactone is transient and is usually limited to a period of 3 months.
Restrictions C-III
Labeled Contraindications Hypersensitivity to testolactone or any component of the formulation; treatment of breast cancer in men
Warnings/Precautions Use with caution in hepatic, renal, or cardiac disease; prolonged use may cause drug-induced hepatic disease; history of porphyria. For use in postmenopausal women or in premenopausal women without ovarian function only. Safety and efficacy in pediatric patients have not been established.
Adverse Reactions Frequency not defined.
Cardiovascular: Edema, blood pressure increased
Central nervous system: Malaise
Dermatologic: Maculopapular rash, alopecia (rare)
Endocrine & metabolic: Hypercalcemia
Gastrointestinal: Anorexia, diarrhea, nausea, edema of the tongue
Neuromuscular & skeletal: Paresthesias, peripheral neuropathies
Miscellaneous: Nail growth disturbance (rare)
Emetic Potential Very low (<10%)
Drug Interactions
Increased Effect/Toxicity: Increased effects of oral anticoagulants.
Pharmacodynamics/Kinetics
Absorption: Well absorbed
Metabolism: Hepatic (forms metabolites)
Excretion: Urine
Dosage Adults: Female: Oral: 250 mg 4 times/day for at least 3 months; desired response may take as long as 3 months
Dosage Forms Tablet: 50 mg
Monitoring Parameters Plasma calcium levels
Patient Information Passive exercises should be maintained throughout therapy to keep patient mobile; report numbness of fingers, toes, or face

♦ **Tetrahydrocannabinol** see Dronabinol on page 292
♦ **Texacort**® see Hydrocortisone on page 419
♦ **TG** see Thioguanine on page 762
♦ **6-TG (error-prone abbreviation)** see Thioguanine on page 762

Thalidomide (tha LI doe mide)

Medication Safety Issues
Sound-alike/look-alike issues:
Thalidomide may be confused with flutamide

Related Information
Safe Handling of Hazardous Drugs on page 1034

U.S. Brand Names Thalomid®

Canadian Brand Names Thalomid®

Generic Available No

Pharmacologic Category Immunosuppressant Agent

Pregnancy Risk Factor X

Lactation Excretion in breast milk unknown/not recommended

Use Treatment and maintenance of cutaneous manifestations of erythema nodosum leprosum

Unlabeled/Investigational Use Treatment of multiple myeloma; Crohn's disease; graft-versus-host reactions after bone marrow transplantation; AIDS-related aphthous stomatitis; Behçet's syndrome; Waldenström's macroglobulinemia; Langerhans cell histiocytosis; may be effective in rheumatoid arthritis, discoid lupus erythematosus, and erythema multiforme

Mechanism of Action A derivative of glutethimide; mode of action for immunosuppression is unclear; inhibition of neutrophil chemotaxis and decreased monocyte phagocytosis may occur; may cause 50% to 80% reduction of tumor necrosis factor - alpha

Restrictions Thalidomide is approved for marketing only under a special distribution program. This program, called the "System for Thalidomide Education and Prescribing Safety" (STEPS) (1-888-423-5436), has been approved by the FDA. No more than a 4-week supply should be dispensed. Blister packs should be dispensed intact (do not repackage capsules). Prescriptions must be filled within 7 days.

Labeled Contraindications Hypersensitivity to thalidomide or any component of the formulation; neuropathy (peripheral); pregnancy or women in childbearing years unless alternative therapies are inappropriate and adequate precautions are taken to avoid pregnancy; patient unable to comply with STEPS™ program.

Warnings/Precautions Effective contraception must be used for at least 4 weeks before initiating therapy, during therapy, and for 4 weeks following discontinuation of thalidomide. May cause sedation, patients must be warned to use caution when performing tasks which require alertness. Use caution in patients with renal or hepatic impairment, neurological disorders, cardiovascular disease, or constipation.

Thalidomide has been associated with the development of peripheral neuropathy, which may be irreversible. Consider immediate discontinuation, if clinically appropriate, in patients who develop neuropathy. Use caution in patients with a history of seizures, concurrent therapy with drugs which alter seizure threshold, or conditions which predispose to seizures. May cause neutropenia; discontinue therapy if absolute neutrophil count decrease to <750/mm^3. Use caution in patients with HIV infection; has been associated with increased viral loads.

May cause orthostasis and/or bradycardia; use with caution in patients with cardiovascular disease or in patients who would not tolerate transient hypotensive episodes. Thrombotic events have been reported (generally in patients with other risk factors for thrombosis [neoplastic disease, inflammatory disease, or concurrent therapy with other drugs which may cause thrombosis]). Safety and efficacy have not been established in children <12 years of age.

Adverse Reactions

Controlled clinical trials: ENL:

>10%:

Central nervous system: Somnolence (37.5%), headache (12.5%)

Dermatologic: Rash (20.8%)

1% to 10%:

Cardiovascular: Peripheral edema

Central nervous system: Dizziness (4.2%), vertigo (8.3%), chills, malaise (8.3%)

Dermatologic: Dermatitis (fungal) (4.2%), nail disorder (4.2%), pruritus (8.3%), rash (maculopapular) (4.2%)

Gastrointestinal (4.2%): Constipation, diarrhea, nausea, moniliasis, tooth pain, abdominal pain

Genitourinary: Impotence (8.2%)

Neuromuscular & skeletal: Asthenia (8.3%), pain (8.3%), back pain (4.2%), neck pain (4.2%), neck rigidity (4.2%), tremor (4.2%)

Respiratory (4.2%): Pharyngitis, rhinitis, sinusitis

HIV-seropositive:

General: An increased viral load has been noted in patients treated with thalidomide. This is of uncertain clinical significance - see Monitoring Parameters

>10%:

Central nervous system: Somnolence (36% to 37%), dizziness (18.7% to 19.4%), fever (19.4% to 21.9%), headache (16.7% to 18.7%)

Dermatologic: Rash (25%), maculopapular rash (16.7% to 18.7%), acne (3.1% to 11.1%)

Gastrointestinal: AST increase (2.8% to 12.5%), diarrhea (11.1% to 18.7%), nausea (≤12.5%), oral moniliasis (6.3% to 11.1%)

Hematologic: Leukopenia (16.7% to 25%), anemia (5.6% to 12.5%)

Neuromuscular & skeletal: Paresthesia (may be severe and/or irreversible) (5.6% to 15.6%), weakness (5.6% to 21.9%)

Miscellaneous: Diaphoresis (≤12.5%), lymphadenopathy (5.6% to 12.5%)

1% to 10%:

Cardiovascular: Peripheral edema (3.1% to 8.3%)

Central nervous system: Nervousness (2.8% to 9.4%), insomnia (≤9.4%), agitation (≤9.4%), chills (≤9.4%), neuropathy (up to 8% in HIV-seropositive patients)

Dermatologic: Dermatitis (fungal) (5.6% to 9.4%), nail disorder (≤3.1%), pruritus (2.8% to 6.3%)

Gastrointestinal: Anorexia (2.8% to 9.4%), constipation (2.8% to 9.4%), dry mouth (8.3% to 9.4%), flatulence (8.3% to 9.4%),

(Continued)

Thalidomide *(Continued)*

multiple abnormalities LFTs (≤9.4%), abdominal pain (2.8% to 3.1%)

Neuromuscular & skeletal: Back pain (≤5%), pain (≤3.1%)

Respiratory: Pharyngitis (6.3% to 8.3%), sinusitis (3.1% to 8.3%)

Miscellaneous: Accidental injury (≤5.6%), infection (6.3% to 8.3%)

Postmarketing and/or case reports (limited to important or life-threatening): Acute renal failure, arrhythmia, bradycardia, CML, dyspnea, electrolyte imbalances, erythema multiforme, erythema nodosum, Hodgkin's disease, hypersensitivity, hyperthyroidism, intestinal perforation, lethargy, lymphopenia, mental status changes, myxedema, neutropenia, orthostatic hypotension, pancytopenia, paresthesia, peripheral neuritis, photosensitivity, pleural effusion, psychosis, Raynaud's syndrome, seizure, Stevens-Johnson syndrome, suicide attempt, syncope, thrombosis, toxic epidermal necrolysis, tumor lysis syndrome

Drug Interactions

Increased Effect/Toxicity: Thalidomide may enhance the sedative activity of other drugs such as ethanol, barbiturates, reserpine, and chlorpromazine. Drugs which may cause peripheral neuropathy should be used with caution in patients receiving thalidomide. Women using any drug which may decrease the serum concentrations and/or efficacy of hormonal contraceptives must use 2 other methods of contraception or abstain from heterosexual contact. Thalidomide may be associated with increased risk of serious infection when used in combination with anakinra.

Ethanol/Nutrition/Herb Interactions

Ethanol: Avoid ethanol (may increase sedation).

Herb/Nutraceutical: Avoid cat's claw (has immunostimulant properties).

Storage/Stability
Store at 15°C to 30°C (50°F to 86°F). Protect from light. Keep in original package.

Pharmacodynamics/Kinetics

Distribution: V_d: 120 L

Protein binding: 55% to 66%

Metabolism: Nonenzymatic hydrolysis in plasma; forms multiple metabolites

Half-life elimination: 5-7 hours

Time to peak, plasma: 2-6 hours

Excretion: Urine (<1%)

Dosage
Oral:

Cutaneous ENL:

Initiate dosing at 100-300 mg/day taken once daily at bedtime with water (at least 1 hour after evening meal)

Patients weighing <50 kg: Initiate at lower end of the dosing range

Severe cutaneous reaction or previously requiring high dose may be initiated at 400 mg/day; doses may be divided, but taken 1 hour after meals

Dosing should continue until active reaction subsides (usually at least 2 weeks), then tapered in 50 mg decrements every 2-4 weeks

Patients who flare during tapering or with a history or requiring prolonged maintenance should be maintained on the minimum dosage necessary to control the reaction. Efforts to taper should be repeated every 3-6 months, in increments of 50 mg every 2-4 weeks.

Behçet's syndrome (unlabeled use): 100-400 mg/day

Graft-vs-host reactions (unlabeled use): 100-1600 mg/day; usual initial dose: 200 mg 4 times/day for use up to 700 days

AIDS-related aphthous stomatitis (unlabeled use): 200 mg twice daily for 5 days, then 200 mg/day for up to 8 weeks

Discoid lupus erythematosus (unlabeled use): 100-400 mg/day; maintenance dose: 25-50 mg

Multiple myeloma: Refer to individual protocols

Combination Regimens

Multiple myeloma:

DTPACE *on page 874*

Thalidomide + Dexamethasone *on page 939*

Administration Oral: Avoid extensive handling of capsules; capsules should remain in blister pack until ingestion. If exposed to the powder content from broken capsules or body fluids from patients receiving thalidomide, the exposed area should be washed with soap and water. Multiple myeloma: Refer to individual protocols.

Dosage Forms Capsule: 50 mg, 100 mg, 200 mg

Monitoring Parameters WBC with differential; signs of neuropathy monthly for the first 3 months, then periodically during treatment; consider monitoring of sensory nerve application potential amplitudes (at baseline and every 6 months) to detect asymptomatic neuropathy. In HIV-seropositive patients: viral load after 1 and 3 months, then every 3 months. Pregnancy testing is required within 24 hours of initiation of therapy, weekly during the first 4 weeks, then every 4 weeks in women with regular menstrual cycles or every 2 weeks in women with irregular menstrual cycles.

Dietary Considerations Should be taken at least 1 hour after the evening meal.

Patient Information Thalidomide must be obtained via "STEPS™ Program" (1-888-423-5436). Effective contraception must be used for at least 1 month prior to beginning therapy, during therapy, and continued for 1 month after thalidomide has been discontinued. Two reliable forms of contraception must be used. Males must use a latex condom during sexual contact with women of childbearing age. Thalidomide may cause drowsiness and/or orthostatic hypotension. Patients should not donate blood. Patients should report signs of tingling, numbness, or pain in hands or feet.

Selected Readings

Bessmertny O and Pham T, "Thalidomide Use in Pediatric Patients," *Ann Pharmacother*, 2002, 36(3):521-5.

Diggle GE, "Thalidomide: 40 years On," *Int J Clin Pract*, 2001, 55(9):627-31.

Eleutherakis-Papaiakovou V, Bamias A, and Dimopoulos MA, "Thalidomide in Cancer Medicine," *Ann Oncol*, 2004, 15(8):1151-60.

Eriksson T, Bjorkman S, and Hoglund P, "Clinical Pharmacology of Thalidomide," *Eur J Clin Pharmacol*, 2001, 57(5):365-76.

Franks ME, Macpherson GR, and Figg WD, "Thalidomide," *Lancet*, 2004, 363(9423):1802-11.

Teo SK, Colburn WA, Tracewell WG, et al, "Clinical Pharmacokinetics of Thalidomide," *Clin Pharmacokinet*, 2004, 43(5):311-27.

♦ **Thalomid**® *see* Thalidomide *on page 758*

♦ **THC** *see* Dronabinol *on page 292*

♦ **TheraCys**® *see* BCG Vaccine *on page 120*

Thioguanine (thye oh GWAH neen)

Medication Safety Issues 6-thioguanine and 6-TG are error-prone abbreviations (associated with six-fold overdoses of thioguanine)

Related Information

Investigational Drug Service *on page 1031*
Management of Nausea and Vomiting *on page 982*
Safe Handling of Hazardous Drugs *on page 1034*

U.S. Brand Names Tabloid®

Canadian Brand Names Lanvis®

Generic Available No

Synonyms 2-Amino-6-Mercaptopurine; NSC-752; TG; 6-TG (error-prone abbreviation); 6-Thioguanine (error-prone abbreviation); Tioguanine

Pharmacologic Category Antineoplastic Agent, Antimetabolite (Purine Antagonist)

Pregnancy Risk Factor D

Lactation Excretion in breast milk unknown

Use Treatment of acute myelogenous (nonlymphocytic) leukemia; treatment of chronic myelogenous leukemia and granulocytic leukemia

Mechanism of Action Purine analog that is incorporated into DNA and RNA resulting in the blockage of synthesis and metabolism of purine nucleotides

Restrictions The I.V. formulation is not available in U.S./Investigational

Labeled Contraindications Hypersensitivity to thioguanine or any component of the formulation; pregnancy

Warnings/Precautions Hazardous agent - use appropriate precautions for handling and disposal. See Safe Handling of Hazardous Drugs *on page 1034* in the Appendix. Use with caution and reduce dose in patients with renal or hepatic impairment. Not recommended for long-term continuous therapy due to potential for hepatotoxicity (hepatic veno-occlusive disease). Discontinue in patients with evidence of hepatotoxicity. Caution with history of previous therapy resistance with either thioguanine or mercaptopurine (there is usually complete cross resistance between these two). Thioguanine is potentially carcinogenic and teratogenic. Patients with genetic deficiency of thiopurine methyltransferase (TPMT) or who are receiving drugs which inhibit this enzyme (mesalazine, olsalazine, sulfasalazine) may be highly sensitive to myelosuppressive effects.

Adverse Reactions

>10%: Hematologic: Myelosuppressive:
  WBC: Moderate
  Platelets: Moderate
  Onset: 7-10 days
  Nadir: 14 days
  Recovery: 21 days

1% to 10%:
  Dermatologic: Skin rash
  Endocrine & metabolic: Hyperuricemia
  Gastrointestinal: Mild nausea or vomiting, anorexia, stomatitis, diarrhea
  Neuromuscular & skeletal: Unsteady gait

<1%: Ascites, esophageal varices, hepatic necrosis, hepatitis, jaundice, LFTs increased, neurotoxicity, photosensitivity, portal hypertension, splenomegaly, thrombocytopenia, veno-occlusive hepatic disease

Vesicant No

Emetic Potential Very low (<10%)

Overdosage/Toxicology Symptoms of overdose include bone marrow suppression, nausea, vomiting, malaise, hypertension, and sweating. Treatment is supportive. Dialysis is not useful.

Drug Interactions

Increased Effect/Toxicity: Allopurinol can be used in full doses with thioguanine unlike mercaptopurine. Use with busulfan may cause hepatotoxicity and esophageal varices. Aminosalicylates (olsalazine, mesalamine, sulfasalazine) may inhibit TPMT, increasing toxicity/myelosuppression of thioguanine.

Ethanol/Nutrition/Herb Interactions Food: Enhanced absorption if administered between meals.

Storage/Stability

Tablet: Store at room temperature.

Injection (investigational in U.S.): Store intact vials under refrigeration (2°C to 8°C). The reconstituted solution is stable for at least 24 hours under refrigeration. Further dilutions for infusion are stable for 24 hours at room temperature or under refrigeration.

Reconstitution Reconstitute parenteral preparation with 5 mL SWFI, NS, or D_5W to yield a 15 mg/mL solution. Dilute in 50-500 mL D_5W or NS for infusion.

Compatibility Compatible: Stable in D_5W, NS

Pharmacodynamics/Kinetics

Absorption: 30% (highly variable)

Distribution: Crosses placenta

Metabolism: Hepatic; rapidly and extensively via TPMT to 2-amino-6-methylthioguanine (active) and inactive compounds

Half-life elimination: Terminal: 11 hours

Time to peak, serum: Within 8 hours

Excretion: Urine

Dosage Total daily dose can be given at one time.

Oral (refer to individual protocols):

Infants and Children <3 years: Combination drug therapy for acute nonlymphocytic leukemia: 3.3 mg/kg/day in divided doses twice daily for 4 days

Children and Adults: 2-3 mg/kg/day calculated to nearest 20 mg or 75-200 mg/m²/day in 1-2 divided doses for 5-7 days or until remission is attained

Dosing comments in renal or hepatic impairment: Reduce dose

Combination Regimens

Leukemia, acute myeloid:

DAT on page 872
TAD on page 938
V-TAD on page 949

Administration Oral; I.V. (investigational) as a short infusion

Dosage Forms

Injection, powder for reconstitution: 75 mg [investigational in U.S.]

Tablet [scored]: 40 mg

Monitoring Parameters CBC with differential and platelet count; liver function tests (weekly when beginning therapy then monthly, more frequently in patients with liver disease or concurrent hepatotoxic drugs); (Continued)

Thioguanine (Continued)

hemoglobin, hematocrit, serum uric acid; some laboratories offer testing for TPMT deficiency

Hepatotoxicity may present with signs of portal hypertension (splenomegaly, esophageal varices, thrombocytopenia) or veno-occlusive disease (fluid retention, ascites, hepatomegaly with tenderness, or hyperbilirubinemia)

Patient Information You may experience nausea and vomiting, diarrhea, or loss of appetite (frequent small meals may help/request medication) or weakness or lethargy (use caution when driving or engaging in tasks requiring alertness until response to drug is known). Use good oral care to reduce incidence of mouth sores. May cause headache (request medication). Report signs or symptoms of infection (eg, fever, chills, sore throat, burning urination, fatigue), bleeding (eg, tarry stools, easy bruising), vision changes, unresolved mouth sores, nausea or vomiting, CNS changes (hallucinations), or respiratory difficulty. Avoid crowds or exposure to infected persons; you will be susceptible to infection. The drug may cause permanent sterility and may cause birth defects. Contraceptive measures should be used during therapy. The drug may be excreted in breast milk, therefore, an alternative form of feeding your baby should be used.

Extemporaneous Preparations A 20 mg/mL oral suspension can be prepared by crushing fifteen 40 mg tablets in a mortar, and then adding 10 mL of methylcellulose 1% (in small amounts). Transfer to a graduate, then add a sufficient quantity of syrup to make 30 mL of suspension. Label "shake well." Room temperature stability is 60 days.

Dressman JB and Poust RI, "Stability of Allopurinol and Five Antineoplastics in Suspension," *Am J Hosp Pharm*, 1983, 40:616-8.

Nahata MC, Morosco RS, and Hipple TF, 4th ed, *Pediatric Drug Formulations*, Cincinnati, OH: Harvey Whitney Books Co, 2000.

Selected Readings

Elgemeie GH, "Thioguanine, Mercaptopurine: Their Analogs and Nucleosides as Antimetabolites," *Curr Pharm Des*, 2003, 9(31):2627-42.

♦ **6-Thioguanine (error-prone abbreviation)** *see* Thioguanine *on page 762*

♦ **Thiophosphoramide** *see* Thiotepa *on page 764*

♦ **Thiosulfuric Acid Disodium Salt** *see* Sodium Thiosulfate *on page 722*

Thiotepa (thye oh TEP a)

Related Information

Safe Handling of Hazardous Drugs *on page 1034*
Transplantation *on page 1019*

Generic Available Yes

Synonyms TESPA; Thiophosphoramide; Triethylenethiophosphoramide; TSPA

Pharmacologic Category Antineoplastic Agent, Alkylating Agent

Pregnancy Risk Factor D

Lactation Enters breast milk/not recommended

Use Treatment of superficial tumors of the bladder; palliative treatment of adenocarcinoma of breast or ovary; lymphomas and sarcomas; controlling intracavitary effusions caused by metastatic tumors; I.T. use: CNS leukemia/lymphoma, CNS metastases

Mechanism of Action Alkylating agent that reacts with DNA phosphate groups to produce cross-linking of DNA strands leading to inhibition of DNA, RNA, and protein synthesis; mechanism of action has not been explored as thoroughly as the other alkylating agents, it is presumed that the aziridine rings open and react as nitrogen mustard; reactivity is enhanced at a lower pH

Labeled Contraindications Hypersensitivity to thiotepa or any component of the formulation; pregnancy

Warnings/Precautions Hazardous agent - use appropriate precautions for handling and disposal. See Safe Handling of Hazardous Drugs *on page 1034* in the Appendix. Potentially mutagenic, carcinogenic, and teratogenic. Reduce dosage and use caution in patients with hepatic, renal, or bone marrow damage. Use should be limited to cases where benefit outweighs risk.

Adverse Reactions

>10%:

Hematopoietic: Dose-limiting toxicity which is dose related and cumulative; moderate to severe leukopenia and severe thrombocytopenia have occurred. Anemia and pancytopenia may become fatal, so careful hematologic monitoring is required; intravesical administration may cause bone marrow suppression as well.

Hematologic: Myelosuppressive:

WBC: Moderate

Platelets: Severe

Onset: 7-10 days

Nadir: 14 days

Recovery: 28 days

Local: Pain at injection site

1% to 10%:

Central nervous system: Dizziness, fever, headache

Dermatologic: Alopecia, rash, pruritus, hyperpigmentation with high-dose therapy

Endocrine & metabolic: Hyperuricemia

Gastrointestinal: Anorexia, nausea and vomiting rarely occur

Emetic potential: Low (<10%)

Genitourinary: Hemorrhagic cystitis

Renal: Hematuria

Miscellaneous: Tightness of the throat, allergic reactions

<1%: Stomatitis, anaphylaxis; like other alkylating agents, this drug is carcinogenic

Vesicant No

Emetic Potential Very low (<10%)

Overdosage/Toxicology Symptoms of overdose include nausea, vomiting, precipitation of uric acid in kidney tubules, bone marrow suppression, and bleeding. Therapy is supportive only. Thiotepa is dialyzable. Transfusions of whole blood or platelets have been proven beneficial.

(Continued)

Thiotepa *(Continued)*

Drug Interactions

Cytochrome P450 Effect: Inhibits CYP2B6 (weak)

Increased Effect/Toxicity: Other alkylating agents or irradiation used concomitantly with thiotepa intensifies toxicity rather than enhancing therapeutic response. Prolonged muscular paralysis and respiratory depression may occur when neuromuscular blocking agents are administered. Succinylcholine and other neuromuscular blocking agents' action can be prolonged due to thiotepa inhibiting plasma pseudocholinesterase.

Ethanol/Nutrition/Herb Interactions

Ethanol: Avoid ethanol (due to GI irritation).

Herb/Nutraceutical: Avoid black cohosh, dong quai in estrogen-dependent tumors.

Storage/Stability

Store intact vials under refrigeration (2°C to 8°C) and protect from light. Reconstituted solutions (10 mg/mL in SWFI) are stable for up to 28 days under refrigeration (4°C to 8°C) or 7 days at room temperature (25°C).

Solutions for infusion in D_5W (≥ 5 mg/mL) are stable for 14 days under refrigeration (4°C) or 3 days at room temperature (23°C).

Solutions for infusion in NS (1, 3, or 5 mg/mL) are stable for 48 hours under refrigeration (4°C to 8°C) or 24 hours at room temperature (25°C). Solutions in NS at a concentration of ≤ 0.5 mg/mL are stable for <1 hour.

Reconstitution

Reconstitute each vial to 10 mg/mL solution. Solutions for infusion should be diluted to a concentration ≥ 5 mg/mL in 5% dextrose or 1, 3, or 5 mg/mL in 0.9% sodium chloride injection. Solutions for intravesicular administration should be diluted in 30-60 mL SWFI or NS. Solutions for intrathecal administration should be diluted in 1-5 mL NS or Elliott's B Solution.

Compatibility

Variable stability (consult detailed reference) in D_5W, NS

Y-site administration: Compatible: Acyclovir, allopurinol, amifostine, amikacin, aminophylline, amphotericin B, ampicillin, ampicillin/sulbactam, aztreonam, bleomycin, bumetanide, buprenorphine, butorphanol, calcium gluconate, carboplatin, carmustine, cefazolin, cefepime, cefoperazone, cefotaxime, cefotetan, cefoxitin, ceftazidime, ceftizoxime, ceftriaxone, cefuroxime, chlorpromazine, cimetidine, ciprofloxacin, clindamycin, co-trimoxazole, cyclophosphamide, cytarabine, dacarbazine, dactinomycin, daunorubicin, dexamethasone sodium phosphate, diphenhydramine,dobutamine, dopamine, doxorubicin, doxycycline, droperidol, enalaprilat, etoposide, etoposide phosphate, famotidine, floxuridine, fluconazole, fludarabine, fluorouracil, furosemide, ganciclovir, gemcitabine, gentamicin, granisetron, haloperidol, heparin, hydrocortisone sodium phosphate, hydrocortisone sodium succinate, hydromorphone, hydroxyzine, idarubicin, ifosfamide, imipenem/cilastatin, leucovorin, lorazepam, magnesium sulfate, mannitol, melphalan, meperidine, mesna, methotrexate, methylprednisolone sodium succinate, metoclopramide, metronidazole, , mitomycin, mitoxantrone, morphine, nalbuphine, netilmicin, ofloxacin, ondansetron, paclitaxel, piperacillin, piperacillin/tazobactam, plicamycin, potassium chloride, prochlorperazine edisylate, promethazine, ranitidine, sodium bicarbonate, streptozocin, teniposide, ticarcillin, ticarcillin/clavulanate, tobramycin, vancomycin, vinblastine, vincristine, zidovudine. **Incompatible:** Cisplatin, filgrastim, minocycline, vinorelbine. **Variable (consult detailed reference):** TPN

Compatibility when admixed: Compatible: Epinephrine, lidocaine. **Incompatible:** Cisplatin

Pharmacodynamics/Kinetics

Absorption: Intracavitary instillation: Unreliable (10% to 100%) through bladder mucosa; I.M.: variable

Metabolism: Extensively hepatic

Half-life elimination: Terminal (dose-dependent clearance): 109 minutes

Excretion: Urine (as metabolites and unchanged drug)

Dosage Refer to individual protocols

Children: Sarcomas: I.V.: 25-65 mg/m^2 as a single dose every 21 days

Adults:

I.M., I.V., SubQ: 30-60 mg/m^2 once weekly

I.V.: 0.3-0.4 mg/kg by rapid I.V. administration every 1-4 weeks, **or** 0.2 mg/kg or 6-8 mg/m^2/day for 4-5 days every 2-4 weeks

High-dose therapy for bone marrow transplant: I.V.: 500 mg/m^2, up to 900 mg/m^2

I.M.: 15-30 mg in various schedules have been given

Intracavitary: 0.6-0.8 mg/kg or 30-60 mg weekly

Intrapericardial: 15-30 mg

Intrathecal: 10-15 mg or 5-11.5 mg/m^2

Dosing comments/adjustment in renal impairment: Use with extreme caution, reduced dose may be warranted.

Combination Regimens

Breast cancer: VATH *on page 944*

Leukemia, acute lymphocytic: TVTG *on page 942*

Leukemia, acute myeloid: TVTG *on page 942*

Administration Thiotepa is usually administered intravenously, either as a short bolus or push, or a 1-hour infusion; or as an intravesical infusion. The drug is occasionally administered as intracavitary, intramuscular, or intrathecal injections. Intrathecal doses are usually diluted to a concentration of 1 mg/mL in preservative-free sterile water or normal saline. Bladder irrigations should be diluted in 50-100 mL of sterile water or normal saline, and retained for at least 2 hours. The patient should be repositioned every 15 minutes for maximal exposure.

Dosage Forms Injection, powder for reconstitution: 15 mg, 30 mg

High Dose Considerations

High Dose: I.V.: 360-1125 mg/m^2 as a single dose or divided into 2 daily doses; generally combined with other high-dose chemotherapeutic drugs.

Unique Toxicities:

Central nervous system: Effect increased with doses >1000 mg/m^2: Confusion, inappropriate behavior, somnolence

Dermatologic: Hyperpigmentation (most common on occluded areas of skin)

Gastrointestinal: Mucositis, mild nausea and vomiting

Hepatic: Serum transaminitis, hyperbilirubinemia

Comments: Administration of thiotepa over 30 minutes, 1 hour before infusion of cyclophosphamide over 60 minutes, reduced bioactivation of cyclophosphamide to 4-hydroxycyclophosphamide in 20 patients. This

(Continued)

767

Thiotepa (Continued)

effect did not occur with administration of thiotepa 1 hour following infusion of cyclophosphamide.

Monitoring Parameters CBC with differential and platelet count, uric acid, urinalysis

Patient Information This drug can only be administered I.V. You will require regular blood tests to assess response to therapy. Avoid alcohol and aspirin or aspirin-containing medications unless approved by prescriber. Maintain adequate hydration (2-3 L/day of fluids unless instructed to restrict fluid intake) to prevent kidney damage. For nausea and vomiting, small frequent meals, chewing gum, or sucking lozenges may help; antiemetics may be prescribed. You may experience amenorrhea or changed sperm production, rash, hair loss, or loss of appetite (maintaining adequate nutrition is important). You may have increased sensitivity to infection (avoid crowds and infected persons). Report unusual bleeding or bruising, persistent fever or chills, sore throat, sores in mouth or vagina, blackened stool, or difficulty breathing. The drug may cause permanent sterility and may cause birth defects. The drug may be excreted in breast milk, therefore, an alternative form of feeding your baby should be used. Contraceptive measures are recommended during therapy.

Additional Information A 1 mg/mL solution is considered isotonic.

Selected Readings

Antman K, Eder JP, Elias A, et al, "High-Dose Thiotepa Alone and in Combination Regimens With Bone Marrow Support," *Semin Oncol*, 1990, 17(1 Suppl 3):33-8.

Badalament RA and Farah RN, "Treatment of Superficial Bladder Cancer With Intravesicle Chemotherapy," *Semin Surg Oncol*, 1997, 13(5):335-41.

Gutin PH, Weiss HD, Wiernik PH, et al, "Intrathecal N,N′,N′′-triethylenethiophosphoramide [thio-TEPA (NSC-6396)] in the Treatment of Malignant Meningeal Disease: Phase I-II Study," *Cancer*, 1976, 38(4):1471-5.

Maanen MJ, Smeets CJ, and Beijnen JH, "Chemistry, Pharmacology and Pharmacokinetics of N,N′,N′ -Triethylenethiophosphoramide (ThioTEPA)," *Cancer Treat Rev*, 2000, 26(4):257-68.

♦ **Thorazine®** [DSC] *see* ChlorproMAZINE *on page 178*
♦ **Thrombate III®** *see* Antithrombin III *on page 94*
♦ **Thymocyte-Stimulating Factor** *see* Aldesleukin *on page 32*
♦ **Thymoglobulin®** *see* Antithymocyte Globulin (Rabbit) *on page 98*

Ticarcillin and Clavulanate Potassium

(tye kar SIL in & klav yoo LAN ate poe TASS ee um)

Related Information
Management of Infections *on page 978*

U.S. Brand Names Timentin®

Canadian Brand Names Timentin®

Generic Available No

Synonyms Ticarcillin and Clavulanic Acid

Pharmacologic Category Antibiotic, Penicillin

Pregnancy Risk Factor B

Lactation Enters breast milk (other penicillins are compatible with breast-feeding)

Use Treatment of infections of lower respiratory tract, urinary tract, skin and skin structures, bone and joint, and septicemia caused by susceptible organisms. Clavulanate expands activity of ticarcillin to include beta-lactamase producing strains of *S. aureus*, *H. influenzae*, *Bacteroides* species, and some other gram-negative bacilli

Mechanism of Action Inhibits bacterial cell wall synthesis by binding to one or more of the penicillin binding proteins (PBPs); which in turn inhibits the final transpeptidation step of peptidoglycan synthesis in bacterial cell walls, thus inhibiting cell wall biosynthesis. Bacteria eventually lyse due to ongoing activity of cell wall autolytic enzymes (autolysins and murein hydrolases) while cell wall assembly is arrested.

Labeled Contraindications Hypersensitivity to ticarcillin, clavulanate, any penicillin, or any component of the formulation

Warnings/Precautions Use with caution and modify dosage in patients with renal impairment. Serious and occasionally fatal hypersensitivity (anaphylactoid) reactions have been reported in patients on penicillin therapy. These reactions are more likely to occur in individuals with a history of cephalosporin hypersensitivity and/or a history of sensitivity to multiple allergens.

Adverse Reactions Frequency not defined.

Central nervous system: Confusion, convulsions, drowsiness, fever, Jarisch-Herxheimer reaction

Dermatologic: Rash, erythema multiforme, toxic epidermal necrolysis, Stevens-Johnson syndrome

Endocrine & metabolic: Electrolyte imbalance

Gastrointestinal: *Clostridium difficile* colitis

Hematologic: Bleeding, hemolytic anemia, leukopenia, neutropenia, positive Coombs' reaction, thrombocytopenia

Hepatic: Hepatotoxicity, jaundice

Local: Thrombophlebitis

Neuromuscular & skeletal: Myoclonus

Renal: Interstitial nephritis (acute)

Miscellaneous: Anaphylaxis, hypersensitivity reactions

Vesicant No

Emetic Potential Very low (<10%)

Overdosage/Toxicology Symptoms of overdose include neuromuscular hypersensitivity and seizures. Hemodialysis may be helpful to aid in removal of the drug from blood; otherwise, treatment is supportive or symptom-directed.

Drug Interactions

Increased Effect/Toxicity: Probenecid may increase penicillin levels. Neuromuscular blockers may have an increased duration of action (neuromuscular blockade). Penicillins may increase the exposure to methotrexate during concurrent therapy; monitor.

Decreased Effect: Tetracyclines may decrease penicillin effectiveness. Aminoglycosides may cause physical inactivation of aminoglycosides in the presence of high concentrations of ticarcillin and potential toxicity in patients with mild-moderate renal dysfunction. Although anecdotal reports suggest oral contraceptive efficacy could be reduced by penicillins, this has been refuted by more rigorous scientific and clinical data.

Storage/Stability Reconstituted solution is stable for 6 hours at room temperature and 72 hours when refrigerated. I.V. infusion in NS is stable for 24 hours at room temperature, 7 days when refrigerated, or 30 days when frozen. Darkening of solution indicates loss of potency of clavulanate potassium.

Compatibility Stable in D_5W, LR, NS, sterile water for injection

(Continued)

Ticarcillin and Clavulanate Potassium *(Continued)*

Y-site administration: Compatible: Allopurinol, amifostine, aztreonam, cefepime, clarithromycin, cyclophosphamide, diltiazem, docetaxel, doxorubicin liposome, etoposide, famotidine, filgrastim, fluconazole, fludarabine, foscarnet, gatifloxacin, gemcitabine, granisetron, heparin, insulin (regular), melphalan, meperidine, morphine, ondansetron, perphenazine, propofol, remifentanil, sargramostim, teniposide, theophylline, thiotepa, vinorelbine. **Incompatible:** Alatrofloxacin, amphotericin B cholesteryl sulfate complex. **Variable (consult detailed reference):** Cisatracurium, topotecan, vancomycin

Compatibility when admixed: Incompatible: Sodium bicarbonate, aminoglycosides

Pharmacodynamics/Kinetics

Clavulanic acid:

Protein binding: 9% to 30%

Metabolism: Hepatic

Half-life elimination: 66-90 minutes

Excretion: Urine (45% as unchanged drug)

Clearance: Does not affect clearance of ticarcillin

Dosage I.V.:

Children and Adults <60 kg: 200-300 mg of ticarcillin component/kg/day in divided doses every 4-6 hours

Children >60 kg and Adults: 3.1 g (ticarcillin 3 g plus clavulanic acid 0.1 g) every 4-6 hours; maximum: 24 g/day

Urinary tract infections: 3.1 g every 6-8 hours

Dosing adjustment in renal impairment:

Cl_{cr} 30-60 mL/minute: Administer 2 g every 4 hours or 3.1 g every 8 hours

Cl_{cr} 10-30 mL/minute: Administer 2 g every 8 hours or 3.1 g every 12 hours

Cl_{cr} <10 mL/minute: Administer 2 g every 12 hours

Moderately dialyzable (20% to 50%)

Continuous arteriovenous or venovenous hemodiafiltration effects: Dose as for Cl_{cr} 10-50 mL/minute

Peritoneal dialysis: 3.1 g every 12 hours

Hemodialysis: 2 g every 12 hours; supplemented with 3.1 g after each dialysis

Dosing adjustment in hepatic dysfunction: Cl_{cr} <10 mL/minute: 2 g every 24 hours

Administration
Infuse over 30 minutes; administer 1 hour apart from aminoglycosides

Dosage Forms

Infusion [premixed, frozen]: Ticarcillin 3 g and clavulanate acid 0.1 g (100 mL) [contains sodium 4.51 mEq and potassium 0.15 mEq per g]

Injection, powder for reconstitution: Ticarcillin 3 g and clavulanate acid 0.1 g (3.1 g, 31 g) [contains sodium 4.51 mEq and potassium 0.15 mEq per g]

Monitoring Parameters
Observe for signs and symptoms of anaphylaxis during first dose.

Dietary Considerations
Sodium content of 1 g: 4.51 mEq; potassium content of 1 g: 0.15 mEq

Special Geriatric Considerations When used as empiric therapy or for a documented pseudomonal pneumonia, it is best to combine with an aminoglycoside such as gentamicin or tobramycin. High sodium content may limit use in patients with congestive heart failure. Adjust dose for renal function.

Selected Readings

Begue P, Quiniou F, Quinet B, "Efficacy and Pharmacokinetics of Timentin® in Paediatric Infections," *J Antimicrob Chemother*, 1986, 17(Suppl C):81-91.

Donowitz GR and Mandell GL, "Beta-Lactam Antibiotics," *N Engl J Med*, 1988, 318(7):419-26 and 318(8):490-500.

Itokazu GS and Danziger LH, "Ampicillin-Sulbactam and Ticarcillin-Clavulanic Acid: A Comparison of Their *In Vitro* Activity and Review of Their Clinical Efficacy," *Pharmacotherapy*, 1991, 11(5):382-414.

Reed MD, Yamashita TS, and Blumer JL, "Pharmacokinetic-Based Ticarcillin/Clavulanic Acid Dose Recommendations for Infants and Children," *J Clin Pharmacol*, 1995, 35(7):658-65.

Stutman HR and Marks MI, "Review of Pediatric Antimicrobial Therapies," *Semin Pediatr Infect Dis*, 1991, 2:3-17.

Wright AJ, "The Penicillins," *Mayo Clin Proc*, 1999, 74(3):290-307.

Tobramycin (toe bra MYE sin)

Medication Safety Issues

Sound-alike/look-alike issues:

Tobramycin may be confused with Trobicin®

AKTob® may be confused with AK-Trol®

Nebcin® may be confused with Inapsine®, Naprosyn®, Nubain®

Tobrex® may be confused with TobraDex®

Related Information

Management of Infections *on page 978*

U.S. Brand Names AKTob®; Nebcin® [DSC]; TOBI®; Tobrex®

Canadian Brand Names Apo-Tobramycin®; Nebcin®; PMS-Tobramycin; TOBI®; Tobrex®; Tomycine™

Generic Available Yes; Excludes ophthalmic ointment, solution for nebulization

Synonyms Tobramycin Sulfate

Pharmacologic Category Antibiotic, Aminoglycoside; Antibiotic, Ophthalmic

Pregnancy Risk Factor D (injection, inhalation); B (ophthalmic)

Lactation Enters breast milk/not recommended

Use Treatment of documented or suspected infections caused by susceptible gram-negative bacilli including *Pseudomonas aeruginosa*; topically used to treat superficial ophthalmic infections caused by susceptible
(Continued)

Tobramycin *(Continued)*

bacteria. Tobramycin solution for inhalation is indicated for the management of cystic fibrosis patients (>6 years of age) with *Pseudomonas aeruginosa*.

Mechanism of Action Interferes with bacterial protein synthesis by binding to 30S and 50S ribosomal subunits resulting in a defective bacterial cell membrane

Labeled Contraindications Hypersensitivity to tobramycin, other aminoglycosides, or any component of the formulation; pregnancy (injection/inhalation)

Warnings/Precautions Use with caution in patients with renal impairment, pre-existing auditory or vestibular impairment, and in patients with neuromuscular disorders. Dosage modification required in patients with impaired renal function (I.M. & I.V.). Aminoglycosides are associated with significant nephrotoxicity or ototoxicity; the ototoxicity is directly proportional to the amount of drug given and the duration of treatment. Tinnitus or vertigo are indications of vestibular injury. Ototoxicity is often irreversible, while renal damage is usually reversible.

Adverse Reactions

Injection: Frequency not defined:

Central nervous system: Confusion, disorientation, dizziness, fever, headache, lethargy, vertigo

Dermatologic: Exfoliative dermatitis, itching, rash, urticaria

Endocrine & metabolic: Serum calcium, magnesium, potassium, and/or sodium decreased

Gastrointestinal: Diarrhea, nausea, vomiting

Hematologic: Anemia, eosinophilia, granulocytopenia, leukocytosis, leukopenia, thrombocytopenia

Hepatic: ALT, AST, bilirubin, and/or LDH increased

Local: Pain at the injection site

Otic: Hearing loss, tinnitus, ototoxicity (auditory), ototoxicity (vestibular), roaring in the ears

Renal: BUN increased, cylindruria, serum creatinine increased, oliguria, proteinuria

Inhalation:
>10%:
Gastrointestinal: Sputum discoloration (21%)
Respiratory: Voice alteration (13%)
1% to 10%:
Central nervous system: Malaise (6%)
Otic: Tinnitus (3%)
Postmarketing and/or case reports: Hearing loss

Ophthalmic: <1%: Ocular: Conjunctival erythema, lid itching, lid swelling

Vesicant No

Emetic Potential Very low (<10%)

Overdosage/Toxicology Symptoms of overdose include ototoxicity, nephrotoxicity, and neuromuscular toxicity. Treatment of choice following a single acute overdose appears to be maintenance of urine output of at least 3 mL/kg/hour during the acute treatment phase. Dialysis is of questionable value in enhancing aminoglycoside elimination. If required, hemodialysis is preferred over peritoneal dialysis in patients with normal renal function. Chelation with penicillins is investigational.

Drug Interactions

Increased Effect/Toxicity: Increased antimicrobial effect of tobramycin with extended spectrum penicillins (synergistic). Neuromuscular blockers may have an increased duration of action (neuromuscular blockade). Amphotericin B, cephalosporins, and loop diuretics may increase the risk of nephrotoxicity.

Storage/Stability

Injection: Stable at room temperature both as the clear, colorless solution and as the dry powder. Reconstituted solutions remain stable for 24 hours at room temperature and 96 hours when refrigerated.

Ophthalmic solution: Store at 8°C to 27°C (46°F to 80°F).

Solution, for inhalation (TOBI®): Store under refrigeration at 2°C to 8°C (36°F to 46°F); may be stored in foil pouch at room temperature of 25°C (77°F) for up to 28 days. Avoid intense light. Solution may darken over time; however, do not use if cloudy or contains particles.

Reconstitution Dilute in 50-100 mL NS, D_5W for I.V. infusion

Compatibility Stable in dextran 40 10% in dextrose, D_5NS, D_5W, $D_{10}W$, mannitol 20%, LR, NS; **variable stability (consult detailed reference)** in peritoneal dialysis solutions

Y-site administration: Compatible: Acyclovir, alatrofloxacin, amifostine, amiodarone, amsacrine, aztreonam, ciprofloxacin, cisatracurium, cyclophosphamide, diltiazem, docetaxel, doxorubicin liposome, enalaprilat, esmolol, etoposide phosphate, filgrastim, fluconazole, fludarabine, foscarnet, furosemide, gatifloxacin, gemcitabine, granisetron, hydromorphone, IL-2, insulin (regular), labetalol, linezolid, magnesium sulfate, melphalan, meperidine, midazolam, morphine, perphenazine, remifentanil, tacrolimus, teniposide, theophylline, thiotepa, tolazoline, vinorelbine, zidovudine. **Incompatible:** Allopurinol, amphotericin B cholesteryl sulfate complex, cefoperazone, heparin, hetastarch, indomethacin, propofol, sargramostim

Compatibility in syringe: Compatible: Doxapram. **Incompatible:** Cefamandole, clindamycin, heparin

Compatibility when admixed: Compatible: Aztreonam, bleomycin, calcium gluconate, cefoxitin, ciprofloxacin, clindamycin, furosemide, metronidazole, metronidazole with sodium bicarbonate, ofloxacin, ranitidine, verapamil. **Incompatible:** Cefamandole, cefepime, cefotaxime, cefotetan, floxacillin, heparin

Pharmacodynamics/Kinetics

Absorption: I.M.: Rapid and complete

Distribution: V_d: 0.2-0.3 L/kg; Pediatrics: 0.2-0.7 L/kg; to extracellular fluid including serum, abscesses, ascitic, pericardial, pleural, synovial, lymphatic, and peritoneal fluids; crosses placenta; poor penetration into CSF, eye, bone, prostate

Protein binding: <30%

Half-life elimination:

Neonates: ≤1200 g: 11 hours; >1200 g: 2-9 hours

Adults: 2-3 hours; directly dependent upon glomerular filtration rate

Adults with impaired renal function: 5-70 hours

Time to peak, serum: I.M.: 30-60 minutes; I.V.: ~30 minutes

Excretion: Normal renal function: Urine (~90% to 95%) within 24 hours

Dosage Individualization is **critical** because of the low therapeutic index.

Use of ideal body weight (IBW) for determining the mg/kg/dose appears to be more accurate than dosing on the basis of total

(Continued)

Tobramycin *(Continued)*

body weight (TBW). In morbid obesity, dosage requirement may best be estimated using a dosing weight of IBW + 0.4 (TBW - IBW).

Initial and periodic plasma drug levels (eg, peak and trough with conventional dosing) should be determined, particularly in critically-ill patients with serious infections or in disease states known to significantly alter aminoglycoside pharmacokinetics (eg, cystic fibrosis, burns, or major surgery).

I.M., I.V.:

Infants and Children <5 years: 2.5 mg/kg/dose every 8 hours

Children >5 years: 2-2.5 g/kg/dose every 8 hours

Cystic fibrosis: 2.5-3.3 mg/kg every 6-8 hours

Note: Some patients may require larger or more frequent doses if serum levels document the need (eg, cystic fibrosis or febrile granulocytopenic patients). Also see "Note" on monitoring and adjustment.

Adults:

Severe life-threatening infections:

Conventional dosing: 2-2.5 mg/kg/dose every 8-12 hours; to ensure adequate peak concentrations early in therapy, higher initial dosages may be considered in selected patients (eg, edema, septic shock, postsurgery, and/or trauma).

Once-daily dosing: Some clinicians suggest a daily dose of 4-7 mg/kg for all patients with normal renal function; this dose is at least as efficacious with similar, if not less, toxicity than conventional dosing.

Urinary tract infection: 1.5 mg/kg/dose

Synergy (for gram-positive infections): 1 mg/kg/dose

Ophthalmic: Children ≥2 months and Adults:

Ointment: Apply 2-3 times/day; for severe infections, apply every 3-4 hours

Solution: Instill 1-2 drops every 4 hours; for severe infections, instill 2 drops every 30-60 minutes initially, then reduce to less frequent intervals

Inhalation: Pulmonary infections:

Standard aerosolized tobramycin:

Children: 40-80 mg 2-3 times/day

Adults: 60-80 mg 3 times/day

High-dose regimen: Children ≥6 years and Adults: 300 mg every 12 hours (do not administer doses >6 hours apart); administer in repeated cycles of 28 days on drug followed by 28 days off drug

Dosing interval in renal impairment: I.M., I.V.:

Conventional dosing:

Cl_{cr} ≥60 mL/minute: Administer every 8 hours

Cl_{cr} 40-60 mL/minute: Administer every 12 hours

Cl_{cr} 20-40 mL/minute: Administer every 24 hours

Cl_{cr} 10-20 mL/minute: Administer every 48 hours

Cl_{cr} <10 mL/minute: Administer every 72 hours

High-dose therapy: Interval may be extended (eg, every 48 hours) in patients with moderate renal impairment (Cl_{cr} 30-59 mL/minute) and/or adjusted based on serum level determinations.

Hemodialysis: Dialyzable; 30% removal of aminoglycosides occurs during 4 hours of HD - administer dose after dialysis and follow levels

Continuous arteriovenous or venovenous hemofiltration: Dose as for Cl_{cr} of 10-40 mL/minute and follow levels

Administration in CAPD fluid:

Gram-negative infection: 4-8 mg/L (4-8 mcg/mL) of CAPD fluid

Gram-positive infection (ie, synergy): 3-4 mg/L (3-4 mcg/mL) of CAPD fluid

Administration IVPB/I.M.: Dose as for Cl_{cr} <10 mL/minute and follow levels

Dosing adjustment/comments in hepatic disease: Monitor plasma concentrations

Administration

I.V.: Infuse over 30-60 minutes; give penicillins or cephalosporins at least 1 hour apart from tobramycin. Flush with saline before and after administration.

Inhalation (TOBI®): To be inhaled over ~15 minutes using a handheld nebulizer.

Ophthalmic solution: Allow 5 minutes between application of "multiple-drop" therapy.

Dosage Forms [DSC] = Discontinued product

Injection, powder for reconstitution (Nebcin® [DSC]): 1.2 g

Injection, solution, as sulfate: 10 mg/mL (2 mL, 8 mL); 40 mg/mL (2 mL, 30 mL, 50 mL) [may contain sodium metabisulfite]

Nebcin®: 40 mg/mL (2 mL) [contains sodium bisulfite] [DSC]

Ointment, ophthalmic (Tobrex®): 0.3% (3.5 g)

Solution for nebulization [preservative free] (TOBI®): 60 mg/mL (5 mL)

Solution, ophthalmic (AKTob®, Tobrex®): 0.3% (5 mL) [contains benzalkonium chloride]

Monitoring Parameters Urinalysis, urine output, BUN, serum creatinine, peak and trough plasma tobramycin levels; be alert to ototoxicity; hearing should be tested before and during treatment

Dietary Considerations May require supplementation of calcium, magnesium, potassium.

Patient Information Report symptoms of superinfection; for eye drops - no other eye drops 5-10 minutes before or after tobramycin; report any dizziness or sensations of ringing or fullness in ears

Additional Information Once-daily dosing: Higher peak serum drug concentration to MIC ratios, demonstrated aminoglycoside postantibiotic effect, decreased renal cortex drug uptake, and improved cost-time efficiency are supportive reasons for the use of once daily dosing regimens for aminoglycosides. Current research indicates these regimens to be as effective for nonlife-threatening infections, with no higher incidence of nephrotoxicity, than those requiring multiple daily doses. Doses are determined by calculating the entire day's dose via usual multiple dose calculation techniques and administering this quantity as a single dose. Doses are then adjusted to maintain mean serum concentrations above the MIC(s) of the causative organism(s). (Example: 2.5-5 mg/kg as a single dose; expected Cp_{max}: 10-20 mcg/mL and Cp_{min}: <1 mcg/mL). Further research is needed for universal recommendation in all patient populations and gram-negative disease; exceptions may include those with known high clearance (eg, children, patients with cystic fibrosis, or burns who may require shorter dosage intervals) and patients with renal function impairment for whom longer than conventional dosage intervals are usually required.

(Continued)

Tobramycin *(Continued)*

Special Geriatric Considerations Aminoglycosides are important therapeutic interventions for susceptible organisms and as empiric therapy in seriously ill patients. Their use is not without risk of toxicity; however, these risks can be minimized if initial dosing is adjusted for estimated renal function and appropriate monitoring is performed. High-dose, once-daily aminoglycosides have been advocated as an alternative to traditional dosing regimens. To date, there is little information on the safety and efficacy of these regimens in persons with a creatinine clearance <60 mL/minute/70 kg. A dosing nomogram based upon creatinine clearance has been proposed. Additional studies comparing high-dose, once-daily aminoglycosides to traditional dosing regimens in the elderly are needed before once-daily aminoglycoside dosing can be routinely adopted to this patient population.

Selected Readings

Smith PF, Ballow CH, Booker BM, et al, "Pharmacokinetics and Pharmacodynamics of Aztreonam and Tobramycin in Hospitalized Patients," *Clin Ther*, 2001, 23(8):1231-44.

♦ **Tobramycin Sulfate** *see* Tobramycin *on page 771*

♦ **Tobrex®** *see* Tobramycin *on page 771*

♦ **Tomudex® (Can)** *see* Raltitrexed *on page 700*

♦ **Tomycine™ (Can)** *see* Tobramycin *on page 771*

♦ **TOPO** *see* Topotecan *on page 776*

♦ **Toposar®** *see* Etoposide *on page 315*

Topotecan *(toe poe TEE kan)*

Medication Safety Issues

Sound-alike/look-alike issues:

Hycamtin® may be confused with Hycomine®

Related Information

Management of Nausea and Vomiting *on page 982*

Safe Handling of Hazardous Drugs *on page 1034*

U.S. Brand Names Hycamtin®

Canadian Brand Names Hycamtin™

Generic Available No

Synonyms Hycamptamine; NSC-609699; SK and F 104864; SKF 104864; SKF 104864-A; TOPO; Topotecan Hydrochloride; TPT

Pharmacologic Category Antineoplastic Agent, Natural Source (Plant) Derivative

Pregnancy Risk Factor D

Lactation Excretion in breast milk unknown/contraindicated

Use Treatment of ovarian cancer, small cell lung cancer

Unlabeled/Investigational Use Investigational: Treatment of nonsmall cell lung cancer, sarcoma (pediatrics)

Mechanism of Action Binds to topoisomerase I and stabilizes the cleavable complex so that religation of the cleaved DNA strand cannot occur. This results in the accumulation of cleavable complexes and single-strand DNA breaks. Topotecan acts in S phase.

Labeled Contraindications Hypersensitivity to topotecan or any component of the formulation; severe bone marrow depression; pregnancy; breast-feeding

Warnings/Precautions Hazardous agent - use appropriate precautions for handling and disposal. See Safe Handling of Hazardous Drugs *on*

page 1034 in the Appendix. Monitor bone marrow function. Should only administer to patients with adequate bone marrow reserves, baseline neutrophils at least 1500 cells/mm³ and platelet counts at least 100,000/mm³. Use caution in renal impairment.

Adverse Reactions

>10%:

Central nervous system: Headache, fatigue, fever, pain

Dermatologic: Alopecia (reversible), rash

Gastrointestinal: Nausea, vomiting, diarrhea, constipation, abdominal pain, stomatitis, anorexia

Hematologic: Myelosuppressive: Principle dose-limiting toxicity; white blood cell count nadir is 8-11 days and is more frequent than thrombocytopenia (at lower doses); recover is usually within 21 days and cumulative toxicity has not been noted.

Neuromuscular & skeletal: Weakness

Respiratory: Dyspnea (22%), cough

1% to 10%:

Hepatic: Transient increases in liver enzymes

Neuromuscular & skeletal: Paresthesia

<1%: Mild erythema and bruising

Postmarketing and/or case reports: Severe bleeding (associated with thrombocytopenia), severe dermatitis or pruritus, allergic reactions, anaphylactoid reactions, angioedema

Vesicant No

Emetic Potential Low (10% to 30%)

Drug Interactions

Increased Effect/Toxicity: Concurrent administration of TPT and G-CSF in clinical trials results in severe myelosuppression. If G-CSF is to be used, manufacturer recommends that it should not be initiated until 24 hours after the completion of treatment with topotecan. Concurrent *in vitro* exposure to TPT and the topoisomerase II inhibitor etoposide results in no altered effect; sequential exposure results in potentiation. Concurrent exposure to TPT and 5-azacytidine results in potentiation both *in vitro* and *in vivo*. Myelosuppression was more severe when given in combination with cisplatin.

Ethanol/Nutrition/Herb Interactions Ethanol: Avoid ethanol (due to GI irritation).

Storage/Stability Store intact vials of lyophilized powder for injection at room temperature and protected from light. Reconstituted solution is stable for 24 hours at room temperature or up to 7 days under refrigeration. Diluted in 50-100 mL D₅W or NS is stable for 24 hours at room temperature or up to 7 days under refrigeration.

Reconstitution Reconstitute vials with 4 mL SWFI, D₅, or NS; may be further diluted in 50-100 mL D₅W or NS for infusion.

Compatibility Stable in D₅W, NS

Y-site administration: **Compatible:** Carboplatin, cimetidine, cisplatin, cyclophosphamide, doxorubicin, etoposide, gemcitabine, granisetron, ifosfamide, methylprednisolone sodium succinate, metoclopramide, ondansetron, paclitaxel, prochlorperazine edisylate, vincristine. **Incompatible:** Dexamethasone sodium phosphate, fluorouracil, mitomycin. **Variable (consult detailed reference):** Ticarcillin/clavulanate

Pharmacodynamics/Kinetics

Absorption: Oral: ~30%

(Continued)

Topotecan *(Continued)*

Distribution: V_{dss} of the lactone is high (mean: 87.3 L/mm^2; range: 25.6-186 L/mm^2), suggesting wide distribution and/or tissue sequestering

Protein binding: 35%

Metabolism: Undergoes a rapid, pH-dependent opening of the lactone ring to yield a relatively inactive hydroxy acid in plasma

Half-life elimination: 2-3 hours

Excretion: Urine (30%) within 24 hours

Dosage Adults (refer to individual protocols):

Metastatic ovarian cancer and small cell lung cancer:

IVPB: 1.5 mg/m^2/day for 5 days; repeated every 21 days (neutrophil count should be >1500/mm^3 and platelet count should be >100,000/mm^3)

I.V. continuous infusion: 0.2-0.7 mg/m^2/day for 7-21 days

Dosage adjustment for hematological effects: If neutrophil count <1500/mm^3, reduce dose by 0.25 mg/m^2/day for 5 days for next cycle

Dosing adjustment in renal impairment:

Cl_{cr} 20-39 mL/minute: Administer 50% of normal dose

Cl_{cr} <20 mL/minute: Do not use, insufficient data available

Hemodialysis: Supplemental dose is not necessary

CAPD effects: Unknown

CAVH effects: Unknown

Dosing adjustment in hepatic impairment: Bilirubin 1.5-10 mg/dL: Adjustment is not necessary

Combination Regimens

Leukemia, acute lymphocytic: TVTG *on page 942*

Leukemia, acute myeloid: TVTG *on page 942*

Administration Administer IVPB over 30 minutes or by 24-hour continuous infusion.

Dosage Forms Injection, powder for reconstitution, as hydrochloride: 4 mg [base]

Monitoring Parameters CBC with differential and platelet count and renal function tests

Patient Information This medication can only be administered I.V. and frequent blood tests may be necessary to monitor effects of the drug. Report pain, swelling, or irritation at infusion site. Do not use alcohol, prescription, and/or OTC medications without consulting prescriber. Maintain adequate hydration (2-3 L/day of fluids unless instructed to restrict fluid intake); maintain good oral hygiene (use a soft toothbrush or cotton applicators several times a day and rinse mouth frequently). You may experience nausea, vomiting, or loss of appetite (frequent small meals, frequent mouth care, sucking lozenges, or chewing gum may help, or consult prescriber). Hair loss may occur (reversible). You will be susceptible to infection; avoid crowds and infected persons and do not receive any vaccinations unless approved by prescriber. Report persistent fever or chills, unhealed sores, oral or vaginal sores, foul-smelling urine, painful urination, easy bruising or bleeding, yellowing of eyes or skin, and change in color of urine or stool. The drug may cause permanent sterility and may cause birth defects. Contraceptive measures should be used during therapy. The drug may be excreted in breast milk, therefore, an alternative form of feeding your baby should be used.

Selected Readings

Arun B and Frenkel EP, "Topoisomerase I Inhibition With Topotecan: Pharmacologic and Clinical Issues," *Expert Opin Pharmacother*, 2001, 2(3):491-505.

Cersosimo RJ, "Topotecan: A New Topoisomerase I Inhibiting Antineoplastic Agent," *Ann Pharmacother*, 1998, 32(12):1334-43.

Dennis MJ, Beijnen JH, Grochow LB, et al, "An Overview of the Clinical Pharmacology of Topotecan," *Semin Oncol*, 1997, 24(1 Suppl 5):5-12, 5-18.

Herben VM, ten Bokkel Huinink WW, and Beijnen JH, "Clinical Pharmacokinetics of Topotecan," *Clin Pharmacokinet*, 1996, 31(2):85-102.

Kollmannsberger C, Mross K, Jakob A, et al, "Topotecan - A Novel Topoisomerase I Inhibitor: Pharmacology and Clinical Experience," *Oncology*, 1999, 56(1):1-12.

Mathijssen RH, Loos WJ, Verweij J, et al, "Pharmacology of Topoisomerase I Inhibitors Irinotecan (CPT-11) and Topotecan," *Curr Cancer Drug Targets*, 2002, 2(2):103-23.

♦ **Topotecan Hydrochloride** *see* Topotecan *on page 776*

Toremifene (TORE em i feen)

Related Information
Safe Handling of Hazardous Drugs *on page 1034*

U.S. Brand Names Fareston®

Canadian Brand Names Fareston®

Generic Available No

Synonyms FC1157a; Toremifene Citrate

Pharmacologic Category Antineoplastic Agent, Estrogen Receptor Antagonist

Pregnancy Risk Factor D

Lactation Excretion in breast milk unknown/contraindicated

Use Treatment of advanced breast cancer; management of desmoid tumors and endometrial carcinoma

Mechanism of Action Nonsteroidal, triphenylethylene derivative. Competitively binds to estrogen receptors on tumors and other tissue targets, producing a nuclear complex that decreases DNA synthesis and inhibits estrogen effects. Nonsteroidal agent with potent antiestrogenic properties which compete with estrogen for binding sites in breast and other tissues; cells accumulate in the G_0 and G_1 phases; therefore, toremifene is cytostatic rather than cytocidal.

Labeled Contraindications Hypersensitivity to toremifene or any component of the formulation; pregnancy

Warnings/Precautions Hazardous agent - use appropriate precautions for handling and disposal. See Safe Handling of Hazardous Drugs *on page 1034* in the Appendix. Hypercalcemia and tumor flare have been reported in some breast cancer patients with bone metastases during the first weeks of treatment. Tumor flare is a syndrome of diffuse musculoskeletal pain and erythema with increased size of tumor lesions that later regress. It is often accompanied by hypercalcemia. Tumor flare does not imply treatment failure or represent tumor progression. Institute appropriate measures if hypercalcemia occurs, and if severe, discontinue treatment. Drugs that decrease renal calcium excretion (eg, thiazide diuretics) may increase the risk of hypercalcemia in patients receiving toremifene. Leukopenia and thrombocytopenia have been reported rarely. Use cautiously in patients with anemia, hepatic failure, or thromboembolic disease.

Adverse Reactions
>10%:
Endocrine & metabolic: Vaginal discharge, hot flashes
Gastrointestinal: Nausea, vomiting

(Continued)

Toremifene *(Continued)*

Miscellaneous: Diaphoresis

1% to 10%:

Cardiovascular: Thromboembolism: Toremifene has been associated with arterial thrombosis and has been described in a few case reports; cardiac failure, MI, edema

Central nervous system: Dizziness

Endocrine & metabolic: Hypercalcemia may occur in patients with bone metastases; galactorrhea and vitamin deficiency, menstrual irregularities

Genitourinary: Vaginal bleeding or discharge, endometriosis, priapism, possible endometrial cancer

Ocular: Ophthalmologic effects (visual acuity changes, cataracts, or retinopathy), corneal opacities, dry eyes

Emetic Potential Moderate (30% to 40%)

Overdosage/Toxicology Theoretically, overdose may manifest as an increase of antiestrogenic effects such as hot flashes; estrogenic effects such as vaginal bleeding; or nervous system disorders such as vertigo, dizziness, ataxia, and nausea. No specific antidote exists and treatment is symptomatic.

Drug Interactions

Cytochrome P450 Effect: Substrate of CYP1A2 (minor), 3A4 (major)

Increased Effect/Toxicity: Concurrent therapy with warfarin results in significant enhancement of anticoagulant effects; has been speculated that a decrease in antitumor effect of tamoxifen may also occur due to alterations in the percentage of active tamoxifen metabolites.

Decreased Effect: CYP3A4 inducers may decrease the levels/effects of toremifene; example inducers include aminoglutethimide, carbamazepine, nafcillin, nevirapine, phenobarbital, phenytoin, and rifamycins.

Storage/Stability Store at 25°C (77°F); excursions permitted to 15°C to 30°C (59°F to 86°F). Protect from heat and light.

Pharmacodynamics/Kinetics

Absorption: Well absorbed

Distribution: V_d: 580 L

Protein binding, plasma: >99.5%, primarily to albumin

Metabolism: Extensively hepatic, principally by CYP3A4 to N-demethyltoremifene, which is also antiestrogenic but with weak *in vivo* antitumor potency

Half-life elimination: ~5 days

Time to peak, serum: ~3 hours

Excretion: Primarily feces; urine (10%) during a 1-week period

Dosage Refer to individual protocols.

Adults: Oral: 60 mg once daily, generally continued until disease progression is observed

Dosage adjustment in renal impairment: No dosage adjustment necessary

Dosage adjustment in hepatic impairment: Toremifene is extensively metabolized in the liver and dosage adjustments may be indicated in patients with liver disease; however, no specific guidelines have been developed

Administration Orally, usually as a single daily dose; occasionally in 2 or 3 divided doses

Dosage Forms Tablet: 60 mg

Monitoring Parameters Obtain periodic complete blood counts, calcium levels, and liver function tests. Closely monitor patients with bone metastases for hypercalcemia during the first few weeks of treatment. Leukopenia and thrombocytopenia have been reported rarely; monitor leukocyte and platelet counts during treatment.

Patient Information Take as directed, without regard to food. You may experience an initial "flare" of this disease (increased bone pain and hot flashes) which will subside with continued use. You may experience nausea, vomiting, or loss of appetite (frequent mouth care, frequent small meals, chewing gum, or sucking lozenges may help); dizziness (use caution when driving, climbing stairs, or engaging in tasks requiring alertness until response to drug is known); or loss of hair (reversible). Report vomiting that occurs immediately after taking medication; chest pain, palpitations or swollen extremities; vaginal bleeding, hot flashes, or excessive perspiration; chest pain, unusual coughing, or difficulty breathing; or any changes in vision or dry eyes.

Additional Information Increase of bone pain usually indicates a good therapeutic response

Selected Readings

Kangas L, "Review of the Pharmacological Properties of Toremifene," *J Steroid Biochem*, 1990, 36(3):191-5.

Taras TL, Wurz GT, Linares GR, et al, "Clinical Pharmacokinetics of Toremifene," *Clin Pharmacokinet*, 2000, 39(5):327-34.

♦ **Toremifene Citrate** *see* Toremifene *on page 779*

Tositumomab and Iodine I 131 Tositumomab

(toe si TYOO mo mab & EYE oh dyne eye one THUR tee one toe si TYOO mo mab)

U.S. Brand Names Bexxar®

Generic Available No

Synonyms Anti-CD20-Murine Monoclonal Antibody I-131; B1; B1 Antibody; 131 I Anti-B1 Antibody; 131 I-Anti-B1 Monoclonal Antibody; Iodine I 131 Tositumomab and Tositumomab; Tositumomab I-131

Pharmacologic Category Antineoplastic Agent, Monoclonal Antibody; Radiopharmaceutical

Pregnancy Risk Factor X

Lactation Enters breast milk/contraindicated

Use Treatment of relapsed or refractory CD20 positive, low-grade, follicular, or transformed non-Hodgkin's lymphoma

Mechanism of Action Tositumomab is a murine IgG2a lambda monoclonal antibody which binds to the CD20 antigen, expressed on B-lymphocytes and on >90% of B-cell non-Hodgkin's lymphomas. Iodine I 131 tositumomab is a radio-iodinated derivative of tositumomab covalently linked to iodine 131. The possible actions of the regimen include apoptosis, complement-dependent cytotoxicity, antibody-dependent cellular cytotoxicity, and cell death. Administration results in depletion of CD20 positive cells.

Labeled Contraindications Hypersensitivity to murine proteins or any component of the formulation; pregnancy; breast-feeding

Warnings/Precautions Hypersensitivity reactions (including anaphylaxis) have been reported. Patients should be screened for human antimouse antibodies (HAMA); may be at increased risk of allergic or (Continued)

Tositumomab and Iodine I 131 Tositumomab
(Continued)

serious hypersensitivity reactions. Hematologic toxicity was reported to be the most common adverse effect with 27% patients requiring supportive care. Severe or life-threatening cytopenias (NCI CTC grade 3 or 4) have been reported in a large number of patients; may be prolonged and severe. Secondary malignancies have been reported following use.

Treatment involves radioactive isotopes; appropriate precautions in handling and administration must be followed. Patients must be instructed in measures to minimize exposure of others. Women of child-bearing potential should be advised of potential fetal risk; effective contraceptive measures should be used for 12 months following treatment (males and females). Treatment may lead to hypothyroidism; patients should receive thyroid-blocking medications prior to the start of therapy. Patients should be premedicated to prevent infusion related reactions. For a single course of therapy only; multiple courses or use in combination with other chemotherapy or irradiation have not been studied.

Safety has not been established in patients with >25% lymphoma marrow involvement, platelet count <100,000 cells/mm^3 or neutrophil count <1500 cells/mm^3. Use caution with cardiovascular disease, renal, or hepatic impairment. Safety and efficacy have not been established with impaired renal function or in pediatric patients.

Adverse Reactions

>10%:

Central nervous system: Fever (37%), pain (19%), chills (18%), headache (16%)

Dermatologic: Rash (17%)

Endocrine & metabolic: Hypothyroidism (7% to 19%)

Gastrointestinal: Nausea (36%), abdominal pain (15%), vomiting (15%), anorexia (14%), diarrhea (12%)

Hematologic:

Neutropenia (grade 3 or 4, 63%); thrombocytopenia (grade 3 or 4, 53%)

Time to nadir: 4-7 weeks

Duration: 30 days (>90 days in 5% to 7% of patients)

Neuromuscular & skeletal: Weakness (46%), myalgia (13%)

Respiratory: Cough (21%), pharyngitis (12%), dyspnea (11%)

Miscellaneous: Infusion-related reactions (26%, occurred within 14 days of infusion, included bronchospasm, chills, dyspnea, fever, hypotension, nausea, rigors, diaphoresis), infection (21%), HAMA-positive seroconversion (11%; up to 21% at 1 year)

1% to 10%:

Cardiovascular: Hypotension (7% to 10%), peripheral edema (9%), chest pain (7%), vasodilation (5%)

Central nervous system: Dizziness (5%), somnolence (5%)

Dermatologic: Pruritus (10%)

Gastrointestinal: Constipation (6%), dyspepsia (6%), weight loss (6%)

Local: Injection site hypersensitivity

Neuromuscular & skeletal: Arthralgia (10%), back pain (8%), neck pain (6%)

Respiratory: Rhinitis (10%), pneumonia (6%), laryngismus

Miscellaneous: Diaphoresis (8%), hypersensitivity reaction (6%), secondary leukemia/myelodysplastic syndrome (3%; up to 6% at 5 years), anaphylactoid reaction, secondary malignancies, serum sickness

Overdosage/Toxicology Grade 4 hematologic toxicity lasting 18 days was reported in one patient accidentally receiving a total body dose of 88 cGy. Monitor for cytopenias and radiation-related toxicity.

Drug Interactions

Increased Effect/Toxicity: No formal drug interaction studies have been conducted.

Decreased Effect: No formal drug interaction studies have been conducted. The ability of patients receiving tositumomab to generate humoral response (primary or anamnestic) to vaccination is unknown; safety of live vaccines has not been established.

Storage/Stability

Tositumomab: Store under refrigeration at 2°C to 8°C (36°F to 46°F); protect from strong light; do not freeze. Following dilution, tositumomab is stable for 24 hour when refrigerated or 8 hours at room temperature.

Iodine I 131 tositumomab: Store frozen at less than or equal to -20°C in the original lead pots. Allow 60 minutes for thawing at ambient temperature. Solutions for infusion are stable for up to 8 hours at 2°C to 8°C (36°F to 46°F) or room temperature.

Reconstitution

Tositumomab: Withdraw and discard 32 mL of saline from a 50 mL bag of NS. Add contents of both 225 mg vials of tositumomab (total 32 mL) to remaining NS to make a final volume of 50 mL. Gently mix by inverting bag, do not shake.

Iodine I 131 tositumomab: Calculate volume required for an iodine I 131 tositumomab activity of 5 mCi (specification sheet provided with product). If the amount of tositumomab contained in the iodine I 131 tositumomab solution contains <35 mg of tositumomab, use the 35 mg vial of tositumomab to prepare a final concentration of tositumomab 35 mg. Using NS, the final volume should equal 30 mL.

Pharmacodynamics/Kinetics

Distribution: Tositumomab: V_d increased with high tumor burden, splenomegaly, or bone marrow involvement

Half-life elimination: Tositumomab:

Elimination: 36-48 hours

Terminal half-life decreased with high tumor burden, splenomegaly, or bone marrow involvement

Clearance: Blood: 68.2 mg/hour

Excretion: Iodine-131: Urine (98%) and decay

Dosage I.V.: Adults: Dosing consists of four components administered in 2 steps. Thyroid protective agents (SSKI, Lugol's solution or potassium iodide), acetaminophen and diphenhydramine should be given prior to or with treatment. Refer to Additional Information.

Step 1: Dosimetric step (Day 0):

Tositumomab 450 mg in NS 50 mL administered over 60 minutes

Iodine I 131 tositumomab (containing I-131 5.0 mCi and tositumomab 35mg) in NS 30 mL administered over 20 minutes

Note: Whole body dosimetry and biodistribution should be determined on Day 0; days 2, 3, or 4; and day 6 or 7 prior to administration of Step 2. If biodistribution is not acceptable, do not administer the

(Continued)

Tositumomab and Iodine I 131 Tositumomab
(Continued)

therapeutic step. On day 6 or 7, calculate the patient specific activity of iodine I 131 tositumomab to deliver 75 cGy TBD or 65 cGy TBD (in mCi).

Step 2: Therapeutic step (Day 7):

Tositumomab 450 mg in NS 50 mL administered over 60 minutes

Iodine I 131 tositumomab:

Platelets ≥150,000/mm^3: Iodine I 131 calculated to deliver 75 cGy total body irradiation and tositumomab 35 mg over 20 minutes

Platelets ≥100,000/mm^3 and <150,000/mm^3: Iodine I 131 calculated to deliver 65 cGy total body irradiation and tositumomab 35 mg over 20 minutes

Administration I.V.:

Tositumomab: Infuse over 60 minutes

Iodine I 131 tositumomab: Infuse over 20 minutes

Reduce the rate of tositumomab or iodine 131 tositumomab infusion by 50% for mild-to-moderate infusion-related toxicities; interrupt for severe toxicity. Once severe toxicity has resolved, infusion may be restarted at half the previous rate. Prior to infusion, patients should be premedicated and a thyroid-protective agent should be started.

Dosage Forms Note: Not all components are shipped from the same facility. When ordering, ensure that all will arrive on the same day.

Kit [dosimetric package] (Bexxar®): Tositumomab 225 mg/16.1 mL [2 vials], tositumomab 35 mg/2.5 mL [1 vial], and iodine I 131 tositumomab 0.1 mg/mL and 0.61mCi/mL (20 mL) [1 vial]

Kit [therapeutic package] (Bexxar®): Tositumomab 225 mg/16.1 mL [2 vials], tositumomab 35 mg/2.5 mL [1 vial], and iodine I 131 tositumomab 1.1 mg/mL and 5.6 mCi/mL (20 mL) [1 or 2 vials]

Monitoring Parameters CBC with differential (prior to therapy and at least weekly for a minimum of 10 weeks); TSH (prior to therapy and yearly); serum creatinine (immediately prior to administration)

Following infusion of the iodine I 131 tositumomab dosimetric dose, the total body gamma camera counts and whole body images should be taken within 1 hour of the infusion and prior to urination, and 2-4 days after the infusion and following urination, and 6-7 days after the infusion and following urination.

Patient Information This medication is given only by injection. Follow instructions to limit exposure of radioactivity to family and friends. Notify prescriber if pregnant or if pregnancy occurs within 12 months after completion of therapy; effective birth control should be used by male and female patients during treatment and for 12 months following therapy. Breast-feeding is not recommended; discontinue and change to formula feedings prior to therapy.

Additional Information Thyroid protective agent: One of the following agents should be used starting at least 24 hours prior to the dosimetric dose and continued for 2 weeks after the therapeutic dose. Therapy should not begin without using one of the following agents:

SSKI: 4 drops 3 times/day

Lugol's solution: 20 drops 3 times/day

Potassium iodide: 130 mg once daily

Selected Readings

Kaminski MS, Zelenetz AD, Press OW, et al, "Pivotal Study of Iodine I 131 Tositumomab for Chemotherapy-Refractory Low-Grade or Transformed Low-Grade B-Cell Non-Hodgkin's Lymphomas," *J Clin Oncol*, 2001, 19(19):3918-28.

Press OW, Eary JF, Appelbaum FR, et al, "Phase II Trial of 131I-B1 (Anti-CD20) Antibody Therapy With Autologous Stem Cell Transplantation for Relapsed B Cell Lymphomas," *Lancet*, 1995, 346(8971):336-40.

Press OW, Eary JF, Appelbaum FR, et al, "Radiolabeled-Antibody Therapy of B-Cell Lymphoma With Autologous Bone Marrow Support," *N Engl J Med*, 1993, 329(17):1219-24.

Zelenetz AD, "A Clinical and Scientific Overview of Tositumomab and Iodine I 131 Tositumomab," *Semin Oncol*, 2003, 30(2 Suppl 4):22-30.

♦ **Tositumomab I-131** see Tositumomab and Iodine I 131 Tositumomab *on page 781*

♦ **tPA** see Alteplase *on page 46*

♦ **TPT** see Topotecan *on page 776*

♦ **tRA** see Tretinoin (Oral) *on page 792*

Tramadol (TRA ma dole)

Medication Safety Issues

Sound-alike/look-alike issues:

Tramadol may be confused with Toradol®, Trandate®, Voltaren®

Ultram® may be confused with Ultane®, Voltaren®

U.S. Brand Names Ultram®

Canadian Brand Names Ultram®

Generic Available Yes

Synonyms Tramadol Hydrochloride

Pharmacologic Category Analgesic, Non-narcotic

Pregnancy Risk Factor C

Lactation Enters breast milk/contraindicated

Use Relief of moderate to moderately-severe pain

Mechanism of Action Binds to μ-opiate receptors in the CNS causing inhibition of ascending pain pathways, altering the perception of and response to pain; also inhibits the reuptake of norepinephrine and serotonin, which also modifies the ascending pain pathway

Labeled Contraindications Hypersensitivity to tramadol, opioids, or any component of the formulation; opioid-dependent patients; acute intoxication with alcohol, hypnotics, centrally-acting analgesics, opioids, or psychotropic drugs

Warnings/Precautions Should be used only with extreme caution in patients receiving MAO inhibitors. May cause CNS depression and/or respiratory depression, particularly when combined with other CNS depressants. Use with caution and reduce dosage when administered to patients receiving other CNS depressants. An increased risk of seizures may occur in patients receiving serotonin reuptake inhibitors (SSRIs or anorectics), tricyclic antidepressants, other cyclic compounds (including cyclobenzaprine, promethazine), neuroleptics, MAO inhibitors, or drugs which may lower seizure threshold. Patients with a history of seizures, or with a risk of seizures (head trauma, metabolic disorders, CNS infection, or malignancy, or during ethanol/drug withdrawal) are also at increased risk.

Elderly patients and patients with chronic respiratory disorders may be at greater risk of adverse events. Use with caution in patients with increased intracranial pressure or head injury. Use with caution and reduce dosage

(Continued)

Tramadol *(Continued)*

in patients with liver disease or renal dysfunction and in patients with myxedema, hypothyroidism, or hypoadrenalism. Not recommended during pregnancy or in nursing mothers. Tolerance or drug dependence may result from extended use (withdrawal symptoms have been reported); abrupt discontinuation should be avoided. Tapering of dose at the time of discontinuation limits the risk of withdrawal symptoms. Safety and efficacy in pediatric patients have not been established.

Adverse Reactions Incidence of some adverse effects may increase over time

>10%:

  Central nervous system: Dizziness, headache, somnolence, vertigo

  Gastrointestinal: Constipation, nausea

1% to 10%:

  Cardiovascular: Vasodilation

  Central nervous system: Agitation, anxiety, confusion, coordination impaired, emotional lability, euphoria, hallucinations, malaise, nervousness, sleep disorder, tremor

  Dermatologic: Pruritus, rash

  Endocrine & metabolic: Menopausal symptoms

  Gastrointestinal: Abdominal pain, anorexia, diarrhea, dry mouth, dyspepsia, flatulence, vomiting

  Genitourinary: Urinary frequency, urinary retention

  Neuromuscular & skeletal: Hypertonia, spasticity, weakness

  Ocular: Miosis, visual disturbance

  Miscellaneous: Diaphoresis

<1%: Abnormal gait, allergic reaction, amnesia, anaphylactoid reactions, anaphylaxis, angioedema, bronchospasm, cognitive dysfunction, concentration difficulty, death, depression, dyspnea, dysuria, hallucinations, menstrual disorder, orthostatic hypotension, paresthesia, seizure, serotonin syndrome, Stevens-Johnson syndrome, suicidal tendency, syncope, taste perversion, tachycardia, toxic epidermal necrolysis, tremor, urticaria, vesicles, weight loss

Postmarketing and/or case reports: Abnormal ECG, cataracts, creatinine increased, deafness, gastrointestinal bleeding, hemoglobin decreased, hepatitis, hyper-/hypotension, liver enzymes elevated, liver failure, migraine, myocardial ischemia, palpitation, proteinuria, pulmonary edema, pulmonary embolism, speech disorders, stomatitis, tinnitus

A withdrawal syndrome may occur with abrupt discontinuation; includes anxiety, diarrhea, hallucinations (rare), nausea, pain, piloerection, rigors, sweating, and tremor. Uncommon discontinuation symptoms may include severe anxiety, panic attacks, or paresthesia.

Overdosage/Toxicology Symptoms of overdose include CNS and respiratory depression, lethargy, coma, seizure, cardiac arrest, and death. Treatment may include naloxone 2 mg I.V. (0.01 mg/kg children) with repeat administration as needed up to 18 mg. Naloxone may increase the risk of seizures in tramadol overdose.

Drug Interactions

Cytochrome P450 Effect: Substrate of CYP2D6 (major), 3A4 (minor)

Increased Effect/Toxicity: Amphetamines may increase the risk of seizures with tramadol. Cimetidine increases the half-life of tramadol by 20% to 25%. SSRIs may increase the risk of seizures with tramadol. Tricyclic antidepressants may increase the risk of seizures. Linezolid may be associated with increased risk of seizures (due to MAO inhibition). MAO inhibitors may increases the risk of seizures. It is not clear if drugs with selective MAO type B inhibition are safer than nonselective agents. Avoid drugs with MAO activity (ie, linezolid). Naloxone may increase the risk of seizures in tramadol overdose. Neuroleptic agents may increase the risk of tramadol-associated seizures and may have additive CNS depressant effects. Opioids may increase the risk of seizures, and may have additive CNS depressant effects. Quinidine (and other inhibitors of CYP2D6) may increase the tramadol serum concentrations.

Decreased Effect: CYP2D6 inhibitors may decrease the effects of tramadol; example inhibitors include chlorpromazine, delavirdine, fluoxetine, miconazole, paroxetine, pergolide, quinidine, quinine, ritonavir, and ropinirole. Carbamazepine may decrease analgesic efficacy of tramadol (half-life decreases 33% to 50%) and may increase the risk of seizures in patients requiring anticonvulsants.

Ethanol/Nutrition/Herb Interactions

Ethanol: Avoid ethanol (may increase CNS depression).

Food: Does not affect the rate or extent of absorption.

Herb/Nutraceutical: Avoid valerian, St John's wort, kava kava, gotu kola (may increase CNS depression).

Storage/Stability Store at controlled room temperature of 25°C (77°F).

Pharmacodynamics/Kinetics

Onset of action: ~1 hour

Duration of action: 9 hours

Absorption: Rapid and complete

Distribution: V_d: 2.5-3 L/kg

Protein binding, plasma: 20%

Metabolism: Extensively hepatic via demethylation, glucuronidation, and sulfation; has pharmacologically active metabolite formed by CYP2D6

Bioavailability: 75%

Half-life elimination: Tramadol: ~6 hours; Active metabolite: 7 hours; prolonged in elderly, hepatic or renal impairment

Time to peak: 2 hours

Excretion: Urine (as metabolites)

Dosage Oral:

Adults: Moderate to severe chronic pain: 50-100 mg every 4-6 hours, not to exceed 400 mg/day

For patients not requiring rapid onset of effect, tolerability may be improved by starting dose at 25 mg/day and titrating dose by 25 mg every 3 days, until reaching 25 mg 4 times/day. Dose may then be increased by 50 mg every 3 days as tolerated, to reach dose of 50 mg 4 times/day.

Elderly: >75 years: 50-100 mg every 4-6 hours (not to exceed 300 mg/day); see dosing adjustments for renal and hepatic impairment

Dosing adjustment in renal impairment: Cl_{cr} <30 mL/minute: Administer 50-100 mg dose every 12 hours (maximum: 200 mg/day)

Dosing adjustment in hepatic impairment: Cirrhosis: Recommended dose: 50 mg every 12 hours

Dosage Forms Tablet, as hydrochloride: 50 mg

Monitoring Parameters Pain relief, respiratory rate, blood pressure, and pulse; signs of tolerance or abuse

Dietary Considerations May be taken with or without food.

(Continued)

Tramadol *(Continued)*

Patient Information Avoid driving or operating machinery until the effect of drug wears off. Report cravings to your prescriber immediately.

Special Geriatric Considerations One study in the elderly found that tramadol 50 mg was similar in efficacy as acetaminophen 300 mg with codeine 30 mg.

Selected Readings

Dayer P, Collart L, and Desmeules J, "The Pharmacology of Tramadol," *Drugs*, 1994, 47(Suppl 1):3-7.

Lewis KS and Han NH, "Tramadol: A New Centrally Acting Analgesic," *Am J Health Syst Pharm*, 1997, 54(6):643-52.

Sunshine A, Olson NZ, Zighelboim I, et al, "Analgesic Oral Efficacy of Tramadol Hydrochloride in Postoperative Pain," *Clin Pharmacol Ther*, 1992; 51(6):740-6.

Sunshine A, "New Clinical Experience With Tramadol," *Drugs*, 1994, 47(Suppl 1):8-18.

Wynn RL, "Tramadol (Ultram) - A New Kind of Analgesic," *Gen Dent*, 1996, 44(3):216-8,220.

♦ **Tramadol Hydrochloride** *see* Tramadol *on page 785*

Tranexamic Acid *(tran eks AM ik AS id)*

Medication Safety Issues

Sound-alike/look-alike issues:

Cyklokapron® may be confused with cycloSPORINE

U.S. Brand Names Cyklokapron®

Canadian Brand Names Cyklokapron®

Generic Available No

Pharmacologic Category Antihemophilic Agent

Pregnancy Risk Factor B

Lactation Enters breast milk/use caution

Use Short-term use (2-8 days) in hemophilia patients during and following tooth extraction to reduce or prevent hemorrhage

Unlabeled/Investigational Use Has been used as an alternative to aminocaproic acid for subarachnoid hemorrhage

Mechanism of Action Forms a reversible complex that displaces plasminogen from fibrin resulting in inhibition of fibrinolysis; it also inhibits the proteolytic activity of plasmin

Labeled Contraindications Acquired defective color vision; active intravascular clotting; subarachnoid hemorrhage; concurrent factor IX complex or anti-inhibitor coagulant concentrates

Warnings/Precautions Dosage modification required in patients with renal impairment; ophthalmic exam before and during therapy required if patient is treated beyond several days; caution in patients with cardiovascular, renal, or cerebrovascular disease; caution in patients with a history of thromboembolic disease (may increase risk of thrombosis); when used for subarachnoid hemorrhage, ischemic complications may occur

Adverse Reactions

>10%: Gastrointestinal: Nausea, diarrhea, vomiting

1% to 10%:

Cardiovascular: Hypotension, thrombosis

Ocular: Blurred vision

<1%: Unusual menstrual discomfort

Postmarketing and/or case reports: Deep venous thrombosis (DVT), pulmonary embolus (PE), renal cortical necrosis, retinal artery obstruction, retinal vein obstruction, ureteral obstruction

Vesicant No

Emetic Potential Low (10% to 30%)

Drug Interactions

  Increased Effect/Toxicity: Chlorpromazine may increase cerebral vasospasm and ischemia. Coadministrations of Factor IX complex or anti-inhibitor coagulant concentrates may increase risk of thrombosis.

Compatibility Incompatible with solutions containing penicillin. **Compatible** with dextrose, saline, and electrolyte solutions

Pharmacodynamics/Kinetics

  Half-life elimination: 2-10 hours

  Excretion: Urine (>90% as unchanged drug)

Dosage Children and Adults: I.V.: 10 mg/kg immediately before surgery, then 25 mg/kg/dose orally 3-4 times/day for 2-8 days

  Alternatively:

    Oral: 25 mg/kg 3-4 times/day beginning 1 day prior to surgery

    I.V.: 10 mg/kg 3-4 times/day in patients who are unable to take oral

  Dosing adjustment/interval in renal impairment:

    Cl_{cr} 50-80 mL/minute: Administer 50% of normal dose or 10 mg/kg twice daily I.V. or 15 mg/kg twice daily orally

    Cl_{cr} 10-50 mL/minute: Administer 25% of normal dose or 10 mg/kg/day I.V. or 15 mg/kg/day orally

    Cl_{cr} <10 mL/minute: Administer 10% of normal dose or 10 mg/kg/dose every 48 hours I.V. or 15 mg/kg/dose every 48 hours orally

Administration May be administered by direct I.V. injection at a maximum rate of 100 mg/minute; compatible with dextrose, saline, and electrolyte solutions; use plastic syringe only for I.V. push

Dosage Forms

  Injection, solution: 100 mg/mL (10 mL)

  Tablet: 500 mg [Not marketed in U.S.; available from manufacturer for select cases]

Patient Information Report any signs of bleeding or myopathy, changes in vision; GI upset usually disappears when dose is reduced

Selected Readings

Astedt B, "Clinical Pharmacology of Tranexamic Acid," *Scand J Gastroenterol Suppl*, 1987, 137:22-5.

Nilsson IM, "Clinical Pharmacology of Aminocaproic and Tranexamic Acids," *J Clin Pathol Suppl* (Royal College of Pathologists), 1980, 14:41-7.

Royston D, "Blood-Sparing Drugs: Aprotinin, Tranexamic Acid, and Epsilon-Aminocaproic Acid," *Int Anesthesiol Clin*, 1995, 33(1):155-79.

Seto AH and Dunlap DS, "Tranexamic Acid in Oncology," *Ann Pharmacother*, 1996, 30(7-8):868-70.

Wellington K and Wagstaff AJ, "Tranexamic Acid: A Review of its Use in the Management of Menorrhagia," *Drugs*, 2003, 63(13):1417-33.

♦ **Transplantation** see page 1019

♦ ***trans*-Retinoic Acid** see Tretinoin (Oral) on page 792

Trastuzumab (tras TU zoo mab)

Related Information

  Safe Handling of Hazardous Drugs on page 1034

U.S. Brand Names Herceptin®

Canadian Brand Names Herceptin®

Generic Available No

Pharmacologic Category Monoclonal Antibody

Pregnancy Risk Factor B

(Continued)

Trastuzumab *(Continued)*

Lactation Excretion in breast milk unknown/not recommended

Use Control of symptoms in patients with metastatic carcinoid and vasoactive intestinal peptide-secreting tumors (VIPomas); pancreatic tumors, gastrinoma, secretory diarrhea, acromegaly

Unlabeled/Investigational Use Treatment of ovarian, gastric, colorectal, endometrial, lung, bladder, prostate, and salivary gland tumors

Mechanism of Action Trastuzumab is a monoclonal antibody which binds to the extracellular domain of the human epidermal growth factor receptor 2 protein (HER-2); it mediates antibody-dependent cellular cytotoxicity against cells which overproduce HER-2

Labeled Contraindications Hypersensitivity to octreotide or any component of the formulation

Warnings/Precautions Hazardous agent - use appropriate precautions for handling and disposal. See Safe Handling of Hazardous Drugs *on page 1034* in the Appendix. Dosage adjustment may be required to maintain symptomatic control; insulin requirements may be reduced as well as sulfonylurea requirements. Monitor patients for cholelithiasis. Use with caution in patients with renal impairment. Somatostatin analogs may affect glucose regulation; in type I diabetes, severe hypoglycemia may occur; in type II diabetes or nondiabetic patients, hyperglycemia may occur.

Adverse Reactions Note: The most common adverse effects are infusion-related, occurring in up to 40% of patients, consisting of fever and chills (mild to moderate, often with other systemic symptoms). Treatment with acetaminophen, diphenhydramine, and/or meperidine is usually effective.

>10%:

    Central nervous system: Pain (47%), fever (36%), chills (32%), headache (26%)

    Dermatologic: Rash (18%)

    Gastrointestinal: Nausea (33%), diarrhea (25%), vomiting (23%), abdominal pain (22%), anorexia (14%)

    Neuromuscular & skeletal: Weakness (42%), back pain (22%)

    Respiratory: Cough (26%), dyspnea (22%), rhinitis (14%), pharyngitis (12%)

    Miscellaneous: Infection (20%); infusion reaction (40%, chills and fever most common)

1% to 10%:

    Cardiovascular: Peripheral edema (10%), CHF (7%), tachycardia (5%)

    Central nervous system: Insomnia (14%), dizziness (13%), paresthesia (9%), depression (6%), peripheral neuritis (2%), neuropathy (1%)

    Dermatologic: Herpes simplex (2%), acne (2%)

    Genitourinary: Urinary tract infection (5%)

    Hematologic: Anemia (4%), leukopenia (3%)

    Neuromuscular & skeletal: Bone pain (7%), arthralgia (6%)

    Respiratory: Sinusitis (9%)

    Miscellaneous: Flu syndrome (10%), accidental injury (6%), allergic reaction (3%)

<1%: Adult respiratory distress syndrome (ARDS), amblyopia, anaphylaxis, anaphylactoid reaction, angioedema, arrhythmia, ascites, bronchospasm, cardiac arrest, cellulitis, coagulopathy, colitis, deafness,

esophageal ulcer, gastroenteritis, hematemesis, hemorrhage, hemorrhagic cystitis, hepatic failure, hepatitis, hydrocephalus, hydronephrosis, hypotension, hypothyroidism, ileus, intestinal obstruction, leukemia (acute), lymphangitis, pancreatitis, pancytopenia, pericardial effusion, pyelonephritis, radiation injury, renal failure, respiratory distress, severe infusion reaction, shock, syncope, stomatitis, vascular thrombosis

Vesicant No

Emetic Potential Moderate (30% to 60%)

Overdosage/Toxicology There is no experience with overdose in human clinical trials. Treatment is supportive.

Drug Interactions

Increased Effect/Toxicity: Paclitaxel may result in a decrease in clearance of trastuzumab, increasing serum concentrations. Combined use with anthracyclines or cyclophosphamide may increase the incidence/severity of cardiac dysfunction. Trastuzumab may increase the incidence of neutropenia and/or febrile neutropenia when used in combination with myelosuppressive chemotherapy.

Storage/Stability Store intact vials under refrigeration (2°C to 8°C/36°F to 46°F) prior to reconstitution. Stable for 28 days after reconstitution if refrigerated; do not freeze. If sterile water for injection without preservative is used for reconstitution, it must be used immediately. After dilution in 0.9% sodium chloride for injection in polyethylene bags, solution is stable for 24 hours.

Reconstitution Reconstitute each vial with 20 mL of bacteriostatic sterile water for injection. Do not shake. If patient has a known hypersensitivity to benzyl alcohol, it may be reconstituted with sterile water for injection.

Compatibility Compatible: Stable in NS

Pharmacodynamics/Kinetics

Distribution: V_d: 44 mL/kg

Half-life elimination: Mean: 5.8 days (range: 1-32 days)

Dosage I.V. infusion: Adults:

Initial loading dose: 4 mg/kg intravenous infusion over 90 minutes

Maintenance dose: 2 mg/kg intravenous infusion over 90 minutes (can be administered over 30 minutes if prior infusions are well tolerated) weekly until disease progression

Dosing adjustment in renal impairment: Data suggest that the disposition of trastuzumab is not altered based on age or serum creatinine (up to 2 mg/dL); however, no formal interaction studies have been performed

Dosing adjustment in hepatic impairment: No data is currently available

Combination Regimens

Breast cancer: Trastuzumab-Paclitaxel *on page 940*

Administration Administered by I.V. infusion; loading doses are infused over 90 minutes; maintenance doses may be infused over 30 minutes if tolerated.

Dosage Forms Injection, powder for reconstitution: 440 mg [packaged with bacteriostatic water for injection; diluent contains benzyl alcohol]

Monitoring Parameters Signs and symptoms of cardiac dysfunction; monitor vital signs during infusion

(Continued)

Trastuzumab *(Continued)*

Selected Readings

Baselga J, Albanell J, Molina MA, et al, "Mechanism of Action of Trastuzumab and Scientific Update," *Semin Oncol*, 2001, 28(5 Suppl 16):4-11.

Jones RL and Smith IE, "Efficacy and Safety of Trastuzumab," *Expert Opin Drug Saf*, 2004, 3(4):317-27.

Treish I, Schwartz R, and Lindley C, "Pharmacology and Therapeutic Use of Trastuzumab in Breast Cancer," *Am J Health Syst Pharm*, 2000, 57(22):2063-76.

Vogel CL and Franco SX, "Clinical Experience With Trastuzumab (Herceptin)," *Breast J*, 2003, 9(6):452-62.

♦ **Trelstar™ Depot** *see* Triptorelin *on page 801*

♦ **Trelstar™ LA** *see* Triptorelin *on page 801*

Tretinoin (Oral) (TRET i noyn, oral)

Medication Safety Issues
Sound-alike/look-alike issues:
Tretinoin may be confused with trientine

U.S. Brand Names Vesanoid®

Canadian Brand Names Vesanoid®

Generic Available No

Synonyms All-*trans*-Retinoic Acid; ATRA; NSC-122758; Ro 5488; tRA; *trans*-Retinoic Acid

Pharmacologic Category Antineoplastic Agent, Miscellaneous

Pregnancy Risk Factor D

Lactation Enters breast milk/not recommended

Use Induction of remission in patients with acute promyelocytic leukemia (APL), French American British (FAB) classification M3 (including the M3 variant)

Mechanism of Action Tretinoin appears to bind one or more nuclear receptors and inhibits clonal proliferation and/or granulocyte differentiation

Labeled Contraindications Sensitivity to parabens, vitamin A, other retinoids, or any component of the formulation; pregnancy

Warnings/Precautions Hazardous agent - use appropriate precautions for handling and disposal. See Safe Handling of Hazardous Drugs *on page 1034* in the Appendix. Patients with acute promyelocytic leukemia (APL) are at high risk and can have severe adverse reactions to tretinoin.

May cause retinoic acid-APL (RA-APL) syndrome (fever, dyspnea, pulmonary infiltrates, pleural/pericardial effusions, cardiac dysfunction). May be treated with high-dose steroids. The majority of patients do not require termination of tretinoin therapy. During treatment, rapidly evolving leukocytosis is associated with a higher risk of life-threatening complications.

Not to be used in women of childbearing potential unless the woman is capable of complying with effective contraceptive measures. Repeat pregnancy testing and contraception counseling monthly throughout the period of treatment.

Retinoids have been associated with pseudotumor cerebri (benign intracranial hypertension), especially in children. Concurrent use of other drugs associated with this effect (eg, tetracyclines) may increase risk. Up to 60% of patients experienced reversible hypercholesterolemia or hypertriglyceridemia. Monitor liver function during treatment.

Adverse Reactions Virtually all patients experience some drug-related toxicity, especially headache, fever, weakness and fatigue. These adverse effects are seldom permanent or irreversible nor do they usually require therapy interruption.

>10%:

Cardiovascular: Peripheral edema (52%), chest discomfort (32%), edema (29%), arrhythmias (23%), flushing (23%), hypotension (14%), hypertension (11%)

Central nervous system: Headache (86%), fever (83%), malaise (66%), pain (37%), dizziness (20%), anxiety (17%), insomnia (14%), depression (14%), confusion (11%)

Dermatologic: Skin/mucous membrane dryness (77%), pruritus (20%), rash (54%), alopecia (14%)

Endocrine & metabolic: Hypercholesterolemia and/or hypertriglyceridemia (60%)

Gastrointestinal: Nausea/vomiting (57%), liver function tests increased (50% to 60%), GI hemorrhage (34%), abdominal pain (31%), mucositis (26%), diarrhea (23%), constipation (17%), dyspepsia (14%), abdominal distention (11%), weight gain (23%), weight loss (17%), xerostomia, anorexia (17%)

Hematologic: Hemorrhage (60%), leukocytosis (40%), disseminated intravascular coagulation (26%)

Local: Phlebitis (11%), injection site reactions (17%)

Neuromuscular & skeletal: Bone pain (77%), myalgia (14%), paresthesia (17%)

Ocular: Visual disturbances (17%)

Otic: Earache/ear fullness (23%)

Renal: Renal insufficiency (11%)

Respiratory: Upper respiratory tract disorders (63%), dyspnea (60%), respiratory insufficiency (26%), pleural effusion (20%), pneumonia (14%), rales (14%), expiratory wheezing (14%), dry nose

Miscellaneous: Infections (58%), shivering (63%), retinoic acid-acute promyelocytic leukemia syndrome (25%), diaphoresis increased (20%)

1% to 10%:

Cardiovascular: Cerebral hemorrhage (9%), pallor (6%), cardiac failure (6%), cardiac arrest (3%), MI (3%), enlarged heart (3%), heart murmur (3%), ischemia, stroke (3%), myocarditis (3%), pericarditis (3%), pulmonary hypertension (3%), secondary cardiomyopathy (3%), Central nervous system: Intracranial hypertension (9%), agitation (9%), hallucination (6%), agnosia (3%), aphasia (3%), cerebellar edema (3%), cerebral hemorrhage (9%), seizures(3%), coma (3%), CNS depression (3%), dysarthria (3%), encephalopathy (3%), hypotaxia (3%), light reflex absent (3%), spinal cord disorder (3%), unconsciousness (3%), dementia (3%), forgetfulness (3%), somnolence (3%), slow speech (3%), hypothermia (3%)

Dermatologic: Cellulitis (8%), photosensitivity

Endocrine & metabolic: Acidosis (3%)

Gastrointestinal: Hepatosplenomegaly (9%), hepatitis (3%), ulcer (3%)

Genitourinary: Dysuria (9%), acute renal failure (3%), micturition frequency (3%), renal tubular necrosis (3%), enlarged prostate (3%)

Hepatic: Ascites (3%), hepatitis

(Continued)

Tretinoin (Oral) *(Continued)*

Neuromuscular & skeletal: Tremor (3%), leg weakness (3%), hyporeflexia, dysarthria, facial paralysis, hemiplegia, flank pain, asterixis, abnormal gait (3%), bone inflammation (3%)

Ocular: Dry eyes, visual acuity change (6%), visual field deficit (3%)

Otic: Hearing loss

Renal: Acute renal failure, renal tubular necrosis

Respiratory: Lower respiratory tract disorders (9%), pulmonary infiltration (6%), bronchial asthma (3%), pulmonary/larynx edema

Miscellaneous: Face edema

<1%: Arterial thrombosis, basophilia, cataracts, conjunctivitis, corneal opacities, erythema nodosum, erythrocyte sedimentation rate increased, gum bleeding, hematocrit decreased, hemoglobin decreased, hypercalcemia, hyperhistaminemia, hyperuricemia, inflammatory bowel syndrome, irreversible hearing loss, mood changes, myositis, optic neuritis, pancreatitis, pseudomotor cerebri, renal infarct, Sweet's syndrome, vasculitis, venous thrombosis

Vesicant No

Emetic Potential Moderate (30% to 60%)

Overdosage/Toxicology Symptoms of overdose include transient headache, facial flushing, cheilosis, abdominal pain, dizziness, and ataxia. All signs or symptoms have been transient and have resolved without apparent residual effects.

Drug Interactions

Cytochrome P450 Effect: Substrate (minor) of CYP2A6, 2B6, 2C8/9; **Inhibits** CYP2C8/9 (weak); **Induces** CYP2E1 (weak)

Increased Effect/Toxicity: Ketoconazole increases the mean plasma AUC of tretinoin. Concurrent use with antifibrinolytic agents (eg, aminocaproic acid, aprotinin, tranexamic acid) may increase risk of thrombosis. Concurrent use with tetracyclines may increase risk of pseudotumor cerebri.

Ethanol/Nutrition/Herb Interactions

Ethanol: Avoid ethanol (may increase CNS depression).

Food: Absorption of retinoids has been shown to be enhanced when taken with food.

Herb/Nutraceutical: St John's wort may decrease tretinoin levels. Avoid dong quai, St John's wort (may also cause photosensitization). Avoid additional vitamin A supplementation. May lead to vitamin A toxicity.

Storage/Stability Store capsule at 15°C to 30°C (59°F to 86°F). Protect from light.

Pharmacodynamics/Kinetics

Protein binding: >95%

Metabolism: Hepatic via CYP; primary metabolite: 4-oxo-all-*trans*-retinoic acid

Half-life elimination: Terminal: Parent drug: 0.5-2 hours

Time to peak, serum: 1-2 hours

Excretion: Urine (63%); feces (30%)

Dosage Oral: Children and Adults:

Remission induction: 45 mg/m^2/day in 2-3 divided doses for up to 30 days after complete remission (maximum duration of treatment: 90 days)

Remission maintenance: 45-200 mg/m^2/day in 2-3 divided doses for up to 12 months

Combination Regimens

Leukemia, acute promyelocytic:

M-3 *on page 906*

Tretinoin/Idarubicin *on page 941*

Administration Administer with meals; do not crush capsules

Dosage Forms Capsule: 10 mg [contains soybean oil and parabens]

Monitoring Parameters Monitor the patient's hematologic profile, coagulation profile, liver function test results and triglyceride and cholesterol levels frequently

Dietary Considerations To enhance absorption, some clinicians recommend giving with a fatty meal. Capsule contains soybean oil.

Patient Information Take with food; do not crush, chew, or dissolve capsules. You will need frequent blood tests while taking this medication. Maintain adequate hydration (2-3 L/day of fluids unless instructed to restrict fluid intake), avoid alcohol and foods containing vitamin A, and foods with high fat content. You may experience lethargy, dizziness, visual changes, confusion, anxiety (avoid driving or engaging in tasks requiring alertness until response to drug is known). For nausea/vomiting, loss of appetite, or dry mouth, small frequent meals, chewing gum, or sucking lozenges may help. You may experience photosensitivity (use sunscreen, wear protective clothing and eyewear, and avoid direct sunlight). You may experience dry, itchy, skin, and dry or irritated eyes (avoid contact lenses). Report persistent vomiting or diarrhea, difficulty breathing, unusual bleeding or bruising, acute GI pain, bone pain, or vision changes immediately.

Selected Readings

Chen GQ, Shen ZX, Wu F, et al, "Pharmacokinetics and Efficacy of Low-*trans* Retinoic Acid in the Treatment of Acute Promyelocytic Leukemia," *Leukemia*, 1996, 10(5):825-8.

Kurzrock R, Estey E, and Talpaz M, "All-*trans* Retinoic Acid: Tolerance and Biologic Effects in Myelodysplastic Syndrome," *J Clin Oncol*, 1993, 11(8):1489-95.

Lazzarino M, Regazzi MB, and Corso A, "Clinical Relevance of All-*trans* Retinoic Acid Pharmacokinetics and Its Modulation in Acute Promyelocytic Leukemia," *Leuk Lymphoma*, 1996, 23(5-6):539-43.

Muindi JR, Frankel SR, Huselton C, et al, "Clinical Pharmacology of Oral All-*trans* Retinoic Acid in Patients With Acute Promyelocytic Leukemia," *Cancer Res*, 1992, 52(8):2138-42.

Smith MA, Adamson PC, Balis FM, et al, "Phase I and Pharmacokinetic Evaluation of All-*trans*-Retinoic Acid in Pediatric Patients With Cancer," *J Clin Oncol*, 1992, 10(11):1666-73.

♦ **Trexall**™ *see* Methotrexate *on page 549*

♦ **Triethylenethiophosphoramide** *see* Thiotepa *on page 764*

♦ **Trikacide (Can)** *see* Metronidazole *on page 568*

Trimethobenzamide (trye meth oh BEN za mide)

Medication Safety Issues

Sound-alike/look-alike issues:

Tigan® may be confused with Tiazac®, Ticar®

Related Information

Management of Nausea and Vomiting *on page 982*

U.S. Brand Names Tigan®

Canadian Brand Names Tigan®

Generic Available Yes: Injection

Synonyms Trimethobenzamide Hydrochloride

Pharmacologic Category Anticholinergic Agent; Antiemetic

Pregnancy Risk Factor C

(Continued)

Trimethobenzamide *(Continued)*

Lactation Excretion in breast milk unknown

Use Treatment of nausea and vomiting

Mechanism of Action Acts centrally to inhibit the medullary chemore-ceptor trigger zone

Labeled Contraindications Hypersensitivity to trimethobenzamide, benzocaine (or similar local anesthetics), or any component of the formulation; injection contraindicated in children; suppositories contraindicated in premature infants or neonates

Warnings/Precautions May mask emesis due to Reye's syndrome or mimic CNS effects of Reye's syndrome in patients with emesis of other etiologies. Use in patients with acute vomiting should be avoided. May cause drowsiness; patient should avoid tasks requiring alertness (eg, driving, operating machinery). May cause extrapyramidal symptoms (EPS) which may be confused with CNS symptoms of primary disease responsible for emesis.

Adverse Reactions Frequency not defined.

Cardiovascular: Hypotension

Central nervous system: Coma, depression, disorientation, dizziness, drowsiness, EPS, headache, opisthotonos, Parkinson-like syndrome, seizure

Hematologic: Blood dyscrasias

Hepatic: Jaundice

Neuromuscular & skeletal: Muscle cramps

Ocular: Blurred vision

Miscellaneous: Hypersensitivity reactions

Vesicant No

Emetic Potential Very low (<10%)

Overdosage/Toxicology Symptoms of overdose include hypotension, seizures, CNS depression, cardiac arrhythmias, disorientation, and confusion. Treatment is symptom-directed and supportive.

Ethanol/Nutrition/Herb Interactions Ethanol: Concomitant use should be avoided.

Storage/Stability Store capsules, injection solution, and suppositories at room temperature.

Pharmacodynamics/Kinetics

Onset of action: Antiemetic: Oral: 10-40 minutes; I.M.: 15-35 minutes

Duration: 3-4 hours

Absorption: Rectal: ~60%

Bioavailability: Oral: 100%

Half-life elimination: 7-9 hours

Time to peak: Oral: 45 minutes; I.M.: 30 minutes

Excretion: Urine (30% to 50%)

Dosage Rectal use is contraindicated in neonates and premature infants

Children:

<14 kg: Oral, rectal: 100 mg 3-4 times/day

14-40 kg: Oral, rectal: 100-200 mg 3-4 times/day

Adults:

Oral: 250-300 mg 3-4 times/day

I.M., rectal: 200 mg 3-4 times/day

Administration Administer I.M. only; inject deep into upper outer quadrant of gluteal muscle

Dosage Forms [DSC] = Discontinued product
Capsule, as hydrochloride: 300 mg
Tigan®: 300 mg
Injection, solution, as hydrochloride: 100 mg/mL (2 mL)
Tigan®: 100 mg/mL (2 mL, 20 mL)
Suppository, rectal, as hydrochloride (Tigan®): 100 mg [DSC], 200 mg [contains benzocaine]

Patient Information May cause drowsiness, impair judgment and coordination; report any restlessness or involuntary movements

Selected Readings
Ginsburg CM and Clahsen J, "Evaluation of Trimethobenzamide Hydrochloride (Tigan®) Suppositories for Treatment of Nausea and Vomiting in Children," *J Pediatr*, 1980, 96(4):767-9.
Hurley JD and Eshelman FN, "Trimethobenzamide HCl in the Treatment of Nausea and Vomiting Associated With Antineoplastic Chemotherapy," *J Clin Pharmacol*, 1980, 20(5-6 Pt1):352-6.
Kaan SK and Eshelman FN, "The Antiemetic Effects of Trimethobenzamide During Chemotherapy: A Controlled Study," *Curr Ther Res*, 1979, 26:210-3.

♦ **Trimethobenzamide Hydrochloride** *see* Trimethobenzamide *on page 795*

Trimethoprim (trye METH oh prim)
Medication Safety Issues
Sound-alike/look-alike issues:
Trimethoprim may be confused with trimethaphan
Proloprim® may be confused with Prolixin®, Protropin®

U.S. Brand Names Primsol®; Proloprim®
Canadian Brand Names Apo-Trimethoprim®; Proloprim®
Generic Available Yes: Tablet
Synonyms TMP
Pharmacologic Category Antibiotic, Miscellaneous
Pregnancy Risk Factor C
Lactation Enters breast milk/use caution (AAP rates "compatible")
Use Treatment of urinary tract infections due to susceptible strains of *E. coli*, *P. mirabilis*, *K. pneumoniae*, *Enterobacter* sp and coagulase-negative *Staphylococcus* including *S. saprophyticus*; acute otitis media in children; acute exacerbations of chronic bronchitis in adults; in combination with other agents for treatment of toxoplasmosis, *Pneumocystis carinii*; treatment of superficial ocular infections involving the conjunctiva and cornea
Mechanism of Action Inhibits folic acid reduction to tetrahydrofolate, and thereby inhibits microbial growth
Labeled Contraindications Hypersensitivity to trimethoprim or any component of the formulation; megaloblastic anemia due to folate deficiency
Warnings/Precautions Use with caution in patients with impaired renal or hepatic function or with possible folate deficiency.
Adverse Reactions Frequency not defined.
Central nervous system: Aseptic meningitis (rare), fever
Dermatologic: Maculopapular rash (3% to 7% at 200 mg/day; incidence higher with larger daily doses), erythema multiforme (rare), exfoliative dermatitis (rare), pruritus (common), phototoxic skin eruptions, Stevens-Johnson syndrome (rare), toxic epidermal necrolysis (rare)
Endocrine & metabolic: Hyperkalemia, hyponatremia
(Continued)

797

Trimethoprim *(Continued)*

Gastrointestinal: Epigastric distress, glossitis, nausea, vomiting

Hematologic: Leukopenia, megaloblastic anemia, methemoglobinemia, neutropenia, thrombocytopenia

Hepatic: Liver enzyme elevation, cholestatic jaundice (rare)

Renal: BUN and creatinine increased

Miscellaneous: Anaphylaxis, hypersensitivity reactions

Emetic Potential Very low (<10%)

Overdosage/Toxicology Symptoms of acute toxicity include nausea, vomiting, confusion, and dizziness. Chronic overdose results in bone marrow suppression. Treatment of acute overdose is supportive following GI decontamination. Use oral leucovorin 5-15 mg/day for treatment of chronic overdose. Hemodialysis is only moderately effective in eliminating drug.

Drug Interactions

Cytochrome P450 Effect: Substrate (major) of CYP2C8/9, 3A4; **Inhibits** CYP2C8/9 (moderate)

Increased Effect/Toxicity: Increased effect/toxicity/levels of phenytoin. Concurrent use with ACE inhibitors increases risk of hyperkalemia. Increased myelosuppression with methotrexate. May increase levels of digoxin. Concurrent use with dapsone may increase levels of dapsone and trimethoprim. Concurrent use with procainamide may increase levels of procainamide and trimethoprim. Trimethoprim may increase the levels/effects of amiodarone, fluoxetine, glimepiride, glipizide, nateglinide, phenytoin, pioglitazone, rosiglitazone, sertraline, warfarin, and other CYP2C8/9 substrates.

Decreased Effect: The levels/effects of trimethoprim may be decreased by aminoglutethimide, carbamazepine, nafcillin, nevirapine, phenobarbital, phenytoin, rifampin, rifapentine, secobarbital, and other CYP2C8/9 or 3A4 inducers.

Storage/Stability Protect the 200 mg tablet from light.

Pharmacodynamics/Kinetics

Absorption: Readily and extensive

Distribution: Widely into body tissues and fluids (middle ear, prostate, bile, aqueous humor, CSF); crosses placenta; enters breast milk

Protein binding: 42% to 46%

Metabolism: Partially hepatic

Half-life elimination: 8-14 hours; prolonged with renal impairment

Time to peak, serum: 1-4 hours

Excretion: Urine (60% to 80%) as unchanged drug

Dosage Oral:

Children: 4 mg/kg/day in divided doses every 12 hours

Adults: 100 mg every 12 hours or 200 mg every 24 hours for 10 days; longer treatment periods may be necessary for prostatitis (ie, 4-16 weeks); in the treatment of *Pneumocystis carinii* pneumonia; dose may be as high as 15-20 mg/kg/day in 3-4 divided doses

Dosing interval in renal impairment:

Cl_{cr} 15-30 mL/minute: Administer 100 mg every 18 hours or 50 mg every 12 hours

Cl_{cr} <15 mL/minute: Administer 100 mg every 24 hours or avoid use

Hemodialysis: Moderately dialyzable (20% to 50%)

Administration Administer with milk or food.

Dosage Forms
  Solution, oral (Primsol®): 50 mg (base)/5 mL (480 mL) [contains sodium benzoate; bubble gum flavor]
  Tablet: 100 mg
    Proloprim®: 100 mg, 200 mg

Dietary Considerations May cause folic acid deficiency, supplements may be needed. Should be taken with milk or food.

Patient Information Take with milk or food; report any skin rash, persistent or severe fatigue, fever, sore throat, or unusual bleeding or bruising; complete full course of therapy

Special Geriatric Considerations Trimethoprim is often used in combination with sulfamethoxazole; it can be used alone in patients who are allergic to sulfonamides; adjust dose for renal function (see Pharmacokinetics and Dosage).

♦ **Trimethoprim and Sulfamethoxazole** *see* Sulfamethoxazole and Trimethoprim *on page 727*

Trimetrexate Glucuronate
  (tri me TREKS ate gloo KYOOR oh nate)

Related Information
  Safe Handling of Hazardous Drugs *on page 1034*

U.S. Brand Names NeuTrexin®

Generic Available No

Synonyms NSC-352122

Pharmacologic Category Antineoplastic Agent, Miscellaneous

Pregnancy Risk Factor D

Lactation Excretion in breast milk unknown/contraindicated

Use Alternative therapy for the treatment of moderate-to-severe *Pneumocystis carinii* pneumonia (PCP) in immunocompromised patients, including patients with acquired immunodeficiency syndrome (AIDS), who are intolerant of, or are refractory to, co-trimoxazole therapy or for whom co-trimoxazole and pentamidine are contraindicated. **Concurrent folinic acid (leucovorin) must always be administered.**

Unlabeled/Investigational Use Treatment of nonsmall cell lung cancer, metastatic colorectal cancer, metastatic head and neck cancer, pancreatic adenocarcinoma

Mechanism of Action Trimetrexate is a folate antimetabolite that inhibits DNA synthesis by inhibition of dihydrofolate reductase (DHFR); DHFR inhibition reduces the formation of reduced folates and thymidylate synthetase, resulting in inhibition of purine and thymidylic acid synthesis.

Labeled Contraindications Hypersensitivity to trimetrexate, methotrexate, leucovorin, or any component of the formulation; severe existing myelosuppression; pregnancy

Warnings/Precautions Hazardous agent - use appropriate precautions for handling and disposal. See Safe Handling of Hazardous Drugs *on page 1034* in the Appendix. **Must be administered with concurrent leucovorin to avoid potentially serious or life-threatening toxicities**. Leucovorin therapy must extend for 72 hours past the last dose of trimetrexate. Hypersensitivity/allergic-type reactions have been reported, primarily when given as a bolus infusion, at higher than recommended doses for PCP, or in combination with fluorouracil or leucovorin. Use with caution in patients with mild myelosuppression, severe hepatic or renal (Continued)

Trimetrexate Glucuronate *(Continued)*

dysfunction, hypoproteinemia, hypoalbuminemia, or previous extensive myelosuppressive therapies.

Adverse Reactions

>10%:

Hematologic: Neutropenia

Hepatic: LFTs increased

1% to 10%:

Central nervous system: Seizures, fever

Dermatologic: Rash

Gastrointestinal: Stomatitis, nausea, vomiting

Hematologic: Thrombocytopenia, anemia

Neuromuscular & skeletal: Peripheral neuropathy

Renal: Increased serum creatinine

Miscellaneous: Flu-like illness, hypersensitivity reactions, anaphylactoid reactions

Vesicant No

Emetic Potential Mild (10% to 30%)

Drug Interactions

Increased Effect/Toxicity: Cimetidine, clotrimazole, and ketoconazole may decrease trimetrexate metabolism, resulting in increased serum levels. Trimetrexate may increase toxicity (infections) of live virus vaccines.

Storage/Stability Prior to reconstitution, vials should stored at controlled room temperature of 20°C to 25°C (68°F to 77°F). Protect from light. Following reconstitution, the solution is stable for 6 hours at room temperature or 24 hours under refrigeration. Diluted solutions for infusion are stable under refrigeration or at room temperature for 24 hours.

Reconstitution Reconstitute with D_5W or SWFI to a concentration of 12.5 mg/mL. Do not use if cloudy or if precipitate forms. Prior to administration, solution should be further diluted with D_5W to a concentration of 0.25 mg/mL to 2 mg/mL.

Compatibility Precipitate occurs with leucovorin or any solution containing chloride ion.

Stable in D_5W, sterile water for injection

Y-site administration: Compatible: Amifostine, zidovudine. **Incompatible:** Foscarnet, indomethacin

Compatibility when admixed: Incompatible: Chloride-containing solutions, leucovorin

Pharmacodynamics/Kinetics

Distribution: V_d: 0.62 L/kg

Metabolism: Extensively hepatic

Half-life elimination: 15-17 hours

Dosage Note: Concurrent leucovorin 20 mg/m^2 every 6 hours must be administered daily (oral or I.V.) during treatment and for 72 hours past the last dose of trimetrexate glucuronate.

Adults: I.V.:

Pneumocystis carinii: 45 mg/m^2 once daily for 21 days; **alternative dosing based on weight:**

<50 kg:Trimetrexate glucuronate 1.5 mg/kg/day; leucovorin 0.6 mg/kg 4 times/day

50-80 kg:Trimetrexate glucuronate 1.2 mg/kg/day; leucovorin 0.5 mg/kg/4 times/day

>80 kg: Trimetrexate glucuronate 1 mg/kg/day; leucovorin 0.5 mg/kg/4 times/day

Note: Oral doses of leucovorin should be rounded up to the next higher 25 mg increment.

Antineoplastic (unlabeled use): 6-16 mg/m^2 once daily for 5 days every 21-28 days **or** 150-200 mg/m^2 every 2 weeks

Dosage adjustment in hepatic impairment: Although it may be necessary to reduce the dose in patients with liver dysfunction, no specific recommendations exist.

Administration I.V. infusion: Over 60-90 minutes; must be used with concurrent leucovorin; trimetrexate and leucovorin solutions **must** be administered separately; intravenous lines should be flushed with at least 10 mL of D$_5$W between trimetrexate and leucovorin

Dosage Forms Injection, powder for reconstitution: 25 mg, 200 mg

Monitoring Parameters Check and record patient's temperature daily; absolute neutrophil counts (ANC), platelet count, renal function tests (serum creatinine, BUN), hepatic function tests (ALT, AST, alkaline phosphatase)

Patient Information Report promptly any fever, rash, flu-like symptoms, numbness or tingling in the extremities, nausea, vomiting, abdominal pain, mouth sores, increased bruising or bleeding, black tarry stools

Additional Information Not a vesicant; methotrexate derivative

Special Geriatric Considerations No specific recommendations are available for the elderly. Use with caution in patients with liver dysfunction (see Dosage).

Selected Readings
Amsden GW, Kowalsky SF, and Morse GD, "Trimetrexate for *Pneumocystis carinii* Pneumonia in Patients With AIDS," *Ann Pharmacother*, 1992, 26(2):218-26.

Bertino JR, "Folate Antagonists: Toward Improving the Therapeutic Index and Development of New Analogs," *J Clin Pharmacol*, 1990, 30(4):291-5.

Bertino JR, "Trimetrexate: Overall Clinical Results," *Semin Oncol*, 1988, 15(2 Suppl 2):50-1.

Donehower RC, "Understanding Trimetrexate Toxicity," *J Natl Cancer Inst*, 1988, 80(16):1268-9.

Fulton B, Wagstaff AJ, and McTavish D, "Trimetrexate. A Review of Its Pharmacodynamic and Pharmacokinetic Properties and Therapeutic Potential in the Treatment of *Pneumocystis carinii* Pneumonia," *Drugs*, 1995, 49(4):563-76.

Ho DH, Covington WP, Legha SS, et al, "Clinical Pharmacology of Trimetrexate," *Clin Pharmacol Ther*, 1987, 42(3):351-6.

Levien TL and Baker DE, "Reviews of Trimetrexate and Oxadrolone," *Hosp Pharm*, 1994, 29:696-708.

Marshall JL and De Lap RJ, "Clinical Pharmacokinetics and Pharmacology of Trimetrexate," *Clin Pharmacokinet*, 1994, 26(3):190-200.

Masur H, "Prevention and Treatment of *Pneumocystis* Pneumonia," *N Engl J Med*, 1992, 327(26):1853-60.

Rogers P, Allegra CJ, Murphy RF, et al, "Bioavailability of Oral Trimetrexate in Patients With Acquired Immunodeficiency Syndrome," *Antimicrob Agents Chemother*, 1988, 32(3):324-6.

♦ **Triptoraline** *see* Triptorelin *on page 801*

Triptorelin (trip toe REL in)

U.S. Brand Names Trelstar™ Depot; Trelstar™ LA

Canadian Brand Names Trelstar™ Depot

Generic Available No

(Continued)

Triptorelin *(Continued)*

Synonyms AY-25650; CL-118,532; D-Trp(6)-LHRH; Triptoraline; Triptorelin Pamoate; Tryptoreline

Pharmacologic Category Gonadotropin Releasing Hormone Agonist

Pregnancy Risk Factor X

Lactation Excretion in breast milk unknown/contraindicated

Use Palliative treatment of advanced prostate cancer as an alternative to orchiectomy or estrogen administration

Unlabeled/Investigational Use Treatment of endometriosis, growth hormone deficiency, hyperandrogenism, *in vitro* fertilization, ovarian carcinoma, pancreatic carcinoma, precocious puberty, uterine leiomyomata

Mechanism of Action Causes suppression of ovarian and testicular steroidogenesis due to decreased levels of LH and FSH with subsequent decrease in testosterone (male) and estrogen (female) levels. After chronic and continuous administration, usually 2-4 weeks after initiation, a sustained decrease in LH and FSH secretion occurs.

Labeled Contraindications Hypersensitivity to triptorelin or any component of the formulation, other LHRH agonists or LHRH; pregnancy

Warnings/Precautions Hazardous agent - use appropriate precautions for handling and disposal. See Safe Handling of Hazardous Drugs *on page 1034* in the Appendix. Transient increases in testosterone can lead to worsening symptoms (bone pain, hematuria, bladder outlet obstruction) of prostate cancer during the first few weeks of therapy. Cases of spinal cord compression have been reported with LHRH agonists. Hypersensitivity reactions including angioedema and anaphylaxis have rarely occurred. Safety and efficacy has not established in pediatric population.

Adverse Reactions As reported with Trelstar™ Depot and Trelstar™ LA; frequency of effect may vary by product:

>10%:

Central nervous system: Headache (30% to 60%)

Endocrine & metabolic: Hot flashes (95% to 100%), glucose increased, hemoglobin decreased, RBC count decreased

Hepatic: Alkaline phosphatase increased, ALT increased, AST increased

Neuromuscular & skeletal: Skeletal pain (12% to 13%)

Renal: BUN increased

1% to 10%:

Cardiovascular: Leg edema (6%), hypertension (4%), chest pain (2%), peripheral edema (1%)

Central nervous system: Dizziness (1% to 3%), pain (2% to 3%), emotional lability (1%), fatigue (2%), insomnia (2%)

Dermatologic: Rash (2%), pruritus (1%)

Endocrine & metabolic: Alkaline phosphatase increased (2%), breast pain (2%), gynecomastia (2%), libido decreased (2%), tumor flare (8%)

Gastrointestinal: Nausea (3%), anorexia (2%), constipation (2%), dyspepsia (2%), vomiting (2%), abdominal pain (1%), diarrhea (1%)

Genitourinary: Dysuria (5%), impotence (2% to 7%), urinary retention (1%), urinary tract infection (1%)

Hematologic: Anemia (1%)

Local: Injection site pain (4%)

Neuromuscular & skeletal: Leg pain (2% to 5%), back pain (3%), arthralgia (2%), leg cramps (2%), myalgia (1%), weakness (1%)

Ocular: Conjunctivitis (1%), eye pain (1%)

Respiratory: Cough (2%), dyspnea (1%), pharyngitis (1%)

Postmarketing and/or case reports: Anaphylaxis, angioedema, hypersensitivity reactions, spinal cord compression, renal dysfunction

Overdosage/Toxicology Accidental or intentional overdose unlikely. If it were to occur, supportive and symptomatic treatment would be indicated.

Drug Interactions

Increased Effect/Toxicity: Not studied. Hyperprolactinemic drugs (dopamine antagonists such as antipsychotics, and metoclopramide) are contraindicated.

Decreased Effect: Not studied. Hyperprolactinemic drugs (dopamine antagonists such as antipsychotics, and metoclopramide) are contraindicated.

Storage/Stability

Trelstar™ Depot: Store at 15°C to 30°C (59°F to 86°F)

Trelstar™ LA: Store at 20°C to 25°C (68°F to 77°F)

Reconstitution Reconstitute with 2 mL sterile water for injection. Shake well to obtain a uniform suspension. Withdraw the entire contents into the syringe and inject immediately.

Pharmacodynamics/Kinetics

Absorption: Oral: Not active

Distribution: V_d: 30-33 L

Protein binding: None

Metabolism: Unknown; unlikely to involve CYP; no known metabolites

Half-life elimination: 2.8 ± 1.2 hours

Moderate to severe renal impairment: 6.5-7.7 hours

Hepatic impairment: 7.6 hours

Time to peak: 1-3 hours

Excretion: Urine (42% as intact peptide); hepatic

Dosage I.M.: Adults: Prostate cancer:

Trelstar™ Depot: 3.75 mg once every 28 days

Trelstar™ LA: 11.25 mg once every 84 days

Dosage adjustment in renal/hepatic impairment: Although this drug is excreted renally, no guidelines for adjustments are available.

Administration Must be administered under the supervision of a physician. Administer by I.M. injection into the buttock; alternate injection sites. Debioclip™: Follow manufacturer's instructions for mixing prior to use.

Dosage Forms Injection, powder for reconstitution, as pamoate [also available packaged with Debioclip™ (prefilled syringe containing sterile water)]:

Trelstar™ Depot: 3.75 mg

Trelstar™ LA: 11.25 mg

Monitoring Parameters Serum testosterone levels, prostate-specific antigen

Patient Information Use as directed. Do not miss monthly appointment for injection. You may experience disease flare (increased bone pain), blood in urine, and urinary retention during early treatment (usually resolves within 1 week). Hot flashes are common; you may feel flushed and hot (wearing layers of clothes or summer clothes and cool environment may help). If it becomes annoying and bothersome, let prescriber know. Report irregular or rapid heartbeat, unresolved nausea or vomiting, (Continued)

Triptorelin *(Continued)*

numbness of extremities, breast swelling or pain, difficulty breathing, or infection at injection sites.

Selected Readings

Anonymous, "Triptorelin Pamoate. Phase III Drug Profiles," 1993, 3:1-8.

Filicor M, "Gonadotrophin-Releasing Hormone Agonists. A Guide to Use and Selection," *Drugs*, 1994, 48(1):41-58.

Swanson LJ, Seely JH, and Garnick MB, "Gonadotropin-Releasing Hormone Analogs and Prostatic Cancer," *Crit Rev Oncol Hematol*, 1988, 8(1):1-26.

♦ **Triptorelin Pamoate** *see* Triptorelin *on page 801*

♦ **Trisenox™** *see* Arsenic Trioxide *on page 102*

♦ **Trivagizole-3® (Can)** *see* Clotrimazole *on page 203*

♦ **Tryptoreline** *see* Triptorelin *on page 801*

♦ **TSPA** *see* Thiotepa *on page 764*

♦ **Tumor Lysis Syndrome** *see page 1002*

UFT

Related Information

Investigational Drug Service *on page 1031*
Safe Handling of Hazardous Drugs *on page 1034*

U.S. Brand Names Orzel®

Generic Available No

Synonyms Uracil and Ftorafur; Uracil and Tegafur; Uracil and Tetrahydrofuranyl-5-Fluorouracil

Pharmacologic Category Antineoplastic Agent, Antimetabolite (Pyrimidine Antagonist)

Unlabeled/Investigational Use Investigational: Treatment of unresectable or metastatic colorectal cancer

Mechanism of Action Tegafur is a prodrug of fluorouracil. It is converted *in vivo* to fluorouracil through hepatic microsomal cytochrome P450, and also via thymidine phosphorylase and spontaneous anabolic conversion. Uracil is a competitive inhibitor of dihydropyrimidine dehydrogenase (DPD), the enzyme responsible for catabolism of approximately 85% of fluorouracil to fluoro-β alanine.

Warnings/Precautions Hazardous agent - use appropriate precautions for handling and disposal. See Safe Handling of Hazardous Drugs *on page 1034* in the Appendix.

Adverse Reactions Frequency not defined.

Central nervous system: Fatigue, cerebellar toxicity (rare)

Dermatologic: Rash, skin pigmentation, photosensitivity, hand-foot syndrome (rare)

Gastrointestinal: Nausea, vomiting, anorexia, diarrhea (may be dose-limiting)

Hematologic: Neutropenia (may be dose-limiting)

Neuromuscular & skeletal: Neurotoxicity (peripheral neuropathy)

Ocular: Lacrimation

Vesicant No

Emetic Potential Moderate (30% to 60%)

Pharmacodynamics/Kinetics

Plasma levels: Tegafur > uracil > fluorouracil

Time to C$_{pmax}$: Tegafur: 0.6-2.1 hours; uracil: 0.6-4.1 hours; fluorouracil: 0.7-2.0 hours; the relationship between UFT dose and fluorouracil C$_{pmax}$ is not linear

Dosage Refer to individual protocols.

Oral: Adults: 300 mg/m^2/day (expressed as tegafur) in combination with oral leucovorin

Administration UFT capsules contain 224 mg uracil + 100 mg tegafur (providing the 4:1 molar ratio). Divided daily dosage (eg, 3 times daily) is recommended over single daily dosage. Cycles of 28-day dosing followed by a 7-day rest period are common.

Dosage Forms Capsule (Orzel®): Tegafur 100 mg and uracil 224 mg

Selected Readings

Ho DH, Covington WP, Pazdur R, et al, "Clinical Pharmacology of Combined Oral Uracil and Ftorafur," *Drug Metab Disp*, 1992, 20(6):936-40.

Hoff PM, Royce M, Medgyesy D, et al, "Oral Fluoropoyrimidines," *Semin Oncol*, 1999, 26(6):640-6.

Kohne CH and Peters GJ, "UFT: Mechanism of Drug Action," *Oncology (Huntingt)*, 2000, 14(10 Suppl 9):13-8.

Pazdur R, Lassere Y, Rhodes V, et al, "Phase II Trial of Uracil and Tegafur Plus Oral Leucovorin: An Effective Oral Regimen in the Treatment of Metastatic Colorectal Carcinoma," *J Clin Oncol*, 1994, 12(11):2296-300.

Saltz LB, Leichman CG, Young CW, et al, "A Fixed-Ration Combination of Uracil and Ftorafur (UFT) With Low Dose Leucovorin: An Active Oral Regimen for Advanced Colorectal Cancer," *Cancer*, 1995, 75(3):782-5.

Sulkes A, Benner SE, and Canetta RM, "Uracil-ftorafur: An Oral Fluoropyrimidine Active in Colorectal Cancer," *J Clin Oncol*, 1998, 16(10):3461-75.

Sun W and Haller D, "UFT in the Treatment of Colorectal and Breast Cancer," *Oncology (Huntingt)*, 2001, 15(1 Suppl 2):49-56.

♦ **Ultram**® *see* Tramadol *on page 785*
♦ **Unipen**® **(Can)** *see* Nafcillin *on page 605*
♦ **Uracil and Ftorafur** *see* UFT *on page 804*
♦ **Uracil and Tegafur** *see* UFT *on page 804*
♦ **Uracil and Tetrahydrofuranyl-5-Fluorouracil** *see* UFT *on page 804*
♦ **Uromitexan (Can)** *see* Mesna *on page 542*

Valacyclovir (val ay SYE kloe veer)

Medication Safety Issues

Sound-alike/look-alike issues:

Valtrex® may be confused with Valcyte™
Valacyclovir may be confused with valganciclovir

Related Information

Management of Infections *on page 978*

U.S. Brand Names Valtrex®

Canadian Brand Names Valtrex®

Generic Available No

Synonyms Valacyclovir Hydrochloride

Pharmacologic Category Antiviral Agent, Oral

Pregnancy Risk Factor B

Lactation Enters breast milk/use caution

Use Treatment of herpes zoster (shingles) in immunocompetent patients; treatment of first-episode genital herpes; episodic treatment of recurrent genital herpes; suppression of recurrent genital herpes and reduction of heterosexual transmission of genital herpes in immunocompetent patients; suppression of genital herpes in HIV-infected individuals; treatment of herpes labialis (cold sores)

(Continued)

Valacyclovir (Continued)

Mechanism of Action Valacyclovir is rapidly and nearly completely converted to acyclovir by intestinal and hepatic metabolism. Acyclovir is converted to acyclovir monophosphate by virus-specific thymidine kinase then further converted to acyclovir triphosphate by other cellular enzymes. Acyclovir triphosphate inhibits DNA synthesis and viral replication by competing with deoxyguanosine triphosphate for viral DNA polymerase and being incorporated into viral DNA.

Labeled Contraindications Hypersensitivity to valacyclovir, acyclovir, or any component of the formulation

Warnings/Precautions Hazardous agent - use appropriate precautions for handling and disposal. See Safe Handling of Hazardous Drugs *on page 1034* in the Appendix. Thrombotic thrombocytopenic purpura/hemolytic uremic syndrome has occurred in immunocompromised patients (at doses of 8 g/day); use caution and adjust the dose in elderly patients or those with renal insufficiency and in patients receiving concurrent nephrotoxic agents. For genital herpes, treatment should begin as soon as possible after the first signs and symptoms (within 72 hours of onset of first diagnosis or within 24 hours of onset of recurrent episodes). For herpes zoster, treatment should begin within 72 hours of onset of rash. For cold sores, treatment should begin at with earliest symptom (tingling, itching, burning). Safety and efficacy in prepubertal patients have not been established.

Adverse Reactions

>10%: Central nervous system: Headache (14% to 35%)

1% to 10%:

Central nervous system: Dizziness (2% to 4%), depression (0% to 7%)

Endocrine: Dysmenorrhea (≤1% to 8%)

Gastrointestinal: Abdominal pain (2% to 11%), nausea (6% to 15%), vomiting (<1% to 6%)

Hematologic: Leukopenia (≤1%), thrombocytopenia (≤1%)

Hepatic: AST increased (1% to 4%)

Neuromuscular & skeletal: Arthralgia (≤1 to 6%)

<1%: Anemia

Postmarketing and/or case reports: Acute hypersensitivity reactions (angioedema, anaphylaxis, dyspnea, pruritus, rash, urticaria); aggression, agitation, alopecia, aplastic anemia, ataxia, creatinine increased, coma, confusion, consciousness decreased, diarrhea, dysarthria, encephalopathy, facial edema, erythema multiforme, hallucinations (auditory and visual), hemolytic uremic syndrome (HUS), hepatitis, hypertension, leukocytoclastic vasculitis, mania, photosensitivity reaction, psychosis, rash, renal failure, seizure, tachycardia, thrombotic thrombocytopenic purpura/hemolytic uremic syndrome, tremor, visual disturbances

Overdosage/Toxicology Precipitation in renal tubules may occur. Treatment is symptomatic and includes hemodialysis, especially if compromised renal function develops.

Drug Interactions

Increased Effect/Toxicity: Valacyclovir and acyclovir have increased CNS side effects with zidovudine and probenecid.

Decreased Effect: Cimetidine and/or probenecid has decreased the rate but not the extent of valacyclovir conversion to acyclovir leading to decreased effectiveness of valacyclovir.

Storage/Stability Store at 15°C to 25°C (59°F to 77°F).

Pharmacodynamics/Kinetics

Absorption: Rapid

Distribution: Acyclovir is widely distributed throughout the body including brain, kidney, lungs, liver, spleen, muscle, uterus, vagina, and CSF

Protein binding: 13.5% to 17.9%

Metabolism: Hepatic; valacyclovir is rapidly and nearly completely converted to acyclovir and L-valine by first-pass effect; acyclovir is hepatically metabolized to a very small extent by aldehyde oxidase and by alcohol and aldehyde dehydrogenase (inactive metabolites)

Bioavailability: ~55% once converted to acyclovir

Half-life elimination: Normal renal function: Adults: Acyclovir: 2.5-3.3 hours, Valacyclovir: ~30 minutes; End-stage renal disease: Acyclovir: 14-20 hours

Excretion: Urine, primarily as acyclovir (88%); **Note:** Following oral administration of radiolabeled valacyclovir, 46% of the label is eliminated in the feces (corresponding to nonabsorbed drug), while 47% of the radiolabel is eliminated in the urine.

Dosage Oral:

Adolescents and Adults: Herpes labialis (cold sores): 2 g twice daily for 1 day (separate doses by ~12 hours)

Adults:

Herpes zoster (shingles): 1 g 3 times/day for 7 days

Genital herpes:

Initial episode: 1 g twice daily for 10 days

Recurrent episode: 500 mg twice daily for 3 days

Reduction of transmission: 500 mg once daily (source partner)

Suppressive therapy:

Immunocompetent patients: 1000 mg once daily (500 mg once daily in patients with <9 recurrences per year)

HIV-infected patients (CD4 ≥100 cells/mm^3): 500 mg twice daily

Dosing interval in renal impairment:

Herpes zoster: Adults:

Cl_{cr} 30-49 mL/minute: 1 g every 12 hours

Cl_{cr} 10-29 mL/minute: 1 g every 24 hours

Cl_{cr} <10 mL/minute: 500 mg every 24 hours

Genital herpes: Adults:

Initial episode:

Cl_{cr} 10-29 mL/minute: 1 g every 24 hours

Cl_{cr} <10 mL/minute: 500 mg every 24 hours

Recurrent episode: Cl_{cr} <10-29 mL/minute: 500 mg every 24 hours

Suppressive therapy: Cl_{cr} <10-29 mL/minute:

For usual dose of 1 g every 24 hours, decrease dose to 500 mg every 24 hours

For usual dose of 500 mg every 24 hours, decrease dose to 500 mg every 48 hours

HIV-infected patients: 500 mg every 24 hours

Herpes labialis: Adolescents and Adults:

Cl_{cr} 30-49 mL/minute: 1 g every 12 hours for 2 doses

Cl_{cr} 10-29 mL/minute: 500 mg every 12 hours for 2 doses

Cl_{cr} <10 mL/minute: 500 mg as a single dose

Hemodialysis: Dialyzable (~33% removed during 4-hour session); administer dose postdialysis

(Continued)

Valacyclovir (Continued)

Chronic ambulatory peritoneal dialysis/continuous arteriovenous hemofiltration dialysis: Pharmacokinetic parameters are similar to those in patients with ESRD; supplemental dose not needed following dialysis

Administration Oral: If GI upset occurs, administer with meals.

Dosage Forms Caplet: 500 mg, 1000 mg

Monitoring Parameters Urinalysis, BUN, serum creatinine, liver enzymes, and CBC

Dietary Considerations May be taken with or without food.

Patient Information

Herpes zoster: Therapy is most effective when started within 48 hours of onset of zoster rash

Recurrent genital herpes: Therapy should be initiated within 24 hours after the onset of signs or symptoms

Special Geriatric Considerations More convenient dosing and increased bioavailability, without increasing side effects, make valacyclovir a favorable choice compared to acyclovir. Has been shown to accelerate resolution of postherpetic pain. Adjust dose for renal impairment.

Selected Readings

Acosta EP and Fletcher CV, "Valacyclovir," *Ann Pharmacother*, 1997, 31(2):185-91.

Perry CM and Faulds D, "Valaciclovir. A Review of Its Antiviral Activity, Pharmacokinetic Properties and Therapeutic Efficacy in Herpesvirus Infections," *Drugs*, 1996, 52(5):754-72.

Weller S, Blum MR, Doucette M, et al, "Pharmacokinetics of the Acyclovir Pro-Drug Valaciclovir After Escalating Single- and Multiple-Dose Administration to Normal Volunteers," *Clin Pharmacol Ther*, 1993, 54(6):595-605.

♦ **Valacyclovir Hydrochloride** *see* Valacyclovir *on page 805*

Valrubicin (val ROO bi sin)

Medication Safety Issues

Sound-alike/look-alike issues:

Valstar® may be confused with valsartan

Related Information

Safe Handling of Hazardous Drugs *on page 1034*

U.S. Brand Names Valstar® [DSC]

Canadian Brand Names Valstar®; Valtaxin®

Generic Available No

Synonyms AD3L; *N*-Trifluoroacetyladriamycin-14-Valerate

Pharmacologic Category Antineoplastic Agent, Anthracycline

Pregnancy Risk Factor C

Lactation Excretion in breast milk unknown/not recommended

Use Intravesical therapy of BCG-refractory carcinoma *in situ* of the urinary bladder

Mechanism of Action Blocks function of DNA topoisomerase II; inhibits DNA synthesis, causes extensive chromosomal damage, and arrests cell development; unlike other anthracyclines, does not appear to intercalate DNA

Labeled Contraindications Hypersensitivity to anthracyclines, Cremophor® EL, or any component of the formulation; concurrent urinary tract infection or small bladder capacity (unable to tolerate a 75 mL instillation)

Warnings/Precautions Hazardous agent - use appropriate precautions for handling and disposal. See Safe Handling of Hazardous Drugs *on page 1034* in the Appendix. If valrubicin contacts the skin, wash and flush thoroughly with water. Do not administer if mucosal integrity of bladder has been compromised or bladder perforation is present. Irritable bladder symptoms may occur during instillation and retention. Caution in patients with severe irritable bladder symptoms. Valrubicin should be used cautiously (if at all) in patients having a history of hypersensitivity reactions to other medications prepared with Cremophor® EL.

Adverse Reactions
>10%: Genitourinary: Frequency (61%), dysuria (56%), urgency (57%), bladder spasm (31%), hematuria (29%), bladder pain (28%), urinary incontinence (22%), cystitis (15%), urinary tract infection (15%)

1% to 10%:
Cardiovascular: Chest pain (2%), vasodilation (2%), peripheral edema (1%)

Central nervous system: Headache (4%), malaise (4%), dizziness (3%), fever (2%)

Dermatologic: Rash (3%)

Endocrine & metabolic: Hyperglycemia (1%)

Gastrointestinal: Abdominal pain (5%), nausea (5%), diarrhea (3%), vomiting (2%), flatulence (1%)

Genitourinary: Nocturia (7%), burning symptoms (5%), urinary retention (4%), urethral pain (3%), pelvic pain (1%), hematuria (microscopic) (3%)

Hematologic: Anemia (2%)

Neuromuscular & skeletal: Weakness (4%), back pain (3%), myalgia (1%)

Respiratory: Pneumonia (1%)

<1%: Tenesmus, pruritus, taste disturbance, skin irritation, decreased urine flow, urethritis

Overdosage/Toxicology Inadvertent paravenous extravasation has not been associated with skin ulceration or necrosis. Myelosuppression is possible following inadvertent systemic administration, or following significant systemic absorption from intravesical instillation.

Drug Interactions
Increased Effect/Toxicity: No specific drug interactions studies have been performed. Systemic exposure to valrubicin is negligible, and interactions are unlikely.

Decreased Effect: No specific drug interactions studies have been performed. Systemic exposure to valrubicin is negligible, and interactions are unlikely.

Storage/Stability Store unopened vials under refrigeration at 2°C to 8°C (36°F to 48°F). Stable for 12 hours when diluted in 0.9% sodium chloride.

Reconstitution Allow vial to warm to room temperature without heating. Dilute 800 mg (20 mL) with 55 mL NS.

Pharmacodynamics/Kinetics
Absorption: Well absorbed into bladder tissue, negligible systemic absorption. Trauma to mucosa may increase absorption, and perforation greatly increases absorption with significant systemic myelotoxicity.

Metabolism: Negligible after intravesical instillation and 2 hour retention

Excretion: Urine when expelled from urinary bladder (98.6% as intact drug; 0.4% as *N*-trifluoroacetyladriamycin)

(Continued)

Valrubicin *(Continued)*

Dosage Adults: Intravesical: 800 mg once weekly for 6 weeks

Dosing adjustment in renal impairment: No specific adjustment recommended

Dosing adjustment in hepatic impairment: No specific adjustment recommended

Administration Valrubicin is administered as an intravesicular bladder lavage, usually in 75 mL of 0.9% sodium chloride injection. The drug is retained in the bladder for 2 hours, then voided. Due to the Cremophor® EL diluent, valrubicin should be administered through non-PVC tubing.

Dosage Forms [DSC] = Discontinued product

Injection, solution [DSC]: 40 mg/mL (5 mL) [contains Cremophor® EL 50% (polyoxyethyleneglycol triricinoleate) and dehydrated alcohol 50%]

Monitoring Parameters Cystoscopy, biopsy, and urine cytology every 3 months for recurrence or progression

Patient Information This medication will be instilled into your bladder through a catheter to be retained for as long as possible. Your urine will be red tinged for the next 24 hours; report promptly if this continues for a longer period. You may experience altered urination patterns (frequency, dysuria, or incontinence), some bladder pain, pain on urination, or pelvic pain; report if these persist. Diabetics should monitor glucose levels closely (may cause hyperglycemia). It is important that you maintain adequate hydration (2-3 L/day of fluids unless instructed to restrict fluid intake). You may experience some dizziness (use caution when driving or engaging in tasks requiring alertness until response to drug is known); or nausea, vomiting, or taste disturbance (small frequent meals, frequent mouth care, chewing gum, or sucking lozenges may help). Report chest pain or palpitations; persistent dizziness; swelling of extremities; persistent nausea, vomiting, diarrhea, or abdominal pain; muscle weakness, pain, or tremors; unusual cough or difficulty breathing; or other adverse effects related to this medication.

Selected Readings

Greenberg RE, Bahnson RR, Wood D, et al, "Initial Report on Intravesical Administration of N-trifluoroacetyldoxorubicin-14-valerate (AD32) to Patients With Refractory Superficial Transitional Cell Carcinoma of the Urinary Bladder," *Urology,* 1997, 49:471-5.

Markman M, Homesley H, Norberts DA, et al, "Phase 1 Trial of Intraperitoneal AD-32 in Gynecologic Malignancies," *Gynecol Oncol,* 1996, 61(1):90-3.

Onrust SV and Lamb, "Valrubicin," *Drug Aging,* 1999, 15(1):69-75.

♦ **Valstar® [DSC]** *see* Valrubicin *on page 808*

♦ **Valtaxin® (Can)** *see* Valrubicin *on page 808*

♦ **Valtrex®** *see* Valacyclovir *on page 805*

♦ **Vancocin®** *see* Vancomycin *on page 810*

Vancomycin *(van koe MYE sin)*

Medication Safety Issues

Sound-alike/look-alike issues:

I.V. vancomycin may be confused with Invanz®

Vancomycin may be confused with vecuronium

Related Information

Management of Infections *on page 978*

U.S. Brand Names Vancocin®

Canadian Brand Names Vancocin®

Generic Available Yes: Injection

Synonyms Vancomycin Hydrochloride

Pharmacologic Category Antibiotic, Miscellaneous

Pregnancy Risk Factor C

Lactation Enters breast milk/use caution

Use Treatment of patients with infections caused by staphylococcal species and streptococcal species; used orally for staphylococcal enterocolitis or for antibiotic-associated pseudomembranous colitis produced by *C. difficile*

Mechanism of Action Inhibits bacterial cell wall synthesis by blocking glycopeptide polymerization through binding tightly to D-alanyl-D-alanine portion of cell wall precursor

Labeled Contraindications Hypersensitivity to vancomycin or any component of the formulation; avoid in patients with previous severe hearing loss

Warnings/Precautions Use with caution in patients with renal impairment or those receiving other nephrotoxic or ototoxic drugs. Dosage modification is required in patients with impaired renal function (especially elderly).

Adverse Reactions
Oral:
>10%: Gastrointestinal: Bitter taste, nausea, vomiting
1% to 10%:
Central nervous system: Chills, drug fever
Hematologic: Eosinophilia
<1%: Vasculitis, thrombocytopenia, ototoxicity, renal failure, interstitial nephritis
Parenteral:
>10%:
Cardiovascular: Hypotension accompanied by flushing
Dermatologic: Erythematous rash on face and upper body (red neck or red man syndrome - infusion rate related)
1% to 10%:
Central nervous system: Chills, drug fever
Dermatologic: Rash
Hematologic: Eosinophilia, reversible neutropenia
<1%: Vasculitis, Stevens-Johnson syndrome, ototoxicity (especially with large doses), thrombocytopenia, renal failure (especially with renal dysfunction or pre-existing hearing loss)

Vesicant No

Overdosage/Toxicology Symptoms of overdose include ototoxicity and nephrotoxicity. There is no specific therapy for overdose with vancomycin. Care is symptomatic and supportive. Peritoneal filtration and hemofiltration (not dialysis) have been shown to reduce the serum concentration of vancomycin. High flux dialysis may remove up to 25% of the drug.

Drug Interactions
Increased Effect/Toxicity: Increased toxicity with other ototoxic or nephrotoxic drugs. Increased neuromuscular blockade with most neuromuscular blocking agents.

Storage/Stability Vancomycin reconstituted intravenous solutions are stable for 14 days at room temperature or refrigeration. Stability of parenteral admixture at room temperature (25°C) or refrigeration temperature (4°C) is 7 days.

(Continued)

Vancomycin *(Continued)*

Reconstitution 10 mL SWFI for 500 mg vial and 20 mL for 1 g vial should be used. Further dilution requires at least 500 mg vancomycin per 100 mL of diluent.

Standard diluent: 500 mg/150 mL D_5W; 750 mg/250 mL D_5W; 1 g/250 mL D_5W

Minimum volume: Maximum concentration is 5 mg/mL to minimize thrombophlebitis.

Compatibility Stable in dextran 6% in NS, D_5LR, D_5NS, D_5W, $D_{10}W$, LR, NS; **variable stability (consult detailed reference)** in peritoneal dialysis solutions, TPN

Y-site administration: Compatible: Acyclovir, alatrofloxacin, allopurinol, amifostine, amiodarone, amsacrine, atracurium, cefpirome, cisatracurium, clarithromycin, cyclophosphamide, diltiazem, docetaxel, doxorubicin liposome, enalaprilat, esmolol, etoposide phosphate, filgrastim, fluconazole, fludarabine, gemcitabine, granisetron, hydromorphone, insulin (regular), labetalol, levofloxacin, linezolid, lorazepam, magnesium sulfate, melphalan, meperidine, meropenem, midazolam, morphine, ondansetron, paclitaxel, pancuronium, perphenazine, propofol, remifentanil, sodium bicarbonate, tacrolimus, teniposide, theophylline, thiotepa, tolazoline, vecuronium, vinorelbine, zidovudine. **Incompatible:** Albumin, amphotericin B cholesteryl sulfate complex, cefepime, gatifloxacin, heparin, idarubicin, omeprazole. **Variable (consult detailed reference):** Ampicillin, ampicillin/sulbactam, aztreonam, cefazolin, cefotaxime, cefotetan, cefoxitin, ceftazidime, ceftizoxime, ceftriaxone, cefuroxime, foscarnet, methotrexate, nafcillin, piperacillin, piperacillin/tazobactam, sargramostim, ticarcillin, ticarcillin/clavulanate, TPN, warfarin

Compatibility in syringe: Incompatible: Heparin

Compatibility when admixed: Compatible: Amikacin, atracurium, calcium gluconate, cefepime, cimetidine, corticotropin, dimenhydrinate, famotidine, hydrocortisone sodium succinate, meropenem, ofloxacin, potassium chloride, ranitidine, verapamil, vitamin B complex with C. **Incompatible:** Amobarbital, chloramphenicol, chlorothiazide, dexamethasone sodium phosphate, penicillin G potassium, pentobarbital, phenobarbital, phenytoin. **Variable (consult detailed reference):** Aminophylline, aztreonam, heparin, sodium bicarbonate

Pharmacodynamics/Kinetics

Absorption: Oral: Poor; I.M.: Erratic; Intraperitoneal: ~38%

Distribution: Widely in body tissues and fluids. except for CSF

Relative diffusion from blood into CSF: Good only with inflammation (exceeds usual MICs)

CSF:blood level ratio: Normal meninges: Nil; Inflamed meninges: 20% to 30%

Protein binding: 10% to 50%

Half-life elimination: Biphasic: Terminal:

Newborns: 6-10 hours

Infants and Children 3 months to 4 years: 4 hours

Children >3 years: 2.2-3 hours

Adults: 5-11 hours; significantly prolonged with renal impairment

End-stage renal disease: 200-250 hours

Time to peak, serum: I.V.: 45-65 minutes

Excretion: I.V.: Urine (80% to 90% as unchanged drug); Oral: Primarily feces

Dosage Initial dosage recommendation:

Neonates: I.V.:

Postnatal age ≤7 days:

<1200 g: 15 mg/kg/dose every 24 hours

1200-2000 g: 10 mg/kg/dose every 12 hours

>2000 g: 15 mg/kg/dose every 12 hours

Postnatal age >7 days:

<1200 g: 15 mg/kg/dose every 24 hours

≥1200 g: 10 mg/kg/dose divided every 8 hours

Infants >1 month and Children: I.V.:

40 mg/kg/day in divided doses every 6 hours

Prophylaxis for bacterial endocarditis:

Dental, oral, or upper respiratory tract surgery: 20 mg/kg 1 hour prior to the procedure

GI/GU procedure: 20 mg/kg plus gentamicin 2 mg/kg 1 hour prior to surgery

Infants >1 month and Children with staphylococcal central nervous system infection: I.V.: 60 mg/kg/day in divided doses every 6 hours

Adults: I.V.:

With normal renal function: 1 g **or** 10-15 mg/kg/dose every 12 hours

Prophylaxis for bacterial endocarditis:

Dental, oral, or upper respiratory tract surgery: 1 g 1 hour before surgery

GI/GU procedure: 1 g plus 1.5 mg/kg gentamicin 1 hour prior to surgery

Dosing interval in renal impairment (vancomycin levels should be monitored in patients with any renal impairment):

Cl_{cr} >60 mL/minute: Start with 1 g or 10-15 mg/kg/dose every 12 hours

Cl_{cr} 40-60 mL/minute: Start with 1 g or 10-15 mg/kg/dose every 24 hours

Cl_{cr} <40 mL/minute: Will need longer intervals; determine by serum concentration monitoring

Hemodialysis: Not dialyzable (0% to 5%); generally not removed; exception minimal-moderate removal by some of the newer high-flux filters; dose may need to be administered more frequently; monitor serum concentrations

Continuous ambulatory peritoneal dialysis (CAPD): Not significantly removed; administration via CAPD fluid: 15-30 mg/L (15-30 mcg/mL) of CAPD fluid

Continuous arteriovenous hemofiltration: Dose as for Cl_{cr} 10-40 mL/minute

Antibiotic lock technique (for catheter infections): 2 mg/mL in SWI/NS or D_5W; instill 3-5 mL into catheter port as a flush solution instead of heparin lock (**Note:** Do not mix with any other solutions)

Intrathecal: Vancomycin is available as a powder for injection and may be diluted to 1-5 mg/mL concentration in preservative-free 0.9% sodium chloride for administration into the CSF

Neonates: 5-10 mg/day

Children: 5-20 mg/day

Adults: Up to 20 mg/day

Oral: Pseudomembranous colitis produced by *C. difficile*:

Neonates: 10 mg/kg/day in divided doses

(Continued)

Vancomycin *(Continued)*

Children: 40 mg/kg/day in divided doses, added to fluids

Adults: 125 mg 4 times/day for 10 days

Administration Administer vancomycin by I.V. intermittent infusion over at least 60 minutes at a final concentration not to exceed 5 mg/mL. If a maculopapular rash appears on the face, neck, trunk, and/or upper extremities (Red man syndrome), slow the infusion rate to over $1\frac{1}{2}$ to 2 hours and increase the dilution volume. Hypotension, shock, and cardiac arrest (rare) have also been reported with too rapid of infusion. Reactions are often treated with antihistamines and steroids.

Dosage Forms

Capsule (Vancocin®): 125 mg, 250 mg

Infusion [premixed in iso-osmotic dextrose] (Vancocin®): 500 mg (100 mL); 1 g (200 mL)

Injection, powder for reconstitution: 500 mg, 1 g, 5 g, 10 g

Monitoring Parameters Periodic renal function tests, urinalysis, serum vancomycin concentrations, WBC, audiogram

Dietary Considerations May be taken with food.

Patient Information Report pain at infusion site, dizziness, fullness or ringing in ears with I.V. use; nausea or vomiting with oral use

Additional Information Because of its long half-life, vancomycin should be dosed on an every 12 hour basis; monitoring of peak and trough serum levels is advisable. The "red man syndrome" characterized by skin rash and hypotension is not an allergic reaction but rather is associated with too rapid infusion of the drug. To alleviate or prevent the reaction, infuse vancomycin at a rate of ≥30 minutes for each 500 mg of drug being administered (eg, 1 g over ≥60 minutes); 1.5 g over ≥90 minutes.

Special Geriatric Considerations As a result of age-related changes in renal function and volume of distribution, accumulation and toxicity are a risk in the elderly. Careful monitoring and dosing adjustment is necessary.

Selected Readings

Abramowicz M, "Antimicrobial Prophylaxis in Surgery," *Medical Letter on Drugs and Therapeutics, Handbook of Antimicrobial Therapy*, 16th ed, New York, NY: Medical Letter, 2002.

Ahkee S, Smith R, and Ritter GW, "Once-Daily Aminoglycoside Dosing in Lower Respiratory Tract Infections," *Pharm Therapeut*, 1995, 20:226-34.

Centers for Disease Control and Prevention, "Recommendations for Preventing the Spread of Vancomycin Resistance - Recommendations of the Hospital Infection Control Practice Advisory Committee (HICPAC)," *MMWR Recomm Rep* 1995, 44(RR-12):1-9.

Chang D, Liem L, and Malogolowkin M, "A Prospective Study of Vancomycin Pharmacokinetics and Dosage Requirements in Pediatric Cancer Patients," *Pediatr Infect Dis J*, 1994, 13(11):969-74.

Cunha BA, "Vancomycin," *Med Clin North Am*, 1995, 79(4):817-31.

♦ **Vancomycin Hydrochloride** *see* Vancomycin *on page 810*

♦ **Vantas**™ *see* Histrelin *on page 415*

♦ **VCR** *see* VinCRIStine *on page 819*

♦ **Velcade**™ *see* Bortezomib *on page 138*

♦ **Venoglobulin®-S [DSC]** *see* Immune Globulin (Intravenous) *on page 458*

♦ **VePesid®** *see* Etoposide *on page 315*

♦ **Veracolate [OTC]** *see* Bisacodyl *on page 133*

♦ **Versiclear**™ *see* Sodium Thiosulfate *on page 722*

♦ **Vesanoid**® *see* Tretinoin (Oral) *on page 792*

♦ **Viadur**® *see* Leuprolide *on page 500*

♦ **Vidaza**™ *see* Azacitidine *on page 110*

VinBLAStine (vin BLAS teen)

Medication Safety Issues

Sound-alike/look-alike issues:

VinBLAStine may be confused with vinCRIStine, vinorelbine

Note: Must be dispensed in overwrap which bears the statement "Do not remove covering until the moment of injection. Fatal if given intrathecally. For I.V. use only." Syringes should be labeled: "Fatal if given intrathecally. For I.V. use only."

Related Information

Management of Drug Extravasations *on page 965*

Management of Nausea and Vomiting *on page 982*

Safe Handling of Hazardous Drugs *on page 1034*

Generic Available Yes

Synonyms NSC-49842; Vinblastine Sulfate; VLB

Pharmacologic Category Antineoplastic Agent, Natural Source (Plant) Derivative; Antineoplastic Agent, Vinca Alkaloid

Pregnancy Risk Factor D

Lactation Enters breast milk/not recommended

Use Treatment of Hodgkin's and non-Hodgkin's lymphoma, testicular, lung, head and neck, breast, and renal carcinomas, Mycosis fungoides, Kaposi's sarcoma, histiocytosis, choriocarcinoma, and idiopathic thrombocytopenic purpura

Mechanism of Action Vinblastine binds to tubulin and inhibits microtubule formation, therefore, arresting the cell at metaphase by disrupting the formation of the mitotic spindle; it is specific for the M and S phases. Vinblastine may also interfere with nucleic acid and protein synthesis by blocking glutamic acid utilization.

Labeled Contraindications For I.V. use only; **I.T. use may result in death**; hypersensitivity to vinblastine or any component of the formulation

Warnings/Precautions Hazardous agent - use appropriate precautions for handling and disposal. See Safe Handling of Hazardous Drugs *on page 1034* in the Appendix. Vinblastine is a moderate vesicant; avoid extravasation. Dosage modification required in patients with impaired liver function and neurotoxicity. Using small amounts of drug daily for long periods may cause neurotoxicity and is therefore not advised. For I.V. use only. **Intrathecal administration results in death**. Use with caution in patients with cachexia or ulcerated skin. Monitor closely for shortness of breath or bronchospasm in patients receiving mitomycin C.

Adverse Reactions

>10%:

Dermatologic: Alopecia

Endocrine & metabolic: SIADH

Gastrointestinal: Diarrhea (less common), stomatitis, anorexia, metallic taste

Hematologic: May cause severe bone marrow suppression and is the dose-limiting toxicity of VLB (unlike vincristine); severe granulocytopenia and thrombocytopenia may occur following the administration of VLB and nadir 5-10 days after treatment

(Continued)

VinBLAStine (Continued)

Myelosuppression (primarily leukopenia, may be dose limiting)
  Onset: 4-7 days
  Nadir: 5-10 days
  Recovery: 4-21 days

1% to 10%:
  Cardiovascular: Hypertension, Raynaud's phenomenon
  Central nervous system: Depression, malaise, headache, seizure
  Dermatologic: Rash, photosensitivity, dermatitis
  Endocrine & metabolic: Hyperuricemia
  Gastrointestinal: Constipation, abdominal pain, nausea (mild), vomiting (mild), paralytic ileus, stomatitis
  Genitourinary: Urinary retention
  Neuromuscular & skeletal: Jaw pain, myalgia, paresthesia
  Respiratory: Bronchospasm

<1%: VLB rarely produces neurotoxicity at clinical doses; however, neurotoxicity may be seen, especially at high doses; if it occurs, symptoms are similar to VCR toxicity (ie, peripheral neuropathy, loss of deep tendon reflexes, headache, weakness, urinary retention, and GI symptoms, tachycardia, orthostatic hypotension, convulsions); hemorrhagic colitis

Vesicant Yes; see Management of Drug Extravasations *on page 965.*

Emetic Potential Very low (<10%)

Overdosage/Toxicology Symptoms of overdose include bone marrow suppression, mental depression, paresthesia, loss of deep tendon reflexes, and neurotoxicity. There are no antidotes for vinblastine. Treatment is supportive and symptomatic, including fluid restriction or hypertonic saline (3% sodium chloride) for drug-induced secretion of inappropriate antidiuretic hormone (SIADH).

Drug Interactions

Cytochrome P450 Effect: Substrate of CYP2D6 (minor), 3A4 (major); **Inhibits** CYP2D6 (weak), 3A4 (weak)

Increased Effect/Toxicity: CYP3A4 inhibitors may increase the levels/effects of vinblastine; example inhibitors include azole antifungals, ciprofloxacin, clarithromycin, diclofenac, doxycycline, erythromycin, imatinib, isoniazid, nefazodone, nicardipine, propofol, protease inhibitors, quinidine, and verapamil.

Previous or simultaneous use with mitomycin-C has resulted in acute shortness of breath and severe bronchospasm within minutes or several hours after *Vinca* alkaloid injection and may occur up to 2 weeks after the dose of mitomycin. Mitomycin-C in combination with administration of VLB may cause acute shortness of breath and severe bronchospasm, onset may be within minutes or several hours after VLB injection.

Decreased Effect: CYP3A4 inducers may decrease the levels/effects of vinblastine; example inducers include aminoglutethimide, carbamazepine, nafcillin, nevirapine, phenobarbital, phenytoin (may reduce vinblastine serum concentrations), and rifamycins.

Ethanol/Nutrition/Herb Interactions Herb/Nutraceutical: St John's wort may decrease vinblastine levels. Avoid black cohosh, dong quai in estrogen-dependent tumors.

Storage/Stability Store intact vials under refrigeration (2°C to 8°C) and protect from light. Solutions reconstituted in bacteriostatic water or bacteriostatic NS are stable for 21 days at room temperature or under refrigeration.

Note: Must be dispensed in overwrap which bears the statement "Do not remove covering until the moment of injection. Fatal if given intrathecally. For I.V. use only." Syringes should be labeled: "Fatal if given intrathecally. For I.V. use only."

Reconstitution Reconstitute to a concentration of 1 mg/mL with bacteriostatic water, bacteriostatic NS, SWFI, NS, or D_5W; for infusion, may be diluted with 50-1000 mL Ns or D_5W.

Compatibility Stable in D_5W, LR, NS, bacteriostatic water

Y-site administration: Compatible: Allopurinol, amifostine, amphotericin B cholesteryl sulfate complex, aztreonam, bleomycin, cisplatin, cyclophosphamide, doxorubicin, doxorubicin liposome, droperidol, etoposide phosphate, filgrastim, fludarabine, fluorouracil, gatifloxacin, gemcitabine, granisetron, heparin, leucovorin, melphalan, methotrexate, metoclopramide, mitomycin, ondansetron, paclitaxel, piperacillin/tazobactam, sargramostim, teniposide, thiotepa, vincristine, vinorelbine. **Incompatible:** Cefepime, furosemide

Compatibility in syringe: Compatible: Bleomycin, cisplatin, cyclophosphamide, droperidol, fluorouracil, leucovorin, methotrexate, metoclopramide, mitomycin, vincristine. **Incompatible:** Furosemide. **Variable (consult detailed reference):** Doxorubicin, heparin

Compatibility when admixed: Compatible: Bleomycin, dacarbazine. **Variable (consult detailed reference):** Doxorubicin

Pharmacodynamics/Kinetics

Distribution: V_d: 27.3 L/kg; binds extensively to tissues; does not penetrate CNS or other fatty tissues; distributes to liver

Protein binding: 99%

Metabolism: Hepatic to active metabolite

Half-life elimination: Biphasic: Initial: 0.164 hours; Terminal: 25 hours

Excretion: Feces (95%); urine (<1% as unchanged drug)

Dosage Refer to individual protocols.

Children and Adults: I.V.: 4-20 mg/m² (0.1-0.5 mg/kg) every 7-10 days **or** 5-day continuous infusion of 1.5-2 mg/m²/day **or** 0.1-0.5 mg/kg/week

Dosing adjustment in hepatic impairment:

Serum bilirubin 1.5-3.0 mg/dL or AST 60-180 units: Administer 50% of normal dose

Serum bilirubin 3.0-5.0 mg/dL: Administer 25% of dose

Serum bilirubin >5.0 mg/dL or AST >180 units: Omit dose

Combination Regimens

Bladder cancer:

CMV *on page 863*

M-VAC (Bladder Cancer) *on page 917*

Breast cancer:

M-VAC (Breast Cancer) *on page 921*

VATH *on page 944*

Cervical cancer: M-VAC (Cervical Cancer) *on page 921*

Endometrial cancer: M-VAC (Endometrial Cancer) *on page 921*

Head and neck cancer: M-VAC (Head and Neck Cancer) *on page 922*

Lymphoma, Hodgkin's:

ABVD *on page 843*

(Continued)

VinBLAStine *(Continued)*

CAD/MOPP/ABV *on page 850*

ChIVPP *on page 859*

EVA *on page 884*

MOPP/ABV Hybrid *on page 913*

MOPP/ABVD *on page 913*

MVPP *on page 922*

Stanford V *on page 937*

Melanoma:

CVD *on page 868*

IL-2 + IFN *on page 902*

Prostate cancer:

Doxorubicin + Ketoconazole/Estramustine + Vinblastine *on page 874*

EV *on page 883*

Testicular cancer:

PVB *on page 935*

VBP *on page 945*

VIP (Vinblastine) (Testicular Cancer) *on page 948*

Administration FATAL IF GIVEN INTRATHECALLY. I.V., usually as a slow (2-3 minutes) push, or a bolus (5- to 15-minute) infusion. It is occasionally given as a 24-hour continuous infusion.

Dosage Forms

Injection, powder for reconstitution, as sulfate: 10 mg

Injection, solution, as sulfate: 1 mg/mL (10 mL) [contains benzyl alcohol]

Monitoring Parameters CBC with differential and platelet count, serum uric acid, hepatic function tests

Patient Information This medication can only be administered by infusion, usually on a cyclic basis. Maintain adequate hydration (2-3 L/day of fluids unless instructed to restrict fluid intake) and nutrition (small frequent meals will help). You will most likely lose your hair (reversible after therapy); experience nausea or vomiting (request antiemetic); photosensitivity (use sunscreen, wear protective clothing and eyewear, and avoid direct sunlight); or feel weak or lethargic (use caution when driving or engaging in tasks requiring alertness until response to drug is known). Use good oral care to reduce incidence of mouth sores. You will be more susceptible to infection; avoid crowds or exposure to infection. Report numbness or tingling in fingers or toes (use care to prevent injury); signs of infection (eg, fever, chills, sore throat, burning urination, fatigue); unusual bleeding (eg, tarry stools, easy bruising, blood in stool, urine, or mouth); unresolved mouth sores; skin rash or itching; or difficulty breathing. The drug may cause permanent sterility and may cause birth defects. Contraceptive measures are recommended during therapy. The drug may be excreted in breast milk, therefore, an alternative form of feeding your baby should be used.

Additional Information Allopurinol may be given to prevent uric acid nephropathy.

Selected Readings

Bonadonna G, Valagussa P, and Santoro A, "Alternating Non-Cross-Resistant Combination Chemotherapy or MOPP in Stage IV Hodgkin's Disease: A Report of 8-Year Results," *Ann Intern Med*, 1986, 104(6):739-46.

Chong CD, Logothetis CJ, Savaraj N, et al, "The Correlation of Vinblastine Pharmacokinetics to Toxicity in Testicular Cancer Patients," *J Clin Pharmacol*, 1998, 28(8):714-8.

Friedman M, Venkatesan TK, and Caldarelli DD, "Intralesional Vinblastine for Treating AIDS-Associated Kaposi's Sarcoma of the Oropharynx and Larynx," *Ann Otol Rhinol Laryngol*, 1996, 105(4):272-4.

Pronzato P, Queirolo P, Vidili MG, et al, "Continuous Venous Infusion of Vinblastine in Metastatic Breast Cancer," *Chemotherapy*, 1991, 37(2):146-9.

Williams SD, Birch R, Einhorn LH, et al, "Treatment of Disseminated Germ-Cell Tumors With Cisplatin, Bleomycin, and Either Vinblastine or Etoposide," *N Engl J Med*, 1987, 316(23):1435-40.

♦ **Vinblastine Sulfate** *see* VinBLAStine *on page 815*

♦ **Vincasar PFS®** *see* VinCRIStine *on page 819*

VinCRIStine (vin KRIS teen)

Medication Safety Issues
Sound-alike/look-alike issues:
VinCRIStine may be confused with vinBLAStine
Oncovin® may be confused with Ancobon®

To prevent fatal inadvertent intrathecal injection, it is recommended that all doses be dispensed in a small minibag; do not dispense in a syringe.

Related Information
Management of Drug Extravasations *on page 965*
Safe Handling of Hazardous Drugs *on page 1034*

U.S. Brand Names Vincasar PFS®

Canadian Brand Names Vincasar® PFS®

Generic Available Yes

Synonyms LCR; Leurocristine Sulfate; NSC-67574; VCR; Vincristine Sulfate

Pharmacologic Category Antineoplastic Agent, Natural Source (Plant) Derivative; Antineoplastic Agent, Vinca Alkaloid

Pregnancy Risk Factor D

Lactation Enters breast milk/not recommended

Use Treatment of leukemias, Hodgkin's disease, non-Hodgkin's lymphomas, Wilms' tumor, neuroblastoma, rhabdomyosarcoma

Mechanism of Action Binds to tubulin and inhibits microtubule formation; therefore arresting the cell at metaphase by disrupting the formation of the mitotic spindle; it is specific for the M and S phases. Vincristine may also interfere with nucleic acid and protein synthesis by blocking glutamic acid utilization.

Labeled Contraindications Hypersensitivity to vincristine or any component of the formulation; **for I.V. use only, fatal if given intrathecally**; patients with demyelinating form of Charcot-Marie-Tooth syndrome; pregnancy

Warnings/Precautions Hazardous agent - use appropriate precautions for handling and disposal. See Safe Handling of Hazardous Drugs *on page 1034* in the Appendix.

Dosage modification required in patients with impaired hepatic function or who have pre-existing neuromuscular disease. Drug is a vesicant. Avoid extravasation. Use with caution in the elderly. Avoid eye contamination. Observe closely for shortness of breath, bronchospasm, especially in patients treated with mitomycin C. Alterations in mental status such as depression, confusion, or insomnia; constipation, paralytic ileus, and urinary tract disturbances may occur. All patients should be on a prophylactic bowel management regimen.
(Continued)

VinCRIStine *(Continued)*

Intrathecal administration of VCR has uniformly caused death; VCR should never be administered by this route. Neurologic effects of VCR may be additive with those of other neurotoxic agents and spinal cord irradiation.

Adverse Reactions

>10%: Dermatologic: Alopecia occurs in 20% to 70% of patients

1% to 10%:

Cardiovascular: Orthostatic hypotension or hypertension, hyper-/hypotension

Central nervous system: Motor difficulties, seizure, headache, CNS depression, cranial nerve paralysis, fever

Dermatologic: Rash

Endocrine & metabolic: Hyperuricemia

SIADH: Rarely occurs, but may be related to the neurologic toxicity; may cause symptomatic hyponatremia with seizure; the increase in serum ADH concentration usually subsides within 2-3 days after onset

Gastrointestinal: Constipation and possible paralytic ileus secondary to neurologic toxicity; oral ulceration, abdominal cramps, anorexia, metallic taste, bloating, nausea (mild), vomiting, weight loss, diarrhea

Local: Phlebitis

Neurologic: Alterations in mental status such as depression, confusion, or insomnia; constipation, paralytic ileus, and urinary tract disturbances may occur. All patients should be on a prophylactic bowel management regimen. Cranial nerve palsies, headaches, jaw pain, optic atrophy with blindness have been reported. Intrathecal administration of VCR has uniformly caused death; VCR should **never** be administered by this route. Neurologic effects of VCR may be additive with those of other neurotoxic agents and spinal cord irradiation.

Neuromuscular & skeletal: Jaw pain, leg pain, myalgia, cramping, numbness, weakness

Peripheral neuropathy: Frequently the dose-limiting toxicity of VCR. Most frequent in patients >40 years of age; occurs usually after an average of 3 weekly doses, but may occur after just one dose. Manifested as loss of the deep tendon reflexes in the lower extremities, numbness, tingling, pain, paresthesia of the fingers and toes (stocking glove sensation), and "foot drop" or "wrist drop"

Ocular: Photophobia

<1%: Stomatitis

Myelosuppressive: Occasionally mild leukopenia and thrombocytopenia may occur

WBC: Rare

Platelets: Rare

Onset: 7 days

Nadir: 10 days

Recovery: 21 days

Vesicant Yes; moderate. See Management of Drug Extravasations *on page 965*.

Emetic Potential Very low (<10%)

Overdosage/Toxicology Symptoms of overdose include bone marrow suppression, mental depression, paresthesia, loss of deep tendon reflexes, alopecia, and nausea. Severe symptoms may occur with 3-4 mg/m^2.

There are no antidotes for vincristine. Treatment is supportive and symptomatic, including fluid restriction or hypertonic saline (3% sodium chloride) for drug-induced secretion of inappropriate antidiuretic hormone (SIADH). Case reports suggest that folinic acid may be helpful in treating vincristine overdose. It is suggested that 100 mg folinic acid be given I.V. every 3 hours for 24 hours, then every 6 hours for 48 hours. This is in addition to supportive care. The use of pyridoxine, leucovorin factor, cyanocobalamin, or thiamine has been used with little success for drug-induced peripheral neuropathy.

Drug Interactions

Cytochrome P450 Effect: Substrate of CYP3A4 (major); **Inhibits** CYP3A4 (weak)

Increased Effect/Toxicity: Vincristine should be given 12-24 hours before asparaginase to minimize toxicity (may decrease the hepatic clearance of vincristine). Acute pulmonary reactions may occur with mitomycin-C. Previous or simultaneous use with mitomycin-C has resulted in acute shortness of breath and severe bronchospasm within minutes or several hours after *Vinca* alkaloid injection and may occur up to 2 weeks after the dose of mitomycin.

CYP3A4 inhibitors may increase the levels/effects of vincristine. Example inhibitors include azole antifungals, ciprofloxacin, clarithromycin, diclofenac, doxycycline, erythromycin, imatinib, isoniazid, nefazodone, nicardipine, propofol, protease inhibitors, quinidine, and verapamil. Digoxin plasma levels and renal excretion may decrease with combination chemotherapy including vincristine.

Decreased Effect: Digoxin levels may decrease with combination chemotherapy. CYP3A4 inducers may decrease the levels/effects of vincristine; example inducers include aminoglutethimide, carbamazepine, nafcillin, nevirapine, phenobarbital, phenytoin, and rifamycins.

Ethanol/Nutrition/Herb Interactions Herb/Nutraceutical: St John's wort may decrease vincristine levels.

Storage/Stability Store intact vials at refrigeration (2°C to 8°C). Protect from light. Solutions reconstituted in NS or D$_5$W are stable for 21 days at room temperature or under refrigeration.

Reconstitution Solutions for I.V. infusion may be mixed in NS or D$_5$W.

Compatibility Stable in D$_5$W, LR, NS

Y-site administration: Compatible: Allopurinol, amifostine, amphotericin B cholesteryl sulfate complex, aztreonam, bleomycin, cisplatin, cladribine, cyclophosphamide, doxorubicin, doxorubicin liposome, droperidol, etoposide phosphate, filgrastim, fludarabine, fluorouracil, gatifloxacin, gemcitabine, granisetron, heparin, leucovorin, linezolid, melphalan, methotrexate, metoclopramide, mitomycin, ondansetron, paclitaxel, piperacillin/tazobactam, sargramostim, teniposide, thiotepa, topotecan, vinblastine, vinorelbine. **Incompatible:** Cefepime, furosemide, idarubicin, sodium bicarbonate

Compatibility in syringe: Compatible: Bleomycin, cisplatin, cyclophosphamide, doxapram, doxorubicin, droperidol, fluorouracil, heparin, leucovorin, methotrexate, metoclopramide, mitomycin, vinblastine. **Incompatible:** Furosemide

(Continued)

VinCRIStine *(Continued)*

Compatibility when admixed: Compatible: Bleomycin, cytarabine, doxorubicin with ondansetron, fluorouracil, methotrexate. **Variable (consult detailed reference):** Doxorubicin with etoposide

Pharmacodynamics/Kinetics

Absorption: Oral: Poor

Distribution: V_d: 163-165 L/m^2; Poor penetration into CSF; rapidly removed from bloodstream and tightly bound to tissues; penetrates blood-brain barrier poorly

Protein binding: 75%

Metabolism: Extensively hepatic

Half-life elimination: Terminal: 24 hours

Excretion: Feces (~80%); urine (<1% as unchanged drug)

Dosage Note: Doses are often capped at 2 mg; however, this may reduce the efficacy of the therapy and may not be advisable. Refer to individual protocols; orders for single doses >2.5 mg or >5 mg/treatment cycle should be verified with the specific treatment regimen and/or an experienced oncologist prior to dispensing. I.V.:

Children ≤10 kg or BSA <1 m^2: Initial therapy: 0.05 mg/kg once weekly then titrate dose; maximum single dose: 2 mg

Children >10 kg or BSA ≥1 m^2: 1-2 mg/m^2, may repeat once weekly for 3-6 weeks; maximum single dose: 2 mg

Neuroblastoma: I.V. continuous infusion with doxorubicin: 1 mg/m^2/day for 72 hours

Adults: 0.4-1.4 mg/m^2, may repeat every week **or**
0.4-0.5 mg/day continuous infusion for 4 days every 4 weeks **or**
0.25-0.5 mg/m^2/day for 5 days every 4 weeks

Dosing adjustment in hepatic impairment:

Serum bilirubin 1.5-3.0 mg/dL or AST 60-180 units: Administer 50% of normal dose

Serum bilirubin 3.0-5.0 mg/dL: Administer 25% of dose

Serum bilirubin >5.0 mg/dL or AST >180 units: Omit dose

Combination Regimens

Brain tumors:
8 in 1 (Brain Tumors) *on page 841*
COPE *on page 866*
MOP *on page 910*
MOPP (Medulloblastoma) *on page 912*
PCV *on page 928*
POC *on page 931*
Gestational trophoblastic tumor:
CHAMOCA *on page 858*
EMA/CO *on page 877*
Head and neck cancer: CABO *on page 849*
Leukemia, acute lymphocytic:
DVP *on page 875*
Larson Regimen *on page 904*
Linker Protocol *on page 904*
MTX/6-MP/VP (Maintenance) *on page 916*
PVA (POG 8602) *on page 932*
PVA (POG 9005) *on page 934*
PVDA *on page 936*

(Continued)

VinCRIStine *(Continued)*

CO *on page 864*

CV *on page 868*

VAC (Retinoblastoma) *on page 942*

Rhabdomyosarcoma:

CEV *on page 857*

VAC (Rhabdomyosarcoma) *on page 943*

VAC Pulse *on page 943*

Sarcoma: CYVADIC *on page 871*

Wilms' tumor:

AAV (DD) *on page 843*

ACAV (J) *on page 844*

AV (EE) *on page 845*

AV (K) *on page 845*

AV (L) *on page 845*

AV (Wilms' Tumor) *on page 846*

AVD *on page 846*

EE *on page 876*

EE-4A *on page 876*

Administration FATAL IF GIVEN INTRATHECALLY.

I.V.: Usually administered as slow (1-2 minutes) push or as short (10-15 minutes) infusion; 24-hour continuous infusions are occasionally used Intralesional injection has been reported for Kaposi's sarcoma.

Dosage Forms Injection, solution, as sulfate: 1 mg/mL (1 mL, 2 mL)

Monitoring Parameters Serum electrolytes (sodium), hepatic function tests, neurologic examination, CBC, serum uric acid

Patient Information This medication can only be administered by infusion, usually on a cyclic basis. Maintain adequate hydration (2-3 L/day of fluids unless instructed to restrict fluid intake) and nutrition (small frequent meals will help). You will most likely lose your hair (reversible after therapy); experience constipation (request medication); or feel weak or lethargic (use caution when driving or engaging in tasks requiring alertness until response to drug is known). Use good oral care to reduce incidence of mouth sores. You will be more susceptible to infection; avoid crowds or exposure to infection. Report pain, numbness, or tingling in fingers or toes (use care to prevent injury); alterations in mental status (eg, confusion, insomnia, headaches, jaw pain, loss of vision); signs of infection (eg, fever, chills, sore throat, burning urination, fatigue); unusual bleeding (eg, tarry stools, easy bruising, or blood in stool, urine, or mouth), unresolved mouth sores; skin rash or itching; nausea; vomiting; abdominal pain; bloating; or difficulty breathing. Contraceptive measures are recommended during therapy.

Selected Readings

Ahn YS, Harrington WJ, Mylvaganam R, et al, "Slow Infusion of Vinca Alkaloids in the Treatment of Idiopathic Thrombocytopenic Purpura," *Ann Intern Med*, 1984, 100(2):192-6.

Camplejohn RS, "A Critical Review of the Use of Vincristine (VCR) as a Tumour Cell Synchronizing Agent in Cancer Therapy," *Cell Tissue Kinet*, 1980, 13(3):327-35.

Joel S, "The Comparative Clinical Pharmacology of Vincristine and Vindesine: Does Vindesine Offer Any Advantage in Clinical Use?" *Cancer Treat Rev*, 1996, 21(6):513-25.

Legha SS, "Vincristine Neurotoxicity. Pathophysiology and Management," *Med Toxicol*, 1986, 1(6):421-7.

McCune JS and Lindley C, "Appropriateness of Maximum-Dose Guidelines for Vincristine," *Am J Health Syst Pharm*, 1997, 54(15):1755-8.

Tajti J, Somogyi I, and Szilard J, "Treatment of Chronic Pain Syndromes With Transcutaneous Iontophoresis of Vinca Alkaloids, With Special Regard to Postherpetic Neuralgia," *Acta Med Hung*, 1989, 46(1):3-12.

♦ **Vincristine Sulfate** *see* VinCRIStine *on page 819*

Vindesine (VIN de seen)

Related Information
Investigational Drug Service *on page 1031*
Safe Handling of Hazardous Drugs *on page 1034*

Generic Available No

Synonyms DAVA; Deacetyl Vinblastine Carboxamide; Desacetyl Vinblastine Amide Sulfate; DVA; Eldisine Lilly 99094; Lilly CT-3231; NSC-245467; Vindesine Sulfate

Pharmacologic Category Antineoplastic Agent, Vinca Alkaloid

Lactation Breast-feeding is not recommended.

Unlabeled/Investigational Use Investigational: Management of acute lymphocytic leukemia, chronic myelogenous leukemia; breast, head, neck, and lung cancers; lymphomas (Hodgkin's and non-Hodgkin's)

Mechanism of Action Vindesine is a semisynthetic vinca alkaloid, having a mechanism of action similar to the other vinca derivatives. It arrests cell division in metaphase through inhibition of microtubular formation of the mitotic spindle. The drug is cell-cycle specific for the S phase.

Restrictions Not available in U.S./Investigational

Labeled Contraindications Hypersensitivity to vindesine, vinca alkaloids, or any component of the formulation

Warnings/Precautions Hazardous agent - use appropriate precautions for handling and disposal. See Safe Handling of Hazardous Drugs *on page 1034* in the Appendix. Vindesine should be used cautiously, if at all in patients with impaired hepatic function or neurologic problems. **Intrathecal administration may be fatal**. Vindesine has been reported to be cross-resistance with vincristine. Vindesine is a moderate vesicant; if extravasation occurs, severe tissue damage leading to ulceration and necrosis, and pain may occur.

Adverse Reactions
>10%:
Central nervous system: Pyrexia, malaise (up to 60%)
Dermatologic: Alopecia (6% to 92%)
Gastrointestinal: Mild nausea and vomiting (7% to 27%), constipation (10% to 17%) - related to the neurotoxicity
Hematologic: Leukopenia (50%) and thrombocytopenia (14% to 26%), may be dose-limiting; thrombocytosis (20% to 28%)
Nadir: 6-12 days
Recovery: Days 14-18
Neuromuscular & skeletal: Paresthesias (40% to 70%); loss of deep tendon reflexes (35% to 60%, may be dose-limiting); myalgia (up to 60%)
1% to 10%:
Dermatologic: Rashes
Gastrointestinal: Loss of taste
Hematologic: Anemia
Local: Phlebitis
Neuromuscular & skeletal: Facial paralysis
(Continued)

Vindesine *(Continued)*

<1%: Acute chest pain, ECG changes, paralytic ileus, jaw pain, photophobia

Vesicant Yes; see Management of Drug Extravasations *on page 965.*

Storage/Stability Reconstituted solutions are stable for 30 days under refrigeration (2°C to 8°C/36°F to 46°F). Solutions diluted in dextrose or saline for I.V. infusion are stable for 24 hours at room temperature (15°C to 30°C/59°F to 86°F). **The drug will precipitate at pH >6.**

Reconstitution The powder is reconstituted to a concentration of 1 mg/mL.

Pharmacodynamics/Kinetics

Distribution: V_d: 8 L/kg; minimal distribution to adipose tissue or CNS

Metabolism: Hepatic

Half-life elimination:

Triphasic; Alpha: 2 minutes; Beta: 1 hour

Terminal: 24 hours

Excretion: Feces; urine (~3% to 25% of dose as unchanged drug)

Dosage Refer to individual protocols. I.V.: Adults:

3-4 mg/m^2 /week **or**

1-2 mg/m^2 days 1 and 2 every 2 weeks **or**

1-2 mg/m^2 days 1-5 (continuous infusion) every 2-4 weeks **or**

1-2 mg/m^2 days 1-5 every 3-4 weeks

Dosage adjustment in hepatic impairment: Dosage reductions of 50% to 75% have been suggested for "severe" hepatic dysfunction; however, specific guidelines have not been published.

Combination Regimens

Lymphoma, Hodgkin's: CAD/MOPP/ABV *on page 850*

Administration Usually administered as a rapid I.V. push (2-3 minutes) or short (15- to 20-minute) infusion; 24-hour continuous infusions are occasionally used

Dosage Forms Injection, powder for reconstitution: 5 mg

Patient Information Hair loss is common but usually reversible. Report any loss of sensation or tingling in hands or feet, constipation, fever, sore throat, bruising, or bleeding.

Selected Readings

Dancey J and Steward WP, "The Role of Vindesine in Oncology - Recommendations After 10 Years' Experience," *Anticancer Drugs*, 1995, 6(5):625-36.

Joel S, "The Comparative Clinical Pharmacology of Vincristine and Vindesine: Does Vindesine Offer Any Advantage in Clinical Use?" *Cancer Treat Rev*, 1996, 21(6):513-25.

Rhomberg W, Eiter H, Soltesz E, et al, "Long-Term Application of Vindesine: Toxicity and Tolerance," *J Cancer Res Clin Oncol*, 1990, 116(6):651-3.

Sorenson JB and Hansen HH, "Is There a Role for Vindesine in the Treatment of Nonsmall Cell Lung Cancer?" *Invest New Drugs*, 1993, 11(2-3):103-33.

♦ **Vindesine Sulfate** *see* Vindesine *on page 825*

Vinorelbine (vi NOR el been)

Medication Safety Issues

Sound-alike/look-alike issues:

Vinorelbine may be confused with vinBLAStine

Related Information

Management of Drug Extravasations *on page 965*

Safe Handling of Hazardous Drugs *on page 1034*

U.S. Brand Names Navelbine®

Canadian Brand Names Navelbine®

Generic Available Yes

Synonyms Dihydroxydeoxynorvinkaleukoblastine; NVB; Vinorelbine Tartrate

Pharmacologic Category Antineoplastic Agent, Natural Source (Plant) Derivative; Antineoplastic Agent, Vinca Alkaloid

Pregnancy Risk Factor D

Lactation Excretion in breast milk unknown/contraindicated

Use Treatment of nonsmall cell lung cancer

Unlabeled/Investigational Use Treatment of breast cancer, ovarian carcinoma, Hodgkin's disease, non-Hodgkin's lymphoma

Mechanism of Action Semisynthetic vinca alkaloid which binds to tubulin and inhibits microtubule formation, therefore, arresting the cell at metaphase by disrupting the formation of the mitotic spindle; it is specific for the M and S phases. Vinorelbine may also interfere with nucleic acid and protein synthesis by blocking glutamic acid utilization.

Labeled Contraindications For I.V. use only; **I.T. use may result in death**; hypersensitivity to vinorelbine or any component of the formulation; severe bone marrow suppression (granulocyte counts <1000 cells/mm^3); pregnancy

Warnings/Precautions Hazardous agent - use appropriate precautions for handling and disposal. See Safe Handling of Hazardous Drugs *on page 1034* in the Appendix. Avoid extravasation; dosage modification required in patients with impaired liver function and neurotoxicity. Frequently monitor patients for myelosuppression both during and after therapy. Granulocytopenia is dose-limiting. **Intrathecal administration may result in death**. Use with caution in patients with cachexia or ulcerated skin.

Acute shortness of breath and severe bronchospasm have been reported, most commonly when administered with mitomycin. Fatal cases of interstitial pulmonary changes and ARDS have also been reported. May cause severe constipation (grade 3-4), paralytic ileus, intestinal obstruction, necrosis, and/or perforation.

Adverse Reactions

>10%:

Central nervous system: Fatigue (27%)

Dermatologic: Alopecia (12%)

Gastrointestinal: Nausea (44%, severe <2%) and vomiting (20%) are most common and are easily controlled with standard antiemetics; constipation (35%), diarrhea (17%)

Emetic potential: Moderate (30% to 60%)

Hematologic: May cause severe bone marrow suppression and is the dose-limiting toxicity of vinorelbine; severe granulocytopenia (90%) may occur following the administration of vinorelbine; leukopenia (92%), anemia (83%)

Myelosuppressive:

WBC: Moderate - severe

Onset: 4-7 days

Nadir: 7-10 days

Recovery: 14-21 days

Hepatic: Elevated SGOT (67%), elevated total bilirubin (13%)

Local: Injection site reaction (28%), injection site pain (16%)

(Continued)

Vinorelbine *(Continued)*

Neuromuscular & skeletal: Weakness (36%), peripheral neuropathy (20% to 25%)

1% to 10%:

Cardiovascular: Chest pain (5%)

Gastrointestinal: Paralytic ileus (1%)

Hematologic: Thrombocytopenia (5%)

Local: Phlebitis (7%)

Neuromuscular & skeletal: Mild to moderate peripheral neuropathy manifested by paresthesia and hyperesthesia, loss of deep tendon reflexes (<5%); myalgia (<5%), arthralgia (<5%), jaw pain (<5%)

Respiratory: Dyspnea (3% to 7%)

<1%: Hemorrhagic cystitis, severe peripheral neuropathy (generally reversible), syndrome of inappropriate ADH secretion

Postmarketing and/or case reports: Angioedema, headache, DVT, flushing, hyper-/hypotension, vasodilation, tachycardia, hyponatremia, abdominal pain, dysphagia, esophagitis, mucositis, back pain, gait instability, muscle weakness, anaphylaxis, tumor pain, pancreatitis, pneumonia, pulmonary edema, pulmonary embolus, radiation recall (dermatitis, esophagitis)

Vesicant Yes; moderate. See Management of Drug Extravasations *on page 965*.

Emetic Potential Moderate (30% to 60%)

Overdosage/Toxicology Symptoms of overdose include bone marrow suppression, mental depression, paresthesia, loss of deep tendon reflexes, and neurotoxicity. There are no antidotes for vinorelbine. Treatment is supportive and symptomatic, including fluid restriction or hypertonic saline (3% sodium chloride) for drug-induced secretion of inappropriate antidiuretic hormone (SIADH).

Drug Interactions

Cytochrome P450 Effect: Substrate of CYP2D6 (minor), 3A4 (major); **Inhibits** CYP2D6 (weak), 3A4 (weak)

Increased Effect/Toxicity: Previous or simultaneous use with mitomycin-C has resulted in acute shortness of breath and severe bronchospasm within minutes or several hours after *Vinca* alkaloid injection and may occur up to 2 weeks after the dose of mitomycin. CYP3A4 inhibitors may increase the levels/effects of vinorelbine; example inhibitors include azole antifungals, ciprofloxacin, clarithromycin, diclofenac, doxycycline, erythromycin, imatinib, isoniazid, nefazodone, nicardipine, propofol, protease inhibitors, quinidine, and verapamil. Incidence of granulocytopenia is significantly higher in cisplatin/vinorelbine combination therapy than with single-agent vinorelbine.

Decreased Effect: CYP3A4 inducers may decrease the levels/effects of vinorelbine; example inducers include aminoglutethimide, carbamazepine, nafcillin, nevirapine, phenobarbital, phenytoin, and rifamycins.

Ethanol/Nutrition/Herb Interactions Herb/Nutraceutical: St John's wort may decrease vinorelbine levels.

Storage/Stability Store intact vials under refrigeration (2°C to 8°C) and protect from light; vials are stable at room temperature for up to 72 hours. Dilutions in D_5W or NS are stable for 24 hours at room temperature.

Reconstitution Dilute in 10-50 mL D_5W or NS.

Compatibility Stable in $D_5^1/_2NS$, D_5W, LR, NS, $^1/_2NS$

Y-site administration: Compatible: Amikacin, aztreonam, bleomycin, bumetanide, buprenorphine, butorphanol, calcium gluconate, carboplatin, carmustine, cefotaxime, ceftazidime, ceftizoxime, chlorpromazine, cimetidine, cisplatin, clindamycin, cyclophosphamide, cytarabine, dacarbazine, dactinomycin, daunorubicin, dexamethasone sodium phosphate, diphenhydramine, doxorubicin, doxorubicin liposome, doxycycline, droperidol, enalaprilat, etoposide, famotidine, filgrastim, floxuridine, fluconazole, fludarabine, gatifloxacin, gemcitabine, gentamicin, granisetron, haloperidol, hydrocortisone sodium phosphate, hydrocortisone sodium succinate, hydromorphone, hydroxyzine, idarubicin, ifosfamide, imipenem/cilastatin, lorazepam, mannitol, mechlorethamine, melphalan, meperidine, mesna, methotrexate, metoclopramide, metronidazole, minocycline, mitoxantrone, morphine, nalbuphine, netilmicin, ondansetron, plicamycin, streptozocin, teniposide, ticarcillin, ticarcillin/clavulanate, tobramycin, vancomycin, vinblastine, vincristine, zidovudine. **Incompatible:** Acyclovir, allopurinol, aminophylline, amphotericin B, amphotericin B cholesteryl sulfate complex, ampicillin, cefazolin, cefoperazone, cefotetan, ceftriaxone, cefuroxime, co-trimoxazole, fluorouracil, furosemide, ganciclovir, methylprednisolone sodium succinate, mitomycin, piperacillin, sodium bicarbonate, thiotepa. **Variable (consult detailed reference):** Heparin

Pharmacodynamics/Kinetics

Absorption: Unreliable; must be given I.V.

Distribution: V_d: 25.4-40.1 L/kg; binds extensively to human platelets and lymphocytes (79.6% to 91.2%)

Protein binding: 80% to 90%

Metabolism: Extensively hepatic to two metabolites, deacetylvinorelbine (active) and vinorelbine N-oxide

Bioavailability: Oral: 26% to 45%

Half-life elimination: Triphasic: Terminal: 27.7-43.6 hours

Excretion: Feces (46%); urine (18%, 10% to 12% as unchanged drug)

Clearance: Plasma: Mean: 0.97-1.26 L/hour/kg

Dosage Refer to individual protocols.

Adults: I.V.:

Single-agent therapy: 30 mg/m^2 every 7 days

Combination therapy with cisplatin: 25 mg/m^2 every 7 days (with cisplatin 100 mg/m^2 every 4 weeks); **Alternatively:** 30 mg/m^2 in combination with cisplatin 120 mg/m^2 on days 1 and 29, then every 6 weeks

Dosage adjustment in hematological toxicity: Granulocyte counts should be ≥1000 cells/mm^3 prior to the administration of vinorelbine. Adjustments in the dosage of vinorelbine should be based on granulocyte counts obtained on the day of treatment as follows:

Granulocytes ≥1500 cells/mm^3 on day of treatment: Administer 100% of starting dose

Granulocytes 1000-1499 cells/mm^3 on day of treatment: Administer 50% of starting dose

Granulocytes <1000 cells/mm^3 on day of treatment: Do not administer. Repeat granulocyte count in one week; if 3 consecutive doses are held because granulocyte count is <1000 cells/mm^3, discontinue vinorelbine

(Continued)

Vinorelbine *(Continued)*

For patients who, during treatment, have experienced fever and/or sepsis while granulocytopenic or had 2 consecutive weekly doses held due to granulocytopenia, subsequent doses of vinorelbine should be:

75% of starting dose for granulocytes ≥1500 cells/mm^3

37.5% of starting dose for granulocytes 1000-1499 cells/mm^3

Dosage adjustment in renal impairment: No dose adjustments are required for renal insufficiency.

Dosing adjustment in hepatic impairment: Vinorelbine should be administered with caution in patients with hepatic insufficiency. In patients who develop hyperbilirubinemia during treatment with vinorelbine, the dose should be adjusted for total bilirubin as follows:

Serum bilirubin ≤2 mg/dL: Administer 100% of starting dose

Serum bilirubin 2.1-3 mg/dL: Administer 50% of starting dose

Serum bilirubin >3 mg/dL: Administer 25% of starting dose

Dosing adjustment in patients with concurrent hematologic toxicity and hepatic impairment: Administer the lower doses determined from the above recommendations

Combination Regimens

Breast cancer:

Paclitaxel-Vinorelbine *on page 927*

PV *on page 932*

Cervical cancer: Cisplatin-Vinorelbine *on page 862*

Leukemia, acute lymphocytic: TVTG *on page 942*

Leukemia, acute myeloid: TVTG *on page 942*

Lung cancer (nonsmall cell):

VC *on page 945*

Gemcitabine-Vinorelbine *on page 897*

Vinorelbine-Cis *on page 946*

Vinorelbine-Gemcitabine *on page 946*

Prostate cancer: Estramustine + Vinorelbine *on page 883*

Administration FATAL IF GIVEN INTRATHECALLY. Administer as a direct intravenous push or rapid bolus, over 6-10 minutes (up to 30 minutes). Longer infusions may increase the risk of pain and phlebitis. Intravenous doses should be followed by 150-250 mL of saline or dextrose to reduce the incidence of phlebitis and inflammation.

Dosage Forms Injection, solution, as tartrate [preservative free]: 10 mg/mL (1 mL, 5 mL)

Monitoring Parameters CBC with differential and platelet count, hepatic function tests

Patient Information This medication can only be administered by infusion, usually on a cyclic basis. Maintain adequate hydration (2-3 L/day of fluids unless instructed to restrict fluid intake) and nutrition (small frequent meals will help). You will most likely lose your hair (reversible after therapy); experience nausea or vomiting (request medication); feel weak or lethargic (use caution when driving or engaging in tasks requiring alertness until response to drug is known). Use good oral care to reduce incidence of mouth sores. You will be more susceptible to infection; avoid crowds or exposure to infection. Report weakness, skeletal pain, or tremors; signs of infection (eg, fever, chills, sore throat, burning urination, fatigue); unusual bleeding (eg, tarry stools, easy bruising, blood in stool, urine, or mouth); numbness, pain, or tingling of fingers or toes; unresolved mouth sores; skin rash or itching; uncontrolled nausea, vomiting, or abdominal pain; or difficulty breathing. The drug may cause permanent sterility and may cause birth defects. Contraceptive measures are recommended during therapy. The drug is excreted in breast milk, therefore, an alternative form of feeding your baby should be used.

Selected Readings
Budman DR, "Vinorelbine (Navelbine®): A Third-Generation Vinca Alkaloid," *Cancer Invest*, 1997, 15(5):475-90.

Johnson SA, Harper P, Hortobagyi GN, et al, "Vinorelbine: An Overview," *Cancer Treat Rev*, 1996, 22(2):127-42.

Jones SF and Burris HA 3d, "Vinorelbine: A New Antineoplastic Drug for the Treatment of Nonsmall Cell Lung Cancer," *Ann Pharmacother*, 1996, 30(5):501-6.

LeVeque D and Jehl F, "Clinical Pharmacokinetics of Vinorelbine," *Clin Pharmacokinet*, 1996, 31(3):184-97.

Toso C and Lindley C, "Vinorelbine: A Novel Vinca Alkaloid," *Am J Health Syst Pharm*, 1995, 52(12):1287-304.

Ziconotide (zi KOE no tide)

U.S. Brand Names Prialt®

Generic Available No

Pharmacologic Category Analgesic, Non-narcotic; Calcium Channel Blocker, N-Type

Pregnancy Risk Factor C

Lactation Excretion in breast milk unknown/not recommended

(Continued)

Ziconotide *(Continued)*

Use Management of severe chronic pain in patients requiring intrathecal (I.T.) therapy and are intolerant or refractory to other therapies

Mechanism of Action Ziconotide selectively binds to N-type voltage sensitive calcium channels located on the afferent nerves of the dorsal horn in the spinal cord. This binding is thought to block N-type calcium channels, leading to a blockade of excitatory neurotransmitter release and reducing sensitivity to painful stimuli.

Labeled Contraindications Hypersensitivity to ziconotide or any component of the formulation; history of psychosis; I.V. administration

I.T. administration is contraindicated in patients with infection at the injection site, uncontrolled bleeding, or spinal canal obstruction that impairs CSF circulation

Warnings/Precautions Severe psychiatric symptoms and neurological impairment have been reported; interrupt or discontinue therapy if cognitive impairment, hallucinations, mood changes, or changes in consciousness occur. Cognitive impairment may appear gradually during treatment and is generally reversible after discontinuation. Use caution in the elderly; may experience confusion. Patients should be instructed to use caution in performing tasks which require alertness (eg, operating machinery or driving). May have additive effects with opiates or other CNS-depressant medications. Does not potentiate opiate-induced respiratory depression. Will not prevent or relieve symptoms associated with opiate withdrawal and opiates should not be abruptly discontinued. Unlike opioids, ziconotide therapy can be interrupted abruptly or discontinued without evidence of withdrawal. Meningitis may occur with use of I.T. pumps and treatment may require removal of system and discontinuation of therapy. Safety and efficacy have not been established with renal or hepatic dysfunction, or in pediatric patients.

Adverse Reactions Percentages reported when using the slow (21-day) titration schedule; frequencies may be higher with faster titration.

>10%:

Central nervous system: Dizziness (47%), somnolence (22%), confusion (18%), ataxia (16%), headache (15%), memory impairment (12%), pain (11%)

Gastrointestinal: Nausea (41%), diarrhea (19%), vomiting (15%)

Neuromuscular & skeletal: Weakness (22%), gait disturbances (15%), hypertonia (11%)

2% to 10%:

Cardiovascular: Chest pain, edema, hyper or hypotension, postural hypotension, tachycardia, vasodilation

Central nervous system: Anxiety (9%), speech disorder (9%), aphasia (8%), dysesthesia (7%), fever (7%), hallucinations (7%), nervousness (7%), vertigo (7%), agitation, chills, depression, dreams abnormal, emotional lability, hostility, hyperesthesia, insomnia, malaise, neuralgia, paranoid reaction, stupor

Dermatologic: Bruising, cellulitis, diaphoresis, dry skin, pruritus, rash

Endocrine & metabolic: Hypokalemia

Gastrointestinal: Anorexia (10%), abdominal pain, constipation, dehydration, dyspepsia, taste perversion, weight loss, xerostomia

Genitourinary: Urinary retention (9%), dysuria, urinary incontinence, urinary tract infection, urination impaired

Hematologic: Anemia

Local: Catheter complication, catheter site pain, pump site complication, pump site mass, pump site pain

Neuromuscular & skeletal: Paresthesia (7%), arthralgia, arthritis, back pain, incoordination, leg cramps, myalgia, myasthenia, neck pain, neck rigidity, reflexes decreased, tremor

Ocular: Vision abnormal (10%), nystagmus (8%), diplopia, photophobia,

Otic: Tinnitus

Renal: CPK increased (<2%)

Respiratory: Bronchitis, cough, dyspnea, pharyngitis, pneumonia, rhinitis, sinusitis

Miscellaneous: Flu-like syndrome, infection, CSF abnormalities, meningitis

<2%: Aspiration pneumonia (<1%), atrial fibrillation, cerebral vascular accident, convulsions, electrocardiogram abnormalities, kidney failure (acute), myoclonus, psychosis, respiratory distress, rhabdomyolysis, sepsis, suicidal ideation, suicide (<1%)

Overdosage/Toxicology Exaggerated pharmacological effects, including ataxia, confusion, dizziness, garbled speech, hypotension, nausea, nystagmus, sedation, spinal myoclonus, stupor, unresponsiveness, vomiting and word-finding difficulty, are reported at doses >19.2 mcg/day. Respiratory depression was not observed. In case of overdose, ziconotide can be discontinued temporarily or withdrawn; additional treatment should be symptom directed and supportive. Opioid antagonists are not effective. Most patients recover within 24 hours of discontinuing ziconotide therapy.

Drug Interactions

Increased Effect/Toxicity: May enhance the adverse/toxic effects of other CNS depressants

Storage/Stability Prior to use, store vials at 2°C to 8°C (36°F to 46°F); once diluted, may be stored at 2°C to 8°C (36°F to 46°F) for 24 hours. Do not freeze. Protect from light.

When using the Medtronic SynchroMed® EL or SynchroMed® II Infusion System, solutions expire as follows:

25 mcg/mL: Undiluted:

Initial fill: Use within 14 days

Refill: use within 60 days

100 mcg/mL

Undiluted: Refill: Use within 60 days

Diluted: Refill: Use within 40 days

Reconstitution Preservative free NS should be used when dilution is needed.

Simms Deltec Cadd Micro® External Microinfusion Device and Catheter: Initial fill: Dilute to final concentration of 5 mcg/mL

Pharmacodynamics/Kinetics

Distribution: I.T.: V_d: ~140 mL

Protein binding: 50%

Metabolism: Metabolized via endopeptidases and exopeptidases present on multiple organs including kidney, liver, lung; degraded to peptide fragments and free amino acids

Half-life elimination: I.V.: 1-1.6 hours (plasma); I.T.: 2.9-6.5 hours (CSF)

Excretion: I.V.: Urine (<1%)

(Continued)

Ziconotide *(Continued)*

Dosage I.T.:

Adults: Chronic pain: Initial dose: 2.4 mcg/day (0.1 mcg/hour)

Dose may be titrated by ≤2.4 mcg/day (0.1 mcg/hour) at intervals ≥2-3 times/week to a maximum dose of 19.2 mcg/day (0.8 mcg/hour) by day 21; average dose at day 21: 6.9 mcg/day (0.29 mcg/hour). A faster titration should be used only if the urgent need for analgesia outweighs the possible risk to patient safety.

Elderly: Refer to Adults dosing; use with caution

Dosage adjustment for toxicity: Cognitive impairment: Reduce dose or discontinue; effects are generally reversible within 2 weeks of discontinuation

Administration Not for I.V. administration. **For I.T. administration only** using a Medtronic SynchroMed® EL, SynchroMed® II Infusion System or Simms Deltec Cadd Micro® External Microinfusion Device and Catheter.

Medtronic SynchroMed® EL or SynchroMed® II Infusion Systems:

Naive pump priming (first time use with ziconotide): Use 2 mL of undiluted ziconotide 25 mcg/mL solution to rinse the internal surfaces of the pump; repeat twice for a total of three rinses

Initial pump fill: Use only undiluted 25 mcg/mL solution and fill pump after priming. Following the initial fill only, adsorption on internal device surfaces will occur, requiring the use of the undiluted solution and refill within 14 days.

Pump refills: Contents should be emptied prior to refill. Subsequent pump refills should occur at least every 40 days if using diluted solution or every 60 days if using undiluted solution

Simms Deltec Cadd Micro® External Microinfusion Device and Catheter: Refer to manufacturers' manual for initial fill and refill instructions

Dosage Forms Injection, solution, as acetate [preservative free]: 100 mcg/mL (1 mL, 2 mL, 5 mL); 25 mcg/mL (20 mL)

Monitoring Parameters Monitor for psychiatric or neurological impairment; signs and symptoms of meningitis or other infection; serum CPK (every other week for first month then monthly); pain relief

Special Geriatric Considerations See Warnings/Precautions, Adverse Reactions, and Dosage. Manufacturer reports that in all trials there was a higher incidence of confusion in the elderly compared to younger adults.

Selected Readings

Jain KK, "An Evaluation of Intrathecal Ziconotide for the Treatment of Chronic Pain," *Expert Opin Investig Drugs*, 2000, 9(10):2403-10.

Miljanich GP, "Ziconotide: Neuronal Calcium Channel Blocker for Treating Severe Chronic Pain," *Curr Med Chem*, 2004, 11(23):3029-40.

♦ **Zinecard**® *see* Dexrazoxane *on page 270*

♦ **ZM-182,780** *see* Fulvestrant *on page 372*

♦ **Zofran**® *see* Ondansetron *on page 622*

♦ **Zofran® ODT** *see* Ondansetron *on page 622*

♦ **Zoladex**® *see* Goserelin *on page 403*

♦ **Zoladex® LA (Can)** *see* Goserelin *on page 403*

♦ **Zoledronate** *see* Zoledronic Acid *on page 834*

Zoledronic Acid *(ZOE le dron ik AS id)*

Related Information

Investigational Drug Service *on page 1031*

U.S. Brand Names Zometa®
Canadian Brand Names Zometa®
Generic Available No
Synonyms CGP-42446; Zoledronate
Pharmacologic Category Adjuvant Analgesic, Bisphosphonate
Pregnancy Risk Factor D
Lactation Excretion in breast milk unknown/not recommended
Use Treatment of hypercalcemia of malignancy and bone metastases of solid tumors
Unlabeled/Investigational Use Investigational: Prevention of bone metastases from breast or prostate cancer; treatment of metabolic bone diseases
Mechanism of Action A bisphosphonate which inhibits bone resorption via actions on osteoclasts or on osteoclast precursors; inhibits osteoclastic activity and skeletal calcium release induced by tumors. Decreases serum calcium and phosphorus, and increases their elimination.
Labeled Contraindications Hypersensitivity to zoledronic acid, other bisphosphonates, or any component of the formulation; pregnancy
Warnings/Precautions Osteonecrosis of the jaw has been reported in patients with cancer who were receiving chemotherapy, corticosteroids, and chronic bisphosphonate therapy; symptoms included nonhealing extraction socket or an exposed jawbone. Dental exams and preventative dentistry should be performed prior to placing patients with risk factors (eg, chemotherapy, corticosteroids, poor oral hygiene) on chronic bisphosphonate therapy. Invasive dental procedures should be avoided during treatment.

Use caution in renal dysfunction; dosage adjustment required. Renal toxicity has been reported with doses >4 mg or infusions administered over 15 minutes. Risk factors for renal deterioration include pre-existing renal insufficiency and repeated doses of zoledronic acid and other bisphosphonates. Dehydration and the use of other nephrotoxic drugs which may contribute to renal deterioration should be identified and managed. Use is not recommended in patients with severe renal impairment (serum creatinine >3 mg/dL) and bone metastases (limited data); use in patients with hypercalcemia of malignancy and severe renal impairment should only be done if the benefits outweigh the risks. Renal function should be assessed prior to treatment; if decreased after treatment, additional treatments should be withheld until renal function returns to within 10% of baseline. Adequate hydration is required during treatment (urine output ~2 L/day); avoid overhydration, especially in patients with heart failure; diuretics should not be used before correcting hypovolemia. Renal deterioration, resulting in renal failure and dialysis has occurred in patients treated with zoledronic acid after single and multiple infusions at recommended doses of 4 mg over 15 minutes.

Use caution in patients with aspirin-sensitive asthma (may cause bronchoconstriction), hepatic dysfunction, and the elderly. Women of childbearing age should be advised against becoming pregnant. Safety and efficacy in pediatric patients have not been established.
Adverse Reactions
>10%:
    Cardiovascular: Leg edema (up to 19%)
(Continued)

Zoledronic Acid *(Continued)*

Central nervous system: Fatigue (36%), fever (30% to 44%), headache (up to 18%), insomnia (15%), anxiety (9% to 14%), dizziness (14%), agitation (13%), depression (12%)

Dermatologic: Alopecia (11%)

Endocrine & metabolic: Hypophosphatemia (13%), hypokalemia (12%), dehydration (up to 12%)

Gastrointestinal: Nausea (29% to 45%), constipation (27% to 28%), vomiting (14% to 30%), diarrhea (17% to 22%), abdominal pain (12% to 16%)

Genitourinary: Urinary tract infection (11% to 14%)

Hematologic: Anemia (22% to 29%), neutropenia (11%)

Neuromuscular & skeletal: Myalgia (21%), paresthesia (18%), arthralgia (up to 18%) skeletal pain (12%)

Respiratory: Dyspnea (22% to 24%), cough (12% to 19%)

Miscellaneous Moniliasis (12%)

1% to 10%:

Cardiovascular: Hypotension (10%), chest pain

Central nervous system: Hypoesthesia (10%)

Dermatologic: Dermatitis (10%)

Endocrine & metabolic: Hypomagnesemia (up to 10%), hypocalcemia, hypophosphatemia (9%), hypermagnesemia (Grade 3: 2%)

Gastrointestinal: Anorexia (9%), mucositis, dysphagia

Genitourinary: Urinary tract infection (14%)

Hematologic: Thrombocytopenia, pancytopenia, granulocytopenia

Neuromuscular & skeletal: Rigors (10%), weakness

Renal: Serum creatinine increased

Respiratory: Pleural effusion, upper respiratory tract infection (8%)

<1%: Conjunctivitis, flu-like symptoms, injection site reactions, pruritus, rash

Postmarketing and/or case reports: Osteonecrosis (primarily of the jaws), renal failure

Symptoms of hypercalcemia include polyuria, nephrolithiasis, anorexia, nausea, vomiting, constipation, weakness, fatigue, confusion, stupor, and coma. These may not be drug-related adverse events, but related to the underlying metabolic condition.

Vesicant No

Emetic Potential Very low (<10%)

Overdosage/Toxicology Clinically significant hypocalcemia, hypophosphatemia, and hypomagnesemia may occur.

Drug Interactions

Increased Effect/Toxicity: Aminoglycosides may also lower serum calcium levels; loop diuretics increase risk of hypocalcemia; thalidomide increases renal toxicity

Storage/Stability Store intact vials at 25°C (77°F).

Reconstitution Dilute solution for injection in 100 mL NS or D_5W prior to administration. Infusion of solution must be completed within 24 hours

Compatibility Incompatible with calcium-containing solutions, such as LR

Pharmacodynamics/Kinetics

Onset of action: Maximum effect may not been seen for 7 days

Distribution: Binds to bone

Protein binding: ~22%

Half-life elimination: Triphasic; Terminal: 146 hours

Excretion: Urine (39% ± 16% as unchanged drug) within 24 hours; feces (<3%)

Dosage I.V.: Adults:

Hypercalcemia of malignancy (albumin-corrected serum calcium ≥12 mg/dL): 4 mg (maximum) given as a single dose. Wait at least 7 days before considering retreatment. Dosage adjustment may be needed in patients with decreased renal function following treatment.

Multiple myeloma or metastatic bone lesions from solid tumors: 4 mg given over 15 minutes every 3-4 weeks

Note: Patients should receive a daily calcium supplement and multivitamin containing vitamin D

Dosage adjustment in renal impairment: Mild-to-moderate renal impairment:

Cl_{cr} >60 mL/minute: 4 mg

Cl_{cr} 50-60 mL/minute: 3.5 mg

Cl_{cr} 40-49 mL/minute: 3.3 mg

Cl_{cr} 30-39 mL/minute: 3 mg

Dosage adjustment for renal toxicity:

Hypercalcemia of malignancy: Evidence of renal deterioration: Evaluate risk versus benefit.

Bone metastases: Evidence of renal deterioration: Discontinue further dosing until renal function returns to within 10% of baseline: renal deterioration defined as follows:

Normal baseline creatinine: Increase of 0.5 mg/dL

Abnormal baseline creatinine: Increase of 1 mg/dL

Reinitiate dose at the same dose administered prior to treatment interruption.

Dosage adjustment in hepatic impairment: Specific guidelines are not available.

Administration Infuse over 15-30 minutes. Infuse in a line separate from other medications. Patients should be appropriately hydrated prior to treatment.

Dosage Forms Injection, solution: 4 mg/5 mL (5 mL) [as monohydrate 4.264 mg]

Monitoring Parameters Prior to initiation of therapy, dental exam and preventative dentistry for patients at risk for osteonecrosis; serum creatinine prior to each dose; serum electrolytes, phosphate, magnesium, and hemoglobin/hematocrit should be evaluated regularly. Monitor serum calcium to assess response and avoid overtreatment.

Dietary Considerations Multiple myeloma or metastatic bone lesions from solid tumors: Take daily calcium supplement (500 mg) and daily multivitamin (with 400 int. units vitamin D).

Patient Information This medication can only be administered intravenously. Avoid food high in calcium or vitamins during infusion or for 2-3 hours after completion. You may experience some nausea or vomiting (small frequent meals, good mouth care, sucking lozenges, or chewing gum may help) or recurrent bone pain (consult prescriber for analgesic). Report unusual muscle twitching or spasms, severe diarrhea/constipation, acute bone pain, or other persistent adverse effects.

(Continued)

Zoledronic Acid *(Continued)*

Selected Readings

Green JR, "Preclinical Pharmacology of Zoledronic Acid," *Semin Oncol,* 2002, 29(6 Suppl 21):3-11.

Li EC and Davis LE, "Zoledronic Acid: A New Parenteral Bisphosphonate," *Clin Ther,* 2003, 25(11):2669-708.

Major P, "The Use of Zoledronic Acid, a Novel, Highly Potent Bisphosphonate, for the Treatment of Hypercalcemia of Malignancy," *Oncologist,* 2002, 7(6):481-91.

Perry CM and Figgitt DP, "Zoledronic Acid: A Review of its Use in Patients With Advanced Cancer," *Drugs,* 2004, 64(11):1197-211.

Theriault RL, "Zoledronic Acid (Zometa) Use in Bone Disease," *Expert Rev Anticancer Ther,* 2003, 3(2):157-66.

Wellington K and Goa KL, "Zoledronic Acid: A Review of its Use in the Management of Bone Metastases and Hypercalcaemia of Malignancy," *Drugs,* 2003, 63(4):417-37.

- **Zometa**® *see* Zoledronic Acid *on page 834*
- **Zosyn**® *see* Piperacillin and Tazobactam Sodium *on page 672*
- **Zovirax**® *see* Acyclovir *on page 26*
- **Zyloprim**® *see* Allopurinol *on page 42*

ALPHABETICAL LISTING OF CHEMOTHERAPY REGIMENS

5 + 2

Use Leukemia, acute myeloid (induction)

Regimen

Cytarabine: I.V.: 100-200 mg/m^2/day continuous infusion days 1 to 5
[total dose/cycle = 500-1000 mg/m^2]

   with

Daunorubicin: I.V.: 45 mg/m^2/day days 1 and 2
[total dose/cycle = 90 mg/m^2]

or

Mitoxantrone: I.V.: 12 mg/m^2/day days 1 and 2
[total dose/cycle = 24 mg/m^2]

References

Rai KR, Holland JF, Glidewell OJ, et al, "Treatment of Acute Myelocytic Leukemia: A Study By Cancer and Leukemia Group B," *Blood*, 1981, 58(6):1203-12.

7 + 3 (Daunorubicin)

Use Leukemia, acute myeloid (induction)

Regimen

Cytarabine: I.V.: 100 mg/m^2/day continuous infusion days 1 to 7
[total dose/cycle = 700 mg/m^2]

Daunorubicin: I.V.: 45 mg/m^2/day days 1 to 3
[total dose/cycle = 135 mg/m^2]

Administer one cycle only

References

Dillman RO, Davis RB, Green MR, et al, "A Comparative Study of Two Different Doses of Cytarabine for Acute Myeloid Leukemia: A Phase III Trial of Cancer and Leukemia Group B," *Blood*, 1991, 78(10):2520-6.

Preisler H, Davis RB, Kirshner J, et al, "Comparison of Three Remission Induction Regimens and Two Postinduction Strategies for the Treatment of Acute Nonlymphocytic Leukemia: A Cancer and Leukemia Group B Study," *Blood*, 1987, 69(5):1441-9.

Rai KR, Holland JF, Glidewell OJ, et al, "Treatment of Acute Myelocytic Leukemia: A Study by Cancer and Leukemia Group B," *Blood*, 1981, 58(6):1203-12.

Vogler WR, Velez-Garcia E, Weiner RS, et al, "A Phase III Trial Comparing Idarubicin and Daunorubicin in Combination With Cytarabine in Acute Myelogenous Leukemia: A Southeastern Cancer Study Group Study," *J Clin Oncol*, 1992, 10(7):1103-11.

Yates J, Glidewell O, Wiernik P, et al, "Cytosine Arabinoside With Daunorubicin or Adriamycin® for Therapy of Acute Myelocytic Leukemia: A CALGB Study," *Blood*, 1982, 60(2):454-62.

Yates JW, Wallace HJ Jr, Ellison RR, et al, "Cytosine Arabinoside (NSC-63878) and Daunorubicin (NSC-83142) Therapy in Acute Nonlymphocytic Leukemia," *Cancer Chemother Rep*, 1973, 57(4):485-8.

7 + 3 (Idarubicin)

Use Leukemia, acute myeloid (induction)

Regimen

Cytarabine: I.V.: 100-200 mg/m^2/day continuous infusion days 1 to 7
[total dose/cycle = 700-1400 mg/m^2]

Idarubicin: I.V.: 12 mg/m^2/day days 1 to 3
[total dose/cycle = 36 mg/m^2]

Administer one cycle only

References

Vogler WR, Velez-Garcia E, Weiner RS, et al, "A Phase III Trial Comparing Idarubicin and Daunorubicin in Combination With Cytarabine in Acute Myelogenous Leukemia: A Southeastern Cancer Study Group Study," *J Clin Oncol*, 1992, 10(7):1103-11.

7 + 3 (Mitoxantrone)

Use Leukemia, acute myeloid (induction)

Regimen

Cytarabine: I.V.: 100-200 mg/m^2/day continuous infusion days 1 to 7
  [total dose/cycle = 700-1400 mg/m^2]

Mitoxantrone: I.V.: 12 mg/m^2/day days 1 to 3
  [total dose/cycle = 36 mg/m^2]

Administer one cycle only

References

Arlin Z, Case DC Jr, Moore J, et al, "Randomized Multicenter Trial of Cytosine Arabinoside With Mitoxantrone or Daunorubicin in Previously Untreated Adult Patients With Acute Nonlymphocytic Leukemia (ANLL). Lederle Cooperative Group, *Leukemia*, 1990, 4(3):177-83.

7 + 3 + 7

Use Leukemia, acute myeloid

Regimen

Cytarabine: I.V.: 100 mg/m^2/day continuous infusion days 1 to 7
  [total dose/cycle = 700 mg/m^2]

Daunorubicin: I.V.: 50 mg/m^2/day days 1 to 3
  [total dose/cycle = 150 mg/m^2]

Etoposide: I.V.: 75 mg/m^2/day days 1 to 7
  [total dose/cycle = 525 mg/m^2]

Repeat cycle every 21 days; up to 3 cycles may be given based on individual response

References

Bishop JF, Lowenthal RM, Joshua D, et al, "Etoposide in Acute Nonlymphocytic Leukemia, Australian Leukemia Study Group," *Blood*, 1990, 75(1):27-32.

8 in 1 (Brain Tumors)

Use Brain tumors

Regimen NOTE: Multiple variations are listed below.

Variation 1:

Methylprednisolone: I.V.: 300 mg/m^2 every 6 hours day 1 (3 doses)
  [total dose/cycle = 900 mg/m^2]

Vincristine: I.V.: 1.5 mg/m^2 (maximum 2 mg) day 1
  [total dose/cycle = 1.5 mg/m^2]

Lomustine: Oral: 75 mg/m^2 day 1
  [total dose/cycle = 75 mg/m^2]

Procarbazine: Oral: 75 mg/m^2 day 1; 1 hour after methylprednisolone and vincristine
  [total dose/cycle = 75 mg/m^2]

Hydroxyurea: Oral: 3000 mg/m^2 day 1; 2 hours after methylprednisolone and vincristine
  [total dose/cycle = 3000 mg/m^2]

Cisplatin: I.V.: 90 mg/m^2 day 1; 3 hours after methylprednisolone and vincristine
  [total dose/cycle = 90 mg/m^2]

Cytarabine: I.V.: 300 mg/m^2 day 1; 9 hours after methylprednisolone and vincristine
  [total dose/cycle = 300 mg/m^2]

Dacarbazine: I.V.: 150 mg/m^2 day 1; 12 hours after methylprednisolone and vincristine
  [total dose/cycle = 150 mg/m^2]

Repeat cycle every 14 days

(Continued)

8 in 1 (Brain Tumors) *(Continued)*

Variation 2:

Methylprednisolone: I.V.: 300 mg/m^2 every 6 hours day 1 (3 doses)
[total dose/cycle = 900 mg/m^2]

Vincristine: I.V.: 1.5 mg/m^2 (maximum 2 mg) day 1
[total dose/cycle = 1.5 mg/m^2]

Lomustine: Oral: 75 mg/m^2 day 1
[total dose/cycle = 75 mg/m^2]

Procarbazine: Oral: 75 mg/m^2 day 1; 1 hour after methylprednisolone
and vincristine
[total dose/cycle = 75 mg/m^2]

Hydroxyurea: Oral: 3000 mg/m^2 day 1; 2 hours after methylprednisolone and vincristine
[total dose/cycle = 3000 mg/m^2]

Cisplatin: I.V.: 60 mg/m^2 day 1; 3 hours after methylprednisolone and
vincristine
[total dose/cycle = 60 mg/m^2]

Cytarabine: I.V.: 300 mg/m^2 day 1; 9 hours after methylprednisolone
and vincristine
[total dose/cycle = 300 mg/m^2]

Cyclophosphamide: I.V.: 300 mg/m^2 day 1; 12 hours after methylprednisolone and vincristine
[total dose/cycle = 300 mg/m^2]

Repeat cycle every 14 days

References

Pendergrass TW, Milstein JM, Geyer JR, et al, "Eight Drugs in One Day Chemotherapy for Brain Tumors: Experience in 107 Children and Rationale for Preradiation Chemotherapy," *J Clin Oncol*, 1987, 5(8):1221-31.

8 in 1 (Retinoblastoma)

Use Retinoblastoma

Regimen

Vincristine: I.V.: 1.5 mg/m^2 day 1
[total dose/cycle = 1.5 mg/m^2]

Methylprednisolone: I.V.: 300 mg/m^2 day 1
[total dose/cycle = 300 mg/m^2]

Lomustine: Oral: 75 mg/m^2 day 1
[total dose/cycle = 75 mg/m^2]

Procarbazine: Oral: 75 mg/m^2 day 1
[total dose/cycle = 75 mg/m^2]

Hydroxyurea: Oral: 1500 mg/m^2 day 1
[total dose/cycle = 1500 mg/m^2]

Cisplatin: I.V.: 60 mg/m^2 day 1
[total dose/cycle = 60 mg/m^2]

Cytarabine: I.V.: 300 mg/m^2 day 1
[total dose/cycle = 300 mg/m^2]

Repeat cycle every 28 days

References

Doz F, Khelfaoui F, Mosseri V, et al, "The Role of Chemotherapy in Orbital Involvement of Retinoblastoma. The Experience of a Single Institution With 33 Patients," *Cancer*, 1994, 74(2):722-32.

AAV (DD)
Use Wilms' tumor
Regimen
Dactinomycin: I.V.: 15 mcg/kg/day days 1 to 5 of weeks 0, 13, 26, 39, 52, and 65
[total dose/cycle = 450 mcg/kg]
Doxorubicin: I.V.: 20 mg/m²/day days 1 to 3 of weeks 6, 19, 32, 45, and 58
[total dose/cycle = 300 mg/m²]
Vincristine: I.V.: 1.5 mg/m² day 1 of weeks 0-10, 13, 14, 26, 27, 39, 40, 52, 53, 65, and 66
[total dose/cycle = 31.5 mg/m²]
References
D'Angio GJ, Breslow N, Beckwith JB, et al, "Treatment of Wilms' Tumor. Results of the Third National Wilms' Tumor Study," *Cancer*, 1989, 64(2):349-60.

ABVD
Use Lymphoma, Hodgkin's disease
Regimen
Doxorubicin: I.V.: 25 mg/m²/day days 1 and 15
[total dose/cycle = 50 mg/m²]
Bleomycin: I.V.: 10 units/m²/day days 1 and 15
[total dose/cycle = 20 units/m²]
Vinblastine: I.V.: 6 mg/m²/day days 1 and 15
[total dose/cycle = 12 mg/m²]
Dacarbazine: I.V.: 375 mg/m²/day days 1 and 15
[total dose/cycle = 750 mg/m²]
Repeat cycle every 28 days
References
Bonadonna G, Zucali R, DeLena M, et al, "Combined Chemotherapy (MOPP or ABVD) - Radiotherapy Approach in Advanced Hodgkin's Disease," *Cancer Treat Rep*, 1977, 61(5):769-77.

AC
Use Breast cancer
Regimen NOTE: Multiple variations are listed below.
Variation 1: AC (conventional):
Doxorubicin: I.V.: 60 mg/m² day 1
[total dose/cycle = 60 mg/m²]
Cyclophosphamide: I.V.: 600 mg/m² day 1
[total dose/cycle = 600 mg/m²]
Repeat cycle every 21 days
Variation 2: AC, Paclitaxel (conventional):
Doxorubicin: I.V.: 60 mg/m² day 1
[total dose/cycle = 60 mg/m²]
Cyclophosphamide: I.V.: 600 mg/m² day 1
[total dose/cycle = 60 mg/m²]
Repeats every 21 days for 4 cycles, then:
Paclitaxel: I.V.: 175 mg/m² day 1
[total dose/cycle = 175 mg/m²]
Repeat cycle every 21 days for 4 cycles
Variation 3: AC + Paclitaxel (dose dense)
Doxorubicin: I.V.: 60 mg/m² day 1
[total dose/cycle = 60 mg/m²]
(Continued)

AC *(Continued)*

Cyclophosphamide: I.V.: 600 mg/m² day 1
[total dose/cycle = 600 mg/m²]

Filgrastim: SubQ: 5 mcg/kg for 7 days, beginning day 3
[total dose/cycle = 35-50 mcg/kg]

Repeat cycle every 14 days for 4 cycles

THEN

Paclitaxel: I.V.: 175 mg/m² day 1
[total dose/cycle = 175 mg/m²]

Filgrastim: SubQ: 5 mcg/kg/day for 7 days, beginning day 3
[total dose/cycle = 350 mcg/kg]

Repeat cycle every 14 days for 4 cycles

References

Variation 1:

Fisher B, Brown AM, Dimitrov NV, et al, "Two Months of Doxorubicin-Cyclophosphamide With and Without Interval Reinduction Therapy Compared With 6 Months of Cyclophosphamide, Methotrexate, and Fluorouracil in Positive-Node Breast Cancer Patients With Tamoxifen-Nonresponsive Tumors: Results From the National Surgical Adjuvant Breast and Bowel Project B-15," *J Clin Oncol*, 1990, 8(9):1483-96.

Variation 2:

Henderson IC, Berry DA, Demetri GD, et al, "Improved Outcomes From Adding Sequential Paclitaxel But Not From Escalating Doxorubicin Dose in an Adjuvant Chemotherapy Regimen for Patients With Node-Positive Primary Breast Cancer," *J Clin Oncol*, 2003, 21(6):976-83.

Variation 3:

Citron ML, Berry DA, Cirrincione C, et al, "Randomized Trial of Dose-Dense Versus Conventionally Scheduled and Sequential Versus Concurrent Combination Chemotherapy as Postoperative Adjuvant Treatment of Node-Positive Primary Breast Cancer: First Report of Intergroup Trial C9741/Cancer Leukemia Group B Trial 9741," *J Clin Oncol*, 2003, 21(8):1431-9.

ACAV (J)

Use Wilms' tumor

Regimen

Dactinomycin: I.V.: 15 mcg/kg/day days 1 to 5 of weeks 0, 13, 26, 39, 52, and 65
[total dose/cycle = 450 mcg/kg]

Cyclophosphamide: I.V.: 10 mg/kg/day days 1 to 3 of weeks 0, 6, 13, 19, 26, 32, 39, 45, 52, 58, and 65
[total dose/cycle = 330 mg/kg]

Doxorubicin: I.V.: 20 mg/m²/day days 1 to 3 of weeks 6, 19, 32, 45, and 58
[total dose/cycle = 300 mg/m²]

Vincristine: I.V.: 1.5 mg/m² day 1 of weeks 0-10, 13, 14, 19, 20, 26, 27, 32, 33, 39, 40, 45, 52, 53, 56, 57, 65, and 66
[total dose/cycle = 42 mg/m²]

References

D'Angio GJ, Breslow N, Beckwith JB, et al, "Treatment of Wilms' Tumor. Results of the Third National Wilms' Tumor Study," *Cancer*, 1989, 64(2):349-60.

AD

Use Soft tissue sarcoma

Regimen

Doxorubicin: I.V.: 60 mg/m²/day day 1
[total dose/cycle = 60 mg/m²]

Dacarbazine: I.V.: 250 mg/m² days 1 to 5
[total dose/cycle = 1250 mg/m²]

Repeat cycle every 21 days

References
Borden EC, Amato DA, Rosenbaum C, et al, "Randomized Comparison of Three Adriamycin Regimens for Metastatic Soft Tissue Sarcomas," *J Clin Oncol*, 1987, 5(6):840-50.

♦ **AlinC 14** *see* PVA (POG 8602) *on page 932*

AP

Use Endometrial cancer
Regimen
Doxorubicin: I.V.: 60 mg/m² day 1
[total dose/cycle = 60 mg/m²]
Cisplatin: I.V.: 60 mg/m² day 1
[total dose/cycle = 60 mg/m²]
Repeat cycle every 21 days
References
Barrett RJ, Blessing JA, Homesley HD, et al, "Circadian-Timed Combination Doxorubicin-Cisplatin Chemotherapy for Advanced Endometrial Carcinoma. A Phase II Study of the Gynecologic Oncology Group," *Am J Clin Oncol*, 1993, 16(6):494-6.

AV (EE)

Use Wilms' tumor
Regimen
Dactinomycin: I.V.: 15 mcg/kg/day days 1 to 5 of weeks 0, 5, 13, and 26
[total dose/cycle = 300 mcg/kg]
Vincristine: I.V.: 1.5 mg/m²/dose day 1 of weeks 0-10, 13, 14, 16, and 17
[total dose/cycle = 22.5 mg/m²]
References
D'Angio GJ, Breslow N, Beckwith JB, et al, "Treatment of Wilms' Tumor. Results of the Third National Wilms' Tumor Study," *Cancer*, 1989, 64(2):349-60.

AV (K)

Use Wilms' tumor
Regimen
Dactinomycin: I.V.: 15 mcg/kg/day days 1 to 5 of weeks 0, 5, 13, 22, 31, 40, 49, and 58
[total dose/cycle = 600 mcg/kg]
Vincristine: I.V.: 1.5 mg/m²/dose day 1 of weeks 0-10, 15-20, 24-29, 33-38, 42-47, 51-56, and 60-65
[total dose/cycle = 70.5 mg/m²]
References
D'Angio GJ, Breslow N, Beckwith JB, et al, "Treatment of Wilms' Tumor. Results of the Third National Wilms' Tumor Study," *Cancer*, 1989, 64(2):349-60.

AV (L)

Use Wilms' tumor
Regimen
Dactinomycin: I.V.: 15 mcg/kg/day days 1 to 5 of weeks 0 and 5
[total dose/cycle = 450 mcg/kg]
Vincristine: I.V.: 1.5 mg/m² day 1 of weeks 0-10
[total dose/cycle = 16.5 mg/m²]
References
D'Angio GJ, Breslow N, Beckwith JB, et al, "Treatment of Wilms' Tumor. Results of the Third National Wilms' Tumor Study," *Cancer*, 1989, 64(2):349-60.

AV (Wilms' Tumor)
Use Wilms' tumor
Regimen
> Dactinomycin: I.V.: 15 mcg/kg/day days 1 to 5 of weeks 0, 13, 26, 39, 52, and 65
> [total dose/cycle = 450 mcg/kg]
> Vincristine: I.V.: 1.5 mg/m^2/dose day 1 of weeks 0-8, 13, 14, 26, 27, 39, 40, 52, 53, 65, and 66
> [total dose/cycle = 28.5 mg/m^2]

References
Green DM, Breslow NE, Evans I, et al, "Treatment of Children With Stage IV Favorable Histology Wilms Tumor: A Report From the National Wilms Tumor Study Group," *Med Pediatr Oncol*, 1996, 26(3):147-52.

AVD
Use Wilms' tumor
Regimen
> Dactinomycin: I.V.: 15 mcg/kg/day days 1 to 5 of weeks 0, 13, 26, 39, 52, and 65
> [total dose/cycle = 450 mcg/kg]
> Doxorubicin: I.V.: 20 mg/m^2/day days 1 to 3 of weeks 6, 19, 32, 45, and 58
> [total dose/cycle = 300 mg/m^2]
> Vincristine: I.V.: 1.5 mg/m^2 day 1 of weeks 0-8, 13, 14, 26, 27, 39, 40, 52, 53, 65, and 66
> [total dose/cycle = 28.5 mg/m^2]

References
Green DM, Breslow NE, Evans I, et al, "Treatment of Children With Stage IV Favorable Histology Wilms Tumor: A Report From the National Wilms Tumor Study Group," *Med Pediatr Oncol*, 1996, 26(3):147-52.

♦ **Baby Brain I** *see* COPE *on page 866*

BEACOPP
Use Lymphoma, Hodgkin's disease
Regimen
> Bleomycin: I.V.: 10 units/m^2 day 8
> [total dose/cycle = 10 units/m^2]
> Etoposide: I.V.: 100 mg/m^2/day days 1 to 3
> [total dose/cycle = 300 mg/m^2]
> Doxorubicin: I.V.: 25 mg/m^2 day 1
> [total dose/cycle = 25 mg/m^2]
> Cyclophosphamide: I.V.: 650 mg/m^2 day 1
> [total dose/cycle = 650 mg/m^2]
> Vincristine: I.V.: 1.4 mg/m^2 (maximum 2 mg) day 1
> [total dose/cycle = 1.4 mg/m^2]
> Procarbazine: Oral: 100 mg/m^2/day days 1 to 7
> [total dose/cycle = 700 mg/m^2]
> Prednisone: Oral: 40 mg/m^2/day days 1 to 14
> [total dose/cycle = 560 mg/m^2]
> Repeat cycle every 21 days

References
Diehl V, Franklin J, Hasenclever D, et al, "BEACOPP, a New Dose-Escalated and Accelerated Regimen, Is at Least as Effective as COPP/ABVD in Patients With Advanced-Stage Hodgkin's Lymphoma: Interim Report From a Trial of the German Hodgkin's Lymphoma Study Group," *J Clin Oncol*, 1998, 16(12):3810-21.

BEP (Ovarian)

Use Ovarian cancer

Regimen

Bleomycin: I.V.: 20 units/m^2 day 1
[total dose/cycle = 20 units/m^2]
Etoposide: I.V.: 75 mg/m^2/day days 1 to 5
[total dose/cycle = 375 mg/m^2]
Cisplatin: I.V.: 20 mg/m^2/day days 1 to 5
[total dose/cycle = 100 mg/m^2]
Repeat cycle every 3 weeks

References

Homesley HD, Bundy BN, Hurteau JA, et al, "Bleomycin, Etoposide, and Cisplatin Combination Therapy of Ovarian Granulosa Cell Tumors and Other Stromal Malignancies: A Gynecologic Oncology Group Study," *Gynecol Oncol*, 1999, 72(2):131-7.

BEP (Ovarian, Testicular)

Use Ovarian cancer; Testicular cancer

Regimen

Bleomycin: I.V.: 30 units/day days 2, 9, and 16
[total dose/cycle = 90 units]
Etoposide: I.V.: 100 mg/m^2/day days 1 to 5
[total dose/cycle = 500 mg/m^2]
or 120 mg/m^2/day days 1 to 3
[total dose/cycle = 360 mg/m^2]
Cisplatin: I.V.: 20 mg/m^2/day days 1 to 5
[total dose/cycle = 100 mg/m^2]
Repeat cycle every 21 days

References

Horwich A, Sleijfer DT, Fossa SD, et al, "Randomized Trial of Bleomycin, Etoposide, and Cisplatin Compared With Bleomycin, Etoposide, and Carboplatin in Good-Prognosis Metastatic Nonseminomatous Germ Cell Cancer: A Multiinstitutional Medical Research Council/European Organization for Research and Treatment of Cancer Trial," *J Clin Oncol*, 1997, 15(5):1844-52.

Nichols CR, Catalano PJ, Crawford ED, et al, "Randomized Comparison of Cisplatin and Etoposide and Either Bleomycin or Ifosfamide in Treatment of Advanced Disseminated Germ Cell Tumors: An Eastern Cooperative Oncology Group, Southwest Oncology Group, and Cancer and Leukemia Group B Study," *J Clin Oncol*, 1998, 16(4):1287-93.

Williams S, Blessing JA, Liao SY, et al, "Adjuvant Therapy of Ovarian Germ Cell Tumors With Cisplatin, Etoposide, and Bleomycin: A Trial of the Gynecologic Oncology Group," *J Clin Oncol*, 1994, 12(4):701-6.

BEP (Testicular)

Use Testicular cancer

Regimen NOTE: Multiple variations are listed below.

Variation 1:

Bleomycin: I.V.: 30 units/day days 2, 9, and 16
[total dose/cycle = 90 units]
Etoposide: I.V.: 100 mg/m^2/day days 1 to 5
[total dose/cycle = 500 mg/m^2]
Cisplatin: I.V.: 20 mg/m^2/day days 1 to 5
[total dose/cycle = 100 mg/m^2]
Repeat cycle every 21 days

(Continued)

BEP (Testicular) *(Continued)*

Variation 2:

Bleomycin: I.V.: 30 units once weekly
[total dose/cycle = 90 units]

Etoposide: I.V.: 120 mg/m^2/day days 1, 3, and 5
[total dose/cycle = 360 mg/m^2]

Cisplatin: I.V.: 20 mg/m^2/day days 1 to 5
[total dose/cycle = 100 mg/m^2]

Repeat cycle every 21 days

Variation 3:

Bleomycin: I.V.: 30 units/day days 1, 8, and 15
[total dose/cycle = 90 units]

Etoposide: I.V.: 165 mg/m^2/day days 1 to 3
[total dose/cycle = 495 mg/m^2]

Cisplatin: I.V.: 50 mg/m^2/day days 1 and 2
[total dose/cycle = 100 mg/m^2]

Repeat cycle every 21 days

References

Variation 1:

Williams SD, Birch R, Einhorn LH, et al, "Treatment of Disseminated Germ-Cell Tumors With Cisplatin, Bleomycin, and Either Vinblastine or Etoposide," *N Engl J Med*, 1987, 316(23):1435-40.

Variation 2:

de Wit R, Stoter G, Sleijfer DT, et al, "Four Cycles of BEP vs Four Cycles of VIP in Patients With Intermediate-Prognosis Metastatic Testicular Nonseminoma: A Randomized Study of the EORTC Genitourinary Tract Cancer Cooperative Group. European Organization for Research and Treatment of Cancer," *Br J Cancer*, 1998, 78(6):828-32.

Variation 3:

de Wit R, Roberts JT, Wilkinson PM, et al, "Equivalence of Three or Four Cycles of Bleomycin, Etoposide, and Cisplatin Chemotherapy and of a 3- or 5-Day Schedule in Good-Prognosis Germ Cell Cancer: A Randomized Study of the European Organization for Research and Treatment of Cancer Genitourinary Tract Cancer Cooperative Group and the Medical Research Council," *J Clin Oncol*, 2001, 19(6):1629-40.

♦ **BI** *see* Bicalutamide + LHRH-A *on page 848*

Bicalutamide + LHRH-A

Synonyms BI; BZ

Use Prostate cancer

Regimen

Bicalutamide: Oral: 50 mg/day
[total dose/cycle = 50 mg]
with

Goserelin acetate: SubQ: 3.6 mg day 1
[total dose/cycle = 3.6 mg]
or

Leuprolide depot: I.M.: 7.5 mg day 1
[total dose/cycle = 7.5 mg]

Repeat cycle every 28 days

References

Schellhammer PF, Sharifi R, Block NL, et al, "A Controlled Trial of Bicalutamide Versus Flutamide, Each in Combination With Luteinizing Hormone-Releasing Hormone Analogue Therapy, in Patients With Advanced Prostate Cancer. Casodex Combination Study Group." *Urology*, 1995, 45(5):745-52.

BOLD

Use Melanoma

Regimen

Dacarbazine: I.V.: 200 mg/m^2/day days 1 to 5
[total dose/cycle = 1000 mg/m^2]
Vincristine: I.V.: 1 mg/m^2/day days 1 and 4
[total dose/cycle = 2 mg/m^2]
Bleomycin: I.V.: 15 units/day days 2 and 5
[total dose/cycle = 30 units]
Lomustine: Oral: 80 mg day 1
[total dose/cycle = 80 mg]
Repeat cycle every 4 weeks

References

Nathan FE, Berd D, Sato T, et al, "BOLD + Interferon in the Treatment of Metastatic Uveal Melanoma: First Report of Active Systemic Therapy," *J Exp Clin Cancer Res*, 1997, 16(2):201-8.

Punt CJ, van Herpen CM, Janasen RL, et al, "Chemoimmunotherapy With Bleomycin, Vincristine, Lomustine, Dacarbazine (BOLD) Plus Interferon Alpha for Metastatic Melanoma: A Multicentre Phase II Study," *Br J Cancer*, 1997, 76(2):266-9.

♦ **BZ** *see Bicalutamide + LHRH-A on page 848*

CA

Use Leukemia, acute myeloid

Regimen

Cytarabine: I.V.: 3000 mg/m^2 every 12 hours days 1 and 2 (4 doses)
[total dose/cycle = 12,000 mg/m^2]
Asparaginase: I.M.: 6000 units/m^2 at hour 42
[total dose/cycle = 6000 units/m^2]
Repeat cycle every 7 days for 2 or 3 cycles

References

Capizzi RL, Davis R, Powell B, et al, "Synergy Between High-Dose Cytarabine and Asparaginase in the Treatment of Adults With Refractory and Relapsed Acute Myelogenous Leukemia: A Cancer and Leukemia Group B Study," *J Clin Oncol*, 1988, 6(3):499-508.

CABO

Use Head and neck cancer

Regimen

Cisplatin: I.V.: 50 mg/m^2 day 4
[total dose/cycle = 50 mg/m^2]
Methotrexate: I.V.: 40 mg/m^2/day days 1 and 15
[total dose/cycle = 80 mg/m^2]
Bleomycin: I.V.: 10 units/day days 1, 8, and 15
[total dose/cycle = 30 units]
Vincristine: I.V.: 2 mg/day days 1, 8, and 15
[total dose/cycle = 6 mg]
Repeat cycle every 21 days

References

Clavel M, Vermorken JB, Cognetti F, et al, "Randomized Comparison of Cisplatin, Methotrexate, Bleomycin, and Vincristine (CABO) Versus Cisplatin and 5-Fluorouracil (CF) Versus Cisplatin in Recurrent or Metastatic Squamous Cell Carcinoma of the Head and Neck. A Phase III Study of the EORTC Head and Neck Cancer Cooperative Group," *Ann Oncol*, 1994, 5(6):521-6.

CAD/MOPP/ABV

Use Lymphoma, Hodgkin's disease

Regimen

CAD:

Lomustine: Oral: 100 mg/m² day 1

[total dose/cycle = 100 mg/m²]

Melphalan: Oral: 6 mg/m²/day days 1 to 4

[total dose/cycle = 24 mg/m²]

Vindesine: I.V.: 3 mg/m²/day days 1 and 8

[total dose/cycle = 6 mg/m²]

MOPP:

Mechlorethamine: I.V.: 6 mg/m²/day days 1 and 8

[total dose/cycle = 12 mg/m²]

Vincristine: I.V.: 1.4 mg/m²/day days 1 and 8

[total dose/cycle = 2.8 mg/m²]

Procarbazine: Oral: 100 mg/m²/day days 1 to 14

[total dose/cycle = 1400 mg/m²]

Prednisone: Oral: 40 mg/m²/day days 1 to 14

[total dose/cycle = 560 mg/m²]

ABV:

Doxorubicin: I.V.: 25 mg/m²/day days 1 and 14

[total dose/cycle = 50 mg/m²]

Bleomycin: SubQ: 6 units/m²/day days 1 and 14

[total dose/cycle = 12 units/m²]

Vinblastine: I.V.: 2 mg/m² continuous infusion days 4 to 12 and 18 to 26

[total dose/cycle = 36 mg/m²]

CAD is administered first, then MOPP begins on day 29 or day 37 following CAD. ABV is administered on day 29 following MOPP; CAD recycles on day 29 following ABV.

References

Straus DJ, Myers J, Koziner B, et al, "Combination Chemotherapy for the Treatment of Hodgkin's Disease in Relapse. Results With Lomustine (CCNU), Melphalan (Alkeran), and Vindesine (DVA) Alone (CAD) and in Alternation With MOPP and Doxorubicin (Adriamycin), Bleomycin, and Vinblastine (ABV)," *Cancer Chemother Pharmacol*, 1983, 11(2):80-5.

CAF

Use Breast cancer

Regimen NOTE: Multiple variations are listed below.

Variation 1:

Cyclophosphamide: Oral: 100 mg/m²/day days 1 to 14

[total dose/cycle = 1400 mg/m²]

Doxorubicin: I.V.: 30 mg/m²/day days 1 and 8

[total dose/cycle = 60 mg/m²]

Fluorouracil: I.V.: 500 mg/m²/day days 1 and 8

[total dose/cycle = 1000 mg/m²]

Repeat cycle every 28 days

Variation 2:

Cyclophosphamide: Oral: 100 mg/m²/day days 1 to 14

[total dose/cycle = 1400 mg/m²]

Doxorubicin: I.V.: 25 mg/m²/day days 1 and 8

[total dose/cycle = 50 mg/m²]

Fluorouracil: I.V.: 500 mg/m²/day days 1 and 8

[total dose/cycle = 1000 mg/m²]

Repeat cycle every 28 days

References
Variation 1:
  Bull JM, Tormey DC, Li SH, et al, "A Randomized Comparative Trial of Adriamycin® Versus Methotrexate in Combination Drug Therapy," *Cancer*, 1978, 41(5):1649-57.
Variation 2:
  Aisner J, Weinberg V, Perloff M, et al, "Chemotherapy Versus Chemoimmunotherapy (CAF v CAFVP v CMF each +/- MER) for Metastatic Carcinoma of the Breast," *J Clin Oncol*, 1987, 5(10):1523-33.

♦ **CAF-IV** *see FAC on page 884*

CAP
Use Bladder cancer
Regimen
Cyclophosphamide: I.V.: 400 mg/m² day 1
  [total dose = 400 mg/m²]
Doxorubicin: I.V.: 40 mg/m² day 1
  [total dose = 40 mg/m²]
Cisplatin: I.V.: 60 mg/m² day 1
  [total dose = 60 mg/m²]
Repeat cycle every 21 days

References
Eagan RT, Frytak S, Creagan ET, et al, "Phase II Study of Cyclophosphamide, Adriamycin, and Cis-Dichlorodiammineplatinum (II) by Infusion in Patients With Adenocarcinoma and Large Cell Carcinoma of the Lung," *Cancer Treat Rep*, 1979, 63(9-10):1589-91.

♦ **CapOx** *see XelOx on page 949*

Carbo-Tax (Adenocarcinoma)
Synonyms Paclitaxel, Carboplatin
Use Adenocarcinoma, unknown primary
Regimen
Paclitaxel: I.V.: 135 mg/m² infused over 24 hours day 1,
  [total dose = 135 mg/m²] **followed by**
Carboplatin: I.V.: Target AUC 7.5
  [total dose = AUC = 7.5]
Repeat cycle every 21 days

References
Sulkes A, Uziely B, Isacson R, et al, "Combination Chemotherapy in Metastatic Tumors of Unknown Origin. 5-Fluorouracil, Adriamycin® and Mitomycin C for Adenocarcinomas and Adriamycin®, Vinblastine and Mitomycin C for Anaplastic Carcinomas," *Isr J Med Sci*, 1988, 24(9-10):604-10.

Carbo-Tax (Nonsmall Cell Lung Cancer)
Use Lung cancer, nonsmall cell
Regimen
Paclitaxel: I.V.: 135-215 mg/m² infused over 24 hours day 1
  [total dose/cycle = 135-215 mg/m²]
or 175 mg/m² infused over 3 hours day 1
  [total dose/cycle = 175 mg/m²]
followed by
Carboplatin: I.V.: Target AUC 7.5
  [total dose/cycle = AUC = 7.5]
Repeat cycle every 21 days
(Continued)

Carbo-Tax (Nonsmall Cell Lung Cancer)
(Continued)

References
Langer CJ, Leighton JC, Comis RL, et al, "Paclitaxel By 24- or 1-hour Infusion in Combination With Carboplatin in Advanced Nonsmall-cell Lung Cancer: The Fox Chase Cancer Center Experience," *Semin Oncol*, 1995, 22(4 Suppl 9):18-29.

Carbo-Tax (Ovarian Cancer)
Use Ovarian cancer

Regimen NOTE: Multiple variations are listed below.

Variation 1:

Paclitaxel: I.V.: 135 mg/m² infused over 24 hours day 1
[total dose/cycle = 135 mg/m²]
or 175 mg/m² over 3 hours day 1
[total dose/cycle = 175 mg/m²]
followed by
Carboplatin: I.V.: Target AUC 5
[total dose/cycle = AUC = 5]
Repeat cycle every 21 days

Variation 2:

Paclitaxel: I.V.: 175 mg/m² day 1
[total dose/cycle = 175 mg/m²]
Carboplatin: I.V.: AUC 7.5 day 1
[total dose/cycle = AUC = 7.5]
Repeat cycle every 21 days

Variation 3:

Paclitaxel: I.V.: 185 mg/m² day 1
[total dose/cycle = 185 mg/m²]
Carboplatin: I.V.: AUC 6 day 1
[total dose/cycle = AUC = 6]
Repeat cycle every 21 days

References
Variation 1:
Ozols RF, "Carboplatin and Paclitaxel in Ovarian Cancer," *Semin Oncol*, 1995, 22(3 Suppl 6):78-83.
Ozols RF, "Update of the NCCN Ovarian Cancer Practice Guidelines," *Oncology (Huntingt)*, 1997, 11(11A):95-105.
Variation 2:
Ozols RF, "Combination Regimens of Paclitaxel and the Platinum Drugs as First-Line Regimens for Ovarian Cancer," *Semin Oncol*, 1995, 22(6 Suppl 15):1-6.
Variation 3:
Meerpohl HG, du Bois A, Kuhnle H, et al, "Paclitaxel Combined With Carboplatin in the First-Line Treatment of Advanced Ovarian Cancer," *Semin Oncol*, 1995, 22(6 Suppl 15):7-12.

CaT (Nonsmall Cell Lung Cancer)
Use Lung cancer, nonsmall cell

Regimen NOTE: Multiple variations are listed below.

Variation 1:

Paclitaxel: I.V.: 175 mg/m² day 1
[total dose/cycle = 175 mg/m²]
or 135 mg/m² continuous infusion day 1
[total dose/cycle = 135 mg/m²]
Carboplatin: I.V.: AUC 7.5 day 1 or 2
[total dose/cycle = AUC = 7.5]

Repeat cycle every 21 days
Variation 2:
    Paclitaxel: I.V.: 225 mg/m² day 1
        [total dose/cycle = 225 mg/m²]
    Carboplatin: I.V.: AUC 6 day 1
        [total dose/cycle = AUC = 6]
    Repeat cycle every 21 days

References

Variation 1:
    Langer CJ, Leighton JC, Comis RL, et al, "Paclitaxel by 24- or 1-Hour Infusion in Combination With Carboplatin in Advanced Nonsmall-Cell Lung Cancer: The Fox Chase Cancer Center Experience," *Semin Oncol*, 1995, 22(4 Suppl 9):18-29.
Variation 2:
    Schiller JH, Harrington D, Belani CP, et al, "Comparison of Four Chemotherapy Regimens for Advanced Nonsmall-Cell Lung Cancer," *N Engl J Med*, 2002, 346(2):92-8.

CaT (Ovarian Cancer)

Use Ovarian cancer

Regimen

Paclitaxel: I.V.: 175 mg/m² day 1
    [total dose/cycle = 175 mg/m²]
or 135 mg/m² continuous infusion day 1
    [total dose/cycle = 135 mg/m²]
Carboplatin: I.V.: AUC 7.5 day 1 or 2
    [total dose/cycle = AUC = 7.5]
Repeat cycle every 21 days

References

Bookman MA, McGuire WP 3rd, Kilpatrick D, et al, "Carboplatin and Paclitaxel in Ovarian Carcinoma: A Phase I Study of the Gynecologic Oncology Group," *J Clin Oncol*, 1996, 14(6):1895-902.

CAVE

Use Lung cancer, small cell

Regimen

Cyclophosphamide: I.V.: 750 mg/m² day 1
    [total dose/cycle = 750 mg/m²]
Doxorubicin: I.V.: 50 mg/m² day 1
    [total dose/cycle = 50 mg/m²]
Vincristine: I.V.: 1.4 mg/m² (maximum 2 mg) day 1
    [total dose/cycle = 1.4 mg/m²]
Etoposide: I.V.: 60-100 mg/m²/day days 1 to 3
    [total dose/cycle = 180-300 mg/m²]
Repeat cycle every 21 days

References

Jett JR, Everson L, Therneau TM, et al, "Treatment of Limited-Stage Small-Cell Lung Cancer With Cyclophosphamide, Doxorubicin, And Vincristine With Or Without Etoposide: A Randomized Trial of the North Central Cancer Treatment Group," *J Clin Oncol*, 1990, 8(1):33-8.
Sufarlan AW and Zainudin BM, "Combination Chemotherapy For Small Cell Lung Cancer," *Med J Malaysia*, 1993, 48(2):166-70.

CAV-P/VP

Use Neuroblastomas

Regimen

Course 1, 2, 4, and 6:
    Cyclophosphamide: I.V.: 70 mg/kg/day days 1 and 2
        [total dose/cycle = 140 mg/kg]
(Continued)

CAV-P/VP *(Continued)*

Doxorubicin: I.V.: 25 mg/m^2/day continuous infusion days 1 to 3
[total dose/cycle = 75 mg/m^2]

Vincristine: I.V.: 0.033 mg/kg/day continuous infusion days 1 to 3
[total dose/cycle = .099 mg/kg]

Vincristine: I.V.: 1.5 mg/m^2 day 9
[total dose/cycle = 1.5 mg/m^2]

Course 3, 5, and 7:

Etoposide: I.V.: 200 mg/m^2/day days 1 to 3
[total dose/cycle = 600 mg/m^2]

Cisplatin: I.V.: 50 mg/m^2/day days 1 to 4
[total dose/cycle = 200 mg/m^2]

References

Kushner BH, LaQuaglia MP, Bonilla MA, et al, "Highly Effective Induction Therapy for Stage 4 Neuroblastoma in Children Over 1 Year of Age," *J Clin Oncol*, 1994, 12(12):2607-13.

CC

Use Ovarian cancer

Regimen

Carboplatin: I.V.: Target AUC 5-7.5 day 1
[total dose/cycle = AUC = 5-7.5]

Cyclophosphamide: I.V.: 600 mg/m^2 day 1
[total dose/cycle = 600 mg/m^2]

Repeat cycle every 28 days

References

Alberts DS, Green S, Hannigan EV, et al, "Improved Therapeutic Index of Carboplatin Plus Cyclophosphamide Versus Cisplatin Plus Cyclophosphamide: Final Report by the Southwest Oncology Group of a Phase III Randomized Trial in Stages III and IV Ovarian Cancer," *J Clin Oncol*, 1992, 10(5):706-17.

Swenerton K, Jeffrey J, Stuart G, et al, "Cisplatin-Cyclophosphamide Versus Carboplatin-Cyclophosphamide in Advanced Ovarian Cancer: A Randomized Phase III Study of the National Cancer Institute of Canada Clinical Trials Group," *J Clin Oncol*, 1992, 10(5):718-26.

CCCDE (Retinoblastoma)

Use Retinoblastoma

Regimen

Cyclophosphamide: I.V.: 150 mg/m^2/day days 1 to 7
[total dose/cycle = 1050 mg/m^2]

Cyclophosphamide: Oral: 150 mg/m^2/day days 22 to 28 and 43 to 49
[total dose/cycle = 2100 mg/m^2]

Doxorubicin: I.V.: 35 mg/m^2/day days 10 and 52
[total dose/cycle = 70 mg/m^2]

Cisplatin: I.V.: 90 mg/m^2/day days 8, 50, and 71
[total dose/cycle = 270 mg/m^2]

Etoposide: I.V.: 150 mg/m^2/day continuous infusion days 29 to 31 and 73 to 75
[total dose/cycle = 900 mg/m^2]

References

Advani SH, Rao SR, Iyer RS, et al, "Pilot Study of Sequential Combination Chemotherapy in Advanced and Recurrent Retinoblastoma," *Med Pediatr Oncol*, 1994, 22(2):125-8.

CCDDT (Neuroblastomas)

Use Neuroblastomas

Regimen

Cyclophosphamide: I.V.: 40 mg/kg/day days 1 and 2
[total dose/cycle = 80 mg/kg]
Cisplatin: I.V.: 20 mg/m^2/day days 1 to 5
[total dose/cycle = 100 mg/m^2]
Teniposide: I.V.: 100 mg/m^2 day 7
[total dose/cycle = 100 mg/m^2]
Doxorubicin: I.V.: 60 mg/m^2 day 1
[total dose/cycle = 60 mg/m^2]
Dacarbazine: I.V.: 250 mg/m^2/day days 1 to 5
[total dose/cycle = 1250 mg/m^2]
Repeat cycle every 21-28 days

References

Ikeda K, Nakagawara A, Yano H, et al, "Improved Survival Rates in Children Over 1 Year of Age With Stage III or IV Neuroblastoma Following an Intensive Chemotherapeutic Regimen," *J Pediatr Surg*, 1989, 24(2):189-93.

CCDT (Melanoma)

Use Melanoma

Regimen

Dacarbazine: I.V.: 220 mg/m^2/day days 1 to 3, every 21 to 28 days
[total dose/cycle = 660 mg/m^2]
Carmustine: I.V.: 150 mg/m^2 day 1, every 42 to 56 days
[total dose/cycle = 150 mg/m^2]
Cisplatin: I.V.: 25 mg/m^2/day days 1 to 3, every 21 to 28 days
[total dose/cycle = 75 mg/m^2]
Tamoxifen: Oral: 20 mg/day (use of tamoxifen is optional)

References

Del Prete SA, Maurer LH, O'Donnell J, et al, "Combination Chemotherapy With Cisplatin, Carmustine, Dacarbazine, and Tamoxifen in Metastatic Melanoma," *Cancer Treat Rep*, 1984, 68(11):1403-5.

Rusthoven JJ, Quirt IC, Iscoe NA, et al, "Randomized, Double-Blind, Placebo-Controlled Trial Comparing the Response Rates of Carmustine, Dacarbazine, and Cisplatin With and Without Tamoxifen in Patients With Metastatic Melanoma. National Cancer Institute of Canada Clinical Trials Group," *J Clin Oncol*, 1996, 14(7):2083-90.

CCT (Neuroblastomas)

Use Neuroblastomas

Regimen

Cyclophosphamide: I.V.: 40 mg/kg/day days 1 and 2
[total dose/cycle = 80 mg/kg]
Cisplatin: I.V.: 20 mg/m^2/day days 22 to 26
[total dose/cycle = 100 mg/m^2]
Teniposide: I.V.: 100 mg/m^2 day 28
[total dose/cycle = 100 mg/m^2]
Repeat every 42 days for 3 cycles

References

Ikeda K, Nakagawara A, Yano H, et al, "Improved Survival Rates in Children Over 1 Year of Age With Stage III or IV Neuroblastoma Following an Intensive Chemotherapeutic Regimen," *J Pediatr Surg*, 1989, 24(2):189-93.

CDDP/VP-16
Use Brain tumors
Regimen
  Cisplatin: I.V.: 90 mg/m² day 1
    [total dose/cycle = 90 mg/m²]
  Etoposide: I.V.: 150 mg/m²/day days 3 and 4
    [total dose/cycle = 300 mg/m²]
  Repeat cycle every 21 days
References
  Kovnar EH, Kellie SJ, Horowitz ME, et al, "Preirradiation Cisplatin and Etoposide in the Treatment of High-Risk Medulloblastoma and Other Malignant Embryonal Tumors of the Central Nervous System: A Phase II Study," *J Clin Oncol*, 1990, 8(2):330-6.

CE (Neuroblastomas)
Use Neuroblastomas
Regimen
  Carboplatin: I.V.: 500 mg/m²/day days 1 and 2
    [total dose/cycle = 1000 mg/m²]
  Etoposide: I.V.: 100 mg/m²/day days 1 to 3
    [total dose/cycle = 300 mg/m²]
  Repeat cycle every 21-28 days
References
  Alvarado CS, Kretschmar C, Joshi VV, et al, "Chemotherapy for Patients With Recurrent or Refractory Neuroblastoma: A POG Phase II Study," *J Pediatr Hematol Oncol*, 1997, 19(1):62-7.

CE (Retinoblastoma)
Use Retinoblastoma
Regimen
  Etoposide: I.V.: 100 mg/m²/day days 1 to 5
    [total dose/cycle = 500 mg/m²]
  Carboplatin: I.V.: 160 mg/m²/day days 1 to 5
    [total dose/cycle = 800 mg/m²]
  Repeat cycle every 21 days
References
  Doz F, Neuenschwander S, Plantaz D, et al, "Etoposide and Carboplatin in Extraocular Retinoblastoma: A Study by the Societe Francaise d'Oncologie Pediatrique," *J Clin Oncol*, 1995, 13(4):902-9.

CE-CAdO
Use Neuroblastomas
Regimen
  Carboplatin: I.V.: 160 mg/m²/day days 1 to 5
    [total dose/cycle = 800 mg/m²]
  Etoposide: I.V.: 100 mg/m²/day days 1 to 5
    [total dose/cycle = 500 mg/m²]
      or
  Carboplatin: I.V.: 200 mg/m²/day days 1 to 3
    [total dose/cycle = 600 mg/m²]
  Etoposide: I.V.: 150 mg/m²/day days 1 to 3
    [total dose/cycle = 450 mg/m²]
    and
  Cyclophosphamide: I.V.: 300 mg/m²/day days 1 to 5
    [total dose/cycle = 1500 mg/m²]

Doxorubicin: I.V.: 60 mg/m^2 day 5
[total dose/cycle = 60 mg/m^2]
Vincristine: I.V.: 1.5 mg/m^2/day days 1 and 5
[total dose/cycle = 3 mg/m^2]
Repeat cycle every 21 days

References
Rubie H, Michon J, Plantaz D, et al, "Unresectable Localized Neuroblastoma: Improved Survival After Primary Chemotherapy Including Carboplatin-Etoposide. Neuroblastoma Study Group of the Societe Francaise d'Oncologie Pediatrique (SFOP)," *Br J Cancer,* 1998, 77(12):2310-7.

CEF

Use Breast cancer
Regimen
Cyclophosphamide: Oral: 75 mg/m^2/day days 1 to 14
[total dose/cycle = 1050 mg/m^2]
Epirubicin: I.V.: 60 mg/m^2/day days 1 and 8
[total dose/cycle = 120 mg/m^2]
Fluorouracil: I.V.: 500 mg/m^2/day days 1 and 8
[total dose/cycle = 1000 mg/m^2]
Repeat cycle every 28 days

References
Levine MN, Bramwell VH, Pritchard KI, et al, "Randomized Trial of Intensive Cyclophosphamide, Epirubicin, and Fluorouracil Chemotherapy Compared With Cyclophosphamide, Methotrexate, and Fluorouracil in Premenopausal Women With Node-Positive Breast Cancer, National Cancer Institute of Canada Clinical Trials Group," *J Clin Oncol,* 1998, 16(8):2651-8.

CEPP(B)

Use Lymphoma, non-Hodgkin's
Regimen
Cyclophosphamide: I.V.: 600-650 mg/m^2/day days 1 and 8
[total dose/cycle = 1200-1300 mg/m^2]
Etoposide: I.V.: 70-85 mg/m^2/day days 1 to 3
[total dose/cycle = 210-255 mg/m^2]
Procarbazine: Oral: 60 mg/m^2/day days 1 to 10
[total dose/cycle = 600 mg/m^2]
Prednisone: Oral: 60 mg/m^2/day days 1 to 10
[total dose/cycle = 600 mg/m^2]
Bleomycin: I.V.: 15 units/m^2/day days 1 and 15 (Bleomycin is sometimes omitted)
[total dose/cycle = 30 units/m^2]
Repeat cycle every 28 days

References
Chao NJ, Rosenberg SA, and Horning SJ, "CEPP(B): An Effective and Well-Tolerated Regimen in Poor-Risk, Aggressive Non-Hodgkin's Lymphoma," *Blood,* 1990, 76(7):1293-8.

CEV

Use Rhabdomyosarcoma
Regimen
Carboplatin: I.V.: 500 mg/m^2 day 1
[total dose/cycle = 500 mg/m^2]
Epirubicin: I.V.: 150 mg/m^2 day 1
[total dose/cycle = 150 mg/m^2]
(Continued)

CEV *(Continued)*

Vincristine: I.V.: 1.5 mg/m²/day days 1 and 7
[total dose/cycle = 3 mg/m²]
Repeat cycle every 21 days

References

Frascella E, Pritchard-Jones K, Modak S, et al, "Response of Previously Untreated Metastatic Rhabdomyosarcoma to Combination Chemotherapy With Carboplatin, Epirubicin and Vincristine," *Eur J Cancer*, 1996, 32A(5):821-5.

CF

Use Head and neck cancer

Regimen

Cisplatin: I.V.: 100 mg/m² day 1
[total dose/cycle = 100 mg/m²]
Fluorouracil: I.V.: 1000 mg/m²/day continuous infusion days 1 to 4
[total dose/cycle = 4000 mg/m²]
or
Fluorouracil: I.V.: 1000 mg/m²/day continuous infusion days 1 to 5
[total dose/cycle = 5000 mg/m²]
Repeat cycle every 21-28 days

References

Kish JA, Ensley JF, Jacobs J, et al, "A Randomized Trial of Cisplatin (CACP) + 5-Fluorouracil (5-FU) Infusion and CACP + 5-FU Bolus for Recurrent and Advanced Squamous Cell Carcinoma of the Head and Neck," *Cancer*, 1985, 56(12):2740-4.

♦ **CFM** *see CNF on page 863*

CHAMOCA

Synonyms Modified Bagshawe

Use Gestational trophoblastic tumor

Regimen

Hydroxyurea: Oral: 500 mg every 6 hours for 4 doses, day 1 (start at 6 AM)
[total dose/cycle = 2000 mg]
Dactinomycin: I.V.: 0.2 mg/day days 1 to 3 (give at 7 PM)
[total dose/cycle = 0.6 mg]
followed by 0.5 mg/day days 4 and 5 (give at 7 PM)
[total dose/cycle = 1 mg]
Cyclophosphamide: I.V.: 500 mg/m²/day days 3 and 8 (give at 7 PM)
[total dose/cycle = 1000 mg/m²]
Vincristine: I.V.: 1 mg/m² (maximum 2 mg) day 2 (give at 7 AM)
[total dose/cycle = 1 mg/m²]
Methotrexate: I.V. push: 100 mg/m² day 2 (give at 7 PM)
[total dose/cycle = 100 mg/m²]
followed by 200 mg/m² over 12 hours day 2
[total dose/cycle = 200 mg/m²]
Leucovorin: I.M.: 14 mg/day every 6 hours for 6 doses days 3 to 5 (begin at 7 PM on day 3)
[total dose/cycle = 84 mg]
Doxorubicin: I.V.: 30 mg/m² day 8 (give at 7 PM)
[total dose/cycle = 30 mg/m²]
Repeat cycle every 18 days or as toxicity permits

References
Weed JC Jr, Barnard DE, Currie JL, et al, "Chemotherapy With the Modified Bagshawe Protocol for Poor Prognosis Metastatic Trophoblastic Disease," *Obstet Gynecol*, 1982, 59(3):377-80.

ChIVPP

Use Lymphoma, Hodgkin's disease

Regimen

Chlorambucil: Oral: 6 mg/m^2/day (maximum 10 mg) days 1 to 14
  [total dose/cycle = 84 mg/m^2]
Vinblastine: I.V.: 6 mg/m^2/day (maximum 10 mg) days 1 and 8
  [total dose/cycle = 12 mg/m^2]
Procarbazine: Oral: 100 mg/m^2/day (maximum 150 mg) days 1 to 14
  [total dose/cycle = 1400 mg/m^2]
Prednisone: Oral: 40-50 mg/day days 1 to 14
  [total dose/cycle = 560-700 mg]
Repeat cycle every 28 days

References
Selby P, Patel P, Milan S, et al, "ChIVPP Combination Chemotherapy for Hodgkin's Disease: Long-Term Results," *Br J Cancer*, 1990, 62(2):279-85.

CHL + PRED

Use Leukemia, chronic lymphocytic

Regimen

Chlorambucil: Oral: 0.4 mg/kg/day for 1 day every other week; increase initial dose of 0.4 mg/kg by 0.1 mg/kg every 2 weeks until toxicity or disease control is achieved
Prednisone: Oral: 100 mg/day for 2 days every other week

References
Han T, Ezdinli EZ, Shimaoka K, et al, "Chlorambucil vs Combined Chlorambucil-Corticosteroid Therapy in Chronic Lymphocytic Leukemia," *Cancer*, 1973, 31(3):502-8.

CHOP

Synonyms Mini-CHOP

Use Lymphoma, non-Hodgkin's

Regimen NOTE: Multiple variations are listed below.

Variation 1:

Cyclophosphamide: I.V.: 750 mg/m^2 day 1
  [total dose/cycle = 750 mg/m^2]
Doxorubicin: I.V.: 50 mg/m^2 day 1
  [total dose/cycle = 50 mg/m^2]
Vincristine: I.V.: 1.4 mg/m^2 (maximum 2 mg) day 1
  [total dose/cycle = 1.4 mg/m^2]
Prednisone: Oral: 100 mg/day days 1 to 5
  [total dose/cycle = 500 mg]
  or 50 mg/m^2/day days 1 to 5
  [total dose/cycle = 250 mg/m^2]
  or 100 mg/m^2/day days 1 to 5
  [total dose/cycle = 500 mg/m^2]
Repeat cycle every 21 days

Variation 2:

Cyclophosphamide: I.V.: 750 mg/m^2 day 1
  [total dose/cycle = 750 mg/m^2]
Doxorubicin: I.V.: 50 mg/m^2 day 1
  [total dose/cycle = 50 mg/m^2]

(Continued)

CHOP *(Continued)*

    Vincristine: I.V.: 2 mg day 1
      [total dose/cycle = 2 mg]
    Prednisone: Oral: 75 mg/day days 1 to 5
      [total dose/cycle = 375 mg]
    Repeat cycle every 21 days
    Variation 3:
    Cyclophosphamide: I.V.: 750 mg/m^2/day days 1 and 8
      [total dose/cycle = 1500 mg/m^2]
    Doxorubicin: I.V.: 25 mg/m^2/day days 1 and 8
      [total dose/cycle = 50 mg/m^2]
    Vincristine: I.V.: 1.4 mg/m^2/day (maximum 2 mg) days 1 and 8
      [total dose/cycle = 2.8 mg/m^2]
    Prednisone: Oral: 50 mg/m^2/day days 1 to 8
      [total dose/cycle = 400 mg/m^2]
    Repeat cycle every 28 days
    Variation 4 - "mini-CHOP":
    Cyclophosphamide: I.V.: 250 mg/m^2/day days 1, 8, and 15
      [total dose/cycle = 750 mg/m^2]
    Doxorubicin: I.V.: 16.7 mg/m^2/day days 1, 8, and 15
      [total dose/cycle = 50.1 mg/m^2]
    Vincristine: I.V.: 0.67 mg/day days 1, 8, and 15
      [total dose/cycle = 2.01 mg]
    Prednisone: Oral: 75 mg/day days 1 to 5
      [total dose/cycle = 375 mg]
    Repeat cycle every 21 days

References

Variation 1:
    Bezwoda W, Rastogi RB, Erazo Valla A, et al, "Long-Term Results of a Multicentre Randomised, Comparative Phase III Trial of CHOP Versus CNOP Regimens in Patients With Intermediate- and High-Grade Non-Hodgkin's Lymphomas, Novantrone International Study Group," *Eur J Cancer*, 1995, 31A(6):903-11.
    McKelvey EM, Gottlieb JA, Wilson HE, et al, "Hydroxyldaunomycin (Adriamycin®) Combination Chemotherapy in Malignant Lymphoma," *Cancer*, 1976, 38(4):1484-93.
    Miller TP, Dahlberg S, Cassady JR, et al, "Chemotherapy Alone Compared With Chemotherapy Plus Radiotherapy for Localized Intermediate- and High-Grade Non-Hodgkin's Lymphoma," *N Engl J Med*, 1998, 339(1):21-6.

Variation 2 and 4:
    Meyer RM, Browman GP, Samosh ML, et al, "Randomized Phase II Comparison of Standard CHOP With Weekly CHOP in Elderly Patients With Non-Hodgkin's Lymphoma," *J Clin Oncol*, 1995, 13(9):2386-93.

Variation 3:
    Linch DC, Vaughan Hudson B, Hancock BW, et al, "A Randomised Comparison of a Third-Generation Regimen (PACEBOM) With a Standard Regimen (CHOP) in Patients With Histologically Aggressive Non-Hodgkin's Lymphoma: A British National Lymphoma Investigation Report," *Br J Cancer*, 1996, 74(2):318-22.

♦ **CHOP-Rituximab** *see* R-CHOP *on page 936*

CI (Neuroblastomas)

Use Neuroblastomas

Regimen

    Ifosfamide: I.V.: 1500 mg/m^2/day days 1 to 3 (with mesna; refer to Mesna monograph *on page 542* for dosing instructions)
      [total dose/cycle = 4500 mg/m^2]

Carboplatin: I.V.: 400 mg/m^2 day 4
[total dose/cycle = 400 mg/m^2]
Repeat cycle every 21-28 days

References
Alvarado CS, Kretschmar C, Joshi VV, et al, "Chemotherapy for Patients With Recurrent or Refractory Neuroblastoma: A POG Phase II Study," *J Pediatr Hematol Oncol*, 1997, 19(1):62-7.

CISCA

Use Bladder cancer

Regimen
Cyclophosphamide: I.V.: 650 mg/m^2 day 1
[total dose = 650 mg/m^2]
Doxorubicin: I.V.: 50 mg/m^2 day 1
[total dose = 50 mg/m^2]
Cisplatin: I.V.: 100 mg/m^2 day 2
[total dose = 100 mg/m^2]
Repeat cycle every 21-28 days

References
Sternberg JJ, Bracken RB, Handel PB, et al, "Combination Chemotherapy (CISCA) for Advanced Urinary Tract Carcinoma. A Preliminary Report," *JAMA*, 1977, 238(21):2282-7.

Cisplatin-Docetaxel

Use Bladder cancer

Regimen
Cisplatin: I.V.: 30 mg/m^2 day 1
[total dose/cycle = 30 mg/m^2]
Docetaxel: I.V.: 40 mg/m^2 day 4
[total dose/cycle = 40 mg/m^2]
Repeat cycle weekly for 8 weeks

References
Varveris H, Delakas D, Anezinis P, et al, "Concurrent Platinum and Docetaxel Chemotherapy and External Radical Radiotherapy in Patients With Invasive Transitional Cell Bladder Carcinoma. A Preliminary Report of Tolerance and Local Control," *Anticancer Res*, 1997, 17(6D):4771-80.

Cisplatin-Fluorouracil

Use Cervical cancer

Regimen NOTE: Multiple variations are listed below.
Variation 1:
Cisplatin: I.V.: 75 mg/m^2 day 1
[total dose/cycle = 75 mg/m^2]
Fluorouracil: I.V.: 1000 mg/m^2/day continuous infusion days 1 to 4 (96 hours)
[total dose/cycle = 4000 mg/m^2]
Repeat cycle every 21 days
Variation 2:
Cisplatin: I.V.: 50 mg/m^2 day 1 starting 4 hours before radiotherapy
[total dose/cycle = 50 mg/m^2]
Fluorouracil: I.V.: 1000 mg/m^2/day continuous infusion days 2 to 5 (96 hours)
[total dose/cycle = 4000 mg/m^2]
Repeat cycle every 28 days
(Continued)

Cisplatin-Fluorouracil *(Continued)*

References

Variation 1:

Morris M, Eifel PJ, Lu J, et al, "Pelvic Radiation With Concurrent Chemotherapy Compared With Pelvic and Para-aortic Radiation for High-Risk Cervical Cancer," *N Engl J Med*, 1999, 340(15):1137-43.

Variation 2:

Whitney CW, Sause W, Bundy BN, et al, "Randomized Comparison of Fluorouracil Plus Cisplatin Versus Hydroxyurea as an Adjunct to Radiation Therapy in Stage IIB-IVA Carcinoma of the Cervix With Negative Para-aortic Lymph Nodes: A Gynecologic Oncology Group and Southwest Oncology Group Study," *J Clin Oncol*, 1999, 17(5):1339-48.

Cisplatin + Pemetrexed

Use Malignant pleural mesothelioma

Regimen

Pemetrexed: I.V.: 500 mg/m^2 infused over 10 minutes day 1
[total dose/cycle = 500 mg/m^2]
Cisplatin: I.V.: 75 mg/m^2 infused over 2 hours (start 30 minutes after pemetrexed)
[total dose/cycle = 75 mg/m^2]
Repeat cycle every 21 days

References

Vogelzang NJ, Rusthoven JJ, Symanowski J, et al, "Phase III Study of Pemetrexed in Combination With Cisplatin Versus Cisplatin Alone in Patients With Malignant Pleural Mesothelioma," *J Clin Oncol*, 2003, 21(14):2636-44.

Cisplatin-Vinorelbine

Use Cervical cancer

Regimen

Cisplatin: I.V.: 80 mg/m^2 day 1
[total dose/cycle = 80 mg/m^2]
Vinorelbine: I.V.: 25 mg/m^2/day days 1 and 8
[total dose/cycle = 50 mg/m^2]
Repeat cycle every 21 days

References

Pignata S, Silvestro G, Ferrari E, et al, "Phase II Study of Cisplatin and Vinorelbine as First-Line Chemotherapy in Patients With Carcinoma of the Uterine Cervix," *J Clin Oncol*, 1999, 17(3):756-60.

CMF

Use Breast cancer

Regimen NOTE: Multiple variations are listed below.

Variation 1:

Methotrexate: I.V.: 40 mg/m^2/day days 1 and 8
[total dose/cycle = 80 mg/m^2]
Fluorouracil: I.V.: 600 mg/m^2/day days 1 and 8
[total dose/cycle = 1200 mg/m^2]
Cyclophosphamide: Oral: 100 mg/m^2/day days 1 to 14
[total dose/cycle = 1400 mg/m^2]
Repeat cycle every 28 days

Variation 2 (older than 60 years):

Methotrexate: I.V.: 30 mg/m^2 days 1 and 8
[total dose/cycle = 60 mg/m^2]
Fluorouracil: I.V.: 400 mg/m^2 days 1 and 8
[total dose/cycle = 800 mg/m^2]

Cyclophosphamide: Oral: 100 mg/m² days 1-14
[total dose/cycle = 1400 mg/m²]
Repeat cycle every 28 days

References

Variations 1 and 2:
Bonadonna G, Brusamolino E, Valagussa P, et al, "Combination Chemotherapy as an Adjuvant Treatment in Operable Breast Cancer," *N Engl J Med*, 1976, 294(8):405-10.
Canellos GP, Pocock SJ, Taylor SG III, et al, "Combination Chemotherapy for Metastatic Breast Carcinoma, Prospective Comparison of Multiple Drug Therapy With L-Phenylalanine Mustard," *Cancer*, 1976, 38(5):1882-6.

CMF-IV

Use Breast cancer

Regimen

Cyclophosphamide: I.V.: 600 mg/m² day 1
[total dose/cycle = 600 mg/m²]
Methotrexate: I.V.: 40 mg/m² day 1
[total dose/cycle = 40 mg/m²]
Fluorouracil: I.V.: 600 mg/m² day 1
[total dose/cycle = 600 mg/m²]
Repeat cycle every 21 or 28 days

References

Bonadonna G, Veronesi U, Brambilla C, et al, "Primary Chemotherapy to Avoid Mastectomy in Tumors With Diameters of Three Centimeters or More," *J Natl Cancer Inst*, 1990, 82(19):1539-45.
Tannock IF, Boyd NF, DeBoer G, et al, "A Randomized Trial of Two Dose Levels of Cyclophosphamide, Methotrexate, and Fluorouracil Chemotherapy for Patients With Metastatic Breast Cancer," *J Clin Oncol*, 1988, 6(9):1377-87.

♦ **C-MOPP** see COPP on page 867

CMV

Use Bladder cancer

Regimen

Cisplatin: I.V.: 100 mg/m² infused over 4 hours (start 12 hours after methotrexate) day 2
[total dose = 100 mg/m²]
Methotrexate: I.V.: 30 mg/m²/day days 1 and 8
[total dose = 60 mg/m²]
Vinblastine: I.V.: 4 mg/m²/day days 1 and 8
[total dose = 8 mg/m²]
Repeat cycle every 21 days

References

Harker WG, Meyers FJ, Freiha FS, et al, "Cisplatin, Methotrexate, and Vinblastine (CMV): An Effective Chemotherapy Regimen for Metastatic Transitional Cell Carcinoma of the Urinary Tract. A Northern California Oncology Group Study," *J Clin Oncol*, 1985, 3(11):1463-70.

CNF

Synonyms CFM; FNC

Use Breast cancer

Regimen NOTE: Multiple variations are listed below.

Variation 1:

Cyclophosphamide: I.V.: 500 mg/m² day 1
[total dose/cycle = 500 mg/m²]
Mitoxantrone: I.V.: 10 mg/m² day 1
[total dose/cycle = 10 mg/m²]

(Continued)

CNF *(Continued)*

Fluorouracil: I.V.: 500 mg/m^2 day 1
[total dose/cycle = 500 mg/m^2]
Repeat cycle every 21 days
Variation 2:
Cyclophosphamide: I.V.: 500-600 mg/m^2 day 1
[total dose/cycle = 500-600 mg/m^2]
Fluorouracil: I.V.: 500-600 mg/m^2 day 1
[total dose/cycle = 500-600 mg/m^2]
Mitoxantrone: I.V.: 10-12 mg/m^2 day 1
[total dose/cycle = 10-12 mg/m^2]
Repeat cycle every 21 days

References

Variation 1:
Bennett JM, Muss HB, Doroshow JH, et al, "A Randomized Multicenter Trial Comparing Mitixantrone, Cyclophosphamide, and Fluorouracil With Doxorubicin, Cyclophosphamide, and Fluorouracil in the Therapy of Metastatic Breast Carcinoma," *J Clin Oncol*, 1988, 6(10):1611-20.
Variation 2:
Alonso MC, Tabernero JM, Ojeda B, "A Phase III Randomized Trial of Cyclophosphamide, Mitoxantrone, and 5-Fluorouracil (CNF) Versus Cyclophosphamide, Adriamycin®, and 5-Fluorouracil (CAF) in Patients With Metastatic Breast Cancer," *Breast Cancer Res Treat*, 1995, 34(1):15-24.
Casciato DA and Lowitz BB, eds, *Manual of Clinical Oncology*, 3rd ed, Boston, MA: Little, Brown, 1995, 596.

CNOP

Use Lymphoma, non-Hodgkin's
Regimen
Cyclophosphamide: I.V.: 750 mg/m^2 day 1
[total dose/cycle = 750 mg/m^2]
Mitoxantrone: I.V.: 10-12 mg/m^2 day 1
[total dose/cycle = 10-12 mg/m^2]
Vincristine: I.V.: 1.4 mg/m^2 day 1
[total dose/cycle = 1.4 mg/m^2]
Prednisone: Oral: 50 mg/m^2/day days 1 to 5
[total dose/cycle = 250 mg/m^2]
Repeat cycle every 21 days

References

Brusamolino E, Bertini M, Guidi S, et al, "CHOP Versus CNOP (N=Mitoxantrone) in non-Hodgkin's Lymphoma: An Interim Report Comparing Efficacy and Toxicity," *Haematologica*, 1988, 73(3):217-22.
Pavlovsky S, Santarelli MT, Erazo A, et al, "Results of a Randomized Study of Previously Untreated Intermediate and High Grade Lymphoma Using CHOP Versus CNOP," *Ann Oncol*, 1992, 3:205-9.

CO

Use Retinoblastoma
Regimen
Cyclophosphamide: I.V.: 10 mg/kg/day days 1 to 3
[total dose/cycle = 30 mg/kg]
Vincristine: I.V.: 1.5 mg/m^2 day 1
[total dose/cycle = 1.5 mg/m^2]
Repeat cycle every 21 days

References

Doz F, Khelfaoui F, Mosseri V, et al, "The Role of Chemotherapy in Orbital Involvement of Retinoblastoma. The Experience of a Single Institution With 33 Patients," *Cancer*, 1994, 74(2):722-32.

CODOX-M

Use Lymphoma, non-Hodgkin's

Regimen

Cytarabine: I.T.: 70 mg/day days 1 and 3
  [total dose/cycle = 140 mg]

Cyclophosphamide: I.V.: 800 mg/m^2 day 1, then 200 mg/m^2 days 2 to 5
  [total dose/cycle = 1600 mg/m^2]

Vincristine: I.V.: 1.5 mg/m^2/day days 1, 8, and 15
  [total dose/cycle = 4.5 mg/m^2]

Doxorubicin: I.V.: 40 mg/m^2 day 1
  [total dose/cycle = 40 mg/m^2]

Methotrexate:

  I.T.: 12 mg day 15
    [total dose/cycle = 12 mg]

  I.V.: 1200 mg/m^2 loading dose then 240 mg/m^2/hour for 23 hours day 10
    [total dose/cycle = 6720 mg/m^2]

Leucovorin: I.V.: 192 mg/m^2 day 11 then 6 mg/m^2 every 6 hours until MTX level <10^{-8}M

Sargramostim: SubQ: 7.5 mcg/kg day 13 until ANC >1000 cells^{-}mm^3
  [total dose/cycle = ANC = >1000 cells/mm^3]

Repeat cycle when ANC >1000 cells/mm^3

References

Magrath I, Adde M, Shad A, et al, "Adults and Children With Small Non-Cleaved-Cell Lymphoma Have a Similar Excellent Outcome When Treated With the Same Chemotherapy Regimen," *J Clin Oncol*, 1996, 14(3):925-34.

COMLA

Use Lymphoma, non-Hodgkin's

Regimen

Cyclophosphamide: I.V.: 1500 mg/m^2 day 1
  [total dose/cycle = 1500 mg/m^2]

Vincristine: I.V.: 1.4 mg/m^2/day (maximum 2 mg) days 1, 8, and 15
  [total dose/cycle = 4.2 mg/m^2]

Methotrexate: I.V.: 120 mg/m^2/day days 22, 29, 36, 43, 50, 57, 64, and 71
  [total dose/cycle = 960 mg/m^2]

Leucovorin: Oral: 25 mg/m^2 every 6 hours for 4 doses (beginning 24 hours after each methotrexate dose)
  [total dose/cycle = 800 mg/m^2]

Cytarabine: I.V.: 300 mg/m^2/day days 22, 29, 36, 43, 50, 57, 64, and 71
  [total dose/cycle = 2400 mg/m^2]

Repeat cycle every 85 days

References

Sweet DL, Golomb HM, Ultmann JE, et al, "Cyclophosphamide, Vincristine, Methotrexate With Leucovorin Rescue, and Cytarabine (COMLA) Combination Sequential Chemotherapy for Advanced Diffuse Histiocytic Lymphoma," *Ann Intern Med*, 1980, 92(6):785-90.

COMP

Use Lymphoma, Hodgkin's disease; Lymphoma, non-Hodgkin's disease

Regimen

Cyclophosphamide: I.V.: 1200 mg/m^2 day 1, cycle 1
[total dose/cycle = 1200 mg/m^2]

followed by 1000 mg/m^2 day 1 on subsequent cycles
[total dose/cycle = 1000 mg/m^2]

Vincristine: I.V.: 2 mg/m^2/day (maximum 2 mg) days 3, 10, 17, 24, cycle 1
[total dose/cycle = 8 mg/m^2]

followed by 1.5 mg/m^2/day days 1 and 4, on subsequent cycles
[total dose/cycle = 3 mg/m^2]

Methotrexate: I.V.: 300 mg/m^2 day 12
[total dose/cycle = 300 mg/m^2]

Prednisone: Oral: 60 mg/m^2/day (maximum 60 mg) days 3 to 30 then taper for 7 days, cycle 1
[total dose/cycle = 1680 mg/m^2 + taper dose over 7 days]

followed by 60 mg/m^2 (maximum 60 mg) days 1 to 5, on subsequent cycles
[total dose/cycle = 300 mg/m^2]

Maintenance cycles repeat every 28 days

References

Anderson JR, Wilson JF, Jenkin DT, et al, "Childhood Non-Hodgkin's Lymphoma. The Results of a Randomized Therapeutic Trial Comparing a 4-drug Regimen (COMP) With a 10-drug Regimen (LSA2-L2)." *N Engl J Med*, 1983, 308(10):559-65.

COP-BLAM

Use Lymphoma, non-Hodgkin's

Regimen

Cyclophosphamide: I.V.: 400 mg/m^2 day 1
[total dose/cycle = 400 mg/m^2]

Vincristine: I.V.: 1 mg/m^2 day 1
[total dose/cycle = 1 mg/m^2]

Prednisone: Oral: 40 mg/m^2/day days 1 to 10
[total dose/cycle = 400 mg/m^2]

Bleomycin: I.V.: 15 mg day 14
[total dose/cycle = 15 mg]

Doxorubicin: I.V.: 40 mg/m^2 day 1
[total dose/cycle = 40 mg/m^2]

Procarbazine: Oral: 100 mg/m^2/day days 1 to 10
[total dose/cycle = 1000 mg/m^2]

References

Salles G, Shipp MA, and Coiffier B, "Chemotherapy of Non-Hodgkin's Aggressive Lymphomas," *Semin Hematol*, 1994, 31(1):46-69.

Urba WJ, Duffey PL, and Longo DL, "Treatment of Patients With Aggressive Lymphomas: An Overview," *J Natl Cancer Inst Monogr*, 1990, (10):29-37.

COPE

Synonyms Baby Brain I

Use Brain tumors

Regimen

Cycle A:

Vincristine: I.V.: 0.065 mg/kg/day (maximum 1.5 mg) days 1 and 8
[total dose/cycle = 0.13 mg/kg]

Cyclophosphamide: I.V.: 65 mg/kg day 1
[total dose/cycle = 65 mg/kg]

Cycle B:
  Cisplatin: I.V.: 4 mg/kg day 1
    [total dose/cycle = 4 mg/kg]
  Etoposide: I.V.: 6.5 mg/kg/day days 3 and 4
    [total dose/cycle = 13 mg/kg]
  Repeat cycle every 28 days in the following sequence: AABAAB

References
Duffner PK, Horowitz ME, Krischer JP, et al "Postoperative Chemotherapy and Delayed Radiation in Children Less Than Three Years of Age With Malignant Brain Tumors," *N Engl J Med*, 1993, 328(24):1725-31.

COPP

Synonyms C-MOPP
Use Lymphoma, non-Hodgkin's
Regimen
  Cyclophosphamide: I.V.: 450-650 mg/m^2/day days 1 and 8
    [total dose/cycle = 900-1300 mg/m^2]
  Vincristine: I.V.: 1.4-2 mg/m^2/day (maximum 2 mg) days 1 and 8
    [total dose/cycle = 2.8-4 mg/m^2]
  Procarbazine: Oral: 100 mg/m^2/day days 1 to 14
    [total dose/cycle = 1400 mg/m^2]
  Prednisone: Oral: 40 mg/m^2/day days 1 to 14
    [total dose/cycle = 560 mg/m^2]
  Repeat cycle every 3 to 4 weeks

References
Brereton HD, Young RC, Longo DL, et al, "A Comparison Between Combination Chemotherapy and Total Body Irradiation Plus Combination Chemotherapy in Non-Hodgkin's Lymphoma," *Cancer*, 1979, 43(6):2227-31.

CP (Leukemia)

Use Leukemia, chronic lymphocytic
Regimen
  Chlorambucil: Oral: 30 mg/m^2 day 1
    [total dose/cycle = 30 mg/m^2]
  Prednisone: Oral: 80 mg/day days 1 to 5
    [total dose/cycle = 400 mg]
  Repeat cycle every 14 days

References
Raphael B, Anderson JW, Silber R, et al, "Comparison of Chlorambucil and Prednisone Versus Cyclophosphamide, Vincristine, and Prednisone as Initial Treatment for Chronic Lymphocytic Leukemia: Long-Term Follow-up of an Eastern Cooperative Oncology Group Randomized Clinical Trial," *J Clin Oncol*, 1991, 9(5):770-6.

CP (Ovarian Cancer)

Use Ovarian cancer
Regimen
  Cyclophosphamide: I.V.: 750 mg/m^2 day 1
    [total dose/cycle = 750 mg/m^2]
  Cisplatin: I.V.: 75 mg/m^2 day 1
    [total dose/cycle = 75 mg/m^2]
  Repeat cycle every 21 days

References
Hainsworth JD, Grosh WW, Burnett LS, et al, "Advanced Ovarian Cancer: Long-Term Results of Treatment With Intensive Cisplatin-Based Chemotherapy of Brief Duration," *Ann Intern Med*, 1988, 108(2):165-70.

(Continued)

CP (Ovarian Cancer) *(Continued)*

Neijt JP, ten Bokkel Huinink WW, van der Burg ME, et al, "Randomized Trial Comparing Two Combination Chemotherapy Regimens (CHAP-5 v CP) in Advanced Ovarian Carcinoma," *J Clin Oncol*, 1987, 5(8):1157-68.

Omura GA, Brady MF, Homesley HD, et al, "Long-Term Follow-Up and Prognostic Factor Analysis in Advanced Ovarian Carcinoma: The Gynecologic Oncology Group Experience," *J Clin Oncol*, 1991, 9(7):1138-50.

CT

Use Ovarian cancer

Regimen

Cisplatin: I.V.: 75 mg/m^2 day 2
[total dose/cycle = 75 mg/m^2]
Paclitaxel: I.V.: 135 mg/m^2 continuous infusion day 1
[total dose/cycle = 135 mg/m^2]
Repeat cycle every 21 days

References

McGuire WP, Hoskins WJ, Brady MF, et al, "Cyclophosphamide and Cisplatin Compared With Paclitaxel and Cisplatin in Patients With Stage III and Stage IV Ovarian Cancer," *N Engl J Med*, 1996, 334(1):1-6.

CV

Use Retinoblastoma

Regimen

Cyclophosphamide: I.V.: 300 mg/m^2
[total dose/cycle = 300 mg/m^2]
Vincristine: I.V.: 1.5 mg/m^2
[total dose/cycle = 1.5 mg/m^2]
Repeat weekly for 6 weeks
followed by
Cyclophosphamide: I.V.: 200 mg/m^2
[total dose/cycle = 200 mg/m^2]
Vincristine: I.V.: 1.5 mg/m^2
[total dose/cycle = 1.5 mg/m^2]
Repeat weekly for 42 weeks

References

Zelter M, Damel A, Gonzalez G, et al, "A Prospective Study on the Treatment of Retinoblastoma in 72 Patients," *Cancer*, 1991, 68(8):1685-90.

CVD

Use Melanoma

Regimen

Cisplatin: I.V.: 20 mg/m^2/day days 2 to 5
[total dose/cycle = 80 mg/m^2]
Vinblastine: I.V.: 1.6 mg/m^2/day days 1 to 5
[total dose/cycle = 8 mg/m^2]
Dacarbazine: I.V.: 800 mg/m^2 day 1
[total dose/cycle = 800 mg/m^2]
Repeat cycle every 21 days

References

Legha SS, Ring S, Papadopoulos N, et al, "A Prospective Evaluation of a Triple-Drug Regimen Containing Cisplatin, Vinblastine, and Dacarbazine (CVD) for Metastatic Melanoma," *Cancer*, 1989, 64(10):2024-9.

CVP (Leukemia)

Use Leukemia, chronic lymphocytic

Regimen NOTE: Multiple variations are listed below.

Variation 1:

Cyclophosphamide: Oral: 400 or 300 mg/m^2/day days 1 to 5
[total dose/cycle = 2000 or 1500 mg/m^2]

Vincristine: I.V.: 1.4 mg/m^2 (maximum 2 mg) day 1
[total dose/cycle = 1.4 mg/m^2]

Prednisone: Oral: 100 mg/m^2/day days 1 to 5
[total dose/cycle = 500 mg/m^2]

Repeat cycle every 21 days

Variation 2:

Cyclophosphamide: I.V.: 800 mg/m^2 day 1
[total dose/cycle = 800 mg/m^2]

Vincristine: I.V.: 1.4 mg/m^2 (maximum 2 mg) day 1
[total dose/cycle = 1.4 mg/m^2]

Prednisone: Oral: 100 mg/m^2/day days 1 to 5
[total dose/cycle = 500 mg/m^2]

Repeat cycle every 21 days

References

Variation 1:

Bagley CM, DeVita VT, Berard CW, et al, "Advanced Lymphosarcoma: Intensive Cyclical Combination Chemotherapy With Cyclophosphamide, Vincristine, and Prednisone," *Ann Int Med*, 1972, 76(2):227-34.

Raphael B, Anderson JW, Silber R, et al, "Comparison of Chlorambucil and Prednisone Versus Cyclophosphamide, Vincristine, and Prednisone as Initial Treatment for Chronic Lymphocytic Leukemia: Long-Term Follow-up of an Eastern Cooperative Oncology Group Randomized Clinical Trial," *J Clin Oncol*, 1991, 9(5):770-6.

Variation 2:

Oken MM and Kaplan ME, "Combination Chemotherapy With Cyclophosphamide, Vincristine, and Prednisone in the Treatment of Refractory Chronic Lymphocytic Leukemia," *Cancer Treat Rep*, 1979, 63(3):441-7.

CVP (Lymphoma, non-Hodgkin's)

Use Lymphoma, non-Hodgkin's

Regimen

Cyclophosphamide: Oral: 400 mg/m^2/day days 1 to 5
[total dose/cycle = 2000 mg/m^2]

Vincristine: I.V.: 1.4 mg/m^2 day 1
[total dose/cycle = 1.4 mg/m^2]

Prednisone: Oral: 100 mg/m^2/day days 1 to 5
[total dose/cycle = 500 mg/m^2]

Repeat cycle every 21 days

References

Bagley CM Jr, Devita VT Jr, Berard CW, et al, "Advanced Lymphosarcoma: Intensive Cyclical Combination Chemotherapy With Cyclophosphamide, Vincristine, and Prednisone," *Ann Intern Med*, 1972, 76(2):227-34.

Portlock CS, Rosenberg SA, Glatstein E, et al, "Treatment of Advanced Non-Hodgkin's Lymphomas With Favorable Histologies: Preliminary Results of a Prospective Trial," *Blood*, 1976, 47(5):747-56.

Cyclophosphamide + Doxorubicin

Use Prostate cancer

Regimen

Doxorubicin: I.V.: 40 mg/m^2 day 1
[total dose/cycle = 40 mg/m^2]

(Continued)

Cyclophosphamide + Doxorubicin *(Continued)*

Cyclophosphamide: I.V.: 800-2000 mg/m² day 1

[total dose/cycle = 800-2000 mg/m²]

Filgrastim: SubQ: 5 mcg/kg/day days 2 to 10 (or until ANC >10,000 cells/µL)

[total dose/cycle = 45 mcg/kg or ANC = >10,000 cells/µL]

Repeat cycle every 21 days

References

Small EJ, Srinivas S, Egan B, et al, "Doxorubicin and Dose-Escalated Cyclophosphamide With Granulocyte Colony-Stimulating Factor for the Treatment of Hormone-Resistant Prostate Cancer," *J Clin Oncol*, 1996, 14(5):1617-25.

Cyclophosphamide + Estramustine

Use Prostate cancer

Regimen

Cyclophosphamide: Oral: 2 mg/kg/day days 1 to 14

[total dose/cycle = 28 mg/kg]

Estramustine: Oral: 10 mg/kg/day days 1 to 14

[total dose/cycle = 140 mg/kg]

Repeat cycle every 28 days

References

Bracarda S, Tonato M, Rosi P, "Oral Estramustine and Cyclophosphamide in Patients With Metastatic Hormone Refractory Prostate Carcinoma: A Phase II Study," *Cancer*, 2000, 88(6):1438-44.

Cyclophosphamide + Etoposide

Use Prostate cancer

Regimen

Cyclophosphamide: Oral: 100 mg/day days 1 to 14

[total dose/cycle = 1400 mg]

Etoposide: Oral: 50 mg/day days 1 to 14

[total dose/cycle = 700 mg]

Repeat cycle every 28 days

References

Maulard-Durdux C, Dufour B, Hennequin C, et al, "Phase II Study of the Oral Cyclophosphamide and Oral Etoposide Combination in Hormone-Refractory Prostate Carcinoma Patients," *Cancer*, 1996, 77(6):1144-8.

Cyclophosphamide + Vincristine + Dexamethasone

Use Prostate cancer

Regimen

Cyclophosphamide: Oral: 250 mg/day days 1 to 14

[total dose/cycle = 3500 mg]

Vincristine: I.V.: 1 mg/day days 1, 8, and 15

[total dose/cycle = 3 mg]

Dexamethasone: Oral: 0.75 mg twice daily days 1 to 14

[total dose/cycle = 21 mg]

Repeat cycle every 28 days

References

Daliani DD, Assikis V, Tu SM, et al, "Phase II Trial of Cyclophosphamide, Vincristine, and Dexamethasone in the Treatment of Androgen-Independent Prostate Carcinoma," *Cancer*, 2003, 97(3):561-7.

CYVADIC
Use Sarcoma
Regimen
Cyclophosphamide: I.V.: 500 mg/m^2 day 1
[total dose/cycle = 500 mg/m^2]
Vincristine: I.V.: 1.4 mg/m^2/day days 1 and 5
[total dose/cycle = 2.8 mg/m^2]
Doxorubicin: I.V.: 50 mg/m^2 day 1
[total dose/cycle = 50 mg/m^2]
Dacarbazine: I.V.: 250 mg/m^2/day days 1 to 5
[total dose/cycle = 1250 mg/m^2]
Repeat cycle every 21 days
References
Pinedo HM, Bramwell VH, Mouridsen HT, et al, "Cyvadic in Advanced Soft Tissue Sarcoma: A Randomized Study Comparing Two Schedules. A study of the EORTC Soft Tissue and Bone Sarcoma Group," *Cancer*, 1984, 53(9):1825-32.

DA
Use Leukemia, acute myeloid (induction)
Regimen Induction:
Daunorubicin: I.V.: 45 mg/m^2/day days 1 to 3
[total dose/cycle = 135 mg/m^2]
Cytarabine: I.V.: 100 mg/m^2/day continuous infusion days 1 to 7
[total dose/cycle = 700 mg/m^2]

Dacarbazine-Carboplatin-Aldesleukin-Interferon
Use Melanoma
Regimen
Dacarbazine: I.V.: 750 mg/m^2/day days 1 and 22
[total dose/cycle = 1500 mg/m^2]
Carboplatin: I.V.: 400 mg/m^2/day days 1 and 22
[total dose/cycle = 800 mg/m^2]
Aldesleukin: SubQ: 4,800,000 units every 8 hours days 36 and 57
[total dose/cycle = 28,800,000 units]
then 4,800,000 units every 12 hours days 37 and 58
[total dose/cycle = 19,200,000 units]
then 4,800,000 units/day days 38 to 40, 43 to 47, 50 to 54, 59 to 61, 65 to 68, 71 to 75
[total dose/cycle = 86,400,000 units]
Interferon alpha-2a: SubQ: 6,000,000 units days 38, 40, 43, 45, 47, 50, 52, 54, 59, 61, 64, 66, 68, 71, 73, and 75
[total dose/cycle = 96,000,000 units]
Repeat cycle every 78 days for 3 cycles
References
Ron IG, Mordish Y, Eisenthal A, et al, "A Phase II Study of Combined Administration of Dacarbazine and Carboplatin With Home Therapy of Recombinant Interleukin-2 and Interferon-alpha 2a in Patients With Advanced Malignant Melanoma," *Cancer Immunol Immunother*, 1994, 38(6):379-84.

Dacarbazine/Tamoxifen
Use Melanoma
Regimen
Dacarbazine: I.V.: 250 mg/m^2/day days 1 to 5, every 21 days
[total dose/cycle = 1250 mg/m^2]
(Continued)

Dacarbazine/Tamoxifen *(Continued)*

Tamoxifen: Oral: 20 mg/day (use of tamoxifen is optional)
[total dose/cycle = 20 mg]

References
Cocconi G, Bella M, Calabresi F, et al, "Treatment Of Metastatic Malignant Melanoma With Dacarbazine Plus Tamoxifen," *N Engl J Med*, 1992, 327(8):516-23.

Dartmouth Regimen

Use Melanoma

Regimen
Cisplatin: I.V.: 25 mg/m^2/day days 1 to 3
[total dose/cycle = 75 mg/m^2]
Dacarbazine: I.V.: 220 mg/m^2/day days 1 to 3
[total dose/cycle = 660 mg/m^2]
Carmustine: I.V.: 150 mg/m^2 day 1 (every other cycle)
[total dose/cycle = 150 mg/m^2]
Repeat cycle every 21 days

References
Creagan ET, Suman VJ, Dalton RJ, et al, "Phase III Clinical Trial of the Combination of Cisplatin, Dacarbazine, and Carmustine With or Without Tamoxifen in Patients With Advanced Malignant Melanoma," *J Clin Oncol*, 1999, 17(6):1884-90.

DAT

Use Leukemia, acute myeloid (induction)

Regimen Induction:
Daunorubicin: I.V. bolus: 45 mg/m^2/day days 1 to 3
[total dose/cycle = 135 mg/m^2]
Cytarabine: I.V. bolus: 200 mg/m^2
[total dose/cycle = 200 mg/m^2]
Thioguanine: Oral: 100 mg/m^2/day days 1 to 7
[total dose/cycle = 700 mg/m^2]

DAV

Use Leukemia, acute myeloid

Regimen
Daunorubicin: I.V.: 60 mg/m^2/day days 3 to 5
[total dose/cycle = 180 mg/m^2]
Cytarabine I.V.: 100 mg/m^2/day continuous infusion days 1 and 2
[total dose/cycle = 200 mg/m^2]
followed by 100 mg/m^2 every 12 hours days 3 to 8 (12 doses)
[total dose/cycle = 1200 mg/m^2]
Etoposide: I.V.: 150 mg/m^2/day days 6 to 8
[total dose/cycle = 450 mg/m^2]
Administer one cycle only

References
Creutzig U, Ritter J, and Schellong G, "Identification of Two Risk Groups in Childhood Acute Myelogenous Leukemia After Therapy Intensification in Study AML-BFM-83 as Compared With Study AML-BFM-78, AML-BFM Study Group," *Blood*, 1990, 75(10):1932-40.

DHAP

Use Lymphoma, non-Hodgkin's
Regimen NOTE: Multiple variations are listed on next page.

Variation 1:

Dexamethasone: I.V. or Oral: 40 mg/day days 1 to 4
[total dose/cycle = 160 mg]

Cisplatin: I.V.: 100 mg/m^2 day 1
[total dose/cycle = 100 mg/m^2]

Cytarabine: I.V.: 2000 mg/m^2 every 12 hours for 2 doses day 2 (begins
at the end of the cisplatin infusion)
[total dose/cycle = 4000 mg/m^2]

Repeat cycle every 3-4 weeks for 6-10 cycles (salvage therapy) or 1-2
cycles (mobilization prior to high-dose therapy with peripheral hematopoietic progenitor cell support)

Variation 2:

Dexamethasone: I.V. or Oral: 40 mg/day days 1 to 4
[total dose/cycle = 160 mg]

Oxaliplatin: I.V.: 130 mg/m^2 day 1
[total dose/cycle = 130 mg/m^2]

Cytarabine: I.V.: 2000 mg/m^2 every 12 hours for 2 doses day 2
[total dose/cycle = 4000 mg/m^2]

Repeat cycle every 3 weeks

References

Variation 1:

Velasquez WS, Cabanillas F, Salvador P, et al, "Effective Salvage Therapy for
Lymphoma With Cisplatin in Combination With High-Dose Ara-C and Dexamethasone
(DHAP)," *Blood*, 1988, 71(1):117-22.

Variation 2:

Chau I, Webb A, Cunningham D, et al, "An Oxaliplatin-Based Chemotherapy in Patients
With Relapsed or Refractory Intermediate and High-Grade Non-Hodgkin's
Lymphoma," *Br J Haematol*, 2001, 115(4):786-92.

Docetaxel-Cisplatin

Use Lung cancer, nonsmall cell

Regimen

Docetaxel: I.V.: 75 mg/m^2 day 1
[total dose/cycle = 75 mg/m^2]

Cisplatin: I.V.: 75 mg/m^2 day 1
[total dose/cycle = 75 mg/m^2]

Repeat cycle every 21 days

References

Zalcberg J, Millward M, Bishop J, et al, "Phase II Study of Docetaxel and Cisplatin in
Advanced Nonsmall-Cell Lung Cancer," *J Clin Oncol*, 1998, 16(5):1948-53.

Doxorubicin + Ketoconazole

Use Prostate cancer

Regimen

Doxorubicin: I.V.: 20 mg/m^2 continuous infusion day 1
[total dose/cycle = 20 mg/m^2]

Ketoconazole: Oral: 400 mg 3 times/day days 1 to 7
[total dose/cycle = 8400 mg]

Repeat cycle every 7 days

References

Sella A, Kilbourn R, Amato R, et al, "Phase II Study of Ketoconazole Combined With
Weekly Doxorubicin in Patients With Androgen-Independent Prostate Cancer," *J Clin
Oncol*, 1994, 12(4):683-8.

Doxorubicin + Ketoconazole/Estramustine + Vinblastine

Use Prostate cancer

Regimen

Doxorubicin: I.V.: 20 mg/m^2/day days 1, 15, and 29

[total dose/cycle = 60 mg/m^2]

Ketoconazole: Oral: 400 mg 3 times/day days 1 to 7, 15 to 21, and 29 to 35

[total dose/cycle = 25,200 mg]

Estramustine: Oral: 140 mg 3 times/day days 8 to 14, 22 to 28, and 36 to 42

[total dose/cycle = 8820 mg]

Vinblastine: I.V.: 5 mg/m^2/day days 8, 22, and 36

[total dose/cycle = 15 mg/m^2]

Repeat cycle every 8 weeks

References

Ellerhorst JA, Tu SM, Amato RJ, et al, "Phase II Trial of Alternating Weekly Chemohormonal Therapy for Patients With Androgen-Independent Prostate Cancer," *Clin Cancer Res*, 1997, 3(12 Pt 1):2371-6.

DTPACE

Use Multiple myeloma

Regimen

Dexamethasone: Oral: 40 mg/day days 1 to 4

[total dose/cycle = 160 mg]

Thalidomide: Oral: 400 mg/day

[total dose/cycle = 11,200-16,800 mg]

Cisplatin: I.V.: 10 mg/m^2/day continuous infusion days 1 to 4

[total dose/cycle = 40 mg/m^2]

Doxorubicin: I.V.: 10 mg/m^2/day continuous infusion days 1 to 4

[total dose/cycle = 40 mg/m^2]

Cyclophosphamide: I.V.: 400 mg/m^2 continuous infusion days 1 to 4

[total dose/cycle = 1600 mg/m^2]

Etoposide: I.V.: 40 mg/m^2 continuous infusion days 1 to 4

[total dose/cycle = 160 mg/m^2]

Repeat cycle every 4-6 weeks

References

Lee CKL, Barlogie B, Munshi N, et al, "DTPACE: An Effective, Novel Combination Chemotherapy With Thalidomide for Previously Treated Patients With Myeloma," *J Clin Oncol*, 2003, 21(14):2732-9.

DVD

Use Multiple myeloma

Regimen

Doxorubicin, liposomal: I.V.: 40 mg/m^2 day 1

[total dose/cycle = 40 mg/m^2]

Vincristine: I.V.: 2 mg day 1

[total dose/cycle = 2 mg]

Dexamethasone: Oral or I.V.: 40 mg/day days 1 to 4

[total dose/cycle = 160 mg]

Repeat cycle every 4 weeks

References

Hussein MA, Wood L, Hsi E, et al, "A Phase II Trial of Pegylated Liposomal Doxorubicin, Vincristine, and Reduced-Dose Dexamethasone Combination Therapy in Newly Diagnosed Multiple Myeloma Patients," *Cancer*, 2002, 95(10):2160-8.

DVP

Use Leukemia, acute lymphocytic

Regimen Induction:

Daunorubicin: I.V.: 25 mg/m^2/day days 1, 8, and 15

[total dose/cycle = 75 mg/m^2]

Vincristine: I.V.: 1.5 mg/m^2/day (maximum 2 mg) days 1, 8, 15, and 22

[total dose/cycle = 6 mg/m^2]

Prednisone: Oral: 60 mg/m^2/day days 1 to 28 then taper over next 14 days

[total dose/cycle = 1680 mg/m^2 + taper over next 14 days]

Administer single cycle; used in conjunction with intrathecal chemotherapy

References

Belasco JB, Luery N, and Scher C, "Multiagent Chemotherapy in Relapsed Acute Lymphoblastic Leukemia in Children," *Cancer*, 1990, 66(12):2492-7.

EAP

Use Gastric cancer

Regimen

Etoposide: I.V.: 120 mg/m^2/day days 4 to 6

[total dose/cycle = 360 mg/m^2]

Doxorubicin: I.V.: 20 mg/m^2/day days 1 and 7

[total dose/cycle = 40 mg/m^2]

Cisplatin: I.V.: 40 mg/m^2/day days 2 and 8

[total dose/cycle = 80 mg/m^2]

Repeat cycle every 28 days

References

Wilke H, Preusser P, Fink U, et al, "New Developments in the Treatment of Gastric Carcinoma," *Semin Oncol*, 1990, 17(1 Suppl 2):61-70.

Wilke H, Preusser P, Fink U, et al, "Preoperative Chemotherapy in Locally Advanced and Nonresectable Gastric Cancer: A phase II Study With Etoposide, Doxorubicin, and Cisplatin," *J Clin Oncol*, 1989, 7(9):1318-26.

ECF

Use Gastric cancer

Regimen

Epirubicin: I.V.: 50 mg/m^2 day 1

[total dose/cycle = 50 mg/m^2]

Cisplatin: I.V.: 60 mg/m^2 day 1

[total dose/cycle = 60 mg/m^2]

Repeat cycle every 3 weeks

Fluorouracil: I.V.: 200 mg/m^2/day continuous infusion for up to 6 months

[total dose/cycle = 36,000 mg/m^2]

References

Webb A, Cunningham D, Scarffe JH, et al, "Randomized Trial Comparing Epirubicin, Cisplatin, and Fluorouracil Versus Fluorouracil, Doxorubicin, and Methotrexate in Advanced Esophagogastric Cancer," *J Clin Oncol*, 1997, 15(1):261-7.

EC (Nonsmall Cell Lung Cancer)

Use Lung cancer, nonsmall cell

Regimen

Etoposide: I.V.: 120 mg/m^2/day days 1 to 3
[total dose/cycle = 360 mg/m^2]

Carboplatin: I.V.: AUC 6 day 1
[total dose/cycle = AUC = 6]

Repeat cycle every 21-28 days

References

Birch R, Weaver CH, Hainsworth JD, et al, "A Randomized Study of Etoposide and Carboplatin With or Without Paclitaxel in the Treatment of Small Cell Lung Cancer," *Semin Oncol*, 1997, 24(4 Suppl 12):S12-135, 137.

EC (Small Cell Lung Cancer)

Use Lung cancer, small cell

Regimen NOTE: Multiple variations are listed below.

Variation 1:

Etoposide: I.V.: 100-120 mg/m^2/day days 1 to 3
[total dose/cycle = 300-360 mg/m^2]

Carboplatin: I.V.: 325-400 mg/m^2 day 1
[total dose/cycle = 325-400 mg/m^2]

Repeat cycle every 28 days

Variation 2:

Etoposide: I.V.: 120 mg/m^2/day days 1 to 3
[total dose/cycle = 360 mg/m^2]

Carboplatin: I.V.: AUC 6 day 1
[total dose/cycle = AUC = 6]

Repeat cycle every 21-28 days

References

Variation 1:

Kosmidis PA, Samantas E, Fountzilas G, et al, "Cisplatin/Etoposide Versus Carboplatin/Etoposide Chemotherapy and Irradiation in Small Cell Lung Cancer: A Randomized Phase III Study. Hellenic Cooperative Oncology Group for Lung Cancer Trials," *Semin Oncol*, 1994, 1(3 Suppl 6):23-30.

Variation 2:

Birch R, Weaver CH, Hainsworth JD, et al, "A Randomized Study of Etoposide and Carboplatin With or Without Paclitaxel in the Treatment of Small Cell Lung Cancer," *Semin Oncol* 1997, 24(4 Suppl 12):S12-135, S12-137.

EE

Use Wilms' tumor

Regimen

Dactinomycin: I.V.: 15 mcg/kg/day days 1 to 5 of weeks 0, 5, 13, and 24
[total dose/cycle = 300 mcg/kg]

Vincristine: I.V.: 1.5 mg/m^2 day 1 of weeks 1-10, 13, 14, 24, and 25
[total dose/cycle = 21 mg/m^2]

References

Green DM, Breslow NE, Beckwith JB, et al, "Effect of Duration of Treatment on Treatment Putcome and Cost of Treatment for Wilms' Tumor: A Report From the National Wilms' Tumor Study Group," *J Clin Oncol*, 16(12):3744-51.

EE-4A

Use Wilms' tumor

Regimen

Dactinomycin: I.V.: 45 mcg/kg day 1 of weeks 0, 3, 6, 9, 12, 15, and 18
[total dose/cycle = 315 mcg/kg]

Vincristine: I.V.: 2 mg/m² day 1 of weeks 1-10, 12, 15, and 18
[total dose/cycle = 26 mg/m²]

References

Green DM, Breslow NE, Beckwith JB, et al, "Effect of Duration of Treatment on Treatment Putcome and Cost of Treatment for Wilms' Tumor: A Report From the National Wilms' Tumor Study Group," *J Clin Oncol*, 16(12):3744-51.

ELF

Use Gastric cancer

Regimen

Leucovorin calcium: I.V.: 300 mg/m²/day days 1 to 3, **followed by**
[total dose/cycle = 900 mg/m²]

Etoposide: I.V.: 120 mg/m²/day days 1 to 3, **followed by**
[total dose/cycle = 360 mg/m²]

Fluorouracil: I.V.: 500 mg/m²/day days 1 to 3
[total dose/cycle = 1500 mg/m²]

Repeat cycle every 21-28 days

References

Wilke H, Preusser P, Fink U, et al, "New Developments in the Treatment of Gastric Carcinoma," *Semin Oncol*, 1990, 17(1 Suppl 2):61-70.

EMA 86

Use Leukemia, acute myeloid

Regimen

Mitoxantrone: I.V.: 12 mg/m²/day days 1 to 3
[total dose/cycle = 36 mg/m²]

Etoposide: I.V.: 200 mg/m²/day continuous infusion days 8 to 10
[total dose/cycle = 600 mg/m²]

Cytarabine: I.V.: 500 mg/m₂/day continuous infusion days 1 to 3 and 8 to 10
[total dose/cycle = 3000 mg/m²]

Administer one cycle only

References

Archimbaud E, Fenaux P, Reiffers J, et al, "Granulocyte-Macrophage Colony-Stimulating Factor in Association to Timed-Sequential Chemotherapy With Mitoxantrone, Etoposide, and Cytarabine for Refractory Acute Myelogenous Leukemia," *Leukemia*, 1993, 7(3):372-7.

EMA/CO

Use Gestational trophoblastic tumor

Regimen

Etoposide: I.V.: 100 mg/m²/day days 1 and 2
[total dose/cycle = 200 mg/m²]

Methotrexate: I.V.: 300 mg/m² infused over 12 hours day 1
[total dose/cycle = 300 mg/m²]

Dactinomycin: I.V. push: 0.5 mg/day days 1 and 2
[total dose/cycle = 1 mg]

Leucovorin: Oral, I.M.: 15 mg twice daily for 2 days (start 24 hours after the start of methotrexate) days 2 and 3
[total dose/cycle = 60 mg]

Alternate weekly with:

Cyclophosphamide: I.V.: 600 mg/m² infused over 30 minutes day 1
[total dose/cycle = 600 mg/m²]

Vincristine: I.V. push: 0.8 mg/m² (maximum 2 mg) day 1
[total dose/cycle = 0.8 mg/m²]

(Continued)

EMA/CO *(Continued)*

References
Bagshawe KD, "High-Risk Metastatic Trophoblastic Disease," *Obstet Gynecol Clin North Am*, 1988, 15(3):531-43.

EP (Adenocarcinoma)
Use Adenocarcinoma, unknown primary

Regimen
Cisplatin: I.V.: 60-100 mg/m² day 1
[total dose = 60-100 mg/m²]
Etoposide: I.V.: 80-100 mg/m²/day days 1 to 3
[total dose = 240-300 mg/m²]
Repeat cycle every 21 days

References
Sulkes A, Uziely B, Isacson R, et al, "Combination Chemotherapy in Metastatic Tumors of Unknown Origin. 5-Fluorouracil, Adriamycin® and Mitomycin C for Adenocarcinomas and Adriamycin®, Vinblastine and Mitomycin C for Anaplastic Carcinomas," *Isr J Med Sci*, 1988, 24(9-10):604-10.

EP (Nonsmall Cell Lung Cancer)
Use Lung cancer, nonsmall cell

Regimen
Etoposide: I.V.: 80-120 mg/m²/day days 1 to 3
[total dose/cycle = 240-360 mg/m²]
Cisplatin: I.V.: 80-100 mg/m² day 1
[total dose/cycle = 80-100 mg/m²]
Repeat cycle every 21-28 days

References
Goldhirsch A, Joss RA, Cavalli F, et al, "Cis-Dichlorodiammineplatinum (II) and VP 16-213 Combination Chemotherapy for Nonsmall-Cell Lung Cancer," *Med Pediatr Oncol*, 1981, 9(3):205-8.

EP (Small Cell Lung Cancer)
Use Lung cancer, small cell

Regimen NOTE: Multiple variations are listed below.
Variation 1:
Etoposide: I.V.: 100 mg/m²/day days 1 to 3
[total dose/cycle = 300 mg/m²]
Cisplatin: I.V.: 100 mg/m² day 1
[total dose/cycle = 100 mg/m²]
Repeat cycle every 21 days
Variation 2:
Etoposide: I.V.: 80 mg/m²/day days 1 to 3
[total dose/cycle = 240 mg/m²]
Cisplatin: I.V.: 80 mg/m² day 1
[total dose/cycle = 80 mg/m²]
Repeat cycle every 21-28 days

References
Variation 1:
Goodman GE, Crowley JJ, Blasko JC, et al, "Treatment of Limited Small-Cell Lung Cancer With Etoposide and Cisplatin Alternating With Vincristine, Doxorubicin, and Cyclophosphamide Versus Concurrent Etoposide, Vincristine, Doxorubicin, and Cyclophosphamide and Chest Radiotherapy: A Southwest Oncology Group Study," *J Clin Oncol*, 1990, 8(1):39-47.

Variation 2:
Perng RP, Chen YM, Ming-Liu J, et al, "Gemcitabine Versus the Combination of Cisplatin and Etoposide in Patients With Inoperable Nonsmall Cell Lung Cancer in a Phase II Randomized Study," *J Clin Oncol*, 1997, 15(5):2097-102.

EP (Testicular Cancer)

Use Testicular cancer

Regimen NOTE: Multiple variations are listed below.

Variation 1:

Etoposide: I.V.: 100 mg/m^2/day days 1 to 5
[total dose/cycle = 500 mg/m^2]
Cisplatin: I.V.: 20 mg/m^2/day days 1 to 5
[total dose/cycle = 100 mg/m^2]
Repeat cycle every 21 days

Variation 2:

Etoposide: I.V.: 120 mg/m^2/day days 1 to 3
[total dose/cycle = 360 mg/m^2]
Cisplatin: I.V.: 20 mg/m^2/day days 1 to 5
[total dose/cycle = 100 mg/m^2]
Repeat cycle every 3 or 4 weeks

Variation 3:

Etoposide: I.V.: 120 mg/m^2/day days 1, 3, and 5
[total dose/cycle = 360 mg/m^2]
Cisplatin: I.V.: 20 mg/m^2/day days 1 to 5
[total dose/cycle = 100 mg/m^2]
Repeat cycle every 3 or 4 weeks

References

Variation 1:
Hainsworth JD, Williams SD, Einhorn LH, et al, "Successful Treatment of Resistant Germinal Neoplasms With VP-16 and Cisplatin: Results of a Southeastern Cancer Study Group Trial," *J Clin Oncol*, 1985, 3(5):666-71.
Variation 2:
Peckham MJ, Horwich A, Blackmore C, et al, "Etoposide and Cisplatin With or Without Bleomycin as First-Line Chemotherapy for Patients With Small-Volume Metastases of Testicular Nonseminoma," *Cancer Treat Rep*, 1985, 69(5):483-8.
Variation 3:
de Wit R, Stoter G, Kaye SB, et al, "Importance of Bleomycin in Combination Chemotherapy for Good-Prognosis Testicular Nonseminoma: A Randomized Study of the European Organization for Research and Treatment of Cancer Genitourinary Tract Cancer Cooperative Group," *J Clin Oncol*, 1997, 15(5):1837-43.

EP/EMA

Use Gestational trophoblastic tumor

Regimen

Etoposide: I.V.: 150 mg/m^2 day 1
[total dose/cycle = 150 mg/m^2]
Cisplatin: I.V.: 25 mg/m^2 infused over 4 hours for 3 consecutive doses, day 1
[total dose/cycle = 75 mg/m^2]

Alternate weekly with:

Etoposide: I.V.: 100 mg/m^2 day 1
[total dose/cycle = 100 mg/m^2]
Methotrexate: I.V.: 300 mg/m^2 infused over 12 hours day 1
[total dose/cycle = 300 mg/m^2]
Dactinomycin: I.V. push: 0.5 mg day 1
[total dose/cycle = 0.5 mg]
(Continued)

EP/EMA *(Continued)*

Leucovorin: Oral, I.M.: 15 mg twice daily for 2 days; start 24 hours after the start of methotrexate, days 2 and 3

[total dose/cycle = 60 mg]

References

Newlands ES, Bower M, Holden L, et al, "Management of Resistant Gestational Trophoblastic Tumors," *J Reprod Med*, 1998, 43(2):111-8.

EP/PE

Use Lung cancer, nonsmall cell

Regimen

Etoposide: I.V.: 120 mg/m^2/day days 1 to 3

[total dose/cycle = 360 mg/m^2]

Cisplatin: I.V.: 60-120 mg/m^2 day 1

[total dose/cycle = 60-120 mg/m^2]

Repeat cycle every 21-28 days

References

Weick JK, Crowley J, Natale RB, et al, "A Randomized Trial of Five Cisplatin-Containing Treatments in Patients With Metastatic NonSmall-Cell Lung Cancer: A Southwest Oncology Group Study," *J Clin Oncol*, 1991, 9(7):1157-62.

EPOCH

Use Lymphoma, non-Hodgkin's

Regimen

Etoposide: I.V.: 50 mg/m^2/day continuous infusion days 1 to 4

[total dose/cycle = 200 mg/m^2]

Vincristine: I.V.: 0.4 mg/m^2/day continuous infusion days 1 to 4

[total dose/cycle = 1.6 mg/m^2]

Doxorubicin: I.V.: 10 mg/m^2/day continuous infusion days 1 to 4

[total dose/cycle = 40 mg/m^2]

Cyclophosphamide: I.V.: 750 mg/m^2 day 6

[total dose/cycle = 750 mg/m^2]

Prednisone: Oral: 60 mg/m^2/day days 1 to 6

[total dose/cycle = 360 mg/m^2]

Repeat cycle every 21 days

References

Wilson WH, Bryant G, Bates S, et al, "EPOCH Chemotherapy: Toxicity and Efficacy in Relapsed and Refractory Non-Hodgkin's Lymphoma," *J Clin Oncol*, 1993, 11(8):1573-82.

ESHAP

Use Lymphoma, non-Hodgkin's

Regimen NOTE: Multiple variations are listed below.

Variation 1:

Etoposide: I.V.: 40 mg/m^2/day days 1 to 4

[total dose/cycle = 160 mg/m^2]

Methylprednisolone: I.V.: 500 mg/day days 1 to 5

[total dose/cycle = 2500 mg]

Cytarabine: I.V.: 2000 mg/m^2 day 1

[total dose/cycle = 2000 mg/m^2]

Cisplatin: I.V.: 25 mg/m^2/day continuous infusion days 1 to 4

[total dose/cycle = 100 mg/m^2]

Repeat cycle every 21-28 days

Variation 2:

Etoposide: I.V.: 40 mg/m^2/day days 1 to 4

[total dose/cycle = 160 mg/m^2]

Methylprednisolone: I.V.: 500 mg/day days 1 to 5
[total dose/cycle = 2500 mg]

Cytarabine: I.V.: 2000 mg/m^2 day 5
[total dose/cycle = 2000 mg/m^2]

Cisplatin: I.V.: 25 mg/m^2/day continuous infusion days 1 to 4
[total dose/cycle = 100 mg/m^2]

Repeat cycle every 21-28 days

Variation 3:

Etoposide: I.V.: 60 mg/m^2/day days 1 to 4
[total dose/cycle = 240 mg/m^2]

Methylprednisolone: I.V.: 500 mg/day days 1 to 4
[total dose/cycle = 2000 mg]

Cytarabine: I.V.: 2000 mg/m^2 day 5
[total dose/cycle = 2000 mg/m^2]

Cisplatin: I.V.: 25 mg/m^2/day continuous infusion days 1 to 4
[total dose/cycle = 100 mg/m^2]

Repeat cycle every 21 days

References

Variation 1:
Velasquez WF, McLaughlin P, Tucker S, et al, "ESHAP - An Effective Chemotherapy Regimen in Refractory and Relapsing Lymphoma: A 4-Year Follow-Up Study," *J Clin Oncol*, 1994, 12(6):1169-76.

Variation 2:
Wang WS, Chiou TJ, Liu JH, et al, "ESHAP as Salvage Therapy for Refractory Non-Hodgkin's Lymphoma: Taiwan Experience," *Jpn J Clin Oncol*, 1999, 29(1):33-7.

Variation 3:
Rodriguez MA, Cabanillas FC, Velasquez W, et al, "Results of a Salvage Treatment Program for Relapsing Lymphoma: MINE Consolidated With ESHAP," *J Clin Oncol*, 1995, 13(7):1734-41.

Estramustine + Docetaxel

Use Prostate cancer

Regimen NOTE: Multiple variations are listed below.

Variation 1:

Docetaxel: I.V.: 20-80 mg/m^2 day 2
[total dose/cycle = 20-80 mg/m^2]

Estramustine: Oral: 280 mg 3 times/day days 1 to 5
[total dose/cycle = 4200 mg]

Repeat cycle every 21 days

Variation 2:

Docetaxel: I.V.: 20-80 mg/m^2 day 2
[total dose/cycle = 20-80 mg/m^2]

Estramustine: Oral: 14 mg/kg/day days 1 to 21
[total dose/cycle = 294 mg/kg]

Repeat cycle every 21 days

Variation 3:

Docetaxel: I.V.: 35 mg/m^2/day days 2 and 9
[total dose/cycle = 70 mg/m^2]

Estramustine: Oral: 420 mg 3 times/day for 4 doses, then 280 mg 3 times/day for 5 doses days 1, 2, 3, 8, 9, and 10
[total dose/cycle = 6160 mg]

Repeat cycle every 21 days

(Continued)

Estramustine + Docetaxel *(Continued)*

References

Variation 1:
Petrylak DP, Macarthur RB, O'Connor J, et al, "Phase I Trial of Docetaxel With Estramustine in Androgen-Independent Prostate Cancer," *J Clin Oncol*, 1999, 17(3):958-67.
Variation 2:
Kreis W, Budman DR, Fetten J, et al, "Phase I Trial of The Combination of Daily Estramustine Phosphate and Intermittent Docetaxel in Patients With Metastatic Hormone Refractory Prostate Carcinoma," *Ann Oncol*, 1999, 10(1):33-8.
Variation 3:
Sitka Copur M, Ledakis P, Lynch J, et al, "Weekly Docetaxel and Estramustine in Patients With Hormone-Refractory Prostate Cancer," *Semin Oncol*, 2001, 28(4 Suppl 15):16-21.

Estramustine + Docetaxel + Carboplatin

Use Prostate cancer

Regimen

Docetaxel: I.V.: 70 mg/m^2 day 2
[total dose/cycle = 70 mg/m^2]
Estramustine: Oral: 280 mg 3 times/day days 1 to 5
[total dose/cycle = 4200 mg]
Carboplatin: I.V.: Target AUC 5 day 2
[total dose/cycle = AUC = 5]
Repeat cycle every 3 weeks

References

Oh WK, Halabi S, Kelly WK, et al, "A Phase II Study of Estramustine, Docetaxel, and Carboplatin (EDC) with G-CSF Support in Men With Hormone Refractory Prostate Cancer: CALGB 99813," *Proc Am Soc Clin Oncol*, 2002, 21:195a.

Estramustine + Docetaxel + Hydrocortisone

Use Prostate cancer

Regimen

Docetaxel: I.V.: 70 mg/m^2 day 2
[total dose/cycle = 70 mg/m^2]
Estramustine: Oral: 10 mg/kg/day days 1 to 5
[total dose/cycle = 50 mg/kg]
Hydrocortisone: Oral: 40 mg daily
[total dose/cycle = 840 mg]
Repeat cycle every 3 weeks

References

Savarese DM, Halabi S, Hars V, et al, "Phase II Study of Docetaxel, Estramustine, and Low-Dose Hydrocortisone in Men With Hormone-Refractory Prostate Cancer: A Final Report of CALGB 9780. Cancer and Leukemia Group B," *J Clin Oncol*, 2001, 19(9):2509-16.

Estramustine + Etoposide

Use Prostate cancer

Regimen NOTE: Multiple variations are listed below.

Variation 1:
Estramustine: Oral: 15 mg/kg/day days 1 to 21
[total dose/cycle = 315 mg/kg]
Etoposide: Oral: 50 mg/m^2/day days 1 to 21
[total dose/cycle = 1050 mg/m^2]
Repeat cycle every 4 weeks

Variation 2:
Estramustine: Oral: 10 mg/kg/day days 1 to 21
[total dose/cycle = 210 mg/kg]

Etoposide: Oral: 50 mg/m^2/day days 1 to 21
[total dose/cycle = 1050 mg/m^2]
Repeat cycle every 4 weeks
Variation 3:
Estramustine: Oral: 140 mg 3 times/day days 1 to 21
[total dose/cycle = 8820 mg]
Etoposide: Oral: 50 mg/m^2/day days 1 to 21
[total dose/cycle = 1050 mg/m^2]
Repeat cycle every 4 weeks

References

Variation 1: Pienta KJ, Redman B, Hussain M, et al, "Phase II Evaluation of Oral Estramustine and Oral Etoposide in Hormone-Refractory Adenocarcinoma of the Prostate," *J Clin Oncol*, 1994, 12(10):2005-12.
Variation 2: Pienta KJ, Redman BG, Bandekar R, et al, "A Phase II Trial of Oral Estramustine and Oral Etoposide in Hormone Refractory Prostate Cancer," *Urology*,1997, 50(3):401-6; discussion 406-7.
Variation 3: Dimopoulos MA, Panopoulos C, Bamia C, et al, "Oral Estramustine and Oral Etoposide for Hormone-Refractory Prostate Cancer," *Urology*,1997, 50(5):754-8.

♦ **Estramustine + Vinblastine** *see* EV *on page 883*

Estramustine + Vinorelbine

Use Prostate cancer
Regimen
Estramustine: Oral: 140 mg 3 times/day days 1 to 14
[total dose/cycle = 5880 mg]
Vinorelbine: I.V.: 25 mg/m^2/day days 1 and 8
[total dose/cycle = 50 mg/m^2]
Repeat cycle every 21 days

References

Smith MR, Kaufman D, Oh W, et al, "Vinorelbine and Estramustine in Androgen-Independent Metastatic Prostate Cancer: A Phase II Study," *Cancer*, 2000, 89(8):1824-8.

EV

Synonyms Estramustine + Vinblastine
Use Prostate cancer
Regimen NOTE: Multiple variations are listed below.
Variation 1:
Estramustine: Oral: 10 mg/kg/day days 1 to 42 (given in 3 divided doses)
[total dose/cycle = 420 mg/kg]
Vinblastine: I.V.: 4 mg/m^2/day days 1, 8, 15, 22, 29, and 36 (weekly for 6 weeks)
[total dose/cycle = 24 mg/m^2]
Repeat cycle every 8 weeks
Variation 2:
Estramustine: Oral: 600 mg/m^2/day days 1 to 42 (given in 3 divided doses)
[total dose/cycle = 25,200 mg/m^2]
Vinblastine: I.V.: 4 mg/m^2/day days 1, 8, 15, 22, 29, and 36 (weekly for 6 weeks)
[total dose/cycle = 24 mg/m^2]
Repeat cycle every 8 weeks
(Continued)

EV (Continued)

References

Variation 1:

Seidman AD, Scher HI, Petrylak D, et al, "Estramustine and Vinblastine: Use of Prostate Specific Antigen as a Clinical Trial End Point for Hormone Refractory Prostatic Cancer," *J Urol*, 1992, 147(3 Pt 2):931-4.

Variation 2:

Hudes GR, Greenberg R, Krigel RL, et al, "Phase II Study of Estramustine and Vinblastine, Two Microtubule Inhibitors, in Hormone-Refractory Prostate Cancer," *J Clin Oncol*, 1992, 10(11):1754-61.

EVA

Use Lymphoma, Hodgkin's disease

Regimen

Etoposide: I.V.: 100 mg/m^2/day days 1 to 3
[total dose/cycle = 300 mg/m^2]
Vinblastine: I.V.: 6 mg/m^2 day 1
[total dose/cycle = 6 mg/m^2]
Doxorubicin: I.V.: 50 mg/m^2 day 1
[total dose/cycle = 50 mg/m^2]
Repeat cycle every 28 days

References

Canellos GP, Petroni GR, Barcos M, et al, "Etoposide, Vinblastine, and Doxorubicin: An Active Regimen for the Treatment of Hodgkin's Disease in Relapse Following MOPP. Cancer and Leukemia Group B," *J Clin Oncol*, 1995, 13(8):2005-11.

FAC

Synonyms CAF-IV; IVCAF

Use Breast cancer

Regimen NOTE: Multiple variations are listed below.

Variation 1:

Fluorouracil: I.V.: 500 mg/m^2/day days 1 and 8
[total dose/cycle = 1000 mg/m^2]
or 500 mg/m^2 day 1
[total dose/cycle = 500 mg/m^2]
Doxorubicin: I.V.: 50 mg/m^2 day 1
[total dose/cycle = 50 mg/m^2]
Cyclophosphamide: I.V.: 500 mg/m^2 day 1
[total dose/cycle = 500 mg/m^2]
Repeat cycle every 21-28 days

Variation 2:

Fluorouracil: I.V.: 200 mg/m^2/day days 1 to 3
[total dose/cycle = 600 mg/m^2]
Doxorubicin: I.V.: 40 mg/m^2 day 1
[total dose/cycle = 40 mg/m^2]
Cyclophosphamide: I.V.: 400 mg/m^2 day 1
[total dose/cycle = 400 mg/m^2]
Repeat cycle every 28 days

Variation 3:

Fluorouracil: I.V.: 400 mg/m^2/day days 1 and 8
[total dose/cycle = 800 mg/m^2]
Doxorubicin: I.V.: 40 mg/m^2 day 1
[total dose/cycle = 40 mg/m^2]
Cyclophosphamide: I.V.: 400 mg/m^2 day 1
[total dose/cycle = 400 mg/m^2]
Repeat cycle every 28 days

Variation 4:

Fluorouracil: I.V.: 600 mg/m^2/day days 1 and 8
[total dose/cycle = 1200 mg/m^2]

Doxorubicin: I.V.: 60 mg/m^2 day 1
[total dose/cycle = 60 mg/m^2]

Cyclophosphamide: I.V.: 600 mg/m^2 day 1
[total dose/cycle = 600 mg/m^2]

Repeat cycle every 28 days

Variation 5:

Fluorouracil: I.V.: 300 mg/m^2/day days 1 and 8
[total dose/cycle = 600 mg/m^2]

Doxorubicin: I.V.: 30 mg/m^2 day 1
[total dose/cycle = 30 mg/m^2]

Cyclophosphamide: I.V.: 300 mg/m^2 day 1
[total dose/cycle = 300 mg/m^2]

Repeat cycle every 28 days

References

Variation 1:

Smalley RV, Carpenter J, Bartolucci A, et al, "A Comparison of Cyclophosphamide, Adriamycin®, 5-Fluorouracil (CAF), and Cyclophosphamide, Methotrexate, 5-Fluorouracil, Vincristine, Prednisone (CMFVP) in Patients With Metastatic Breast Cancer: A Southeastern Cancer Study Group Project," *Cancer*, 1977, 40(2):625-32.

Swenerton KD, Legha SS, Smith T, et al, "Prognostic Factors in Metastatic Breast Cancer Treated With Combination Chemotherapy," *Cancer Res*, 1979, 39(5):1552-62.

Variation 2:

Nemoto T, Horton J, Simon R, et al, "Comparison of Four-Combination Chemotherapy Programs in Metastatic Breast Cancer: Comparison of Multiple Drug Therapy With Cytoxan, 5-FU, and Prednisone, Versus Cytoxan and Adriamycin, Versus Cytoxan, 5-FU, and Adriamycin, Versus Cytoxan, 5-FU, and Prednisone Alternation With Cytoxan and Adriamycin," *Cancer*, 1982, 49(10):1988-93.

Variation 3-5:

Wood WC, Budman DR, Korzun AH, et al, "Dose and Dose Intensity of Adjuvant Chemotherapy for State II, Node-Positive Breast Carcinoma," *N Engl J Med*, 1994, 330(18):1253-9.

FAM

Use Gastric cancer; Pancreatic cancer

Regimen

Fluorouracil: I.V.: 600 mg/m^2/day days 1, 8, 29, and 36
[total dose/cycle = 2400 mg/m^2]

Doxorubicin: I.V.: 30 mg/m^2/day days 1 and 29
[total dose/cycle = 60 mg/m^2]

Mitomycin C: I.V.: 10 mg/m^2 day 1
[total dose/cycle = 10 mg/m^2]

Repeat cycle every 8 weeks

References

Cullinan SA, Moertel CG, Fleming TR, et al, "A Comparison of Three Chemotherapeutic Regimens in the Treatment of Advanced Pancreatic and Gastric Carcinoma. Fluorouracil vs Fluorouracil and Doxorubicin vs Fluorouracil, Doxorubicin, and Mitomycin," *JAMA*, 1985, 253(14):2061-7.

Preusser P, Achterrath W, Wilke H, et al, "Chemotherapy of Gastric Cancer," *Cancer Treat Rev*, 1988, 15(4):257-77.

FAMTX

Use Gastric cancer

Regimen

Methotrexate: I.V.: 1500 mg/m^2 day 1

[total dose/cycle = 1500 mg/m^2]

Fluorouracil: I.V.: 1500 mg/m^2 day 1

[total dose/cycle = 1500 mg/m^2]

Leucovorin: Oral: 15 mg/m^2 every 6 hours for 8 doses (start 24 hours after methotrexate)

[total dose/cycle = 120 mg/m^2]

followed by 30 mg/m^2 every 6 hours for 8 more doses if 24-hour methotrexate level ≥2.5 mol/L (start 24 hours after methotrexate)

[total dose/cycle = 240 mg/m^2]

Doxorubicin: I.V.: 30 mg/m^2 day 15

[total dose/cycle = 30 mg/m^2]

Repeat cycle every 28 days

References

Webb A, Cunningham D, Scarffe JH, et al, " Randomized Trial Comparing Epirubicin, Cisplatin, and Fluorouracil Versus Fluorouracil, Doxorubicin, and Methotrexate in Advanced Esophagogastric Cancer," *J Clin Oncol*, 1997, 15(1):261-7.

Wils J, Bleiberg H, Dalesio O, et al, "An EORTC Gastrointestinal Group Evaluation of the Combination of Sequential Methotrexate and 5-Fluorouracil, Combined With Adriamycin in Advanced Measurable Gastric Cancer," *J Clin Oncol*, 1986, 4(12):1799-803.

F-CL

Synonyms FU/Leucovorin; FU-LV

Use Colorectal cancer

Regimen NOTE: Multiple variations are listed below.

Variation 1 (Mayo Regimen):

Fluorouracil: I.V.: 425 mg/m^2/day days 1 to 5

[total dose/cycle = 2125 mg/m^2]

Leucovorin: I.V.: 20 mg/m^2/day days 1 to 5

[total dose/cycle = 100 mg/m^2]

Repeat cycle every 28 days

Variation 2:

Fluorouracil: I.V.: 400 mg/m^2/day days 1 to 5

[total dose/cycle = 2000 mg/m^2]

Leucovorin: I.V.: 20 mg/m^2/day days 1 to 5

[total dose/cycle = 100 mg/m^2]

Repeat cycle every 28 days

Variation 3:

Fluorouracil: I.V.: 500 mg/m^2 day 1

[total dose/cycle = 500 mg/m^2]

Leucovorin: I.V.: 20 mg/m^2 (2-hour infusion) day 1

[total dose/cycle = 20 mg/m^2]

or 500 mg/m^2 (2-hour infusion) day 1

[total dose/cycle = 500 mg/m^2]

Repeat cycle weekly

Variation 4:

Fluorouracil: I.V.: 600 mg/m^2 weekly for 6 weeks

[total dose/cycle = 3600 mg/m^2]

Leucovorin: I.V.: 500 mg/m^2 (3-hour infusion) weekly for 6 weeks

[total dose/cycle = 3000 mg/m^2]

Repeat cycle every 8 weeks

Variation 5:
  Fluorouracil: I.V.: 600 mg/m^2 weekly for 6 weeks
    [total dose/cycle = 3600 mg/m^2]
  Leucovorin: I.V.: 500 mg/m^2 weekly for 6 weeks
    [total dose/cycle = 3000 mg/m^2]
  Repeat cycle every 8 weeks
Variation 6:
  Fluorouracil: I.V.: 600 mg/m^2 weekly
  Leucovorin: I.V.: 500 mg/m^2 (2-hour infusion) weekly
  Repeat cycle weekly
Variation 7:
  Fluorouracil: I.V.: 2600 mg/m^2 continuous infusion day 1
    [total dose/cycle = 2600 mg/m^2]
  Leucovorin: I.V.: 500 mg/m^2 continuous infusion day 1
    [total dose/cycle = 500 mg/m^2]
  Repeat cycle weekly
Variation 8:
  Fluorouracil: I.V.: 2600 mg/m^2 continuous infusion day 1
    [total dose/cycle = 2600 mg/m^2]
  Leucovorin: I.V.: 300 mg/m^2 (maximum 500 mg) continuous infusion
    day 1
    [total dose/cycle = 300 mg/m^2]
  Repeat cycle weekly
Variation 9:
  Fluorouracil: I.V.: 2600 mg/m^2 continuous infusion once weekly for 6
    weeks
    [total dose/cycle = 15,600 mg/m^2]
  Leucovorin: I.V.: 500 mg/m^2 weekly for 6 weeks
    [total dose/cycle = 3000 mg/m^2]
  Repeat cycle every 8 weeks
Variation 10:
  Fluorouracil: I.V.: 2300 mg/m^2 continuous infusion day 1
    [total dose/cycle = 2300 mg/m^2]
  Leucovorin: I.V.: 50 mg/m^2 continuous infusion day 1
    [total dose/cycle = 50 mg/m^2]
  Repeat cycle weekly
Variation 11:
  Fluorouracil: I.V.: 200 mg/m^2/day continuous infusion days 1 to 14
    [total dose/cycle = 2800 mg/m^2]
  Leucovorin: I.V.: 5 mg/m^2/day days 1 to 14
    [total dose/cycle = 70 mg/m^2]
  Repeat cycle every 28 days
Variation 12:
  Fluorouracil: I.V.: 200 mg/m^2 continuous infusion daily for 4 weeks
    followed by (starting week 5): 200 mg/m^2 continuous infusion days
    1-21
    [total dose/cycle = 4200 mg/m^2]
  Leucovorin: I.V.: 20 mg/m^2/day days 1, 8, and 15
    [total dose/cycle = 60 mg/m^2]
  Repeat cycle every 4 weeks
(Continued)

F-CL *(Continued)*

References

Variation 1:
  Poon MA, O'Connell MJ, Moertel CG, et al, "Biochemical Modulation of Fluorouracil: Evidence of Significant Improvement of Survival and Quality of Life in Patients With Advanced Colorectal Carcinoma," *J Clin Oncol*, 1989 7(10):1407-18.

Variation 2:
  Borner MM, Castiglione M, Bacchi M, et al "The Impact of Adding Low-Dose Leucovorin to Monthly 5-Fluorouracil in Advanced Colorectal Carcinoma: Results of a Phase III Trial. Swiss Group for Clinical Cancer Research (SAKK)," *Ann Oncol*, 1998, 9(5):535-41.

Variation 3:
  Jager E, Heike M, Bernhard H, et al, "Weekly High-Dose Leucovorin Versus Low-Dose Leucovorin Combined With Fluorouracil in Advanced Colorectal Cancer: Results of a Randomized Multicenter Trial. Study Group for Palliative Treatment of Metastatic Colorectal Cancer Study Protocol 1," *J Clin Oncol*, 1996, 14(8):2274-9.

Variation 4:
  Leichman CG, Fleming TR, Muggia FM, et al, "Phase II Study of Fluorouracil and its Modulation in Advanced Colorectal Cancer: A Southwest Oncology Group Study," *J Clin Oncol*, 1995, 13(6):1303-11.

Variation 5:
  Buroker TR, O'Connell MJ, Wieand HS, et al, "Randomized Comparison of Two Schedules of Fluorouracil and Leucovorin in the Treatment of Advanced Colorectal Cancer," *J Clin Oncol*, 1994, 12(1):14-20.

Variation 6:
  Nobile MT, Rosso R, Sertoli MR, et al, "Randomised Comparison of Weekly Bolus 5-Fluorouracil With or Without Leucovorin in Metastatic Colorectal Carcinoma," *Eur J Cancer*, 1992, 28A(11):1823-7.

Variation 7:
  Ardalan B, Chua L, Tian EM, et al, "A Phase II Study of Weekly 24-Hour Infusion With High-Dose Fluorouracil With Leucovorin in Colorectal Carcinoma," *J Clin Oncol*, 1991, 9(4):625-30.

Variation 8:
  Yeh KH, Cheng AL, Lin MT, et al, "A Phase II Study of Weekly 24-Hour Infusion of High-Dose 5-Fluorouracil and Leucovorin (HDFL) in the Treatment of Recurrent or Metastatic Colorectal Cancers," *Anticancer Res*, 1997, 17(5B):3867-72.

Variation 9:
  Kohne CH, Schoffski P, Wilke H, et al, "Effective Biomodulation by Leucovorin of High-Dose Infusion Fluorouracil Given as a Weekly 24-Hour Infusion: Results of a Randomized Trial in Patients With Advanced Colorectal Cancer," *J Clin Oncol*, 1998, 16(2):418-26.

Variation 10:
  Haas NB, Schilder RJ, Nash S, et al, "A Phase II Trial of Weekly Infusional 5-Fluorouracil in Combination With Low-Dose Leucovorin in Patients With Advanced Colorectal Cancer," *Invest New Drugs*, 1995, 13(3):229-33.

Variation 11:
  Falcone A, Allegrini G, Lencioni M, et al, "Protracted Continuous Infusion of 5-Fluorouracil and Low-Dose Leucovorin in Patients With Metastatic Colorectal Cancer Resistant to 5-Fluorouracil Bolus-Based Chemotherapy: A Phase II Study," *Cancer Chemother Pharmacol*, 1999, 44(2):159-63.

Variation 12:
  Leichman CG, Leichman L, Spears CP, et al, "Prolonged Continuous Infusion of Fluorouracil With Weekly Bolus Leucovorin: A Phase II Study in Patients With Disseminated Colorectal Cancer," *J Natl Cancer Inst*, 1993, 85(1):41-4.

FEC

Use Breast cancer

Regimen

Fluorouracil: I.V.: 500 mg/m^2 day 1
  [total dose/cycle = 500 mg/m^2]
Cyclophosphamide: I.V.: 500 mg/m^2 day 1
  [total dose/cycle = 500 mg/m^2]

Epirubicin: I.V.: 100 mg/m² day 1
  [total dose/cycle = 100 mg/m²]
Repeat cycle every 21 days

References
Bonneterre J, Roché H, Bremond A, et al, "Results of a Randomized Trial of Adjuvant Chemotherapy With FEC 50 vs FEC 100 in High Risk Node-Positive Breast Cancer Patients," *Proc Am Soc Clin Oncol*, 1998, 17:124a (abstract 473).

FIS-HAM

Use Leukemia, acute lymphocytic; Leukemia, acute myeloid
Regimen
Fludarabine: I.V.: 15 mg/m²/day every 12 hours days 1, 2, 8, and 9
  [total dose/cycle = 120 mg/m²]
Cytarabine: I.V.: 750 mg/m²/day every 3 hours days 1, 2, 8, and 9
  [total dose/cycle = 24,000 mg/m²]
Mitoxantrone: I.V.: 10 mg/m²/day days 3, 4, 10, and 11
  [total dose/cycle = 40 mg/m²]

References
Kern W, Schleyer E, Braess J, et al, "Efficacy of Fludarabine, Intermittent Sequential High-Dose Cytosine Arabinoside, and Mitoxantrone (FIS-HAM) Salvage Therapy in Highly Resistant Acute Leukemias," *Ann Hematol*, 2001, 80(6):334-9.

FL

Synonyms Flutamide + Leuprolide
Use Prostate cancer
Regimen NOTE: Multiple variations are listed below.
Variation 1:
  Flutamide: Oral: 250 mg every 8 hours
    [total dose/cycle = 21,000 mg]
  Leuprolide acetate: SubQ: 1 mg/day
    [total dose/cycle = 28 mg]
  or
  Leuprolide depot: I.M.: 7.5 mg day 1
    [total dose/cycle = 7.5 mg]
  Repeat cycle every 28 days
Variation 2:
  Flutamide: Oral: 250 mg every 8 hours
    [total dose/cycle = 67,500 mg]
  Leuprolide acetate depot: I.M.: 22.5 mg day 1
    [total dose/cycle = 22.5 mg]
  Repeat cycle every 3 months

References
Variation 1: Crawford ED, Eisenberger MA, McLeod DG, et al, "A Controlled Trial of Leuprolide With and Without Flutamide in Prostatic Carcinoma," *N Engl J Med*, 1989, 17:321(7):419-24.
Variation 2: McLeod DG, Schellhammer PF, Vogelzang NJ, et al, "Exploratory Analysis on the Effect of Race on Clinical Outcome in Patients With Advanced Prostate Cancer Receiving Bicalutamide or Flutamide, Each in Combination With LHRH Analogues. The Casodex Combination Study Group." *Prostate*, 1999, 1:40(4):218-24.

FLAG

Use Leukemia, acute myeloid
Regimen
Fludarabine: I.V.: 30 mg/m²/day days 1 to 5
  [total dose/cycle = 150 mg/m²]
(Continued)

FLAG *(Continued)*

Cytarabine: I.V.: 2000 mg/m^2/day days 1 to 5 (3.5 hours after end of fludarabine infusion)
[total dose/cycle = 10,000 mg/m^2]

Filgrastim: SubQ: 5 mcg/kg day 1
[total dose/cycle = 5 mcg/kg]

followed by 300 mcg daily until ANC >500-1000 cells/mcL postnadir
[total dose/cycle = 40-7800 mcg/kg]

Repeat cycle every 3-4 weeks

References
Clavio M, Carrara P, Miglino M, et al, "High Efficacy of Fludarabine-Containing Therapy (FLAG-FLANG) in Poor Risk Acute Myeloid Leukemia," *Haematologica*, 1996, 81(6):513-20.

FLe

Use Colorectal cancer

Regimen

Fluorouracil: I.V.: 450 mg/m^2/day for 5 days
[total dose/cycle = 2250 mg/m^2]

After a pause of 4 weeks: 450 mg/m^2/week for 48 weeks
[total dose/cycle = 21.6 g/m^2]

Levamisole: Oral: 50 mg 3 times/day for 3 days, repeated every 2 weeks for 1 year
[total dose/cycle = 11.7 g/m^2]

References
Laurie JA, Moertel CG, Fleming TR, et al, "Surgical Adjuvant Therapy of Large-Bowel carcinoma: An Evaluation of Levamisole and the Combination of Levamisole and Fluorouracil. The North Central Cancer Treatment Group and the Mayo Clinic," *J Clin Oncol*, 1989, 7(10):1447-56.

Fludarabine-Rituximab

Use Leukemia, chronic lymphocytic

Regimen

Rituximab: I.V.: 375 mg/m^2/day days 1 and 4 (cycle 1)
[total dose/cycle 1 = 750 mg/m^2]

Rituximab: I.V.: 375 mg/m^2/day day 1 (cycles 2-6)
[total dose/cycle = 375 mg/m^2]

Fludarabine: I.V.: 25 mg/m^2/day days 1 to 5
[total dose/cycle = 125 mg/m^2]

Repeat cycle every 4 weeks

References
Byrd JC, Peterson BL, Morrison VA, et al, "Randomized Phase 2 Study of Fludarabine With Concurrent vs Sequential Treatment With Rituximab in Symptomatic, Untreated Patients With B-Cell Chronic Lymphocytic Leukemia: Results from Cancer and Leukemia Group B 9712 (CALGB 9712)," *Blood*, 2003, 101(1):6-14.

- ♦ **Flutamide + Goserelin** *see FZ on page 895*
- ♦ **Flutamide + Leuprolide** *see FL on page 889*
- ♦ **FNC** *see CNF on page 863*

FOIL

Use Colorectal cancer

Regimen

Irinotecan: I.V.: 175 mg/m^2 day 1
[total dose/cycle = 175 mg/m^2]

Oxaliplatin: I.V.: 100 mg/m^2 day 1
 [total dose/cycle = 100 mg/m^2]
Leucovorin: I.V.: 200 mg/m^2 day 1
 [total dose/cycle = 200 mg/m^2]
Fluorouracil: I.V.: 3800 mg/m^2/day continuous infusion days 1 and 2
 [total dose/cycle = 7600 mg/m^2]
Repeat cycle every 14 days

References

Falcone A, Masi G, Allegrini G, et al, "Biweekly Chemotherapy With Oxaliplatin, Irinotecan, Infusional Fluorouracil, and Leucovorin: A Pilot Study in Patients With Metastatic Colorectal Cancer," *J Clin Oncol*, 2002, 20(19):4006-14.

FOLFOX 1

Use Colorectal cancer

Regimen

Oxaliplatin: I.V.: 130 mg/m^2 day 1 (every other cycle)
 [total dose/cycle = 130 mg/m^2]
Leucovorin: I.V.: 500 mg/m^2/day days 1 and 2
 [total dose/cycle = 1000 mg/m^2]
Fluorouracil: I.V.: 1.5-2 g/m^2/day continuous infusion days 1 and 2
 [total dose/cycle = 3-4 g/m^2]
Repeat cycle every 14 days

References

de Gramont A, Tournigand C, Louvet C, et al, "Oxaliplatin, Folinic Acid and 5-Fluorouracil (Folfox) in Pretreated Patients With Metastatic Advanced Cancer, The GERCOD," *Rev Med Interne*, 1997, 18(10):769-75.

FOLFOX 2

Use Colorectal cancer

Regimen

Oxaliplatin: I.V.: 100 mg/m^2 day 1
 [total dose/cycle = 100 mg/m^2]
Leucovorin: I.V.: 500 mg/m^2/day days 1 and 2
 [total dose/cycle = 1000 mg/m^2]
Fluorouracil: I.V.: 1.5-2 g/m^2/day continuous infusion days 1 and 2
 [total dose/cycle = 3-4 g/m^2]
Repeat cycle every 14 days

References

de Gramont A, Vignoud J, Tournigand C, et al, "Oxaliplatin With High-Dose Leucovorin and 5-Fluorouracil 48-Hour Continuous Infusion in Pretreated Metastatic Colorectal Cancer," *Eur J Cancer*, 1997, 33(2):214-9.

FOLFOX 3

Use Colorectal cancer

Regimen

Oxaliplatin: I.V.: 85 mg/m^2 day 1
 [total dose/cycle = 85 mg/m^2]
Leucovorin: I.V.: 500 mg/m^2/day days 1 and 2
 [total dose/cycle = 1000 mg/m^2]
Fluorouracil: I.V.: 1.5-2 g/m^2/day continuous infusion days 1 and 2
 [total dose/cycle = 3-4 g/m^2]
Repeat cycle every 14 days
(Continued)

FOLFOX 3 *(Continued)*

References
de Gramont A, Tournigand C, Louvet C, et al, "Oxaliplatin, Folinic Acid and 5-Fluorouracil (Folfox) in Pretreated Patients With Metastatic Advanced Cancer, The GERCOD," *Rev Med Interne*, 1997, 18(10):769-75.

FOLFOX 4

Use Colorectal cancer

Regimen

Oxaliplatin: I.V.: 85 mg/m^2 day 1
[total dose/cycle = 85 mg/m^2]
Leucovorin: I.V.: 200 mg/m^2/day days 1 and 2
[total dose/cycle = 400 mg/m^2]
Fluorouracil: I.V. bolus: 400 mg/m^2/day days 1 and 2
[total dose/cycle = 800 mg/m^2]
followed by 600 mg/m^2 CIVI (over 22 hours) days 1 and 2
[total dose/cycle = 1200 mg/m^2]
Note: Bolus fluorouracil and CIVI are both given on each day.
Repeat cycle every 14 days

References
André T, Bensmaine MA, Louvet C, et al, "Multicenter Phase II Study of Bimonthly High-Dose Leucovorin, Fluorouracil Infusion, and Oxaliplatin for Metastatic Colorectal Cancer Resistant to the Same Leucovorin and Fluorouracil Regimen," *J Clin Oncol*, 1999, 17(11):3560-8.

FOLFOX 6

Use Colorectal cancer

Regimen

Oxaliplatin: I.V.: 100 mg/m^2 day 1
[total dose/cycle = 100 mg/m^2]
Leucovorin: I.V.: 400 mg/m^2 day 1
[total dose/cycle = 400 mg/m^2]
Fluorouracil: I.V. bolus: 400 mg/m^2 day 1
[total dose/cycle = 400 mg/m^2]
followed by 2.4-3 g/m^2 CIVI (46 hours) continuous infusion extending over days 1 and 2
[total dose/cycle = 2.4-3 g/m^2]
Repeat cycle every 14 days

References
Maindrault-Goebel F, Louvet C, Andre T, et al, "Oxaliplatin Added to the Simplified Bimonthly Leucovorin and 5-Fluorouracil Regimen as Second-Line Therapy for Metastatic Colorectal Cancer (FOLFOX6), GERCOR," *Eur J Cancer*, 1999, 35(9):1338-42.

FOLFOX 7

Use Colorectal cancer

Regimen

Oxaliplatin: I.V.: 130 mg/m^2 day 1
[total dose/cycle = 130 mg/m^2]
Leucovorin: I.V.: 400 mg/m^2 day 1
[total dose/cycle = 400 mg/m^2]
Fluorouracil: I.V. bolus: 400 mg/m^2 day 1
[total dose/cycle = 400 mg/m^2]
followed by 2.4 g/m^2 CIVI (46 hours) continuous infusion extending over days 1 and 2
[total dose/cycle = 2.4 g/m^2]
Repeat cycle every 14 days

References
Maindrault-Goebel F, de Gramont A, Louvet C, et al, "High-Dose Intensity Oxaliplatin Added to the Simplified Bimonthly Leucovorin and 5-Fluorouracil Regimen as Second-Line Therapy for Metastatic Colorectal Cancer (FOLFOX 7)," *Eur J Cancer*, 2001, 37(8):1000-5.

FU HURT

Use Head and neck cancer

Regimen

Hydroxyurea: Oral: 1000 mg every 12 hours for 11 doses days 0 to 5
[total dose/cycle = 11,000 mg]

Fluorouracil: I.V.: 800 mg/m^2/day continuous infusion (start AM after admission) days 1 to 5
[total dose/cycle = 4000 mg/m^2]

Paclitaxel: I.V.: 5-25 mg/m^2/day continuous infusion days 1 to 5
[total dose/cycle = 25-125 mg/m^2]

5-7 cycles may be administered

References
"Induction Chemotherapy Plus Radiation Compared With Surgery Plus Radiation in Patients With Advanced Laryngeal Cancer. The Department of Veterans Affairs Laryngeal Cancer Study Group," *N Engl J Med*, 1991, 324(24):1685-90.

♦ **FU/Leucovorin** *see* F-CL *on page 886*

♦ **FU-LV** *see* F-CL *on page 886*

FU/LV/CPT-11

Use Colorectal cancer

Regimen NOTE: Multiple variations are listed below.

Variation 1:

Irinotecan: I.V.: 350 mg/m^2 day 1
[total dose/cycle = 350 mg/m^2]

Leucovorin: I.V.: 20 mg/m^2/day days 22 to 26
[total dose/cycle = 100 mg/m^2]

Fluorouracil: I.V.: 425 mg/m^2/day days 22 to 26
[total dose/cycle = 2125 mg/m^2]

Repeat cycle every 6 weeks

Variation 2:

Irinotecan: I.V.: 80 mg/m^2 day 1
[total dose/cycle = 80 mg/m^2]

Fluorouracil: I.V.: 2300 mg/m^2 continuous infusion day 1
[total dose/cycle = 2300 mg/m^2]

Leucovorin: I.V.: 500 mg/m^2 day 1
[total dose/cycle = 500 mg/m^2]

Repeat cycle weekly

or

Irinotecan: I.V.: 180 mg/m^2 day 1
[total dose/cycle = 180 mg/m^2]

Leucovorin: I.V.: 200 mg/m^2/day days 1 and 2
[total dose/cycle = 400 mg/m^2]

Fluorouracil: I.V.: 400 mg/m^2/day days 1 and 2
[total dose/cycle = 800 mg/m^2]

followed by 600 mg/m^2/day continuous infusion days 1 and 2
[total dose/cycle = 1200 mg/m^2]

Repeat cycle every 2 weeks

(Continued)

FU/LV/CPT-11 *(Continued)*

Variation 3:

Irinotecan: I.V.: 175 mg/m² day 1
[total dose/cycle = 175 mg/m²]

Leucovorin: I.V.: 250 mg/m² day 2
[total dose/cycle = 250 mg/m²]

Fluorouracil: I.V.: 950 mg/m² day 2
[total dose/cycle = 950 mg/m²]

or

Irinotecan: I.V.: 200 mg/m² day 1
[total dose/cycle = 200 mg/m²]

Leucovorin: I.V.: 250 mg/m² day 2
[total dose/cycle = 250 mg/m²]

Fluorouracil: I.V.: 850 mg/m² day 2
[total dose/cycle = 850 mg/m²]

Repeat cycle every other week

References

Variation 1:

Van Cutsem E, Pozzo C, Starkhammar H, et al, "A Phase II Study of Irinotecan Alternated With Five Days Bolus of 5-Fluorouracil and Leucovorin in First-Line Chemotherapy of Metastatic Colorectal Cancer," *Ann Oncol*, 1998, 9(11):1199-204.

Variation 2:

Douillard JY, Cunningham D, Roth AD, et al, "Irinotecan Combined With Fluorouracil Compared With Fluorouracil Alone as First-Line Treatment for Metastatic Colorectal Cancer: A Multicentre Randomised Trial," *Lancet*, 2000, 355(9209):1041-7.

Variation 3:

Comella P, Casaretti F, De Vita F, et al, "Concurrent Irinotecan and 5-Fluorouracil Plus Levo-Folinic Acid Given Every Other Week in the First-Line Management of Advanced Colorectal Carcinoma: A Phase I Study of the Southern Italy Cooperative Oncology Group," *Ann Oncol*, 1999, 10(8):915-21.

FU/LV/CPT-11 (Saltz Regimen)

Synonyms Saltz Regimen

Use Colorectal cancer

Regimen

Fluorouracil: I.V.: 500 mg/m²/day days 1, 8, 15, and 22
[total dose/cycle = 2000 mg/m²]

Leucovorin: I.V.: 20 mg/m²/day days 1, 8, 15, and 22
[total dose/cycle = 80 mg/m²]

Irinotecan: I.V.: 125 mg/m²/day days 1, 8, 15, and 22
[total dose/cycle = 500 mg/m²]

Repeat cycle every 42 days

References

Saltz LB, Cox JV, Blanke C, et al, "Irinotecan Plus Fluorouracil and Leucovorin for Metastatic Colorectal Cancer, Irinotecan Study Group," *N Engl J Med*, 2000, 343(13):905-14.

FUP

Use Gastric cancer

Regimen

Fluorouracil: I.V.: 1000 mg/m²/day continuous infusion days 1 to 5
[total dose/cycle = 5000 mg/m²]

Cisplatin: I.V.: 100 mg/m² day 2
[total dose/cycle = 100 mg/m²]

Repeat cycle every 28 days

References

Vanhoefer U, Rougier P, Wilke H, et al, "Final Results of a Randomized Phase III Trial of Sequential High-Dose Methotrexate, Fluorouracil, and Doxorubicin Versus Etoposide, Leucovorin, and Fluorouracil Versus Infusional Fluorouracil and Cisplatin in Advanced Gastric Cancer: A Trial of the European Organization for Research and Treatment of Cancer Gastrointestinal Tract Cancer Cooperative Group," *J Clin Oncol*, 2000, 18(14):2648-57.

FZ

Synonyms Flutamide + Goserelin

Use Prostate cancer

Regimen NOTE: Multiple variations are listed below.

Variation 1:

Flutamide: Oral: 250 mg every 8 hours
[total dose/cycle = 21,000 mg]

Goserelin acetate: SubQ: 3.6 mg day 1
[total dose/cycle = 3.6 mg]

Repeat cycle every 28 days

Variation 2:

Flutamide: Oral: 250 mg every 8 hours
[total dose/cycle = 67,500 mg]

Goserelin acetate: SubQ: 10.8 mg day 1
[total dose/cycle = 10.8 mg]

Repeat cycle every 3 months

References

McLeod DG, Schellhammer PF, Vogelzang NJ, et al, "Exploratory Analysis on the Effect of Race on Clinical Outcome in Patients With Advanced Prostate Cancer Receiving Bicalutamide or Flutamide, Each in Combination With LHRH Analogues. The Casodex Combination Study Group," *Prostate*, 1999, 40(4):218-24.

GC

Use Lung cancer, nonsmall cell

Regimen

Gemcitabine: I.V.: 1000 mg/m^2/day days 1, 8, and 15
[total dose/cycle = 3000 mg/m^2]

Cisplatin: I.V.: 100 mg/m^2 day 1 **or** 2 **or** 15
[total dose/cycle = 100 mg/m^2]

Repeat cycle every 28 days for 2-6 cycles

References

Comella P, Frasci G, Panza N, et al, "Randomized Trial Comparing Cisplatin, Gemcitabine, and Vinorelbine With Either Cisplatin and Gemcitabine or Cisplatin and Vinorelbine in Advanced Nonsmall-Cell Lung Cancer: Interim Analysis of a Phase III Trial of the Southern Italy Cooperative Oncology Group," *J Clin Oncol*, 2000, 18(7):1451-7.

Sandler AB, Nemunaitis J, Denham C, et al, "Phase III Trial of Gemcitabine Plus Cisplatin Versus Cisplatin Alone in Patients With Locally Advanced or Metastatic Nonsmall-Cell Lung Cancer," *J Clin Oncol*, 2000, 18(1):122-30.

Gemcitabine/Capecitabine

Use Pancreatic cancer

Regimen

Gemcitabine: I.V.: 1000 mg/m^2/day days 1 and 8
[total dose/cycle = 2000 mg/m^2]

Capecitabine: Oral: 650 mg/m^2 twice daily days 1 to 14
[total dose/cycle = 18,200 mg/m^2]

Repeat cycle every 21 days

(Continued)

Gemcitabine/Capecitabine *(Continued)*

References

Hess V, Salzberg M, Borner M, et al, "Combining Capecitabine and Gemcitabine in Patients With Advanced Pancreatic Carcinoma: A Phase I/II Trial," *J Clin Oncol*, 2003, 21(1):66-8.

Gemcitabine-Carboplatin

Use Lung cancer, nonsmall cell

Regimen

Gemcitabine: I.V.: 1000 or 1100 mg/m^2/day days 1 and 8

[total dose/cycle = 2000 or 2200 mg/m^2]

Carboplatin: I.V.: AUC 5 day 8

[total dose/cycle = AUC = 5]

Repeat cycle every 28 days

References

Iaffaioli RV, Tortoriello A, Facchini G, et al, "Phase I-II Study of Gemcitabine and Carboplatin in Stage IIIB-IV Nonsmall-Cell Lung Cancer," *J Clin Oncol*, 1999, 17(3):921-6.

Gemcitabine-Cis

Use Lung cancer, nonsmall cell

Regimen

Gemcitabine: I.V.: 1000-1200 mg/m^2/day days 1, 8, and 15

[total dose/cycle = 3000-3600 mg/m^2]

Cisplatin: I.V.: 100 mg/m^2 day 1 **or** 2 **or** 15

[total dose/cycle = 100 mg/m^2]

Repeat cycle every 28 days

References

Anton A, Diaz-Fernandez N, Gonzalez Larriba JL, et al, "Phase II Trial Assessing the Combination of Gemcitabine and Cisplatin in Advanced Non-Small Cell Lung Cancer (NSCLC)," *Lung Cancer*, 1998, 22(2):139-48.

Gemcitabine-Cisplatin

Use Bladder cancer

Regimen

Gemcitabine: I.V.: 1000 mg/m^2/day days 1, 8, and 15

[total dose/cycle = 3000 mg/m^2]

Cisplatin: I.V.: 70 mg/m^2 day 2

[total dose/cycle = 70 mg/m^2]

Repeat cycle every 28 days for 6 cycles

References

von der Maase H, Hansen SW, Roberts JT, et al, "Gemcitabine and Cisplatin Versus Methotrexate, Vinblastine, Doxorubicin, and Cisplatin in Advanced or Metastatic Bladder Cancer: Results of a Large, Randomized, Multinational, Multicenter, Phase III Study," *J Clin Oncol*, 2000, 18(17):3068-77.

Gemcitabine-Docetaxel

Use Bony sarcoma; Soft tissue sarcoma

Regimen

Gemcitabine: I.V.: 675 mg/m^2/day days 1 and 8

[total dose/cycle = 1350 mg/m^2]

Docetaxel: I.V.: 100 mg/m^2 day 8

[total dose/cycle = 100 mg/m^2]

Repeat cycle every 21 days

References

Leu KM, Ostruszka LJ, Shewach D, et al, "Laboratory and Clinical Evidence of Synergistic Cytotoxicity of Sequential Treatment With Gemcitabine Followed by Docetaxel in the Treatment of Sarcoma," *J Clin Oncol*, 2004, 22(9):1706-12.

Gemcitabine/Irinotecan

Use Pancreatic cancer

Regimen

Gemcitabine: I.V.: 1000 mg/m^2/day days 1 and 8
[total dose/cycle = 2000 mg/m^2]
Irinotecan: I.V.: 100 mg/m^2/day days 1 and 8
[total dose/cycle = 200 mg/m^2]
Repeat cycle 21 days

References

Rocha Lima CM, Savarese D, Bruckner H, et al, "Irinotecan Plus Gemcitabine Induces Both Radiographic and CA 19-9 Tumor Marker Responses in Patients With Previously Untreated Advanced Pancreatic Cancer," *J Clin Oncol*, 2002, 20(5):1182-91.

Gemcitabine-Paclitaxel

Use Ovarian cancer

Regimen

Paclitaxel: I.V.: 80 mg/m^2 infused over 60 minutes days 1, 8, and 15
[total dose/cycle = 240 mg/m^2]
Gemcitabine: I.V.: 1000 mg/m^2/day (start at end of paclitaxel infusion) days 1, 8, and 15
[total dose/cycle = 3000 mg/m^2]
Repeat cycle every 4 weeks

References

Garcia AA, O'Meara A, Bahador A, et al, "Phase II Study of Gemcitabine and Weekly Paclitaxel in Recurrent Platinum-Resistant Ovarian Cancer," *Gynecol Oncol*, 2004, 93(2):493-8.

Gemcitabine-Vinorelbine

Use Lung cancer, nonsmall cell

Regimen NOTE: Multiple variations are listed below.

Variation 1:

Gemcitabine: I.V.: 1200 mg/m^2/day days 1 and 8
[total dose/cycle = 2400 mg/m^2]
Vinorelbine: I.V.: 30 mg/m^2/day days 1 and 8
[total dose/cycle = 60 mg/m^2]
Repeat cycle every 21 days for 6 cycles

Variation 2:

Gemcitabine: I.V.: 1000 mg/m^2/day days 1, 8, and 15
[total dose/cycle = 3000 mg/m^2]
Vinorelbine: I.V.: 20 mg/m^2/day days 1, 8, and 15
[total dose/cycle = 60 mg/m^2]
Repeat cycle every 28 days for 6 cycles

References

Variation 1 and 2:

Frasci G, Lorusso V, Panza N, et al, "Gemcitabine Plus Vinorelbine vs Vinorelbine Alone in Elderly Patients With Advanced Nonsmall Cell Lung Cancer," *J Clin Oncol*, 2000, 18(13):2529-36.

Hainsworth JD, Burris HA 3rd, Litchy S, et al, "Gemcitabine and Vinorelbine in the Second-Line Treatment of Nonsmall Cell Lung Carcinoma Patients: A Minnie Pearl Cancer Research Network Phase II Trial," *Cancer*, 2000, 88(6):1353-8.

HDMTX (Osteosarcoma)
Use Osteosarcoma
Regimen
Methotrexate: I.V.: 12 g/m^2/week for 2-12 weeks
[total dose/cycle = 24-144 g/m^2]
Leucovorin calcium rescue: Oral, I.V.: 15 mg/m^2 every 6 hours (beginning 30 hours after the beginning of the 4-hour methotrexate infusion) for 10 doses; **serum methotrexate levels must be monitored**
[total dose/cycle = 150 mg/m^2]
References
Camitta BM and Holcenberg JS, "Safety of Delayed Leucovorin "Rescue" Following High-Dose Methotrexate in Children," *Med Pediatr Oncol*, 1978, 5(1):55-9.

HIPE-IVAD
Use Neuroblastomas
Regimen
Cisplatin: I.V.: 40 mg/m^2/day days 1 to 5
[total dose/cycle = 200 mg/m^2]
Etoposide: I.V.: 100 mg/m^2/day days 1 to 5
[total dose/cycle = 500 mg/m^2]
Ifosfamide: I.V.: 3 g/m^2/day days 21 to 23
[total dose/cycle = 9 g/m^2]
Mesna: I.V.: 3 g/m^2/day continuous infusion days 21 to 23
[total dose/cycle = 9 g/m^2]
Vincristine: I.V.: 1.5 mg/m^2 day 21
[total dose/cycle = 1.5 mg/m^2]
Doxorubicin: I.V.: 60 mg/m^2 day 23
[total dose/cycle = 60 mg/m^2]
Repeat cycle every 28 days
References
Pinkerton CR, Zucker JM, Hartmann O, et al, "Short Duration, High Dose, Alternating Chemotherapy in Metastatic Neuroblastoma. (ENSG 3C Induction Regimen). The European Neuroblastoma Study Group," *Br J Cancer*, 1990, 62(2):319-23.

Hyper-CVAD
Related Information POMP *on page 931*
Use Multiple myeloma; Lymphoma, non-Hodgkin's (Burkitt's); Leukemia, acute lymphocytic
Regimen
Course 1, 3, 5, and 7:
Cyclophosphamide: I.V.: 300 mg/m^2/day every 12 hours days 1 to 3
[total dose/cycle = 1.8 g/m^2]
Mesna: I.V.: 3600 mg/m^2/day continuous infusion days 1 to 3
[total dose/cycle = 10,800 mg/m^2]
Methotrexate: I.T.: 12 mg day 2
[total dose/cycle = 12 mg]
Vincristine: I.V.: 2 mg/day days 4 and 11
[total dose/cycle = 4 mg]
Doxorubicin: I.V.: 50 mg/m^2 day 4
[total dose/cycle = 50 mg/m^2]
Cytarabine: I.T.: 100 mg day 8
[total dose/cycle = 100 mg]
Dexamethasone: Oral or I.V.: 40 mg/day days 1 to 4 and 11 to 14
[total dose/cycle = 320 mg]

Course 2, 4, 6, and 8:
Methotrexate: I.V.: 200 mg/m^2 day 1
[total dose/cycle = 200 mg/m^2]
followed by 800 mg/m^2 continuous infusion day 1
[total dose/cycle = 800 mg/m^2]
Cytarabine: I.V.: 3 g/m^2 every 12 hours days 2 and 3
[total dose/cycle = 12 g/m^2]
Methotrexate: I.T.: 12 mg day 2
[total dose/cycle = 12 mg]
Leucovorin: I.V.: 15 mg every 6 hours days 3 and 4
[total dose/cycle = 120 mg]
Methylprednisolone: I.V.: 50 mg twice daily days 1 to 3
[total dose/cycle = 300 mg]
Cytarabine: I.T.: 100 mg day 8
[total dose/cycle = 100 mg]
Cycles are given when WBC is ≥3000 mm^3, Plt ≥60,000 mm^3

References

Dimopoulos MA, Weber D, Kantarjian H, et al, "Hyper-CVAD for VAD-Resistant Multiple Myeloma," *Am J Hematol*, 1996, 52(2):77-81.

Kantarjian HM, O'Brien S, Smith TL, et al, "Results of Treatment With Hyper-CVAD, a Dose-Intensive Regimen, in Adult Acute Lymphocytic Leukemia," *J Clin Oncol*, 2000, 18(3):547-61.

Thomas DA, Cortes J, O'Brien S, et al, "Hyper-CVAD Program in Burkitt's-Type Adult Acute Lymphoblastic Leukemia," *J Clin Oncol*, 1999, 17(8):2461-70.

♦ **ICE (Leukemia)** *see* Idarubicin, Cytarabine, Etoposide (ICE Protocol) *on page 900*

ICE (Lymphoma, non-Hodgkin's)

Use Lymphoma, non-Hodgkin's
Regimen
Etoposide: I.V.: 100 mg/m^2/day days 1 to 3
[total dose/cycle = 300 mg/m^2]
Carboplatin: I.V.: AUC 5 day 2 (maximum 800 mg)
[total dose/cycle = AUC = 5]
Ifosfamide: I.V.: 5000 mg/m^2 continuous infusion day 2
[total dose/cycle = 5000 mg/m^2]
Mesna: I.V.: 5000 mg/m^2 continuous infusion day 2
[total dose/cycle = 5000 mg/m^2]
Filgrastim: SubQ: 5 mcg/kg days 5 and 12
[total dose/cycle = 10 mcg/kg]
Repeat cycle every 2 weeks

References

Moskowitz CH, Bertino JR, Glassman JR, et al, "Ifosfamide, Carboplatin, and Etoposide: A Highly Effective Cytoreduction and Peripheral-Blood Progenitor-Cell Mobilization Regimen for Transplant-Eligible Patients With Non-Hodgkin's Lymphoma," *J Clin Oncol*, 1999, 17(12):3776-85.

ICE (Sarcoma)

Use Osteosarcoma; Soft tissue sarcoma
Regimen
Ifosfamide: I.V.: 1250-1500 mg/m^2/day days 1 to 3
[total dose/cycle = 3750-4500 mg/m^2]
Carboplatin: I.V.: 300-635 mg/m^2 day 3
[total dose/cycle = 300-635 mg/m^2]
(Continued)

ICE (Sarcoma) *(Continued)*

Etoposide: I.V.: 80-100 mg/m^2/day days 1 to 3

[total dose/cycle = 240-300 mg/m^2]

Mesna: I.V.: 1250 mg/m^2/day days 1 to 3

[total dose/cycle = 3750 mg/m^2]

or 20% of ifosfamide dose before, 4 and 8 hours after each ifosfamide infusion

[total dose/cycle = 60% of ifosfamide dose]

Repeat cycle every 21-28 days

References

Kung FH, Desai SJ, Dickerman JD, et al, " Ifosfamide/Carboplatin/Etoposide (ICE) for Recurrent Malignant Solid Tumors of Childhood: A Pediatric Oncology Group Phase I/II Study," *J Pediatr Hematol Oncol*, 1995, 17(3):265-9.

ICE-T

Use Soft tissue sarcoma

Regimen

Ifosfamide: I.V.: 1250 mg/m^2/day days 1, 2, and 3

[total dose/cycle = 3750 mg/m^2]

Carboplatin: I.V.: 300 mg/m^2 day 1

[total dose/cycle = 300 mg/m^2]

Etoposide: I.V.: 80 mg/m^2/day days 1, 2, and 3

[total dose/cycle = 240 mg/m^2]

Paclitaxel: I.V.: 175 mg/m^2 day 4

[total dose/cycle = 175 mg/m^2]

Mesna: I.V.: 20% of ifosfamide dose before

followed by: Oral: 40% of ifosfamide dose 4 and 8 hours after ifosfamide

[total dose/cycle = 100% of ifosfamide dose]

or

Mesna: I.V.: 1250 mg/m^2/day days 1, 2, and 3

[total dose/cycle = 3750 mg/m^2]

Repeat cycle every 28 days

References

Chang AY, Boros L, Garrow GC, et al, "Ifosfamide, Carboplatin, Etoposide, and Paclitaxel Chemotherapy: A Dose-Escalation Study," *Semin Oncol*, 1996, 23(3 Suppl 6):74-7.

Idarubicin, Cytarabine, Etoposide (ICE Protocol)

Synonyms ICE (Leukemia)

Use Leukemia, acute myeloid

Regimen

Idarubicin: I.V.: 6 mg/m^2/day days 1 to 5

[total dose/cycle = 30 mg/m^2]

Cytarabine: I.V.: 600 mg/m^2/day days 1 to 5

[total dose/cycle = 3000 mg/m^2]

Etoposide: I.V.: 150 mg/m^2/day days 1 to 3

[total dose/cycle = 450 mg/m^2]

Administer one cycle only

References

Carella AM, Carlier P, Pungolino E, et al, "Idarubicin in Combination With Interme-diate-Dose Cytarabine and VP-16 in the Treatment of Refractory or Rapidly Relapsed Patients With Acute Myeloid Leukemia," *Leukemia*, 1993, 7(2):196-9.

Idarubicin, Cytarabine, Etoposide (IDA-Based BF12)

Use Leukemia, acute myeloid

Regimen Induction:

Idarubicin: I.V.: 5 mg/m^2/day days 1 to 5
[total dose/cycle = 25 mg/m^2]

Cytarabine: I.V.: 2000 mg/m^2 every 12 hours days 1 to 5 (10 doses)
[total dose/cycle = 20,000 mg/m^2]

Etoposide: I.V.: 100 mg/m^2/day days 1 to 5
[total dose/cycle = 500 mg/m^2]

Second cycle may be given based on individual response; time between cycles not specified

References

Mehta J, Powles R, Singhal S, et al, "Idarubicin, High-Dose Cytarabine, and Etoposide for Induction of Remission in Acute Leukemia," *Semin Hematol*, 1996, 33(4 Suppl 3):18-23.

IDMTX/6-MP

Use Leukemia, acute lymphocytic

Regimen Intensification:

Week 1:

Methotrexate: I.V.: 200 mg/m^2
[total dose/cycle = 200 mg/m^2]
followed by 800 mg/m^2 continuous infusion day 1
[total dose/cycle = 800 mg/m^2]

Mercaptopurine: I.V.: 200 mg/m^2
[total dose/cycle = 200 mg/m^2]
followed by 800 mg/m^2 over 8 hours day 1
[total dose/cycle = 800 mg/m^2]

Leucovorin: Oral or I.V.: 5 mg/m^2 every 6 hours for 5 to 13 doses beginning 24 hours after end of methotrexate infusion
[total dose/cycle = 30-65 mg/m^2]

Week 2:

Methotrexate: I.M.: 20 mg/m^2 day 8
[total dose/cycle = 20 mg/m^2]

Mercaptopurine: Oral: 50 mg/m^2/day days 8 to 14
[total dose/cycle = 350 mg/m^2]

Repeat cycle every 2 weeks up to 12 cycles

References

Camitta B, Mahoney D, Leventhal B, et al, "Intensive Intravenous Methotrexate and Mercaptopurine Treatment of Higher-Risk Non-T, Non-B Acute Lymphocytic Leukemia: A Pediatric Oncology Group Study," *J Clin Oncol*, 1994, 12(7):1383-9.

IE

Use Soft tissue sarcoma

Regimen

Etoposide: I.V.: 100 mg/m^2/day days 1 to 3
[total dose/cycle = 300 mg/m^2]

Ifosfamide: I.V.: 2500 mg/m^2/day days 1 to 3
[total dose/cycle = 7500 mg/m^2]

Mesna: I.V.: 20% of ifosfamide dose prior to and at 4-, 8-, and 12 hours after ifosfamide administration
[total dose/cycle = 80% ifosfamide dose]

Repeat cycle every 28 days
(Continued)

IE *(Continued)*

References
Edmonson JH, Buckner JC, Long HJ, et al, "Phase II Study of Ifosfamide-Etoposide-Mesna in Adults With Advanced Nonosseous Sarcomas," *J Natl Cancer Inst*, 1989, 81(11):863-6.

IL-2 + IFN

Use Melanoma

Regimen

Cisplatin: I.V.: 20 mg/m^2/day days 1 to 4
[total dose/cycle = 80 mg/m^2]
Vinblastine: I.V.: 1.6 mg/m^2/day days 1 to 4
[total dose/cycle = 6.4 mg/m^2]
Dacarbazine: I.V.: 800 mg/m^2 day 1
[total dose/cycle = 800 mg/m^2]
Aldesleukin: I.V.: 9 million units/m^2/day continuous infusion days 1 to 4
[total dose/cycle = 36 million units/m^2]
Interferon alfa-2b: SubQ: 5 million units/m^2/day days 1 to 5, 7, 9, 11, and 13
[total dose/cycle = 45 million units/m^2]
Repeat cycle every 21 days

References
McDermott DF, Mier JW, Lawrence DP, et al, "A Phase II Pilot Trial of Concurrent Biochemotherapy With Cisplatin, Vinblastine, Dacarbazine, Interleukin 2, and Interferon Alpha-2B in Patients With Metastatic Melanoma," *Clin Cancer Res*, 2000, 6(6):2201-8.

IMVP-16

Use Lymphoma, non-Hodgkin's

Regimen

Ifosfamide: I.V.: 4 g/m^2 continuous infusion over 24 hours day 1
[total dose/cycle = 4 g/m^2]
Mesna: I.V.: 800 mg/m^2 bolus prior to ifosfamide, then 4 g/m^2 continuous infusion over 12 hours concurrent with ifosfamide, then 2.4 g/m^2 continuous infusion over 12 hours after ifosfamide infusion day 1
[total dose/cycle = 7.2 g/m^2]
Methotrexate: I.V.: 30 mg/m^2/day days 3 and 10
[total dose/cycle = 60 mg/m^2]
Etoposide: I.V.: 100 mg/m^2/day days 1 to 3
[total dose/cycle = 300 mg/m^2]
Repeat cycle every 21-28 days

References
Cabanillas F, Hagemeister FB, Bodey GP, et al, "IMVP-16: An Effective Regimen for Patients With Lymphoma Who Have Relapsed After Initial Combination Chemotherapy," *Blood*, 1982, 60(3):693-7.

Interleukin 2-Interferon Alfa 2

Use Renal cell cancer

Regimen

Weeks 1 and 4:
Aldesleukin: SubQ: 20 million units/m^2 3 times weekly
[total dose/cycle = 120 million units/m^2]
Interferon alfa: SubQ: 6 million units/m^2 once weekly
[total dose/cycle = 12 million units/m^2]

Weeks 2, 3, 5, and 6:
> Aldesleukin: SubQ: 5 million units/m² 3 times weekly
> > [total dose/cycle = 60 million units/m²]
> Interferon alfa: SubQ: 6 million units/m² 3 times weekly
> > [total dose/cycle = 72 million units/m²]

Repeat cycle every 56 days

References
Atzpodien J, Kirchner H, Hanninen EL, et al, "European Studies of Interleukin-2 In Meta-static Renal Cell Carcinoma," *Semin Oncol*, 1993, 20(6 Suppl 9):22-6.

Interleukin 2-Interferon Alfa 2-Fluorouracil
Use Renal cell cancer
Regimen
Weeks 1 and 4:
> Aldesleukin: SubQ: 20 million units/m² 3 times weekly
> > [total dose/cycle = 120 million units/m²]
> Interferon alfa: SubQ: 6 million units/m² once weekly
> > [total dose/cycle = 12 million units/m²]

Weeks 2 and 3:
> Aldesleukin: SubQ: 5 million units/m² 3 times weekly
> > [total dose/cycle = 30 million units/m²]

Weeks 5-8:
> Interferon alfa: SubQ: 9 million units/m² 3 times weekly
> > [total dose/cycle = 108 million units/m²]
> Fluorouracil: I.V.: 750 mg/m² once weekly
> > [total dose/cycle = 3000 mg/m²]

Repeat cycle every 56 days

References
Atzpodien J, Kirchner H, Hanninen EL, et al, "European Studies of Interleukin-2 In Meta-static Renal Cell Carcinoma," *Semin Oncol*, 1993, 20(6 Suppl 9):22-6.

IPA
Use Hepatoblastoma
Regimen
Ifosfamide: I.V.: 500 mg/m² day 1
> [total dose/cycle = 500 mg/m²]

followed by 1000 mg/m²/day continuous infusion days 1 to 3
> [total dose/cycle = 3000 mg/m²]

Cisplatin: I.V.: 20 mg/m²/day days 4 to 8
> [total dose/cycle = 100 mg/m²]

Doxorubicin: I.V.: 30 mg/m²/day continuous infusion days 9 and 10
> [total dose/cycle = 60 mg/m²]

Repeat cycle every 21 days

References
von Schweinitz D, Byrd DJ, Hecker H, et al, "Efficiency and Toxicity of Ifosfamide, Cisplatin, and Doxorubicin in the Treatment of Childhood Hepatoblastoma. Study Committee of the Cooperative Paediatric Liver Tumour Study HB89 of the German Society for Paediatric Oncology and Haematology," *Eur J Cancer*, 1997, 33(8):1243-9.

Irinotecan/Cisplatin
Use Esophageal cancer
Regimen
Cisplatin: I.V.: 30 mg/m²/day days 1, 8, 15 and 22
> [total dose/cycle = 120 mg/m²]

Irinotecan: I.V.: 65 mg/m²/day days 1, 8, 15 and 22
> [total dose/cycle = 260 mg/m²]

(Continued)

Irinotecan/Cisplatin *(Continued)*

Repeat cycle every 6 weeks

References

Ilson DH, Saltz L, Enzinger P, et al, "Phase II Trial of Weekly Irinotecan Plus Cisplatin in Advanced Esophageal Cancer," *J Clin Oncol*, 1999, 17(10):3270-5.

IVAC

Use Lymphoma, non-Hodgkin's

Regimen

Ifosfamide: I.V.: 1500 mg/m^2/day days 1 to 5
[total dose/cycle = 7500 mg/m^2]

Etoposide: I.V.: 60 mg/m^2/day days 1 to 5
[total dose/cycle = 300 mg/m^2]

Cytarabine: I.V.: 2000 mg/m^2 every 12 hours days 1 and 2
[total dose/cycle = 8000 mg/m^2]

Mesna: I.V.: 360 mg/m^2 every 3 hours days 1 to 5
[total dose/cycle = 14,400 mg/m^2]

Methotrexate: I.T.: 12 mg day 5
[total dose/cycle = 12 mg]

Repeat when ANC >1000 cells/mm^3

References

Magrath I, Adde M, Shad A, et al, "Adults and Children With Small Non-Cleaved-Cell Lymphoma Have a Similar Excellent Outcome When Treated With the Same Chemotherapy Regimen," *J Clin Oncol*, 1996, 14(3):925-34.

♦ **IVCAF** *see FAC on page 884*

Larson Regimen

Use Leukemia, acute lymphocytic

Regimen Induction:

Cyclophosphamide: I.V.: 1200 mg/m^2 day 1
[total dose/cycle = 1200 mg/m^2]

Daunorubicin: I.V.: 45 mg/m^2/day days 1 to 3
[total dose/cycle = 135 mg/m^2]

Vincristine: I.V.: 2 mg/day days 1, 8, 15, and 22
[total dose/cycle = 8 mg]

Prednisone: Oral or I.V.: 60 mg/m^2/day days 1 to 21
[total dose/cycle = 1260 mg/m^2]

Asparaginase: SubQ: 6000 units/m^2/day days 5, 8, 11, 15, 18, and 22
[total dose/cycle = 36,000 units/m^2]

Administer one cycle only

References

Larson RA, Dodge RK, Burns CP, et al, "A Five-Drug Remission Induction Regimen With Intensive Consolidation for Adults With Acute Lymphoblastic Leukemia: Cancer and Leukemia Group B Study 8811," *Blood*, 1995, 85(8):2025-37.

Linker Protocol

Use Leukemia, acute lymphocytic

Regimen

Remission induction:

Daunorubicin: I.V.: 50 mg/m^2/day days 1 to 3
[total dose/cycle = 150 mg/m^2]

Vincristine: I.V.: 2 mg/day days 1, 8, 15, and 22
[total dose/cycle = 8 mg]

Prednisone: Oral: 60 mg/m²/day days 1 to 28
[total dose/cycle = 1680 mg/m²]
Asparaginase: I.M.: 6000 units/m²/day days 17 to 28
[total dose/cycle = 72,000 units/m²]

If residual leukemia in bone marrow on day 14:
Daunorubicin: I.V.: 50 mg/m² day 15
[total dose/cycle = 50 mg/m²]

If residual leukemia in bone marrow on day 28:
Daunorubicin: I.V.: 50 mg/m²/day days 29 and 30
[total dose/cycle = 100 mg/m²]
Vincristine: I.V.: 2 mg/day days 29 and 36
[total dose/cycle = 4 mg]
Prednisone: Oral: 60 mg/m²/day days 29 to 42
[total dose/cycle = 840 mg/m²]
Asparaginase: I.M.: 6000 units/m²/day days 29 to 35
[total dose/cycle = 42,000 units/m²]

Consolidation therapy:
Treatment A (cycles 1, 3, 5, and 7)
Daunorubicin: I.V.: 50 mg/m²/day days 1 and 2
[total dose/cycle = 100 mg/m²]
Vincristine: I.V.: 2 mg/day days 1 and 8
[total dose/cycle = 4 mg]
Prednisone: Oral: 60 mg/m²/day days 1 to 14
[total dose/cycle = 840 mg/m²]
Asparaginase: I.M.: 12,000 units/m²/day days 2, 4, 7, 9, 11, and 14
[total dose/cycle = 72,000 units/m²]
Treatment B (cycles 2, 4, 6, and 8)
Teniposide: I.V.: 165 mg/m²/day days 1, 4, 8, and 11
[total dose/cycle = 660 mg/m²]
Cytarabine: I.V.: 300 mg/m²/day days 1, 4, 8, and 11
[total dose/cycle = 1200 mg/m²]
Treatment C (cycle 9)
Methotrexate: I.V.: 690 mg/m² continuous infusion day 1 (over 42 hours)
[total dose/cycle = 690 mg/m²]
Leucovorin: I.V.: 15 mg/m² every 6 hours for 12 doses (start at end of methotrexate infusion)
[total dose/cycle = 180 mg/m²]
Administer remission induction regimen for one cycle only. Repeat consolidation cycle every 28 days.

References
Linker CA, Levitt LJ, O'Donnell M, et al, "Treatment of Adult Acute Lymphoblastic Leukemia With Intensive Cyclical Chemotherapy: A Follow-up Report," *Blood*, 1991 78(11):2814-22.

LOPP

Use Lymphoma, Hodgkin's disease
Regimen
Chlorambucil: Oral: 10 mg/day days 1 to 10
[total dose/cycle = 100 mg]
Vincristine: I.V.: 1.4 mg/m²/day (maximum 2 mg) days 1 and 8
[total dose/cycle = 2.8 mg/m²]
Procarbazine: Oral: 100 mg/m²/day days 1 to 10
[total dose/cycle = 1000 mg/m²]
(Continued)

LOPP *(Continued)*

Prednisone: Oral: 25 mg/m²/day (maximum 60 mg) days 1 to 14
[total dose/cycle = 350 mg/m²]
or
Prednisolone: Oral: 25 mg/m²/day (maximum 60 mg) days 1 to 14
[total dose/cycle = 350 mg/m²]
Repeat cycle every 28 days

References

Hancock BW, "Randomised Study of MOPP (Mustine, Oncovin, Procarbazine, Prednisone) Against LOPP (Leukeran Substituted for Mustine) in Advanced Hodgkin's Disease. British National Lymphoma Investigation," *Radiother Oncol*, 1986, 7(3):215-21.

M-2

Use Multiple myeloma

Regimen

Vincristine: I.V.: 0.03 mg/kg (maximum 2 mg) day 1
[total dose/cycle = 0.03 mg/kg]
Carmustine: I.V.: 0.5 mg/kg day 1
[total dose/cycle = 0.5 mg/kg]
Cyclophosphamide: I.V.: 10 mg/kg day 1
[total dose/cycle = 10 mg/kg]
Melphalan: Oral: 0.25 mg/kg/day days 1 to 4
[total dose/cycle = 1 mg/kg]
or 0.1 mg/kg/day days 1 to 7 or 1 to 10
[total dose/cycle = 0.7 or 1 mg/kg]
Prednisone: Oral: 1 mg/kg/day days 1 to 7 (taper over 14 days)
[total dose/cycle = 7 mg/kg + taper over 14 days]
Repeat cycle every 5 weeks

References

Case DC Jr, Lee DJ 3rd, and Clarkson BD, "Improved Survival Times in Multiple Myeloma Treated With Melphalan, Prednisone, Cyclophosphamide, Vincristine and BCNU: M-2 Protocol," *Am J Med*, 1977, 63(6):897-903.

M-3

Use Leukemia, acute promyelocytic)

Regimen NOTE: Multiple variations are listed below.

Induction:

Variation 1:
Tretinoin: Oral: 45 mg/m²/day day 1 up to 90 days
[total dose/cycle = 45-4050 mg/m²]
≤ 20 years: 25 mg/m²/day day 1 up to 90 days
[total dose/cycle = 25-2250 mg/m²]
Idarubicin: I.V.: 12 mg/m²/day days 2, 4, 6, and 8
[total dose/cycle = 48 mg/m²]

Consolidation:

Course 1:
Idarubicin: I.V.: 5 mg/m²/day days 1 to 4
[total dose/cycle = 20 mg/m²]
or 7 mg/m²/day days 1 to 4
[total dose/cycle = 28 mg/m²]
Tretinoin: Oral: 45 mg/m²/day days 1 to 15
[total dose/cycle = 675 mg/m²]
Course 2:
Mitoxantrone: I.V.: 10 mg/m²/day days 1 to 5
[total dose/cycle = 50 mg/m²]

   or 10 mg/m^2/day days 1 to 5
     [total dose/cycle = 50 mg/m^2]
  Tretinoin: Oral: 45 mg/m^2/day days 1 to 15
     [total dose/cycle = 675 mg/m^2]
Course 3:
  Idarubicin: I.V.: 12 mg/m^2 on day 1
     [total dose/cycle = 12 mg/m^2]
  or 12 mg/m^2/day on days 1 and 2
     [total dose/cycle = 24 mg/m^2]
  Tretinoin: Oral: 45 mg/m^2/day days 1 to 15
     [total dose/cycle = 675 mg/m^2]
  Repeat course at one month intervals.

Maintenance:
  Mercaptopurine: Oral: 50 mg/m^2 daily
     [total dose/cycle = 4.5 g/m^2]
  Methotrexate: I.M.: 15 mg/m^2 weekly
     [total dose/cycle = 180 mg/m^2]
  Tretinoin: Oral: 45 mg/m^2/day days 1 to 15
     [total dose/cycle = 675 mg/m^2]
  Repeat cycle every 3 months for 2 years

Variation 2:
Induction:
  Tretinoin: Oral: 45 mg/m^2/day day 1 up to 90 days
     [total dose/cycle = 45-4050 mg/m^2]
  ≤ 15 years: 25 mg/m^2/day day 1 up to 90 days
     [total dose/cycle = 25-2250 mg/m^2]
  Idarubicin: I.V.: 12 mg/m^2/day days 2, 4, 6, and 8
     [total dose/cycle = 48 mg/m^2]

Consolidation:
Course 1:
  Idarubicin: I.V.: 5 mg/m^2/day days 1 to 4
     [total dose/cycle = 20 mg/m^2]
Course 2:
  Mitoxantrone: I.V.: 10 mg/m^2/day days 1 to 5
     [total dose/cycle = 50 mg/m^2]
Course 3:
  Idarubicin: I.V.: 12 mg/m^2 day 1
     [total dose/cycle = 12 mg/m^2]
  Repeat course at one month intervals

Maintenance:
  Mercaptopurine: Oral: 90 mg/m^2 daily
     [total dose/cycle = 8.1 g/m^2]
  Methotrexate: I.M.: 15 mg/m^2 weekly
     [total dose/cycle = 60 mg/m^2]
  Tretinoin: Oral: 45 mg/m^2/day days 1 to 15
     [total dose/cycle = 675 mg/m^2]
  Repeat cycle every 3 months for 2 years

References
Sanz MA, Martin G, Gonzalez M, et al, "Risk-Adapted Treatment of Acute Promyelocytic Leukemia With All-Trans-Retinoic Acid and Anthracycline Monochemotherapy: A Multicenter Study by the PETHEMA Group," *Blood*, 2004, 103(4):1237-43.

Sanz MA, Martin G, Rayon C, et al, "A Modified AIDA Protocol With Anthracycline-Based Consolidation Results in High Antileukemic Efficacy and Reduced Toxicity in Newly Diagnosed PML/RARalpha-Positive Acute Promyelocytic Leukemia," *Blood* 1999, 94(9):3015-21.

MACOP-B

Use Lymphoma, non-Hodgkin's

Regimen

Methotrexate: I.V.: 400 mg/m^2 weeks 2, 6, and 10
  [total dose/cycle = 1200 mg/m^2]
Doxorubicin: I.V.: 50 mg/m^2 weeks 1, 3, 5, 7, 9, and 11
  [total dose/cycle = 300 mg/m^2]
Cyclophosphamide: I.V.: 350 mg/m^2 weeks 1, 3, 5, 7, 9, and 11
  [total dose/cycle = 2100 mg/m^2]
Vincristine: I.V.: 1.4 mg/m^2 (maximum 2 mg) weeks 2, 4, 8, 10, and 12
  [total dose/cycle = 7 mg/m^2]
Bleomycin: I.V.: 10 units/m^2 weeks 4, 8, and 12
  [total dose/cycle = 30 units/m^2]
Prednisone: Oral: 75 mg/day for 12 weeks, taper over last 2 weeks
Leucovorin calcium: Oral: 15 mg/m^2 every 6 hours for 6 doses (beginning
  24 hours after methotrexate) weeks 2, 6, and 10
  [total dose/cycle = 270 mg/m^2]
Administer one cycle

References

Fisher RI, "Cyclophosphamide, Doxorubicin, Vincristine, and Prednisone Versus Intensive Chemotherapy in Non-Hodgkin's Lymphoma," *Cancer Chemother Pharmacol*, 1997, 40 Suppl:S42-6.

Klimo P and Connors JM, "MACOP-B Chemotherapy for the Treatment of Diffuse Large-Cell Lymphoma," *Ann Intern Med*, 1985, 102(5):596-602.

MAID

Use Soft tissue sarcoma

Regimen

Mesna: I.V.: 2500 mg/m^2/day continuous infusion days 1 to 4
  [total dose/cycle = 10,000 mg/m^2]
Doxorubicin: I.V.: 20 mg/m^2/day continuous infusion days 1 to 3
  [total dose/cycle = 60 mg/m^2]
Ifosfamide: I.V.: 2500 mg/m^2/day continuous infusion days 1 to 3
  [total dose/cycle = 7500 mg/m^2]
Dacarbazine: I.V.: 300 mg/m^2/day continuous infusion days 1 to 3
  [total dose/cycle = 900 mg/m^2]
Repeat cycle every 21-28 days

References

Elias A, Ryan L, Sulkes A, et al, "Response to Mesna, Doxorubicin, Ifosfamide, and Dacarbazine in 108 Patients With Metastatic or Unresectable Sarcoma and No Prior Chemotherapy," *J Clin Oncol*, 1989, 7(9):1208-16.

m-BACOD

Use Lymphoma, non-Hodgkin's

Regimen

Methotrexate: I.V.: 200 mg/m^2/day days 8 and 15
  [total dose/cycle = 400 mg/m^2]
Leucovorin calcium: Oral: 10 mg/m^2 every 6 hours for 8 doses (beginning
  24 hours after each methotrexate dose) days 9 and 16
  [total dose/cycle = 160 mg/m^2]
Bleomycin: I.V.: 4 units/m^2 day 1
  [total dose/cycle = 4 units/m^2]

Doxorubicin: I.V.: 45 mg/m² day 1
[total dose/cycle = 45 mg/m²]
Cyclophosphamide: I.V.: 600 mg/m² day 1
[total dose/cycle = 600 mg/m²]
Vincristine: I.V.: 1 mg/m² day 1
[total dose/cycle = 1 mg/m²]
Dexamethasone: Oral: 6 mg/m²/day days 1 to 5
[total dose/cycle = 30 mg/m²]
Repeat cycle every 21 days

References

Salles G, Shipp MA, and Coiffier B, "Chemotherapy of Non-Hodgkin's Aggressive Lymphomas," *Semin Hematol*, 1994, 31(1):46-69.

Urba WJ, Duffey PL, and Longo DL, "Treatment of Patients With Aggressive Lymphomas: An Overview," *J Natl Cancer Inst Monogr*, 1990, (10):29-37.

MINE

Use Lymphoma, non-Hodgkin's

Regimen

Mesna: I.V.: 1.33 g/m²/day concurrent with ifosfamide dose, then 500 mg orally (4 hours after each ifosfamide infusion) days 1 to 3
[total dose/cycle = 3.99 g/m²/1500 mg]
Ifosfamide: I.V.: 1.33 g/m²/day days 1 to 3
[total dose/cycle = 3.99 mg/m²]
Mitoxantrone: I.V.: 8 mg/m² day 1
[total dose/cycle = 8 mg/m²]
Etoposide: I.V.: 65 mg/m²/day days 1 to 3
[total dose/cycle = 195 mg/m²]
Repeat cycle every 28 days

References

Rodriguez-Monge EJ and Cabanillas F, "Long-Term Follow-Up of Platinum-Based Lymphoma Salvage Regimens. The M.D. Anderson Cancer Center Experience," *Hematol Oncol Clin North Am*, 1997, 11(5):937-47.

MINE-ESHAP

Use Lymphoma, non-Hodgkin's

Regimen

Mesna: I.V.: 1.33 g/m² concurrent with ifosfamide dose, then 500 mg orally (4 hours after ifosfamide) days 1 to 3
[total dose/cycle = 3.99 g/m²/1500 mg]
Ifosfamide: I.V.: 1.33 g/m²/day days 1 to 3
[total dose/cycle = 3.99 mg/m²]
Mitoxantrone: I.V.: 8 mg/m² day 1
[total dose/cycle = 8 mg/m²]
Etoposide: I.V.: 65 mg/m²/day days 1 to 3
[total dose/cycle = 195 mg/m²]
Repeat cycle every 21 days for 6 cycles, followed by 3-6 cycles of ESHAP

References

Rodriguez MA, Cabanillas FC, Velasquez W, et al, "Results of a Salvage Treatment Program for Relapsing Lymphoma: MINE Consolidated With ESHAP," *J Clin Oncol*, 1995, 13(7):1734-41.

mini-BEAM
Use Lymphoma, Hodgkin's disease
Regimen
Carmustine: I.V.: 60 mg/m^2 day 1
[total dose/cycle = 60 mg/m^2]
Etoposide: I.V.: 75 mg/m^2/day days 2 to 5
[total dose/cycle = 300 mg/m^2]
Cytarabine: I.V.: 100 mg/m^2 every 12 hours days 2 to 5 (8 doses)
[total dose/cycle = 800 mg/m^2]
Melphalan: I.V.: 30 mg/m^2 day 6
[total dose/cycle = 30 mg/m^2]
Repeat cycle every 4-6 weeks
References
Colwill R, Crump M, Couture F, et al, "Mini-BEAM as Salvage Therapy for Relapsed or Refractory Hodgkin's Disease Before Intensive Therapy and Autologous Bone Marrow Transplantation," *J Clin Oncol*, 1995, 13(2):396-402.

♦ **Mini-CHOP** see CHOP on page 859

Mitoxantrone + Hydrocortisone
Use Prostate cancer
Regimen
Mitoxantrone: I.V.: 14 mg/m^2 day 1
[total dose/cycle = 14 mg/m^2]
Hydrocortisone: Oral: 40 mg daily
[total dose/cycle = 840 mg]
Repeat cycle every 3 weeks
References
Kantoff PW, Halabi S, Conaway M, et al, "Hydrocortisone With or Without Mitoxantrone in Men With Hormone-Refractory Prostate Cancer: Results of the Cancer and Leukemia Group B 9182 Study." *J Clin Oncol*, 1999, 17(8):2506-13.

♦ **Mitoxantrone + Prednisone** see MP (Prostate Cancer) on page 916

MM
Use Leukemia, acute lymphocytic (maintenance)
Regimen
Mercaptopurine: Oral: 50-75 mg/m^2/day days 1 to 7
[total dose/cycle = 350-525 mg/m^2]
Methotrexate: Oral, I.V.: 20 mg/m^2 day 1
[total dose/cycle = 20 mg/m^2]
Repeat cycle every 7 days

♦ **Modified Bagshawe** see CHAMOCA on page 858

MOP
Use Brain tumors
Regimen
Mechlorethamine: I.V.: 6 mg/m^2/day days 1 and 8
[total dose/cycle = 12 mg/m^2]
Vincristine: I.V.: 1.5 mg/m^2/day (maximum 2 mg) days 1 and 8
[total dose/cycle = 3 mg/m^2]
Procarbazine: Oral: 100 mg/m^2/day days 1 to 14
[total dose/cycle = 1400 mg/m^2]
Repeat cycle every 28 days

References
Kretschmar CS, Tarbell NJ, Kupsky W, et al, "Preirradiation Chemotherapy for Infants and Children With Medulloblastoma: A Preliminary Report," *J Neurosurg*, 1989, 71(6):820-5.

MOPP (Lymphoma, Hodgkin's Disease)

Use Lymphoma, Hodgkin's disease

Regimen NOTE: Multiple variations are listed below.

Variation 1:

Mechlorethamine: I.V.: 6 mg/m^2/day days 1 and 8
[total dose/cycle = 12 mg/m^2]

Vincristine: I.V.: 1.4 mg/m^2/day days 1 and 8
[total dose/cycle = 2.8 mg/m^2]

Procarbazine: Oral: 100 mg/m^2/day days 1 to 14
[total dose/cycle = 1400 mg/m^2]

Prednisone: Oral: 40 mg/m^2/day days 1 to 14 (cycles 1 and 4)
[total dose/cycle = 560 mg/m^2]

Repeat cycle every 28 days for 6-8 cycles

Variation 2:

Mechlorethamine: I.V.: 6 mg/m^2/day (maximum 15 mg) days 1 and 8
[total dose/cycle = 12 mg/m^2]

Vincristine: I.V.: 1.4 mg/m^2/day (maximum 2 mg) days 1 and 8
[total dose/cycle = 2.8 mg/m^2]

Procarbazine: Oral: 100 mg/m^2/day days 1 to 10
[total dose/cycle = 1000 mg/m^2]

Prednisone: Oral: 25 mg/m^2/day (maximum 60 mg) days 1 to 14
[total dose/cycle = 350 mg/m^2]
or
Prednisolone: Oral: 25 mg/m^2/day (maximum 60 mg) days 1 to 14
[total dose/cycle = 350 mg/m^2]

Repeat cycle every 28 days

Variation 3:

Mechlorethamine: I.V.: 6 mg/m^2/day days 1 and 8
[total dose/cycle = 12 mg/m^2]

Vincristine: I.V.: 1.4 mg/m^2/day days 1 and 8
[total dose/cycle = 2.8 mg/m^2]

Procarbazine: Oral: 50 mg day 1, 100 mg day 2, 100 mg/m^2/day days 3 to 14
[total dose/cycle = 150 mg / 1200 mg/m^2]

Prednisone: Oral: 40 mg/m^2/day days 1 to 14
[total dose/cycle = 560 mg/m^2]

Repeat cycle every 28 days

Variation 4:

Mechlorethamine: I.V.: 6 mg/m^2/day days 1 and 8
[total dose/cycle = 12 mg/m^2]

Vincristine: I.V.: 1.4 mg/m^2/day days 1 and 8
[total dose/cycle = 2.8 mg/m^2]

Procarbazine: Oral: 50 mg day 1, 100 mg day 2, 100 mg/m^2/day days 3 to 10
[total dose/cycle = 150 mg / 800 mg/m^2]

Prednisone: Oral: 40 mg/m^2/day days 1 to 14
[total dose/cycle = 560 mg/m^2]

Repeat cycle every 28 days

Variation 5:

Mechlorethamine: I.V.: 6 mg/m^2/day days 1 and 8
[total dose/cycle = 12 mg/m^2]

(Continued)

MOPP (Lymphoma, Hodgkin's Disease)
(Continued)

Vincristine: I.V.: 1.4 mg/m^2/day days 1 and 8
[total dose/cycle = 2.8 mg/m^2]
Procarbazine: Oral: 50 mg/m^2 day 1, then 100 mg/m^2/day days 2 to 14
[total dose/cycle = 1350 mg/m^2]
Prednisone: Oral: 40 mg/m^2/day days 1 to 14
[total dose/cycle = 560 mg/m^2]
Repeat cycle every 28 days

References

Variation 1:
Devita VT Jr, Serpick AA, and Carbone PP, "Combination Chemotherapy in the Treatment of Advanced Hodgkin's Disease," *Ann Intern Med*, 1970, 73(6):881-95.

Variation 2:
Hancock BW, "Randomised Study Of MOPP (Mustine, Oncovin, Procarbazine, Prednisone) Against LOPP (Leukeran Substituted for Mustine) in Advanced Hodgkin's Disease. British National Lymphoma Investigation," *Radiother Oncol*, 1986, 7(3):215-21.

Variation 3:
Nissen NI, Pajak TF, Glidewell O, et al, "A Comparative Study of a BCNU Containing 4-Drug Program Versus MOPP Versus 3-Drug Combinations in Advanced Hodgkin's Disease: A Cooperative Study by the Cancer and Leukemia Group B," *Cancer*, 1979, 43(1):31-40.

Variation 4:
Huguley CM Jr, Durant JR, Moores RR, et al, "A Comparison of Nitrogen Mustard, Vincristine, Procarbazine, and Prednisone (MOPP) vs Nitrogen Mustard In Advanced Hodgkin's Disease," *Cancer*, 1975, 36(4):1227-40.

Variation 5:
Bakemeier RF, Anderson JR, Costello W, et al, "BCVPP Chemotherapy for Advanced Hodgkin's Disease: Evidence for Greater Duration of Complete Remission, Greater Survival, and Less Toxicity Than With a MOPP Regimen. Results of the Eastern Cooperative Oncology Group Study," *Ann Intern Med*, 1984, 101(4):447-56.

MOPP (Medulloblastoma)

Use Brain tumors

Regimen

Mechlorethamine: I.V.: 3 mg/m^2/day days 1 and 8
[total dose/cycle = 6 mg/m^2]
Vincristine: I.V.: 1.4 mg/m^2/day (maximum 2 mg) days 1 and 8
[total dose/cycle = 2.8 mg/m^2]
Prednisone: Oral: 40 mg/m^2/day days 1 to 10
[total dose/cycle = 400 mg/m^2]
Procarbazine: Oral: 50 mg day 1
[total dose = 50 mg]
followed by 100 mg day 2
[total dose = 100 mg]
followed by 100 mg/m^2/day days 3 to 10
[total dose = 800 mg/m^2]
Repeat cycle every 28 days

References

Krischer JP, Ragab AH, Kun L, et al, "Nitrogen Mustard, Vincristine, Procarbazine, and Prednisone as Adjuvant Chemotherapy in the Treatment of Medulloblastoma. A Pediatric Oncology Group Study," *J Neurosurg*, 1991, 74(6):905-9.

MOPP/ABV Hybrid

Use Lymphoma, Hodgkin's disease

Regimen

Mechlorethamine: I.V.: 6 mg/m² day 1
  [total dose/cycle = 6 mg/m²]
Vincristine: I.V.: 1.4 mg/m² (maximum 2 mg) day 1
  [total dose/cycle = 1.4 mg/m²]
Procarbazine: Oral: 100 mg/m²/day days 1 to 7
  [total dose/cycle = 700 mg/m²]
Prednisone: Oral: 40 mg/m²/day days 1 to 14
  [total dose/cycle = 560 mg/m²]
Doxorubicin: I.V.: 35 mg/m² day 8
  [total dose/cycle = 35 mg/m²]
Bleomycin: I.V.: 10 units/m² day 8
  [total dose/cycle = 10 units/m²]
Vinblastine: I.V.: 6 mg/m² day 8
  [total dose/cycle = 6 mg/m²]
Repeat cycle every 28 days

References

Klimo P and Connors JM, "MOPP/ABV Hybrid Program: Combination Chemotherapy Based on Early Introduction of Seven Effective Drugs for Advanced Hodgkin's Disease," *J Clin Oncol*, 1985, 3(9):1174-82.

MOPP/ABVD

Use Lymphoma, Hodgkin's disease

Regimen NOTE: Multiple variations are listed below.

Variation 1:

Mechlorethamine: I.V.: 6 mg/m²/day days 1 and 8
  [total dose/cycle = 12 mg/m²]
Vincristine: I.V.: 1.4 mg/m²/day (maximum 2 mg) days 1 and 8
  [total dose/cycle = 2.8 mg/m²]
Procarbazine: I.V.: 100 mg/m²/day days 1 to 14
  [total dose/cycle = 1400 mg/m²]
Prednisone: Oral: 40 mg/m²/day days 1 to 14 (during cycles 1, 4, 7, and 10 only)
  [total dose/cycle = 560 mg/m²]
Doxorubicin: Oral: 25 mg/m²/day days 29 and 43
  [total dose/cycle = 50 mg/m²]
Bleomycin: I.V.: 10 units/m²/day days 29 and 43
  [total dose/cycle = 20 units/m²]
Vinblastine: I.V.: 6 mg/m²/day days 29 and 43
  [total dose/cycle = 12 mg/m²]
Dacarbazine: I.V.: 375 mg/m²/day days 29 and 43
  [total dose/cycle = 750 mg/m²]
Repeat cycle every 56 days

Variation 2:

Mechlorethamine: I.V.: 6 mg/m²/day days 1 and 8
  [total dose/cycle = 12 mg/m²]
Vincristine: I.V.: 1.4 mg/m²/day (maximum 2 mg) days 1 and 8
  [total dose/cycle = 2.8 mg/m²]
Procarbazine: I.V.: 100 mg/m²/day days 1 to 14
  [total dose/cycle = 1400 mg/m²]
Prednisone: Oral: 40 mg/m2/day days 1 to 14 (during cycles 1 and 7 only)
  [total dose/cycle = 560 mg/m²]

(Continued)

MOPP/ABVD *(Continued)*

Doxorubicin: Oral: 25 mg/m^2/day days 29 and 43
  [total dose/cycle = 50 mg/m^2]
Bleomycin: I.V.: 10 units/m^2/day days 29 and 43
  [total dose/cycle = 20 units/m^2]
Vinblastine: I.V.: 6 mg/m^2/day days 29 and 43
  [total dose/cycle = 12 mg/m^2]
Dacarbazine: I.V.: 375 mg/m^2/day days 29 and 43
  [total dose/cycle = 750 mg/m^2]
Repeat cycle every 56 days
Variation 3:
  Mechlorethamine: I.V.: 6 mg/m^2/day days 1 and 8
    [total dose/cycle = 12 mg/m^2]
  Vincristine: I.V.: 1.4 mg/m^2/day (maximum 2 mg) days 1 and 8
    [total dose/cycle = 2.8 mg/m^2]
  Procarbazine: I.V.: 100 mg/m^2/day days 1 to 14
    [total dose/cycle = 1400 mg/m^2]
  Prednisone: Oral: 40 mg/m^2/day days 1 to 14 (every cycle)
    [total dose/cycle = 560 mg/m^2]
  Doxorubicin: Oral: 25 mg/m^2/day days 29 and 43
    [total dose/cycle = 50 mg/m^2]
  Bleomycin: I.V.: 10 units/m^2/day days 29 and 43
    [total dose/cycle = 20 units/m^2]
  Vinblastine: I.V.: 6 mg/m^2/day days 29 and 43
    [total dose/cycle = 12 mg/m^2]
  Dacarbazine: I.V.: 375 mg/m^2/day days 29 and 43
    [total dose/cycle = 750 mg/m^2]
  Repeat cycle every 56 days
Variation 4:
  MOPP Regimen:
  Mechlorethamine: I.V.: 6 mg/m^2/day days 1 and 8
    [total dose/cycle = 12 mg/m^2]
  Vincristine: I.V.: 1.4 mg/m^2/day (maximum 2 mg) days 1 and 8
    [total dose/cycle = 2.8 mg/m^2]
  Procarbazine: I.V.: 100 mg/m^2/day days 1 to 14
    [total dose/cycle = 1400 mg/m^2]
  Prednisone: Oral: 25 mg/m^2/day days 1 to 14
    [total dose/cycle = 350 mg/m^2]
  ABVD Regimen:
  Doxorubicin: Oral: 25 mg/m^2/day days 1 and 15
    [total dose/cycle = 50 mg/m^2]
  Bleomycin: I.V.: 6 units/m^2/day days 1 and 15
    [total dose/cycle = 12 units/m^2]
  Vinblastine: I.V.: 6 mg/m^2/day days 1 and 15
    [total dose/cycle = 12 mg/m^2]
  Dacarbazine: I.V.: 250 mg/m^2/day days 1 and 15
    [total dose/cycle = 500 mg/m^2]
  Each regimen cycle is 28 days. Administer regimens in alternating
    fashion as follows: 2 cycles of MOPP alternating with 2 cycles of
    ABVD for a total of 8 cycles
Variation 5 (pediatrics):
  Mechlorethamine: I.V.: 6 mg/m^2/day days 1 and 8
    [total dose/cycle = 12 mg/m^2]

Vincristine: I.V.: 1.4 mg/m^2/day days 1 and 8
[total dose/cycle = 2.8 mg/m^2]

Procarbazine: Oral: 100 mg/m^2/day days 1 to 14
[total dose/cycle = 1400 mg/m^2]

Prednisone: Oral: 40 mg/m^2/day days 1 to 14
[total dose/cycle = 560 mg/m^2]

Doxorubicin: Oral: 25 mg/m^2/day days 29 and 42
[total dose/cycle = 50 mg/m^2]

Bleomycin: I.V.: 10 units/m^2/day days 29 and 42
[total dose/cycle = 20 units/m^2]

Vinblastine: I.V.: 6 mg/m^2/day days 29 and 42
[total dose/cycle = 12 mg/m^2]

Dacarbazine: I.V.: 150 mg/m^2/day days 29 to 33
[total dose/cycle = 750 mg/m^2]

Repeat cycle every 56 days for 4 cycles

Variation 6 (pediatrics):

Mechlorethamine: I.V.: 6 mg/m^2/day days 1 and 8
[total dose/cycle = 12 mg/m^2]

Vincristine: I.V.: 1.4 mg/m^2/day days 1 and 8
[total dose/cycle = 2.8 mg/m^2]

Procarbazine: Oral: 100 mg/m^2/day days 1 to 14
[total dose/cycle = 1400 mg/m^2]

Prednisone: Oral: 40 mg/m^2/day days 1 to 14
[total dose/cycle = 560 mg/m^2]

Doxorubicin: Oral: 25 mg/m^2/day days 29 and 42
[total dose/cycle = 50 mg/m^2]

Bleomycin: I.V.: 10 units/m^2/day days 29 and 42
[total dose/cycle = 20 units/m^2]

Vinblastine: I.V.: 6 mg/m^2/day days 29 and 42
[total dose/cycle = 12 mg/m^2]

Dacarbazine: I.V.: 375 mg/m^2/day days 29 and 43
[total dose/cycle = 750 mg/m^2]

Repeat cycle every 56 days for 4 cycles

References

Variation 1:

Bonadonna G, Valagussa P, and Santoro A, "Alternating Noncross-Resistant Combination Chemotherapy or MOPP in State IV Hodgkin's Disease. A Report of 8-Year Results," *Ann Int Med*, 1986, 104(6):739-46.

Variation 2:

Canellos, GP, Anderson JR, Propert KJ, et al, "Chemotherapy of Advanced Hodgkin's Disease With MOPP, ABVD, or MOPP Alternating With ABVD," *N Engl J Med*, 1992, 327(21):1478-84.

Variation 3:

Glick JH, Young ML, Harrington D, et al, "MOPP/ABV Hybrid Chemotherapy for Advanced Hodgkin's Disease Significantly Improves Failure-Free and Overall Survival. The 8-Year Results of the Intergroup Trial," *J Clin Oncol* 1998, 16(1):19-26.

Variation 4:

Somers R, Carde P, Henry-Amar M, et al, "A Randomized Study in State IIIB and IV Hodgkin's Disease Comparing Eight Courses of MOPP Versus an Alternation of MOPP With ABVD. A European Organization for Research and Treatment of Cancer Lymphoma Cooperative Group and Groupe Pierre-et-Marie-Curie Controlled Clinical Trial," *J Clin Oncol*, 1994, 12(2):279-87.

Variation 5 (pediatrics):

Weiner MA, Leventhal BG, Marcus R, et al, "Intensive Chemotherapy and Low-Dose Radiotherapy for the Treatment of Advanced-Stage Hodgkin's Disease in Pediatric Patients. A Pediatric Oncology Group Study," *J Clin Oncol*, 1991, 9(9):1591-8.

(Continued)

MOPP/ABVD *(Continued)*

Variation 6 (pediatrics):

Weiner MA, Leventhal B, Brecher ML, et al, "Randomized Study of Intensive MOPP-ABVD With or Without Low-Dose Total-Nodal Radiation Therapy in the Treatment of Stages IIB, IIIA2, IIIB, and IV Hodgkin's Disease in Pediatric Patients. A Pediatric Oncology Group Study," *J Clin Oncol*, 1997, 15(8):2769-79.

MP (Multiple Myeloma)

Use Multiple myeloma

Regimen

Melphalan: Oral: 8-10 mg/m^2/day days 1 to 4
[total dose/cycle = 32-40 mg/m^2]
Prednisone: Oral: 40-60 mg/m^2/day days 1 to 4
[total dose/cycle = 160-240 mg/m^2]
Repeat cycle every 28-42 days

References

Southwest Oncology Group Study, "Remission Maintenance Therapy for Multiple Myeloma," *Arch Intern Med*, 1975, 135(1):147-52.

MP (Prostate Cancer)

Synonyms Mitoxantrone + Prednisone

Use Prostate cancer

Regimen

Mitoxantrone: I.V.: 12 mg/m^2 day 1
[total dose/cycle = 12 mg/m^2]
Prednisone: Oral: 5 mg twice daily
[total dose/cycle = 210 mg]
Repeat cycle every 21 days

References

Moore MJ, Osoba D, Murphy K, et al, "Use of Palliative End Points to Evaluate the Effects of Mitoxantrone and Low-Dose Prednisone in Patients With Hormonally Resistant Prostate Cancer," *J Clin Oncol*, 1994, 12(4):689-94.

MTX/6-MP/VP (Maintenance)

Use Leukemia, acute lymphocytic

Regimen

Methotrexate: Oral: 20 mg/m^2 weekly
[total dose/cycle = 80 mg/m^2]
Mercaptopurine: Oral: 75 mg/m^2/day
[total dose/cycle = 2250 mg/m^2]
Vincristine: I.V.: 1.5 mg/m^2 day 1
[total dose/cycle = 1.5 mg/m^2]
Prednisone: Oral: 40 mg/m^2/day days 1 to 5
[total dose/cycle = 200 mg/m^2]
Repeat monthly for 2-3 years

References

Bleyer WA, Sather HN, Nickerson HJ, et al, "Monthly Pulses of Vincristine and Prednisone Prevent Bone Marrow and Testicular Relapse in Low-Risk Childhood Acute Lymphoblastic Leukemia: A Report of the CCG-161 Study by the Childrens Cancer Study Group," *J Clin Oncol*, 1991, 9(6):1012-21.

MTX-CDDPAdr

Use Osteosarcoma

Regimen

Cisplatin: I.V.: 75 mg/m^2 day 1 of cycles 1-7
[total dose/cycle = 75 mg/m^2]

Cisplatin: I.V.: 120 mg/m^2 day 1 cycles 8-10
[total dose/cycle = 120 mg/m^2]
Doxorubicin: I.V.: 25 mg/m^2/day days 1 to 3 of cycles 1 to 7
[total dose/cycle = 75 mg/m^2]
Methotrexate: I.V.: 12 g/m^2/day days 21 and 28
[total dose/cycle = 24 g/m^2]
Leucovorin calcium rescue: I.V.: 20 mg/m^2 every 3 hours (beginning 16 hours after completion of methotrexate) for 8 doses, then orally every 6 hours for 8 doses
[total dose/cycle = 640 mg/m^2]

References

Meyers PA, Heller G, Healey J, et al, "Chemotherapy for Nonmetastatic Osteogenic Sarcoma: The Memorial Sloan-Kettering Experience," *J Clin Oncol*, 1992, 10(1):5-15.

MV

Use Leukemia, acute myeloid

Regimen

Mitoxantrone: I.V.: 10 mg/m^2/day days 1 to 5
[total dose/cycle = 50 mg/m^2]
Etoposide: I.V.: 100 mg/m^2/day days 1 to 5
[total dose/cycle = 500 mg/m^2]
Second cycle may be given based on individual response; time between cycles not specified

References

Ho AD, Lipp T, Ehninger G, et al, "Combination of Mitoxantrone and Etoposide in Refractory Acute Myelogenous Leukemia an Active and Well-Tolerated Regimen," *J Clin Oncol*, 1988, 6(2):213-17.

M-VAC (Bladder Cancer)

Use Bladder cancer

Regimen NOTE: Multiple variations are listed below.

Variation 1:

Methotrexate: I.V.: 30 mg/m^2/day days 1, 15, and 22
[total dose/cycle = 90 mg/m^2]
Vinblastine: I.V.: 3 mg/m^2/day days 2, 15, and 22
[total dose/cycle = 9 mg/m^2]
Doxorubicin: I.V.: 30 mg/m^2 day 2
[total dose/cycle = 30 mg/m^2]
Cisplatin: I.V.: 70 mg/m^2 day 2
[total dose/cycle = 70 mg/m^2]
Repeat cycle every 4 weeks

Variation 2:

Methotrexate: I.V.: 40 or 50 mg/m^2/day days 1, 15, and 22
[total dose/cycle = 120 or 150 mg/m^2]
Vinblastine: I.V.: 4 or 5 mg/m^2/day days 2, 15, and 22
[total dose/cycle = 12 or 15 mg/m^2]
Doxorubicin: I.V.: 40 or 50 mg/m^2 day 2
[total dose/cycle = 40 or 50 mg/m^2]
Cisplatin: I.V.: 100 mg/m^2 day 2
[total dose/cycle = 100 mg/m^2]
Repeat cycle every 4 weeks

Variation 3:

Methotrexate: I.V.: 30 mg/m^2/day days 1, 15, and 22
[total dose/cycle = 90 mg/m^2]

(Continued)

M-VAC (Bladder Cancer) *(Continued)*

Vinblastine: I.V.: 3 mg/m² day 2
[total dose/cycle = 3 mg/m²]
Doxorubicin: I.V.: 30 mg/m² day 2
[total dose/cycle = 30 mg/m²]
Cisplatin: I.V.: 70 mg/m² day 2
[total dose/cycle = 70 mg/m²]
Repeat cycle every 4 weeks

Variation 4:
Methotrexate: I.V.: 60 mg/m² day 1
[total dose/cycle = 60 mg/m²]
followed by 30 mg/m² day 16
[total dose/cycle = 30 mg/m²]
Vinblastine: I.V.: 4 mg/m²/day days 2 and 16
[total dose/cycle = 8 mg/m²]
Doxorubicin: I.V.: 60 mg/m² day 2
[total dose/cycle = 60 mg/m²]
Cisplatin: I.V.: 100 mg/m² day 2
[total dose/cycle = 100 mg/m²]
Repeat cycle every 23 days

Variation 5:
Methotrexate: I.V.: 30 mg/m²/day days 1, 16, and 23
[total dose/cycle = 90 mg/m²]
Vinblastine: I.V.: 4 mg/m²/day days 1, 16, and 23
[total dose/cycle = 12 mg/m²]
Doxorubicin: I.V.: 60 mg/m² day 2
[total dose/cycle = 60 mg/m²]
Cisplatin: I.V.: 100 mg/m² day 2
[total dose/cycle = 100 mg/m²]
Repeat cycle every 23 days

Variation 6:
Methotrexate: I.V.: 30 or 35 mg/m² day 1
[total dose/cycle = 30 or 35 mg/m²]
Vinblastine: I.V.: 3 or 3.5 mg/m² day 2
[total dose/cycle = 3 or 3.5 mg/m²]
Doxorubicin: I.V.: 30 or 35 mg/m² day 2
[total dose/cycle = 30 or 35 mg/m²]
Cisplatin: I.V.: 70 or 80 mg/m² day 2
[total dose/cycle = 70 or 80 mg/m²]
Repeat cycle every 2 weeks

Variation 7:
Methotrexate: I.V.: 30 mg/m² day 1
[total dose/cycle = 30 mg/m²]
Vinblastine: I.V.: 3 mg/m² day 2
[total dose/cycle = 3 mg/m²]
Doxorubicin: I.V.: 30 mg/m² day 2
[total dose/cycle = 30 mg/m²]
Cisplatin: I.V.: 70 mg/m² day 2
[total dose/cycle = 70 mg/m²]
Repeat cycle every 14 days

Variation 8:
Methotrexate: I.V.: 30 mg/m²/day days 1, 15, and 22
[total dose/cycle = 90 mg/m²]

Vinblastine: I.V.: 3 mg/m^2/day days 1, 15, and 22
 [total dose/cycle = 9 mg/m^2]
Doxorubicin: I.V.: 45 mg/m^2 day 2
 [total dose/cycle = 45 mg/m^2]
Cisplatin: I.V.: 70 mg/m^2 day 2
 [total dose/cycle = 70 mg/m^2]
Repeat cycle every 4 weeks
Variation 9:
 Methotrexate: I.V.: 40 mg/m^2/day days 1 and 15
  [total dose/cycle = 80 mg/m^2]
 Vinblastine: I.V.: 4 mg/m^2/day days 1, 16, and 23
  [total dose/cycle = 12 mg/m^2]
 Doxorubicin: I.V.: 60 mg/m^2 day 2
  [total dose/cycle = 60 mg/m^2]
 Cisplatin: I.V.: 100 mg/m^2 day 2
  [total dose/cycle = 100 mg/m^2]
 Repeat cycle every 23 days
Variation 10:
 Methotrexate: I.V.: 30 mg/m^2/day days 1, 15, and 22
  [total dose/cycle = 90 mg/m^2]
 Vinblastine: I.V.: 3 mg/m^2/day days 1, 16, and 22
  [total dose/cycle = 9 mg/m^2]
 Doxorubicin: I.V.: 30 mg/m^2 day 1
  [total dose/cycle = 30 mg/m^2]
 Cisplatin: I.V.: 70 mg/m^2 day 1
  [total dose/cycle = 70 mg/m^2]
 Repeat cycle every 4 weeks
Variation 11:
 Methotrexate: I.V.: 30 mg/m^2/day days 1, 15, and 22
  [total dose/cycle = 90 mg/m^2]
 Vinblastine: I.V.: 3 mg/m^2/day days 2, 15, and 22
  [total dose/cycle = 9 mg/m^2]
 Doxorubicin: I.V.: 30 mg/m^2 day 2
  [total dose/cycle = 30 mg/m^2]
 Cisplatin: I.V.: 70 mg/m^2 day 2
  [total dose/cycle = 70 mg/m^2]
 Leucovorin: Oral: 15 mg every 6 hours for 4 doses, days 2, 16, and 23
  [total dose/cycle = 180 mg]
 Repeat cycle every 4 weeks
Variation 12:
 Methotrexate: I.V.: 30 mg/m^2/day days 1 and 15
  [total dose/cycle = 60 mg/m^2]
 Vinblastine: I.V.: 3 mg/m^2/day days 2 and 15
  [total dose/cycle = 6 mg/m^2]
 Doxorubicin: I.V.: 30 or 40 mg/m^2 day 3
  [total dose/cycle = 30 or 40 mg/m^2]
 Cisplatin: I.V.: 70 mg/m^2 day 2
  [total dose/cycle = 70 mg/m^2]
 Repeat cycle every 4 weeks
Variation 13:
 Methotrexate: I.V.: 30 mg/m^2/day days 1 and 15
  [total dose/cycle = 60 mg/m^2]
 Vinblastine: I.V.: 3 mg/m^2/day days 2 and 15
  [total dose/cycle = 6 mg/m^2]
(Continued)

M-VAC (Bladder Cancer) *(Continued)*

Doxorubicin: I.V.: 30 or 40 mg/m^2 day 2
[total dose/cycle = 30 or 40 mg/m^2]

Cisplatin: I.V.: 70 mg/m^2 day 2
[total dose/cycle = 70 mg/m^2]

Repeat cycle every 4 weeks

References

Variation 1:

Sternberg CN, Yagoda A, Scher HI, et al, "Preliminary Results of M-VAC (Methotrexate, Vinblastine, Doxorubicin, and Cisplatin) for Transitional Cell Carcinoma of the Urothelium," *J Urol*, 1985, 133(3):403-7.

Variation 2:

Loehrer PJ Sr, Elson P, Dreicer R, et al, "Escalated Dosages of Methotrexate, Vinblastine, Doxorubicin, and Cisplatin Plus Recombinant Human Granulocyte Colony-Stimulating Factor in Advanced Urothelial Carcinoma: An Eastern Cooperative Oncology Group Trial," *J Clin Oncol*, 1994, 12(3):483-8.

Variation 3:

Loehrer PJ Sr, Einhorn LH, Elson PJ, et al, "A Randomized Comparison of Cisplatin Alone or in Combination With Methotrexate, Vinblastine, and Doxorubicin in Patients With Metastatic Urothelial Carcinoma: A Cooperative Group Study," *J Clin Oncol*, 1992, 10(7):1066-73.

Variation 4:

Logothetis CJ, Finn LD, Smith T, et al, "Escalated MVAC With or Without Recombinant Human Granulocyte-Macrophage Colony-Stimulating Factor for the Initial Treatment of Advanced Malignant Urothelial Tumors: Results of a Randomized Trial," *J Clin Oncol*, 1995, 13(9):2272-7.

Variation 5:

Logothetis CJ, Dexeus FH, Sella A, et al, "Escalated Therapy for Refractory Urothelial Tumors: Methotrexate-Vinblastine-Doxorubicin-Cisplatin Plus Unglycosylated Recombinant Human Granulocyte-Macrophage Colony-Stimulating Factor," *J Natl Cancer Inst*, 1990, 82(8):667-72.

Variation 6:

Sternberg CN, de Mulder PH, van Oosterom AT, et al, "Escalated M-VAC Chemotherapy and Recombinant Human Granulocyte-Macrophage Colony Stimulating Factor (rhGM-CSF) in Patients With Advanced Urothelial Tract Tumors," *Ann Oncol*, 1993, 4(5):403-7.

Variation 7:

Sternberg CN, de Mulder PH, Schornagel JH, et al, "Randomized Phase III Trial of High-Dose-Intensity Methotrexate, Vinblastine, Doxorubicin, and Cisplatin (M-VAC) Chemotherapy and Recombinant Human Granulocyte Colony-Stimulating Factor Versus Classic M-VAC in Advanced Urothelial Tract Tumors: European Organization for Research and Treatment of Cancer Protocol no. 30924," *J Clin Oncol*, 2001, 19(10):2638-46.

Variation 8 and 9:

Seidman AD, Scher HI, Gabrilove JL, et al, "Dose-Intensification of MVAC With Recombinant Granulocyte Colony-Stimulating Factor as Initial Therapy in Advanced Urothelial Cancer," *J Clin Oncol*, 1993, 11(3):408-14.

Variation 10:

Bamias A, Aravantinos G, Deliveliotis C, et al, "Docetaxel and Cisplatin With Granulocyte Colony-Stimulating Factor (G-CSF) Versus M-VAC With G-CSF in Advanced Urothelial Carcinoma: A Multicenter, Randomized, Phase III Study From the Hellenic Cooperative Oncology Group," *J Clin Oncol*, 2004, 22(2):220-8.

Variation 11:

Simon SD and Srougi M, "Neoadjuvant M-VAC Chemotherapy and Partial Cystectomy for Treatment of Locally Invasive Transitional Cell Carcinoma of the Bladder," *Prog Clin Biol Res*, 1990, 353:169-74.

Variation 12:

Farah R, Chodak GW, Vogelzang NJ, et al, "Curative Radiotherapy Following Chemotherapy for Invasive Bladder Carcinoma (A Preliminary Report)," *Int J Radiat Oncol Biol Phys*, 1991, 20(3):413-7.

Variation 13:

Vogelzang NJ, Moormeier JA, Awan AM, et al, "Methotrexate, Vinblastine, Doxorubicin, and Cisplatin Followed by Radiotherapy or Surgery for Muscle Invasive Bladder Cancer: The University of Chicago Experience," *J Urol*, 1993, 149(4):753-7.

M-VAC (Breast Cancer)

Use Breast cancer

Regimen

Methotrexate: I.V.: 30 mg/m^2/day days 1, 15, and 22
  [total dose/cycle = 90 mg/m^2]
Vinblastine: I.V.: 3 mg/m^2/day days 2, 15, and 22
  [total dose/cycle = 9 mg/m^2]
Doxorubicin: I.V.: 30 mg/m^2 day 2
  [total dose/cycle = 30 mg/m^2]
Cisplatin: I.V.: 70 mg/m^2 day 2
  [total dose/cycle = 70 mg/m^2]
Leucovorin: Oral: 10 mg every 6 hours for 6 doses days 2, 16, and 23
  [total dose/cycle = 180 mg]
Repeat cycle every 4 weeks

References

Morrell LE, Lee YJ, Hurley J, et al, "A Phase II Trial of Neoadjuvant Methotrexate, Vinblastine, Doxorubicin, and Cisplatin in the Treatment of Patients With Locally Advanced Breast Carcinoma," *Cancer*, 1998, 82(3):503-11.

M-VAC (Cervical Cancer)

Use Cervical cancer

Regimen

Methotrexate: I.V.: 30 mg/m^2/day days 1, 15, and 22
  [total dose/cycle = 90 mg/m^2]
Vinblastine: I.V.: 3 mg/m^2/day days 2, 15, and 22
  [total dose/cycle = 9 mg/m^2]
Doxorubicin: I.V.: 30 mg/m^2 day 2
  [total dose/cycle = 30 mg/m^2]
Cisplatin: I.V.: 70 mg/m^2 day 2
  [total dose/cycle = 70 mg/m^2]
Repeat cycle every 4 weeks

References

Wilson TO, "Neoadjuvant MVAC (Methotrexate, Vinblastine, Doxorubicin, Cisplatin) Chemotherapy for Locally Advanced or Metastatic Cervical and Vaginal Cancer," *Adjuvant Therapy of Cancer VII*, Salmon SE, ed, Philadelphia, PA: J B Lipincott Co, 1997, 366-71.

M-VAC (Endometrial Cancer)

Use Endometrial cancer

Regimen

Methotrexate: I.V.: 30 mg/m^2/day days 1, 15, and 22
  [total dose/cycle = 90 mg/m^2]
Vinblastine: I.V.: 3 mg/m^2/day days 2, 15, and 22
  [total dose/cycle = 9 mg/m^2]
Doxorubicin: I.V.: 30 mg/m^2/day day 2
  [total dose/cycle = 30 mg/m^2]
Cisplatin: I.V.: 70 mg/m^2/day day 2
  [total dose/cycle = 70 mg/m^2]
Repeat cycle every 4 weeks
(Continued)

M-VAC (Endometrial Cancer) *(Continued)*

References
Long HJ 3rd, Langdon RM Jr, Cha SS, et al, "Phase II Trial of Methotrexate, Vinblastine, Doxorubicin, and Cisplatin in Advanced/Recurrent Endometrial Carcinoma," *Gynecol Oncol*, 1995, 58(2):240-3.

M-VAC (Head and Neck Cancer)
Use Head and neck cancer
Regimen
Methotrexate: I.V.: 30 mg/m^2/day days 1, 15, and 22
[total dose/cycle = 90 mg/m^2]
Vinblastine: I.V.: 3 mg/m^2/day days 2, 15, and 22
[total dose/cycle = 9 mg/m^2]
Doxorubicin: I.V.: 30 mg/m^2 day 2
[total dose/cycle = 30 mg/m^2]
Cisplatin: I.V.: 70 mg/m^2 day 2
[total dose/cycle = 70 mg/m^2]
Repeat cycle every 4 weeks
References
Okuno SH, Mailliard JA, Suman VJ, et al, "Phase II Study of Methotrexate, Vinblastine, Doxorubicin, and Cisplatin in Patients With Squamous Cell Carcinoma of the Upper Respiratory or Alimentary Passages of the Head and Neck," *Cancer*, 2002, 94(8):2224-31.

MVPP
Use Lymphoma, Hodgkin's disease
Regimen
Mechlorethamine: I.V.: 6 mg/m^2/day days 1 and 8
[total dose/cycle = 12 mg/m^2]
Vinblastine: I.V.: 4 mg/m^2/day days 1 and 8
[total dose/cycle = 8 mg/m^2]
Procarbazine: Oral: 100 mg/m^2/day days 1 to 14
[total dose/cycle = 1400 mg/m^2]
Prednisone: Oral: 40 mg/m^2/day days 1 to 14
[total dose/cycle = 560 mg/m^2]
Repeat cycle every 4-6 weeks
References
Cooper MR, Pajak TF, Nissen NI, et al, "A New Effective Four-Drug Combination of CCNU (1-[2-Chloroethyl]-3-Cyclohexyl-1-Nitrosourea) (NSC-79038), Vinblastine, Prednisone, and Procarbazine for the Treatment of Advanced Hodgkin's Disease," *Cancer*, 1980, 46(4):654-62.

N4SE Protocol
Use Neuroblastomas
Regimen
Vincristine: I.V.: 0.05 mg/kg/day days 1 and 2
[total dose/cycle = 0.1 mg/kg]
Doxorubicin: I.V.: 15 mg/m^2/day days 1 and 2
[total dose/cycle = 30 mg/m^2]
Cyclophosphamide: I.V.: 30 mg/kg/day days 1 and 2
[total dose/cycle = 60 mg/kg]
Fluorouracil: I.V.: 1 mg/kg/day days 3, 8, and 9
[total dose/cycle = 3 mg/kg]
Cytarabine: I.V.: 3 mg/kg/day days 3, 8, and 9
[total dose/cycle = 9 mg/kg]

Hydroxyurea: Oral: 40 mg/kg/day days 3, 8, and 9
[total dose/cycle = 120 mg/kg]
Repeat cycle every 21-28 days

References
Kushner BH and Helson L, "Coordinated Use of Sequentially Escalated Cyclophosphamide and Cell-Cycle-Specific Chemotherapy (N4SE Protocol) for Advanced Neuroblastoma: Experience With 100 Patients," *J Clin Oncol*, 1987, 5(11):1746-51.

N6 Protocol

Use Neuroblastomas

Regimen

Course 1, 2, 4, and 6:
Cyclophosphamide: I.V.: 70 mg/kg/day days 1 and 2
[total dose/cycle = 140 mg/kg]
Doxorubicin: I.V.: 25 mg/m²/day continuous infusion days 1 to 3
[total dose/cycle = 75 mg/m²]
Vincristine: I.V.: 0.033 mg/kg/day continuous infusion days 1 to 3
[total dose/cycle = 0.099 mg/kg]
Vincristine: I.V.: 1.5 mg/m² day 9
[total dose/cycle = 1.5 mg/m²]
Course 3, 5, and 7:
Etoposide: I.V.: 200 mg/m²/day days 1 to 3
[total dose/cycle = 600 mg/m²]
Cisplatin: I.V.: 50 mg/m²/day days 1 to 4
[total dose/cycle = 200 mg/m²]

References
Kushner BH, LaQuaglia MP, Bonilla MA, et al, "Highly Effective Induction Therapy for Stage 4 Neuroblastoma in Children Over 1 Year of Age," *J Clin Oncol*, 1994, 12(12):2607-13.

NFL

Use Breast cancer

Regimen NOTE: Multiple variations are listed below.

Variation 1:
Mitoxantrone: I.V.: 12 mg/m² day 1
[total dose/cycle = 12 mg/m²]
Fluorouracil: I.V.: 350 mg/m²/day days 1 to 3
[total dose/cycle = 1050 mg/m²]
Leucovorin: I.V.: 300 mg/m²/day days 1 to 3
[total dose/cycle = 900 mg/m²]
Repeat cycle every 21 days
Variation 2:
Mitoxantrone: I.V.: 10 mg/m² day 1
[total dose/cycle = 10 mg/m²]
Fluorouracil: I.V.: 1000 mg/m²/day continuous infusion days 1 to 3
[total dose/cycle = 3000 mg/m²]
Leucovorin: I.V.: 100 mg/m²/day days 1 to 3
[total dose/cycle = 300 mg/m²]
Repeat cycle every 21 days

References
Variation 1:
Hainsworth JD, Andrews MB, Johnson DH, et al, "Mitoxantrone, Fluorouracil, and High-Dose Leucovorin: An Effective, Well-Tolerated Regimen for Metastatic Breast Cancer," *J Clin Oncol*, 1991, 9(10):1731-5.

(Continued)

NFL *(Continued)*

Variation 2:
Jones SE, Mennel RG, Brooks B, et al, "Phase II Study of Mitoxantrone, Leucovorin, and Infusional Fluorouracil for Treatment of Metastatic Breast Cancer," *J Clin Oncol*, 1991, 9(10):1736-9.

OPA

Use Lymphoma, Hodgkin's disease

Regimen

Vincristine: I.V.: 1.5 mg/m^2/day (maximum 2 mg) days 1, 8, and 15
[total dose/cycle = 4.5 mg/m^2]

Prednisone: Oral: 60 mg/m^2/day days 1 to 15 in 3 divided doses
[total dose/cycle = 900 mg/m^2]

Doxorubicin: I.V.: 40 mg/m^2/day days 1 and 15
[total dose/cycle = 80 mg/m^2]

Second cycle may be given based on individual response; time between cycles not specified

References

Schellong G, Riepenhausen M, Creutzig U, et al, "Low Risk of Secondary Leukemias After Chemotherapy Without Mechlorethamine in Childhood Hodgkin's Disease. German-Austrian Pediatric Hodgkin's Disease Group," *J Clin Oncol*, 1997, 15(6):2247-53.

OPEC

Use Neuroblastomas

Regimen

Vincristine: I.V.: 1.5 mg/m^2 day 1
[total dose/cycle = 1.5 mg/m^2]

Cyclophosphamide: I.V.: 600 mg/m^2 day 1
[total dose/cycle = 600 mg/m^2]

Cisplatin: I.V.: 100 mg/m^2 day 2
[total dose/cycle = 100 mg/m^2]

Teniposide: I.V.: 150 mg/m^2 day 4
[total dose/cycle = 150 mg/m^2]

Repeat cycle every 21 days

References

Shafford EA, Rogers DW, Pritchard J, et al, "Advanced Neuroblastoma: Improved Response Rate Using a Multiagent Regimen (OPEC) Including Sequential Cisplatin and VM-26," *J Clin Oncol*, 1984, 2(7):742-7.

OPEC-D

Use Neuroblastomas

Regimen

Vincristine: I.V.: 1.5 mg/m^2 day 1
[total dose/cycle = 1.5 mg/m^2]

Cyclophosphamide: I.V.: 600 mg/m^2 day 1
[total dose/cycle = 600 mg/m^2]

Doxorubicin: I.V.: 40 mg/m^2 day 1
[total dose/cycle = 40 mg/m^2]

Cisplatin: I.V.: 100 mg/m^2 day 2
[total dose/cycle = 100 mg/m^2]

Teniposide: I.V.: 150 mg/m^2 day 4
[total dose/cycle = 150 mg/m^2]

Repeat cycle every 21 days

References

Shafford EA, Rogers DW, Pritchard J, et al, "Advanced Neuroblastoma: Improved Response Rate Using a Multiagent Regimen (OPEC) Including Sequential Cisplatin and VM-26," *J Clin Oncol*, 1984, 2(7):742-7.

OPPA

Use Lymphoma, Hodgkin's disease

Regimen

Vincristine: I.V.: 1.5 mg/m^2/day (maximum 2 mg) days 1, 8, and 15
[total dose/cycle = 4.5 mg/m^2]
Prednisone: Oral: 60 mg/m^2/day days 1 to 15 in 3 divided doses
[total dose/cycle = 900 mg/m^2]
Doxorubicin: I.V.: 40 mg/m^2/day days 1 and 15
[total dose/cycle = 80 mg/m^2]
Procarbazine: Oral: 100 mg/m^2/day days 1 to 15 in 2 or 3 divided doses
[total dose/cycle = 1500 mg/m^2]
Second cycle may be given based on individual response; time between cycles not specified

References

Schellong G, Riepenhausen M, Creutzig U, et al, "Low Risk of Secondary Leukemias After Chemotherapy Without Mechlorethamine in Childhood Hodgkin's Disease. German-Austrian Pediatric Hodgkin's Disease Group," *J Clin Oncol*, 1997, 15(6):2247-53.

♦ **Oxaliplatin/Capecitabine** *see* XelOx *on page 949*

PAC (CAP)

Use Ovarian cancer

Regimen

Cisplatin: I.V.: 50 mg/m^2 day 1
[total dose/cycle = 50 mg/m^2]
Doxorubicin: I.V.: 50 mg/m^2 day 1
[total dose/cycle = 50 mg/m^2]
Cyclophosphamide: I.V.: 1000 mg/m^2 day 1
[total dose/cycle = 1000 mg/m^2]
Repeat cycle every 21 days for 8 cycles

References

Omura GA, Bundy BN, Berek JS, et al, "Randomized Trial of Cyclophosphamide Plus Cisplatin With or Without Doxorubicin in Ovarian Carcinoma: A Gynecologic Oncology Group Study," *J Clin Oncol*, 1989, 7(4):457-65.

PA-Cl

Use Hepatoblastoma

Regimen NOTE: Multiple variations are listed below.

Variation 1:
Cisplatin: I.V.: 90 mg/m^2 day 1
[total dose/cycle = 90 mg/m^2]
Doxorubicin: I.V.: 20 mg/m^2/day continuous infusion days 2 to 5
[total dose/cycle = 80 mg/m^2]
Repeat cycle every 21 days
Variation 2:
Cisplatin: I.V.: 20 mg/m^2/day days 1 to 4
[total dose/cycle = 80 mg/m^2]
Doxorubicin: I.V.: 100 mg/m^2 continuous infusion day 1
[total dose/cycle = 100 mg/m^2]
Repeat cycle every 21-28 days
(Continued)

PA-CI *(Continued)*

References

Variation 1:

Ortega JA, Douglass EC, Feusner JH, et al, "Randomized Comparison of Cisplatin/ Vincristine/Fluorouracil and Cisplatin/Continuous Infusion Doxorubicin for Treatment of Pediatric Hepatoblastoma: A Report From the Children's Cancer Group and the Pediatric Oncology Group," *J Clin Oncol*, 2000, 18(14):2665-75.

Variation 2:

Ortega JA, Krailo MD, Haas JE, et al, "Effective Treatment of Unresectable or Metastatic Hepatoblastoma With Cisplatin and Continuous Infusion Doxorubicin Chemotherapy: A Report From the Childrens Cancer Study Group," *J Clin Oncol*, 1991, 9(12):2167-76.

♦ **Paclitaxel, Carboplatin** *see* Carbo-Tax (Adenocarcinoma) *on page 851*

Paclitaxel, Carboplatin, Etoposide

Use Adenocarcinoma, unknown primary

Regimen

Paclitaxel: I.V.: 200 mg/m² infused over 1 hour day 1
[total dose/cycle = 200 mg/m²]
followed by
Carboplatin: I.V.: Target AUC 6
[total dose/cycle = AUC = 6]
Etoposide: Oral: 50 mg/day, alternate with 100 mg/day, days 1 to 10
[total dose/cycle = 750 mg/day]
Repeat cycle every 21 days

References

Hainsworth JD, Erland JB, Kalman LA, et al, "Carcinoma of Unknown Primary Site: Treatment With 1-Hour Paclitaxel, Carboplatin, and Extended-Schedule Etoposide," *J Clin Oncol*, 1997, 15(6):2385-93.

♦ **Paclitaxel + Estramustine** *see* PE *on page 928*

Paclitaxel + Estramustine + Carboplatin

Use Prostate cancer

Regimen

Paclitaxel: I.V.: 100 mg/m² day 3 each week
[total dose/cycle = 400 mg/m²]
Estramustine: Oral: 10 mg/kg/day days 1 to 5 each week
[total dose/cycle = 200 mg/kg]
Carboplatin: I.V.: Target AUC 6 day 3
[total dose/cycle = AUC = 6]
Repeat cycle every 28 days

References

Kelly WK, Curley T, Slovin S, et al, "Paclitaxel, Estramustine Phosphate, and Carboplatin in Patients With Advanced Prostate Cancer," *J Clin Oncol*, 2001, 19(1):44-53.

Paclitaxel + Estramustine + Etoposide

Use Prostate cancer

Regimen

Paclitaxel: I.V.: 135 mg/m² day 2
[total dose/cycle = 135 mg/m²]
Estramustine: Oral: 280 mg 3 times/day days 1 to 14
[total dose/cycle = 11,760 mg]
Etoposide: Oral: 100 mg/day days 1 to 14
[total dose/cycle = 1400 mg]
Repeat cycle every 21 days

References
Smith DC, Esper P, Strawderman M, et al, "Phase II Trial of Oral Estramustine, Oral Etoposide, and Intravenous Paclitaxel in Hormone-Refractory Prostate Cancer," *J Clin Oncol*, 1999, 17(6):1664-71.

Paclitaxel-Vinorelbine
Use Breast cancer
Regimen
Paclitaxel: I.V.: 135 mg/m^2 day 1
[total dose/cycle = 135 mg/m^2]
Vinorelbine: I.V.: 30 mg/m^2/day days 1 and 8
[total dose/cycle = 60 mg/m^2]
Repeat cycle every 28 days
References
Romero Acuna LR, Langhi M, Perez J, et al, "Vinorelbine and Paclitaxel as First-Line Chemotherapy in Metastatic Breast Cancer," *J Clin Oncol*, 1999, 17(1):74-81.

PC (Bladder Cancer)
Use Bladder cancer
Regimen
Paclitaxel: I.V.: 200 mg/m^2 or 225 mg/m^2 day 1
[total dose/cycle = 200 or 225 mg/m^2]
Carboplatin: I.V.: AUC 5-6 day 1
[total dose/cycle = AUC = 5-6
Repeat cycle every 21 days
References
Vaughn DJ, Malkowicz SB, Zoltick B, et al, "Paclitaxel Plus Carboplatin in Advanced Carcinoma of the Urothelium: An Active and Tolerable Outpatient Regimen," *J Clin Oncol*, 1998, 16(1):255-60.

PC (Nonsmall Cell Lung Cancer)
Use Lung cancer, nonsmall cell
Regimen NOTE: Multiple variations are listed below.
Variation 1:
Paclitaxel: I.V.: 175-225 mg/m^2 day 1
[total dose/cycle = 175-225 mg/m^2]
Carboplatin: I.V.: Target AUC 5-7 day 1
[total dose/cycle = AUC = 5-7]
Repeat cycle every 21 days for 2-8 cycles
Variation 2:
Paclitaxel: I.V.: 175 mg/m^2 day 1
[total dose/cycle = 175 mg/m^2]
Cisplatin: I.V.: 80 mg/m^2 day 1
[total dose/cycle = 80 mg/m^2]
Repeat cycle every 21 days
Variation 3:
Paclitaxel: I.V.: 135 mg/m^2 continuous infusion day 1
[total dose/cycle = 135 mg/m^2]
Carboplatin: I.V.: AUC 7.5 day 2
[total dose/cycle = AUC = 7.5]
Repeat cycle every 21 days
Variation 4:
Paclitaxel: I.V.: 135 mg/m^2 continuous infusion day 1
[total dose/cycle = 135 mg/m^2]
(Continued)

PC (Nonsmall Cell Lung Cancer) *(Continued)*

Cisplatin: I.V.: 75 mg/m² day 2
[total dose/cycle = 75 mg/m²]
Repeat cycle every 21 days

References

Variation 1:

Hainsworth JD, Urba WJ, Hon JK, et al, "One-Hour Paclitaxel Plus Carboplatin in the Treatment of Advanced Nonsmall-Cell Lung Cancer: Results of a Multicentre, Phase II Trial," *Eur J Cancer*, 1998, 34(5):654-8.

Helsing M, Thaning L, Sederholm C, et al, "Treatment With Paclitaxel 1-h Infusion and Carboplatin of Patients With Advanced Nonsmall-Cell Lung Cancer: A Phase II Multicentre Trial. Joint Lung Cancer Study Group," *Lung Cancer*, 1999, 24(2):107-13.

Kosmidis PA, Mylonakis N, Fountzilas G, et al, "Paclitaxel and Carboplatin in Inoperable Nonsmall-Cell Lung Cancer: A Phase II Study," *Ann Oncol*, 1997, 8(7):697-9.

Laohavinij S, Maoleekoonpairoj S, Cheirsilpa A, et al, "Phase II Study of Paclitaxel and Carboplatin for Advanced Nonsmall-Cell Lung Cancer," *Lung Cancer*, 1999, 26(3):175-85.

Variation 2:

Giaccone G, Splinter TA, Debruyne C, et al, "Randomized Study of Paclitaxel-Cisplatin Versus Cisplatin-Teniposide in Patients With Advanced Nonsmall-Cell Lung Cancer. The European Organization for Research and Treatment of Cancer Lung Cancer Cooperative Group," *J Clin Oncol*, 1998, 16(6):2133-41.

Variation 3:

Langer CJ, Leighton JC, Comis RL, et al, "Paclitaxel by 24- or 1-Hour Infusion in Combination With Carboplatin in Advanced Nonsmall Cell Lung Cancer: The Fox Chase Cancer Center Experience," *Semin Oncol*, 1995, 22(4 Suppl 9):18-29.

Variation 4:

Schiller JH, Harrington D, Belani CP, et al, "Comparison of Four Chemotherapy Regimens for Advanced Nonsmall-Cell Lung Cancer," *N Engl J Med*, 2002, 346(2):92-8.

PCV

Use Brain tumors

Regimen

Lomustine: Oral: 110 mg/m² day 1
[total dose/cycle = 110 mg/m²]
Procarbazine: Oral: 60 mg/m²/day days 8 to 21
[total dose/cycle = 840 mg/m²]
Vincristine: I.V.: 1.4 mg/m²/day (maximum 2 mg) days 8 and 29
[total dose/cycle = 2.8 mg/m²]
Repeat cycle every 6-8 weeks

References

Levin VA, Silver P, Hannigan J, et al, "Superiority of Post-Radiotherapy Adjuvant Chemotherapy With CCNU, Procarbazine, and Vincristine (PCV) Over BCNU for Anaplastic Gliomas: NCOG 6G61 Final Report," *Int J Radiat Oncol Biol Phys*, 1990, 18(2):321-4.

PE

Synonyms Paclitaxel + Estramustine

Use Prostate cancer

Regimen NOTE: Multiple variations are listed below.

Variation 1:

Paclitaxel: I.V.: 30-35 mg/m²/day continuous infusion days 2 to 5 (given in 2-3 divided doses daily)
[total dose/cycle = 120-140 mg/m²]
Estramustine: Oral: 600 mg/m²/day days 1 to 21
[total dose/cycle = 12,600 mg/m²]
Repeat cycle every 21 days

Variation 2:

Paclitaxel: I.V. 60-107 mg/m² infused over 3 hours weekly
[total dose/cycle = 180-321 mg/m²]

Estramustine: Oral: 280 mg twice daily 3 days/week
  [total dose/cycle = 5040 mg]
Variation 3:
  Paclitaxel: I.V. 150 mg/m^2 weekly
    [total dose/cycle = 450 mg/m^2]
  Estramustine: Oral: 280 mg 3 times/day 3 days/week
    [total dose/week = 7560 mg/m^2]
Variation 4:
  Paclitaxel: I.V.: 100 mg/m^2/day days 1, 8, and 15
    [total dose/cycle = 300 mg/m^2]
  Estramustine: Oral: 280 mg 3 times/day days 1, 2, and 3 every week
    [total dose/cycle = 10,080 mg]
  Repeat cycle every 4 weeks

References

Variation 1:
  Hudes GR, Nathan FE, Khater C, et al, "Paclitaxel Plus Estramustine in Metastatic Hormone-Refractory Prostate Cancer," *Semin Oncol*, 1995, 22(5 Suppl 12):41-5.
  Hudes GR, Nathan F, Khater C, et al, "Phase II Trial of 96-Hour Paclitaxel Plus Oral Estramustine Phosphate in Metastatic Hormone-Refractory Prostate Cancer," *J Clin Oncol*, 1997, 15(9):3156-63.
Variation 2: Haas N, Roth B, Garay C, et al, "Phase I Trial of Weekly Paclitaxel Plus Oral Estramustine Phosphate in Patients With Hormone-Refractory Prostate Cancer," *Urology*, 2001, 58(1):59-64
Variation 3: Vaishampayan U, Fontana J, Du W, et al, "An Active Regimen of Weekly Paclitaxel and Estramustine in Metastatic Androgen-Independent Prostate Cancer," *Urology*, 2002, 60(6):1050-4.
Variation 4: Berry W, Gregurich M, Dakhil S, et al, "Phase II Randomized Trial of Weekly Paclitaxel With or Without Estramustine Phosphate in Patients With Symptomatic, Hormone-Refractory Metastatic Carcinoma of the Prostate." *Proc Am Soc Clin Oncol*, 2001, 20:175a.

PE-CAdO

Use Neuroblastomas

Regimen

Cisplatin: I.V.: 100 mg/m^2 day 1
  [total dose/cycle = 100 mg/m^2]
Teniposide: I.V.: 160 mg/m^2 day 3
  [total dose/cycle = 160 mg/m^2]

alternating with

Cyclophosphamide: I.V.: 300 mg/m^2/day days 1 to 5
  [total dose/cycle = 1500 mg/m^2]
Doxorubicin: I.V.: 60 mg/m^2 day 5
  [total dose/cycle = 60 mg/m^2]
Vincristine: I.V.: 1.5 mg/m^2/day days 1 and 5
  [total dose/cycle = 3 mg/m^2]
Repeat cycle every 21 days

References

Bernard JL, Philip T, Zucker JM, et al, "Sequential Cisplatin/VM-26 and Vincristine/Cyclophosphamide/Doxorubicin in Metastatic Neuroblastoma: An Effective Alternating Non-Cross-Resistant Regimen?" *J Clin Oncol*, 1987, 5(12):1952-9.

PFL (Colorectal Cancer)

Use Colorectal cancer

Regimen

Cisplatin: I.V.: 25 mg/m^2/day continuous infusion days 1 to 5
  [total dose/cycle = 125 mg/m^2]
(Continued)

PFL (Colorectal Cancer) *(Continued)*

Fluorouracil: I.V.: 800 mg/m^2/day continuous infusion days 2 to 5
  [total dose/cycle = 3200 mg/m^2]
Leucovorin calcium: I.V.: 500 mg/m^2/day continuous infusion days 1 to 5
  [total dose/cycle = 2500 mg/m^2]
Repeat cycle every 28 days

References

Dreyfuss AI, Clark JR, Wright JE, et al, "Continuous Infusion High-Dose Leucovorin With 5-Fluorouracil and Cisplatin for Untreated Stage IV Carcinoma of the Head and Neck," *Ann Intern Med*, 1990, 112(3):167-72.

PFL (Head and Neck Cancer)

Use Head and neck cancer

Regimen NOTE: Multiple variations are listed below.

Variation 1:
  Cisplatin: I.V.: 25 mg/m^2/day continuous infusion days 1 to 5
    [total dose/cycle = 125 mg/m^2]
  Fluorouracil: I.V.: 800 mg/m^2/day continuous infusion days 2 to 6
    [total dose/cycle = 4000 mg/m^2]
  Leucovorin: I.V.: 500 mg/m^2/day continuous infusion days 1 to 6
    [total dose/cycle = 3000 mg/m^2]
  Repeat cycle every 28 days

Variation 2:
  Cisplatin: I.V.: 100 mg/m^2 day 1
    [total dose/cycle = 100 mg/m^2]
  Fluorouracil: I.V.: 600-1000 mg/m^2/day continuous infusion days 1 to 5
    [total dose/cycle = 3000-5000 mg/m^2]
  Leucovorin: Oral: 50 mg/m^2 every 4-6 hours days 1 to 6
    [total dose/cycle = 1200-1800 mg/m^2]
  Repeat cycle every 21 days

References

Variation 1:
  Dreyfuss AI, Clark JR, Wright JE, et al, "Continuous Infusion High-Dose Leucovorin With 5-Fluorouracil and Cisplatin for Untreated State IV Carcinoma of the Head and Neck," *Ann Intern Med*, 1990, 112(3):167-72.
Variation 2:
  Vokes EE, Schilsky RL, Weichselbaum RR, et al, "Cisplatin, 5-Fluorouracil, and High-Dose Oral Leucovorin for Advanced Head and Neck Cancer," *Cancer*, 1989, 63(6 Suppl):1048-53.

PFL + IFN

Use Head and neck cancer

Regimen

Cisplatin: I.V.: 100 mg/m^2 day 1
  [total dose/cycle = 100 mg/m^2]
Fluorouracil: I.V.: 640 mg/m^2/day continuous infusion days 1 to 5
  [total dose/cycle = 3200 mg/m^2]
Leucovorin calcium: Oral: 100 mg every 4 hours days 1 to 5
  [total dose/cycle = 3000 mg/m^2]
Interferon alfa-2b: SubQ: 2 x 10^6 units/m^2 days 1 to 6
  [total dose/cycle = 12 x 10^6 units/m^2]

References

Brockstein BE, Weichselbaum RW, and Vokes EE, "Concomitant and Rapidly Alternating Chemoradiotherapy for Head and Neck Cancer," *Advances in Oncology*, 1998, 14:8-15.

Kies MS, Haraf DJ, Athanasiadis I, et al, "Induction Chemotherapy Followed by Concurrent Chemoradiation for Advanced Head and Neck Cancer: Improved Disease Control And Survival," *J Clin Oncol*, 1998, 16(8):2715-21.

POC

Use Brain tumors

Regimen

Prednisone: Oral: 40 mg/m^2/day days 1 to 14
  [total dose/cycle = 560 mg/m^2]
Vincristine: I.V.: 1.5 mg/m^2/day (maximum 2 mg) days 1, 8, and 15
  [total dose/cycle = 4.5 mg/m^2]
Lomustine: Oral: 100 mg/m^2 day 1
  [total dose/cycle = 100 mg/m^2]
Repeat cycle every 6 weeks

References

Finlay JL, Boyett JM, Yates AJ, et al, "Randomized Phase III Trial in Childhood High-Grade Astrocytoma Comparing Vincristine, Lomustine, and Prednisone With the Eight-Drugs-In-1-Day Regimen. Childrens Cancer Group," *J Clin Oncol*, 1995, 13(1):112-23.

POMP

Related Information

Hyper-CVAD *on page 898*

Use Leukemia, acute lymphocytic

Regimen Maintenance:

Mercaptopurine: Oral: 50 mg 3 times a day
  [total dose/cycle = 4.5 g]
Methotrexate: Oral: 20 mg/m^2 once weekly
  [total dose/cycle = 80 mg/m^2]
Vincristine: I.V.: 2 mg day 1
  [total dose/cycle = 2 mg]
Prednisone: Oral: 200 mg/day days 1 to 5
  [total dose/cycle = 1000 mg]
Repeat cycle monthly for 2 years

References

Kantarjian HM, O'Brien S, Smith TL, et al, "Results of Treatment With Hyper-CVAD, a Dose-Intensive Regimen, in Adult Acute Lymphocytic Leukemia," *J Clin Oncol*, 2000, 18(3):547-61.

Pro-MACE-CytaBOM

Use Lymphoma, non-Hodgkin's

Regimen

Prednisone: Oral: 60 mg/m^2/day days 1 to 14
  [total dose/cycle = 840 mg/m^2]
Doxorubicin: I.V.: 25 mg/m^2 day 1
  [total dose/cycle = 25 mg/m^2]
Cyclophosphamide: I.V.: 650 mg/m^2 day 1
  [total dose/cycle = 650 mg/m^2]
Etoposide: I.V.: 120 mg/m^2 day 1
  [total dose/cycle = 120 mg/m^2]
Cytarabine: I.V.: 300 mg/m^2 day 8
  [total dose/cycle = 300 mg/m^2]
Bleomycin: I.V.: 5 units/m^2 day 8
  [total dose/cycle = 5 units/m^2]
Vincristine: I.V.: 1.4 mg/m^2 (maximum 2 mg) day 8
  [total dose/cycle = 1.4 mg/m^2]
(Continued)

Pro-MACE-CytaBOM *(Continued)*

Methotrexate: I.V.: 120 mg/m² day 8
[total dose/cycle = 120 mg/m²]

Leucovorin: Oral: 25 mg/m² every 6 hours (start 24 hours after methotrexate) for 4 doses day 9
[total dose/cycle = 100 mg/m²]

Repeat cycle every 21 days

References

Longo DL, DeVita VT Jr, Duffey PL, et al, "Superiority of ProMACE-CytaBOM Over ProMACE-MOPP in the Treatment of Advanced Diffuse Aggressive Lymphoma: Results of a Prospective Randomized Trial," *J Clin Oncol*, 1991, 9(1):25-38.

PV

Use Breast cancer

Regimen NOTE: Multiple variations are listed below.

Variation 1:

Paclitaxel: I.V.: 135 mg/m² day 1
[total dose/cycle = 135 mg/m²]

Vinorelbine: I.V.: 30 mg/m² day 1
[total dose/cycle = 30 mg/m²]

Repeat cycle every 21 days

Variation 2:

Paclitaxel: I.V.: 150 mg/m² day 1
[total dose/cycle = 150 mg/m²]

Vinorelbine: I.V.: 25 mg/m² day 1
[total dose/cycle = 25 mg/m²]

Repeat cycle every 21 days

References

Variation 1:
Martin M, Lluch A, Casado A, et al, "Paclitaxel Plus Vinorelbine: An Active Regimen in Metastatic Breast Cancer Patients With Prior Anthracycline Exposure," *Ann Oncol*, 2000, 11(1):85-9.
Variation 2:
Vici P, Amodio A, Di Lauro L, et al, "First-Line Chemotherapy With Vinorelbine and Paclitaxel As Simultaneous Infusion in Advanced Breast Cancer," *Oncology*, 2000, 58(1):3-7.

PVA (POG 8602)

Synonyms AlinC 14

Use Leukemia, acute lymphocytic

Regimen

Induction:

Prednisone: Oral: 40 mg/m²/day (maximum 60 mg) days 0 to 28 (given in 3 divided doses)
[total dose/cycle = 1160 mg/m²]

Vincristine: I.V.: 1.5 mg/m²/day (maximum 2 mg) days 0, 7, 14, and 21
[total dose/cycle = 6 mg/m²]

Asparaginase: I.M.: 6000 units/m² 3 times per week for 2 weeks
[total dose/cycle = 36,000/units/m²]

Intrathecal therapy: Days 0 and 22

Administer one cycle only

CNS consolidation:

Mercaptopurine: Oral: 75 mg/m²/day days 29 to 42
[total dose/cycle = 1050 mg/m²]

Intrathecal therapy: Days 29 and 36

Administer one cycle only

Intensification:

Regimen A:

Methotrexate: I.V.: 1000 mg/m^2 continuous infusion day 1

[total dose/cycle = 1000 mg/m^2]

Cytarabine: I.V.: 1000 mg/m^2 continuous infusion day 1 (start 12 hours after methotrexate)

[total dose/cycle = 1000 mg/m^2]

Leucovorin: I.M., I.V., or Oral: 30 mg/m^2 24 and 36 hours after the **start** of methotrexate

[total dose/cycle = 60 mg/m^2]

followed by 3 mg/m^2 48, 60, and 72 hours after the **start** of methotrexate

[total dose/cycle = 9 mg/m^2]

Intrathecal therapy: Weeks 9, 12, 15, and 18

Repeat cycle every 3 weeks for 6 cycles

or

Regimen B:

Methotrexate: I.V.: 1000 mg/m^2 continuous infusion day 1

[total dose/cycle = 1000 mg/m^2]

Cytarabine: I.V.: 1000 mg/m^2 continuous infusion day 1 (start 12 hours after methotrexate)

[total dose/cycle = 1000 mg/m^2]

Leucovorin: I.M., I.V., or Oral: 30 mg/m^2 24 and 36 hours after the **start** of methotrexate

[total dose/cycle = 60 mg/m^2]

followed by 3 mg/m^2 48, 60, and 72 hours after the **start** of methotrexate

[total dose/cycle = 9 mg/m^2]

Intrathecal therapy: Weeks 9, 12, 15, and 18

Repeat cycle every 12 weeks for 6 cycles

Maintenance:

Regimen A:

Methotrexate: I.M.: 20 mg/m^2 weekly

[total dose/cycle = 2640 mg/m^2]

Mercaptopurine: Oral: 75 mg/m^2 daily

[total dose/cycle = 69,300 mg/m^2]

Intrathecal therapy: Day 1 every 8 weeks for 10 doses

Weeks 25-156

Prednisone: Oral: 40 mg/m^2/day (maximum 60 mg) days 1 to 7 (given in 3 divided doses)

[total dose/cycle = 2240 mg/m^2]

Vincristine: I.V.: 1.5 mg/m^2/day (maximum 2 mg) days 1 and 8

[total dose/cycle = 24 mg/m^2]

Weeks 8, 17, 25, 41, 57, 73, 89, and 105

or

Regimen B:

Methotrexate: I.M.: 20 mg/m^2 weekly for 7 weeks

[total dose/cycle = 140 mg/m^2]

Mercaptopurine: Oral: 75 mg/m^2 daily for 7 weeks

[total dose/cycle = 3675 mg/m^2]

Repeat cycle every 12 weeks for 4 cycles (begins weeks 22, 34, 46, 58, and 70)

followed by

(Continued)

PVA (POG 8602) *(Continued)*

Methotrexate: I.M.: 20 mg/m^2 weekly
[total dose/cycle = 1720 mg/m^2]
Mercaptopurine: Oral: 75 mg/m^2 daily
[total dose/cycle = 45,150 mg/m^2]
Weeks 70-156
Intrathecal therapy: Day 1 every 8 weeks for 10 doses
Weeks 25-156
Prednisone: Oral: 40 mg/m^2/day (maximum 60 mg) days 1 to 7 (given in 3 divided doses)
[total dose/cycle = 2240 mg/m^2]
Vincristine: I.V.: 1.5 mg/m^2/day (maximum 2 mg) days 1 and 8
[total dose/cycle = 24 mg/m^2]
Weeks 8, 17, 25, 41, 57, 73, 89, and 105

References

Land VJ, Shuster JJ, Crist WM, et al, "Comparison of Two Schedules of Intermediate-Dose Methotrexate and Cytarabine Consolidation Therapy for Childhood B-Precursor Cell Acute Lymphoblastic Leukemia: A Pediatric Oncology Group Study," *J Clin Oncol*, 1994, 12(9):1939-45.

PVA (POG 9005)

Use Leukemia, acute lymphocytic

Regimen

Induction:
Prednisone: Oral: 40 mg/m^2/day (maximum 60 mg) days 1 to 28 (given in 3 divided doses)
[total dose/cycle = 1120 mg/m^2]
Vincristine: I.V.: 1.5 mg/m^2/day (maximum 2 mg) days 1, 8, 15, and 22
[total dose/cycle = 6 mg/m^2]
Asparaginase: I.M.: 6000 units/m^2/day days 2, 5, 8, 12, 15, and 19
[total dose/cycle = 36,000 units/m^2]
Intrathecal therapy: Day 1
Administer one cycle only

Intensification:

Regimen A:
Methotrexate: I.V.: 1000 mg/m^2 continuous infusion day 1
[total dose/cycle = 1000 mg/m^2]
Mercaptopurine: I.V.: 1000 mg/m^2 day 2
[total dose/cycle = 1000 mg/m^2]
Leucovorin: I.M., I.V., or Oral: 5 mg/m^2 every 6 hours for 5 doses day 3 (start 48 hours after the **start** of methotrexate)
[total dose/cycle = 25 mg/m^2]
Repeat cycle every 2 weeks for 12 cycles

or

Regimen B:
Methotrexate: Oral: 30 mg/m^2 every 6 hours for 6 doses day 1
[total dose/cycle = 180 mg/m^2]
Mercaptopurine: I.V.: 1000 mg/m^2 day 2 (start after last methotrexate dose)
[total dose/cycle = 1000 mg/m^2]
Leucovorin: I.M., I.V., or Oral: 5 mg/m^2 every 6 hours for 5 doses day 3 (start 48 hours after the **start** of methotrexate)
[total dose/cycle = 25 mg/m^2]
Repeat cycle every 2 weeks for 12 cycles

Maintenance:
Methotrexate: I.M.: 20 mg/m^2 weekly
[total dose/cycle = 2120 mg/m^2]
Mercaptopurine: Oral: 50 mg/m^2 daily
[total dose/cycle = 37,100 mg/m^2]
Intrathecal therapy: Day 1 every 12 weeks
Weeks 25-130

References

Mahoney DH Jr, Shuster J, Nitschke R, et al, "Intermediate-Dose Intravenous Methotrexate With Intravenous Mercaptopurine is Superior to Repetitive Low-Dose Oral Methotrexate With Intravenous Mercaptopurine for Children With Lower-Risk B-Lineage Acute Lymphoblastic Leukemia: A Pediatric Oncology Group Phase III Trial," *J Clin Oncol*, 1998, 16(1):246-54.

PVB

Use Testicular cancer

Regimen NOTE: Multiple variations are listed below.
Variation 1:
Cisplatin: I.V.: 20 mg/m^2/day days 1 to 5
[total dose/cycle = 100 mg/m^2]
Vinblastine: I.V.: 0.2 mg/kg/day days 1 and 2
[total dose/cycle = 0.4 mg/kg]
Bleomycin: I.V.: 30 units/day days 2, 9, and 16
[total dose/cycle = 90 units]
Repeat cycle every 3 weeks
Variation 2:
Cisplatin: I.V.: 20 mg/m^2/day days 1 to 5
[total dose/cycle = 100 mg/m^2]
Vinblastine: I.V.: 0.15 mg/kg/day days 1 and 2
[total dose/cycle = 0.3 mg/kg]
Bleomycin: I.V.: 30 units/day days 2, 9, and 16
[total dose/cycle = 90 units]
Repeat cycle every 3 weeks
Variation 3:
Cisplatin: I.V.: 20 mg/m^2/day days 1 to 5
[total dose/cycle = 100 mg/m^2]
Vinblastine: I.V.: 6 mg/m^2/day days 1 and 2
[total dose/cycle = 12 mg/m^2]
Bleomycin: I.M.: 30 units/day days 2, 9, and 16
[total dose/cycle = 90 units]
Repeat cycle every 3 weeks

References

Variation 1:
Einhorn LH and Donohue J, "Cis-Diamminedichloroplatinum, Vinblastine, and Bleomycin Combination Chemotherapy in Disseminated Testicular Cancer," *Ann Intern Med*, 1977, 87(3):293-8.
Variation 2:
Williams SD, Birch R, Einhorn LH, et al, "Treatment of Disseminated Germ-Cell Tumors With Cisplatin, Bleomycin, and Either Vinblastine or Etoposide," *N Engl J Med*, 1987, 316(23):1435-40.
Variation 3:
Bodrogi I, Baki M, Horti J, et al, "Vinblastine, Cisplatin and Bleomycin Treatment of Advanced Nonseminomatous Testicular Tumors," *Neoplasma*, 1990, 37(4):445-50.

♦ **PVB** *see* VBP *on page 945*

PVDA

Use Leukemia, acute lymphocytic

Regimen

Prednisone: Oral: 60 mg/m^2/day days 1 to 28
[total dose/cycle = 1680 mg/m^2]

Vincristine: I.V.: 1.5 mg/m^2/day days 1, 8, 15, and 22
[total dose/cycle = 6 mg/m^2]

Daunorubicin: I.V.: 25 mg/m^2/day days 1, 8, 15, and 22
[total dose/cycle = 100 mg/m^2]

Asparaginase: I.M., SubQ, or I.V.: 5000 units/m^2/day days 1 to 14
[total dose/cycle = 70,000 units/m^2]

Administer one cycle only; used in conjunction with intrathecal chemotherapy

References

Hoelzer D, Thiel E, Loffler H, et al, "Intensified Therapy in Acute Lymphoblastic and Acute Undifferentiated Leukemia in Adults," *Blood*, 1984, 64(1):38-47.

R-CHOP

Synonyms CHOP-Rituximab

Use Lymphoma, non-Hodgkin's

Regimen

Rituximab: I.V.: 375 mg/m^2 day 1
[total dose/cycle = 375 mg/m^2]

Cyclophosphamide: I.V.: 750 mg/m^2 day 3
[total dose/cycle = 750 mg/m^2]

Doxorubicin: I.V.: 50 mg/m^2 day 3
[total dose/cycle = 50 mg/m^2]

Vincristine: I.V.: 1.4 mg/m^2 (maximum 2 mg) day 3
[total dose/cycle = 1.4 mg/m^2]

Prednisone: Oral: 40 mg/m^2/day days 1 to 5
[total dose/cycle = 200 mg/m^2]

Repeat cycle every 21 days

References

Coiffier B, Lepage E, Briere J, et al, "CHOP Chemotherapy Plus Rituximab Compared With CHOP Alone in Elderly Patients With Diffuse Large-B-Cell Lymphoma," *N Engl J Med*, 2002, 346(4):235-42.

R-CVP

Use Lymphoma, non-Hodgkin's

Regimen

Rituximab: I.V.: 375 mg/m^2 day 1
[total dose/cycle = 375 mg/m^2]

Cyclophosphamide: I.V.: 750 mg/m^2 day 1
[total dose/cycle = 750 mg/m^2]

Vincristine: I.V.: 1.4 mg/m^2 day 1
[total dose/cycle = 1.4 mg/m^2]

Prednisolone: Oral: 40 mg/m^2/day days 1 to 5
[total dose/cycle = 200 mg/m^2]

Repeat cycle every 21 days

References

Marcus R, Imrie K, Belch A, et al, "An International Multi-Centre, Randomized, Open-Label, Phase III Trial Comparing Rituximab Added to CVP Chemotherapy to CVP Chemotherapy Alone in Untreated State III/IV Follicular Non-Hodgkin's Lymphoma," *Proc Am Soc Hematol*, 2003, abstract 2003.

Regimen A1
Use Neuroblastomas
Regimen
Cyclophosphamide: I.V.: 1.2 g/m^2 day 1
[total dose/cycle = 1.2 g/m^2]
Vincristine: I.V.: 1.5 mg/m^2 day 1
[total dose/cycle = 1.5 mg/m^2]
Doxorubicin: I.V.: 40 mg/m^2 day 3
[total dose/cycle = 40 mg/m^2]
Cisplatin: I.V.: 90 mg/m^2 day 5
[total dose/cycle = 90 mg/m^2]
Repeat cycle every 28 days
References
Kaneko M, Nishihira H, Mugishima H, et al, "Stratification of Treatment of Stage 4 Neuro-blastoma Patients Based on N-myc Amplification Status. Study Group of Japan for Treatment of Advanced Neuroblastoma, Tokyo, Japan." *Med Pediatr Oncol*, 1998, 31(1):1-7.

Regimen A2
Use Neuroblastomas
Regimen
Cyclophosphamide: I.V.: 1.2 g/m^2 day 1
[total dose/cycle = 1.2 g/m^2]
Etoposide: I.V.: 100 mg/m^2/day days 1 to 5
[total dose/cycle = 500 mg/m^2]
Doxorubicin: I.V.: 40 mg/m^2 day 3
[total dose/cycle = 40 mg/m^2]
Cisplatin: I.V.: 90 mg/m^2 day 5
[total dose/cycle = 90 mg/m^2]
Repeat cycle every 28 days
References
Kaneko M, Nishihira H, Mugishima H, et al, "Stratification of Treatment of Stage 4 Neuro-blastoma Patients Based on N-myc Amplification Status. Study Group of Japan for Treatment of Advanced Neuroblastoma, Tokyo, Japan." *Med Pediatr Oncol*, 1998, 31(1):1-7.

♦ **Saltz Regimen** *see* FU/LV/CPT-11 (Saltz Regimen) *on page 894*

Sequential Dox-CMF
Use Breast cancer
Regimen
Doxorubicin: I.V.: 75 mg/m^2 every 21 days for 4 cycles followed by 21- or 28-day CMF for 8 cycles
References
Bonadonna G, Zambetti M, and Valagussa P, "Sequential or Alternating Doxorubicin and CMF Regimens in Breast Cancer With More Than Three Positive Nodes. Ten-Year Results," *JAMA*, 1995, 273(7):542-7.

Stanford V
Use Lymphoma, Hodgkin's disease
Regimen
Mechlorethamine: I.V.: 6 mg/m^2 day 1
[total dose/cycle = 6 mg/m^2]
Doxorubicin: I.V.: 25 mg/m^2/day days 1 and 15
[total dose/cycle = 50 mg/m^2]
(Continued)

Stanford V *(Continued)*

Vinblastine: I.V.: 6 mg/m^2/day days 1 and 15
[total dose/cycle = 12 mg/m^2]

Vincristine: I.V.: 1.4 mg/m^2/day (maximum 2 mg) days 8 and 22
[total dose/cycle = 2.8 mg/m^2]

Bleomycin: I.V.: 5 units/m^2/day days 8 and 22
[total dose/cycle = 10 units/m^2]

Etoposide: I.V.: 60 mg/m^2/day days 15 and 16
[total dose/cycle = 120 mg/m^2]

Prednisone: Oral: 40 mg/m^2 every other day for 10 weeks
[total dose/cycle = 1400 mg/m^2]
followed by tapering of dose by 10 mg every other day for next 14 days

Repeat cycle every 28 days

References

Bartlett NL, Rosenberg SA, Hoppe RT, et al, "Brief Chemotherapy, Stanford V, and Adjuvant Radiotherapy for Bulky or Advanced-Stage Hodgkin's Disease: A Preliminary Report," *J Clin Oncol*, 1995, 13(5):1080-8.

TAC

Use Breast cancer

Regimen

Docetaxel: I.V.: 75 mg/m^2 day 1
[total dose/cycle = 75 mg/m^2]

Doxorubicin: I.V.: 50 mg/m^2 day 1
[total dose/cycle = 50 mg/m^2]

Cyclophosphamide: I.V.: 500 mg/m^2 day 1
[total dose/cycle = 500 mg/m^2]

Repeat cycle every 3 weeks

References

Nabholtz JM, Smylie M, Mackey JR, et al, "Docetaxel/Doxorubicin/Cyclophosphamide in the Treatment of Metastatic Breast Cancer," *Oncology (Huntingt)*, 1997, 11(8 Suppl 8):37-41.

TAD

Use Leukemia, acute myeloid

Regimen

Daunorubicin: I.V.: 60 mg/m^2/day days 3 to 5
[total dose/cycle = 180 mg/m^2]

Cytarabine: I.V.: 100 mg/m^2/day continuous infusion days 1 and 2
[total dose/cycle = 200 mg/m^2]
followed by 100 mg/m^2/day every 12 hours days 3 to 8
[total dose/cycle = 1200 mg/m^2]

Thioguanine: Oral: 100 mg/m^2/day every 12 hours days 3 to 9
[total dose/cycle = 1400 mg/m^2]

Administer one cycle only

References

Buchner T, Hiddemann W, Wormann B, et al, "Double Inductions Strategy for Acute Myeloid Leukemia: The Effect of High-Dose Cytarabine With Mitoxantrone Instead of Standard-Dose Cytarabine With Daunorubicin and 6-Thioguanine: A Randomized Trial by the German AML Cooperative Group," *Blood*, 1999, 93(12):4116-24.

Tamoxifen-Epirubicin

Use Breast cancer

Regimen

Tamoxifen: Oral: 20 mg daily

[total dose/cycle = 560 mg]

Epirubicin: I.V.: 50 mg/m²/day days 1 and 8

[total dose/cycle = 100 mg/m²]

Repeat epirubicin cycle every 28 days for 6 cycles; continue tamoxifen for 4 years

References

Wils JA, Bliss JM, Marty M, et al, "Epirubicin Plus Tamoxifen Versus Tamoxifen Alone in Node-Positive Postmenopausal Patients With Breast Cancer: A Randomized Trial of the International Collaborative Cancer Group." *J Clin Oncol*, 1999, 17(7):1988-98.

TCF

Use Esophageal cancer

Regimen

Paclitaxel: I.V.: 175 mg/m² day 1

[total dose/cycle = 175 mg/m²]

Cisplatin: I.V.: 20 mg/m²/day days 1 to 5

[total dose/cycle = 100 mg/m²]

Fluorouracil: I.V.: 750 mg/m²/day continuous infusion days 1 to 5

[total dose/cycle = 3750 mg/m²]

Repeat cycle every 28 days

References

Ajani JA, Ilson D, Bhalla K, et al, "Taxol, Cisplatin, and 5-FU (TCF): A Multi-institutional Phase II Study in Patients With Carcinoma of the Esophagus," *Proc AM Soc Clin Oncol*, 1995, 14:203.

Thalidomide + Dexamethasone

Use Multiple myeloma

Regimen NOTE: Multiple variation are listed below.

Variation 1:

Thalidomide: Oral: 100 mg/day days 1 to 28

[total dose/cycle = 2800 mg]

Dexamethasone: Oral: 40 mg/day days 1 to 4

[total dose/cycle = 160 mg]

Repeat cycle every 28 days

Variation 2:

Thalidomide: Oral: 200 mg/day days 1 to 14 cycle 1

followed by 400 mg/day days 15 to 28 cycle 1

[total dose/cycle = 8400 mg]

Thalidomide: Oral: 400 mg/day days 1 to 28 (subsequent cycles)

[total dose/cycle = 11,200 mg]

Dexamethasone: Oral: 20 mg/m²/day days 1 to 4, 9 to 12, and 17 to 20 cycle 1

[total dose/cycle = 240 mg/m²]

Dexamethasone: Oral: 20 mg/m²/day days 1 to 4 (subsequent cycles)

[total dose/cycle = 80 mg/m²]

Repeat cycle every 28 days

Variation 3:

Thalidomide: Oral: 100 mg/day days 1 to 7, 150 mg/day days 8 to 14, 200 mg/day days 15 to 21, 250 mg/day days 22 to 28, and 300 mg/day days 29 to 35 (cycle 1)

[total dose/cycle = 7000 mg]

(Continued)

Thalidomide + Dexamethasone *(Continued)*

Thalidomide: Oral: 300 mg/day days 1 to 35 (subsequent cycles)
[total dose/cycle = 10,500 mg]
Dexamethasone: Oral: 20 mg/m²/day days 1 to 4, 9 to 12, and 17 to 20
[total dose/cycle = 240 mg/m²]
Repeat cycle every 35 days
Variation 4:
Thalidomide: Oral: 200 mg/day days 1 to 28
[total dose/cycle = 5600 mg]
Dexamethasone: Oral: 40 mg/day days 1 to 4, 9 to 12, and 17 to 20
(odd cycles)
[total dose/cycle = 480 mg]
Dexamethasone: Oral: 40 mg/day days 1 to 4 (even cycles)
[total dose/cycle = 160 mg]

References
Variation 1:
Palumbo A, Giaccone L, Bertola A, et al, "Low-Dose Thalidomide Plus Dexamethasone is an Effective Salvage Therapy for Advanced Myeloma," *Haematologica*, 2001, 86(4):399-403.
Variation 2:
Dimopoulos MA, Zervas K, Kouvatseas G, et al, "Thalidomide and Dexamethasone Combination for Refractory Multiple Myeloma," *Ann Oncol*, 2001, 12(7):991-5.
Variation 3:
Alexanian R, Weber D, Giralt S, et al, "Consolidation Therapy of Multiple Myeloma With Tthalidomide-Dexamethasone After Intensive Chemotherapy," *Ann Oncol*, 2002, 13(7):1116-9.
Variation 4:
Rajkumar SV, Hayman S, Gertz MA, et al, "Combination Therapy With Thalidomide Plus Dexamethasone for Newly Diagnosed Myeloma," *J Clin Oncol*, 2002, 20(21):4319-23.

TIP

Use Esophageal cancer; Head and neck cancer
Regimen
Paclitaxel: I.V.: 175 mg/m² day 1
[total dose/cycle = 175 mg/m²]
Ifosfamide: I.V.: 1000 mg/m²/day days 1 to 3
[total dose/cycle = 3000 mg/m²]
Mesna: I.V.: 400 mg/m²/day before ifosfamide days 1 to 3
[total dose/cycle = 1200 mg/m²]
followed by 200 mg/m² 4 hours after ifosfamide days 1 to 3
[total dose/cycle = 600 mg/m²]
Cisplatin: I.V.: 60 mg/m² day 1
[total dose/cycle = 60 mg/m²]
Repeat cycle every 21-28 days

References
Shin DM, Glisson BS, Khuri FR, et al, "Phase II Trial of Paclitaxel, Ifosfamide, and Cisplatin in Patients With Recurrent Head and Neck Squamous Cell Carcinoma," *J Clin Oncol*, 1998, 16(4):1325-30.

Trastuzumab-Paclitaxel

Use Breast cancer
Regimen
Paclitaxel: I.V.: 175 mg/m² day 1
[total dose/cycle = 175 mg/m²]
Trastuzumab: I.V.: 4 mg/kg (loading dose) day 1 cycle 1
[total dose/cycle = 4 mg/kg]

Trastuzumab: I.V.: 2 mg/kg/day days 8 and 15 cycle 1
 [total dose/cycle = 4 mg/kg]
followed by 2 mg/kg/day days 1, 8, and 15 (subsequent cycles)
 [total dose/cycle = 6 mg/kg]
Repeat cycle every 21 days for at least 6 cycles

References

Slamon DJ, Leyland-Jones B, Shak S, et al, "Use of Chemotherapy Plus a Monoclonal Antibody Against HER2 for Metastatic Breast Cancer That Overexpresses HER2," *N Engl J Med*, 2001, 344(11):783-92.

Tretinoin/Idarubicin

Use Leukemia, acute promyelocytic

Regimen

Induction:

Tretinoin: Oral: >20 years: 45 mg/m^2/day day 1 up to 90 days
 [total dose/cycle = 4050 mg/m^2]
Tretinoin Oral: ≤20 years: 25 mg/m^2/day day 1 up to 90 days
 [total dose/cycle = 2250 mg/m^2]
Idarubicin: I.V.: 12 mg/m^2/day days 2, 4, 6, and 8
 [total dose/cycle = 48 mg/m^2]

Consolidation Course 1:

Idarubicin: I.V.: 5 mg/m^2/day days 1 to 4
 [total dose/cycle = 20 mg/m^2]
 or
Idarubicin: I.V.: 7 mg/m^2/day days 1 to 4
 [total dose/cycle = 28 mg/m^2]
Tretinoin: Oral: 45 mg/m^2/day days 1 to 15
 [total dose/cycle = 675 mg/m^2]

Consolidation Course 2:

Mitoxantrone: I.V.: 10 mg/m^2/day days 1 to 5
 [total dose/cycle = 50 mg/m^2]
Tretinoin: Oral: 45 mg/m^2/day days 1 to 15
 [total dose/cycle = 675 mg/m^2]

Consolidation Course 3:

Idarubicin: I.V.: 12 mg/m^2 day 1
 [total dose/cycle = 12 mg/m^2]
 or
Idarubicin: I.V.: 12 mg/m^2/day days 1 and 2
 [total dose/cycle = 24 mg/m^2]
Tretinoin: Oral: 45 mg/m^2/day days 1 to 15
 [total dose/cycle = 675 mg/m^2]
Given at 1 month intervals

Maintenance:

Mercaptopurine: Oral: 50 mg/m^2 daily
 [total dose/cycle = 4200 mg/m^2]
Methotrexate: I.M.: 15 mg/m^2 weekly
 [total dose/cycle = 180 mg/m^2]
Tretinoin: Oral: 45 mg/m^2/day days 1 to 15
 [total dose/cycle = 675 mg/m^2]
Repeat every 3 months for 2 years

TVTG

Use Leukemia, acute lymphocytic; Leukemia, acute myeloid

Regimen

Topotecan: I.V.: 1 mg/m^2/day continuous infusion days 1 to 5
[total dose/cycle = 5 mg/m^2]

Vinorelbine: I.V.: 20 mg/m^2/day days 0, 7, 14, and 21
[total dose/cycle = 80 mg/m^2]

Thiotepa: I.V.: 15 mg/m^2 day 2
[total dose/cycle = 15 mg/m^2]

Gemcitabine: I.V.: 3600 mg/m^2 day 7
[total dose/cycle = 3600 mg/m^2]

Dexamethasone: Oral or I.V.: 45 mg/m^2/day days 7 to 14 (given in 3 divided doses)
[total dose/cycle = 315 mg/m^2]

Repeat cycle when ANC >500 cells/mcL and platelet count >75,000 cells/mcL

References

Kolb EA and Steinherz PG, "A New Multidrug Reinduction Protocol With Topotecan, Vinorelbine, Thiotepa, Dexamethasone, and Gemcitabine for Relapsed or Refractory Acute Leukemia," *Leukemia*, 2003, 17(10):1967-72.

VAC (Ovarian Cancer)

Use Ovarian cancer

Regimen

Vincristine: I.V.: 1.2-1.5 mg/m^2 (maximum 2 mg) weekly for 10-12 weeks
[total dose/cycle = 12-15 mg/m^2 to 14.4-18]

or every 2 weeks for 12 doses
[total dose/cycle = 14.4-18 mg/m^2]

Dactinomycin: I.V.: 0.3-0.4 mg/m^2/day days 1 to 5
[total dose/cycle = 1.5-2 mg/m^2]

Cyclophosphamide: I.V.: 150 mg/m^2/day days 1 to 5
[total dose/cycle = 750 mg/m^2]

Repeat every 28 days

References

Gershenson DM, Copeland LJ, Kavanagh JJ, et al, "Treatment of Malignant Nondysgerminomatous Germ Cell Tumors of the Ovary With Vincristine, Dactinomycin, and Cyclophosphamide," *Cancer*, 1985, 56(12):2756-61.

VAC (Retinoblastoma)

Use Retinoblastoma

Regimen

Vincristine: I.V.: 1.5 mg/m^2 day 1
[total dose/cycle = 1.5 mg/m^2]

Dactinomycin: I.V.: 0.015 mg/kg/day days 1 to 5
[total dose/cycle = 0.075 mg/kg]

Cyclophosphamide: I.V.: 200 mg/m^2/day days 1 to 5
[total dose/cycle = 1000 mg/m^2]

References

Doz F, Khelfaoui F, Mosseri V, et al, "The Role of Chemotherapy in Orbital Involvement of Retinoblastoma. The Experience of a Single Institution With 33 Patients," *Cancer*, 1994, 74(2):722-32.

VAC (Rhabdomyosarcoma)

Use Rhabdomyosarcoma

Regimen

Induction:

Vincristine: I.V. push: 1.5 mg/m^2 (maximum 2 mg) weekly for 12 weeks, then at week 16

[total dose/cycle = 19.5 mg/m^2]

Dactinomycin: I.V. push: 0.015 mg/kg/day (maximum 0.5 mg) days 1 to 5, repeat every 3 weeks for 3 cycles, then stop for 2 cycles; repeat at week 16

Cyclophosphamide: I.V.: 10 mg/kg/day days 1 to 3 (alternately: 2.2 g/m^2 day 1), repeat every 3 weeks for 5 cycles; then at week 16

Continuation:

Vincristine: I.V. push: 1.5 mg/m^2 (maximum 2 mg) weeks 20 to 25, 29 to 34, and 38 to 43

[total dose/cycle = 27 mg/m^2]

Dactinomycin: I.V. push: 0.015 mg/kg (maximum 0.5 mg) weeks 20 and 23, 29 and 32, 38 and 41

[total dose/cycle = .18 mg/kg]

Cyclophosphamide: I.V.: 2.2 g/m^2 weeks 20 and 23, 29 and 32, 38 and 41

[total dose/cycle = 26.4 g/m^2]

References

Baker KS, Anderson JR, Link MP, et al, "Benefit of Intensified Therapy for Patients With Local or Regional Embryonal Rhabdomyosarcoma: Results From the Intergroup Rhabdomyosarcoma Study IV," *J Clin Oncol*, 2000, 18(12):2427-34.

VAC Pulse

Use Rhabdomyosarcoma

Regimen

Vincristine: I.V.: 2 mg/m^2/dose (maximum 2 mg/dose) every 7 days for 12 weeks

[total dose/cycle = 24 mg/m^2]

Dactinomycin: I.V.: 0.015 mg/kg/day (maximum 0.5 mg/day) days 1 to 5, weeks 1 and 13

[total dose/cycle = 0.15 mg/kg]

Cyclophosphamide: Oral, I.V.: 10 mg/kg/day for 7 days, repeat every 6 weeks

References

Wilbur JR, Sutow WW, Sullivan MP, et al, "Chemotherapy of Sarcomas," *Cancer*, 1975, 36(3):765-9.

VAD

Use Multiple myeloma

Regimen

Vincristine: I.V.: 0.4 mg/day continuous infusion days 1 to 4

[total dose/cycle = 1.6 mg]

Doxorubicin: I.V.: 9 mg/m^2/day continuous infusion days 1 to 4

[total dose/cycle = 36 mg/m^2]

Dexamethasone: Oral: 40 mg/day days 1 to 4, 9 to 12, and 17 to 20

[total dose/cycle = 480 mg]

Repeat cycle every 28-35 days

(Continued)

VAD *(Continued)*

References
Barlogie B, Smith L, and Alexanian R, "Effective Treatment of Advanced Multiple Myeloma Refractory to Alkylating Agents," *N Engl J Med*, 1984, 310(21):1353-6.

VAD/CVAD
Use Leukemia, acute lymphocytic

Regimen Induction:

Vincristine: I.V.: 0.4 mg continuous infusion/day days 1 to 4 and 24 to 27
[total dose/cycle = 3.2 mg]

Doxorubicin: I.V.: 12 mg/m^2/day continuous infusion days 1 to 4 and 24 to 27
[total dose/cycle = 96 mg/m^2]

Dexamethasone: Oral: 40 mg/day days 1 to 4, 9 to 12, and 17 to 20
[total dose/cycle = 480 mg]

Cyclophosphamide: I.V.: 1 g/m^2 day 24
[total dose/cycle = 1 g/m^2]

Dexamethasone: Oral: 40 mg/day days 24 to 27, 32 to 35, and 40 to 43
[total dose/cycle = 480 mg]

Administer one cycle only

References
Kantarjian H, Walters RS, Keating MJ, et al, "Results of the Vincristine, Doxorubicin, and Dexamethasone Regimen in Adults With Standard and High-Risk Acute Lymphocytic Leukemia," *J Clin Oncol*, 1990, 8(6):994-1004.

VATH
Use Breast cancer

Regimen

Vinblastine: I.V.: 4.5 mg/m^2 day 1
[total dose/cycle = 4.5 mg/m^2]

Doxorubicin: I.V.: 45 mg/m^2 day 1
[total dose/cycle = 45 mg/m^2]

Thiotepa: I.V.: 12 mg/m^2 day 1
[total dose/cycle = 12 mg/m^2]

Fluoxymesterone: Oral: 10 mg 3 times/day days 1 to 21
[total dose/cycle = 630 mg]

Repeat cycle every 21 days

References
Hart RD, Perloff M, and Holland JF, "One-Day VATH (Vinblastine, Adriamycin®, Thiotepa, and Halotestin®) Therapy for Advanced Breast Cancer Refractory to Chemotherapy," *Cancer*, 1981, 48(7):1522-7.

VBAP
Use Multiple myeloma

Regimen

Vincristine: I.V.: 1 mg day 1
[total dose/cycle = 1 mg]

Carmustine: I.V.: 30 mg/m^2 day 1
[total dose/cycle = 30 mg/m^2]

Doxorubicin: I.V.: 30 mg/m^2 day 1
[total dose/cycle = 30 mg/m^2]

Prednisone: Oral: 100 mg/day days 1 to 4
[total dose/cycle = 400 mg]

Repeat cycle every 21 days

References
Bonnet J, Alexanian R, Salmon S, et al, "Vincristine, BCNU, Doxorubicin, and Prednisone (VBAP) Combination in the Treatment of Relapsing or Resistant Multiple Myeloma: A Southwest Oncology Group Study," *Cancer Treat Rep*, 1982, 66(6):1267-71.

VBMCP

Use Multiple myeloma

Regimen

Vincristine: I.V.: 1.2 mg/m^2 (maximum 2 mg) day 1
[total dose/cycle = 1.2 mg/m^2]

Carmustine: I.V.: 20 mg/m^2 day 1
[total dose/cycle = 20 mg/m^2]

Melphalan: Oral: 8 mg/m^2/day days 1 to 4
[total dose/cycle = 32 mg/m^2]

Cyclophosphamide: I.V.: 400 mg/m^2 day 1
[total dose/cycle = 400 mg/m^2]

Prednisone: Oral: 40 mg/m^2/day days 1 to 7 (all cycles)
[total dose/cycle = 280 mg/m^2]

followed by 20 mg/m^2/day days 8 to 14 (first 3 cycles only)
[total dose/cycle = 140 mg/m^2]

Repeat cycle every 35 days

References
Oken MM, Harrington DP, Abramson N, et al, "Comparison of Melphalan and Prednisone With Vincristine, Carmustine, Melphalan, Cyclophosphamide, and Prednisone in the Treatment of Multiple Myeloma: Results of Eastern Cooperative Oncology Group Study E2479," *Cancer*, 1997, 79(8):1561-7.

VBP

Synonyms PVB

Use Testicular cancer

Regimen

Vinblastine: I.V.: 6 mg/m^2/day days 1 and 2
[total dose/cycle = 12 mg/m^2]

Bleomycin: I.V.: 30 units/day days 1, 8, 15, and (22)
[total dose/cycle = 120 units]

Cisplatin: I.V.: 20 mg/m^2/day days 1 to 5
[total dose/cycle = 100 mg/m^2]

Repeat cycle every 21-28 days

References
Williams SD, Birch R, Einhorn LH, et al, "Treatment of Disseminated Germ-Cell Tumors With Cisplatin, Bleomycin, and Either Vinblastine or Etoposide," *N Engl J Med*, 1987, 316(23):1435-40.

VC

Use Lung cancer, nonsmall cell

Regimen

Vinorelbine: I.V.: 30 mg/m^2 weekly
[total dose/cycle = 180 mg/m^2]

Cisplatin: I.V.: 120 mg/m^2/day days 1 and 29 (cycle 1); day 1 only on subsequent cycles
[total dose/cycle = 240 mg/m^2 cycle 1 only, 120 mg/m^2 (subsequent cycles)]

Repeat cycle every 6 weeks

(Continued)

VC (Continued)

References
Le Chevalier T, Pujol JL, Douillard JY, et al, "A Three-Arm Trial of Vinorelbine (Navelbine) Plus Cisplatin, Vindesine Plus Cisplatin, and Single-Agent Vinorelbine in the Treatment of Nonsmall Cell Lung Cancer: An Expanded Analysis," *Semin Oncol*, 1994, 21(5 Suppl 10):28-33; discussion 33-4.

VCAP
Use Multiple myeloma

Regimen
Vincristine: I.V.: 1 mg day 1
  [total dose/cycle = 1 mg]
Cyclophosphamide: Oral: 100 mg/m^2/day days 1 to 4
  [total dose/cycle = 400 mg/m^2]
Doxorubicin: I.V.: 25 mg/m^2 day 2
  [total dose/cycle = 25 mg/m^2]
Prednisone: Oral: 60 mg/m^2/day days 1 to 4
  [total dose/cycle = 240 mg/m^2]
Repeat cycle every 28 days

References
Salmon SE, Haut A, Bonnet JD, et al, "Alternating Combination Chemotherapy and Levamisole Improves Survival in Multiple Myeloma: A Southwest Oncology Group Study," *J Clin Oncol*, 1983, 1(8):453-61.

Vinorelbine-Cis
Use Lung cancer, nonsmall cell

Regimen
Vinorelbine: I.V.: 30 mg/m^2 every 7 days
Cisplatin: I.V.: 120 mg/m^2/day day 1 and 29, then every 6 weeks

References
Le Chevalier T, Brisgand D, Douillard JY, et al, "Randomized Study of Vinorelbine and Cisplatin Versus Vindesine and Cisplatin Versus Vinorelbine Alone in Advanced Nonsmall-Cell Lung Cancer: Results of a European Multicenter Trial Including 612 Patients," *J Clin Oncol*, 1994, 12(2):360-7.

Vinorelbine-Gemcitabine
Use Lung cancer, nonsmall cell

Regimen
Vinorelbine: I.V.: 20 mg/m^2/day days 1, 8, and 15
  [total dose/cycle = 60 mg/m^2]
Gemcitabine: I.V.: 800 mg/m^2/day days 1, 8, and 15
  [total dose/cycle = 2400 mg/m^2]
Repeat cycle every 28 days

References
Chen YM, Perng RP, Yang KY, et al, "A Multicenter Phase II Trial of Vinorelbine Plus Gemcitabine in Previously Untreated Inoperable (Stage IIIB/IV) Non-Small Cell Lung Cancer," *Chest*, 2000, 117(6):1583-9.

VIP (Etoposide) (Testicular Cancer)
Use Testicular cancer

Regimen NOTE: Multiple variations are listed below.
Variation 1:
Etoposide: I.V.: 75 mg/m^2/day days 1 to 5
  [total dose/cycle = 375 mg/m^2]
Ifosfamide: I.V.: 1200 mg/m^2/day days 1 to 5
  [total dose/cycle = 6000 mg/m^2]

Cisplatin: I.V.: 20 mg/m^2/day days 1 to 5
  [total dose/cycle = 100 mg/m^2]
Repeat cycle every 21 days
Variation 2:
  Etoposide: I.V.: 100 mg/m^2/day days 1 to 5
    [total dose/cycle = 500 mg/m^2]
  Ifosfamide: I.V.: 1200 mg/m^2/day days 1 to 5
    [total dose/cycle = 6000 mg/m^2]
  Cisplatin: I.V.: 20 mg/m^2/day days 1 to 5
    [total dose/cycle = 100 mg/m^2]
  Repeat cycle every 21 days
Variation 3:
  Ifosfamide: I.V.: 2500 mg/m^2/day days 1 and 2
    [total dose/cycle = 5000 mg/m^2]
  Mesna: I.V.: 2400 mg/m^2/day days 1 and 2
    [total dose/cycle = 4800 mg/m^2]
  Etoposide: I.V.: 100 mg/m^2/day days 3, 4, and 5
    [total dose/cycle = 300 mg/m^2]
  Cisplatin: I.V.: 40 mg/m^2/day days 3, 4, and 5
    [total dose/cycle = 120 mg/m^2]
  Repeat cycle every 21 days
Variation 4:
  Etoposide: I.V.: 75 mg/m^2/day days 1 to 5
    [total dose/cycle = 375 mg/m^2]
  Ifosfamide: I.V.: 1200 mg/m^2/day days 1 to 5
    [total dose/cycle = 6000 mg/m^2]
  Cisplatin: I.V.: 20 mg/m^2/day days 1 to 5
    [total dose/cycle = 100 mg/m^2]
  Mesna: I.V.: 120 mg/m^2 day 1 only, then 1200 mg/m^2 continuous infusion days 1 to 5
    [total dose/cycle = 6120 mg/m^2]
  Repeat cycle every 21 days

References

Variation 1:
  Loehrer PJ Sr, Lauer R, Roth BJ, et al, "Salvage Therapy in Recurrent Germ Cell Cancer: Ifosfamide and Cisplatin Plus Either Vinblastine or Etoposide," *Ann Intern Med*, 1988 109(7):540-6.
Variation 2:
  Harstrick A, Schmoll HJ, Wilke H, et al, "Cisplatin, Etoposide, and Ifosfamide Salvage Therapy for Refractory or Relapsing Germ Cell Carcinoma." *J Clin Oncol*, 1991 9(9):1549-55.
Variation 3:
  Pizzocaro G, Salvioni R, Piva L, et al, "Modified Cisplatin, Etoposide (or Vinblastine) and Ifosfamide Salvage Therapy for Male Germ-cell Tumors. Long-term Results." *Ann Oncol*, 1992 3(3):211-6.
Variation 4:
  Nichols CR, Catalano PJ, Crawford ED, et al, "Randomized Comparison of Cisplatin and Etoposide and Either Bleomycin or Ifosfamide in Treatment of Advanced Disseminated Germ Cell Tumors: An Eastern Cooperative Oncology Group, Southwest Oncology Group, and Cancer and Leukemia Group B Study," *J Clin Oncol*, 1998, 16(4):1287-93.

VIP (Small Cell Lung Cancer)

Use Lung cancer, small cell

Regimen

Etoposide: I.V.: 75 mg/m^2/day days 1 to 4
  [total dose/cycle = 300 mg/m^2]
(Continued)

VIP (Small Cell Lung Cancer) *(Continued)*

Ifosfamide: I.V.: 1200 mg/m²/day days 1 to 4
[total dose/cycle = 4800 mg/m²]
Cisplatin: I.V.: 20 mg/m²/day days 1 to 4
[total dose/cycle = 80 mg/m²]
Mesna: I.V.: 300 mg/m² day 1
[total dose/cycle = 300 mg/m²]
followed by 1200 mg/m²/day continuous infusion days 1 to 4
[total dose/cycle = 4800 mg/m²]
Repeat cycle every 21 days

References
Loehrer PJ Sr, Ansari R, Gonin R, et al, "Cisplatin Plus Etoposide With and Without Ifosfamide in Extensive Small Cell Lung Cancer: A Hoosier Oncology Group Study," *J Clin Oncol*, 1995, 13(10):2594-9.

VIP (Vinblastine) (Testicular Cancer)

Use Testicular cancer
Regimen NOTE: Multiple variations are listed below.
Variation 1:
Vinblastine: I.V.: 0.11 mg/kg/day days 1 and 2
[total dose/cycle = 0.22 mg/kg]
Ifosfamide: I.V.: 1200 mg/m²/day days 1 to 5
[total dose/cycle = 6000 mg/m²]
Cisplatin: I.V.: 20 mg/m²/day days 1 to 5
[total dose/cycle = 100 mg/m²]
Repeat cycle every 21 days
Variation 2:
Vinblastine: I.V.: 6 mg/m²/day days 1 and 2
[total dose/cycle = 12 mg/m²]
Ifosfamide: I.V.: 1500 mg/m²/day days 1 to 5
[total dose/cycle = 7500 mg/m²]
Cisplatin: I.V.: 20 mg/m²/day days 1 to 5
[total dose/cycle = 100 mg/m²]
Repeat cycle every 21 days

References
Variation 1:
Loehrer PJ Sr, Lauer R, Roth BJ, et al, "Salvage Therapy in Recurrent Germ Cell Cancer: Ifosfamide and Cisplatin Plus Either Vinblastine or Etoposide," *Ann Intern Med*, 1988 109(7):540-6.
Variation 2:
Clemm C, Hartenstein R, Willich N, et al, "Vinblastine-Ifosfamide-Cisplatin Treatment of Bulky Seminoma," *Cancer*, 1986, 58(10):2203-7.

VP (Small Cell Lung Cancer)

Use Lung cancer, small cell
Regimen
Etoposide: I.V.: 100 mg/m²/day days 1 to 4
[total dose/cycle = 400 mg/m²]
Cisplatin: I.V.: 20 mg/m²/day days 1 to 4
[total dose/cycle = 80 mg/m²]
Repeat cycle every 21 days

References
Loehrer PJ Sr, Ansari R, Gonin R, et al, "Cisplatin Plus Etoposide With and Without Ifosfamide in Extensive Small Cell Lung Cancer: A Hoosier Oncology Group Study," *J Clin Oncol*, 1995, 13(10):2594-9.

V-TAD

Use Leukemia, acute myeloid

Regimen Induction:

Etoposide: I.V.: 50 mg/m^2/day days 1 to 3
[total dose/cycle = 150 mg/m^2]

Thioguanine: Oral: 75 mg/m^2/day every 12 hours days 1 to 5
[total dose/cycle = 750 mg/m^2]

Daunorubicin: I.V.: 20 mg/m^2/day days 1 and 2
[total dose/cycle = 40 mg/m^2]

Cytarabine: I.V.: 75 mg/m^2/day continuous infusion days 1 to 5
[total dose/cycle = 375 mg/m^2]

Up to 3 cycles may be given based on individual response; time between cycles not specified

References

Bigelow CL, Kopecky K, Files JC, et al, "Treatment of Acute Myelogenous Leukemia in Patients Over 50 Years of Age With V-TAD: A Southwest Oncology Group Study," *Am J Hematol*, 1995, 48(4)228-32.

XelOx

Synonyms CapOx; Oxaliplatin/Capecitabine

Use Colorectal cancer

Regimen NOTE: Multiple variations are listed below.

Variation 1:

Oxaliplatin: I.V.: 130 mg/m^2 day 1
[total dose/cycle = 130 mg/m^2]

Capecitabine: Oral: 2500 mg/m^2/day days 1 to 14
[total dose/cycle = 35,000 mg/m^2]

Repeat cycle every 21 days

Variation 2:

Oxaliplatin: I.V.: 85 mg/m^2/day days 1 and 14
[total dose/cycle = 170 mg/m^2]

Capecitabine: Oral: 3500 mg/m^2/day days 1 to 7 and 14 to 21
[total dose/cycle = 52,500 mg/m^2]

Repeat cycle every 28 days

Variation 3:

Oxaliplatin: I.V.: 50 mg/m^2/day days 1, 8, 22, and 29
[total dose/cycle = 200 mg/m^2]

Capecitabine: Oral: 1650 mg/m^2/day days 1 to 14 and 22 to 35
[total dose/cycle = 46,200 mg/m^2]

Variation 4:

Oxaliplatin: I.V.: 70 mg/m^2/day days 1 and 8
[total dose/cycle = 140 mg/m^2]

Capecitabine: Oral: 2000 mg/m^2/day days 1 to 14
[total dose/cycle = 28,000 mg/m^2]

Variation 5:

Oxaliplatin: I.V.: 120 mg/m^2 day 1
[total dose/cycle = 120 mg/m^2]

Capecitabine: Oral: 2500 mg/m^2/day days 1 to 14
[total dose/cycle = 35,000 mg/m^2]

Variation 6:

Oxaliplatin: I.V.: 85 mg/m^2 day 1
[total dose/cycle = 85 mg/m^2]

Capecitabine: Oral: 2500 mg/m^2/day days 1 to 7
[total dose/cycle = 17,500 mg/m^2]

(Continued)

XelOx *(Continued)*

    or Capecitabine: Oral: 3000 mg/m^2/day days 1 to 7
       [total dose/cycle = 21,000 mg/m^2]
    or Capecitabine: Oral: 3500 mg/m^2/day days 1 to 7
       [total dose/cycle = 24,500 mg/m^2]
    or Capecitabine: Oral: 4000 mg/m^2/day days 1 to 7
       [total dose/cycle = 28,00 mg/m^2]
    Repeat cycle every 14 days

References

Variation 1:
    Borner MM, Dietrich D, Stupp R, et al, "Phase II Study of Capecitabine and Oxaliplatin in First- and Second-Line Treatment of Advanced or Metastatic Colorectal Cancer," *J Clin Oncol*, 2002, 20(7):1759-66.

Variation 2:
    Scheithauer W, Kornek GV, Raderer M, et al, "Randomized Multicenter Phase II Trial of Two Different Schedules of Capecitabine Plus Oxaliplatin as First-Line Treatment in Advanced Colorectal Cancer," *J Clin Oncol*, 2003, 21(7):1307-12.

Variation 3:
    Rodel C, Grabenbauer GG, Papadopoulos T, et al, "Phase I/II Trial of Capecitabine, Oxaliplatin, and Radiation for Rectal Cancer," *J Clin Oncol*, 2003, 21(16):3098-104.

Variation 4:
    Jordan K, Grothey A, Kellner O, et al, "Randomized Phase II Trial of Capecitabine Plus Irinotecan vs Capecitabine Plus Oxaliplatin as First-Line Therapy in Advanced Colorectal Cancer (ACRC): Results of an Interim Analysis," *Proc Annu Meet Am Soc Clin Oncol*, 2002, 21:2225.

Variation 5:
    Zeuli M, Nardoni C, Pino MS, et al, "Phase II Study of Capecitabine and Oxaliplatin as First-Line Treatment in Advanced Colorectal Cancer," *Ann Oncol*, 2003, 14(9):1378-82.

Variation 6:
    Scheithauer W, Kornek GV, Raderer M, et al, "Intermittent Weekly High-Dose Capecitabine in Combination With Oxaliplatin: A Phase I/II Study in First-Line Treatment of Patients With Advanced Colorectal Cancer," *Ann Oncol*, 2002, 13(10):1583-9.

CHEMOTHERAPY REGIMEN INDEX

ADENOCARCINOMA, UNKNOWN PRIMARY

BRAIN

Neuroblastomas

BREAST

CHEMOTHERAPY REGIMEN INDEX *(Continued)*

EYE

GASTROINTESTINAL

GENITOURINARY

CHEMOTHERAPY REGIMEN INDEX *(Continued)*

HEAD AND NECK CANCER

HEMATOLOGIC/LEUKEMIA

CHEMOTHERAPY REGIMEN INDEX *(Continued)*

LYMPHOID TISSUE (LYMPHOMA)

SPECIAL TOPICS

CHEMOTHERAPY AND PREGNANCY

INTRODUCTION

The occurrence of cancer and pregnancy at the same time is reportedly rare. The cancers most often described in pregnancy women include breast cancer, cervical cancer, hematologic cancers, melanoma, thyroid cancer, and colorectal cancer. There is no apparent link between these malignancies and pregnancy; rather, these cancers are those most common in women of child-bearing age. Obviously, the decision to continue or terminate a pregnancy encompasses a host of factors, including the effects of chemotherapy on the fetus.

EFFECTS OF CHEMOTHERAPY

As a rapidly proliferating tissue, the fetus would be expected to be a target for cytotoxic agents. Exposure to cytotoxic drugs during the first week of pregnancy is thought to present an "all or none" phenomenon – that is, spontaneous abortion or a normal fetus. Exposure during the remainder of the first trimester can lead to spontaneous abortion or to teratogenicity. Teratogenicity (ie, congenital abnormalities) occurs at this time, as this is the period of organ development. Indeed, teratogenicity is thought to be negligible when cytotoxic agents are given in the second and third trimesters. However, during the second and third trimesters, cytotoxic agents can interfere with fetal growth and functional development (eg, low birth weight, intrauterine growth retardation).

In addition to the timing of chemotherapy, the occurrence of an adverse outcome of pregnancy is influenced by the particular class of cytotoxic agent, as well as the dose. The literature suggests that antimetabolites, and in particular, methotrexate, are the most likely teratogens. The "aminopterin syndrome" of congenital abnormalities is characterized by dysostosis (delay in ossification of the bones of the skull), hypertelorism (a wide nasal bridge), anomalies of the external ears, and micrognathia (smallness of the jaws). Interestingly, a recent review noted no congenital abnormalities among fetuses exposed to low-dose methotrexate used in mothers with rheumatologic disorders. Methotrexate was used before or during the first trimester in 15 of 16 pregnancies described; six spontaneous abortions occurred, and none of the live births displayed congenital abnormalities. This would seem to underscore the influence of degree of exposure (ie, dose). Numerous case reports document successful pregnancies with no teratogenicity when chemotherapy was administered after the first trimester. Alkylating agents are reported to be "safer" than antimetabolites, and the vinca alkaloids are reportedly the "safest" even during the first trimester.

Long-term complications following *in utero* exposure to cytotoxic drugs might include abnormal physical and/or mental development, carcinogenesis, and teratogenicity in subsequent generation(s). Some adverse long-term outcomes have been described, but there are few systematic long-term follow-up studies.

CONCLUSION

Given the toxicity associated with most cytotoxic drugs, the likelihood of adverse outcomes of pregnancy seems lower than one might expect, especially after the first trimester. In addition to the effects of chemotherapy on the fetus, multiple other factors (eg, ability to stage cancer in the pregnant female; interactions, if any, of pregnancy and a particular cancer; prognosis) must be considered in the pregnant cancer patient.

Selected Readings

Caligiuri MA, "Leukemia and Pregnancy: Treatment and Outcome," *Adv Oncol*, 1992, 8:10-7.

Fisher PM and Hancock BW, "Hodgkin's Disease in the Pregnant Patient," *Br J Hosp Med*, 1996, 56(10):529-32.

Shapiro CL and Mayer RJ, "Breast Cancer During Pregnancy," *Adv Oncol*, 1992, 8:25-9.

Ward FT and Weiss RB, "Managing Lymphoma During Pregnancy," *Adv Oncol*, 1992, 8:18-22.

FERTILITY AND CANCER THERAPY

Antineoplastic therapy (chemotherapy, radiation, surgery) or cancer itself may affect fertility and/or sexual function in both men and women. They may also effect pregnancy outcomes, neonatal development or pubertal development and gonadal function in children. These effects on fertility may be temporary or permanent; and are dependent on a variety of factors including: Intensity of therapy; duration of therapy; age; gender.

Antineoplastic Agents Associated With Sterility

Women	Men
Alkylating agents	Alkylating agents
Busulfan	Busulfan
Chlorambucil	Chlorambucil
Cyclophosphamide	Cisplatin
Mechlorethamine	Cyclophosphamide
Melphalan	Mechlorethamine
Procarbazine	Nitrosoureas
	Procarbazine

FEMALES

Females are born with a set number of ova that are arrested in the meiotic prophase stage. Following sexual maturation, growth of these oocytes is stimulated by follicle stimulating hormone (FSH). Each follicle produces estrogen, which inhibits the secretion of FSH and luteinizing hormone (LH). In midcycle, estrogen levels rise and a surge of LH and increased release of FSH cause the follicle to swell and induce ovulation. After release of the ovum, the corpus luteum is formed which secretes progesterone, estrogen, and inhibin. LH, FSH, and inhibin act as negative feedback to the hypothalamus and pituitary to decrease secretion of LH and FSH. If fertilization does not occur, progesterone levels decrease, the corpus luteum involutes, and the cycle begins again.

Antineoplastic drugs may stop the development of follicles or may damage oocytes. Prepubertal gonads may be more resistant than postpubertal gonads, possibly due to a larger number of follicles as compared to ovaries in older patients. Gonadal destruction causes clinical findings associated with estrogen deficiency such as amenorrhea, endometrial hypoplasia, vaginal atrophy and dryness, and hot flashes. FSH levels are elevated and estrogen levels decreased. The onset and duration of symptoms is dose- and age-related. Younger patients are able to tolerate higher doses of chemotherapy before symptoms develop and have a higher likelihood of the return of menses when therapy is stopped.

Radiation therapy can cause ovarian damage, but the ovaries are more radioresistant than the testes and can tolerate higher doses of radiation. The effect on the ovaries depends on the age of the patient, the number of remaining oocytes at the time of radiation, and the exposure dose and field. Irradiation fields that do not include the pelvis generally do not cause infertility as evidenced by follow-up of Hodgkin's disease patients who received nodal irradiation.

For women, there is little available to protect against gonadal damage, and few options for preservation of ova. Although cryopreservation of ova is possible, it is experimental and has a low success rate. Standard *in vitro* fertilization and freezing of the embryo is another alternative, but there is little data to support this and it brings up many ethical issues. Other experimental approaches to preserving ovarian function that have been suggested include diminishing ovarian function during the period of treatment by use of gonadotropin-releasing hormone (GnRH) agonists or oral contraceptives; and implantation of cryopreserved ovarian cortical strips after chemotherapy.

MALES

Seminiferous tubules make up 75% of testicular mass. Their epithelium is composed of two cell types: Spermatogenic cells and Sertoli cells. Sertoli cells help regulate the release of mature spermatozoa. In males, gonadotropin-releasing hormone (GnRH) causes the release of FSH and LH from the anterior pituitary. LH stimulates Leydig cells in the testis to produce testosterone, which in turn has a negative feedback on the secretion of LH. FSH stimulates Sertoli cells that assist in spermatogenesis. Spermatogenesis occurs constantly. It takes about 64-90 days to progress from spermatogonia stem-cell mitosis to spermatocytes, spermatids, and finally spermatozoa.

Antineoplastic drugs and radiation destroy epithelial germ cells in a dose-dependent fashion. This damage results in increased FSH levels, decreased testosterone levels, oligospermia, or azoospermia. Spermatogenesis is more susceptible than testosterone production; and postpubertal testes are more susceptible to damage than prepubertal testes. Azoospermia may or may not be reversible. When it does recover, return of spermatogenesis may take up to 49 months.

Effects of radiation therapy on the testes are dependent on the dose, stage of development of the germ cell, and pubertal stage of the patient. Spermatogonia are the most sensitive to radiation damage, followed in decreasing sensitivity by spermatocytes and spermatids. Prepubertal boys may have oligo- or azoospermia once they reach sexual maturation. They may also have delayed sexual maturation due to destruction of Leydig cells and thus decreased testosterone production.

Surgery can affect male sexuality and fertility. Surgery for testicular cancer includes orchiectomy and retroperitoneal lymph node resection which has resulted in decreased semen volume, erectile dysfunction, and low sexual desire. Prostate cancer surgery can also produce erectile dysfunction and changes in semen volume or ejaculatory problems.

Interestingly, patients with testicular cancer may be at increased risk for fertility problems before treatment is started. Patients with testicular cancer are more likely to have impaired semen quality even before orchiectomy, and may have lower semen counts than would be expected following orchiectomy. This could be due to abnormal pathology in the contralateral testis. There is some evidence to suggest that exposure to abnormal hormone levels during development (eg, high progesterone levels associated with morning sickness) may be at risk for developing testicular cancer.

FERTILITY AND CANCER THERAPY *(Continued)*

In men, cryopreservation of sperm is a viable alternative and should be offered. Advances in *in vitro* fertilization using intracytoplasmic sperm injection may be helpful. There has also been some work done looking at suppressing spermatogenesis and Leydig cell function using LHRH analogues with either antiandrogens or testosterone to protect against chemotherapy-induced damage. Finally, cooling of the testes during radiation therapy has shown some promising results.

OUTCOMES OF PREGNANCY

Most studies of parents who have been treated for childhood cancer with chemotherapy, radiation therapy, or both suggest these individuals are not at increased risk of having children with congenital or chromosomal anomalies. However, one report of patients treated for Wilms' Tumor did suggest a trend toward increased risk of congenital malformations, fetal malposition, or early labor in previously irradiated women.

Available data do not show increased risk of miscarriage, fetal demise, or birth weight following chemotherapy. One small study of pregnancy outcome found no significant differences between patients who had received chemotherapy and controls. The same investigators also compared pregnancy outcome in the partners of male survivors of childhood cancer to outcome in the partners of their male siblings. The percent of live births in the male cancer survivors' partners was higher than among female cancer survivors, but was significantly lower than in the partners of male siblings. Rate of miscarriage, stillbirth, and birthweight distribution was similar in both cases and controls. In women who have received pelvic irradiation complications such as preterm labor and delivery, low birth weight, and placenta accrete have been reported.

Generally, there is no increased risk of cancer in the offspring of cancer survivors. Nor, with the possible exception of gestational trophoblastic disease, does pregnancy seem to affect the risk of cancer recurrence.

Selected Readings

Bahadur G, "Fertility Issues for Cancer Patients," *Mol Cell Endocrinol*, 2000, 169(1-2):117-22.

Goldman S and Johnson FL, "Effects of Chemotherapy and Irradiation on the Gonads," *Endocrinol Metab Clin North Am*, 1993, 22(3):617-29.

Gulati SC and Van Poznak C, "Pregnancy After Bone Marrow Transplantation," *J Clin Oncol*, 1998, 16(5):1978-85.

Kwon JS and Case AM, "Effects of Cancer Treatment on Reproduction and Fertility," *J Obstet Gynaecol Can*, 2002, 24(8):619-27.

Petersen PM, Giwercman A, Skakkebaek NE, et al, "Gonadal Function in Men With Testicular Cancer," *Sem Oncol*, 1998, 25(2):224-33.

Pont J and Albrecht W, "Fertility After Chemotherapy for Testicular Cancer," *Fertil Steril*, 1997, 68:1-5.

Shahin MS and Puscheck E, "Reproductive Sequelae of Cancer Treatment," *Obstet Gynecol Clin North Am*, 1998, 25(2):423-33.

MANAGEMENT OF DRUG EXTRAVASATIONS

Vesicant: An agent that causes tissue destruction.

Irritant: An agent that causes aching, tightness, and phlebitis with or without inflammation.

Extravasation: Unintentional leakage of fluid out of a blood vessel into surrounding tissue.

Vesicant extravasation: Leakage of a drug that causes pain, necrosis, or tissue sloughing.

Delayed extravasation: Symptoms occur 48 hours, or later, after drug administration.

Flare: Local, nonpainful, possibly allergic reaction often accompanied by reddening along the vein.

A potential, and potentially highly morbid, complication of drug therapy is soft tissue damage caused by leakage of the drug solution out of the vein. A variety of complications, including erythema, ulceration, pain, tissue sloughing, and necrosis are possible. This problem is not unique to antineoplastic therapy; a variety of drugs have been reported to cause tissue damage if extravasated. See table.

Vesicant Agents

Hyperosmotic Agents (>280 mOsm/L)	Ischemia Inducers	Direct Cellular Toxins	
		Nonantineoplastic Agents	Antineoplastic Agents
Calcium chloride (>10%)	Aminophylline	Chlordiazepoxide	Amsacrine[1]
Calcium gluconate	Dobutamine	Diazepam	Dactinomycin
Calcium gluceptate	Dopamine	Digoxin	Daunorubicin
Contrast media	Epinephrine	Ethanol	Doxorubicin
Crystalline amino acids (4.25%)	Esmolol	Nafcillin	Epirubicin
Dextrose (>10%)	Metaraminol	Nitroglycerine	Esorubicin[1]
Mannitol (>5%)	Metoprolol	Phenytoin	Idarubicin
Potassium acetate (>2 mEq/mL)	Norepinephrine	Propylene glycol	Mechlorethamine
Potassium chloride (>2 mEq/mL)	Phenylephrine	Sodium thiopental	Mitomycin
Sodium bicarbonate (≥8.4%)	Vasopressin	Tetracycline	Streptozocin (?)
Sodium chloride (>1%)			Valrubicin
Thiopentone			Vinblastine
Urea (30%)			Vincristine
			Vindesine[1]
			Vinorelbine

[1]In addition to the known vesicants, a number of other antineoplastic agents, not generally considered to be vesicants, have been associated with isolated reports of tissue damage following extravasation.

MANAGEMENT OF DRUG EXTRAVASATIONS
(Continued)

Agents Associated With Occasional Extravasation Reactions

Aclarubicin[1]
Arsenic trioxide
Bleomycin
Carboplatin ≥10 mg/mL
Carmustine
Cisplatin
Cyclophosphamide
Dacarbazine
Daunorubicin citrate
(liposomal)
Dexrazoxane
Docetaxel
Doxorubicin, liposomal

Etoposide
Floxuridine
Fluorouracil
Gemcitabine
Gemtuzumab
Ifosfamide
Irinotecan
Menogaril[1]
Mitoxantrone
Oxaliplatin
Paclitaxel
Teniposide
Topotecan

[1]Not commercially available in the U.S.

The actual incidence of drug extravasations is unknown. Some of the uncertainty stems from varying definitions of incidence. Incidence rates have been reported based on total number of drug doses administered, number of vesicant doses administered, number of treatments, number of patients treated with vesicants, and total number of patients treated. Most estimates place the incidence of extravasations with cytotoxic agents in the range of 1% to 7%.

The optimal treatment of drug extravasations is uncertain. A variety of antidotes have been proposed; however, objective clinical evidence to support these recommendations frequently is not available. There are no well done randomized prospective trials of potential treatments. Controlled clinical trials are not feasible, limiting efforts to identify optimal management of these reactions. Extant reports are based on animal models, anecdotal cases, and/or small uncontrolled series of patients. Many of the existing reports, both animal and human, used more than one therapeutic intervention simultaneously, adding to the difficulty of identifying the efficacy of any single approach.

The best "treatment" for extravasation reactions is prevention. Although it is not possible to prevent all accidents, a few simple precautions can minimize the risk to the patient. The vein used should be a large, intact vessel with good blood flow. To minimize the risk of dislodging the catheter, veins in the hands and in the vicinity of joints (eg, antecubital) should be avoided. Veins in the forearm (ie, the basilic, cephalic, and median antebrachial, basilic and cephalic) are usually good options for peripheral infusions. Prior to drug administration, the patency of the I.V. line should be verified. The line should be flushed with 5-10 mL of a saline or dextrose solution; and the drug(s) infused through the side of a free-flowing isotonic saline or dextrose infusion.

A frequently recommended precaution against drug extravasation is the use of a central venous catheter. Use of a central line has several advantages, including high patient satisfaction, reliable venous access, high flow rates, and rapid dilution of the drug. A wide variety of devices are readily available. Many institutions encourage or require use of a vascular access device for administration of vesicant agents.

Despite their benefit, central lines are not an absolute solution. Vascular access devices are subject to a number of complications. The catheter tip may not be properly positioned in the superior vena cava/right atrium, or may migrate out of position. Additionally, these catheters require routine care to maintain patency and avoid infections. Finally, extravasation of drugs from venous access devices is possible. Misplacement/migration of the catheter tip, improper placement of the needle in accessing injection ports, and cuts, punctures, or rupture of the catheter itself have all been reported. Reports of extravasation from central catheters range from 0.3% to 50%, and are similar to extravasation rates reported from peripheral lines.

When a drug extravasation does occur, a variety of immediate actions have been recommended. Although there is considerable uncertainty regarding the value of some potential treatments, a few initial steps seem to be generally accepted.

1. **Stop the infusion.** At the first suspicion of infiltration, the drug infusion should be stopped. If infiltration is not certain, the line can be tested by attempting to aspirate blood, and careful infusion of a few milliliters of saline or dextrose solution.

2. **Do NOT remove the catheter/needle.** The infiltrated catheter should not be removed immediately. It should be left in place to facilitate aspiration of fluid from the extravasation site, and, if appropriate, administration of an antidote directly into the extravasation site.

3. **Aspirate fluid.** To the extent possible, the extravasated drug solution should be removed from the subcutaneous tissues.

4. **Do NOT flush the line.** Flooding the infiltration site with saline or dextrose in an attempt to dilute the drug solution generally is not recommended. Rather than minimizing damage, such a procedure may have the opposite effect by distributing the vesicant solution over a wider area.

5. **Remove the catheter/needle.** If an antidote is not going to be injected into the extravasation site, the infiltrated catheter should be removed. If an antidote is to be injected into the area, it should be injected through the catheter to ensure delivery of the antidote to the infiltration site. When this has been accomplished, the catheter should then be removed.

Two issues for which there is less consensus are the application of heat or cold, and the use of various antidotes. A variety of recommendations exist for each of these concerns; there is no consensus concerning the proper approach.

Cold. Intermittent cooling of the area of infiltration results in vasoconstriction, which tends to restrict the spread of the drug. It may also inhibit the local effects of some drugs (eg, anthracyclines). Application of cold is usually

MANAGEMENT OF DRUG EXTRAVASATIONS
(Continued)

recommended as immediate treatment for most drug extravasations, except the vinca alkaloids. In one report of antineoplastic drug extravasation treatment, almost 90% of the extravasations treated only with topical cold required no further therapy.

The largest single published series of antineoplastic drug extravasations was 175 patients reported by Larson in 1985. This series includes some of the more commonly used vesicants, including the anthracyclines, mechlorethamine, mitomycin, and the vinca alkaloids. For 119 patients, local application of cold (15 minutes four times a day for 3 days) and close observation was the sole treatment. The remaining 56 patients received a variety of antidotes. In 89% of the patients treated with cold alone, the extravasation resolved without further treatment. Of the patients treated by other methods, only 53% resolved without further treatment.

Helpful as it may be, Larson's report does have some limitations. Agents such as the epipodophyllotoxins and taxanes which are occasionally associated with soft tissue damage were not included, nor were extravasations of non-antineoplastic agents mentioned. The report included infiltrations of the vinca alkaloids, even though the literature recommends use of heat to treat these. Also, except for doxorubicin extravasations in the group treated with ice and observation, responses for the individual drugs were not indicated. In this group, 72% of the doxorubicin extravasations resolved completely.

Heat. Application of heat results in a localized vasodilation and increased blood flow. Increased circulation is believed to facilitate removal of the drug from the area of infiltration. The data supporting use of heat are less convincing than for cold. One report of the application of heat for nonantineoplastic drug extravasations suggested application of heat increased the risk of skin maceration and necrosis. Most data are from animal studies, with relatively few human case reports. Animal models indicate application of heat exacerbates the damage from anthracycline extravasations. No large series of extravasations managed with the application of heat has been published. Heat is generally recommended for treatment for vinca alkaloid extravasations; a few reports recommend it for treatment of amino acid solutions, aminophylline, calcium, contrast media, dextrose, mannitol, nafcillin, paclitaxel, phenytoin, podophyllotoxin, potassium and vinca alkaloid infiltrations. There are conflicting reports on the initial management of paclitaxel infiltrations.

For some agents, such as cisplatin, epipodophyllotoxins, mechlorethamine and paclitaxel, there are conflicting recommendations. Some reports recommend application of cold, others recommend heat. At least one report suggests neither cold nor heat is effective for paclitaxel extravasations.

ANTIDOTES

A very wide variety of agents have been reported as possible antidotes for extravasated drugs, with no consensus on their proper use. For a number of reasons, evaluation of the various reports is difficult.

1. Mechanism of action. For many drugs, the underlying mechanism responsible for the tissue damage is not certain. For some of the

antidotes, the purported mechanism of action of the antidote is also unclear.

2. Controlled trials. Prospective, randomized controlled trials are not practical. Information concerning treatment of extravasations is based almost exclusively on animal models, anecdotal reports, and small, uncontrolled studies.

3. Outcome definitions. Published reports use a number of different end-points and outcomes to define efficacy of a given treatment.

4. Confounding factors. A number of confounding factors exist which make assessment of various antidotes difficult. Among these are:

    a. Response to nonpharmacologic therapy. Application of heat or cold alone, especially the latter, appears to have a significant protective effect.

    b. Multiple therapies. A number of reports used more than one therapeutic modality to treat drug extravasations. In many cases, cold or heat is applied along with the antidote. In some cases, more than one antidote is used, sometimes in conjunction with heat or cold. Use of multiple approaches further complicates the determination of the possible effect of a particular antidote, or the additive effect of various combinations.

    c. Variable applications. For some proposed antidotes, a wide variety of different doses, concentrations, methods of application, and duration of therapy have been reported, making determination of the optimal treatment regimen difficult.

Agents Used as Antidotes

Albumin	Iron dextran
Antihistamines	Isoproterenol
Antioxidants	Nitroglycerine paste
Beta-adrenergics	Phentolamine
Carnitine	Radical dimer
Corticosteroids[1]	Saline
Dexrazoxane	Sodium bicarbonate
Dextranomer	Sodium hypochlorite
Dimethyl sulfoxide	Sodium thiosulfate[1]
Dopamine	Terbutaline
Fluorescein	Vitamin E
Hyaluronidase[1]	

[1]Listed in the package insert of at least one agent.

Sodium bicarbonate. An 8.4% solution of sodium bicarbonate was briefly recommended for treatment of anthracycline extravasations. The recommendation was based on a case report of its use in a single patient. The proposed mechanism of action was that the high pH of the bicarbonate solution would break the glycosidic bond of the anthracycline; thereby, inactivating it. Follow-up studies in a variety of animal models failed to confirm the original report. Also, the concentrated sodium bicarbonate may itself be a vesicant. See the Vesicant Agents table *on page 965*. At present, most reviews and guidelines discourage its use for treating extravasations.

MANAGEMENT OF DRUG EXTRAVASATIONS
(Continued)

Corticosteroids. Steroids are most commonly used to treat anthracycline extravasations. Hydrocortisone is the steroid most frequently recommended, although dexamethasone has also been used. It is suggested that steroids reduce local inflammation from the extravasated drug. Such activity has not been confirmed; nor has it been demonstrated that the tissue damage from drug infiltrations is the result of an inflammatory process. Interpretation of steroid efficacy is complicated by the multiple doses, routes of administration, duration of therapy, and outcome measurements used. Reports of animal trials offer little additional information, being plagued by many of the limitations of the clinical case reports. The official labeling of only one of the three suppliers of doxorubicin includes a steroid as part of the treatment for drug extravasations. The product labeling from two doxorubicin suppliers, as well as the suppliers of daunorubicin, idarubicin, and liposome-encapsulated anthracyclines do not mention corticosteroids to treat drug infiltrations. Most reports question the efficacy of steroids for treatment of drug extravasations; they are not recommended by most guidelines.

Dexrazoxane. Dexrazoxane, a derivative of EDTA, is an intracellular chelating agent often used as a cardioprotective agent in patients receiving anthracycline therapy. It is believed that dexrazoxane's cardioprotective effect is a result by chelating iron following intracellular hydrolysis. Dexrazoxane is not an effective chelator itself, but is hydrolyzed intracellularly to an open-ring chelator form, which complexes with iron, other heavy metals, and doxorubicin complexes to inhibit the generation of free radicals. It has been postulated that dexrazoxane's chelating effect, or its ability to inhibit topoisomerase II, may be useful in preventing tissue damage from anthracycline infiltrations. There have been individual case reports of dexrazoxane being used to reduce tissue damage after extravasation of doxorubicin and epirubicin. Tests in mice suggest it might also be effective for treatment of daunorubicin and idarubicin.

Dimethyl sulfoxide (DMSO). A number of reports have suggested application of DMSO is an effective treatment for infiltrations of a number of different drugs. It is believed DMSO's protective effect is due to its ability to act as a free radical scavenger (one theory suggests tissue damage from vesicants, particularly anthracyclines, is due to formation of hydroxyl free radicals). Results in animal models have been equivocal, with some reports indicating DMSO is beneficial, and some showing little or no effect. Clinical reports of its use are extremely difficult to interpret due to variations in DMSO concentration, number of applications/day, duration of therapy, and concomitant treatments. A number of different treatments, including cold, steroids, vitamin E, and sodium bicarbonate have been used in conjunction with DMSO. Also, most reports that suggest DMSO is effective in preventing tissue damage used DMSO concentrations >90% which is not available for clinical use in the United States.

A further complication to interpretation of DMSO's efficacy is that some series included infiltrations of agents not generally considered to be vesicants. The largest clinical series included infiltrations in 75 patients; but only 31 of the extravasations involved vesicants (doxorubicin, epirubicin, or mitomycin). The remaining incidents involved drugs not usually associated with tissue damage (cisplatin, ifosfamide, and mitoxantrone). Application of 99% DMSO for 7 days and cold for 3 days resulted in a 93.5% success rate in the patients with vesicant extravasations. Only two patients (6.5%) had complications requiring further therapy. Whether the addition of DMSO represented a real improvement over cold alone is difficult to assess.

Hyaluronidase. Hyaluronidase is an enzyme that destroys hyaluronic acid, an essential component of connective tissue. This results in increased permeability of the tissue, facilitating diffusion and absorption of fluids. It is postulated that increasing the diffusion of extravasated fluids results in more rapid absorption, thereby limiting tissue damage. In individual case reports, hyaluronidase has been reported effective in preventing tissue damage from a wide variety of agents, including amino acid solutions, aminophylline, calcium, contrast media, dextrose, mannitol, nafcillin, phenytoin, potassium and vinca alkaloids. Other reports suggest it might also be useful in managing extravasations of epipodophyllotoxins and taxanes, although not all guidelines recommend its use for these agents.

Phentolamine. Phentolamine is an alpha$_1$ adrenergic antagonist which produces peripheral vasodilation. It has been reported to reduce tissue necrosis following extravasation of pressor (vasoconstrictor) agents such as dobutamine, dopamine, epinephrine and norepinephrine.

Sodium thiosulfate. A freshly prepared $1/6$M (~4%) solution of sodium thiosulfate has been recommended for treatment of mechlorethamine and cisplatin infiltrations. A 2% solution has been recommended for doxorubicin, epirubicin, mitomycin and vinblastine extravasations. This recommendation is based on *in vitro* data demonstrating an interaction between sodium thiosulfate and cisplatin, dacarbazine, and mechlorethamine; and very limited animal data on thiosulfate's ability to inactivate dacarbazine and mechlorethamine. At present, no clinical reports of its efficacy for treating cisplatin or dacarbazine extravasations have been published. Since cisplatin and dacarbazine are generally not considered to be vesicants, the use of thiosulfate to treat infiltrations of these drugs may not be required.

The use of sodium thiosulfate to treat mechlorethamine infiltrations is based almost exclusively on the *in vitro* and animal data. A single case report of successful thiosulfate treatment of an accidental intramuscular mechlorethamine injection has been published. Thus far, no reports of thiosulfate treatment of mechlorethamine infiltrations have been published.

One study of thiosulfate therapy of antineoplastic drug extravasations has been published. In a series of 63 patients with extravasation of doxorubicin, epirubicin, mitomycin, or vinblastine, 31 were treated with subcutaneous hydrocortisone and topical dexamethasone. The remaining 32 patients received subcutaneous injection of a 2% thiosulfate solution in addition to the subcutaneous and topical steroids. No patient in either group developed skin ulceration or required surgery; but the patients who received the thiosulfate healed in about half the time as the patients who received only the steroid therapy.

MANAGEMENT OF DRUG EXTRAVASATIONS
(Continued)

Reported Treatment Regimens for Vesicant Drug Extravasations

Treatment	Dose	Route	Duration	Concomitant Therapy	Used to Treat	Preparation	Administration
Cold[1]	15 min qid	Topical	3-4 days	None	All agents[2]	N/A	N/A
Heat[1]	15 min on; 15 min off	Topical	1 day	None	Vinca alkaloids	N/A	N/A
Heat	NS	Topical	NS	None	Epipodophyllotoxins, taxanes[3]	N/A	N/A
Dexrazoxone	1000 mg/m^2 500 mg/m^2	I.V.	Days 1 and 2 Day 3	Cold	Daunorubicin, doxorubicin, epirubicin, idarubicin	NS	NS
Dexrazoxone	1000 mg	I.V.	Day 1	Cold, DMSO, topical hydrocortisone	Epirubicin	NS	NS
Dexamethasone	4 mg	SubQ, I.D.	One time	Cold	Daunorubicin, doxorubicin	NS	Inject into several sites surrounding the area of extravasation.
Dexamethasone	8 mg I.D.	Topical	3 days	Dexamethasone	Doxorubicin	N/A	N/A
Dimethyl sulfoxide[4]	50%-99% q2-4h	Topical	3 days	Sodium bicarbonate SubQ, dexamethasone 4 mg SubQ	Daunorubicin	N/A	N/A
Dimethyl sulfoxide[4]	70% q3-4h	Topical	10 days	Vitamin E 10% topical	Doxorubicin, epirubicin, mitomycin	N/A	N/A
Dimethyl sulfoxide[4]	90% q12h	Topical	2 days			N/A	N/A

Reported Treatment Regimens for Vesicant Drug Extravasations *(continued)*

Treatment	Dose	Route	Duration	Concomitant Therapy	Used to Treat	Preparation	Administration
Dimethyl sulfoxide[4]	99% q8h for up to 1 week	Topical	1 week	Cold for 3 days	Doxorubicin, mitomycin, mitoxantrone	N/A	Apply 4 drops/10 cm² of skin surface over an area twice the size of the extravasation; allow to air dry without dressings.
Dimethyl sulfoxide[4]	99% q2-4h	Topical	3 days	None	Doxorubicin	N/A	N/A
Dimethyl sulfoxide[4]	99% q6-24h	Topical	14 days	None	Doxorubicin, daunorubicin	N/A	N/A
Dimethyl sulfoxide[4]	99% q6-12h	Topical	1-5 weeks	None	Mitomycin	N/A	N/A
Hyaluronidase[1]	15 units	SubQ	One time	Heat	Amino acid solutions, aminophylline, calcium, contrast media[5], dextrose, mannitol, nafcillin, phenytoin, potassium, vinca alkaloids	Reconstitute vial with NS to a concentration of 150 units/mL. Dilute 0.1 mL (15 units) with 0.9 mL NS for a final concentration of 15 units/mL	4-5 injections (0.2 mL) into area of extravasation

MANAGEMENT OF DRUG EXTRAVASATIONS
(Continued)

Reported Treatment Regimens for Vesicant Drug Extravasations *(continued)*

Treatment	Dose	Route	Duration	Concomitant Therapy	Used to Treat	Preparation	Administration
Hyaluronidase[1]	150 units	SubQ	One time	Heat	Amino acid solutions, aminophylline, calcium, contrast media[5] dextrose, mannitol, nafcillin, phenytoin, potassium, vinca alkaloids	Reconstitute with 1 mL NS	5-10 injections (0.5-1 mL) into area of extravasation
Hyaluronidase[1]	250 units	SubQ	One time	None	Amino acid solutions, aminophylline, calcium, contrast media[5] dextrose, mannitol, nafcillin, phenytoin, potassium, vinca alkaloids	Reconstitute with 6 mL NS	Inject directly through the original needle; OR 6 SubQ injections into area of extravasation.
Hydrocortisone	50-200 mg	I.V., SubQ, I.D.	NS	Cold	All agents except *vinca alkaloids*	NS	Inject into several sites surrounding the area of extravasation
Hydrocortisone	500 mg	SubQ	One time	Betamethasone and gentamycin ointment q12h for 2 days, then qd	Doxorubicin, epirubicin, vinblastine, mitomycin	500 mg in 10 mL NS	Inject at 1 cm intervals around the area of extravasation.

Reported Treatment Regimens for Vesicant Drug Extravasations *(continued)*

Treatment	Dose	Route	Duration	Concomitant Therapy	Used to Treat	Preparation	Administration
Nitroglycerin paste	NS	Topical	NS	NS	Vasopressors (dobutamine, dopamine, epinephrine, norepinephrine, phenylephrine)	N/A	N/A
Phentolamine	5 mg	SubQ	1 day	None	Vasopressors (dobutamine, dopamine, epinephrine, norepinephrine, phenylephrine)	Mix 5 mg with 9 mL NS	Inject a small amount into extravasated area. Blanching should reverse immediately. If blanching should recur, additional injections may be needed.
Sodium thiosulfate[1,5]	2%	SubQ	One time	Hydrocortisone 500 mg SubQ, betamethasone and gentamycin ointment q12h for 2 days, then qd	Doxorubicin, epirubicin, vinblastine, mitomycin	NS	Inject at 1 cm intervals around the area of extravasation.

MANAGEMENT OF DRUG EXTRAVASATIONS
(Continued)

Reported Treatment Regimens for Vesicant Drug Extravasations *(continued)*

Treatment	Dose	Route	Duration	Concomitant Therapy	Used to Treat	Preparation	Administration
Sodium thiosulfate[1,5]	1/6 M (~4%)	I.V., SubQ	One time	Cold or heat	Mechlorethamine, cisplatin	Mix 4 mL of 10% sodium thiosulfate with 6 mL sterile water	Inject 2 mL for each 1 mg of mechlorethamine or 100 mg cisplatin
Terbutaline	1 mg	SubQ	NS	NS	Vasopressors (dobutamine, dopamine, epinephrine, norepinephrine, phenylephrine)	NS	NS

N/A = Not applicable; NS = Not specified; I.V. = Intravenous; SubQ = Subcutaneous; I.D. = Intradermal.

[1]Listed in the package insert of at least one product.

[2]Most guidelines discourage application of cold to treat infiltrations of vinca alkaloids. Some reports discourage its use to treat infiltrations of epipodophyllotoxins and/or taxanes.

[3]There are conflicting data on the efficacy or heat or cold for infiltrations of epipodophyllotoxins and taxanes. Each approach has been reported to be effective, harmful, and of no discernable effect.

[4]DMSO concentrations >50% are not available for human use in the U.S.

[5]Large extravasations only.

Selected Readings

Bertelli G, "Prevention and Management of Extravasation of Cytotoxic Drugs," *Drug Safety*, 1995, 12(4):245-55.

Boyle DM and Engelking C, "Vesicant Extravasation: Myths and Realities," *Oncol Nurs Forum*, 1995, 22(1):57-67.

Kurul S, Saip P, and Aydin T, "Totally Implantable Venous-Access Ports: Local Problems and Extravasation Injury," *Lancet Oncol*, 2002, 3(11):684-92.

Larson DL, "What Is the Appropriate Management of Tissue Extravasation by Antitumor Agents?," *J Plast Reconstr Surg*, 1985, 75(3):397-402.

Larson DL, "Treatment of Tissue Extravasation by Antitumor Agents," *Cancer*, 1982, 49(9):1796-9.

Larson DL, "Alterations in Wound Healing Secondary to Infusion Injury," *Clin Plast Surg*, 1990, 17(3):509-17.

MacCara ME, "Extravasation: A Hazard of Intravenous Therapy," *Drug Intell Clin Pharm*, 1983, 17(10):713-7.

Schrijvers DL, "Extravasation: A Dreaded Complication of Chemotherapy," *Ann Oncol*, 2003, 14 Suppl 3:iii26-30.

Schulmeister L and Camp-Sorrell D, "Chemotherapy Extravasation From Implanted Ports," *Oncol Nurs Forum*, 2000, 27(3):531-8.

MANAGEMENT OF INFECTIONS

Certain oncology patients are at increased risk of morbidity and mortality from infectious complications secondary to disease- or treatment-related loss of immunity (see table). Impaired immunity is associated with malignancies that arise from hematologic cells and lymphoid tissues. Iatrogenic reasons for impaired immunity include splenectomy during staging of Hodgkin's disease and repeated courses of chemotherapy or radiation. Patients undergoing allogeneic bone marrow (stem cell) transplantation are at great risk for infectious complications because they generally have a hematologic malignancy, receive intensive chemotherapy prior to the bone marrow transplant, and require chronic immunosuppression to prevent graft-versus-host disease.

Disease-Related Risks for Infections

Cancer	Corresponding Normal Cell	Infectious Risk
Hodgkin's disease	Lymphoid?	Encapsulated bacteria; *Pneumocystis pneumoniae*; herpes simplex virus and varicella zoster virus; extensive chemotherapy/radiation
Non-Hodgkin's lymphoma	B cells (90%) T cells (10%)	*Pneumocystis pneumoniae*; herpes simplex virus and varicella zoster virus; extensive chemotherapy/radiation
Acute lymphoblastic leukemia	B cells (90%) T cells (10%)	Extensive chemotherapy/radiation
Acute myelogenous leukemia	Myelogenous cell	Extensive chemotherapy/radiation
Chronic lymphocytic leukemia	B cells (90%) T cells (10%)	Atypical infections secondary to chronic immune impairment with indolent course of disease

Treatment-related neutropenia increases the risk of developing infection. The likelihood of morbidity or mortality from infection increases as the depth and duration of neutropenia increase. An absolute neutrophil count (ANC) <500 cells/μL blood increases the risk of infectious complications. In fact, patients are considered "high-risk" neutropenics when the ANC is <500 cells/μL blood for more than 7 days. The ANC is calculated as follows.

$$ANC = \frac{WBC \times (\% \text{ segmented neutrophils} + \% \text{ band neutrophils})}{100\%}$$

The most frequent source of opportunistic pathogens is the patient or close human contacts. Common causes of gram-positive bacterial infections include *Staphylococcus aureus*, *Staphylococcus epidermidis*, *Streptococcus pneumoniae*, *Streptococcus pyogenes*, *Streptococcus viridans*, *Enterococcus faecalis*, *Enterococcus faecium*, and *Corynebacterium* spp. Common causes of gram-negative bacterial infections include *Escherichia coli*, *Klebsiella pneumoniae*, and *Pseudomonas* spp. *Candida albicans* generally colonizes mucous membranes of the gastrointestinal and urogenital tract. Environmental sources of opportunistic pathogens include the surface of fresh fruits and vegetables (bacteria), dried foliage, tobacco, marijuana leaves (*Aspergillus* spp); recent construction or renovation (*Aspergillus* spp); and tap water (*Legionella* spp). Rarely, viruses can be transmitted by blood products (packed red blood cells, platelets, stem cells) or plasma-derived products (intravenous immune globulin).

Thorough and frequent handwashing reduces the risk of transmitting opportunistic pathogens to neutropenic patients. In addition, limitation of the number of visitations and personal contacts also reduces opportunity for transmission of opportunistic pathogens. Additional preventive measures which are generally implemented to reduce the risk of infection in patients at greatest risk (eg, allogeneic bone marrow transplant patients) include hospital room-specific instrumentation, HEPA filtration of patient rooms or nursing units, total room clean following discharge, low microbial diets, and diligent mouth care. HEPA filtration involves circulation of room air through a filter 8-12 times per hour to remove small airborne particles. Low microbial diets prohibit ingestion of fresh fruits and vegetables, or undercooked meat. Diligent mouth care requires swishing and expectoration of mouthwash 4-6 times daily. Mouthwashes may be 0.9% NaCl or dilute bicarbonate solution (sodium bicarbonate 50 mEq/L in sterile water), because the greatest utility of mouth care is to remove oral debris and thereby prohibit microbial growth. However, chlorhexidine 0.12% may also be used as a mouthwash.

Selective gut decontamination using co-trimoxazole or a fluoroquinolone is used to reduce gram-negative colonization in patient undergoing intensive chemotherapy. Selective gut decontamination allows continued colonization of the lower gastrointestinal tract with anaerobic bacteria, which reduces the possibility of fungal overgrowth. High-risk patients undergoing treatment with intensive chemotherapy, such as allogeneic bone marrow transplant recipients, or patients with acute myelogenous leukemia undergoing induction chemotherapy, may also receive prophylactic acyclovir and fluconazole. Allogeneic bone marrow transplant recipients at risk for cytomegalovirus infection may receive prophylactic ganciclovir following engraftment.

Fever is frequently the only sign of infection in the neutropenic patient. Febrile neutropenic patients are empirically managed for presumed infection. Fever is defined as single oral temperature exceeding 38.3°C (101°F), or oral temperature 38°C (100.4°F) for at least 60 minutes. Evaluation of the febrile neutropenic patient should include history and physical examination, chest radiograph, blood cultures drawn from the central venous line (all ports), blood cultures drawn by peripheral venipuncture, specimens of urine and diarrheal stool, plus additional specimens as indicated by history and physical examination. Blood cultures must be drawn prior to initiation of antibiotics to increase the likelihood of acquiring a positive culture; although, blood cultures generally remain negative due to the small inoculum of microbes needed to cause infection in the neutropenic host and due to the early initiation of broad spectrum antibacterials. Empiric treatment with aggressive intravenous doses of broad spectrum, bactericidal antibiotics should be initiated as soon as possible after blood cultures have been collected. Antibiotics should be infused through alternating central venous line ports.

Antibiotic selection should include vancomycin for patients with severe mucositis, history of quinolone prophylaxis, colonization with methicillin-resistant *S. aureus*, or penicillin/cephalosporin-resistant *S. pneumoniae*, obvious central venous line involvement, hypotension, and

MANAGEMENT OF INFECTIONS *(Continued)*

sepsis. Vancomycin should be used in combination with a bactericidal agent with activity against gram-negative organisms, including *Pseudomonas* spp (eg, ceftazidime or aztreonam for penicillin-allergic patients). When criteria for use of vancomycin are not met, the patient may receive monotherapy (ceftazidime or imipenem), or dual therapy (aminoglycoside plus and antipseudomonal beta lactam or aztreonam for penicillin allergic patients) should be initiated. The choice for monotherapy versus dual therapy is determined by the patient's history and physical examination. The effect of antimicrobial therapy should be assessed in 72 hours or as indicated by the patient's clinical status.

The low-risk febrile neutropenic patient who defervesces within 72 hours following appropriate antibiotic therapy and is free of signs and symptoms of infection, may be converted to oral antibiotics (second generation cephalosporin or quinolone). Criteria for considering a patient high risk and continuing intravenous antibiotics include signs and symptoms of sepsis at presentation, additional signs of infection such as pneumonia or endocarditis, moderate-to-severe mucositis, dermal or mucosal loss of integrity, impending invasive procedure(s), or impending immunosuppressive therapy. If the patient remains febrile despite 72 hours of broad spectrum antibiotic coverage, the selection of antibiotics can be changed or additional antibiotics can be started. Vancomycin can be discontinued in patients who are clinically stable. Additional antibiotics should be added to patients who appear acutely ill from infection or are at high risk for infectious complications. The choice of antibiotic, which is dependant on current antimicrobial therapy in addition to the patient's history and physical examination, may include vancomycin, second gram-negative agent, amphotericin B, or antianaerobic agent. Treatment with amphotericin B should be started for patients with persistent fevers despite 5-7 days of appropriate empiric antibiotic therapy. Atypical pathogens, including invasive *Legionella pneumoniae*, molds (*Aspergillus* spp, *Fusarium* spp, mucormycoses), and viruses (cytomegalovirus, adenovirus), should be considered in the chronically immunosuppressed patient.

Positive cultures and antibiotic sensitivity reports may streamline therapy in the stable patient. However, the high-risk patient may continue receiving broad spectrum antibacterials because the finding of a specific pathogen does not exclude the possibility of additional infecting organisms in the neutropenic patient. Amphotericin B is the antifungal drug of choice for treatment of presumed fungal infection in the neutropenic patient. Central venous line removal is done judiciously due to the ongoing need for intravenous fluids, drugs, and blood products in the neutropenic and thrombocytopenic patient, and the risk of infection or bleeding with insertion of a new central venous line. Empiric antibiotics should be continued until the patient is afebrile and clinically stable. Empiric antibiotics can be discontinued after 7 days in the low-risk neutropenic patient. One may consider discontinuation of empiric antibiotics in the high-risk neutropenic patient following 5-7 days without fever. Antibiotics should be continued until neutrophil recovery for patients with ANC >100 cells/μL, severe mucositis, or signs and symptoms of sepsis. Four to 5 days following resolution of neutropenia, discontinuation of antibiotics may be considered in the low-risk, neutropenic, clinically stable patient with persistent fevers. With close observation and follow-up, antibiotics may be discontinued after 2 weeks of therapy in the clinically stable patient with persistent fever and persistent neutropenia.

Colony stimulating factors, which reduce the duration of neutropenia, are helpful in reducing hospital admission for neutropenic fevers in patients with a history of febrile neutropenia or prolonged neutropenia following outpatient chemotherapy.

Selected Readings

Hughes WT, Armstrong D, Bodey GP, et al, "1997 Guidelines for the Use of Antimicrobial Agents in Neutropenic Patients With Unexplained Fever," *Clin Infect Dis*, 1997, 25:551-73.

Maki DG, Alvarado CJ, Hassemer CA, et al, "Relation of the Inanimate Hospital Environment to Endemic Nosocomial Infection," *N Engl J Med*, 1982, 307(25):1562-5.

Pizzo PA, Hathorn JW, Hiemenz J, et al, "A Randomized Trial Comparing Ceftazidime Alone With Combination Antibiotic Therapy in Cancer Patients With Fever and Neutropenia," *N Engl J Med*, 1986, 315(9):552-8.

MANAGEMENT OF NAUSEA AND VOMITING

> **Nausea:** The feeling or sensation of an imminent desire to vomit.
>
> **Vomiting:** The forceful upward expulsion of gastric contents.
>
> **Retching:** Rhythmic, labored, spasmodic respiratory movements involving the diaphragm, chest wall, and abdominal muscles.

Nausea and vomiting are common side effects of many antineoplastic agents and are often the effects patients fear most. Uncontrolled nausea and vomiting can have a significant impact on a patient's overall therapy and response to treatment. In addition to the deleterious effect on the patient's attitude and quality of life, nausea and vomiting can cause significant, potentially fatal complications. Uncontrolled nausea and vomiting can result in dehydration, electrolyte imbalances, weight loss, and malnutrition. Prolonged vomiting and retching can cause esophageal and/or gastric ruptures (Mallory-Weiss tears, Boerhaave's syndrome) and bleeding. Patients with poorly-controlled nausea or vomiting often require interruptions or delays in therapy. This can also lead to development of anticipatory nausea and vomiting, the patient's loss of confidence in the overall therapy, noncompliance, and refusal of further therapy.

Table 1. Causes of Nausea or Vomiting

Abdominal Emergencies
    Appendicitis
    Cholecystitis
    Peritonitis
    GI obstruction

Acute Systemic Infections
    Bacterial
    Parasitic
    Viral

Cardiovascular Disorders
    Congestive heart failure
    Myocardial infarction

CNS Disorders
    Hypotension
    Increased intracranial pressure
    Mènière's disease
    Otitis interna
    Syncope

Drugs
    Antibiotics
    Antineoplastics
    Aspirin
    Cardiac glycosides
    Levodopa
    Nonsteroidal anti-inflammatory agents
    Opiates
    Quinidine
    Steroids
    Theophylline

Endocrine Disorders
    Adrenal insufficiency
    Diabetes mellitus

Gastrointestinal Disorders

Pregnancy

Psychogenic Stimuli

Uremia

Emesis is controlled by a complex system, centering on the vomiting (or emetic) center in the medulla, and the chemoreceptor trigger zone (CTZ) located in the area postrema in the fourth ventricle of the brain. A network of various neuroreceptors, located throughout the gastrointestinal tract and CNS, processes signals to and from the emetic center and CTZ. When stimulated by impulses from visceral afferents, vestibular or limbic systems, cerebral cortex, or chemoreceptor trigger zone, the emetic center transmits signals that initiate the vomiting cascade. These impulses from the emetic center stimulate the salivary, vasomotor, respiratory centers, and cranial nerves, and initiate the vomiting reflex. Activation of the vomiting center appears to be crucial to initiation of vomiting. Elimination of the vomiting center, or failure to stimulate it, completely eliminates vomiting.

Receptors for a large number of different neurotransmitters, including dopamine, serotonin, acetylcholine, histamine, opiates, and benzodiazepines, are involved in the vomiting reflex. Blockade of one or more of these receptors is the basic mechanism of action of most antiemetic agents. Most drug-induced nausea, including that provoked by the antineoplastic drugs, appears to be caused by activation of the emetic center by impulses from the peripheral afferents and/or the CTZ. Blockade of these impulses is a primary focus of antiemetic therapy.

Patterns of Drug-Induced Nausea / Vomiting

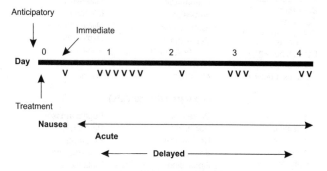

Nausea and vomiting caused by cytotoxic therapy generally falls into one of three categories: immediate, acute, or delayed. While not drug-induced *per se*, a fourth syndrome, anticipatory nausea and vomiting, is also a relatively common complication of antineoplastic therapy. Immediate nausea/vomiting occurs within the first 30-120 minutes of drug administration. Acute nausea/vomiting is seen within the first 24 hours of drug administration. These two syndromes are often grouped together under the term acute nausea/vomiting. Delayed nausea/vomiting begins after the first 24 hours of drug administration; however, in some cases, onset may be delayed for as long as 3-5 days. Even in the absence of actual emesis, patients may experience varying degrees of nausea, often accompanied by anorexia.

MANAGEMENT OF NAUSEA AND VOMITING
(Continued)

Table 2 describes the emetogenic potential of many of the antineoplastic agents. Several factors affect the emetic potential of these agents. For some drugs, such as cyclophosphamide or methotrexate, the dose given has a significant effect on the drug's emetogenicity. Higher doses of these agents are much more emetogenic than low doses. The method of administration can also affect the incidence of nausea. Cytarabine, when given as a continuous infusion, is generally moderately emetogenic; higher doses given as short infusions usually produce a much higher incidence and severity of nausea and vomiting.

Table 2. Emetogenic Potential of Antineoplastic Agents

Very High (>90%)

Cisplatin	Didemnin-B	Melphalan (I.V.)
Cytarabine (>2 g)	JM-216	Streptozocin
Dacarbazine	Mechlorethamine	

High (60% to 90%)

Aldesleukin	Elsamitrucin	Irinotecan
Amifostine	Epirubicin	Lomustine
Arsenic trioxide	Estramustine	Mitomycin
Bortezomib	Etoposide	Mitotane
Carmustine	Gemcitabine	Mitoxantorone
Cyclophosphamide (>1 g)	Gemtuzumab ozogamicin	Oxaliplatin
Cytarabine (<2 g)	Hydroxyurea	Pemetrexed
Dactinomycin	Idarubicin	Toremifene
Denileukin diftitox		Tretinoin

Moderate (30% to 60%)

Alemtuzumab	Diazequone	Pegaspargase
Altretamine	Docetaxel	Pentostatin
Aminocamptothecin	Doxorubicin	Plicamycin
Amonafide	Epirubicin	Procarbazine
Amsacrine	Floxuridine	Raltitrexed
Asparaginase	Flutamide	Temozolomide
Azacitidine	Fulvestrant	Teniposide
Bevacizumab	Gefitinib	Tomudex
Carboplatin	Ibritumomab	Topotecan
Cetuximab	Ifosfamide	Tositumomab
Cladribine	Imatinib	Trastuzumab
Cyclophosphamide (<1 g)	Interferons	Trimetrexate
Daunorubicin	Interleukin-6	UFT
Daunorubicin (liposomal)	Mitoguazone	Vinblastine
Dexrazoxane	PALA	Vinorelbine

Low (10% to 30%)

Abarelix	Flutamide	Nilutamide
BCG vaccine	Fulvestrant	Porfimer
Bexarotene	Gefitinib	Rituximab
Cetuximab	Gemcitabine	Steroids
Cytarabine (liposomal)	Letrozole	Suramin
Doxorubicin (liposomal)	Levamisole	Tamoxifen
Etoposide phosphate	Melphalan (oral)	Thioguanine
Exemestane	Methotrexate	Vindesine
Floxuridine	(high dose)	
Fluorouracil		

Very Low (<10%)

Alitretinoin	Estrogens	Mesna
Androgens	Fludarabine	Methotrexate (low dose)
Aminoglutethimide	Goserelin	Paclitaxel
Anastrozole	Homoharringtonine	Thalidomide
Bicalutamide	Leucovorin	Thiotepa
Bleomycin	Leuprolide	Triptorelin
Busulfan	Megestrol	Valrubicin
Chlorambucil	Mercaptopurine	Vincristine

Drugs With a High Incidence But Low Severity of Nausea / Vomiting

Amonafide	Hydroxyurea
Carboplatin	Interferons
Cyclophosphamide (<1 g)	Mitoguazone
Dexrazoxane	Mitoxantrone
Docetaxel	Tretinoin
Gemcitabine	Vinblastine

Drugs With a Low Incidence But High Severity of Nausea / Vomiting

Lomustine	Semustine
Methotrexate (high dose)	

DELAYED NAUSEA AND VOMITING

The problem of delayed nausea and vomiting has become more obvious within the last few years. As more effective drugs and combination regimens were developed to control acute nausea/vomiting, the delayed syndrome has emerged as a more significant problem. Although it is most commonly associated with cisplatin, delayed nausea may also be seen in patients receiving mitomycin, cyclophosphamide, or ifosfamide. The nausea or vomiting generally begins within 48-72 hours after chemotherapy administration, but may be seen as early as 16-18 hours after drug administration, or as late as 4 or 5 days. The nausea/vomiting usually resolves over 2 or 3 days. The exact cause of this effect is not clear; however, it is believed to have a separate mechanism from acute nausea or vomiting. Gastritis, tissue destruction, electrolyte fluctuations, or effects on the central or peripheral nervous system have all been postulated as possible mechanisms for delayed nausea.

MANAGEMENT OF NAUSEA AND VOMITING
(Continued)

Appropriate therapy for delayed nausea and vomiting remains problematic. Current information seems to support early prophylactic therapy with a steroid, steroid/serotonin antagonist, or steroid/dopamine antagonist combination as the most effective therapy for delayed nausea and vomiting. In patients refractory to a steroid/serotonin regimen, aprepitant, a neurokinin receptor antagonist, may be added. The current approach to delayed nausea and vomiting tends to favor a scheduled, prophylactic regimen of dexamethasone, or dexamethasone/serotonin or dopamine antagonist combination, beginning 16-24 hours after administration of the chemotherapy, and continuing for 2-5 days. This approach is more advantageous than intermittent intervention with a $5HT_3$ antagonist.

BREAKTHROUGH NAUSEA AND VOMITING

Continuing the same regimen that failed to prevent vomiting usually is not desirable. There is little evidence that breakthrough vomiting may respond to an additional dose(s) of a serotonin blocker. A scheduled regimen of "conventional" antiemetics is probably more effective than intermittent administration of a $5HT_3$ antagonist. Merely increasing the dose of the serotonin antagonist may not be an option either. The currently available serotonin antagonists have relatively flat dose/response curves. Dose response studies have demonstrated that granisetron's efficacy seems to reach a plateau at 10 mcg/kg. There appears to be no difference in efficacy between granisetron doses of 10 mcg/kg and 40 mcg/kg. A similar limitation exists for dolasetron, ondansetron, and palonosetron. A number of reports suggests that ondansetron doses between 20-32 mg have comparable efficacy in preventing nausea induced by a variety of antineoplastic drugs. Daily doses >32 mg seem to provide no increase in response. Data are also lacking on the value of using a different serotonin antagonist to treat nausea/vomiting resulting from the failure of the initial serotonin antagonist regimen.

Likewise, there is minimal information regarding the appropriate prophylactic antiemetic regimen for subsequent chemotherapy cycles, both in patients who responded well during the initial treatment cycle, and in patients who do not respond well to the initial serotonin antagonist/steroid regimen. Several reports suggest the efficacy of the initial antiemetic regimen diminishes over time. Patients often experience gradual increased incidences of nausea and vomiting during subsequent treatment cycles. A number of possible alternatives exist, including switching to another serotonin antagonist, switching to a nonserotonin modulating antiemetic, adding a nonserotonin blocking antiemetic to the original regimen, and altering the schedule of drug administration. The addition of a neurokinin receptor antagonist (eg, aprepitant) to the previous serotonin antagonist/steroid regimen is recommended. One study suggests that the addition of low-dose propofol to the steroid/serotonin antagonist may be useful.

Table 3. Classification of Antiemetic Agents

Antihistamines	Diphenhydramine, hydroxyzine, promethazine
Anticholinergics	Scopolamine
Benzodiazepines	Diazepam, lorazepam
Butyrophenones	Droperidol, haloperidol
Cannabinoids	Dronabinol, nabilone
Corticosteroids	Dexamethasone, methylprednisolone
Neurokinin antagonists	Aprepitant, ezlopitant,[1] vofopitant,[1] L-758298,[1] CP-122721[1]
Phenothiazines	Chlorpromazine, perphenazine, prochlorperazine, thiethylperazine,[1] triflupromazine, (promethazine)
Serotonin antagonists	Dolasetron, granisetron, ondansetron, palonosetron, tropesitron[1]
Substituted benzamides	Metoclopramide, trimethobenzamide

[1]Not commercially available in the U.S.

Table 4. Site of Action of Antiemetic Agents

Emetic center	Antihistamines, anticholinergics, serotonin antagonists
Chemoreceptor trigger zone (CTZ)	Benzamides, butyrophenones, phenothiazines
Cerebral cortex	Antihistamines, benzodiazepines, cannabinoids, (corticosteroids), neurokinin antagonists(?)
Peripheral	Metoclopramide, neurokinin antagonists, serotonin antagonists
Unknown	Corticosteroids

Table 5. Equitherapeutic Serotonin Antagonist Doses

Drug	Oral	I.V.
Dolasetron	100-200 mg	1.8 mg/kg or 100 mg
Granisetron	2 mg	10 mcg/kg or 1 mg
Ondansetron	8-24 mg	8-10 mg
Palonosetron	–	0.25 mg

Anticholinergics. Alkaloids (eg, atropine and scopolamine) exhibit some antiemetic activity, primarily postoperative nausea and vomiting, and motion sickness. The apparent mechanism of action is blockage of central muscarinic receptors. Toxicities such as sedation, restlessness, blurred vision, and dry mouth limit the systemic use of these agents. Transdermal application of scopolamine is sometimes helpful as an adjunct in delayed nausea, or in treating prolonged mild nausea seen occasionally. The recent lack of availability of the transdermal scopolamine formulation effectively precludes use of this drug for chemotherapy-induced nausea.

Antihistamines. The antihistamines block H_1 receptors both centrally and in the middle ear. A number of drugs in this class are effective against motion

MANAGEMENT OF NAUSEA AND VOMITING
(Continued)

sickness and labyrinth disorders; but only diphenhydramine, hydroxyzine, and promethazine seem to have any activity against chemotherapy-induced nausea or vomiting. The major toxicities seen with these drugs are drowsiness, sedation, and dry mouth. These agents are most commonly used to enhance the efficacy of combination antiemetic regimens, although hydroxyzine or promethazine are occasionally used to treat mild-to-moderate nausea in patients who cannot tolerate, or are refractory to, other antiemetics. Diphenhydramine is frequently used in combination with dopamine antagonists to prevent extrapyramidal reactions often seen with those agents.

Benzodiazepines. The exact antiemetic mechanism or location of action of the benzodiazepines is unclear. An inhibitory effect on the vomiting center, anxiolytic activity, and general CNS depression have all been postulated. Possible sites of action include the limbic system, vomiting center, cerebrum, and brain stem. The most common side effects include sedation, drowsiness, and amnesia. Lorazepam is the most commonly used benzodiazepine, but midazolam and diazepam have also been used. As single agents, the benzodiazepines have only mild antiemetic activity. Benzodiazepines are commonly used as adjuncts to conventional antiemetics in the prophylaxis and treatment of acute nausea and vomiting. In this setting, the anterograde amnesia induced by the benzodiazepine is usually considered a desired therapeutic effect rather than an adverse reaction. The benzodiazepines are also highly effective in the prevention of anticipatory nausea and vomiting, possibly due to their anxiolytic effect.

Butyrophenones. A group of dopamine antagonists that is occasionally useful in treating chemotherapy-induced nausea and vomiting is the butyrophenones. Both haloperidol and droperidol have been reported to have antiemetic activity against moderate-to-highly emetogenic chemotherapy. Domperidone, a related drug, is also reported to have antiemetic activity; however, significant cardiovascular toxicities have limited trials with this drug. As with most other antiemetics, the optimum response to the butyrophenones is seen in multidrug regimens. Like other dopamine blockers, extrapyramidal reactions, restlessness, sedation, and hypotension are relatively common side effects.

Cannabinoids. Proper evaluation of the antiemetic activity of cannabinoid derivatives has been hindered by social and political stigmas associated with marijuana use. Tetrahydrocannabinol, levonantradol, and nabilone are all reported to be effective in treating chemotherapy-induced nausea and vomiting. The specific site and mechanism of activity is unclear. Inhibition of endorphins in the emetic center, suppression of prostaglandin synthesis, and inhibition of medullary activity through an unspecified cortical action have all been postulated. Cannabinoids can inhibit buildup of cyclic adenosine monophosphate, and cannabinoid receptors have been identified in the hippocampus, hypothalamus, and cortex. What role, if any, these have in the control of nausea and vomiting is not known. Cannabinoids seem to be most effective against mild-to-moderately emetogenic chemotherapy. Blurred vision, hypotension, and tachycardia, and a number of CNS complications, including euphoria, dysphoria, hallucinations, and sedation are seen with cannabinoid therapy. Cannabinoids are not often used as initial antiemetic therapy, but do offer an alternative in patients unable to tolerate, or who are refractory to, other antiemetic agents.

Corticosteroids. The mechanism of antiemetic activity for the steroids is unknown, although alterations of cell permeability and inhibition of prostaglandin activity have been postulated. In spite of this uncertainty, corticosteroids, particularly dexamethasone, are frequent components of combination antiemetic regimens for high-to-moderately emetogenic chemotherapy. As a single agent, dexamethasone appears to be equal to, or more effective than, $5HT_3$ antagonists for delayed nausea and vomiting. For patients in whom a corticosteroid is not clearly contraindicated, these agents are an important component of antiemetic therapy.

Neurokinin-1 (NK_1) Receptor Antagonists. Neurokinin, or substance P, antagonists are the latest class of antiemetics. Substance P is a tachykinin (neurokinin) located in neurons of the central and peripheral nervous system. It is associated with a variety of functions, including emesis, depression, inflammatory pain and inflammatory/immune responses in asthma, and other diseases. Substance P's activity is mediated by the NK_1 receptor, a G-protein receptor coupled to the inositol phosphate signal pathway. Blocking this receptor is a mechanism to treat conditions mediated at least in part by substance P. Several neurokinin receptor antagonists, including aprepitant (MK-869, L-754030), its prodrug L-758298, ezlopitant (CJ-11974), vofopitant (GR-205171), and CP-122721 have been studied, but aprepitant is the only one that has been approved for marketing. NK_1 antagonists are effective in preventing cisplatin-induced nausea and vomiting, when used in conjunction with a serotonin antagonist and steroid. Addition of a neurokinin antagonist to a serotonin ($5HT_3$) antagonist and steroid combination increases control of acute nausea by 10% to 15%, and control of delayed nausea by 20% to 30%. Most studies indicate the neurokinin receptors are less effective then serotonin antagonists, particularly for prevention of acute nausea within the first 8-12 hours. However, the neurokinin antagonists appear to be more effective than serotonin antagonists in preventing delayed nausea (days 2-5). Although the National Cancer Coordinating Network (NCCN) and Multinational Association of Supportive Cancer Care (MASCC) guidelines include use of aprepitant as initial therapy for highly emetogenic regimens, other guidelines [American Society of Clinical Oncology (ASCO), American Society of Health-System Pharmacists (ASHP)], and most practitioners reserve these agents for patients who develop vomiting after receiving an appropriate serotonin antagonist and steroid antiemetic regimen.

Phenothiazines. Phenothiazines were the first class of drugs accepted as antiemetic therapy for antineoplastic chemotherapy. Blockade of dopamine (D_2) receptors in the area postrema (chemoreceptor trigger zone and vomiting center) appears to be their primary mechanism of action. A number of different drugs, including chlorpromazine, perphenazine, prochlorperazine, promethazine, and thiethylperazine (no longer marketed in the United States), have antiemetic activity. Common toxicities such as extrapyramidal reactions, restlessness, sedation, and hypotension limit the use of these drugs. In generally tolerated doses, the phenothiazines are most effective against mild-to-moderate nausea or vomiting, but have little impact on emesis from highly emetogenic agents such as dacarbazine or cisplatin. Higher doses of these agents may have increased activity, but the increased

MANAGEMENT OF NAUSEA AND VOMITING
(Continued)

incidence and severity of side effects usually prohibits their use. Since the serotonin antagonists became available, use of the phenothiazines generally has been limited to prevention of nausea from mildly emetogenic chemotherapy, treatment of breakthrough nausea/vomiting in patients refractory to a serotonin blocker, or in association with dexamethasone to treat delayed nausea.

Serotonin (5HT$_3$) Antagonists. A major advance in antiemetic therapy was the introduction of the serotonin (5HT$_3$) antagonists. The high efficacy rate of these agents in preventing acute nausea and vomiting, coupled with their low incidence of side effects, has made them the preferred choice in this setting. The major limitation to their use has been economic. The high cost of serotonin antagonists has resulted in many institutions placing severe limitations on their use. Most comparisons have shown that a serotonin antagonist/steroid combination is significantly better than either agent alone. For prevention of acute nausea and vomiting caused by highly emetogenic antineoplastic regimens, a serotonin antagonist/steroid combination usually represents the most effective antiemetic therapy. Since there seems to be little difference in efficacy or toxicity among the available serotonin antagonists, selection of a specific agent is a matter of institutional or prescriber preference.

In spite of their popularity, the serotonin antagonists are not the complete solution to treatment-induced emesis. Some trials have found no difference in efficacy between serotonin antagonist-based regimens and previously used combinations, leaving toxicity, convenience, and economic issues as the discriminating factors in drug selection. Two particular questions concerning serotonin antagonist use remain unanswered: appropriate second-line therapy for treatment failures, and use in noncisplatin regimens.

Like any medication, serotonin antagonists are not 100% effective. Approximately 40% to 60% of patients receiving serotonin antagonist monotherapy will experience some nausea, or have at least one episode of vomiting. Addition of a steroid to the regimen reduces the failure rate significantly, with some trials reporting only 10% to 15% of patients failing the initial therapy. Regardless of the initial antiemetic therapy, some patients will experience one or more episodes of vomiting following administration of the cytotoxic therapy. Choice of a salvage antiemetic regimen for these patients is problematic. Controlled trials of the serotonin antagonists have focused primarily on prevention of nausea/vomiting. Only a few small uncontrolled reports relate to their utility as salvage therapy to terminate vomiting once it begins.

Most studies in patients receiving chemotherapy over several consecutive days suggest the serotonin antagonists have their greatest protective effect in the initial 24 hours, and possibly the initial 16-18 hours, of a chemotherapy cycle. These factors further limit the usefulness of serotonin antagonists in patients who experience nausea/vomiting following prophylactic antiemetic therapy with one of these agents.

Substituted Benzamides. Metoclopramide is the most commonly used antiemetic drug in this category. Prior to introduction of the 5HT$_3$ antagonists, high-dose (2-3 mg/kg) metoclopramide was the preferred drug for prevention of nausea/vomiting from highly emetogenic chemotherapy. Metoclopramide's ability to block central and peripheral dopamine receptors was believed to be the mechanism of it's antiemetic activity. Recognition that high doses also blocked serotonin receptors led to identification of the role serotonin inhibition has in preventing nausea/vomiting, and, ultimately, to development of the $5HT_3$ antagonists. Like the phenothiazines, use of metoclopramide is complicated by extrapyramidal reactions, restlessness, sedation, and hypotension. Diarrhea is also a significant side effect, especially with the high doses used for antiemetic therapy. Also like the phenothiazines, the current use of metoclopramide is generally limited to prevention of nausea from mild-to-moderately emetogenic chemotherapy, treatment of breakthrough nausea/vomiting, or to treat delayed nausea.

REPRESENTATIVE ANTIEMETIC REGIMENS

HIGHLY EMETOGENIC CHEMOTHERAPY

Dexamethasone 10-20 mg P.O. or I.V. + a serotonin antagonist daily 15-30 minutes before treatment on each day of chemotherapy

> Recommended serotonin antagonist regimens:
> > **Dolasetron 100-200 mg P.O.** once daily
> > **Dolasetron 1.8 mg/kg I.V.** once daily
> > **Dolasetron 100 mg I.V.** once daily
> > **Granisetron 2 mg P.O.** once daily
> > **Granisetron 1 mg P.O.** q12h
> > **Granisetron 10 mcg/kg I.V.** once daily
> > **Granisetron 1 mg I.V.** once daily
> > **Ondansetron 0.45 mg/kg I.V.** once daily
> > **Ondansetron 8-16 mg I.V.** once daily
> > **Ondansetron 8-10 mg I.V.** q8h
> > **Ondansetron 16-24 mg P.O.** q12-24h
> > **Palonosetron 0.25 mg I.V.** day 1 of each cycle
> > *(doses should not be given more than once weekly)*

For continuous infusion therapy, carboplatin and high-dose (>1 g/m^2) cyclophosphamide regimens, the following regimen may be preferred:

> **Dexamethasone 10 mg P.O. or I.V. + a serotonin antagonist** q12h

> Recommended serotonin antagonist regimens:
> > **Granisetron 1 mg P.O.**
> > **Granisetron 10 mcg/kg I.V.**
> > **Ondansetron 8-16 mg I.V.**
> > **Ondansetron 16-24 mg P.O.**
> > **Palonosetron 0.25 mg I.V.** day 1 of each cycle
> > *(doses should not be given more than once weekly)*

Refractory patients: Add:
> **Aprepitant 125 mg** P.O. 30-60 minutes before treatment, then
> **Aprepitant 80 mg** P.O. days 2 and 3

MANAGEMENT OF NAUSEA AND VOMITING
(Continued)

MODERATELY EMETOGENIC CHEMOTHERAPY

Dexamethasone 10 mg P.O. or I.V. + a serotonin antagonist daily 15-30 minutes before treatment on each day of chemotherapy

Recommended serotonin antagonist regimens:
> **Ondansetron 8-16 mg P.O.** once daily
> **Ondansetron 8 mg P.O.** q12h
> **Ondansetron 8-10 mg I.V.** once daily

For continuous infusion therapy, the following regimen may be preferred:

> **Dexamethasone 4 mg P.O. or I.V. + ondansetron 8 mg P.O. or I.V.** q12h on each day of chemotherapy

MILDLY EMETOGENIC CHEMOTHERAPY

All agents are given 15-30 minutes before treatment and may be repeated every 4-6 hours, if necessary. With the exceptions of dexamethasone (given over 5-15 minutes) and droperidol (given by I.V. push), intravenous doses should be given over 30 minutes.

> **Dexamethasone 4 mg P.O./I.V./I.M.**
> **Droperidol 1.25-5 mg I.M./I.V. push**
> **Haloperidol 2 mg P.O./I.V./I.M.**
> **Metoclopramide 20-40 mg P.O./I.V./I.M.**
> **Prochlorperazine 10-20 mg P.O./I.V./I.M.**

DELAYED NAUSEA AND VOMITING

Dexamethasone + a dopamine, neurokinen, or serotonin antagonist. Therapy should start within 12-24 hours of administration of the emetogenic chemotherapy.

Recommended regimens:
> **Dexamethasone**
> 8 mg P.O. q12h for 2 days, then 4 mg P.O. q12h for 2 days
> **or**
> 20 mg P.O. 1 hour before chemotherapy; 10 mg P.O. 12 hours after chemotherapy, then 8 mg P.O. q12h for 4 doses, then 4 mg P.O. q12h for 4 doses

Recommended dopamine/neurokinin/serotonin antagonist regimens:
> **Droperidol 1.25-2.5 mg I.V./I.M. q4h** for 2-4 days
> **Metoclopramide 0.5 mg/kg P.O. q6h** for 2-4 days
> **Ondansetron 8 mg P.O. q8h** for 2-4 days
> **Prochlorperazine 10 mg P.O. q6h** for 2-4 days
> **Aprepitant 125 mg P.O.** day 1, **80 mg P.O.** days 2 and 3

GENERAL PRINCIPLES FOR MANAGING NAUSEA AND VOMITING

1. **Prophylaxis is *MUCH* better than treatment of actual vomiting**. For agents with a moderate-to-high (30% to 100%) incidence of nausea, patients should be pretreated with an antiemetic. Depending on the antiemetic agent(s) and route(s) of administration, pretreatment may range from 1 hour to 5 minutes prior to administration of the antineoplastic agent(s).

2. **Doses and intervals of the antiemetic regimen need to be individualized for each patient**. "PRN" regimens should **not** be used. A fixed schedule of drug administration is preferable.

3. **If a patient has had no nausea for 24 hours** while on their scheduled antiemetic regimen, **it is usually possible to switch to a "PRN" regimen**. The patient should be advised to resume the fixed schedule *at the FIRST sign of recurrent nausea*, and continue it until they have had at least 24 hours without nausea.

4. **Titrate antiemetic dose to patient tolerance**.

5. In most cases, **combination regimens are required for optimum control of nausea**. Do not be afraid to use two or more agents, *from different pharmacologic categories*, to achieve optimal results.

6. To the extent possible, **avoid duplication of agents from the same pharmacologic category**.

7. **Anticipatory nausea and vomiting can often be minimized if the patient receives effective prophylaxis against nausea from the first cycle of therapy**.

8. **If anticipatory nausea does develop, an anxiolytic agent is usually the drug of choice**.

9. **"If it's not broken – DON'T fix it!"** Regardless of your own preferences, if the patient's current antiemetic regimen is working, don't change it.

10. **For moderately emetogenic regimens, a steroid and dopamine blocker** (eg, metoclopramide, prochlorperazine) **is usually the most cost-effective regimen**.

11. **For highly emetogenic regimens, a steroid and serotonin receptor blocker** (eg, dolasetron, granisetron, ondansetron) **combination is the preferred regimen**.

12. **A neurokinin blocker** (eg, aprepitant) **is a good first alternative if the serotonin blocker fails**. A dopamine antagonist (eg, metoclopramide, prochlorperazine) may also be effective.

13. Although most nausea or vomiting develops within the first 24 hours after treatment, **delayed reactions (1-7 days after chemotherapy) are not uncommon**.

14. **Other antiemetics, such as cannabinoids, antihistamines, or anticholinergics) have limited use as initial therapy**. They are best used in combination with more effective agents (steroids, dopamine, or serotonin blockers); or, as second- or third-line therapy.

MANAGEMENT OF NAUSEA AND VOMITING
(Continued)

15. **Serotonin and neurokinin blockers are most effective in scheduled prophylactic regimens**; rather than in "PRN" regimens to chase existing vomiting.

16. **Serotonin and neurokinin antagonists have limited efficacy in stopping nausea or vomiting once it has begun.** A dopamine blocker may be more effective.

17. **The serotonin blockers appear to have a "ceiling" dose**, above which there is little or no added antiemetic effect.

18. **Serotonin antagonists are most effective within the first 24-48 hours.** Most studies of multiple day dosing show a sharp decline in the efficacy of the serotonin antagonists after the second or third day.

19. **Neurokinin antagonists are not very effective as single agents**, and should only be used in combination with a serotonin antagonist and steroid.

Selected References

"ASHP Therapeutic Guidelines on the Pharmacologic Management of Nausea and Vomiting in Adult and Pediatric Patients Receiving Chemotherapy or Radiation Therapy or Undergoing Surgery", *Am J Health Syst Pharm*, 1999, 56(8):729-64.

De Wit R, "Current Position of 5HT$_3$ Antagonists and the Additional Value of NK$_1$ Antagonists; A New Class of Antiemetics," *Br J Cancer*, 2003, 88(12):1823-7.

Gralla RJ, Osoba D, Kris MG, et al, "Recommendations for the Use of Antiemetics: Evidence-Based, Clinical Practice Guidelines," *J Clin Oncol*, 1999, 17(9):2971-94.

Graves T, "Emesis as a Complication of Cancer Chemotherapy: Pathophysiology, Importance, and Treatment," *Pharmacotherapy*, 1992, 12(4):337-45.

Grunberg SM and Hesketh PJ, —Control of Chemotherapy-Induced Emesis," *N Engl J Med*, 1993, 329(24):1790-6.

Hesketh PJ, Kris MG, Grunberg SM, et al, "Proposal for Classifying the Acute Emetogenicity of Cancer Chemotherapy," *J Clin Oncol*, 1997, 15(1):103-9.

Hesketh PJ, Van Belle S, Aapro M, et al, "Differential Involvement of Neurotransmitters Through the Time Course of Cisplatin-Induced Emesis as Revealed by Therapy With Specific Receptor Antagonists," *Eur J Cancer*, 2003, 39(8):1074-80.

Holdsworth MT, "Ethical Issues Regarding Study Designs Used in Serotonin-Antagonist Drug Development," *Ann Pharmacother*, 1996, 30(10):1182-4.

NCCN Antiemesis Practice Guidelines, The Complete Library of NCCN Oncology Practice Guidelines, Rockledge, PA: National Comprehensive Cancer Network, 2004; www.nccn.org.

"Prevention of Chemotherapy- and Radiotherapy-Induced Emesis: Results of Perugia Consensus Conference. Antiemetic Subcommittee of the Multinational Association of Supportive Care in Cancer (MASCO)," *Ann Oncol*, 1998, 9(8):811-9.

MUCOSITIS/STOMATITIS

Mucositis and stomatitis are general terms for the erythema, edema, desquamation, and ulceration of the gastrointestinal tract caused by many antineoplastic drugs and external beam radiation therapy (radiotherapy). Stomatitis refers to the finding of mucositis in the mouth or oropharynx. Gastrointestinal complications of mucositis include pain, xerostomia, bloating, diarrhea, malabsorption, and dysmotility. Severe mucositis increases the risk of infectious complications and airway compromise. In addition, severe and prolonged mucositis contributes to anticancer treatment dosage reductions and delays and increases the cost of therapy.

The severity of chemotherapy-associated mucositis is related to drug selection, increased dose, combination versus single agent chemotherapy, extended infusion of cell cycle-specific chemotherapy drugs, and concurrent radiotherapy. The frequency of severe mucositis for patients undergoing standard dose therapy and high dose therapy is 5% to 40% and 60% to 100%, respectively. The risk of mucositis from methotrexate administration is increased in patients with Down syndrome or carriers of the methylenetetrahydrofolate reductase *677 TT* genotype. The severity of mucositis secondary to radiotherapy is related to the anatomic site of radiation exposure, radiation dose, and dosage fractionation. Grade 3 to 4 mucositis occurs in more than 50% of patients undergoing radiotherapy to the head and neck, abdomen, or pelvis. Table 1 lists various anticancer treatments associated with severe mucositis. The duration and severity of regimen-related mucositis can be increased by concurrent infections from opportunistic bacterial or viral pathogens affecting the gastrointestinal tract. Moreover, graft-versus-host disease can worsen regimen-related mucositis following allogeneic hematopoietic stem cell transplantation.

MUCOSITIS/STOMATITIS *(Continued)*

Standard Dose Regimens Associated With Grade 3-4 Mucositis

Occurring in ≥30% of Patients	Occurring in ≥10% of Patients
Anthracycline + docetaxel + fluorouracil	Anthracycline + cyclophosphamide
	Anthracycline + taxane
Taxane + radiotherapy	
	Anthracycline + cyclophosphamide + docetaxel
Docetaxel + fluorouracil	
Paclitaxel + fluorouracil + radiotherapy	Anthracycline + docetaxel + platinum
Taxane + platinum + radiotherapy	Docetaxel
Taxane + platinum + fluorouracil	Platinum + radiotherapy
Oxaliplatin + radiotherapy	
	Platinum + gemcitabine + taxane
Platinum + taxane + radiotherapy	
	Platinum + taxane + irinotecan
Fluorouracil CIV[1] +	
	Platinum + methotrexate + leucovorin
platinum + radiotherapy	
	Fluorouracil CIV[1]
Fluorouracil + leucovorin + taxane	
	Fluorouracil CIV[1] + radiotherapy
Irinotecan	
	Fluorouracil CIV[1] + platinum
Irinotecan + fluorouracil + radiotherapy	
	Fluorouracil + leucovorin
Irinotecan + fluorouracil + leucovorin	
	Fluorouracil + leucovorin + mitomycin
Irinotecan + fluorouracil + leucovorin + platinum	
	Irinotecan + taxane

[1] CIV, continuous intravenous infusion; adapted from Sonis ST, Elting LS, Keefe D, et al, "Perspectives on Cancer Therapy-Induced Mucosal Injury: Pathogenesis, Measurement, Epidemiology, and Consequences for Patients," *Cancer*, 2004, 100(9 Suppl):1995-2025.

Palifermin is a recombinant human keratinocyte growth factor that works in a receptor-mediated manner to reduce the duration and severity of mucositis by promoting epithelial cell proliferation, differentiation, and migration. At the time this chapter was written, palifermin was a newly approved product indicated to decrease the incidence and duration of severe oral mucositis in patients with hematologic malignancies receiving myelotoxic therapy requiring hematopoietic stem cell support. Studies evaluating the efficacy and safety of palifermin for reduction of mucositis in other patient groups undergoing treatment of malignant disease are ongoing. Clinical trials suggest that amifostine pretreatment reduces pharyngeal and esophageal mucositis in patients receiving radiotherapy to the head and neck. Amifostine has been studied for reduction of chemotherapy-associated mucositis; however, the findings are equivocal. Additional pharmaceutical agents and interventions that have been employed to reduce the duration and severity of mucositis, but lack sufficient evidence to support routine use, include allopurinol-cryotherapy, chlorhexidine, glutamine suspension, pilocarpine, sargramostim, and zinc sulfate.

Therapy of stomatitis consists primarily of symptomatic support. Good oral hygiene is essential in the prevention of infections. Routine, gentle brushing with a soft toothbrush or cotton swab several times a day is helpful in removing dental plaque. Rinsing the mouth with a saline/bicarbonate solution helps remove debris and increases the pH, slowing the growth of oral flora. Use of mouthwashes containing alcohol may be painful or dry the oral mucosa; phenol may promote mucosal ulceration.

Pain control is a crucial part of stomatitis therapy. In addition to making the patient more comfortable, adequate pain control allows the patient to communicate and eat normally, thereby improving quality of life and reducing nutritional complications. Narcotic analgesia is frequently required for management of moderate-to-severe pain from mucositis. Topical application of local anesthetics is the most common approach to management of mild-to-moderate pain from stomatitis. Local application of cold sometimes provides adequate relief. Diphenhydramine has been used, but may cause drying of local tissues and sedation. Most products also contain significant amounts of alcohol which can exacerbate symptomatology. Local anesthetics (eg, benzocaine, lidocaine, tetracaine) are more potent than diphenhydramine, and are not associated with significant drying of local tissues. However, the numbing effect of these agents can impair swallowing. In addition, most of these products are unpalatable, and some are relatively expensive. The following table lists some of the commonly used agents.

Various Mouth Care Products

Product	Concentration(s)	Dosage
Anesthetics		
Benzocaine	5% to 20%	1-5 mL; swish and expectorate q4-6h
Diphenhydramine	12.5 mg/5 mL	5 mL; swish and expectorate (or swallow) q4-6h
Lidocaine	1%	5 mL; swish and expectorate (or swallow) q2-3 h
Antibiotics		
Amphotericin B	100 mg/mL	1 mL qid; swish in mouth as long as possible; swallow or expectorate
Chlorhexidine gluconate	0.12%	15 mL q4-6h; swish and expectorate
Clotrimazole	10 mg	1 tid (prophylaxis) One 5 times/day for 14 days (treatment)
Nystatin	100,000 units/mL	5 mL; swish and expectorate (or swallow) q4-6h
	100,000 units (vaginal tablet)	1 q4-6h (dissolve in mouth)

MUCOSITIS/STOMATITIS *(Continued)*

Various Mouth Care Products *(continued)*

Product	Concentration(s)	Dosage
Mouth Rinses		
Sodium bicarbonate (8.4 g/50 mEq/ 0.9% NaCl [1000 mL] mixture)	0.5 mEq/10 mL	5-15 mL q3-4h
Sodium chloride	0.9%	5-15 mL q3-4h

Many institutions and prescribers use locally compounded anesthetic formulations for treatment of stomatitis pain. Although the exact formulae vary tremendously, the general rubric includes a local anesthetic to which one or more of the following are added: a second anesthetic, aluminum hydroxide/magnesium hydroxide suspension, diphenhydramine, kaolin/pectin suspension, sucralfate suspension, nystatin, or water. Controlled trials comparing various formulations with each other, or with the various individual ingredients are not available. However, these products often form the mainstay of symptomatic treatment for stomatitis. Examples of recipes for a few such formulations are found in Table 3.

Sucralfate is basic aluminum sucrose sulfate, a sulfate disaccharide, used primarily as an antiulcer agent. The activity of sucralfate appears to be local, rather than systemic. The drug forms a viscous material that adheres to the surface of gastric and duodenal ulcers, forming a protective barrier over the ulcer. Protected from the activity of gastric enzymes and acid, ulcers are able to heal naturally. This local activity stimulated investigation of sucralfate as a treatment for oral ulcers. A number of groups have studied sucralfate as a therapy for various oral ulcerative conditions with equivocal results. Although the results published to date do not demonstrate a real advantage to sucralfate therapy, some patients may benefit from its use. Sucralfate is commercially available as a tablet (1 g) or suspension (1 g/10 mL). When placed into water, the tablet readily absorbs the fluid and forms a gelatinous suspension.

Examples of Extemporaneously Compounded Oral Stomatitis Products

Anesthetics

Diphenhydramine syrup 5 mL +
Lidocaine 2% 10 mL
Aluminum/magnesium hydroxide suspension 15 mL
(Maalox®/Mylanta®)

Diphenhydramine elixir 5 mL +
Lidocaine 2% 5 mL +
Aluminum/magnesium hydroxide suspension 5 mL
(Maalox®/Mylanta®)

Lidocaine 2% 45 mL
Diphenhydramine elixir 30 mL
Sodium bicarbonate 8.4 g
0.9% sodium chloride qs 1000 mL

Capsaicin, the active component of various peppers, is occasionally used as a topical counterirritant in the treatment of neuritic pain, rheumatoid and inflammatory conditions. A study by Berger, et al used oral capsaicin in a candy base to treat oral stomatitis caused by cancer chemotherapy or radiation. All eleven patients achieved some pain relief, although the benefit was only temporary. Side effects of the capsaicin candy were minimal. The capsaicin concentration in the candy formulation was estimated to be 5-9 parts per million (ppm); roughly 0.0005% to 0.001%. The formula used in this trial is as follows.

Capsaicin taffy

1 cup	sugar
3/4 cup	light corn syrup
2/3 cup	water
1 Tbsp	cornstarch
2 Tbsp	butter or margarine
1 tsp	salt
2 tsp	vanilla (or other flavor)
1/2 tsp	cayenne pepper

Combine all ingredients except flavor and cayenne and cook over medium heat, stirring constantly, to 256°F or to hard-ball stage. Remove from heat, stir in flavor and cayenne. When cool, pull taffy. When stiff, pull into strips and cut into pieces.

Xerostomia often accompanies stomatitis, particularly in patients who have received radiation to the neck and lower jaw. The condition can result in severe pain, dysphagia, malnutrition, and secondary infections. Subcutaneous or intravenous push administration of amifostine 200 mg/m^2 15 to 30 minutes prior to radiotherapy of the head and neck reduces acute and chronic xerostomia. Clinical trials suggest that amifostine pretreatment reduces pharyngeal and esophageal mucositis in patients receiving radiotherapy to the head and neck. The dose of amifostine for reduction of radiation-associated xerostomia and mucositis can be standardized to 500 mg in 0.9% sodium chloride 2.5 mL.

In spite of good oral hygiene, some patients develop oral infections. This is particularly common in the patient with additional sources of immunosuppression, such as neutropenia, treatment with exogenous immunosuppressions, or disease-related immune impairment. The organism most commonly seen in such infections is *Candida albicans*. Topical treatment with nystatin or clotrimazole is usually sufficient to control these infections. Such treatments are usually well tolerated and produce minimal systemic effects. Nystatin 400,000-600,000 units (4-6 mL) four times a day, swished in the mouth for at least 2 minutes, then swallowed is recommended. Alternatively, nystatin vaginal tablets can be used orally. Clotrimazole 10 mg five times a day is another effective treatment for these infections. Troches are placed under the tongue or in a buccal cavity and allowed to dissolve. In some patients, clotrimazole used three times a day is an effective prophylaxis against oral *Candida* infections. Patients with significant xerostomia may have trouble dissolving the nystatin or clotrimazole tablets, and may require an artificial saliva product to moisten the mouth. Oral or intravenous administration of fluconazole 100 to 200 mg daily may be necessary for treatment of

MUCOSITIS/STOMATITIS *(Continued)*

microbiologically documented or presumed oromucosal candidiasis in the patient with moderate-to-severe mucositis extending proximally beyond the mouth or the patient with additional sources of immune suppression. The fluconazole should be continued for at least 2 weeks, and until microbiologic and clinical evidence of infectious disease have resolved and the patient's immune recovery is considered adequate. Alternative systemic antifungal agents that can be considered for treatment of oromucosal and esophageal candidiasis include caspofungin, itraconazole, voriconazole, and amphotericin B products.

Herpes simplex virus is another common pathogen causing oral and other gastrointestinal infections in the patient with moderate-to-severe mucositis. The risk for oral Herpes simplex infection is greatest in patients with an additional source of immune compromise. Systemic treatment with acyclovir, famciclovir, or valacyclovir is required for oromucosal or gastrointestinal Herpes simplex infection. Alternative systemic antiviral agents for treatment of resistant Herpes simplex infections include ganciclovir and foscarnet.

Nondepolarizing neuromuscular blockade should be used for the patient with sever mucositis requiring intubation to support the airway. One case report describes succinylcholine-induced hyperkalemia in a patient with severe mucositis following treatment chemotherapy.

Selected Readings

Al-Khafaji AH, Dewhirst WE, Cornell CJ Jr, et al, "Succinylcholine-Induced Hyperkalemia in a Patient With Mucositis Secondary to Chemotherapy," *Crit Care Med*, 2001, 29(6):1274-6.

Awidi A, Homsi U, Kakail RI, et al, "Double-Blind, Placebo-Controlled Cross-Over Study of Oral Pilocarpine for the Prevention of Chemotherapy-Induced Oral Mucositis in Adult Patients With Cancer," *Eur J Cancer*, 2001, 37(16):2010-4.

Berger A, Henderson M, Nadoolman W, et al, "Oral Capsaicin Provides Temporary Relief for Oral Mucositis Pain Secondary to Chemotherapy/Radiation Therapy," *J Pain Symptom Manage*, 1995, 10(3):243-8.

Chiara S, Nobile MT, Vincenti M, et al, "Sucralfate in the Treatment of Chemotherapy-Induced Stomatitis: A Double-Blind, Placebo-Controlled Pilot Study," *Anticancer Res*, 2001, 21(5):3707-10.

Dodd MJ, Miaskowski C, Greenspan D, et al, "Radiation-Induced Mucositis: A Randomized Clinical Trial of Micronized Sucralfate Versus Salt & Soda Mouthwashes," *Cancer Invest*, 1988, 2003, 21(1):21-33.

Ertekin MV, Koc M, Karslioglu I, et al, "Zinc Sulfate in the Prevention of Radiation-Induced Oropharyngeal Mucositis: A Prospective, Placebo-Controlled, Randomized Study," *Int J Radiat Oncol Biol Phys*, 2004, 58(1):167-74.

Franzen L, Henriksson R, Littbrand B, et al, "Effects of Sucralfate on Mucositis During and Following Radiotherapy of Malignancies in the Head and Neck Region, A Double-Blind Placebo-Controlled Study" *Acta Oncol*, 1995, 34(2):219-23.

Garre ML, Relling MV, Kalwinsky D, et al, "Pharmacokinetics and Toxicity of Methotrexate in Children With Down Syndrome and Acute Lymphocytic Leukemia," *J Pediatr*, 1987, 111(4):606-12.

Huang EY, Leung SW, Wang CJ, et al, "Oral Glutamine to Alleviate Radiation-Induced Oral Mucositis: A Pilot Randomized Trial," *Int J Radiat Oncol Biol Phys*, 2000, 46(3):535-9.

Kinzie BJ, "Treatment of Stomatitis Associated With Antineoplastic-Drug Therapy," *Clinical Pharmacy*, 1988, 7:14-7.

Makkonen TA, Bostrom P, Vilja P, et al, "Sucralfate Mouth Washing in the Prevention of Radiation-Induced Mucositis: A Placebo-Controlled Double-Blind Randomized Study," *Int J Radiat Oncol Biol Phys*, 1994, 30:177-82.

Okuno SH, Woodhouse CO, Loprinzi CL, et al, "Phase III Controlled Evaluation of Glutamine for Decreasing Stomatitis in Patients Receiving Fluorouracil (5-FU)-Based Chemotherapy," *Am J Clin Oncol*, 1999, 22(3):258-61.

Pfeiffer P, Madsen EL, Hansen O, et al, "Effect of Prophylactic Sucralfate Suspension on Stomatitis Induced by Cancer Chemotherapy: A Randomized, Double-Blind Cross-Over Study," *Acta Oncol*, 1990, 29(2):171-3.

Pitten FA, Kiefer T, Buth C, et al, "Do Cancer Patients With Chemotherapy-Induced Leukopenia Benefit From an Antiseptic Chlorhexidine-Based Oral Rinse? A Double-Blind, Block-Randomized, Controlled Study," *J Hosp Infect*, 2003, 53(4):283-91.

Quintiliani R, Owens NJ, Quercia RA, et al, "Treatment and Prevention of Oropharyngeal Candidiasis," *Am J Med*, 1984, 77(4D):44-8.

Rattan J, Schneider M, Arber N, et al, "Sucralfate Suspension as a Treatment of Recurrent Aphthous Stomatitis," *J Intern Med*, 1994, 236(3):341-3.

Rossi A, Rosati G, Colarusso D, et al, "Subcutaneous Granulocyte-Macrophage Colony-Stimulating Factor in Mucositis Induced by an Adjuvant 5-Fluorouracil Plus Leucovorin Regimen. A Phase II Study and Review of the Literature," *Oncology*, 2003, 64(4):353-60.

Rubenstein EB, Peterson DE, Schubert M, et al, "Clinical Practice Guidelines for the Prevention and Treatment of Cancer Therapy-Induced Oral and Gastrointestinal Mucositis," *Cancer*, 2004, 100(9 Suppl):2026-46.

Saarilahti K, Kajanti M, Joensuu T, et al, "Comparison of Granulocyte-macrophage Colony-Stimulating Factor and Sucralfate Mouthwashes in the Prevention of Radiation-Induced Mucositis: A Double-Blind Prospective Randomized Phase III Study," *Int J Radiat Oncol Biol Phys*, 2002, 54(2):479-85.

Sonis ST, Elting LS, Keefe D, et al, "Perspectives on Cancer Therapy-Induced Mucosal Injury: Pathogenesis, Measurement, Epidemiology, and Consequences for Patients," *Cancer*, 2004, 100 (9 Suppl):2026-46.

Ulrich CM, Yasui Y, Storb R, et al, "Pharmacogenetics of Methotrexate: Toxicity Among Marrow Transplantation Patients Varies With the Methylenetetrahydrofolate Reductase C677T Polymorphism," *Blood*, 2001, 98(1):231-4.

Yokomizo H, Yoshimatsu K, Hashimoto M, et al, "Prophylactic Efficacy of Allopurinol Ice Ball for Leucovorin/5-Fluorouracil Therapy-Induced Stomatitis," *Anticancer Res*, 2004, 24(2C):1131-4.

TUMOR LYSIS SYNDROME

INTRODUCTION

Tumor lysis syndrome (TLS) is characterized as an acute metabolic disturbance resulting from the rapid destruction of tumor cells. Destruction of tumor cells releases cellular breakdown products that overwhelm the body's normal mechanisms for excretion and utilization. The result is acute renal failure due to deposition of either uric acid crystals or calcium phosphate solubility products. Although most commonly reported in patients with leukemias and other lymphoproliferative malignancies (Burkitt's and non-Burkitt's lymphomas), it has also been reported with nonhematologic malignancies such as breast, small-cell lung and testicular cancers.

PREDISPOSING FACTORS

1. Bulky disease
2. Marked sensitivity of the tumor to a particular treatment modality
3. Renal impairment, including pre-existing volume depletion
4. Elevated pretreatment lactic dehydrogenase serum levels
5. Elevated pretreatment uric acid serum levels independent of renal impairment

CLINICAL FEATURES AND TREATMENT

General Principles

Prevention and early management of TLS is aimed at decreasing the risk of development of acute oliguric renal failure. Vigorous hydration with intravenous fluids and sodium bicarbonate helps to expand volume, dilute serum concentrations of potassium, phosphate, and uric acid, and alkalinizes the urine. Increasing the urine pH to 7.0 increases the solubility of uric acid but may also increase the tendency for calcium phosphate nephrocalcinosis. Allopurinol in doses of 300-600 mg/day should be given to decrease uric acid production. Clinical features and treatment for specific metabolic disorders are discussed in the following sections.

Hyperuricemia

Breakdown of cells releases free nucleotides. Purines are metabolized to uric acid via the oxidation of hypoxanthine and xanthine. Uric acid, hypoxanthine, and xanthine all have independent solubilities. A high concentration of uric acid and an acidic urine pH cause uric acid crystals to precipitate in the renal tubules, resulting in oliguric renal failure. Maintenance of urine flow and alkalinization of the urine may prevent precipitation of these purines. Allopurinol blocks the production of uric acid by inhibiting the enzyme xanthine oxidase, which oxidizes hypoxanthine and xanthine to uric acid, and should be used prophylactically and during the early treatment of TLS. Rasburicase, an alternative to allopurinol, decreases uric acid by converting it to an inactive and soluble metabolite (allentoin). Despite quicker onset and unique mechanism of action, rasburicase has not replaced allopurinol as the standard of care. Rasburicase is presently only approved for use in pediatric patients.

Hyperkalemia

Potassium is primarily an intracellular ion that is released during massive cellular breakdown. Increasing levels of serum potassium can be dangerous, leading to cardiac arrhythmias or sudden death, especially in the presence of hypocalcemia (see following discussion). Standard treatment to remove potassium from the body should be initiated. Routine volume expansion with forced diuresis and/or shifting of potassium intracellularly by administering glucose and insulin may not be sufficient and should not be used alone. Potassium intake from nutritional sources and intravenous solutions should be restricted and administration of Kayexalate® orally (15 g every 6 hours) or by a retention enema (50-100 g) should be initiated immediately. The use of hemodialysis should be considered in patients with deteriorating organ function.

Hyperphosphatemia and Hypocalcemia

The release of intracellular inorganic phosphate following massive cellular breakdown sets into motion several important clinical features. Serum phosphate levels will quickly exceed the threshold for normal renal excretion, with phosphate excretion becoming limited to the glomerular filtration rate. Any azotemia that develops during therapy will aggravate phosphate excretion. Treatment includes the use of aluminum hydroxide orally to reduce phosphate levels and dialysis, if necessary. High phosphate levels will also cause reciprocal hypocalcemia. Although generally asymptomatic, hypocalcemia may cause neuromuscular irritation, tetany, and cardiac dysrhythmias. Symptomatic patients may receive calcium gluconate 10%, 10 mL intravenously, or calcitriol to increase serum calcium levels. However, despite hypocalcemia, the solubility product of calcium and phosphate may be exceeded, resulting in metastatic tissue calcification and acute nephrocalcinosis, resulting in renal failure.

Hemodialysis

Due to the unpredictability of TLS, hemodialysis may be needed and can be life-saving. Hemodialysis may be used to control and maintain fluid volume and/or to remove uric acid, phosphate, and potassium from serum. This may be important in a patient who is clinically unstable, with an inadequate urine output, and rapidly rising serum electrolyte abnormalities, despite preventative therapy.

CONCLUSION

Tumor lysis syndrome is characterized by massive cell breakdown resulting in metabolic disturbances such as hyperkalemia, hyperphosphatemia, hypocalcemia, and hyperuricemia which may lead to an acute, but reversible, oliguric renal failure. Appropriate prevention and treatment with adequate hydration, maintenance of high urine flow, and alkalinization of urine. Renal dialysis should be considered early if the patient is clinically unstable despite preventative therapies.

TUMOR LYSIS SYNDROME *(Continued)*

Selected Readings

Arrambide K and Toto RD, "Tumor Lysis Syndrome," *Semin Nephrol*, 1993, 13(3):273-80.

Chasty RC and Liu-Yin JA, "Acute Tumor Lysis Syndrome," *Br J Hosp Med*, 1993, 49(7):488-92.

Drakos P, Bar-Ziv J, and Catane R, "Tumor Lysis Syndrome in Nonhematologic Malignancies. Report of a Case and Review of the Literature," *Am J Clin Oncol*, 1994, 17(6):502-5.

Yim BT, Sims-McCallum RP, and Chong PH, "Rasburicase for the Treatment and Prevention of Hyperuricemia," *Ann Pharmacother*, 2003, 37(7-8):1047-54.

HYPERCALCEMIA

INTRODUCTION

Hyperparathyroidism and cancer are the most frequent causes of hypercalcemia. In cancer patients, hypercalcemia is the most frequently occurring life-threatening metabolic disorder. The incidence varies with the specific type of cancer; the highest incidence is seen in multiple myeloma and breast cancer. The etiology of cancer-associated hypercalcemia is multifactorial. The immediate cause is increased bone resorption. Bone resorption is stimulated by mediators released from tumor cells. The most common mediator of osteoclastic bone resorption, in patients with and without bone metastases, is thought to be parathyroid hormone-related protein (PTH-RP). PTH-RP mimics some, but not all, of the effects of parathyroid hormone. Other mediators or presumed mediators of bone resorption include vitamin D_3, prostaglandins, and a variety of cytokines. Hypercalcemia leads to polyuria and resultant volume depletion and decreased glomerular filtration rate. Attempts by the kidney to increase intravascular volume by increasing proximal tubular reabsorption of water and sodium are accompanied by increased tubular reabsorption of calcium. This perpetuates the hypercalcemia. The median survival for cancer patients with hypercalcemia who are not receiving chemotherapy is reported to be 30 days. Treatment of hypercalcemia, however, can lead to improvement of symptoms (eg, confusion, constipation, malaise, nausea, vomiting, polyuria, polydipsia). Although treatment of the underlying malignancy may correct hypercalcemia, the late and/or refractory stage of cancer at which hypercalcemia occurs often precludes successful antitumor therapy.

TREATMENT

The urgency with which cancer-associated hypercalcemia is approached/treated is determined by the presence/severity of symptoms and the level of calcium. Most guidelines suggest that serum calcium be corrected for albumin in order to estimate the level of ionized (free or active) calcium. Although ionized calcium may in fact not be accurately estimated by the formulae that correct for albumin [eg, corrected Ca^{++} = measured Ca^{++} (mg/dL) + 0.8 mg/dL for each g albumin <4 g/dL, corrected Ca^{++} = measured Ca^{++} (mg/dL) - albumin (g/dL) + 4.0], many studies of treatments for hypercalcemia have used corrected rather than total calcium in determining study entry and/or endpoints.

Several treatments exist for the management of hypercalcemia. They have not all been compared to each other, or have not been compared at doses that reflect clinical usage, etc. Thus, treatment remains somewhat empiric.

0.9% NaCl

Sodium chloride provides replacement of intravascular volume. Following rehydration, proximal tubular reabsorption of sodium, and therefore calcium, will decrease. Further, other treatments for hypercalcemia require prior volume replacement in order to minimize toxicities. Sodium chloride can lower serum calcium by approximately 2 mg/dL. The rate of administration of

HYPERCALCEMIA *(Continued)*

sodium chloride depends on the degree of dehydration, the degree of hyper-calcemia, and the cardiovascular status of the patient. Even if normocalcemia is achieved, without further treatment calcium will rise again. In many studies, rehydration has been continued for 48 hours before adding another calcium-lowering agent. In hospitalized patients, sodium chloride can be continued while other agents are administered.

FUROSEMIDE

The major use of furosemide *on page 374* in the management of cancer-associated hypercalcemia is to prevent/treat fluid overload in order to facilitate the administration of sodium chloride for volume replacement. Although high doses of furosemide (eg, 100 mg) have been used to promote calcium excretion, such high doses require the use of strict monitoring of input and output and replacement of fluid and electrolytes. The possibility of further dehydration and worsening of hypercalcemia with furosemide should be considered.

BISPHOSPHONATES

Bisphosphonates bind to hydroxyapatite in bone and inhibit osteoclastic bone resorption. Pamidronate *on page 650* is reported to bring calcium to the normocalcemic range in 70% to 100% of patients. Although there appears to be a dose-response relationship, it is not clear that 90 mg is clinically superior to 60 mg. It is recommended that use of pamidronate be weighed carefully in patients with serum creatinine ≥3 mg/dL. This is primarily because of lack of data in this population. Rehydration usually precedes administration of pamidronate, and elevated creatinine values are often corrected. Side effects of pamidronate are mild and include fever and infusion site reactions such as phlebitis. Etidronate *on page 313* is reported to bring calcium to the normo-calcemic range in 40% to 100% of patients. Etidronate is generally thought to be less potent as a calcium-lowering agent than pamidronate. The usual dose of etidronate is 7.5 mg/kg/day for 3 days. Like pamidronate, etidronate is not recommended for use in patients with serum creatinine >5 mg/dL. Also, like pamidronate, etidronate is generally given after rehydration. Side effects of etidronate include occasional mild elevations in creatinine and a metallic taste. Because of the multiple daily dose regimens of etidronate, pamidronate is more convenient for outpatient administration. Oral etidronate has been used to maintain normocalcemia with minimal clinical benefit.

CALCITONIN

Calcitonin *on page 145* inhibits bone resorption and enhances urinary excretion of calcium. It is the fastest acting of the agents used to treat hypercalcemia and may be given safely before rehydration is complete. The usual dose of calcitonin is 4 units/kg every 12 hours. Side effects are mild and infrequent and include nausea, abdominal cramps, and flushing. Calcitonin lowers serum calcium by approximately 2 mg/dL. As is the case for saline hydration, this may or may not result in normocalcemia. However, rebound hypercalcemia develops quickly (within days), limiting the usefulness of calci-tonin in the treatment of hypercalcemia.

GALLIUM NITRATE

Gallium *on page 380* decreases serum calcium by adsorbing to hydroxyapatite and inhibiting bone resorption. It is given as a continuous infusion at a dose of 200 mg/m^2/day for 5 days. Gallium is reported to result in normocalcemia in 75% of patients. Nephrotoxicity has been seen with the use of gallium. Although nephrotoxicity reportedly occurs with doses higher than those used to treat hypercalcemia, it has been noted in patients treated for hypercalcemia. Nephrotoxicity may be potentiated by other nephrotoxic drugs. Gallium should not be used in patients with serum creatinine >2.5 mg/dL. Because of the potential for nephrotoxicity and the inconvenient dosing schedule relative to other agents, gallium should not be considered a first-line treatment for hypercalcemia.

MISCELLANEOUS

Other agents have been evaluated or used to treat hypercalcemia. Cisplatin *on page 190* is known to lower serum calcium and may be effective in hypercalcemia independent of tumor response. Amifostine *on page 53* has been associated with hypocalcemia and was effective in lowering serum calcium in at least one report. Intravenous alendronate as well as other bisphosphonates not available in the United States have also been reported to be effective in the management of hypercalcemia.

Drug	Usual Dose	Onset of Effect (h)	Duration of Effect
Calcitonin	4 units/kg q12h	3	Median 1 day (1-6)
Etidronate	7.5 mg/kg/d x 3 d	24-48	Median 5 days (2-30)
Gallium	200 mg/m^{2}d x 5 d	24-48	Median 6 days
NaCl	2-5 L/24 h	24-48	Transient
Pamidronate	60 or 90 mg	24-48	Median 10 days (1-30)
Plicamycin	25 mcg/kg	12	3-21 days

Selected Readings

Bilezikian JP, "Management of Acute Hypercalcemia," *N Engl J Med*, 1992, 326(18):1196-203.

Glover DJ, Shaw L, Glick JH, et al, "Treatment of Hypercalcemia in Parathyroid Cancer With WR-2721, S-2-(3-Aminopropylamino)Ethyl-Phosphorothioic Acid," *Ann Intern Med*, 1985, 103(1):55-7.

Lad TE, Mishoulam HM, Shevrin DH, et al, "Treatment of Cancer-Associated Hypercalcemia With Cisplatin," *Arch Intern Med*, 1987, 147(2):329-32.

Ladenson JH, Lewis JW, and Boyd JC, "Failure of Total Calcium Corrected for Protein, Albumin, and pH to Correctly Assess Free Calcium Status," *J Clin Endocrinol Metab*, 1978, 46:986-93.

Nakashima L, "Guidelines for the Treatment of Hypercalcemia Associated With Malignancy," *J Oncol Pharm Pract*, 1997, 3:31-7.

Nussbaum SR, Warrell RP Jr, Rude R, et al, "Dose-Response Study of Alendronate Sodium for the Treatment of Cancer-Associated Hypercalcemia," *J Clin Oncol*, 1993, 11(8):1618-23.

Nussbaum SR, Younger J, Vandepol CJ, et al, "Single-Dose Intravenous Therapy With Pamidronate for the Treatment of Hypercalcemia of Malignancy: Comparison of 30-, 60-, and 90-mg Dosages," *Am J Med*, 1993, 95(3):297-304.

Perlia CP, Gubisch NJ, Wolter J, et al, "Mithramycin Treatment of Hypercalcemia," *Cancer*, 1970, 25:389-94.

HYPERCALCEMIA *(Continued)*

Ralston SH, Gallacher SJ, Patel U, et al, "Cancer-Associated Hypercalcemia: Morbidity and Mortality. Clinical Experience in 126 Treated Patients," *Ann Intern Med*, 1990, 112(7):499-504.

Ringenberg QS and Ritch PS, "Efficacy of Oral Administration of Etidronate Disodium in Maintaining Normal Serum Calcium Levels in Previously Hypercalcemic Cancer Patients," *Clin Ther*, 1987, 9(3):318-25.

Schaiff RA, Hall TG, and Bar RS, "Medical Treatment of Hypercalcemia," *Clin Pharm*, 1989, 8(2):108-21.

Shemerdiak WP, Kukreja SC, Lad TE, et al, "Evaluation of Routine Ionized Calcium Determination in Cancer Patients," *Clin Chem*, 1981, 27:1621-2.

Shevrin DH, Bressler LR, McGuire WP, et al, "Treatment of Cancer-Associated Hypercalcemia With Mithramycin and Oral Etidronate Disodium," *Clin Pharm*, 1985, 4(2):204-5.

Stewart AF, "Clinical Practice. Hypercalcemia Associated With Cancer, "*N Engl J Med*, 2005, 352(4):373-9.

Thiebaud D, Jaeger PH, Jacquet AF, et al, "Dose-Response in the Treatment of Hypercalcemia of Malignancy by a Single Infusion of the Bisphosphonate AHPrBP," *J Clin Oncol*, 1988, 6(5):762-8.

Warrell RP, "Metabolic Emergencies: Hypercalcemia", *Cancer: Principles and Practice of Oncology*, 5th ed, DeVita, Hellman, and Rosenberg, eds, Lippincott-Raven, 1997, 2486-93.

Warrell RP Jr, Israel R, Frisone M, et al, "Gallium Nitrate for Acute Treatment of Cancer-Related Hypercalcemia. A Randomized, Double-Blind Comparison to Calcitonin," *Ann Intern Med*, 1988, 108(5):699-74.

MALIGNANT EFFUSIONS

Malignant effusions occur when fluid accumulates in the pleural space secondary to direct extension of a tumor or because of metastatic dissemination. Carcinoma of the breast, carcinoma of the lung, and lymphomas account for two-thirds of malignant effusions but they are also found with gastric or ovarian carcinomas. A malignant effusion may be the presenting sign of cancer, but most often it is a complication of a diagnosed malignancy.

PATHOPHYSIOLOGY

The pleura is a thin membrane that covers the lungs and chest wall. It is composed of the visceral pleura (covering the surface of the lungs) and the parietal pleura (covering the thoracic cavity). The space between the visceral pleura and parietal pleura is the pleural space. Normally, pleural fluid production is <100 mL/day. Movement of fluid within the pleural space is governed by hydrostatic and oncotic pressures and follows Starling's law of transcapillary exchange. Hydrostatic pressure in the parietal capillaries is higher, causing a net movement into the pleural space. Reabsorption of the fluid occurs primarily through lymphatics on the parietal surface and less importantly via lymphatics on the visceral surface. Changes in pleural fluid production, reabsorption, or both produce a pleural effusion.

Malignancies can cause an imbalance within the pleural space in several ways. Pleural implantation of malignant cells can cause an inflammatory response that increases capillary permeability and increases the net filtration of fluid into the pleural space. Obstruction of lymphatic channels and changes in pleural fluid protein content can impair reabsorption of fluid. Any of these changes can result in a net accumulation of fluid.

Normally, pleural fluid is produced through a passive process and the ion content is similar to serum concentrations while the protein content is <2%. The resulting fluid is transudative. Neoplastic processes, which increase capillary permeability and obstruct lymphatic drainage, often produce an exudative pleural fluid with an increased protein and cell content. Typically, the characteristics of the exudative fluid include increased protein content, glucose level lower than the serum, variable number of identifiable tumor cells, and an absence of eosinophils.

CLINICAL SYMPTOMS

Many patients with pleural effusions are asymptomatic. The most common symptom is dyspnea, often in conjunction with cough, chest pain, and tachypnea. Symptoms are often related not to the amount of fluid present, but to the rate of fluid accumulation. A diagnosis often begins with a chest x-ray, which will demonstrate fluid accumulation on the PA and lateral decubitus film. Physical findings include dullness to percussion, decreased breath sounds, decreased diaphragmatic excursion, and possible contralateral tracheal deviation.

MALIGNANT EFFUSIONS *(Continued)*

TREATMENT

The goal of treatment is to provide a cost-efficient, effective therapy that provides symptomatic relief with the least amount of discomfort to the patient. Not all patients with pleural effusions need to be treated. Some patients with effusions are asymptomatic and may not require treatment until symptoms develop. Patients with a life expectancy of less than 1 month might only require oxygen, narcotics, and possibly thoracentesis. Patients with tumors highly sensitive to chemotherapy may have resolution of the effusion with systemic treatment of the tumor.

LOCAL THERAPY

1. Thoracentesis is utilized frequently for symptomatic patients, but it is ineffective for any long-term control of the effusion. Recurrence is frequent, and repeated procedures carry a risk of increased complications such as pneumothorax.

2. Tube thoracostomy (chest tube) is effective in controlling a malignant effusion for a short period of time. Its 30-day success rate is approximately 70%. However, it is ineffective in the long-term control of effusions. It is most useful in draining the fluid from the pleural space prior to instilling a sclerosing agent.

3. Pleurectomy involves stripping the parietal and visceral pleura and it carries a high mortality and morbidity rate as compared to less invasive procedures.

4. Pleuroperitoneal shunts are used to manually pump fluid from the pleural space into the peritoneal cavity. The pumps must be manually operated daily and are prone to blockage by the high protein content of the fluid.

PLEURODESIS

Pleurodesis, or sclerosis, should be considered in symptomatic patients who have symptomatic relief from thoracentesis with complete lung re-expansion and a life expectancy of weeks to months. Sclerosing agents act by causing an inflammatory response in the pleura, which resolves to cause adhesions of the visceral and parietal pleura, resulting in obliteration of the pleural space. Sclerosing agents are administered via a thoracostomy tube following adequate drainage (<100 mL/day). Factors affecting the success of the agent include uniform distribution in the pleural space, the presence of loculations that interfere with distribution, and the dose of the selected drug.

GENERAL METHOD OF ADMINISTRATION

Fluid is drained via a chest tube until the production is <100 mL/day. The patient is premedicated with a parenteral narcotic. Since pleurodesis is associated with pleuritic chest pain, instillation of 10-25 mL of 1% lidocaine (3-4 mg/kg) is recommended 10-15 minutes prior to the sclerosing agent. The sclerosing agent is instilled through the chest tube and the tube is clamped for 30 minutes to 2 hours with frequent repositioning of the patient to assure uniform distribution, although this repositioning is controversial. Then the tube is unclamped, reconnected to water-seal suction until production is <100-150 mL/day, and the chest tube is removed.

DRUGS

1. Doxycycline and minocycline: Tetracycline was one of the most widely used sclerosing agents with a success rate of 30% to 80%. It was inexpensive, caused few side effects, and was moderately effective. However, it was removed from the market in the mid-1990s and an effective replacement has been sought. In three noncomparative studies, doxycycline 500-1000 mg mixed in 50-100 mL NS, was found to be moderately effective in controlling effusions but generally required 1-4 instillations to achieve results similar to tetracycline. Comparative studies are needed to confirm these results. Minocycline has only been studied in two small noncomparative trials with good results. It is inexpensive and may offer an alternative to tetracycline but larger comparative trials are needed to fully assess its usefulness.

2. Bleomycin 30-180 units in 100 mL of 0.9% sodium chloride or dextrose 5% in water has been studied and found to be an effective agent in controlling malignant effusions. Because of a lack of increased efficacy at doses >60 units, some authors have recommended limiting the dose to 60 units or 1 unit/kg body weight. Also, report of 2 deaths in elderly patients who may have had decreased clearance of the drug has prompted the recommendation to limit the dose to 40 units/m^2 in the elderly. Although 40% to 50% of the dose may enter the systemic circulation, toxicity is generally low. Adverse effects include nausea, vomiting, diarrhea, febrile reactions, and chest pain. Myelosuppression has not been clinically important but is theoretically a potential side effect. A disadvantage is the high cost of therapy due to the cost of the drug.

3. Talc is one of the oldest and most effective treatments for malignant effusions. Its use is somewhat controversial because of the costs associated with preparation and administration. Although the talc itself is relatively inexpensive, in the past the talc (asbestos-free only) had to be sterilized (ethylene oxide gas, dry heat, or irradiation) and was administered via a thoracostomy tube while the patient was under general anesthesia. The talc (5-10 g) was either insufflated or instilled as a slurry. Talc sclerosis is associated with pain, hypotension, fever, and adult respiratory distress syndrome as well as complications of general anesthesia. The cost of sterilization, use of the operating room, and anesthesia drive the costs of this therapy up, despite its nearly 100% efficacy. Use of small-bore pigtail catheters for sclerosis in the ambulatory setting, insertion of chest tubes under local anesthesia, and the recent availability of an aerosolized talc product may make this an attractive alternative.

OTHER AGENTS

A number of other agents including aldesleukin, doxorubicin, mitoxantrone, cisplatin, cytarabine, interferon, aldesleukin-2, *Cornybacterium parvum*, fluorouracil, mechlorethamine, methylprednisone acetate, and quinacrine have been used with varying degrees of success in small numbers of patients. Routine use cannot be recommended although some have shown promising results.

MALIGNANT EFFUSIONS *(Continued)*

COMPLICATIONS

Management of malignant effusions is associated with several complications. Pain from insertion of the chest tube or instillation of the sclerosing agent should be pretreated with parenteral narcotics. Traction pneumothorax results from repeated attempts to re-expand the lung. Cough is caused by lung re-expansion and is self-limiting. Fluid loculation is associated with drainage and pleurodesis. Lysis of adhesions may be necessary prior to pleurodesis. Empyema (purulent fluid) formation from contamination or bronchopulmonary communication should be treated with appropriate antibiotics.

CHOICE OF THERAPY

Although there have been many clinical trials documenting the efficacy of a number of agents for sclerosis, comparing efficacy is difficult. Flaws in the studies, such as different eligibility criteria, the use of concomitant therapies, and the lack of uniform response criteria make the task of choosing a therapy almost impossible. Talc is the least expensive and most effective therapy, but the cost of instillation under general anesthesia drives up hospital costs. The use of local anesthesia to insert chest tubes, the use of small-bore pigtail catheters, and the availability of aerosolized talc may provide alternatives in the future. Bleomycin is effective, requires one instillation allowing the chest tube to be removed earlier, and is well tolerated but is quite expensive. Doxycycline or minocycline may be alternatives but the lack of good dosing information and the small number of clinical trials make these agents alternatives to talc or bleomycin.

Selected Readings

Andrew CO and Gora ML, "Pleural Effusions: Pathophysiology and Management," *Ann Pharmcother*, 1994, 28:894-902.

Belani CP, Pajeau TS, and Bennett CL, "Treating Malignant Pleural Effusions Cost Consciously," *Chest*, 1998, 113:78S-85S.

Grossi F, Pennucci MC, Tixi L, et al, "Management of Malignant Pleural Effusions," *Drugs*, 1998, 55:47-58.

Hausheer FH and Yarbro JW, "Diagnosis and Treatment of Malignant Pleural Effusion," *Semin Oncol*, 1985, 12:54-75.

Putnam JB Jr., "Malignant Pleural Effusions," *Surg Clin North Am*, 2002, 82(4):867-83.

Walker-Renard PB, Vaughan LM, and Salm SA, "Chemical Pleurodesis for Malignant Pleural Effusions," *Ann Intern Med*, 1994, 120:56-64.

PAIN MANAGEMENT

DEFINITION AND INCIDENCE

Pain is defined by the International Society for the Study of Pain as "an unpleasant sensory and emotional experience associated with actual or potential tissue damage, or described in terms of such damage". The reported incidence of pain in cancer patients varies with the method used to determine the presence of pain, and the type and stage of cancer. It is estimated that 51% of patients with various stages of cancer experience pain, and patients with advanced disease are more likely to have severe pain. Pain in cancer patients may be due to the disease itself (eg, metastatic bone disease); it may be secondary to some treatments (eg, painful neuropathy from vincristine or paclitaxel, or postoperative pain); it may result from complications associated with cancer (eg, postherpetic neuralgia); or it may have been present prior to the diagnosis of cancer and be unrelated to cancer (eg, arthritis). Most often, treatment guidelines and discussions are directed against chronic pain associated with progressive disease.

NONOPIOID ANALGESICS

The World Health Organization recommends a stepwise approach to the management of cancer pain (see figure).

WHO Three-Step Analgesic Ladder

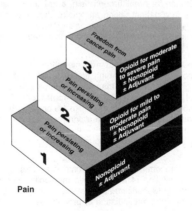

This approach recommends that the choice of therapy match the severity of pain (ie, strong opioids for moderate to severe pain). Nonopioids for (mild) cancer pain include aspirin, nonsteroidal anti-inflammatory drugs (NSAIDs), and acetaminophen. All of these have a ceiling above which increasing the dose will not enhance pain relief and will increase the likelihood of side effects.

PAIN MANAGEMENT *(Continued)*

Aspirin is frequently avoided because of the potential for gastropathy and inhibition of platelet aggregation. Concerns regarding the use of NSAIDs in chronic cancer pain also include the reversible inhibition of platelet aggregation, and the potential for gastropathy and nephrotoxicity. Nonacetylated salicylates do not inhibit platelet aggregation.

Although probably more of a potential than actual concern, it is recommended that the daily dose of acetaminophen not exceed 4-6 grams to minimize the likelihood of hepatotoxicity. Thus, when nonopioids are no longer effective or for pain of increased severity, opioids should be used. Tramadol, although having weak opioid activity in addition to inhibiting reuptake of monoamines, may be classified clinically with nonopioids. That is, its role or effectiveness in the management of chronic, severe pain is not well documented. Similarly, propoxyphene is a weak opioid not generally recommended for chronic cancer pain.

OPIOID ANALGESICS

Opioid analgesics for severe, persistent pain should be given "around-the-clock", not on an "as needed" or "PRN" basis. It is easier to prevent pain from recurring than to treat it once it has recurred. Titration of opioids to pain relief is easiest using short-acting drugs (average duration of pain relief of 4 hours) or a continuous parenteral infusion. Once adequate pain relief is achieved, the 24-hour opioid dose can be given as a long-acting preparation (eg, sustained release morphine or oxycodone, transdermal fentanyl). Medication for breakthrough pain, a transient worsening of otherwise stable pain in a patient taking an opioid, should always be available. Doses for breakthrough pain (ie, rescue doses) are commonly 5% to 15% of the 24-hour opioid dose, and may be administered every 1-2 hours as needed.

When possible, the oral route of administration of opioids is generally preferred. All opioids undergo a high first-pass effect, making them more effective when given parenterally than orally. The parenteral to oral ratios for effectiveness of the different opioids vary from 1:2 to 1:6. The 1:6 ratio reported with morphine is probably more like 1:3 or 1:2 with chronic oral use. A convenient "rule of thumb" is to use a parenteral to oral ratio of 1:3 for all opioids. Unlike the nonopioid analgesics, there is no ceiling on effectiveness of opioids, and, as tolerance develops to respiratory depression, there is no maximum dose.

Meperidine is not recommended for chronic use. This is because of the potential for accumulation of a neurotoxic metabolite, normeperidine (see following information). Meperidine administration is best reserved for incident pain (ie, before a painful manipulation or procedure).

Partial opioid agonists (eg, buprenorphine) or agonist-antagonists (eg, pentazocine, butorphanol, dezocine, nalbuphine) are generally not recommended for use in chronic cancer pain management. They have a ceiling for analgesic effectiveness, above which side effects are much more likely to increase, and they may precipitate withdrawal in patients receiving opioid agonists (eg, morphine).

Tolerance is characterized by the requirement for a higher dose of opioid in order to produce the same effect previously seen with a lower dose. Tolerance develops to many side effects of opioids: respiratory depression, sedation, nausea, and vomiting. Tolerance does not usually develop to constipation. It is not clear that tolerance develops, clinically, to the analgesic effect of opioids. When a given dose of opioid is not effective, for whatever reason, and if side effects are tolerable, the dose can be increased. Physical dependence occurs with regular use of opioids, but is only of clinical importance if the opioid is abruptly discontinued or an opioid antagonist (eg, naloxone) administered, in which cases a withdrawal syndrome can be seen. Opioids should be tapered in patients whose pain improves. Withdrawal can be avoided by maintaining 25% of the previous day's opioid dose. The opioid can be discontinued when the total daily dose is the equivalent of 10-15 mg of intramuscular morphine. Psychological dependence is defined as a "pattern of compulsive drug use characterized by a continued craving for an opioid and the need to use the opioid for effects other than pain relief." Unlike tolerance and physical dependence, psychological dependence is a characteristic of the patient, and is a function of environmental, social, economic, and personality factors. Psychological dependence, or "addiction", does not result from legitimate exposure to opioids for medical reasons.

The most troublesome side effect associated with chronic opioid use is constipation, and, as noted above, tolerance to constipation does not occur. Regular use of stimulant laxatives is often required.

Tolerance does develop to respiratory depression, allowing safe dose escalation. In the event of an acute overdose, or in the case of respiratory depression not responding to supportive measures, naloxone may be used. In general, naloxone use is not encouraged, as it precipitates withdrawal and the prompt return of pain in patients physically dependent on opioids. For life-threatening respiratory depression, naloxone may be administered by preparing a dilute solution (0.4 mg in 10 mL 0.9% NaCl) and injecting intravenous boluses of 0.5-1 mL (20-40 mcg) every minute, titrating to respiratory rate. Alternatively, a naloxone infusion (0.8 mg in 250 mL) may be titrated similarly. Other side effects include nausea and vomiting, sedation, sweating and itching, dry mouth, and seizures. Tolerance develops to nausea and vomiting, and these effects are more likely to be seen when opioid therapy is initiated. Phenothiazines may be used to treat nausea and vomiting until they disappear. Because there may be a vestibular component to nausea and vomiting, dimenhydrinate or meclizine can also be used to treat this side effect. Tolerance also usually develops to sedation. For those patients in whom sedation continues to be a problem, limiting opioid dose escalation and therefore pain relief, the use of stimulants (eg, dextroamphetamine, methylphenidate) should be considered. Sweating and itching are thought to be due to histamine release. If they are intolerable, switching to another opioid should be considered. Seizures associated with opioids are seen primarily with large overdoses or with neurotoxic metabolites. Normeperidine, a metabolite of meperidine *on page 535* that can accumulate with frequent repeated doses or in patients with renal insufficiency, is the most well known of these neurotoxic metabolites. Propoxyphene (a very weak opioid analgesic not generally recommended for treatment of cancer pain) also forms potentially neurotoxic metabolites. Distinct from seizures, myoclonic jerks may be seen with the use of high doses of opioids. Occasional reports indicate that

PAIN MANAGEMENT *(Continued)*

they may also be seen with relatively lower doses. Benzodiazepines have been suggested to treat this side effect.

As noted above, the oral route of administration for opioids is generally preferred. When this is impossible, several other routes are available (see following table). When patients suddenly become unable to take medication by mouth, opioids intended for oral administration have been administered rectally or vaginally. Morphine and hydromorphone are also available in rectal suppositories. The recommended rectal dose is the same as the oral dose. Continuous subcutaneous or intravenous infusions administered with an infusion control device are useful when oral administration is impossible and intermittent injections result in peaks and valleys of pain relief or side effects. Continuous infusions also allow for quick titration of opioid in patients with uncontrolled pain. Patient-controlled analgesia provides a continuous infusion of opioid with a capacity for patient-administered bolus injections for breakthrough pain. This is not unlike the concept of regularly scheduled sustained release oral opioid with immediate release tablets for breakthrough, as discussed above. Assessment of the use of breakthrough doses, whether oral or parenteral, provides a basis for adjusting the dose/rate of the underlying opioid. Transdermal fentanyl is another alternative, long-acting, analgesic for patients unable to take oral opioids. As is the case with sustained release oral opioids, it is preferable to titrate to pain relief using short-acting drugs, and then switch to transdermal fentanyl. Spinal opioids should be reserved for patients in whom systemic administration of opioids results in unacceptable or unmanageable toxicity. Epidural morphine is 5-10 times more potent than parenteral morphine, and intrathecal morphine is 10 times more potent than epidural morphine. Bupivicaine and clonidine have been added to epidural morphine infusions to enhance effectiveness.

Opioid Analgesics

Drug	Route of Administration	Approx Equianalgesic Dose (mg)	Approx Duration (h)
Codeine	Oral, parenteral	120	4-6
Fentanyl	Transdermal, parenteral	0.1	48-72*
Hydrocodone	Oral	15	4-6
Hydromorphone	Oral, parenteral, rectal	2	2-5
Levorphanol	Oral, parenteral	2	4-6
Meperidine	Oral, parenteral	100	2-4
Methadone	Oral, parenteral	10	6-12
Morphine	Oral, parenteral, rectal	10	3-4†
Oxycodone	Oral	15	4-6†

*Duration for transdermal fentanyl.

†Duration for sustained release dosage forms is 8-12 hours (MS Contin®, Oramorph SR®), 24 hours (Kadian®), 12 hours (Oxycontin®).

ADJUVANT ANALGESICS

Adjuvant analgesics are frequently used in addition to, rather than instead of, opioid analgesics. Adjuvants are often drugs which have primary indications other than pain, but may provide pain relief in certain situations. NSAIDs are commonly used for pain due to bone metastases (see individual NSAID monographs). Tricyclic antidepressants (eg, amitriptyline, nortriptyline), anticonvulsants (eg, carbamazepine, gabapentin), steroids, and antiarrhythmics (eg, lidocaine, mexiletine) are often recommended for treatment of neuropathic pain. Neuropathic pain, often characterized by sharp, shooting, lancinating sensations, may result from nerve compression, infiltration, or destruction by tumor or from other associated conditions (eg, postherpetic neuralgia). Pain relief is usually not complete and, as is the case with NSAIDs in bone pain, these drugs are generally used in addition to opioids. Baclofen has also been used as an adjuvant analgesic for various types of neuropathic pain. Strontium-89 is a radiopharmaceutical that is reported to decrease the need for analgesics in patients with osteoblastic bone metastases. Prostate cancer is the most frequent malignancy associated with painful osteoblastic lesions. Monthly administration of pamidronate, a bisphosphonate, has been demonstrated to decrease pain and adverse skeletal events in patients with multiple myeloma and breast cancer. Calcitonin has also been reported to be effective in cancer pain. Capsaicin is a topically applied adjuvant analgesic that depletes substance P, a "painful" neurotransmitter. Capsaicin is recommended for use in postherpetic neuralgia and other painful neuropathies.

Selected Readings

American Pain Society, *Principles of Analgesic Use in the Treatment of Acute Pain and Chronic Cancer Pain*, 3rd ed, Skokie, IL: American Pain Society, 1992.

Berenson JR, Lichtenstein A, Porter L, et al, "Efficacy of Pamidronate in Reducing Skeletal Events in Patients With Advanced Multiple Myeloma," *N Engl J Med*, 1996, 334(8):488-93.

Bressler LR, "Cancer Pain Management in Ambulatory Patients," *J Pharm Pract*, 1995, 8:260-8.

Bressler LR, Geraci MC, and Schatz BS, "Misperceptions and Inadequate Pain Management in Cancer Patients," *DICP*, 1991, 25(11):1225-30.

Chapman CR and Bonica JJ, "Cancer Pain," *Scope*, 1992.

Cherny NI and Portenoy RK, "Cancer Pain Management. Current Strategy," *Cancer*, 1993, 72(11):3393-415.

Cordell GA and Araujo OE, "Capsaicin: Identification, Nomenclature, and Pharmacotherapy," *Ann Pharmacother*, 1993, 27(3):330-6.

Foley KM, "The Treatment of Cancer Pain," *N Engl J Med*, 1985, 313(2):84-95.

Fromm GH, "Baclofen as an Adjuvant Analgesic," *J Pain Symptom Manage*, 1994, 9(8):500-9.

Holdsworth MT, Adams VR, and Chavez CM, "Continuous Midazolam Infusion for the Management of Morphine-Induced Myoclonus," *Ann Pharmacother*, 1995, 29(1):25-9.

IASP Subcommittee on Classification, "Pain Terms: A Current List With Definitions and Notes on Usage," *Pain*, 1986, 25(Suppl 3):S215-21.

Jacox A, Carr DB, Payne R, et al, "Management of Cancer Pain," *Clinical Practice Guideline No. 9, AHCPR Publication No. 94-0592*, Rockville, MD: Agency for Health Care Policy and Research, U.S. Department of Health and Human Services, Public Health Service, March 1994.

Kaiko RF, Foley KM, Grabinski PY, et al, "Central Nervous System Excitatory Effects of Meperidine in Cancer Patients," *Ann Neurol*, 1983, 13:180-5.

Laizure SC, "Considerations in Morphine Therapy," *Am J Hosp Pharm*, 1994, 51(16):2042-3.

Levy MH, "Pharmacologic Treatment of Cancer Pain," *N Engl J Med*, 1996, 335(15):1124-32.

Portenoy RK and Hagen NA, "Breakthrough Pain: Definition, Prevalence, and Characteristics," *Pain*, 1990, 41(3):273-81.

Potter JM, Reid DB, Shaw RJ, et al, "Myoclonus Associated With Treatment With High Doses of Morphine: The Role of Supplemental Drugs," *BMJ*, 1989, 299(6692):150-3.

Robinson RG, Preston DF, Baxter KG, et al, "Clinical Experience With Strontium-89 in Prostatic and Breast Cancer Patients," *Semin Oncol*, 1993, 20(3 Suppl 2):44-8.

PAIN MANAGEMENT *(Continued)*

Steinberg RB, Gilman DE, and Johnson F 3d, "Acute Toxic Delirium in a Patient Using Transdermal Fentanyl," *Anesth Analg*, 1992, 75(6):1014-6.

Szeto HH, Inturrisi CE, Houde R, et al, "Accumulation of Normeperidine, an Active Metabolite of
Meperidine in Patients With Renal Failure or Cancer," *Ann Intern Med*, 1977, 86:738-41.

Watson CP, "Antidepressant Drugs as Adjuvant Analgesics," *J Pain Symptom Manage*, 1994,
9(6):392-405.

TRANSPLANTATION

Hematopoietic stem cell transplantation (SCT) involves the infusion of hema-topoietic progenitor cells into a patient in order to treat certain hematologic or immunologic malignant and nonmalignant diseases. Hematopoietic progen-itor cells are immature cells that mature and differentiate into the various functional myelogenous cells (eg, neutrophils, monocytes, macrophages, megakaryocytes, erythrocytes) and lymphoid cells (eg, T lymphocytes, B lymphocytes, natural killer cells) of the hematopoietic system. Hematopoietic progenitor cells are transplanted in order to replace diseased hematopoietic cells or reduce the duration of pancytopenia following administration of high dose chemotherapy. Stem cell transplants are classified according to the familial relationship of the donor and recipient, the immunologic likeness of the donor and recipient, and the intensity of pretransplant preparative treat-ment. Allogeneic stem cell transplants require donation of stem cells from a healthy donor; whereas, autologous transplantation uses stem cells previ-ously collected from the patient undergoing treatment. Allogeneic stem cell transplants are further classified as related transplants (donor and recipient are siblings), unrelated transplants (donor and recipient are not related), or syngeneic transplants (donor and recipient are identical twins). Immunologic likeness of the donor and recipient is determined by comparison of the genotype and phenotype of donor and recipient class I and class II major histocompatibility (MHC) antigens. MHC Class I proteins (HLA-A, HLA-B, HLA-C) are present on all nucleated cells in the body and provide a means for the immune system to differentiate self versus nonself. MHC Class II proteins (HLA-DP, HLA-DQ, HLA-DR) are present on antigen presenting cells, such as macrophages, dendritic cells, and B lymphocytes, and acti-vated endothelial cells. Classification of stem cell transplants according to the intensity of the pretransplant preparative regimen differentiates myeloablative versus nonmyeloablative regimens. Myeloablative chemotherapy regimens administer the highest possible dose of chemotherapy, with the doses limited by regimen-related nonhematologic toxicity. The goal of the myeloablative regimen is to achieve the maximum anticancer effect and complete immuno-suppression through the effects of the high dose cytotoxic agents. The goal of the nonmyeloablative preparative regimen is to inhibit the recipient immune system adequately to allow chimeric engraftment of the donated hematopoi-etic cells. Complete donor engraftment following nonmyeloablative transplan-tation is associated with disease response and may be mediated by a graft-versus-malignancy effect. Less regimen-related morbidity occurs following treatment with nonmyeloablative preparative regimens in comparison to myeloablative preparative regimens.

Terms that are synonymous with hematopoietic stem cell transplantation include stem cell transplantation, peripheral stem cell transplantation, bone marrow transplantation, peripheral blood cell transplantation, and peripheral blood cell rescue. The following table lists clinical uses for allogeneic and autologous myeloablative hematopoietic stem cell transplantation.

TRANSPLANTATION *(Continued)*

Condition	Allogeneic	Autologous
Acute lymphocytic leukemia (ALL)	+	+
Acute myelogenous leukemia (AML)	+	+
Myelodysplastic syndrome	+	-
Chronic myelogenous leukemia (CML)	+	+
Non-Hodgkin's lymphoma (NHL)	+	+
Hodgkin's lymphoma	-	+
Multiple myeloma (MM)	+	+
Severe aplastic anemia (SAA)	+	-
Sickle cell disease (SCD)	+	-
Congenital immunodeficiency syndromes	+	-
Adult autoimmune disorders, eg, scleroderma, multiple sclerosis, rheumatoid arthritis	-	+
Breast cancer	-	+
Ovarian cancer	-	+
Germ cell/testicular cancer	-	+
Neuroblastoma	-	+

SOURCES, COLLECTION, AND PROCESSING OF HEMATOPOIETIC PROGENITOR CELLS

Peripheral blood is generally the site for obtaining the hematopoietic progenitor cells for transplantation. The hematopoietic progenitor cells are removed via leukapheresis, which is easily done in an ambulatory setting and requires no anesthesia. Cells collected for autologous transplantation are processed and frozen in the same manner as bone marrow cells. Cells collected for allogeneic transplantation are generally processed and infused immediately; however, cells for allogeneic transplantation have been frozen and stored prior to transplantation. Leukapheresis involves the processing of approximately 10 liters of peripheral blood over a 2-6 hour period. The usual goal is a product containing at least 2×10^6/kg of CD34$^+$ cells. This may require just 1 day of leukopheresis or several days. Patients may require calcium supplementation during leukopheresis due to the citrate anticoagulant used during the procedure. Hematopoietic engraftment (normalization of the peripheral white blood cell count) occurs earlier following peripheral stem cell transplantation than following bone marrow transplantation. Common medical risks to the allogeneic donor of peripheral hematopoietic stem cells include adverse effects from treatment with a colony-stimulating factor, and adverse events associated with plasmapheresis (acute hypocalcemia, catheter-related discomfort).

The peripheral blood concentration of hematopoietic stem cells and progenitor cells must be increased to facilitate successful product collection. This process is known as peripheral progenitor cell mobilization. After administration of chemotherapy, colony-stimulating factors, or a combination of the two agents, the numbers of circulating early and late progenitor cells becomes greatly increased. A colony-stimulating factor, such as filgrastim or sargramostim, is used for this purpose in the healthy allogeneic donor. For the autologous donor, a colony-stimulating factor is administered alone or prescribed following chemotherapy. Mobilization of hematopoietic progenitor cells can be more difficult in patients with hematologic malignancies, or a history of extensive treatment with chemotherapy and radiation. The following table provides the dosage and schedule for some of the more commonly used mobilization regimens. Selection of the chemotherapy for mobilization in the autologous donor is primarily based on the type of cancer being treated. Cytokines such as stem cell factor (SCF), interleukin-3 (IL-3), and PIXY 321 have been used investigationally for mobilization of progenitor cells.

Mobilization Agent	Dosage and Duration
Filgrastim (G-CSF)	10 mcg/kg/day SubQ for 5-7 days or until target WBC; dose escalation to 16-32 mcg/kg/day has been used to improve inadequate mobilization
Sargramostim (GM-CSF)	250 mg/m^2/day SubQ for 5-7 days or until target WBC
Etoposide (VP-16)	2 g/m^2 I.V. over 2 hours followed in 24 hours by G-CSF or GM-CSF until target WBC
Cyclophosphamide	4 g/m^2 (range of 1.5-7 g/m^2) I.V. over 2 hours followed at 24 hours by G-CSF 5-10 mcg/kg/day until target WBC
Doxorubicin	90 mg/m^2 every 2 wk + G-CSF 5 mcg/kg/day
Paclitaxel plus cyclophosphamide	170 mg/m^2 (P) plus 4 g/m^2 (C) followed by G-CSF
Cytarabine plus etoposide	2 g/m^2 I.V. q12h x 8 doses + 40 mg/kg VP-16 over 4 days then G-CSF 10 mcg/kg/day from day 14 until cells collected

Historically, the bone marrow was the primary source of hematopoietic stem cells for transplantation. The bone marrow contains populations of hematopoietic cells ranging from the pluripotent stem cell, early progenitor cells, and later, more differentiated progenitor cells that all exist within and are supported by the bone marrow stroma (matrix composed of connective tissue, reticuloendothelial cells, adipose cells). Bone marrow can be harvested by removing an adequate volume of marrow (approximately 10 mL/kg) from the posterior iliac crests of the donor or patient. This is generally done in an operating room and requires general or local anesthesia. Bone marrow collected for autologous transplantation is processed in a cryopreservation laboratory and frozen until the day of transplantation. Common medical risks to the donor of bone marrow include the risks of undergoing anesthesia, and transient moderate pain in the area of cell harvesting. The frequency of life-threatening complications, which have included thromboembolic disorders, aspiration pneumonia, and cardiac dysrhythmias, is ≤0.3%.

Umbilical cord blood (UCB) is another source of hematopoietic progenitor cells. The product, which is harvested from UCB immediately after birth, can be processed and transplanted or frozen for future use. The product obtained from UCB contains a high proportion of pluripotent stem cells, and natural

TRANSPLANTATION *(Continued)*

killer cells, and a low proportion of mature lymphocytes. The time to engraftment is generally longer following UCB transplantation than following hematopoietic stem cell transplantation when peripheral blood or bone marrow is harvested and infused. Moreover, UCB transplantation is generally reserved for children and small adults because the number of stem cells that can be collected from cord blood may be inadequate to support timely engraftment for larger patients. The process of harvesting UCB does not present a medical risk to the donor, because the actual collection of cells is done after the placenta is extruded as part of the birthing process.

The hematopoietic progenitor cells may be treated prior to transplantation to eradicate tumor cell contamination in the product following autologous donation or reduce the number of T lymphocytes that may promote graft-versus-host disease in an allogeneic recipient. The term purging refers to the removal of tumor cells from the bone marrow by various techniques such as binding to specific monoclonal antibodies or incubation with cytotoxic drugs, such as 4-hydroperoxycyclophosphamide, that spare the immature progenitor cells. Ex-vivo T lymphocyte reduction, also known as T cell depletion, is generally achieved using monoclonal antibodies directed against surface proteins expressed on T lymphocytes. An alternative to purging or T lymphocyte depletion is the application of positive selection techniques, which remove the CD34$^+$ cells (CD34 is a marker for the pluripotent hematopoietic stem cell) for use and discards the remaining cells. Engraftment is generally delayed following transplantation of hematopoietic progenitor cells that have undergone ex-vivo purging, T cell depletion, or positive selection of CD34$^+$ cells.

AUTOLOGOUS MYELOABLATIVE TRANSPLANTATION

Chemotherapy selection for this type of SCT is based on three important principles:

1. Certain drugs such as alkylating agents and etoposide exhibit steep dose-response curves when used to treat susceptible malignancies. Therefore, when the dose-limiting adverse effect of these drugs is myelosuppression, high doses can be administered with hematopoietic stem cell rescue to achieve high response rates.

2. High doses of chemotherapy with nonoverlapping major organ toxicity can be combined without compromising dose.

3. Cryopreserved bone marrow and/or blood progenitor cells can rescue the patient from the myeloablative effects of the high-dose chemotherapy.

Administration of filgrastim or sargramostim following reinfusion of the autologous hematopoietic progenitor cells can significantly shorten the duration of neutropenia associated with myeloablative chemotherapy (refer to filgrastim or sargramostim monographs for dosing, etc). The hematopoietic recovery period following autologous SCT is generally 1-2 weeks, which is shorter than that for allogeneic or UCB transplants which require 2-4 weeks. The monocytes and neutrophils engraft first followed by the platelets about a week later. The most common complications associated with autologous SCT are febrile neutropenia, serum electrolyte abnormalities, infection, bleeding, gastrointestinal toxicities (mucositis, nausea, vomiting, and diarrhea), and less commonly, other organ toxicities that are related to the specific chemotherapy administered. The following table lists commonly used chemotherapy agents with their dose-limiting toxicities in SCT.

Chemotherapy	Standard Dose	Maximum SCT Dose as Single Agent	Maximum SCT Dose in Combination	Dose-Limiting Toxicity
Busulfan	4 mg/d	16 mg/kg	16 mg/kg	GI, liver
Carboplatin	400 mg/m²	2000 mg/m²	1800 mg/m²	Liver, renal
Carmustine	200 mg/m²	800 mg/m²	600 mg/m²	Liver, lungs
Cisplatin	75-100 mg/m²	180 mg/m²	165 mg/m²	Renal, neuropathy
Cyclophosphamide	50 mg/kg or 600-1875 mg/m²	200 mg/kg or 7.5 g/m²	200 mg/kg or 7.5 g/m²	Cardiac, hemorrhagic cystitis
Etoposide	360 mg/m²	2400 mg/m²	2400 mg/m²	GI
Ifosfamide	5 g/m²	18 g/m²	16 g/m²	CNS, renal
Melphalan	40 mg/m²	220 mg/m²	140-180 mg/m²	GI
Mitoxantrone	12 mg/m²/d x 3	90 mg/m²	60 mg/m²	GI, cardiac
Thiotepa	30-50 mg/m²	1500 mg/m²	900 mg/m²	CNS, GI

ALLOGENEIC MYELOABLATIVE TRANSPLANTATION

The principle behind allogeneic myeloablative hematopoietic stem cell transplantation is that hematological disease can be cured by complete marrow ablation with profound immunosuppression such that the donor cells can engraft and successfully replace the patient's diseased hematopoietic system. Prolonged immunosuppressive therapy is essential for successful engraftment of donor cells and prevention of graft versus host disease (GVHD). Preparative regimens for allogeneic transplantation are based on the need for both marrow ablation and immunosuppression. The most commonly used regimens are listed below.

Acronym	Chemotherapy Drugs (Total Dose)	Dosages and Scheduling
BuCy	Busulfan (12-16 mg/kg)	0.875-1 mg/kg/dose P.O. q6h x 16 doses; or 1 mg/kg/dose P.O. q6h x 12 doses; or 0.8 mg/kg I.V. q6h x 16 doses
	Cyclophosphamide (120 mg/kg)	60 mg/kg/dose I.V. q24h x 2 doses
FTBI/Cy, or CyTBI	Fractionated total body irradiation	1200-1500 cGy divided bid over 3-5 days
	Cyclophosphamide (120-200 mg/kg)	50 mg/kg/dose I.V. q24h x 4 doses or 60 mg/kg/dose I.V. q24h x 2 doses
Bu/Mel	Busulfan (16 mg/kg)	1 mg/kg/dose P.O. q6h x 16 doses
	Melphalan (135-140 mg/m²)	45 mg/m²/dose I.V. q24h x 3, or 140 mg/m² once
FTBI/Mel	Fractionated total body irradiation	1200-1500 cGy divided bid over 3-5 days
	Melphalan (135-140 mg/m²)	45 mg/m²/dose I.V. q24h x 2, or 70 mg/m²/dose I.V. q24h x 2; or 140 mg/m² once

TRANSPLANTATION (Continued)

(continued)

Acronym	Chemotherapy Drugs (Total Dose)	Dosages and Scheduling
CyATG	Cyclophosphamide (200 mg/kg)	50 mg/kg/dose I.V. q24h x 4
	Lymphocyte immune globulin (90-160 mg/kg)	30-40 mg/kg/dose I.V. q24-48h x 3-4 doses

Lymphocyte immune globulin or antithymocyte globulin is included in the preparative regimen for patients with severe aplastic anemia. Lymphocyte immune globulin or antithymocyte globulin is often added to the preparative regimen for allogeneic transplants when the donor and recipient are immunologically mismatched or unrelated, and for umbilical cord blood transplants. This added immunosuppression improves engraftment and may decrease acute GVHD.

Graft versus host disease (GVHD) is an immune-mediated reaction initiated by donor T-cell recognition of recipient tissues as nonself. GVHD which occurs before 100 days post-transplant is called acute GVHD, and after this time it is called chronic GVHD. Acute GVHD primarily affects the skin, gastrointestinal tract, and liver. It is graded based on extent of organ involvement from grade I (mild) to grade IV (life-threatening). Chronic GVHD affects the skin, gastrointestinal tract, liver, and other organs and tissues including the lungs, lacrimal glands, and connective tissue. Chronic GVHD is generally graded as limited or extensive disease. Mortality from this toxicity ranges from 10% to 30%. An effect of acute or chronic mild-to-moderate GVHD is the graft vs malignancy effect which can occur.

The goal of therapy is to prevent severe GVHD. A combination of 2-3 immunosuppressants is used to prevent GVHD. The selection of prophylactic immunosuppressants used is based on the degree of risk for GVHD and the risk of malignant relapse. In general, as the depth and duration of immunosuppression increase so does the risk of malignant relapse, and infectious disease. Commonly used prophylactic immunosuppressants include cyclosporine or tacrolimus plus methotrexate, with addition of a methylprednisolone for patients at high risk for GVHD.

GVHD Prophylactic Agents	Usual Dose and Schedule
Cyclosporine	2.5-4 mg/kg/day I.V. continuous infusion or divided q12h over 2-6 hours. Dose adjust according to toxicity and blood concentrations. Convert to oral dose when appropriate.
Tacrolimus	0.03 mg/kg/day continuous infusion. Adjust dose according to toxicity and blood concentrations. Convert to oral dose when appropriate.
Methotrexate	15 mg/m^2/day on day + 1, 10 mg/m^2 on days +3, +6, and +11; give I.V. push, or "mini methotrexate" 5 mg/m^2/day I.V.P. on days +1, +3, +6

(continued)

GVHD Prophylactic Agents	Usual Dose and Schedule
Methylprednisolone	Variable; 0.5-1 mg/kg/day divided q6-12h then taper. May start +1 up to +7; increase dose for acute GVHD reactions.
Mycophenolate Mofetil	1 g/dose I.V. or P.O. q12h; or 15 mg/kg/dose I.V. or P.O. q12h

Initial treatment of GVHD includes addition of a corticosteroid or a dosage increase of ongoing corticosteroid treatment. Additional agents used for the treatment of steroid-refractory acute GVHD include lymphocyte immune globulin or antithymocyte globulin, interleukin-2 receptor antagonists (basiliximab, daclizumab), tumor necrosis factor antagonists (etanercept, infliximab), sirolimus, pentostatin, and muromonab CD3. Additional agents used for the treatment of steroid-refractory chronic GVHD include thalidomide, pentostatin, PUVA (8-methoxypsoralen plus UV-A radiation), and sirolimus.

Allogeneic stem cell transplantation is associated with a wide range of infectious complications that occur during identifiable time periods after the transplant. The early period of neutropenia is most commonly associated with bacterial infections, yeast (*Candida* species), and possibly herpes simplex virus (HSV) reactivation. Pneumocystis pneumonia (PCP) risk increases with duration of immunosuppressive therapy. Other life-threatening infections typically occurring 2-3 months post-transplant include aspergillosis and CMV (disseminated or pneumonitis). Other serious atypical viral and fungal infections can also be seen at this later time.

Prophylaxis for certain infections is routine while others are treated when they are diagnosed. Trimethoprim-sulfamethoxazole is given during the preparative regimen as a selective gut decontaminant, and then restarted after hematopoietic recovery on a 2-3 times weekly schedule as PCP prophylaxis. The major concern with this drug is the myelosuppressive effect. Flouroquinolones may be used as selective gut decontamination. Some type of fungal prophylaxis is routinely given as well. This consists of either a daily low dose amphotericin-B (0.15-0.25 mg/kg) or fluconazole 100-400 mg daily. Inhalation amphotericin B can also be used to decrease risk of pulmonary aspergillosis. Acyclovir is routinely used to prevent HSV reinfection. The role of acyclovir for prevention of CMV infection is controversial. Some centers routinely prescribe acyclovir immediately following the transplant for prevention of CMV or HSV infection. After cellular recovery, the patient may be switched to ganciclovir therapy. Ganciclovir is not used earlier due to the risk of graft failure. The role of antibacterial prophylaxis or gut decontamination varies with transplant centers but is often used in some form.

Hematopoietic growth factors (filgrastim or sargramostim) are usually but not always administered after infusion of allogeneic donor blood cells. The doses range from 5-10 mcg/kg/day and administration is begun either on day 0 or +1 or may be delayed up to 6 days post cell infusion. Concerns that leukemia cells would be stimulated have been largely unfounded. The colony

TRANSPLANTATION *(Continued)*

stimulating factors are discontinued when neutrophil recovery reaches some target number (5000-10,000/μL has been used).

NONMYELOABLATIVE TRANSPLANTS

Nonmyeloablative hematopoietic stem cell transplants are a new and largely investigational approach to the treatment of malignant and nonmalignant diseases. Clinical trials and case series describe use of nonmyeloablative hematopoietic stem cell transplantation for the following diseases: congenital immunodeficiency syndromes, acute myelogenous leukemia, myelodysplastic syndrome, acute lymphocytic leukemia, multiple myeloma, non-Hodgkin's lymphoma, Hodgkin's disease, sickle cell disease, renal cell carcinoma, and various advanced solid tumors. Most of the published studies and case series report use of this procedure in patients with relapsed or refractory disease, elderly patients, or those unable to tolerate myeloablative preparative regimens.

The theory supporting nonmyeloablative transplantation is that chimeric engraftment will support a graft-versus-malignancy effect. The preparative regimens used for nonmyeloablative hematopoietic stem cell transplantation, which are termed "reduced-intensity preparative regimens", induce profound immunosuppression without total obliteration of the recipient's bone marrow. This supports chimeric engraftment, which involves engraftment of transplanted allogeneic hematopoietic progenitor cells in the presence of recipient hematopoietic cells. Complete donor engraftment, also known as 100% donor chimerism, occurs when all of the detectable hematopoietic cells are of donor origin. Complete donor chimerism occurring within 30-90 days following transplantation is generally associated with disease response.

The preparative regimens used for nonmyeloablative hematopoietic stem cell transplantation are associated with less regimen-related toxicity than myeloablative preparative regimens. This provides the impetus for studying use of nonmyeloablative hematopoietic stem cell transplantation in patients unable to tolerate the myeloablative preparative regimens, such as the elderly, or patients with an extensive history of chemotherapy treatment, impaired major organ function, or comorbid conditions. Examples of reduced-intensity preparative regimens are listed in the following table.

Acronym	Chemotherapy Drugs (Total Dose)	Dosages and Scheduling
Flu/ATG	Lymphocyte immune globulin 40 mg/kg (Atgam)	10 mg/kg/day I.V. on 4 consecutive days
	Antithymoglobulin 10 mg/kg (Thymoglobulin)	2.5 mg/kg/day I.V. on 4 consecutive days
	Fludarabine 125 mg/m^2	2.5 mg/m^2/day I.V.on 5 consecutive days
FC-ATG	Fludarabine 125 mg/m^2	25 mg/m^2/day I.V. on days -6 to -2
	Cyclophosphamide 120 mg/kg	60 mg/kg/day I.V. on days -3 and -2
	Lymphocyte immune globulin 60 mg/kg (Atgam)	20 mg/kg/day I.V. on 3 consecutive days
TBI/Flu	Total body irradiation 4 Gy	2 Gy/day on days -8 and -7
	Fludarabine 125 mg/m^2	25 mg/m^2/day I.V. on days -6 to -2

(continued)

Acronym	Chemotherapy Drugs (Total Dose)	Dosages and Scheduling
Flu/Mel/ATG	Fludarabine 125 mg/m^2	25 mg/m^2/day I.V. on days -6 to -2
	Melphalan 140-180 mg/m^2	70-90 mg/m^2/day I.V. on days -3 and -2
	Lymphocyte immune globulin 120 mg/kg (Atgam)	30 mg/kg/day I.V. on days -4 to -1
Bu/Flu/ATG	Busulfan 8 mg/kg	1 mg/kg/dose P.O. q6h X8 doses on days -6 and -5
	Fludarabine 125 mg/m^2	25 mg/m^2/day I.V. on days -6 to -2
	Antithymocyte globulin (Fresnius) 10 mg/kg	2.5 mg/kg/day I.V. on 4 consecutive days

GVHD prophylaxis generally includes cyclosporine or tacrolimus plus mycophenolate mofetil. Treatment of moderate-to-severe GVHD is similar to the approach taken for treatment of GVHD following myeloablative allogeneic hematopoietic stem cell transplantation. Most complications following nonmyeloablative hematopoietic stem cell transplantation are related to GVHD and the immunosuppression required for treatment of GVHD. Infectious complications from Cytomegalovirus, herpes virus, candidiasis, aspergillosis, and other atypical infections are common.

Selected Readings

Bacigalupo A, "Second EBMT Workshop on Reduced Intensity Allogeneic Hemopoietic Stem Cell Transplants (RI-HSCT)," *Bone Marrow Transplant*, 2002, 29:191-5.

Cairo MS and Wagner JE, "Placental and/or Umbilical Cord Blood: An Alternative Source of Hematopoietic Stem Cells for Transplantation," *Blood*, 1997, 90:4665-78.

Champlin R, Khouri I, Anderlini P, et al, "Nonmyeloablative Preparative Regimens for Allogeneic Hematopoietic Transplantation," *Bone Marrow Transplant*, 2001, 27 Suppl 2:S13-22.

Ho VT and Soiffer RJ, "The History and Future of T-Cell Depletion as Graft-Versus-Host Disease Prophylaxis for Allogeneic Hematopoietic Stem Cell Transplantation," *Blood*, 2001, 98:3192-204.

Klingebiel T and Schlegel PG, "GVHD: Overview on Pathophysiology, Incidence, Clinical and Biological Features," *Bone Marrow Transplant*, 1998, 21 (Suppl 2):S45-9.

Mogul MJ, "Unrelated Cord Blood Transplantation Vs Matched Unrelated Donor Bone Marrow Transplantation: The Risks and Benefits of Each Choice," *Bone Marrow Transplant*, 2000, 25 (Suppl 2):S58-60.

Rowe JM, Ciobanu N, Ascensao J, et al, "Recommended Guidelines for the Management of Autologous and Allogeneic Bone Marrow Transplantation. A Report From the Eastern Cooperative Oncology Group (ECOG)," *Ann Intern Med*, 1994, 120:143-58.

Stiff P, "Mucositis Associated With Stem Cell Transplantation: Current Status and Innovative Approaches to Management," *Bone Marrow Transplant* , 2001, 27 (Suppl 2):S3-S11.

Storb R, Deeg HJ,,Whitehead J, et al, "Methotrexate and Cyclosporine Compared With Cyclosporine Alone for Prophylaxis of Acute Graft Versus Host Disease After Marrow Transplantation for Leukemia," *N Engl J Med*, 1986, 314:729-35.

Vogelsang GB and Arai S, "Mycophenolate Mofetil for the Prevention and Treatment of Graft-Versus-Host Disease Following Stem Cell Transplantation: Preliminary Findings," *Bone Marrow Transplant*, 2001, 27:1255-62.

DRUG DEVELOPMENT PROCESS

DRUG SYNTHESIS

A rational and empiric approach is used in the discovery of drugs. Compounds may be selected which inhibit certain molecular targets. These compounds may be modified based on target inhibitor interactions. Increasingly, natural products are being studied as suitable compounds for anti-cancer therapy through molecular target screenings. Another screening technique is the use of human tumor cell lines, which have known characteristics with respect to drug response, growth factor dependence, oncogene expression, and other factors. The response patterns of these compounds is then compared against other agents.

PRECLINICAL PHARMACOLOGY

Studies in mice, rats, and dogs are conducted to provide pharmacokinetic and pharmacologic information prior to testing in humans. Pharmacokinetic studies provide a rationale for dose escalation in humans. Simultaneously, drug formulation studies begin, looking at solubility issues and drug delivery systems. Animal toxicology studies must occur before testing in humans. Initially, acute toxicity in mice is studied to determine the LD 10, the dose that is lethal to 10% of the mice. Then, organ-specific toxicity is studied in rodents. Toxicology studies must use the same drug schedule that will be utilized in humans.

INVESTIGATIONAL NEW DRUG (IND) APPLICATION (FDA 1571)

An IND must be submitted prior to clinical trials. It contains all of the preclinical data, proposed clinical protocol, investigator's brochure, and manufacturing information. There is a waiting period of 30 days after submission, after which clinical trials may start unless the FDA asks for changes. Emergency Use or Compassionate IND makes investigational drugs available before IND submission. This is used only for life-saving therapy in refractory patients. Treatment IND (group C drugs) makes investigational drugs available for use under an approved protocol before a new drug application is approved.

An institutional review board (IRB) must approve all phases of clinical drug trials. The purpose of an IRB is to review clinical trials to assure that patients will not be exposed to unnecessary risks and that there is a scientific basis for the research protocol.

PHASE I STUDIES

A protocol for drug administration that will be used in the Phase I trial is required in the IND. Additionally, an informed consent document is required. The purpose of the Phase I study is to characterize pharmacology, pharmacokinetics, pharmacodynamics, maximum tolerated dose (MTD), drug-related toxicity, and dose-limiting toxicity (DLT). Unlike other Phase I trials in normal human subjects, patients with advanced cancer refractory to treatment and with normal organ function, are utilized for Phase I oncology studies. The most common Phase I oncology study involves a new cytotoxic drug at a starting dose $\frac{1}{10}$ the LD10 dose in the most sensitive animal model. The dose is increased in a stepwise fashion until the DLT is reached in >33% of a patient cohort. The dose at which <33% of patients have DLT is utilized in Phase II studies.

PHASE II STUDIES

Phase II trials look at drug safety and efficacy in a group of patients with a disease the drug is intended to treat. Data is collected on adverse effects and response to the therapy, although tumor response is not the objective. The starting dose is the safest dose found in Phase I trials as detailed above.

PHASE III STUDIES

Phase III studies involve a larger number of patients with a particular tumor. Patients are randomized to the new treatment or the current standard of care. A placebo arm is used for Phase III analysis of novel treatments for which there is no comparable standard of care. Data is collected on efficacy, safety, drug interactions, affect on survival curve, etc. As was the case with gemcitabine in pancreatic cancer, a clinical benefit response may be an endpoint that is measured.

NEW DRUG APPLICATION (NDA)

All of the data collected from these trials is collated and submitted as a New Drug Application (NDA). The FDA has 60 days after an NDA filing to reject the NDA due to gross deficiencies. It then has 180 days (sometimes longer) to complete a full review.

PHASE IV STUDIES

Phase IV studies are postmarketing studies which look at a drug's performance in a clinical setting. An IND is not necessary unless the drug is being studied for an indication not present in the package labeling. Phase IV studies are large, multicenter studies that study a drug's use for a specific labeled indication. These studies may provide valuable information on long-term effects of the drug and potential adverse reactions that were not well documented in the limited number of patients in preclinical trials. In addition, restrictions on eligibility criteria will be less strict than in preclinical trials, providing information on efficacy and safety in a wide population.

ACCELERATED NDA REVIEW

In order to decrease the approval process for drugs with significant therapeutic gains, the FDA has instituted some short-track approval mechanisms. The FDA and sponsor may begin meeting as soon as Phase I trials are completed. NDA approval may be based on expanded Phase II trials. Parallel tracks may collect data from open-label noncontrolled studies as well as Phase II studies. Preclinical data from Europe and Japan may be submitted in some cases. Using surrogate endpoints, which may improve the patient's quality of life but do not show measurable disease improvement, may accelerate the approval process especially in diseases with little treatment options.

The FDA, whose purpose is to regulate drug development and manufacturing, and sales and marketing, oversees this entire process. The IND

DRUG DEVELOPMENT PROCESS *(Continued)*

requires FDA approval before the drug is tested in humans. The NDA is reviewed and approved, often with the help of advisory committees composed of non-FDA members. Postmarketing surveillance which includes voluntary reporting of adverse drug reactions and drug recalls are also of great interest to the FDA. It is important to recognize that this entire approval process is constantly changing to help both patients and investigators.

Selected Readings

Dunsworth T, "Drug Regulatory Process," *Pharmacotherapy Self-Assessment Program*, 2nd ed, Carter BL, Angaran DM, Lake KD, et al, eds, Kansas City, KS: American College of Clinical Pharmacy, 1996.

Grever MR and Chabner BA, "Cancer Drug Discovery and Development," *Cancer: Principles & Practice of Oncology*, 5th ed, DeVita VT, Hellman S, Rosenberg SA, eds, Philadelphia, PA: Lippincott-Raven Publishers, 1997.

Simon RM, "Design and Analysis of Clinical Trials," *Cancer: Principles & Practice of Oncology*, 5th ed, DeVita VT, Hellman S, Rosenberg SA, eds, Philadelphia, PA: Lippincott-Raven Publishers, 1997.

INVESTIGATIONAL DRUG SERVICE

An Investigational Drug Service (IDS) is an organized pharmacy-based service that controls the inventory, preparation, and dispensation of investigational drugs. Investigational drugs are administered only to patients who have, in an informed manner, signed a consent form to participate in the particular study using these investigational drugs. A patient formally enrolled to participate in a clinical study is known as a "subject". Investigational drugs used in this manner are frequently new drugs undergoing Phase I, Phase II, or Phase III evaluation prior to FDA approval for a medical purpose. However, investigational drugs can be commercially available drugs used under the direction of a protocol for a nonlabeled indication or as a supportive measure for a new drug. An IDS should be under the direction of an appropriately trained pharmacist with technical support as appropriate for the workload.

A study protocol is the document describing the scientific background providing the basis for doing the study, specific study objectives and endpoints, treatments and tests done as part of the study, study drug information, statistical methodology, means for assurance of patient confidentiality, and the subject consent form. Some studies provide an Investigator's Drug Brochure, which presents very detailed and comprehensive study drug information. Each study is assigned a unique study number, eg, SWOG 9923, that is frequently a truncation of the year of study development and its position within a series of studies. Study protocols and Investigator's Drug Brochures are confidential, and frequently proprietary documents. Prior to study activation at an institution, it must be approved by the institutional investigational review board. All departments needed to provide personnel or resources for study implementation should review the protocol prior to study implementation to ensure that study activities can reasonably be supported with available resources. The IDS pharmacist should scrutinize each study protocol prior to study activation to determine the impact of study implementation on pharmacy department personnel and resources.

Investigational drug inventory must be stored at the appropriate conditions, and separate from commercial drug inventory. An ongoing drug-specific inventory must be maintained for all investigational drugs housed within a pharmacy. Some studies will require lot number-specific, or subject-specific inventory for study drugs. Minimal inventory documentation should include study identification number, study drug dosage form and lot number, study drug expiration date or date of preparation, transaction date, transaction type (receipt, dispensation, return, waste), and current number of dosage forms available. Although it may be kept separately from individual study drug inventories, the pharmacy must maintain an ongoing refrigerator, freezer, and ambient temperature log for study drug storage facilities. All inventory records should be kept in a secure and accessible location by the pharmacy, even after study closure. In addition, study drug should be shipped directly to the Pharmacy Department rather than the Principal Investigator's office. This will ensure that the Pharmacy Department has shipping receipts and shipment invoices to verify receipt of the packaged contents. This will also reduce the possibility of prolonged study drug storage at inappropriate conditions, such as the institutional loading dock.

INVESTIGATIONAL DRUG SERVICE *(Continued)*

Study drug preparation should be described in the protocol or Investigator's Drug Brochure. Unfortunately, extensive admixture stability and compatibility information is not available for many injectable study drugs. Subsequently, these may have to be prepared on a dose-by-dose basis. Departmental inservices to acquaint professional and technical personnel with each new study are helpful tools for increasing staff familiarity with new studies and study drug preparation. Pharmacy department personnel should have 24-hour access to information about study drug preparation. Ideally, this is in the form of an easy-to-read and readily accessible fast facts sheet. Study protocols and Investigator's Drug Brochures should also be available to Pharmacy Department personnel around the clock for questions that arise outside of standard business hours. The Investigational Drug Service must develop a plan such that study drug doses are labeled in the manner directed by the study, are consistent with institutional policies and procedures, and are in accordance with state and federal regulations.

Study drug doses prepared for administration within a hospital or clinic should be dispensed directly to the study or institutional nurse for delivery to the patient's bedside, or placed directly into the subject's medication bin for delivery to the nursing unit. Generally, study drug doses should not be intermixed with standard medication doses transported via the routine intra-institutional delivery system. Although the risk of inadvertent misplacement of a study drug dose may be low, the consequences can have ethical and legal implications. As an example, a study drug dose inadvertently transported to the wrong nursing unit may be mistakenly administered to a patient with a name similar to that of the actual study subject. In other words, the study drug dose could be administered to a person who did not consent to receive an investigational drug.

Pharmacy support of blinded studies can involve additional responsibilities and challenges. Pharmacy-related activities may include randomization (treatment assignment) of subjects when the Principal Investigator and other study personnel are blinded to the study treatment. Randomization for treatment assignment can be done for some studies by simply following a list of treatment assignments sequentially for consecutive subjects. However, randomization for some multicenter studies may require contacting a central randomization center with provision of patient-specific information. When pharmacy activities include randomization, it is important for the Investigational Drug Service to ensure that a workable plan is in place prior to study activation. Moreover, labeling of blinded study drug doses can be challenging since the traditional role of pharmacy labeling is to provide a completely clear description of the dosage form. In contrast, to maintain a study blind, the specific contents of a study dosage form must be omitted from the pharmacy label. Several approaches have been taken to balance study methods with institutional and legislative requirements. As an example, for a blinded study, protocol #9872, evaluating the efficacy of fluconazole 200 mg versus placebo (0.9% NaCl 100 mL), the following labeling techniques can be utilized to identify the dosage form: "fluconazole 200 mg or placebo", "fluconazole study drug", "protocol #9872 study drug". Nursing personnel should be consulted regarding the proposed labeling of blinded study drug to ensure that the labeling used is compatible with medication administration records maintained by nursing staff.

The Investigational Drug Service determines fair charges for Pharmacy Department personnel time and resources utilized in the support of study activities. As a rule, routine pharmacy charges to the patient's bill, cannot be generated for investigational new drugs, or study drugs provided free-of-charge by the study sponsor. The Investigation Drug Service must charge the study funds. This is generally achieved at the institutional level by generating charges to the local Principal Investigator or Clinical Trials Office.

SAFE HANDLING OF
HAZARDOUS DRUGS

Due to their inherent toxicity, particularly mutagenicity and carcinogenicity, there is concern about the risks of long-term, low level exposure to a number of drugs, particularly antineoplastic agents. The possible risk to healthcare providers who are responsible for preparation and administration of such agents has been a subject of much debate, but few definite answers. Despite more than 20 years of research and literally thousands of publications on the topic, there is no definitive evidence of a causal relationship between prolonged exposure to low levels of antineoplastic agents in the workplace and development of malignancies. Neither is there conclusive evidence that such exposure is not hazardous. In the absence of convincing evidence that healthcare personnel are not at risk, prudence requires the presumption that there is some degree of risk, and employees should employ appropriate protective measures.

The potential for many antineoplastic agents to cause secondary malignancies in patients was identified in the 1960s and 1970s. Coupled with evidence of some drugs' carcinogenicity in animals, this information raised the question of possible adverse effects from prolonged low level exposure. In the late 1970s and 1980s, a large number of anecdotal reports of various side effects and adverse reactions in nurses, pharmacists, and pharmacy technicians involved in preparation and administration of antineoplastic therapy began to appear in the literature. These were followed by reports of increased urine mutagenicity, chromosome abnormalities, changes in immune function, and detectable blood or urine drug levels in personnel who routinely handled antineoplastic agents. As a result of these concerns, a number of groups issued guidelines intended to minimize exposure to antineoplastic agents in the workplace. By the end of the 1980s, a variety of organizations, including the Occupational Safety and Health Administration (OSHA), American Society of Hospital (now Health-System) Pharmacists (ASHP), the National Institutes of Health (NIH), and the National Study Commission on Cytotoxic Exposure had all issued documents addressing the proper handling of cytotoxic agents by healthcare personnel. Most of the early guidelines acknowledged the paucity and low quality of the available data, and recommended further research to define the actual risks.

During the remainder of the 1980s and 1990s, a number of studies and reports attempting to delineate the nature of the risk, and the appropriate safety measures to be taken were published. The vast majority of these were uncontrolled trials involving very small numbers of individuals, usually at a single institution. The nature and magnitude of the risk has never been properly delineated. Due to the nature of the problem, there has never been a large scale, prospective controlled trial to determine the efficacy of the various protective measures employed. As a result, there is no known threshold of safety for exposure to these agents; nor have any reliable monitoring techniques to assess exposure been developed. Most guidelines are therefore based on an assumption of "zero tolerance" - any exposure is hazardous, and must be avoided. Achieving the appropriate balance between necessary protection for personnel who must work with these agents and over-reaction to the threat remains a challenge.

Defining hazardous agents and identifying effective protective measures remains a problem. There is no agreement among various agencies as to the definition of a hazardous agent or which agents should be classified as hazardous. The Environmental Protection Agency (EPA), National Institute for Occupational Safety and Health (NIOSH), and American Society of Health-System Pharmacists all have guidelines for handling hazardous agents, but there is little agreement, and considerable variation among these guidelines. The EPA lists 723 chemicals as hazardous. Only eight are antineoplastic agents; an additional 16 non-antineoplastic agents are listed as hazardous. NIOSH has 60 drugs on its list (which it states is incomplete and "not all-inclusive"), including 13 nonantineoplastic agents. (see Tables 1 and 2 on the following pages). Some manufacturers also recommend special precautions for handling specific drugs (eg, mycophenolate, ganciclovir).

SAFE HANDLING OF
HAZARDOUS DRUGS *(Continued)*

Table 1: Criteria for Defining Hazardous Agents

EPA	NIOSH	ASHP
Meets one of the following criteria: Ignitability: Create fire under certain conditions or are spontaneously combustible and have a flash point <600°C Corrosivity: Acids or bases (pH >2 or ≤12.5) capable of corroding metal containers Reactivity: Unstable under "normal" conditions; can cause explosions, toxic fumes, gases, or vapors when mixed with water Toxicity characteristic: When disposed of on land, contaminated liquid may drain or leach from the waste and pollute ground water	Designated as therapeutic category 10:00 (Antineoplastic Agent) in the American Hospital Formulary Service Drug Information	Genotoxic
	Manufacturer suggests use of special techniques in handling administration, or disposal	Carcinogenic
	Mutagenic	Teratogenic or impairs fertility
	Carcinogenic	Causes serious organ or other toxic manifestation at low doses
	Teratogenic or reproductive toxicant	
OR	Acutely toxic to an organ system	
Appears on one of the following lists: F: Wastes from certain common or industrial manufacturing processes from nonspecific sources K: Wastes from certain specific industries from specific sources P: Wastes from pure or commercial grade formulations of certain specific unused chemicals U: Wastes from pure or commercial grade formulations of certain specific unused chemicals	Investigational drugs	

Table 2: Drugs Listed as Hazardous by EPA or NIOSH

EPA		NIOSH	
Antineoplastic	**Nonantineoplastic**	**Antineoplastic**	**Nonantineoplastic**
Arsenic Trioxide	Dichlorodifluoromethane	Altretamine	Anesthetic, agents
Chlorambucil	Diethylstilbesterol	Aminoglutethimide	Cyclosporine
Cyclophosphamide	Epinephrine	Azathioprine	Diethylstilbestrol
Daunomycin	Hexachlorophene	Asparaginase	Estradiol
Malphalan	Lindane	Bleomycin	Ethinyl Estradiol
Mitomycin	Nitroglycerin	Busulfan	Ganciclovir
Streptozocin	Paraldehyde	Carboplatin	Isotretinoin
Uracil Mustard	Phenacetin	Carmustine	Medroxyprogesterone
	Physostigmine	Chlorambucil	Nafarelin
	Physostigmine Salicylate	Chloramphenicol	Pentamidine
	Reserpine	Chlorozotocin	Plicamycin
	Resorcinol	Cisplatin	Ribavirin
	Saccharin	Cyclophosphamide	Testolactone
	Selenium Sulfide	Cytarabine	Vidarabine
	Trichloromono-fluoromethane	Dacarbazine	Zidovudine
	Warfarin	Dactinomycin	
		Daunorubicin	
		Doxorubicin	
		Estramustine	
		Etoposide	
		Floxuridine	
		Fluorouracil	
		Flutamide	
		Hydroxyurea	
		Idarubicin	
		Ifosfamide	
		Interferon A	
		Leuprolide	
		Levamisole	
		Lomustine	
		Mechlorethamine	
		Megestrol	
		Melphalan	
		Mercaptopurine	
		Methotrexate	
		Mitomycin	
		Mitotane	
		Mitoxantrone	
		Pipobroman	
		Procarbazine	
		Streptozocin	
		Tamoxifen	
		Thioguanine	
		Thiotepa	
		Uracil Mustard	
		Vinblastine	
		Vincristine	

SAFE HANDLING OF
HAZARDOUS DRUGS *(Continued)*

In addition to the differences among the available guidelines, some criteria are extremely vague or broad, adding to the uncertainty. The NIOSH criterion "Acutely toxic to an organ system" could be applied to almost any drug. ASHP's "Causes serious organ or other toxic manifestation at low doses" could also apply to a large number of drugs not commonly considered "hazardous" to persons handling them. The EPA standard "Appears on one of the following lists" seems to be particularly subjective. Drugs appear on, and are removed from, the EPA lists in what appears a purely arbitrary manner. For example, cisplatin and dexamethasone have appeared on previous lists, but are not on the current one. Daunomycin and cyclophosphamide are listed as hazardous; other anthacyclines and ifosfamine are not. Inquiries to EPA have failed to identify why these changes were made; or why one drug in a class is considered hazardous, but other agents in that category are not.

Analysis of the problem has not completely clarified the risks. Rather, previously accepted practices are subject to question. A 1992 report on exposure of healthcare personnel to hazardous agents suggested that the standard biologic safety cabinets recommended for use when compounding hazardous drugs may not provided the desired level of protection. There is evidence suggesting rather than forming particles or aerosol droplets that could be trapped in a standard HEPA filter, some antineoplastic agents vaporize, yielding particles that cannot be trapped in the filter. This potential for vaporization may be a partial explanation for recent reports indicating detectable contamination of work surfaces in, and near, hazardous drug preparation areas. This information has led some institutions to begin investigating use of isolator cabinets and sealed preparation systems as replacements for the biologic cabinets.

A 1996 review of 64 studies of workplace exposure to cytotoxic drugs noted numerous methodologic flaws in study design and procedures. The report concluded the methods used to assess exposure in these studies were too nonspecific and insensitive to be reliable measures of exposure. One disturbing aspect of this is the fact that the studies and procedures found to be not sensitive enough to assess routine levels of exposure were the ones used as the basis for development of the existing handling guidelines.

Several studies have found containers have detectable amounts of drug residue on them when they arrive in the pharmacy. These reports raise the concern that exposure may be a hazard originating at least partially outside the pharmacy; and that additional procedures for decontaminating drug containers upon arrival at the pharmacy may be necessary.

Guidelines and institutional policies for minimizing exposure to hazardous materials have been based on the presumption that environmental exposure to hazardous drugs occurs through three mechanisms:

- **inhalation** of drug dust or aerosolized droplets
- **absorption** through the skin
- **ingestion** of contaminated food or drink

Accordingly, the existing recommendations are heavily weighted toward the use of physical barriers as the primary means of reducing exposure. Among the commonly employed precautions are:

- **Separation:** Hazardous agents are often prepared in a limited number of areas which are separated, to the extent possible, from other drug preparation areas. Almost all institutions have a separate biologic safety cabinet reserved solely for the preparation of antineoplastic agents. Many institutions have a separate "oncology" drug preparation area or satellite pharmacy.

- **Biologic safety cabinets:** Use of a Class IIA or B biologic safety cabinet for the preparation of hazardous agents. Recent reports have questioned the efficacy of these cabinets, and some institutions have adopted the use of Isolator® systems or special closed preparation systems for compounding hazardous agents.

- **Protective clothing:** Another almost universal precaution is the used of protective gloves, gowns, and eye protection while handling antineoplastic agents. If drug preparation is performed in a biologic safety cabinet equipped with a glass front, many institutions dispense with the requirement for wearing safety goggles.

- **Training:** Some of the early reports attributed lower, or undetectable, levels of exposure to hazardous drugs to the experience level, or skill at aseptic technique, of the individual worker. Many institutions require some degree of training before personnel are allowed to handle hazardous agents. Although most of the published guidelines recommend personnel who handle hazardous agents have "appropriate" training and experience, none specify what should be included in such a program. Accordingly, the exact nature and length of the required training programs vary widely among institutions.

- **Monitoring:** Appropriate physical parameters for assessing exposure to hazardous drugs are not available. Although some institutions require periodic health monitoring, the definition of what constitutes an appropriate screening program is a matter of some debate. Attempts to monitor the existence of hazardous materials in the work area has been slightly more successful. Assessment of airborne drug levels and surface contamination, in preparation cabinets, "secure" work areas and areas outside the hazardous drug area has been reported. Additionally, techniques for using ultraviolet light to detect occult drug spills, and assess individual's handling technique have been reported. Most of these techniques have not been developed sufficiently to be used in routine practice, and are still limited to the research setting.

- **Decontamination:** Drug containers should be examined upon their arrival at the pharmacy. Containers that show signs of damage should be handled carefully, and may require quarantine and decontamination before being placed in stock. Consideration should be given to the possible need to quarantine and decontaminate all containers of hazardous agents as a routine precaution.

SAFE HANDLING OF
HAZARDOUS DRUGS *(Continued)*

Selected Readings

American Society of Hospital Pharmacists, "ASHP Technical Assistance Bulletin on Handling Cytotoxic and Hazardous Drugs," *Am J Hosp Pharm*, 1990, 47:1033-49.

Baker ES and Connor TH, "Monitoring Occupational Exposure to Cancer Chemotherapy Drugs," *Am J Health Syst Pharm*, 1996, 53(22):2713-23.

Bos RP and Sessink PJ, "Biomonitoring of Occupational Exposures to Cytostatic Anticancer Drugs," *Rev Environ Health*, 1997, 12(1):43-58.

Connor TH, "Permeability of Nitrile Rubber, Latex, Polyurethane, and Neoprene Gloves to 18 Antineoplastic Drugs," *Am J Health Syst Pharm*, 1999, 56(23):2450-3.

Connor TH, Anderson RW, Sessink PJ, et al, "Surface Contamination With Antineoplastic Agents in Six Cancer Treatment Centers in Canada and the United States," *Am J Health Syst Pharm*, 1999, 56(14):1427-32.

Connor TH, Sessink PJ, Harrison BR, et al, "Surface Contamination of Chemotherapy Drug Vials and Evaluation of New Vial-Cleaning Techniques: Results of Three Studies," *Am J Health Syst Pharm*, 2005, 62(5):475-84.

"Preventing Occupational Exposure to Antineoplastic and Other Hazardous Drugs in Health Care Settings," Available at http://www.cdc.gov/niosh/docs/2004-165. Accessed February 6, 2005.

Sessink PJ, Anzion RB, Van den Broek PH, et al, "Detection of Contamination With Antineoplastic Agents in a Hospital Pharmacy Department," *Pharm Weekbl Sci*, 1992, 14(1):16-22.

Sessink PJ, Boer KA, Scheefhals AP, et al, "Occupational Exposure to Antineoplastic Agents at Several Departments in a Hospital. Environmental Contamination and Excretion of Cyclophosphamide and Ifosfamide in Urine of Exposed Workers," *Int Arch Occup Environ Health*, 1992, 64(2):105-12.

Sessink PJ and Bos RP, "Drugs Hazardous to Healthcare Workers. Evaluation of Methods for Monitoring Occupational Exposure to Cytostatic Drugs," *Drug Saf*, 1999, 20(4):347-59.

Solimando D and Wilson J, "Demonstration of Skin Fluorescence Following Exposure to Doxorubicin," *Cancer Nursing*, 1983, 6(4):313-5.

Sorsa M and Anderson D, "Monitoring of Occupational Exposure to Cytostatic Anticancer Agents," *Mutat Res*, 1996, 355(1-2):253-61.

Wilson J and Solimando D, "Aseptic Technique as a Safety Precaution in the Preparation of Antineoplastic Agents," *Hospital Pharmacy*, 1981, 16(11):575-81.

APPENDIX TABLE OF CONTENTS

MILLIEQUIVALENT AND MILLIMOLE CALCULATIONS AND CONVERSIONS

DEFINITIONS AND CALCULATIONS

Definitions

mole	=	gram molecular weight of a substance (aka molar weight)
millimole (mM)	=	milligram molecular weight of a substance (a millimole is 1/1000 of a mole)
equivalent weight	=	gram weight of a substance which will combine with or replace 1 gram (1 mole) of hydrogen; an equivalent weight can be determined by dividing the molar weight of a substance by its ionic valence
milliequivalent (mEq)	=	milligram weight of a substance which will combine with or replace 1 milligram (1 millimole) of hydrogen (a milliequivalent is 1/1000 of an equivalent)

Calculations

moles	=	$\dfrac{\text{weight of a substance (grams)}}{\text{molecular weight of that substance (grams)}}$
millimoles	=	$\dfrac{\text{weight of a substance (milligrams)}}{\text{molecular weight of that substance (milligrams)}}$
equivalents	=	moles x valence of ion
milliequivalents	=	millimoles x valence of ion
moles	=	$\dfrac{\text{equivalents}}{\text{valence of ion}}$
millimoles	=	$\dfrac{\text{milliequivalents}}{\text{valence of ion}}$
millimoles	=	moles x 1000
milliequivalents	=	equivalents x 1000

Note: Use of equivalents and milliequivalents is valid only for those substances which have fixed ionic valences (eg, sodium, potassium, calcium, chlorine, magnesium bromine, etc). For substances with variable ionic valences (eg, phosphorous), a reliable equivalent value cannot be determined. In these instances, one should calculate millimoles (which are fixed and reliable) rather than milliequivalents.

MILLIEQUIVALENT CONVERSIONS

To convert mg/100 mL to mEq/L the following formula may be used:

$$\frac{(\text{mg/100 mL}) \times 10 \times \text{valence}}{\text{atomic weight}} = \text{mEq/L}$$

To convert mEq/L to mg/100 mL the following formula may be used:

$$\frac{(\text{mEq/L}) \times \text{atomic weight}}{10 \times \text{valence}} = \text{mg/100 mL}$$

To convert mEq/L to volume of percent of a gas the following formula may be used:

$$\frac{(mEq/L) \times 22.4}{10} = \text{volume percent}$$

Valences and Atomic Weights of Selected Ions

Substance	Electrolyte	Valence	Molecular Wt
Calcium	Ca^{++}	2	40
Chloride	Cl^-	1	35.5
Magnesium	Mg^{++}	2	24
Phosphate	HPO_4^{--} (80%)	1.8	96[1]
pH = 7.4	$H_2PO_4^-$ (20%)	1.8	96[1]
Potassium	K^+	1	39
Sodium	Na^+	1	23
Sulfate	SO_4^{--}	2	96[1]

[1]The molecular weight of phosphorus only is 31, and sulfur only is 32.

Approximate Milliequivalents — Weights of Selected Ions

Salt	mEq/g Salt	mg Salt/mEq
Calcium carbonate [$CaCO_3$]	20	50
Calcium chloride [$CaCl_2 \bullet 2H_2O$]	14	74
Calcium gluceptate [$Ca(C_7H_{13}O_8)_2$]	4	245
Calcium gluconate [$Ca(C_6H_{11}O_7)_2 \bullet H_2O$]	5	224
Calcium lactate [$Ca(C_3H_5O_3)_2 \bullet 5H_2O$]	7	154
Magnesium gluconate [$Mg(C_6H_{11}O_7)_2 \bullet H_2O$]	5	216
Magnesium oxide [MgO]	50	20
Magnesium sulfate [$MgSO_4$]	17	60
Magnesium sulfate [$MgSO_4 \bullet 7H_2O$]	8	123
Potassium acetate [$K(C_2H_3O_2)$]	10	98
Potassium chloride [KCl]	13	75
Potassium citrate [$K_3(C_6H_5O_7) \bullet H_2O$]	9	108
Potassium iodide [KI]	6	166
Sodium acetate [$Na(C_2H_3O_2)$]	12	82
Sodium acetate [$Na(C_2H_3O_2) \bullet 3H_2O$]	7	136
Sodium bicarbonate [$NaHCO_3$]	12	84
Sodium chloride [$NaCl$]	17	58
Sodium citrate [$Na_3(C_6H_5O_7) \bullet 2H_2O$]	10	98
Sodium iodine [NaI]	7	150
Sodium lactate [$Na(C_3H_5O_3)$]	9	112
Zinc sulfate [$ZnSO_4 \bullet 7H_2O$]	7	144

CORRECTED SODIUM

Corrected Na^+ = measured Na^+ + [1.5 x (glucose − 150 divided by 100)]

Note: Do not correct for glucose <150.

MILLIEQUIVALENT AND MILLIMOLE CALCULATIONS AND CONVERSIONS (Continued)

WATER DEFICIT

Water deficit = 0.6 x body weight [1 − (140 divided by Na^+)]

Note: Body weight is estimated weight in kg when fully hydrated; **Na^+** is serum or plasma sodium. Use corrected Na^+ if necessary. Consult medical references for recommendations for replacement of deficit.

TOTAL SERUM CALCIUM CORRECTED FOR ALBUMIN LEVEL

[(Normal albumin − patient's albumin) x 0.8] + patient's measured total calcium

ACID-BASE ASSESSMENT

Henderson-Hasselbalch Equation

$$pH = 6.1 + \log (HCO_3^- / (0.03) (pCO_2))$$

Alveolar Gas Equation

$$PIO_2 = FiO_2 \text{ x (total atmospheric pressure − vapor pressure of } H_2O \text{ at } 37°C)$$
$$= FiO_2 \text{ x (760 mm Hg − 47 mm Hg)}$$
$$PAO_2 = PIO_2 − PACO_2 / R$$

Alveolar/arterial oxygen gradient = $PAO_2 − PaO_2$

Normal ranges:

Children	15-20 mm Hg
Adults	20-25 mm Hg

where:

PIO_2	=	oxygen partial pressure of inspired gas (mm Hg) (150 mm Hg in room air at sea level)
FiO_2	=	fractional pressure of oxygen in inspired gas (0.21 in room air)
PAO_2	=	alveolar oxygen partial pressure
$PACO_2$	=	alveolar carbon dioxide partial pressure
PaO_2	=	arterial oxygen partial pressure
R	=	respiratory exchange quotient (typically 0.8, increases with high carbohydrate diet, decreases with high fat diet)

Acid-Base Disorders

Acute metabolic acidosis:
 $PaCO_2$ expected = 1.5 (HCO_3^-) + 8 ± 2 **or**
 Expected decrease in $PaCO_2$ = 1.3 (1-1.5) x decrease in HCO_3^-

Acute metabolic alkalosis:
 Expected increase in $PaCO_2$ = 0.6 (0.5-1) x increase in HCO_3^-

Acute respiratory acidosis (<6 h duration):
 For every $PaCO_2$ increase of 10 mm Hg, HCO_3 increases by 1 mEq/L

Chronic respiratory acidosis (>6 h duration):

For every $PaCO_2$ increase of 10 mm Hg, HCO_3 increases by 4 mEq/L

Acute respiratory alkalosis (<6 h duration):

For every $PaCO_2$ decrease of 10 mm Hg, HCO_3 decreases by 2 mEq/L

Chronic respiratory alkalosis (>6 h duration):

For every $PaCO_2$ decrease of 10 mm Hg, HCO_3 increases by 5 mEq/L

ACID-BASE EQUATION

H^+ (in mEq/L) = (24 x $PaCO_2$) divided by HCO_3^-

Aa GRADIENT

Aa gradient $[(713)(FiO_2 - (PaCO_2 \text{ divided by } 0.8))] - PaO_2$

Aa gradient	=	alveolar-arterial oxygen gradient
FiO_2	=	inspired oxygen (expressed as a fraction)
$PaCO_2$	=	arterial partial pressure carbon dioxide (mm Hg)
PaO_2	=	arterial partial pressure oxygen (mm Hg)

OSMOLALITY

Definition: The summed concentrations of all osmotically active solute particles.

Predicted serum osmolality =

$$mOsm/L = (2 \times \text{serum } Na^{++}) + \frac{\text{serum glucose}}{18} + \frac{BUN}{2.8}$$

The normal range of serum osmolality is 285-295 mOsm/L.

Calculated Osm

Note: Osm is a term used to reconcile osmolality and osmolarity

Osmol gap = measured Osm − calculated Osm

0 to +10: Normal

>10: Abnormal

<0: Probable lab or calculation error

Drugs Causing Osmolar Gap

(by freezing-point depression, gap is >10 mOsm)

Ethanol	Isopropanol (acetone)
Ethylene glycol	Mannitol
Glycerol	Methanol
Hypermagnesemia (>9.5 mEq/L)	Sorbitol
Iodine (questionable)	

MILLIEQUIVALENT AND MILLIMOLE CALCULATIONS AND CONVERSIONS *(Continued)*

BICARBONATE DEFICIT

HCO_3^- deficit = (0.4 x wt in kg) x (HCO_3^- desired − HCO_3^- measured)

Note: In clinical practice, the calculated quantity may differ markedly from the actual amount of bicarbonate needed or that which may be safely administered.

ANION GAP

Definition: The difference in concentration between unmeasured cation and anion equivalents in serum.

Anion gap = Na^+ − (Cl^- + HCO_3^-)
(The normal anion gap is 10-14 mEq/L)

Differential Diagnosis of Increased Anion Gap Acidosis

Organic anions

Lactate (sepsis, hypovolemia, seizures, large tumor burden)
Pyruvate
Uremia
Ketoacidosis (β-hydroxybutyrate and acetoacetate)
Amino acids and their metabolites
Other organic acids

Inorganic anions

Hyperphosphatemia
Sulfates
Nitrates

Differential Diagnosis of Decreased Anion Gap

Organic cations

Hypergammaglobulinemia

Inorganic cations

Hyperkalemia
Hypercalcemia
Hypermagnesemia

Medications and toxins

Lithium

Hypoalbuminemia

RETICULOCYTE INDEX

(% retic divided by 2) x (patient's Hct divided by normal Hct) **or**
(% retic divided by 2) x (patient's Hgb divided by normal Hgb)

Normal index: 1.0
Good marrow response: 2.0-6.0

BODY SURFACE AREA

Body Surface Area (BSA) – Adults and Pediatric

$$\text{BSA (m}^2) = \frac{kg^{0.425} \times cm^{0.725} \times 71.84}{10,000}$$

or

$$\log \text{BSA (m}^2) = \frac{(\log kg \times 0.425) + (\log cm \times 0.725) + 1.8564}{10,000}$$

DuBois D and DuBois EF, "A Formula to Estimate the Approximate Surface Area if Height and Weight Be Known," *Arch Intern Med*, 1916, 17:863-71.

$$\text{BSA (m}^2) = \sqrt{\frac{\text{ht (in) x wt (lb)}}{3131}} \quad \textit{or} \quad \text{BSA (m}^2) = \sqrt{\frac{\text{ht (cm) x wt (kg)}}{3600}}$$

Lam TK and Leung DT, "More on Simplified Calculation of Body-Surface Area," *N Engl J Med*, 1988, 318(17):1130 (letter).

Mosteller RD, "Simplified Calculation of Body Surface Area," *N Engl J Med*, 1987, 317:1098 (letter).

Ideal Body Weight

Men:	50 kg + 2.3 kg/inch >5 ft
Women:	45 kg + 2.3 kg/in >5 ft

Devine BJ, "Gentamicin Therapy," *Drug Intelligence and Clinical Pharmacy*, 1974, 8:650-5.

or

Men:	51.65 kg + 1.85 kg/in >5 ft
Women:	48.67 kg + 1.7 kg/in >5 ft

Robinson JD, Lupkiewicz SM, Palenik L, et al, "Determination of Ideal Body Weight for Drug Dosage Calculations,"*Am J Hosp Pharm*, 1983, 40(6): 1016-9.

Adjusted Body Weight

Adjusted wt (kg) = actual weight (kg) – 0.4 [actual wt (kg) – ideal weight (kg)]

Notari EE, "Biopharmaceuticals and Clinical Pharmacokinetics," New York, Basel, 1987, 380.

Area Under the Curve (AUC) for Carboplatin Dosing

Carboplatin (mg) = desired AUC x (25 + GFR)

GFR = creatinine clearance (measured or estimated)

Calvert AH, Newell DR, Gumbrell LA, et al, "Carboplatin Dosage: Prospective Evaluation of a Simple Formula Based on Renal Function," *J Clin Oncol*, 1989, 7(11):1748-56.

CREATININE CLEARANCE ESTIMATING METHODS IN PATIENTS WITH STABLE RENAL FUNCTION

These formulas provide an acceptable estimate of the patient's creatinine clearance **except** in the following instances.

- Patient's serum creatinine is changing rapidly (either up or down).
- Patients are markedly emaciated.

In above situations, certain assumptions have to be made.

- In patients with rapidly rising serum creatinine (ie, >0.5-0.7 mg/dL/day), it is best to assume that the patient's creatinine clearance is probably <10 mL/minute.
- In emaciated patients, although their actual creatinine clearance is less than their calculated creatinine clearance (because of decreased creatinine production), it is not possible to easily predict how much less.

Infants

Estimation of creatinine clearance using serum creatinine and body length (to be used when an adequate timed specimen cannot be obtained). **Note:** This formula may not provide an accurate estimation of creatinine clearance for infants younger than 6 months of age and for patients with severe starvation or muscle wasting.

$$Cl_{cr} = K \times L/S_{cr}$$

where:

Cl_{cr}	=	creatinine clearance in mL/minute/1.73 m^2
K	=	constant of proportionality that is age specific

Age	K
Low birth weight ≤1 y	0.33
Full-term ≤1 y	0.45
2-12 y	0.55
13-21 y female	0.55
13-21 y male	0.70

L	=	length in cm
S_{cr}	=	serum creatinine concentration in mg/dL

Reference

Schwartz GJ, Brion LP, and Spitzer A, "The Use of Plasma Creatinine Concentration for Estimating Glomerular Filtration Rate in Infants, Children and Adolescents," *Pediatr Clin North Am*, 1987, 34(3):571-90.

Children (1-18 years)

Method 1: (Traub SL and Johnson CE, *Am J Hosp Pharm*, 1980, 37(2):195-201)

$$Cl_{cr} = \frac{0.48 \times (height)}{S_{cr}}$$

where:

Cl_{cr}	=	creatinine clearance in mL/min/1.73 m^2
S_{cr}	=	serum creatinine in mg/dL
Height	=	height in cm

Method 2: Nomogram (Traub SL and Johnson CE, *Am J Hosp Pharm*, 1980, 37(2):195-201)

Children 1-18 Years

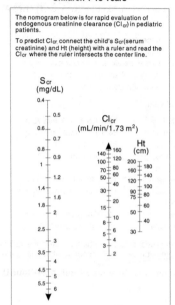

The nomogram below is for rapid evaluation of endogenous creatinine clearance (Cl_{cr}) in pediatric patients.

To predict Cl_{cr} connect the child's S_{cr} (serum creatinine) and Ht (height) with a ruler and read the Cl_{cr} where the ruler intersects the center line.

Adults (18 years and older)

Method 1: (Cockroft DW and Gault MH, *Nephron*, 1976, 16:31-41)

Estimated creatinine clearance (Cl_{cr}) (mL/min):

$$\text{Male} = \frac{(140 - \text{age}) \times \text{BW (kg)}}{72 \times S_{cr}}$$
$$\text{Female} = \text{male} \times 0.85$$

Note: Use of actual body weight (BW) in obese patients (and possibly patients with ascites) may significantly overestimate creatinine clearance. Some clinicians prefer to use an adjusted ideal body weight (IBW) in such cases [eg, IBW + 0.4(ABW-IBW)], especially when calculating dosages for aminoglycoside antibiotics.

Method 2: (Jelliffe RW, *Ann Intern Med*, 1973, 79:604)

Estimated creatinine clearance (Cl_{cr}) (mL/min/1.73 m²):

$$\text{Male} = \frac{98 - 0.8 \,(\text{age} - 20)}{S_{cr}}$$
$$\text{Female} = \text{male} \times 0.90$$

RENAL FUNCTION TESTS

Endogenous Creatinine Clearance vs Age (timed collection)

Creatinine clearance (mL/min/1.73 m²) = $(Cr_u V / Cr_s T)$ (1.73/A)

where:

Cr_u	=	urine creatinine concentration (mg/dL)
V	=	total urine collected during sampling period (mL)
Cr_s	=	serum creatinine concentration (mg/dL)
T	=	duration of sampling period (min) (24 h = 1440 min)
A	=	body surface area (m²)

Age-specific normal values

5-7 d	50.6 ± 5.8 mL/min/1.73 m²
1-2 mo	64.6 ± 5.8 mL/min/1.73 m²
5-8 mo	87.7 ± 11.9 mL/min/1.73 m²
9-12 mo	86.9 ± 8.4 mL/min/1.73 m²
≥18 mo	
male	124 ± 26 mL/min/1.73 m²
female	109 ± 13.5 mL/min/1.73 m²
Adults	
male	105 ± 14 mL/min/1.73 m²
female	95 ± 18 mL/min/1.73 m²

Note: In patients with renal failure (creatinine clearance <25 mL/min), creatinine clearance may be elevated over GFR because of tubular secretion of creatinine.

Calculation of Creatinine Clearance From a 24-Hour Urine Collection

Equation 1:

$$Cl_{cr} = \frac{U \times V}{P}$$

where:

Cl_{cr}	=	creatinine clearance
U	=	urine concentration of creatinine
V	=	total urine volume in the collection
P	=	plasma creatinine concentration

Equation 2:

$$Cl_{cr} = \frac{\text{(total urine volume [mL]) x (urine Cr concentration [mg/dL])}}{\text{(serum creatinine [mg/dL]) x (time of urine collection [minutes])}}$$

Occasionally, a patient will have a 12- or 24-hour urine collection done for direct calculation of creatinine clearance. Although a urine collection for 24 hours is best, it is difficult to do since many urine collections occur for a much shorter period. A 24-hour urine collection is the desired duration of urine collection because the urine excretion of creatinine is diurnal and thus the measured creatinine clearance will vary throughout the day as the creatinine in the urine varies. When the urine collection is less than 24 hours, the total excreted creatinine will be affected by the time of the day during which the collection is performed. A 24-hour urine collection is sufficient to be able to accurately average the diurnal creatinine excretion variations. If a patient has 24 hours of urine collected for creatinine clearance, equation 1 can be used for calculating the creatinine clearance. To use equation 1 to calculate the creatinine clearance, it will be necessary to know the duration of urine collection, the urine collection volume, the urine creatinine concentration, and the serum creatinine value that reflects the urine collection period. In most cases, a serum creatinine concentration is drawn anytime during the day, but it is best to have the value drawn halfway through the collection period.

Amylase:Creatinine Clearance Ratio

$$\frac{Amylase_u \times creatinine_p}{Amylase_p \times creatinine_u} \times 100$$

u = urine; p = plasma

Serum BUN:Serum Creatinine Ratio

Serum BUN (mg/dL:serum creatinine (mg/dL))

Normal BUN:creatinine ratio is 10-15

BUN:creatinine ratio >20 suggests prerenal azotemia (also seen with high urea-generation states such as GI bleeding)

BUN:creatinine ratio <5 may be seen with disorders affecting urea biosynthesis such as urea cycle enzyme deficiencies and with hepatitis.

Fractional Sodium Excretion

Fractional sodium secretion (FENa) = $Na_uCr_s/Na_sCr_u \times 100\%$

where:

Na_u	=	urine sodium (mEq/L)
Na_s	=	serum sodium (mEq/L)
Cr_u	=	urine creatinine (mg/dL)
Cr_s	=	serum creatinine (mg/dL)

FENa <1% suggests prerenal failure
FENa >2% suggest intrinsic renal failure
    (for newborns, normal FENa is approximately 2.5%)

Note: Disease states associated with a falsely elevated FENa include severe volume depletion (>10%), early acute tubular necrosis, and volume depletion in chronic renal disease. Disorders associated with a lowered FENa include acute glomerulonephritis, hemoglobinuric or myoglobinuric renal failure, nonoliguric acute tubular necrosis, and acute urinary tract obstruction. In addition, FENa may be <1% in patients with acute renal failure **and** a second condition predisposing to sodium retention (eg, burns, congestive heart failure, nephrotic syndrome).

Urine Calcium:Urine Creatinine Ratio (spot sample)

Urine calcium (mg/dL): urine creatinine (mg/dL)

Normal values <0.21 (mean values 0.08 males, 0.06 females)

Premature infants show wide variability of calcium:creatinine ratio, and tend to have lower thresholds for calcium loss than older children. Prematures without nephrolithiasis had mean Ca:Cr ratio of 0.75 ± 0.76. Infants with nephrolithiasis had mean Ca:Cr ratio of 1.32 ± 1.03 (Jacinto JS, Modanlou HD, Crade M, et al, "Renal Calcification Incidence in Very Low Birth Weight Infants," *Pediatrics*, 1988, 81:31.)

RENAL FUNCTION TESTS *(Continued)*

Urine Protein:Urine Creatinine Ratio (spot sample)

P_u/Cr_u	Total Protein Excretion $(mg/m^2/d)$
0.1	80
1	800
10	8000

where:

P_u = urine protein concentration (mg/dL)
Cr_u = urine creatinine concentration (mg/dL)

REFERENCE VALUES FOR ADULTS

Automated Chemistry (CHEMISTRY A)

Test	Values	Remarks
SERUM / PLASMA		
Acetone	Negative	
Albumin	3.2-5 g/dL	
Alcohol, ethyl	Negative	
Aldolase	1.2-7.6 IU/L	
Ammonia	20-70 mcg/dL	Specimen to be placed on ice as soon as collected.
Amylase	30-110 units/L	
Bilirubin, direct	0-0.3 mg/dL	
Bilirubin, total	0.1-1.2 mg/dL	
Calcium	8.6-10.3 mg/dL	
Calcium, ionized	2.24-2.46 mEq/L	
Chloride	95-108 mEq/L	
Cholesterol, total	≤200 mg/dL	Fasted blood required – normal value affected by dietary habits. This reference range is for a general adult population.
HDL cholesterol	40-60 mg/dL	Fasted blood required – normal value affected by dietary habits.
LDL cholesterol	<160 mg/dL	If triglyceride is >400 mg/dL, LDL cannot be calculated accurately (Friedewald equation). Target LDL-C depends on patient's risk factors.
CO_2	23-30 mEq/L	
Creatine kinase (CK) isoenzymes		
CK-BB	0%	
CK-MB (cardiac)	0%-3.9%	
CK-MM (muscle)	96%-100%	
CK-MB levels must be both ≥4% and 10 IU/L to meet diagnostic criteria for CK-MB positive result consistent with myocardial injury.		
Creatine phosphokinase (CPK)	8-150 IU/L	
Creatinine	0.5-1.4 mg/dL	
Ferritin	13-300 ng/mL	
Folate	3.6-20 ng/dL	
GGT (gamma-glutamyltranspeptidase)		
male	11-63 IU/L	
female	8-35 IU/L	
GLDH	To be determined	
Glucose (preprandial)	<115 mg/dL	Goals different for diabetics.
Glucose, fasting	60-110 mg/dL	Goals different for diabetics.
Glucose, nonfasting (2-h postprandial)	<120 mg/dL	Goals different for diabetics.
Hemoglobin A_{1c}	<8	
Hemoglobin, plasma free	<2.5 mg/100 mL	
Hemoglobin, total glycosolated (Hb A_1)	4%-8%	
Iron	65-150 mcg/dL	

REFERENCE VALUES FOR ADULTS *(Continued)*

Automated Chemistry (CHEMISTRY A) *(continued)*

Test	Values	Remarks
Iron binding capacity, total (TIBC)	250-420 mcg/dL	
Lactic acid	0.7-2.1 mEq/L	Specimen to be kept on ice and sent to lab as soon as possible.
Lactate dehydrogenase (LDH)	56-194 IU/L	
Lactate dehydrogenase (LDH) isoenzymes		
LD$_1$	20%-34%	
LD$_2$	29%-41%	
LD$_3$	15%-25%	
LD$_4$	1%-12%	
LD$_5$	1%-15%	
Flipped LD$_1$/LD$_2$ ratios (>1 may be consistent with myocardial injury) particularly when considered in combination with a recent CK-MB positive result.		
Lipase	23-208 units/L	
Magnesium	1.6-2.5 mg/dL	Increased by slight hemolysis.
Osmolality	289-308 mOsm/kg	
Phosphatase, alkaline		
adults 25-60 y	33-131 IU/L	
adults 61 y or older	51-153 IU/L	
infancy-adolescence	Values range up to 3-5 times higher than adults	
Phosphate, inorganic	2.8-4.2 mg/dL	
Potassium	3.5-5.2 mEq/L	Increased by slight hemolysis.
Prealbumin	>15 mg/dL	
Protein, total	6.5-7.9 g/dL	
SGOT (AST)	<35 IU/L (20-48)	
SGPT (ALT) (10-35)	<35 IU/L	
Sodium	134-149 mEq/L	
Transferrin	>200 mg/dL	
Triglycerides	45-155 mg/dL	Fasted blood required.
Troponin I	<1.5 ng/mL	
Urea nitrogen (BUN)	7-20 mg/dL	
Uric acid		
male	2-8 mg/dL	
female	2-7.5 mg/dL	

CEREBROSPINAL FLUID

Glucose	50-70 mg/dL	
Protein		
adults and children	15-45 mg/dL	CSF obtained by lumbar puncture.
newborn infants	60-90 mg/dL	

On CSF obtained by cisternal puncture: About 25 mg/dL

On CSF obtained by ventricular puncture: About 10 mg/dL

Note: Bloody specimen gives erroneously high value due to contamination with blood proteins

Automated Chemistry (CHEMISTRY A) *(continued)*

Test	Values	Remarks
URINE		
(24-hour specimen is required for all these tests unless specified)		
Amylase	32-641 units/L	The value is in units/L and **not** calculated for total volume.
Amylase, fluid (random samples)		Interpretation of value left for physician, depends on the nature of fluid.
Calcium	Depends upon dietary intake	
Creatine		
male	150 mg/24 h	Higher value on children and during pregnancy.
female	250 mg/24 h	
Creatinine	1000-2000 mg/24 h	
Creatinine clearance (endogenous)		
male	85-125 mL/min	A blood sample must accompany urine specimen.
female	75-115 mL/min	
Glucose	1 g/24 h	
5-hydroxyindoleacetic acid	2-8 mg/24 h	
Iron	0.15 mg/24 h	Acid washed container required.
Magnesium	146-209 mg/24 h	
Osmolality	500-800 mOsm/kg	With normal fluid intake.
Oxalate	10-40 mg/24 h	
Phosphate	400-1300 mg/24 h	
Potassium	25-120 mEq/24 h	Varies with diet; the interpretation of urine electrolytes and osmolality should be left for the physician.
Sodium	40-220 mEq/24 h	
Porphobilinogen, qualitative	Negative	
Porphyrins, qualitative	Negative	
Proteins	0.05-0.1 g/24 h	
Salicylate	Negative	
Urea clearance	60-95 mL/min	A blood sample must accompany specimen.
Urea N	10-40 g/24 h	Dependent on protein intake.
Uric acid	250-750 mg/24 h	Dependent on diet and therapy.
Urobilinogen	0.5-3.5 mg/24 h	For qualitative determination on random urine, send sample to urinalysis section in Hematology Lab.
Xylose absorption test		
children	16%-33% of ingested xylose	
FECES		
Fat, 3-day collection	<5 g/d	Value depends on fat intake of 100 g/d for 3 days preceding and during collection.
GASTRIC ACIDITY		
Acidity, total, 12 h	10-60 mEq/L	Titrated at pH 7.

REFERENCE VALUES FOR ADULTS *(Continued)*

Blood Gases

	Arterial	Capillary	Venous
pH	7.35-7.45	7.35-7.45	7.32-7.42
pCO_2 (mm Hg)	35-45	35-45	38-52
pO_2 (mm Hg)	70-100	60-80	24-48
HCO_3 (mEq/L)	19-25	19-25	19-25
TCO_2 (mEq/L)	19-29	19-29	23-33
O_2 saturation (%)	90-95	90-95	40-70
Base excess (mEq/L)	-5 to +5	-5 to +5	-5 to +5

HEMATOLOGY

Complete Blood Count

Age	Hgb (g/dL)	Hct (%)	RBC (mill/mm³)	RDW
0-3 d	15.0-20.0	45-61	4.0-5.9	<18
1-2 wk	12.5-18.5	39-57	3.6-5.5	<17
1-6 mo	10.0-13.0	29-42	3.1-4.3	<16.5
7 mo to 2 y	10.5-13.0	33-38	3.7-4.9	<16
2-5 y	11.5-13.0	34-39	3.9-5.0	<15
5-8 y	11.5-14.5	35-42	4.0-4.9	<15
13-18 y	12.0-15.2	36-47	4.5-5.1	<14.5
Adult male	13.5-16.5	41-50	4.5-5.5	<14.5
Adult female	12.0-15.0	36-44	4.0-4.9	<14.5

Age	MCV (fL)	MCH (pg)	MCHC (%)	Plts (x 10³/mm³)
0-3 d	95-115	31-37	29-37	250-450
1-2 wk	86-110	28-36	28-38	250-450
1-6 mo	74-96	25-35	30-36	300-700
7 mo to 2 y	70-84	23-30	31-37	250-600
2-5 y	75-87	24-30	31-37	250-550
5-8 y	77-95	25-33	31-37	250-550
13-18 y	78-96	25-35	31-37	150-450
Adult male	80-100	26-34	31-37	150-450
Adult female	80-100	26-34	31-37	150-450

WBC and Differential

Age	WBC (x 10³/mm³)	Segs	Bands	Lymphs	Monos
0-3 d	9.0-35.0	32-62	10-18	19-29	5-7
1-2 wk	5.0-20.0	14-34	6-14	36-45	6-10
1-6 mo	6.0-17.5	13-33	4-12	41-71	4-7
7 mo to 2 y	6.0-17.0	15-35	5-11	45-76	3-6
2-5 y	5.5-15.5	23-45	5-11	35-65	3-6
5-8 y	5.0-14.5	32-54	5-11	28-48	3-6
13-18 y	4.5-13.0	34-64	5-11	25-45	3-6
Adults	4.5-11.0	35-66	5-11	24-44	3-6

Age	Eosinophils	Basophils	Atypical Lymphs	No. of NRBCs
0-3 d	0-2	0-1	0-8	0-2
1-2 wk	0-2	0-1	0-8	0
1-6 mo	0-3	0-1	0-8	0
7 mo to 2 y	0-3	0-1	0-8	0
2-5 y	0-3	0-1	0-8	0
5-8 y	0-3	0-1	0-8	0
13-18 y	0-3	0-1	0-8	0
Adults	0-3	0-1	0-8	0

Segs = segmented neutrophils.
Bands = band neutrophils.
Lymphs = lymphocytes.
Monos = monocytes.

Erythrocyte Sedimentation Rates and Reticulocyte Counts

Sedimentation rate, Westergren	Children	0-20 mm/hour
	Adult male	0-15 mm/hour
	Adult female	0-20 mm/hour
Sedimentation rate, Wintrobe	Children	0-13 mm/hour
	Adult male	0-10 mm/hour
	Adult female	0-15 mm/hour
Reticulocyte count	Newborns	2%-6%
	1-6 mo	0%-2.8%
	Adults	0.5%-1.5%

PHARMACOLOGIC CATEGORY INDEX

Antifungal Agent, Oral *(Continued)*

Antifungal Agent, Oral Nonabsorbed

Antifungal Agent, Parenteral

Antifungal Agent, Topical

Antifungal Agent, Vaginal

Antihemophilic Agent

Antihistamine

Anti-inflammatory Agent

Anti-inflammatory Agent, Ophthalmic

Antineoplastic Agent

Antineoplastic Agent, Alkylating Agent

NOTES

NOTES

NOTES

NOTES

NOTES

NOTES

NOTES

Products offered by LEXI-COMP

DRUG INFORMATION HANDBOOK (International edition available)
by Charles Lacy, RPh, PharmD, FCSHP; Lora L. Armstrong, RPh, PharmD, BCPS;
Morton P. Goldman, RPh, PharmD, BCPS; and Leonard L. Lance, RPh, BSPharm

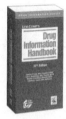

Specifically compiled and designed for the healthcare professional requiring quick access to concisely-stated comprehensive data concerning clinical use of medications.

The Drug Information Handbook is an ideal portable drug information resource, providing the reader with up to 34 key points of data concerning clinical use and dosing of the medication. Material provided in the Appendix section is recognized by many users to be, by itself, well worth the purchase of the handbook.

PEDIATRIC DOSAGE HANDBOOK (International edition available)
by Carol K. Taketomo, PharmD; Jane Hurlburt Hodding, PharmD; and Donna M. Kraus, PharmD

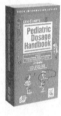

Special considerations must frequently be taken into account when dosing medications for the pediatric patient. This highly regarded quick reference handbook is a compilation of recommended pediatric doses based on current literature, as well as the practical experience of the authors and their many colleagues who work every day in the pediatric clinical setting.

Includes neonatal dosing, drug administration, and (in select monographs) extemporaneous preparations for medications used in pediatric medicine.

GERIATRIC DOSAGE HANDBOOK
by Todd P. Semla, PharmD, BCPS, FCCP; Judith L. Beizer, PharmD, FASCP; and
Martin D. Higbee, PharmD, CGP

2000 "Book of the Year" — American Journal of Nursing

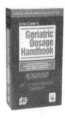

Many physiologic changes occur with aging, some of which affect the pharmacokinetics or pharmacodynamics of medications. Strong consideration should also be given to the effect of decreased renal or hepatic functions in the elderly, as well as the probability of the geriatric patient being on multiple drug regimens.

Healthcare professionals working with nursing homes and assisted living facilities will find the drug information contained in this handbook to be an invaluable source of helpful information.

An International Brand Name Index with names from 58 different countries is also included.

To order call toll free anywhere in the U.S.: 1-866-EXP-DIFF (397-3433)
Outside of the U.S. call: 330-650-6506 or online at www.lexi.com

Products offered by LEXI-COMP

DRUG INTERACTIONS HANDBOOK

by Bachmann, Lewis, Fuller, Bonfiglio

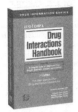

The new standard for evaluating drug and herbal interactions. A comprehensive table of Cytochrome P450 enzyme substrates, inducers and inhibitors. Each interaction monograph contains the following ratings: Reliability Rating - indicating the quantity and nature of documentation for an interaction: A - No Known Interaction, B - No Action Needed, C - Monitor Therapy, D - Consider Therapy Modification, and X - Avoid Combination; Severity Rating - indicating the reported or possible magnitude of an interaction outcome. This book also contains the following: detailed patient management suggestions, full reference citations, discussion of published reports and potential mechanisms, identifies the greatest number of potential interactions compared to any other available references, user-friendly structure, over 3,000 brand names, includes interactions data on the most commonly used herbs, and "tall man" letters to identify between "look-a-like" medications.

NATURAL THERAPEUTICS POCKET GUIDE

by Daniel L. Krinsky, RPh, MS; James B. LaValle, RPh, DHM, NMD, CCN; Ernest B. Hawkins, RPh, MS; Ross Pelton, RPh, PhD, CCN; Nancy Ashbrook Willis, BA, JD

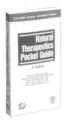

Provides condition-specific information on common uses of natural therapies. Each condition discussed includes the following: review of condition, decision tree, list of commonly recommended herbals, nutritional supplements, homeopathic remedies, lifestyle modifications, and special considerations.

Provides herbal/nutritional/nutraceutical monographs with over 10 fields including references, reported uses, dosage, pharmacology, toxicity, warnings & interactions, and cautions & contraindications.

The Appendix includes: drug-nutrient depletion, herb-drug interactions, drug-nutrient interaction, herbal medicine use in pediatrics, unsafe herbs, and reference of top herbals.

DRUG-INDUCED NUTRIENT DEPLETION HANDBOOK

by Ross Pelton, RPh, PhD, CCN; James B. LaValle, RPh, DHM, NMD, CCN; Ernest B. Hawkins, RPh, MS; Daniel L. Krinsky, RPh, MS

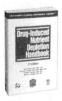

A complete and up-to-date listing of all drugs known to deplete the body of nutritional compounds.

This book is alphabetically organized and provides extensive cross-referencing to related information in the various sections of the book. Drug monographs identify the nutrients depleted and provide cross-references to the nutrient monographs for more detailed information on effects of depletion, biological function & effect, side effects & toxicity, RDA, dosage range, and dietary sources. this book also contains a studies & abstracts section, a valuable appendix, and alphabetical & pharmacological indexes.

Products offered by LEXI-COMP

DRUG INFORMATION HANDBOOK FOR ADVANCED PRACTICE NURSING
by Beatrice B. Turkoski, RN, PhD; Brenda R. Lance, RN, MSN; and Mark F. Bonfiglio, PharmD Foreword by: Margaret A. Fitzgerald, MS, RN, CS-FNP

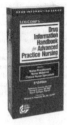

Designed specifically to meet the needs of nurse practitioners, clinical nurse specialists, nurse midwives, and graduate nursing students. The handbook is a unique resource for detailed, accurate information, which is vital to support the advanced practice nurse's role in patient drug therapy management. Over 4750 U.S., Canadian, and Mexican medications are covered in the 1000 monographs. Drug data is presented in an easy-to-use, alphabetically-organized format covering up to 46 key points of information (including dosing for pediatrics, adults, and geriatrics). Appendix contains over 230 pages of valuable comparison tables and additional information. Also included are two indexes, Pharmacologic Category and Controlled Substance, which facilitate comparison between agents.

DRUG INFORMATION HANDBOOK FOR NURSING
by Beatrice B. Turkoski, RN, PhD; Brenda R. Lance, RN, MSN; and Mark F. Bonfiglio, PharmD

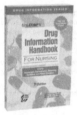

Registered professional nurses and upper-division nursing students involved with drug therapy will find this handbook provides quick access to drug data in a concise easy-to-use format.

Over 4000 U.S., Canadian, and Mexican medications are covered with up to 43 key points of information in each monograph. The handbook contains basic pharmacology concepts and nursing issues such as patient factors that influence drug therapy (ie, pregnancy, age, weight, etc) and general nursing issues (ie, assessment, administration, monitoring, and patient education). The Appendix contains over 230 pages of valuable information.

DRUG INFORMATION HANDBOOK FOR THE ALLIED HEALTH PROFESSIONAL
by Leonard L. Lance, RPh, BSPharm; Charles Lacy, RPh, PharmD, FCSHP; Lora L. Armstrong, RPh, PharmD, BCPS; and Morton P. Goldman, PharmD, BCPS

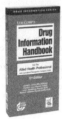

Working with clinical pharmacists, hospital pharmacy and therapeutics committees, and hospital drug information centers, the authors have assisted hundreds of hospitals in developing institution-specific formulary reference documentation.

The most current basic drug and medication data from those clinical settings have been reviewed, coalesced, and cross-referenced to create this unique handbook. The handbook offers quick access to abbreviated monographs for generic drugs.

This is a great tool for physician assistants, medical records personnel, medical transcriptionists and secretaries, pharmacy technicians, and other allied health professionals.

To order call toll free anywhere in the U.S.: 1-866-EXP-DIFF (397-3433)
Outside of the U.S. call: 330-650-6506 or online at www.lexi.com

Products offered by LEXI-COMP

INFECTIOUS DISEASES HANDBOOK

by Carlos M. Isada, MD; Bernard L. Kasten Jr., MD; Morton P. Goldman, PharmD; Larry D. Gray, PhD; and Judith A. Aberg, MD

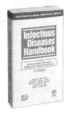

A four-in-one quick reference concerned with the identification and treatment of infectious diseases. Each of the four sections of the book contains related information and cross-referencing to one or more of the other three sections. The Disease Syndrome section provides the clinical presentation, differential diagnosis, diagnostic tests, and drug therapy recommended for treatment of more common infectious diseases. The Organism section presents the microbiology, epidemiology, diagnosis, and treatment of each organism. The Laboratory Diagnosis section describes performance of specific tests and procedures. The Antimicrobial Therapy section presents important facts and considerations regarding each drug recommended for specific diseases of organisms. Also contains an International Brand Name Index with names from 58 different countries.

PHARMACOGENOMICS HANDBOOK

by Humma, Ellingrod, Kolesar

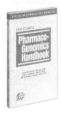

This exciting new title by Lexi-Comp, introduces Pharmacogenomics to the forward-thinking healthcare professional and student! It presents information concerning key genetic variations that may influence drug disposition and/or sensitivity. Brief introductions to fundamental concepts in genetics and genomics are provided in order to bring the reader up-to-date on these rapidly emerging sciences. This book provides a foundation for all clinicians who will be called on to integrate rapidly expanding genomic knowledge into the management of drug therapy. A great introduction to pharmacogenetic principles as well as a concise reference on key polymorphisms known to influence drug response!

ANESTHESIOLOGY & CRITICAL CARE DRUG HANDBOOK

by Andrew J. Donnelly, PharmD; Francesca E. Cunningham, PharmD; Verna L. Baughman, MD

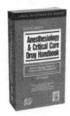

Contains the most common perioperative drugs in the critical care setting and also contains Special Issues and Topics including: Allergic Reaction, Cardiac Patients in Noncardiac Surgery, Obstetric Patients in Nonobstetric Surgery, Patients With Liver Disease, Chronic Pain Management, Chronic Renal Failure, Conscious Sedation, Perioperative Management of Patients on Antiseizure Medication, and more.

The Appendix includes Abbreviations & Measurements, Anesthesiology Information, Assessment of Liver & Renal Function, Comparative Drug Charts, Infectious Disease-Prophylaxis & Treatment, Laboratory Values, Therapy Re-commendations, Toxicology information, and much more.

International Brand Name Index with names from over 58 different countries is also included.

Products offered by LEXI-COMP

CLINICIAN'S GUIDE TO LABORATORY MEDICINE
—A Practical Approach by Samir P. Desai, MD and Sana Isa-Pratt, MD

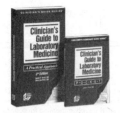

When faced with the patient presenting with abnormal laboratory tests, the clinician can now turn to the Clinician's Guide to Laboratory Medicine: A Practical Approach. This source is unique in its ability to lead the clinician from laboratory test abnormality to clinical diagnosis. Written for the busy clinician, this concise handbook will provide rapid answers to the questions that busy clinicians face in the care of their patients. No longer does the clinician have to struggle in an effort to find this information - it's all here.

Included is a **FREE** copy of Clinician's Guide to Laboratory Medicine - Pocket. Great to carry in your pocket! Perfect for use "in the trenches."

CLINICIAN'S GUIDE TO INTERNAL MEDICINE—A Practical Approach by Samir P. Desai, MD

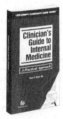

Provides quick access to essential information covering diagnosis, treatment, and management of commonly encountered patient problems in Internal Medicine. Contains up-to-date, clinically-relevant information in an easy-to-read format and is easily accessible. Contains practical approaches that are not readily available in standard textbooks. Contains algorithms to help you establish the diagnosis and select the appropriate therapy. There are numerous tables and boxes that summarize diagnostic and therapeutic strategies. It is an ideal reference for use at the point-of-care. This is a reference companion that will provide you with the tools necessary to tackle even the most challenging problems in Internal Medicine.

CLINICIAN'S GUIDE TO DIAGNOSIS—A Practical Approach by Samir P. Desai, MD

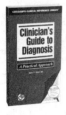

Symptoms are what prompt patients to seek medical care. In the evaluation of a patient's symptom, it is not unusual for healthcare professionals to ask "What do I do next?" This is precisely the question for which the Clinician's Guide to Diagnosis: A Practical Approach provides the answer. It will lead you from symptom to diagnosis through a series of steps designed to mimic the logical thought processes of seasoned clinicians. For the young clinician, this is an ideal book to help bridge the gap between the classroom and actual patient care. For the experienced clinician, this concise handbook offers rapid answers to the questions that are commonly encountered on a day-to-day basis. Let this guide become your companion, providing you with the tools necessary to tackle even the most challenging symptoms.

Products offered by LEXI-COMP

POISONING & TOXICOLOGY HANDBOOK
by Jerrold B. Leikin, MD and Frank P. Paloucek, PharmD

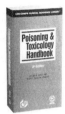

It's back by popular demand! The small size of our Poisoning & Toxicology Handbook is once again available. Better than ever, this comprehensive, portable reference contains 80 antidotes and drugs used in toxicology with 694 medicinal agents, 287 nonmedicinal agents, 291 biological agents, 57 herbal agents, and more than 200 laboratory tests. Monographs are extensively referenced and contain valuable information on overdose symptomatology and treatment considerations, as well as, admission criteria and impairment potential of select agents. Designed for quick reference with monographs arranged alphabetically, plus a cross-referencing index. The authors have expanded current information on drugs of abuse and use of antidotes, while providing concise tables, graphics, and other pertinent toxicology text.

LABORATORY TEST HANDBOOK & CONCISE version
by David S. Jacobs MD, FACP; Wayne R. DeMott, MD, FACP; and Dwight K. Oxley, MD, FACP

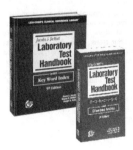

Contains over 900 clinical laboratory tests and is an excellent source of laboratory information for physicians of all specialties, nurses, laboratory professionals, students, medical personnel, or anyone who needs quick access to most routine and many of the more specialized testing procedures available in today's clinical laboratory. Each monograph contains test name, synonyms, patient care, specimen requirements, reference ranges, and interpretive information with footnotes, references, and selected web sites. The Laboratory Test Handbook Concise is a portable, abridged (800 tests) version and is an ideal, quick reference for anyone requiring information concerning patient preparation, specimen collection and handling, and test result interpretation.

DIAGNOSTIC PROCEDURES HANDBOOK   by Frank Michota, MD

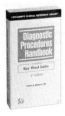

A comprehensive, yet concise, quick reference source for physicians, nurses, students, medical records personnel, or anyone needing quick access to diagnostic procedure information. This handbook is an excellent source of information in the following areas: allergy, rheumatology, and infectious disease; cardiology; computed tomography; diagnostic radiology; gastroenterology; invasive radiology; magnetic resonance imaging; nephrology, urology, and hematology; neurology; nuclear medicine; pulmonary function; pulmonary medicine and critical care; ultrasound; and women's health.

Products offered by LEXI-COMP

DRUG INFORMATION HANDBOOK FOR PSYCHIATRY
by Matthew A. Fuller, PharmD and Martha Sajatovic, MD

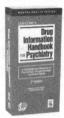

The source for comprehensive and clinically-relevant drug information for the mental health professional. Alphabetically arranged by generic and brand name for ease-of-use. There are up to 35 key fields of information including these unique fields: "Effect on Mental Status" and "Effect on Psychiatric Treatment."

A special topics/issues section includes psychiatric assessment, major psychiatric disorders, major classes of psychotropic medications, psychiatric emergencies, special populations, enhanced patient education information section, and DSM-IV classification. Also contains a valuable appendix section, Pharmacologic Index, and Alphabetical Index.

RATING SCALES IN MENTAL HEALTH
by Martha Sajatovic, MD and Luis F. Ramirez, MD

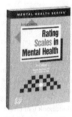

A basic guide to the rating scales in mental health, this is an ideal reference for psychiatrists, nurses, residents, psychologists, social workers, healthcare administrators, behavioral healthcare organizations, and outcome committees. It is designed to assist clinicians in determining the appropriate rating scale when assessing their client. A general concepts section provides text discussion on the use and history of rating scales, statistical evaluation, rating scale domains, and two clinical vignettes. Information on over 100 rating scales used in mental health is organized by condition. Appendix contains tables and charts in a quick reference format allowing clinicians to rapidly identify categories and characteristics of rating scales.

PSYCHOTROPIC DRUG INFORMATION HANDBOOK
by Matthew A. Fuller, PharmD and Martha Sajatovic, MD

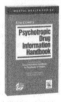

This portable, yet comprehensive guide to psychotropic drugs provides healthcare professionals with detailed information on use, drug interactions, pregnancy risk factors, warnings/precautions, adverse reactions, mechanism of action, and contraindications. Alphabetically organized by brand and generic name, this concise handbook provides quick access to the information you need and includes patient education sheets on the psychotropic medications. It is the perfect pocket companion to the Drug Information for Psychiatry.

Products offered by LEXI-COMP

DRUG INFORMATION HANDBOOK FOR DENTISTRY
by Richard L. Wynn, BSPharm, PhD; Timothy F. Meiller, DDS, PhD; Harold L. Crossley, DDS, PhD

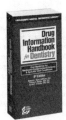

For all dental professionals requiring quick access to concisely-stated drug information pertaining to medications commonly prescribed by dentists and physicians.

Designed and written by dentists for all dental professionals as a portable, chair-side resource. Includes drugs commonly prescribed by dentists or being taken by dental patients and written in an easy-to-understand format. There are 24 key points of information for each drug including **Local Anesthetic/Vasoconstrictor, Precautions, Effects on Dental Treatment,** and **Drug Interactions**. Includes information on dental treatment for medically-compromised patients and dental management of specific oral conditions.

Also contains Canadian & Mexican brand names.

MANUAL OF DENTAL IMPLANTS
by David P. Sarment, DDS, MS and Beth Peshman, RDH

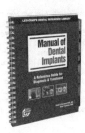

Contains over 220 quality color photos, plus diagrams and decision trees. The diagnosis and treatment plans are explained in detail. Restorative step-by-step illustrations are included for each case type. Hygiene techniques and protocols are also included as well as assistant and staff training guidelines.

8 Tabbed Sections for Ease-of-Use:

① Basic Principles
② Diagnosis
③ Treatment Planning
④ Restoration Sequences
⑤ Maintenance
⑥ Implants and Your Practice
⑦ Appendix
⑧ Index

MANUAL OF CLINICAL PERIODONTICS
by Francis G. Serio, DMD, MS and Charles E. Hawley, DDS, PhD

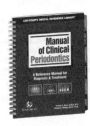

A reference manual for diagnosis and treatment including sample treatment plans. It is organized by basic principles and is visually-cued with over 220 high quality color photos. The presentation is in a "question & answer" format. There are 12 chapters tabbed for easy access: 1) Problem-based Periodontal Diagnosis; 2) Anatomy, Histology, and Physiology; 3) Etiology and Disease Classification; 4) Assessment, Diagnosis, and Treatment Planning; 5) Prevention and Maintenance; 6) Nonsurgical Treatment; 7) Surgical Treatment: Principles; 8) Repair, Resection, and Regeneration; 9) Periodontal Plastic Surgery; 10) Periodontal Emergencies; 11) Implant Considerations; 12) Appendix

Products offered by LEXI-COMP

ORAL SOFT TISSUE DISEASES

by J. Robert Newland, DDS, MS; Timothy F. Meiller, DDS, PhD; Richard L. Wynn, BSPharm, PhD; and Harold L.Crossley, DDS, PhD

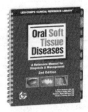

Designed for all dental professionals, a pictorial reference to assist in the diagnosis and management of oral soft tissue diseases (over 160 photos). Easy-to-use, sections include: Diagnosis process: obtaining a history, examining the patient, establishing a differential diagnosis, selecting appropriate diagnostic tests, interpreting the results, etc.; white lesions; red lesions; blistering-sloughing lesions; ulcerated lesions; pigmented lesions; papillary lesions; soft tissue swelling (each lesion is illustrated with a color representative photograph); specific medications to treat oral soft tissue diseases; sample prescriptions; and special topics.

ORAL HARD TISSUE DISEASES

by J. Robert Newland, DDS, MS

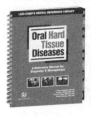

A reference manual for radiographic diagnosis, visually-cued with over 130 high quality radiographs is designed to require little more than visual recognition to make an accurate diagnosis. Each lesion is illustrated by one or more photographs depicting the typical radiographic features and common variations. There are 12 chapters tabbed for easy access: 1) Periapical Radiolucent Lesions; 2) Pericoronal Radiolucent Lesions; 3) Inter-Radicular Radiolucent Lesions; 4) Periodontal Radiolucent Lesions; 5) Radiolucent Lesions Not Associated With Teeth; 6) Radiolucent Lesions With Irregular Margins; 7) Periapical Radiopaque Lesions; 8) Periocoronal Radiopaque Lesions; 9) Inter-Radicular Radiopaque Lesions; 10) Radiopaque Lesions Not Associated With Teeth; 11) Radiopaque Lesions With Irregular Margins; 12) Selected Readings / Alphabetical Index

DENTAL OFFICE MEDICAL EMERGENCIES

by Timothy F. Meiller, DDS, PhD; Richard L. Wynn, BSPharm, PhD; Ann Marie McMullin, MD; Cynthia Biron, RDH, EMT, MA; and Harold L. Crossley, DDS, PhD

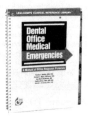

Designed specifically for general dentists during times of emergency. A tabbed paging system allows for quick access to specific crisis events. Created with urgency in mind, it is spiral bound and drilled with a hole for hanging purposes. Contains the following: Basic Action Plan for Stabilization; Allergic / Drug Reactions; Loss of Consciousness / Respiratory Distress / Chest Pain; Altered Sensation / Changes in Affect; Management of Acute Bleeding; Office Preparedness / Procedures and Protocols; Automated External Defibrillator (AED); Oxygen Delivery

Products offered by LEXI-COMP

ADVANCED PROTOCOLS FOR MEDICAL EMERGENCIES

by Donald P. Lewis, Jr, DDS, Ann Marie McMullin, MD, Timothy Meiller, DDS, PhD, Richard L. Wynn BSPharm, PhD, Cynthia Biron, RDH, EMT, MA, Harold L. Crossley, DDS, PhD

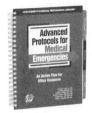

An Action Plan for Office Response!

A must for all offices that practice the use and safety of the administration of local anesthesia, nitrous oxide analgesia, conscious sedation, deep sedation, and general anesthesia. Occasionally, medical emergencies can become life threatening. This book is designed to facilitate advanced medical emergency protocols. Includes all of our popular Dental Office Medical Emergencies and introduces the following chapters in an easy-to-understand and tabbed manner: Loss of Conciousness; Respiratory Distress; Chest Pain; Cardiac Dysrhythmias; Venipuncture Complications; Malignant Hyperthermia; Allergic/Drug Reaction; Altered Sensation/Changes in Effect; Blood Pressure Abnormalities; Management of Acute Bleeding; Emesis and Aspiration; Drug Monographs. Additional Sections Include: Office Preparedness; Glossary of Terms; Appendix

YOUR ROADMAP TO FINANCIAL INTEGRITY IN THE DENTAL OFFICE by Donald P. Lewis, Jr., DDS, CFE

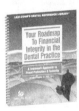

A Teamwork Approach to Fraud Protection & Security

Ideal practice management reference, designed and written by a dentist in private practice. Covers 4 basic areas of financial security. Utilizes tabbed paging system with 8 major tabs for quick reference. **Part I: Financial Transactions   Incoming:** Financial Arrangements, Billing, Accounts Receivable, Banking, Cash, Checks, and Credit Cards; **Part II: Financial Transactions Outgoing:** Accounts Payable, Supplies, Cash-on-hand, Payroll; **Part III: Internal Controls:** Banking, General Office Management, Human Resource (H/R) issues; **Part IV: Employees:** Employee Related Issues and Employees Manual Topics **Part V: Report Checklist:** Daily, Weekly, Monthly, Quarterly, Semi-annually, Annually; **Additional Features:** Glossary terms for clarification, alphabetical index for quick reference, 1600 bulleted points of interest, over 180 checklist options, 12 real-life stories (names changed to protect the innocent!), 80-boxed topics of special interest for quick review.

DENTAL INSURANCE AND REIMBURSEMENT

by Tom M. Limoli DDS and Associates & Atlanta Dental Consultants

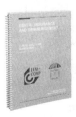

Accurately and appropriately identify the procedure code for the complete procedure using this book! This reference not only gives you the up-to-date codes, it provides you the knowledge on how to use the codes appropriately. With this reference text, your office will begin to simplify the reimbursement process by first utilizing the most appropriate procedure code. The text is fully tabbed, indexed, and color coded to simplify code identification. This books includes: no nonsense approaches to accurate benefit plan coding; 25 years of streamlining the reimbursement process; thousands of Dental Practices have implemented this approach to third party reimbursement; text is fully tabbed and color coded [Black: Word for word CDT coding; Purple: Includes coding descriptors, comments, and sample narrative; Green: Additions and changes from previous versions of the "Code on Dental Procedure and Nomenclature"; Red: Deletions from previous versions of the "CODE"].

To order call toll free anywhere in the U.S.: 1-866-EXP-DIFF (397-3433)
Outside of the U.S. call: 330-650-6506 or online at www.lexi.com

Products offered by LEXI-COMP

Patient Education Flip Charts

A PATIENT GUIDE TO MENTAL HEALTH ISSUES

- ▸ Alzheimer's Disease
- ▸ Anxiety (GAD)
- ▸ Bipolar Disorder (BD)
- ▸ Depression
- ▸ Insomnia
- ▸ Obsessive-Compulsive Disorder (OCD)
- ▸ Panic Attacks (PD)
- ▸ Schizophrenia

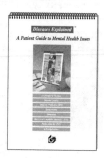

A PATIENT GUIDE TO ROOT CANAL THERAPY
Contributor Thom C. Dumsha, M.S., D.D.S., M.S.

- • An ideal tool used to educate and explain to your patients about root canals

- • 8 1/2" x 11" colorful tabbed flip chart explaining each of the steps involved in a root canal

- • Actual clinical photographs, radiographs, and diagrams

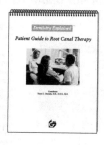

PATIENT GUIDE TO DENTAL IMPLANTS
Contributor Marvin L. Baer, D.D.S., M.Sc.

- • An ideal tool used to educate and explain to your patients about dental implants

- • 8 1/2" x 11" colorful tabbed flip chart explaining each of the steps involved in:

    1.) Single tooth restoration
    2.) Replacement of several teeth
    3.) Implants supported overdenture
        (4 implants/2 implants)
    4.) Screw-retained denture

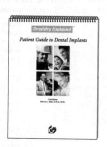

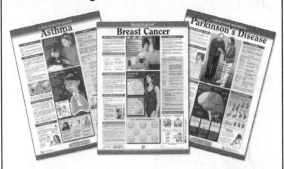

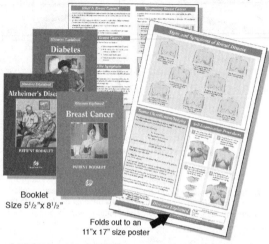

Outside of the U.S. call: 330-650-6506

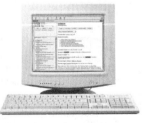

LEXI-COMP ON-HAND™ SOFTWARE LIBRARY

For Palm OS® and
Windows™ Powered Pocket PC Devices

Lexi-Comp's handheld software solutions provide quick, portable access to clinical information needed at the point-of-care. Whether you need laboratory test or diagnostic procedure information, to validate a dose, or to check multiple medications and natural products for drug interactions, Lexi-Comp has the information you need in the palm of your hand. Lexi-Comp also provides advanced linking technology to allow you to hyperlink to related information topics within a title or to the same topic in another title for more extensive information. No longer will you have to exit one database (such as Griffith's 5-Minute Clinical Consult) to look up a drug dose in Lexi-Drugs® or lab test information in Lexi-Lab & Diagnostic Procedures™. Seamless linking between all databases to **saves valuable time and helps to improve patient care.**

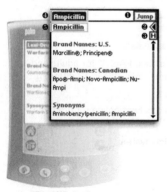

Palm OS® Device shown

Navigational Tools:

❶ **"Jump"** provides a drop down list of available fields to easily navigate through information.

❷ **Back arrow** returns to the index from a monograph or to the "Installed Books" menu from the Index.

❸ **"H"** provides a linkable History to return to any of the last 12 Topics viewed during your session.

❹ **Title bar:** Tap the monograph or topic title bar to activate a menu to "Edit a Note" or return to the "Installed Books" menu.

❺ **Linking:** Link to another companion database by clicking the topic or monograph title link or within a database noted by various hyperlinked (colorized and underlined) text.